Therapeutic Drug Monitoring

PUBLICATION AND ADVERTISING STAFF
RAVEN PRESS, NEW YORK

Janis E. Hoagland *Production Editor*
Susan Weiser Liebegott *Advertising Manager*

CONTENTS

61 **Assessment of Cyclosporin A in Whole Blood and Plasma in Five Patients with Different Hematocrits**
R. P. Agarwal, R. A. McPherson, and G. A. Threatte

66 **Computer-Assisted Drug Assay Interpretation Based on Bayesian Estimation of Individual Pharmacokinetics: Application to Lidocaine**
S. Vozeh, R. Hillman, M. Wandell, T. Ludden, and L. Sheiner

74 **Comparison of Eight Phenytoin Dosing Methods in Institutionalized Patients**
Nora Flint, Larry M. Lopez, J. Daniel Robinson, Charles Williams, and Ronald B. Salem

81 **Therapeutic Blood Levels of Phenytoin in Treatment of Paroxysmal Choreoathetosis**
Bor-Jeng Wang and Yang-Chyuan Chang

83 **Steady-State Serum Levels of Anticonvulsant Drugs in Chinese Epileptic Patients Living in Taiwan**
Ming-Liang Lai

87 **Monitoring Drug Noncompliance in Epileptic Patients: Assessing Phenobarbital Plasma Levels**
Seiichiro Takaki, Toru Kurokawa, and Toshinobu Aoyama

92 **No Influence of Doxycycline on Theophylline Pharmacokinetics**
J. H. G. Jonkman, W. J. V. van der Boon, R. Schoenmaker, A. Holtkamp, and J. Hempenius

95 **Evaluation of the Du Pont Theophylline Assay Adapted to a Centrifugal Analyzer**
Roger L. Boeckx and Sara T. Munson

101 **Dual-Label Fluoroimmunoassay for Simultaneous Determination of Primidone and Phenobarbital**
A. M. Sidki, D. S. Smith, and J. Landon

108 **Evaluation of an Automated System (Optimate) for Substrate-Labeled Fluorescent Immunoassays**
Michael Sheehan and Geoffrey Caron

115 **Determination of Free Valproic Acid Concentrations Using the Amicon Micropartition MPS-1 Ultrafiltration System**
Clark March and Robert V. Blanke

121 **Interference with High Performance Liquid Chromatographic Chloramphenicol Assay in a Patient Receiving Dobutamine**
M. Beth Powel, C. Andrew Robinson, and Raymond L. Furner

(continued on next page)

Therapeutic Drug Monitoring

VOLUME 7, NUMBER 1
MARCH 1985

CONTENTS

EDITORIAL

1 **Cyclosporine: Right or Wrong?**
C. E. Pippenger

REVIEWS

2 **Clinical Pharmacology of Pediatric Antipyretic Drugs**
John T. Wilson

12 **An Overview of Amikacin**
Angela M. Ristuccia and Burke A. Cunha

26 **Oral Contraceptive Drug Interactions**
Anne M. Baciewicz

ARTICLES

36 **Simultaneous Plasma Carbamazepine and Carbamazepine-Epoxide Concentrations in Pharmacokinetic and Bioavailability Studies**
W. D. Hooper, A. R. King, M. Patterson, R. G. Dickinson, and M. J. Eadie

41 **Fallacious Results from Measuring Salivary Carbamazepine Concentrations**
R. G. Dickinson, W. D. Hooper, A. R. King, and M. J. Eadie

46 **Determination of Total and Free Plasma Carbamazepine Concentrations by Enzyme Multiplied Immunoassay: Interference with the 10,11-Epoxide Metabolite**
Manuela Contin, Roberto Riva, Fiorenzo Albani, Emilio Perucca, and Agostino Baruzzi

51 **Carbamazepine–Phenytoin Interaction: Elevation of Plasma Phenytoin Concentrations Due to Carbamazepine Comedication**
Janusz J. Zielinski, Dan Haidukewych, and Boris J. Leheta

54 **Investigations of Long-Term Treatment with Perhexiline Maleate Using Therapeutic Monitoring and Electromyography**
J. Pilcher, J. D. H. Cooper, D. C. Turnell, J. Matenga, R. Paul, and J. D. F. Lockhart

(continued on next page)

Listed in INDEX MEDICUS, CURRENT CONTENTS, and BIOLOGICAL ABSTRACTS

Therapeutic Drug Monitoring (ISSN 0163-4356) is published quarterly in March, June, September, and December by Raven Press Books, Ltd., 1140 Avenue of the Americas, New York, N.Y. 10036. Second class postage paid at New York, N.Y., and at additional mailing offices. *Subscription rates for Vol. 7, 1985:* Personal subscriptions $75 in U.S., $89 elsewhere; institutional subscriptions $109 in U.S., $124 elsewhere. Single copies $32. Journal issues prior to the current volume, when available, may be ordered at the single copy rate. Air delivery included for European and Mediterranean countries; for air delivery elsewhere, add $25. Payment should accompany all orders. Please enclose present mailing label with all change of address requests. Address advertising inquiries to Advertising Manager, Raven Press. **Postmaster:** Send change of address to *Therapeutic Drug Monitoring,* Subscription Department, Raven Press, 1140 Avenue of the Americas, New York, NY 10036.

When citing this journal, abbreviate as *Ther Drug Monit.*

CONTENTS

LETTERS TO THE EDITOR

123 **On the Interaction Between Phenytoin and Antineoplastic Agents**
Roberto Riva, Fiorenzo Albani, and Agostino Baruzzi

123 **Measurement of Cyclosporine: A Challenge to the Professional Laboratory Organizations**
Thomas P. Moyer

124 **Extraction of Interfering Substance from the Sera of Uremic Subjects Prior to Homogeneous Enzyme Immunoassay**
Clark A. Rundell and Sue Ellen Tupper

127 **Book Reviews**

Conversion Formula

Readers who wish to convert drug concentrations to or from SI units may apply the following formulas.

$$\text{To determine the conversion factor (CF): CF} = \frac{1{,}000}{\text{mol wt}}$$

To convert *to* SI units: (μg/ml) × CF = (μmol/liter)
To convert *from* SI units: (μmol/liter) ÷ CF = (μg/ml)

Example: Phenytoin conversion

$$\text{Conversion factor: CF} = \frac{1{,}000}{\text{mol wt}} = \frac{1{,}000}{252.3} = 3.96$$

Conversion: (μg/ml) × 3.96 = (10 μg/ml) × 3.96 = 39.6 μmol/liter (39.6 μmol/liter) ÷ 3.96 = 10 μg/ml

Therapeutic Drug Monitoring

PUBLICATION AND ADVERTISING STAFF
RAVEN PRESS, NEW YORK

Janis E. Hoagland *Production Editor*

Susan Weiser Liebegott *Advertising Manager*

Therapeutic Drug Monitoring

VOLUME 7, NUMBER 2
JUNE 1985

CONTENTS

EDITORIAL

129 **Cyclosporine Quality Control Program is a Reality**

130 **Clinical Pharmacokinetics of Sulfonamides in Children: Relationship Between Maturing Kidney Function and Renal Clearance of Sulfonamides**
Tom B. Vree, Yechiel A. Hekster, and Rob J. J. Lippens

148 **Therapeutic Drug Monitoring in Pediatric Acute Drug Intoxications**
Kent E. Opheim and Vidmantas A. Raisys

159 **Chloramphenicol: Clinical Pharmacology in Pediatrics**
Angela M. Ristuccia

ARTICLES

168 **Theophylline Serum Concentrations in Ambulatory Patients with Chronic Obstructive Pulmonary Disease**
James W. Bredon, J. Lyle Bootman, William N. Jones, William F. McGhan, Donald G. Perrier, and Sammy C. Campbell

174 **Bayesian Pharmacokinetic/Pharmacodynamic Forecasting of Prothrombin Response to Warfarin Therapy: Preliminary Evaluation**
Jennifer M. Svec, Robert W. Coleman, Dennis R. Mungall, and Thomas M. Ludden

181 **Influence of High-Dose Pentobarbital on Theophylline Pharmacokinetics: A Case Report**
Gene A. Gibson, Robert A. Blouin, Larry A. Bauer, Robert P. Rapp, and Phillip A. Tibbs

(continued on next page)

Listed in INDEX MEDICUS, CURRENT CONTENTS, BIOLOGICAL ABSTRACTS, and PASCAL/CNRS

Therapeutic Drug Monitoring (ISSN 0163-4356) is published quarterly in March, June, September, and December by Raven Press Books, Ltd., 1140 Avenue of the Americas, New York, N.Y. 10036. Second class postage paid at New York, N.Y., and at additional mailing offices. *Subscription rates for Vol. 7, 1985:* Personal subscriptions $75 in U.S., $89 elsewhere; institutional subscriptions $109 in U.S., $124 elsewhere. Single copies $32. Journal issues prior to the current volume, when available, may be ordered at the single copy rate. Air delivery included for European and Mediterranean countries; for air delivery elsewhere, add $25. Payment should accompany all orders. Please enclose present mailing label with all change of address requests. Address advertising inquiries to Advertising Manager, Raven Press. **Postmaster:** Send change of address to *Therapeutic Drug Monitoring,* Subscription Department, Raven Press, 1140 Avenue of the Americas, New York, NY 10036.
When citing this journal, abbreviate as *Ther Drug Monit.*

CONTENTS

185 **Effect of Associated Antiepileptic Treatment on Valproate-Induced Hyperammonemia**
G. Zaccara, M. Paganini, R. Campostrini, F. Moroni, T. Valenza, A. Messori, M. Bartelli, G. Arnetoli, and R. Zappoli

191 **Red Blood Cell Electrolytes for Monitoring Digoxin Therapy in Adults**
C. J. van Boxtel, R. Koopmans, B. Oosterhuis, and F. J. Hoek

197 **Influence of Body Fat on the Volume of Distribution of Theophylline**
Peter J. Jewesson and Robin J. Ensom

202 **Falsely Elevated Digoxin Concentrations in Patients with Liver Disease**
Bernd Rosenkranz and Jürgen C. Frölich

207 **Determination of Chloroquine and its Desethyl Metabolite in Whole Blood: An Application for Samples Collected in Capillary Tubes and Dried on Filter Paper**
Björn Lindström, Örjan Ericsson, Gunnar Alván, Lars Rombo, Lena Ekman, Margareta Rais, and Folke Sjöqvist

211 **Chloroquine and Desethylchloroquine in Plasma, Serum, and Whole Blood: Problems in Assay and Handling of Samples**
Lars Rombo, Örjan Ericsson, Gunnar Alván, Björn Lindström, Lars L. Gustafsson, and Folke Sjöqvist

216 **A Sensitive Liquid Chromatographic Assay for Plasma Aspirin and Salicylate Concentrations After Low Doses of Aspirin**
Roslyn A. Brandon, Mervyn J. Eadie, and Maree T. Smith

222 **Therapeutic Monitoring of Chlorpromazine I: Pitfalls in Plasma Analysis**
J. W. Hubbard, J. K. Cooper, E. M. Hawes, D. J. Jenden, P. R. A. May, M. Martin, G. McKay, T. Van Putten, and K. K. Midha

229 **Comparative Determination of Flupentixol in Plasma by Gas Chromatography and Radioimmunoassay in Schizophrenic Patients**
A. E. Balant-Gorgia, L. P. Balant, Ch. Genet, and R. Eisele

236 **Evaluation of Valproic Acid Fluoroimmunoassay and Comparison with a Gas Liquid Chromatographic Method**
Sandra Tosoni, Costantino Signorini, and Alberto Albertini

(continued on next page)

CONTENTS

CASE REPORT

239 **Desmethylimipramine Overdose: Nonlinear Kinetics in a Slow Hydroxylator**
Edoardo Spina, Thomas K. Henthorn, Lennart Eleborg, Conny Nordin, and Juliette Säwe

SHORT COMMUNICATION

242 **Analysis of Tricyclic Antidepressants in Serum and Plasma Yields Similar Results**
E. Spina, Ö. Ericsson, and C. Nordin

244 **Book Reviews**

Conversion Formula

Readers who wish to convert drug concentrations to or from SI units may apply the following formulas.

$$\text{To determine the conversion factor (CF): CF} = \frac{1{,}000}{\text{mol wt}}$$

To convert *to* SI units: (μg/ml) × CF = (μmol/liter)
To convert *from* SI units: (μmol/liter) ÷ CF = (μg/ml)

Example: Phenytoin conversion

$$\text{Conversion factor: CF} = \frac{1{,}000}{\text{mol wt}} = \frac{1{,}000}{252.3} = 3.96$$

Conversion: (μg/ml) × 3.96 = (10 μg/ml) × 3.96 = 39.6 μmol/liter (39.6 μmol/liter) ÷ 3.96 = 10 μg/ml

Therapeutic Drug Monitoring

PUBLICATION AND ADVERTISING STAFF
RAVEN PRESS, NEW YORK

Wendy Middlemiss Ross *Production Editor*
Susan Weiser Liebegott *Advertising Manager*

Therapeutic Drug Monitoring

VOLUME 7, NUMBER 3
SEPTEMBER 1985

CONTENTS

247 **Blood–Brain Barrier Transport of CI-912: Single-Passage Equilibration of Erythrocyte-Borne Drug**
Eain M. Cornford and Kristin P. Landon

255 **Evaluation of Amitriptyline Pharmacokinetics During Peritoneal Dialysis**
Jerry J. Tasset, Satwant Singh, and Amadeo J. Pesce

258 **Experience with a Computer-Based Technique for Estimating Pharmacokinetic Constants from Limited Data**
K. Bachmann, V. Pongsin, R. Forney Jr., and G. Gronau

265 **Nomogram for Bretylium Dosing in Renal Impairment**
Joseph Adir, Prem K. Narang, and John Josselson

269 **Carbamazepine Protein Binding and Disposition in Pregnancy**
M. S. Yerby, P. N. Friel, and D. Q. Miller

274 **Carbamazepine and Carbamazepine-Epoxide Serum Protein Binding in Newborn Infants**
James B. Groce III, Daniel T. Casto, and Peter Gal

277 **Lateral Gaze Nystagmus in Carbamazepine-Treated Epileptic Patients: Correlation with Total and Free Plasma Concentrations of Parent Drug and Its 10,11-Epoxide Metabolite**
R. Riva, M. Contin, F. Albani, E. Perucca, G. Ambrosetto, G. Procaccianti, M. Santucci, and A. Baruzzi

283 **Extent of Urinary Excretion of *p*-Hydroxyphenytoin in Healthy Subjects Given Phenytoin**
R. G. Dickinson, W. D. Hooper, M. Patterson, M. J. Eadie, and B. Maguire

(continued on next page)

Listed in INDEX MEDICUS, CURRENT CONTENTS, BIOLOGICAL ABSTRACTS, and PASCAL/CNRS

Therapeutic Drug Monitoring (ISSN 0163-4356) is published quarterly in March, June, September, and December by Raven Press Books, Ltd., 1140 Avenue of the Americas, New York, N.Y. 10036. Second class postage paid at New York, N.Y., and at additional mailing offices. *Subscription rates for Vol. 7, 1985:* Personal subscriptions $75 in U.S., $89 elsewhere; institutional subscriptions $109 in U.S., $124 elsewhere. Single copies $32. Journal issues prior to the current volume, when available, may be ordered at the single copy rate. Air delivery included for European and Mediterranean countries; for air delivery elsewhere, add $25. Payment should accompany all orders. Please enclose present mailing label with all change of address requests. Address advertising inquiries to Advertising Manager, Raven Press. **Postmaster:** Send change of address to *Therapeutic Drug Monitoring*, Subscription Department, Raven Press, 1140 Avenue of the Americas, New York, NY 10036.

When citing this journal, abbreviate as *Ther Drug Monit*.

CONTENTS

290 **Chronic Valproic Acid Therapy and Incidence of Increases in Venous Plasma Ammonia**
Dan Haidukewych, Geetha John, Janusz J. Zielinski, and Ernst A. Rodin

295 **Organization and Efficacy of a Therapeutic Drug Monitoring Consultation Service in a Pediatric Hospital**
Gideon Koren, Steven J. Soldin, and Stuart M. MacLeod

299 **Experience with a Specific Request Form for Antidepressant Drug Monitoring**
Albert D. Fraser

303 **Aminoglycoside Monitoring: Timing of Peak Levels Is Critical**
Jürg Blaser, Hans Peter Simmen, Hans Ruedi Gonzenbach, Wolfgang Sonnabend, and Ruedi Lüthy

CASE REPORT
308 **Evidence Supporting 3(S)-3-Hydroxyquinidine-Associated Cardiotoxicity**
Larry D. Bowers, Kay M. Nelson, Robert Connor, Cynthia J. Lais, and Elliot Krauss

313 **Rapid Protein Determinations on Ultrafiltrates Prepared for Free Phenytoin Quantification**
Charles P. Turley and Tammy Milligan

315 **Analysis of 6-Mercaptopurine in Serum or Plasma Using High Performance Liquid Chromatography**
C. E. Whalen, H. Tamary, M. Greenberg, A. Zipursky, and S. J. Soldin

321 **Reversed-Phase High Performance Liquid Chromatographic Determination of Nifedipine in Human Plasma**
B. J. Gurley, Robert G. Buice, and Paramjeet Sidhu

324 **Quantitative Liquid Chromatography of Allopurinol and Oxypurinol in Human Plasma and Urine**
J. M. Failler, R. Farinotti, and A. Dauphin

329 **Determination of Warfarin in Human Plasma by High Performance Liquid Chromatography and Photodiode Array Detector**
Per Magne Ueland, Gry Kvalheim, Per Eystein Lønning, and Stener Kvinnsland

336 **Determination of Valproic Acid in Plasma or Serum by Solid-Phase Column Extraction and Gas-Liquid Chromatography**
Wen-nuei Lin and Annetta R. Kelly

344 **Radioimmunoassay for Clonidine in Human Plasma and Urine Using a Solid Phase Second Antibody Separation**
Peter R. Farina, Carol A. Homon, Chien T. Chow, James J. Keirns, Paul A. Zavorskas, and Henry J. Esber

(continued on next page)

CONTENTS

351 **Evaluation of Fluorescence Polarization Immunoassay for Quantitation of Serum Salicylates**
H. Thomas Karnes and Larry A. Beightol

355 **Evaluation of a Mouse Monoclonal Antibody for the Determination of Serum Theophylline by Fluorescence Polarization Immunoassay**
Catherine A. Ross, Cheryl J. Kraft, Min Hwa Lee, and David B. Haughey

358 **Assessment of Blood Collection Systems for the High Performance Liquid Chromatography Measurement of Propranolol**
Steven H. Y. Wong, William B. White, Rosinda Fernandes, Robert Holden, F. C. Lin, and S. Narayanan

364 **Measurement of Vitamin E in Serum and Plasma by High Performance Liquid Chromatography with Electrochemical Detection**
M. C. Castle and W. J. Cooke

SHORT COMMUNICATION
369 **Daily Variations in Plasma Levels of Lidocaine During Local Anaesthesia in Dental Practice**
Bernard Bruguerolle and Roger Isnardon

Conversion Formula

Readers who wish to convert drug concentrations to or from SI units may apply the following formulas.

To determine the conversion factor (CF): $CF = \frac{1{,}000}{\text{mol wt}}$

To convert *to* SI units: (μg/ml) × CF = (μmol/liter)
To convert *from* SI units: (μmol/liter) ÷ CF = (μg/ml)

Example: Phenytoin conversion

Conversion factor: $CF = \frac{1{,}000}{\text{mol wt}} = \frac{1{,}000}{252.3} = 3.96$

Conversion: (μg/ml) × 3.96 = (10 μg/ml) × 3.96 = 39.6 μmol/liter (39.6 μmol/liter) ÷ 3.96 = 10 μg/ml

Therapeutic Drug Monitoring

PUBLICATION AND ADVERTISING STAFF
RAVEN PRESS, NEW YORK

Wendy Middlemiss Ross *Production Editor*
Susan Weiser Liebegott *Advertising Manager*

Therapeutic Drug Monitoring

VOLUME 7, NUMBER 4
DECEMBER 1985

CONTENTS

EDITORIAL

371 **Cyclosporine Quality Control Program**
C. E. Pippenger

372 **Interaction Between Digoxin and Nifedipine at Steady State in Patients with Atrial Fibrillation**
C. H. Kleinbloesem, P. van Brummelen, J. Hillers, A. J. Moolenaar, and D. D. Breimer

377 **New and Simple Method to Predict Dosage of Drugs Obeying Simple Michaelis-Menten Elimination Kinetics and to Distinguish Such Kinetics from Simple First Order and from Parallel Michaelis-Menten and First Order Kinetics**
John G. Wagner

387 **Serum Concentrations of Valproic Acid: Influence of Dose and Comedication**
T. May and B. Rambeck

391 **A New Approach to Establishing Individualized Maintenance Doses of Phenytoin**
K. Bachmann, T. J. Sullivan, J. Schwartz, and L. Jauregui

401 **Effect of Phenothiazines on Serum Antiepileptic Drug Concentrations in Psychiatric Patients with Seizure Disorder**
Dan Haidukewych and Ernst A. Rodin

405 **Michaelis-Menten Kinetics and the Steady-State Serum Phenytoin/Hydroxyphenytoin Ratio**
Blaise F. D. Bourgeois and Nils Wad

411 **Plasma Flupentixol Concentrations and Clinical Response in Acute Schizophrenia**
A. E. Balant-Gorgia, R. Eisele, J. M. Aeschlimann, L. P. Balant, and G. Garrone

(continued on next page)

Listed in INDEX MEDICUS, CURRENT CONTENTS, BIOLOGICAL ABSTRACTS, and PASCAL/CNRS

Therapeutic Drug Monitoring (ISSN 0163-4356) is published quarterly in March, June, September, and December by Raven Press Books, Ltd., 1140 Avenue of the Americas, New York, N.Y. 10036. Second class postage paid at New York, N.Y., and at additional mailing offices. *Subscription rates for Vol. 8, 1986:* Personal subscriptions $81 in U.S., $95 elsewhere; institutional subscriptions $125 in U.S., $139 elsewhere. Single copies $36. Journal issues prior to the current volume, when available, may be ordered at the single copy rate. Air delivery is included for European and Mediterranean countries; for air delivery elsewhere, add $25. Payment should accompany all orders. Please enclose present mailing label with all change of address requests. Address advertising inquiries to Advertising Manager, Raven Press. **Postmaster:** Send change of address to *Therapeutic Drug Monitoring*, Subscription Department, Raven Press, P.O. Box 2046, Mahopac, NY 10541.
When citing this journal, abbreviate as *Ther Drug Monit.*

415 **Simultaneous Estimation of Serum Concentrations of Dapsone, Monoacetyldapsone, and Pyrimethamine in Chinese Men on Maloprim for Malaria Prophylaxis Using Reversed-Phase High Performance Liquid Chromatography**
H. S. Lee, T. Y. Ti, P. S. Lee, and C. L. Yap

421 **Computer Prediction of Serum Theophylline Concentrations in Ambulatory Patients**
Paul A. Deci, Larry M. Lopez, J. Daniel Robinson, and Ken Grauer

426 **Cimetidine-Theophylline Interaction: Effects of Age and Cimetidine Dose**
Ira A. Cohen, Cary E. Johnson, Rosemary R. Berardi, Martha L. Hyneck, and Sami R. Achem

435 **Effects of Salsalate (Nonacetylated Salicylate) and Aspirin on Serum Prostaglandins in Humans**
H. G. Morris, N. A. Sherman, C. McQuain, M. B. Goldlust, S. F. Chang, and L. I. Harrison

439 **Sensitive High Performance Liquid Chromatographic Analysis of Ethmozin in Plasma**
J. M. Poirier

442 **Comparison of High Pressure Liquid Chromatography and Fluorescence Polarization Immunoassay Methods in a Theophylline Pharmacokinetic Study**
Richard L. Lalonde, Michael B. Bottorff, and Arthur B. Straughn

447 **Stability of Bupropion and its Major Metabolites in Human Plasma**
S. Casey Laizure and C. Lindsay DeVane

451 **Determination of Serum Theophylline by Apoenzyme Reactivation Immunoassay System**
Mario Plebani and Angelo Burlina

455 **Loop-Column Extraction and Liquid Chromatographic Analysis of Doxorubicin and Three Metabolites in Plasma**
Cynthia A. Riley, William R. Crom, and William E. Evans

461 **Ultrafiltration Compared with Equilibrium Dialysis in the Determination of Unbound Phenytoin in Plasma**
Yuichi Koike, Anita Magnusson, Eugen Steiner, Anders Rane, and Folke Sjöqvist

466 **Determination of Free Disopyramide Plasma Concentrations Using Ultrafiltration and Enzyme Multiplied Immunoassay**
Gursharan Raghow, Marvin C. Meyer, and Arthur B. Straughn

(continued on next page)

472 **Therapeutic Monitoring of Chlorpromazine II: Pitfalls in Whole Blood Analysis**
G. McKay, J. K. Cooper, E. M. Hawes, J. W. Hubbard, M. Martin, and K. K. Midha

SHORT COMMUNICATION
478 **Extremely Rapid Hydroxylation of Debrisoquine: A Case Report with Implication for Treatment with Nortriptyline and Other Tricyclic Antidepressants**
Leif Bertilsson, Anna Åberg-Wistedt, Lars L. Gustafsson, and Conny Nordin

CASE REPORT
481 **Phenytoin/Clonazepam Interaction**
Ivan N. Saavedra, Ledda I. Aguilera, Evelyng Faure, and Daniel G. Galdames

CASE REPORT
485 **Hemodialysis Clearance of Pentobarbital During Continuous Infusion**
Daniel Wermeling, Kenneth Record, Richard Bell, William Porter, and Robert Blouin

LETTERS TO THE EDITOR
488 **An Interactive Opinion on the Rationalization of Therapeutic Cyclosporine Monitoring**
R. Camsonne and X. Troussard

489 **Caffeine Interference with the CANAM-Theophylline Reagent Kit**
Ingo S. Kampa and Jean I. Jarzabek

491 **Announcement**

492 **Subject and Author Indexes, Volume 7, 1985**

Conversion Formula

Readers who wish to convert drug concentrations to or from SI units may apply the following formulas.

$$\text{To determine the conversion factor (CF): CF} = \frac{1{,}000}{\text{mol wt}}$$

To convert *to* SI units: (μg/ml) × CF = (μmol/liter)
To convert *from* SI units: (μmol/liter) ÷ CF = (μg/ml)

Example: Phenytoin conversion

$$\text{Conversion factor: CF} = \frac{1{,}000}{\text{mol wt}} = \frac{1{,}000}{252.3} = 3.96$$

Conversion: (μg/ml) × 3.96 = (10 μg/ml) × 3.96 = 39.6 μmol/liter (39.6 μmol/liter) ÷ 3.96 = 10 μg/ml

Therapeutic Drug Monitoring

PUBLICATION AND ADVERTISING STAFF
RAVEN PRESS, NEW YORK

Wendy Middlemiss Ross *Production Editor*

Susan Weiser Liebegott *Advertising Manager*

Therapeutic Drug Monitoring
7:1 © 1985 Raven Press, New York

Editorial

Cyclosporine: Right or Wrong?

In this issue of *Therapeutic Drug Monitoring*, we wish to call your attention to the Letter to the Editor from Dr. Thomas P. Moyer, which raises the issue of the desperate need to establish some uniformity throughout the scientific community with respect to cyclosporine drug monitoring. We all recognize the importance of cyclosporine drug monitoring. Yet it appears that each laboratory group monitoring cyclosporine has chosen to go its own way. Consequently, a great deal of confusion exists within the medical community today, not only concerning the utility of routine cyclosporine drug monitoring, but also with respect to the interpretation of the various published studies, each of which seems to utilize a different analytical technique and different optimal concentration range.

Our current problems with cyclosporine are certainly reminiscent of the problems that were encountered 15 years ago in the monitoring of antiepileptic drugs. The same issues need to be faced. It is of interest to note that the confusion that existed in the early 1970s with respect to therapeutic drug monitoring of antiepileptic drugs was not due to a failure on the part of any individual laboratory to perform the assays to the best of its ability, but rather to a failure of communication between the various laboratories with respect to analytical techniques, quality control, interpretation of the results, and the dissemination of information throughout the medical community, especially the practical aspects of drug monitoring.

I agree with Dr. Moyer's challenge. The appropriate organizations should respond quickly to provide guidelines for monitoring cyclosporine. Responding quickly does not mean a year or two down the road, but within the next 6 months. We certainly would be willing to provide the space in *Therapeutic Drug Monitoring* for the dissemination of their criteria. One must also recognize that we need an interlaboratory quality control scheme for cyclosporine, in addition to a consensus as to what is the most clinically useful way to monitor cyclosporine drug concentrations. We urge all of you to contact both the College of American Pathologists Therapeutic Drug Monitoring Resource Committee and the American Association for Clinical Chemistry Therapeutic Drug Monitoring Committee to express your opinions and urge that action be taken. We commend and support Dr. Moyer's efforts to bring rationality to the monitoring of cyclosporine concentrations. Only a rational approach and solution to our cyclosporine problems will assure the best possible patient care, and that is our responsibility.

C. E. Pippenger
Cleveland, Ohio

Therapeutic Drug Monitoring
7:2–11 © 1985 Raven Press, New York

Review

Clinical Pharmacology of Pediatric Antipyretic Drugs

John T. Wilson

Departments of Pharmacology and Pediatrics, and Section on Clinical Pharmacology, Louisiana State University Medical School, Shreveport, Louisiana, U.S.A.

The decision to treat fever with antipyretic drugs remains controversial (1). Some believe that fever is a useful adjunct of host defense against an infecting organism. Fever may have prognostic value for monitoring of efficacy of other treatments, or it may have diagnostic importance, especially with regard to occurrence of rheumatic diseases. Anticipatory use of antipyretic drugs (APDs) may decrease the frequency of febrile seizures (2). The most frequent use of APDs, however, pertains to infectious diseases outside the hospital and often outside medical attention. The APDs are given for fever and also for analgesic purposes (3). These drugs are widely available as over-the-counter (OTC) and prescription items. The controversy surrounding appropriateness of fever treatment will continue but probably will have little impact on the current widespread use of APDs. This use will continue until a definitive study clarifies indications for treatment of fever. In the interim, it could be argued that children are entitled to the same relief of discomfort (i.e., fever) and pain as offered to adults. This "benefit" needs to be weighed against the risk of adverse drug effects in febrile children. Both the nature and extent of these risks and also the effective dose of APDs for children need to be known.

Two APDs have been extensively used in children. An adult dose of aspirin was given to children in 1901 (4) and an antipyretic response was observed. Division of the adult tablet produced the 1-¼ grain (80-mg) dose; this appears to be the basis for subsequent use of this dosing unit in children. The recent U.S. Food and Drug Administration (FDA) report on OTC drugs (5) underscored the lack of dosing data for children even though studies had shown repeatedly an absolute and relative efficacy for aspirin (6). Literature data were analyzed by Done et al. (7,8), to provide rationale for changing the aspirin dosage interval to 4 h and for increasing the age-related dose at each interval. This analysis and the FDA report on APDs (5) produced the current label directions for aspirin. Acetaminophen was shown in 1956 (9) to be an effective antipyretic in children. Until recently acetaminophen has been dosed in an amount similar to that for aspirin. There are apparently no published reports in this country on the single- or multiple-dosage antipyretic efficacy of aspirin or acetaminophen in children with regard to assessment of the optimum dose. We recently described the dose–plasma level efficacy relationship for a single dose of aspirin and acetaminophen (6). An effective plasma level for febrile children was proposed. Plasma level profiles and associated efficacy were predicted for multiple-dose regimens of aspirin and acetaminophen. Until our proposed dosage regimens are tested in febrile children, the use of both drugs will remain on an empiric basis—as it has for at least a quarter of a century.

Information on specific antipyretic drug formulations available for children has been summarized (2). Drugs such as phenacetin, antipyrine, aminopyrine, or dipyrone have antipyretic activity but are not suitable for pediatric use. Indomethacin is not a first-line drug for antipyresis. The use of salicylamide has decreased over the last 5 years. Multiple approaches to antipyresis are often necessary such that physical and pharmacologic agents are used (2,10). Information on

Address correspondence and reprint requests to Dr. J. T. Wilson at Departments of Pharmacology and Pediatrics, and Section on Clinical Pharmacology, Louisiana State University Medical School, P.O. Box 33932, Shreveport, LA 71130, U.S.A.

This review will be published in the forthcoming book: *Pediatric Clinical Pharmacology* (Handbook of Therapeutic Drug Monitoring Series). P. L. Morselli and C. E. Pippenger, eds. New York: Raven Press, 1985.

pediatric efficacy, safety, and disposition, however, can be reviewed for some drugs.

ASPIRIN

Children's aspirin is available in the fixed-dose tablet of 1-¼ grain (80 mg), which is the FDA recommended dosing unit for pediatric ADPs (5). Prior to 1979 the dose was given every 3 h, but the recommended interval is now every 4 h (5,7,8). The age-related dose and corresponding body weight-adjusted dose both for aspirin and for salicylic acid are given in Table 1. An age-related dose delivers more drug (mg/kg) to the younger children in the age range. Thus, the higher weight-adjusted dose shown is for younger children. The average weight-adjusted dose currently recommended for ages 2–8 years is 13.2 mg/kg of aspirin. A high dose is shown in Table 1 for the purpose of the following discussion about loading dose regimens. A high dose should not be used for maintenance therapy, since it and the corresponding interval have not been evaluated. As reviewed in the following discussion, our computer simulations (6) reveal that a revised dose and dosing interval of aspirin may provide plasma levels effective for antipyresis and with less risk of toxicity.

Both the absolute (decrease from initial temperature) and relative (compared with acetaminophen and other drugs) efficacy of aspirin have been established (6,11–21). The milligram doses of aspirin and acetaminophen appear equipotent for maximum antipyresis, but no graded-dose comparative study of both drugs has been done in febrile children. Differences in the onset and duration of antipyretic response may also exist for different doses of aspirin and acetaminophen. Comparison of a similar dose of each drug, however, revealed a similar onset time (0.6–0.9 h) and a duration of at least 3 h (6).

A single-dose (9.4 ± 0.34 mg/kg as salicylic acid) disposition study of aspirin in febrile children aged 2–7 years revealed the following for plasma salicylic acid (6): k_{el} = 0.214 ± 0.044 h^{-1}, $t_{1/2}$ = 3.2 h, and V_d = 113 ± 4.7 ml/kg. The k_{el} and $t_{1/2}$ are described for the observed salicylic acid terminal elimination profile and are not necessarily indicative of first-order conditions. A pharmacokinetic model was developed

TABLE 1. *Dose of aspirin adjusted for age and corresponding body weight*[a]

		Units/dose[b]					Units/dose[b]				
Age (yr)	Body wt (kg)	1	2	3	4	5	1	2	3	4	5
		mg/dose as ASA (or as SA)					mg/kg/dose as ASA (or as SA)				
2–3	13–15	80(62)	160(124)	240(186)			6.2–5.3 (4.8–4.1)	12.3–10.7 (9.5–8.3)	18.5–16.0 (14.3–12.4)		
4–5	16–19		160(124)	240(186)	320(248)			10.0–8.4 (7.8–6.5)	15.0–12.6 (11.6–9.8)	20.0–16.8 (15.5–13.1)	
6–8	20–26			240(186)	320(248)	400(310)			12.0–9.2 (9.3–7.2)	16.0 12.3 (12.4–9.54)	20.0–15.4 (15.5–11.9)
Average single dose:											
Prior to 1979			160(124)				ASA range		9.4–7.6		
							mean		8.5		
							SA range		(7.3–5.9)		
							mean		(6.7)		
Current				240(186)			ASA range			14.4–11.9	
							mean			13.2	
							SA range			(11.2–9.2)	
							mean			(10.2)	
High					320(248)		ASA range				19.5–16.1
							mean				17.8
							SA range				(15.1–12.5)
							mean				(13.8)

ASA, aspirin; SA, salicylic acid.

[a]The body weight-adjusted dose shows the range for young (low body weight) and older (higher body weight) children included in the defined age groups. The range and the mean are shown for the mg/kg/dose, whereas only the mean is shown for the mg/dose. See text for caveat about high dose. The high dose is shown for information purposes as it relates to the discussion about loading doses. The high dose should not be used for repeated administration without appropriate adjustment of dosage interval.

[b]Units/dose: ASA, 80 mg/tablet (or as SA, 62 mg/tablet) = 1 dosing unit.

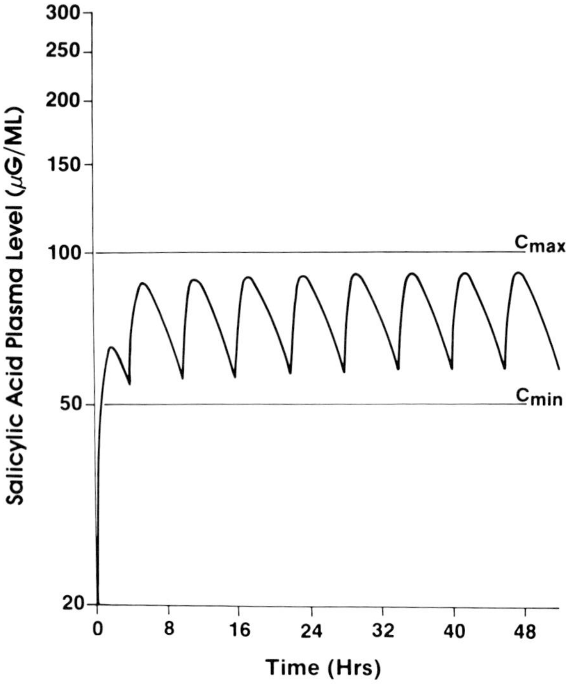

FIG. 1. Predicted average plasma level profile for a revised aspirin dose. Simulated plasma levels are based on the single-dose model described by Wilson et al. (6). A loading dose of one tablet more (total average dose 13.3 mg/kg aspirin or 10.2 mg/kg salicylic acid) than the age-related maintenance dose was given. The loading dose followed in 4 h by an average maintenance dose of 8.5 mg/kg aspirin or 6.7 mg/kg salicylic acid given every 6 h. This maintenance dosage corresponds to one tablet of aspirin less at each age range than that currently recommended. C_{max} and C_{min} depict the proposed range for antipyretic efficacy.

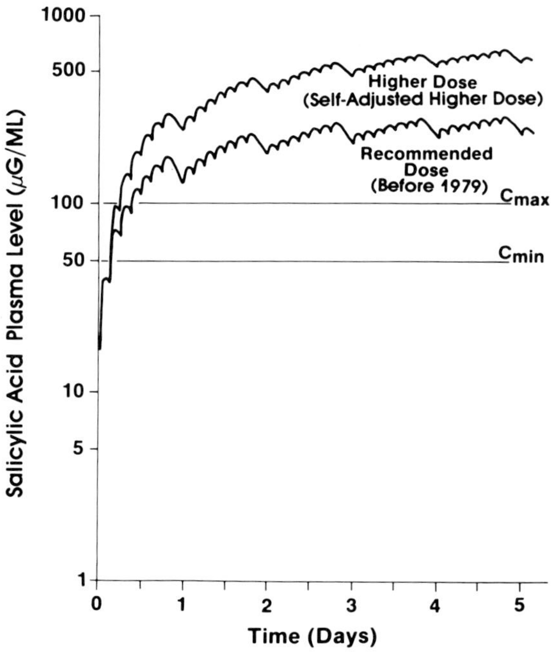

FIG. 2. Predicted average plasma levels for previous (before 1979) aspirin dose recommendations. Simulations are based on the model described for single-dose data in Wilson et al. (6). The recommended dose was 8.7 mg/kg aspirin or 6.7 mg/kg salicylic acid, and the higher dose was twofold higher, beginning after the first dose. Dosing interval was 3 h, and one nighttime dose was omitted at each 24-h period. C_{max} and C_{min} represent an estimate of therapeutic plasma drug levels for an average 70% Eff_{maxN}.

to incorporate both the first-order and Michaelis-Menten expressions. Data from febrile children and from those intoxicated with salicylic acid closely fit plasma salicylic acid simulations derived from the model (6).

The plasma level range to achieve about 70% antipyretic efficacy was estimated as 50–100 μg/ml salicylic acid. This estimate was based on maximum efficacy observed, corresponding plasma levels, and our pharmacodynamic analysis of probable mechanisms responsible for aspirin antipyresis. Briefly, in children given a single aspirin dose, antipyresis occurred during a phase temporally related to drug distribution. The plasma levels associated with this phase and the observed plateau of decreased temperature were used to estimate the therapeutic range.

Aspirin dose revisions were used to simulate plasma levels in accordance with our model (6). A regimen of doses lower than that now used as well as longer dosing intervals was proposed to keep plasma salicylic acid oscillations within the desired range. Two revisions have practical utility. In Fig. 1, a loading dose of aspirin is given, and the maintenance dose every 6 h is begun 4 h after the loading dose. If this schedule is modified slightly such that the dose interval is 6 h between loading and maintenance doses, then dosing instructions are simplified and could be similar to a proposed acetaminophen dose schedule (see below). An aggressive approach, with the first loading dose of two tablets more (instead of one more) than the maintenance dose shown in the legend of Fig. 1, produces predicted average plasma salicylic acid levels within the proposed range after the first and subsequent doses for 5 days of treatment when the loading and maintenance intervals were 6 h. These simulations require prospective testing for efficacy and predicted plasma salicylic acid levels in children before therapeutic recommendations can be made.

Adverse effects from aspirin are predominately hematologic and metabolic (22) and occur from iatrogenic causes in children as well as after single overdose (23–27). A pharmacokinetic basis for toxicity with repeated, self-directed doses is apparent. Application of our model produced simulations of plasma levels that were above the proposed range and within those associated with toxicity (17) (Fig 2). This applies to simulated levels for doses prior to 1979 (17) (Fig. 2) and also for those currently on the package label. This plasma salicylic acid accumulation pattern is a result of saturation kinetics for salicylic acid elimination (20,28–30). The current dosage regimen produced an average predicted plasma salicylic acid peak of 370 μg/ml and a trough of 270 μg/ml after 5 days of dosing. The peak level of salicylic was above the proposed therapeutic range after the second dose of aspirin. This simulation reveals the need to evaluate a lower dosage regimen so that a safer dose of aspirin can be used. Such use may not only lessen iatrogenic problems with aspirin, but also clarify the proposed association with Reye's syndrome. A functional association has not been demonstrated in spite of the statistical association (i.e., relative risk) found by epidemiologic studies (31). The plasma levels of salicylic acid found in some cases of Reye's syndrome and controls (32) have not been suitable for pharmacokinetic analysis of peak after last dose or for detection of differences in metabolite profile. Information on the Reye's syndrome issue as it relates to an adverse effect of aspirin requires that we have data on salicylic acid disposition in control children properly matched to those with Reye's syndrome. Until then, the relative risk of epidemiologic studies will be difficult to interpret for purposes of therapeutic decisions (33).[1]

ACETAMINOPHEN

The liquid formulation of acetaminophen for children enables a more flexible approach to dosing. However, doses were (and are) indexed to aspirin dosing, since no chronic graded dose–response study has been reported for either drug in febrile children. The manufacturer of Tylenol (McNeil Consumer Products) has recently changed the Tylenol Elixir to 160 mg/tsp from 120 mg/tsp. This conforms to the FDA recommendation of 80 mg as a standard dosing unit of APDs for children. An age-related and corresponding body weight-adjusted dose of acetaminophen is shown in Tables 2 and 3 for the 120-mg and the 160-mg/tsp formulation, respectively. Acetaminophen tablets are also available for children aged 2–8 years, and a summary of doses is similar to that shown in Table 3, with the exception that one unit is 80 mg/tablet. Comments made for aspirin with regard to average doses for the ages shown and for young versus older children doses pertain also to acetaminophen doses given in these tables.

[1]See footnote 2 on page 9.

The absolute and relative antipyretic efficacy of acetaminophen has been established for febrile children (see aspirin efficacy and references). A graded dose study of acetaminophen efficacy in children has been done in the Federal Republic of Germany recently by Windorfer and Vogel (34). They found a dose-dependent efficacy for single doses of 5, 10, and 20 mg/kg. Data are not sufficient to calculate a time of onset, but the rate of initial antipyresis [estimated by use of a modified ESTRIP program (6,35)] was dose dependent. Their rates of antipyresis as calculated by us were higher than for our children given a similar acetaminophen dose. Our study (6), however, had more data points available prior to the maximum decrease in temperature. The duration of acetaminophen antipyresis was at least 4 h in our study and about 6 h in their study (34). It is possible that a longer duration would be found for aspirin and acetaminophen if a chronic graded-dose study were done. Dose predictions will necessarily be based on available information from current doses and the derived simulations (see below) until such information is available.

A single-dose (9.1 ± 0.62 mg/kg) disposition study of acetaminophen in febrile children aged 2–7 years revealed the following average values for plasma acetaminophen (6): k_{el} = 0.376 ± 0.052 h^{-1}, $t_{1/2}$ = 1.8 h, V_d = 859 ± 69 ml/kg, Cl = 277 ± 20 ml/kg/h. The V_d and Cl were adjusted for the presystemic clearance effect described for adults (36).

The plasma level range to achieve 70% antipyretic efficacy was estimated at 4–18 μg/ml acetaminophen. This estimate was derived according to the criteria described above for aspirin. This range also encompasses antipyresis observed with a slightly higher single dose of acetaminophen (12.4 ± 0.82 mg/kg) (6).

Dose revisions for acetaminophen were calculated from plasma levels simulated by use of a model for acetaminophen in febrile children (6). It was apparent that the prior to 1982 dose and dosage interval (6–8 h) for acetaminophen produced plasma levels that were subtherapeutic for the entire interval. Plasma levels predicted for a dosage interval of 4 h and a higher dose are shown in Fig. 3. Interestingly, this dose is that attained with the new formulation of Tylenol Elixir (160 mg/tsp), and the manufacturer has also recently adjusted the dosage interval for both Tylenol Children's Tablets and Elixir to 4 h. The plasma acetaminophen levels and efficacy predicted in Fig. 3, however, have not been confirmed by prospective clinical evaluation. To simplify dosing instructions such that both aspirin and acetaminophen would have sim-

TABLE 2. *Dose of acetaminophen adjusted for age and corresponding body weight*[a]

Age (yr)	Body wt (kg)	Tsp/dose[b] 1 (mg/dose)	1.5	2	2.5	3	Tsp/dose[b] 1 (mg/kg/dose)	1.5	2	2.5	3
2–3	13–15	120	180	240			9.2–8.0	13.8–12.0	18.5–16.0		
4–5	16–19		180	240	300			11.3–9.5	15.0–12.6	18.8–15.8	
6–8	20–26			240	300	360		9.0–6.9	12.0–9.2	15.0–11.5	18.0–13.8
Average single dose:			180								
Prior to 1982							APAP range	10.8–8.9			
							mean	9.9			
				240			APAP range		14.6–12.0		
							mean		13.3		
High					300		APAP range			18.5–15.1	
							mean			16.8	

APAP, acetaminophen.
[a]See Table 1 footnote regarding range for younger and older children and for caveat about high doses.
[b]Units/dose for APAP: 120 mg/tsp, 24 mg/ml.

TABLE 3. *Dose of acetaminophen adjusted for age and corresponding body weight*[a]

Age (yr)	Body wt (kg)	Tsp/dose[b] 1 (mg/dose)	1.5	2	2.5	3	Tsp/dose[b] 1 (mg/kg/dose)	1.5	2	2.5	3
2–3	13–15	160	240	320			12.3–10.7	18.5–16.0	24.6–21.3		
4–5	16–19		240	320	400			15.0–12.6	20.0–16.8	25.0–21.0	
6–8	20–26			320	400	480			16.0–12.3	20.0–15.4	24.0–18.5
Average single dose:			240								
							APAP range	14.4–11.9			
							mean	13.3			
				320			APAP range		19.5–16.1		
							mean		17.8		
High					400		APAP range			24.5–20.3	
							mean			22.4	

APAP, acetaminophen.
[a]See Table 1 footnote regarding range for younger and older children and for caveat about high doses.
[b]Units/dose for APAP: 160 mg/tsp, 32 mg/ml.

ilar instructions, a higher dose of acetaminophen given every 6 h was simulated. As seen in Fig. 4, the first plasma acetaminophen peak level is above the proposed range, but subsequent peaks and troughs remain in the range for most of the dosage interval. As for aspirin, these dose–plasma level efficacy predictions require prospective evaluation.

Liver toxicity of acetaminophen has been described in children given a single dose (23,37,38) or repeated (39) large doses. In contrast to aspirin, single overdose rather than unexpected accumulation of acetaminophen to toxic levels has been responsible for the majority of hepatic toxicity. Saturation kinetics for acetaminophen elimination have been described (40), but do not appear to have a significant effect at plasma levels proposed for antipyresis. The acetaminophen sulfate metabolite predominates in the young infant (41). The age-related (or fever-influenced) rate and route of acetaminophen metabolite formation is not known for children 2–8 years old or older. While this information can be obtained in children, the long-term mutagenic or carcinogenic potential of reactive acetaminophen metabolites requires careful and extended observation.

CHOLINE SALICYLATE

Choline salicylic acid is a liquid salicylate formulation available for children. It has an amount of salicylic acid in each teaspoon equivalent to the amount of salicylic acid in a children's aspirin tablet.

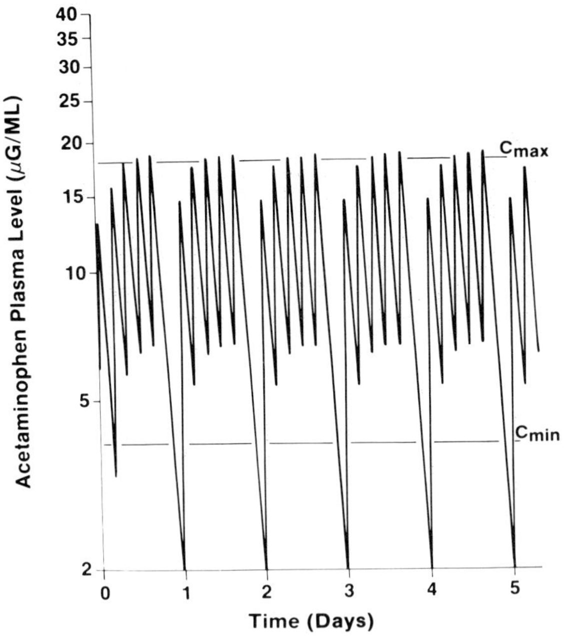

FIG. 3. Predicted average plasma level profile for a revised acetaminophen dose given every 4 h. See Wilson et al. (6) for simulation parameters. The dosage of acetaminophen is 13.3 mg/kg given every 4 h, and a nightly dose was deleted during each 24-h period. This dose corresponds to 1.5, 2, and 2.5 tsp/dose of acetaminophen (120 mg/tsp) on an age-related basis. (See Table 2.)

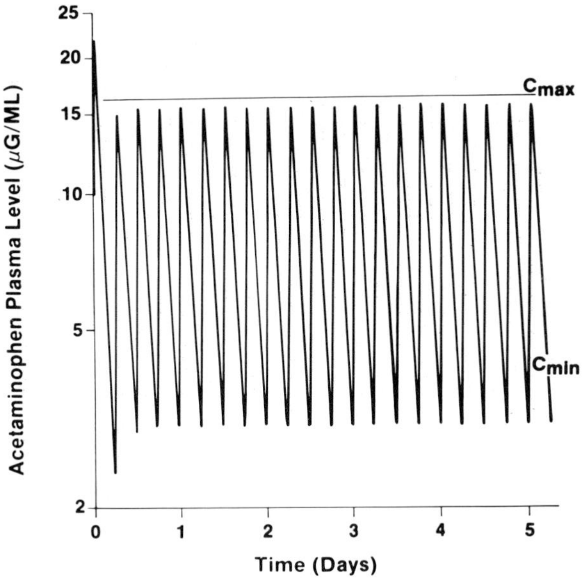

FIG. 4. Predicted plasma levels of acetaminophen for a revised acetaminophen dose (new dose strength of 160 mg/5 ml). See Wilson et al. (6) for pharmacokinetic parameters, as derived from single-dose data, which were used to prepare this simulation. The average loading dose was 17.8 mg/kg, and this corresponds to 1.5, 2, and 2.5 tsp for children aged 2–3, 4–5, and 6–8 years, respectively. The average maintenance dose was 13.3 mg/kg, and this corresponds to 1, 1.5, and 2 tsp for children aged 2–3, 4–5, and 6–8 years, respectively. The dosage interval was 6 h. (See Table 3.)

Absolute efficacy of choline salicylic acid as shown in an earlier pediatric study (42,43) has been confirmed (6). However, the average extent of temperature reduction was 28%, as compared with about 70% for similar single doses of aspirin and acetaminophen [see $\%Eff_{max_N}$ expression in Wilson et al. (6)]. The onset of antipyresis was similar for aspirin and choline salicylic acid These findings and our pharmacodynamic interpretation of salicylate antipyresis raise questions about the role of aspirin per se in antipyresis observed with aspirin.

The disposition of salicylic acid from choline salicylic acid appeared similar to that of salicylic acid from aspirin (6). The k_{abs} for choline salicylic acid was 6.96 ± 1.75 h^{-1} as compared with 1.46 ± 0.20 h^{-1} for that from aspirin. This contributed to an earlier t_{max} for choline salicylate (0.67 ± 0.12 h) as compared with aspirin (2.26 ± 0.31 h). The k_{abs} and t_{max} of choline salicylate were similar to those for acetaminophen. It is unfortunate that the time of onset of fever reduction and the maximum extent of temperature decrease were not found to be greater for choline salicylate, since an earlier t_{max} and similar C_{max} were found for plasma salicylic acid as compared with aspirin.

The dose revisions for aspirin may apply to choline salicylate if one restricts estimates to salicylic acid only. Similar disposition kinetics for the two drugs reveal this as a likely possibility. Graded doses of choline salicylate have not been examined in children. This drug should not be discarded from a useful list of pediatric APDs until such studies are done.

The adverse effects of salicylic acid from choline salicylate are presumed to be the same as those for salicylic acid in children. Information from studies or from widespread use, however, is not available to confirm this assumption.

NONSTEROID ANTIINFLAMMATORY DRUGS

Ibuprofen

Ibuprofen (2-[-4-isobutylphenyl]propionic acid) is available as a liquid formulation in Europe. Efficacy of ibuprofen syrup was compared with acetaminophen syrup in febrile children aged 2–8 years (44). A single dose was calculated for children by application of Young's Rule to an adult dose of 400 and 300 mg ibuprofen and acetaminophen, respectively. The exact dose was not stated for the age range studied. Both rectal and axillary temperatures were monitored. The rate of temperature fall was similar for both drugs, and the maximum decrease was at about 4–6 h. The magnitude of this decrease was similar for both drugs. Duration of antipyresis was at least 12 h (with regard to values less than initial temperature), but the temperature decrease with ibuprofen was greater than that of acetaminophen at 6–8 h after the dose. The antipyretic plateau ended at about 5 and 8 h for acetaminophen and ibuprofen, respectively.

A previous study used ibuprofen tablets in febrile children aged 3 months to 13 years (45) and compared antipyretic efficacy to that of acetaminophen and aspirin. Body weight–adjusted doses (by use of crushed tablets) were 5 mg/kg ibuprofen, 10 mg/kg aspirin, and 12.5 mg/kg acetaminophen as a single oral dose. The maximum antipyretic response was at 4 h for all drugs, and the plateau of effect ended at about 6 h. The mass potency (i.e., dose) of ibuprofen was about twofold that of aspirin with regard to assessed parameters for antipyresis. A graded dosage regimen for optimal antipyresis in febrile children has not been studied.

The disposition of ibuprofen in febrile children has not been evaluated. We have recently adapted our high performance liquid chromatography (HPLC) method (46) for application to pediatric blood samples. It is hoped that pharmacokinetic information on ibuprofen in plasma will soon be available for febrile children. However, a recent study of ibuprofen disposition in children with juvenile chronic arthritis contains some pharmacokinetic information that may be useful for developing studies of ibuprofen in febrile children (47). Children (aged 1.5–15 years) with arthritis received a mean ibuprofen dose of 37.1 mg/kg/day divided in three doses. The mean peak plasma level at 1–2 h was 31 μg/ml and at 12 h it was 4 μg/ml. The average $t_{1/2}$ was 2.3 ± 0.5 h. Interindividual variation in plasma levels was marked. This may be indicative of age-dependent differences in drug disposition if the data were segregated into ranges more narrow than 1.5–15 years. Synovial fluid concentrations were less than those of serum until 10 h after a dose of ibuprofen. Disposition of serum ibuprofen found in this study is apparently similar to the results reported previously for adults and children (47–50).

A single-dose study of febrile children given ibuprofen showed no changes in serum alanine aminotransferase (GOT) or aspartate aminotransferase (GPT) (45). Chronic toxicity remains unknown for such children, although side effects have been described for children with chronic juvenile arthritis (51) and may be as high as 18% in such children (52). Stempel and Miller (53) reported fever, lymphopenia, and liver dysfunction in a 12-year old child who had received long-term treatment with ibuprofen for arthritis.

Naproxen

Naproxen [(+)-6-methoxy-α-methyl-2-naphthalene acetic acid] was placed in suspension for administration to febrile children aged 3–12 years (54). A dose of 2.5 and 7.5 mg/kg was compared with a 15 mg/kg dose of aspirin and a placebo, all given in a double-blind manner. Both aspirin and naproxen showed an antipyretic effect maximum at about 4 h. After about 4 h, the temperature in those receiving aspirin increased, whereas in those given naproxen (higher dose), it remained lower until 9 h and then decreased further until 12 h. An antipyretic dose response was shown for naproxen. When this study is reviewed, it is important to note that high fever required children to be removed from the placebo group, thereby giving an apparent efficacy to placebo. Comments here are restricted to comparisons to initial (predose) temperature. In general, the duration of antipyresis was longer for naproxen, and dose potency was about twofold as compared with aspirin. The recommended dose of naproxen for treatment of juvenile rheumatoid arthritis is 10 mg/kg/day divided in two daily doses (55).

Disposition of naproxen in febrile children is not known. This must await development of suitable technology for analysis of blood and urine samples. Such are needed to establish a therapeutic range for antipyresis when graded and long-term dose studies are undertaken with naproxen. It is also important to have such information for assessment of the drug accumulation profile. A detailed study of naproxen in animals and adult men revealed general disposition characteristics (56). Plasma $t_{1/2}$ was 10–17 h, and the majority of naproxen was eliminated as metabolites and conjugates in the urine. Prior treatment in a limited number of individuals showed no enzyme induction effects on its own metabolism. Dose-dependent changes in $t_{1/2}$ were not found. The human V_d was about twice that of the plasma compartment, and plasma protein binding was 99.9%. A large amount of the drug was restricted to the vascular compartment. While this information is useful for naproxen dosing in adults, similar pharmacokinetic information needs to be obtained for children.

Single-dose toxicity of naproxen was evaluated in febrile children (54). Gastrointestinal complaints were more frequent in children given naproxen (7.5 mg/kg) as compared with children given placebo or aspirin. Laboratory analyses of blood count and chemistries showed no differences between groups treated with placebo, aspirin, or naproxen. In children with juvenile rheumatoid arthritis, who were treated with repeated dosing of naproxen, gastrointestinal disturbance and central nervous system symptoms were found and were reported to disappear when the drug was discontinued (55).

Diclofenac

Suppositories of diclofenac [2-[(2,6-dichlorophenyl)amino]benzeneacetic acid monosodium salt] were given to febrile children aged 2–10 years (57). The dose was 25 mg for ages 2–5 years and 50 mg for ages 6–10 years. Temperature returned to normal by 2 h with a maximum decrease seen at 2–4 h as compared with placebo or initial temperature. Duration of antipyresis was for at least 6 h. Similar efficacy results were obtained in another study (58) of febrile children.

Disposition of diclofenac has not been studied in febrile children who have no underlying chronic illness. In those with chronic juvenile arthritis (aged 2–7 years), the urinary profile of the drug was similar to that of adults (5). It is apparent that information on diclofenac disposition is needed for dosing and efficacy purposes in febrile children.

Single-dose and long-term studies for adverse effects from diclofenac in febrile children are needed if this drug is considered for antipyretic use.

INDICATIONS FOR ANTIPYRETIC DRUG USE

The role of fever has been analyzed from a phylogenetic or comparative standpoint (59,60). Results from ectothermic and endothermic animals appear to support a beneficial role of initial fever in the host response to infection. From an evolutionary perspective fever may be adaptive. A physiologic and biochemical review of fever production during an infection suggests prostaglandin synthesis as one site for APD action (60,61,61a). Stern (61) has contrasted the specificity of APD action in conditions with altered hypothalamic set point as compared with application of physical methods to lower body temperature. The latter methods may provide increased stress and discomfort with little sustained antipyresis in such conditions. The prevalent use of APDs in children with mild fever has been termed "fever phobia" (62). About 85% of parents gave APDs before the temperature was 38.9°C (102°F). Discomfort from fever was described at about 39.5–40.0°C (103–104°F), and temperatures over 42°C (107.6°F) have been harmful. Hyperpyrexia was defined by Schmidtt (62) as a temperature of more than 41°C (105.8°F), but this was rare, with an occurrence of 1 in 2,100 patient visits. Occurrence among hospitalized patients was higher, especially in those with a central nervous system infection. From these reviews we conclude that indiscriminate use of APDs in all febrile children cannot be justified. APDs, however, cannot be withheld from certain febrile children[2] if, in the individual case, the use is considered appropriate because of concern for harmful elevations of temperatures, febrile seizures, or for alleviation of discomfort. Benefit–risk decisions await answers to the important question about fever and the host defense mechanism in man. Regardless of the reason for their use, the dosage regimen for APDs should be one to provide optimum antipyresis and minimum risk of toxicity.

CONCLUDING REMARKS

If APDs are used in children then they must be tested in them. A single- and multiple-dosage finding study should include design features sufficient to provide efficacy and pharmacokinetic information necessary to make practical and safe dose recommendations. A model and simulations for such a design have been proposed (6). Attention to adverse effects must include risks posed by developing systems and by the age-related changes in drug disposition. Ethical and technical limitations heretofore cited as impediments to data acquisition in children can be handled sufficiently to perform a carefully planned study. Indeed, technical advancements have allowed ethically feasible studies to go forward in children (63). Therapeutic indications and dosage regimens of APDs (i.e., label directions) for children must be based on similar criteria demanded for drug use in adults.

---

[2]The functional meaning of the epidemiologic findings about aspirin and Reye's syndrome was being debated at the time this report was prepared. The reader is advised to refer to current aspirin package labelling as it reflects emerging guidelines about aspirin and Reye's syndrome.

Note added in proof: Two recent publications (64,65) utilized a somewhat different approach to arrive at recommendations similar to ours (6) for the dosing of acetaminophen in young children.

Acknowledgment: This work was supported in part by a Clinical Pharmacology Program Development Grant from the Pharmaceutical Manufacturers Association Foundation. The secretarial assistance of Mrs. Carole Webb is appreciated. I thank my coauthors on a previous publication (6) for their help with excerpts from that work.

REFERENCES

1. Done AK. Antipyretics: should fever be reduced? *Pediatr Clin North Am* 1972;19:167–77.
2. Wilson JT. Antipyretic management of febrile seizures. In: Nelson KB, Ellenberg JH, eds. *Febrile seizures*, New York: Raven Press, 1981:231–9.
3. MacKintosh DA, Bowie J, Baird-Lambert J, Buchanan N. Febrile children and antipyretic drugs [Letter to Editor]. *Med J Aust* 1982;18:264–6.
4. Landau J, Schudmak A. Der therapeutische wert des aspirins in der kinderpraxis. *Heilkunde* 1901;14:509.
5. Federal Register. Over-the-counter drugs (proposed rules). *Fed Reg* 1977; 42:35346.
6. Wilson JT, Brown RD, Bocchini JA, Kearns GL. Efficacy, disposition and pharmacodynamics of aspirin, acetaminophen and choline salicylate in young febrile children. *Ther Drug Monit* 1982;4:147–80.
7. Done AK, Yaffe SJ, Clayton JM. Aspirin dosage for infants and children. *J Pediatr* 1979;95:617.
8. Done AK, Yaffe SJ, Clayton JM. New dosage for aspirin—long overdue, but wrong. *Pediatr Alert* 1979;4:93–4.
9. Cornely DA, Ritter JA. N-Acetyl-P-Aminophenol (Tylenol® Elixir) as a pediatric antipyretic-analgesic. *JAMA* 1956; 160:1219–21.
10. Steele RW, Tanaka PT, Lara RP, Bass JW. Evaluation of sponging and of oral antipyretic therapy to reduce fever. *J Pediatr* 1970;77:824–9.
11. Colgan MT, Mintz AA. The comparative antipyretic effect of N-acetyl-p-aminophenol and acetylsalicylic acid. *J Pediatr* 1957;50:552–5.
12. Mintz AA. Management of the febrile child. *Ken Acad Gen Pract J* 1959;5:26.
13. Steele RW, Young FSH, Bass JW, Shirkey HC. Oral antipyretic therapy. Evaluation of aspirin–acetaminophen combination. *Am J Dis Child* 1972;123:204–6.
14. Eden AN, Kauffman A. Clinical comparison of three antipyretic agents. *AM J Dis Child* 1967;114:284–7.
15. Tarlin L, Landrigan P. A comparison of the antipyretic effect of acetaminophen and aspirin. *Am J Dis Child* 1972;124:880–2.
16. Hunter J. Study of antipyretic therapy in current use. *Arch Dis Child* 1973;48:313–5.
17. Vignec AJ, Gasparik M. Antipyretic effectiveness of salicylamide and acetylsalicylic acid in infants. *JAMA* 1958;167:1821–6.
18. Borovsky MP. Antipyretic activity of acetylsalicylic acid and salicylamide suspension in pediatrics. *Am J Dis Child* 1960;100:47–54.
19. Mintz AA. Antipyretic effect of acetophenetidin. *Clin Med* 1964; 71:865–70.
20. Levy G. Clinical pharmacokinetics of aspirin. *Pediatrics* 1978;62:867–72.
21. Yaffe SJ. Comparative efficacy of aspirin and acetaminophen in the reduction of fever in children. *Arch Intern Med* 1981;141:286–92.
22. Gilman AG, Goodman LS, Gilman A, eds. *The pharmacological basis of therapeutics, 6th ed*, New York: Macmillan, 1980:126.
23. Wilson JT, Ksantikul V, Harbison R, Martin D. Death in an adolescent following an overdose of acetaminophen and phenobarbital. *Am J Dis Child* 1978;132:466–73.
24. Wilson JT. Special problems for drugs used in children. *South Med J* 1976;69:779–86.
25. Levy G, Yaffe SJ. The study of salicylate pharmacokinetics in intoxicated infants and children. *Clin Toxicol* 1968;1:409–24.
26. Done AK. Salicylate intoxication. Significance of measurements of salicylate in blood in cases of acute ingestion. *Pediatrics* 1960;26:800–7.
27. Done AK. Treatment of salicylate poisoning: review of personal and published experiences. *Clin Toxicol* 1968;1:451–67.
28. Levy G. Pharmacokinetics of salicylate elimination in man. *J Pharm Sci* 1965;54:959–67.
29. Levy G, Tsuchiya T, Amsel LP. Limited capacity for salycil phenolic glucuronide formation and its effect on the kinetics of salicylate elimination in man. *Clin Pharmacol Ther* 1972;13:258–68.
30. Levy G, Tsuchiya T. Salicylate accumulation kinetics in man. *N Engl J Med* 1972;287:430–2.
31. Reye's Syndrome. Report from Ohio and Michigan. *Morbidity and mortality report*. 1980;29:532–8, 1982;31:53–6, 61–3.
32. Partin JS, Partin JC, Schubert WK, Hammond JG. Serum salicylate concentrations in Reye's Disease. A study of 130 biopsy-proven cases. *Lancet* 1982; 1;191–4.
33. Wilson JT, Brown RD. Reye Syndrome and aspirin use: the role of prodromal illness severity in the assessment of relative risk. *Pediatrics* 1982;69:822–5.
34. Windorfer A, Vogel C. Investigations concerning serum concentration and temperature following oral application of a new paracetamol preparation. *Klin Padiatr* 1976;188:430–4.
35. Brown RD, Manno JE. ESTRIP, A BASIC computer program for obtaining initial polyexponential parameter estimates. *J Pharm Sci* 1978;67:1687–91.
36. Rawlins MD, Henderson DB, Hijab AR. Pharmacokinetics of paracetamol (acetaminophen) after intravenous and oral administration. *Eur J Clin Pharmacol* 1977;11:283–6.
37. Arena JM, Rourk MH, Sibrack CD. Acetaminophen: report of an unusual poisoning. *Pediatrics* 1978;61:68–72.
38. Rumack BH, Peterson RG. Acetaminophen overdose: incidence, diagnosis, and management in 416 patients. *Pediatrics* 1978;62(suppl):898–903.
39. Nogen AG, Bremner JE. Fatal acetaminophen overdosage in a young child. *J Pediatr* 1978;92:832–3.
40. Slattery JT, Levy G. Acetaminophen kinetics in acutely poisoned patients. *Clin Pharmacol Ther* 1979;25:185–95.
41. Alam SN, Roberts RJ, Fischer LJ. Age-related differences in salicylamide and acetaminophen conjugation in man. *J Pediatr* 1977;90:130–5.
42. Hunt WD. Choline salicylate as an antipyretic and analgesic in pediatric practice. *Clin Med* 1962; 69(12):2688–93.
43. Tupper JA. Choline salicylate in pediatric practice. *Northwest Med* 1963;62:122–4.
44. Sheth UK, Gupta K, Paul T, Pispati PK. Measurement of antipyretic activity of ibuprofen and paracetamol in children. *J Clin Pharmacol* 1980;20:672–4.
45. Simila S, Kouvalainen K, Keinanen S. Oral antipyretic therapy: evaluation of ibuprofen. *Scand J Rheumatol* 1976;5: 81–3.
46. Kearns GL, Wilson JT. Determination of ibuprofen in serum by high-performance liquid chromatography and application to ibuprofen disposition. *J Chromatogr* 1981;226:183–90.
47. Makela AL, Lempiainen M, Yrjana T. Ibuprofen in the treatment of juvenile rheumatoid arthritis metabolism and concentrations in synovial fluid. *Br J Clin Pract* 1980;6(suppl):23.
48. Adams SS, Bough RG, Cliffe EE, Lessel B, Mills RFN.

Absorption, distribution and toxicity of ibuprofen. *Toxicol Appl Pharmacol* 1969;15:310–30.
49. Adams SS, Bough RG, Cliffe EE, et al. Some aspects of the pharmacology, metabolism, and toxicology of Ibuprofen. I. Pharmacology and metabolism. *Rheumatol Phys Med* 1970;10(suppl):9–22.
50. Mills RFN, Adams SS, Cliffe EE, Dickinson W, Nicholson JS. The metabolism of ibuprofen. *Xenobiotica* 1973;3:589.
51. Makela AL, Lempiainen M, Ylijoki H. Ibuprofen levels in serum and synovial fluid. *Scand J Rheumatol* 1981;39:15–7.
52. Brewer EJ. Nonsteroidal anti-inflammatory agents. *Arthritis Rheum* 1977;20:513–25.
53. Stempel DA, Miller JJ. Lymphopenia and hepatic toxicity with ibuprofen. *J Pediatr* 1977;90:657–8.
54. Cashman TM, Starns RJ, Johnson J, Oren J. Comparative effects of naproxen and aspirin on fever in children. *J Pediatr* 1979;95:626–9.
55. Ansell BM, Hanna B, Moran H, et al. Naproxen in juvenile chronic polyarthritis. *Eur J Rheum Inflam* 1979;2:79.
56. Runkel R, Chaplin M, Boost G, Segre E, Forchielli E. Absorption, distribution, metabolism, and excretion of naproxen in various laboratory animals and human subjects. *J Pharm Sci* 1972;61(5):703–8.
57. Polman HA, Huijbers WAR, Augusteijn R. The use of diclofenac sodium (Voltaren®) suppositories as an antipyretic in children with fever due to acute infections: a double-blind, between-patient, placebo-controlled study. *J Int Med Res* 1981;9:343–8.
58. Keinanen-Kiukaanniemi S, Simila S, Kapyla H. Antipyretic therapy: evaluation of diclofenac sodium as an antipyretic agent. *Clin Ther* 1980;2:421.
59. Donaldson JF. Therapy of acute fever: a comparative approach. *Hosp Pract* 1981;16(9):125–38.
60. Kluger MJ. Fever. *Pediatrics* 1980;66:720–24.
61. Stern RC. Pathophysiologic basis for symptomatic treatment of fever. *Pediatrics* 1977;59:92–8.
61a. Dinarello C, Wolff S. Pathogenesis of fever in man. *N Engl J Med* 1978;298:607–12.
62. Schmidtt BD. Fever phobia. *Am J Dis Child* 1980;134:176–81.
63. Wilson JT. Pediatric pharmacology: who will test the drugs? *J Pediatr* 1972;80:855–7.
64. Temple AR. Pediatric dosing of acetaminophen. *Pediatr Pharmacol* 1983;3:321–7.
65. Lewis JM. Pediatric dosing of acetaminophen [Letter to the Editor]. *Pediatr Pharmacol* 1984;4:253–4.

Therapeutic Drug Monitoring
7:12–25

Review

An Overview of Amikacin

Angela M. Ristuccia and Burke A. Cunha

Infectious Disease Division, Department of Medicine, Nassau Hospital, Mineola, New York, U.S.A.

Amikacin, a semisynthetic derivative of kanamycin A, was developed in an effort to chemically modify the basic kanamycin structure to protect it from the inactivating mechanisms of resistant organisms. The structure of amikacin is shown in Fig. 1. Amikacin differs in structure from kanamycin by the acylation at the C-1 amino group of the deoxystreptamine nucleus. The selective acylation of the amino group with an amino acid (L-(−)-4-amino-2-hydroxybutyric acid) proved to greatly widen the antimicrobial spectrum and increase the activity of kanamycin.

Physicochemically, amikacin is a white, crystalline, basic, water-soluble antibiotic with a melting point of 201–204°C. The specific optical rotation of amikacin is +97° to +105°. The molecular formula for the compound in its free base form is $C_{22}H_{43}N_5O_{13}$ (1).

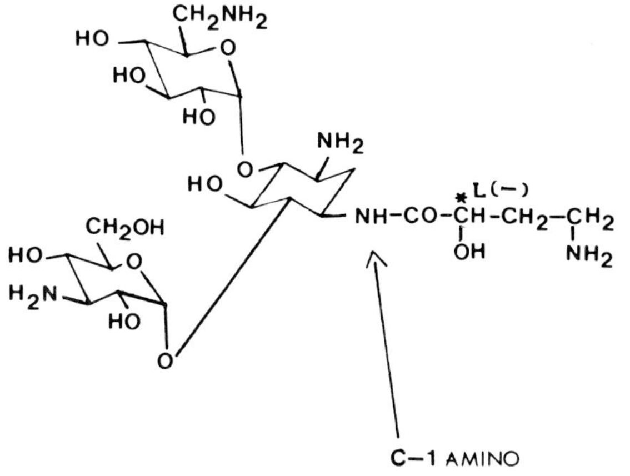

FIG. 1. Structure of amikacin.

MECHANISM OF ACTION

Amikacin, like other aminoglycoside antibiotics, is bactericidal, acting directly on the 30S and 50S bacterial ribosomal subunits to inhibit protein synthesis. Since the drug is highly polar, it is actively transported across the cell membrane in two distinct transport phases (2,3). The first is relatively inefficient and involves binding of the drug to respiratory energization complexes transported through the cell membrane. The second phase is energy dependent (oxygen-generated active transport). With marked accumulation of the drug within the cell, inhibition of protein synthesis begins. Binding irreversibly to the bacterial ribosomes, amikacin blocks the recognition step in protein synthesis, causing the misreading of the genetic code and production of defective proteins. The ribosomes prematurely separate from mRNA and cell death ensues.

The rate of transport of the aminoglycoside across the bacterial cell membrane can be altered significantly by the presence of divalent cations (Mg^{2+}, Ca^{2+}), the pH of the environment, and the amount of oxygen present. This observation explains the significant decrease in antimicrobial activity seen in an anaerobic or an acidic environment (4).

SPECTRUM

Studies have shown that amikacin is active in vitro and in vivo against a wide variety of gram-negative organisms (4–11). The spectrum of amikacin includes activity against *Citrobacter* spp., *Enterobacter* spp., *Escherichia coli, Haemophilus influenzae, Klebsiella pneumoniae, Morganella morganii (Proteus morganii), Proteus vulgaris, Providencia* spp., and *Pseudomonas aeruginosa*.

Comparative studies of the aminoglycosides have shown that on a weight basis amikacin is less active than gentamicin or tobramycin (4,12). However, a clinical decision about the choice of an aminoglycoside should not be made on a weight basis but rather

Address correspondence and reprint requests to Dr. A. M. Ristuccia at Infectious Disease Division, Nassau Hospital, Mineola, NY 11501, U.S.A.

the achievable concentrations of each aminoglycoside should be considered. This apparent disadvantage of amikacin is no longer as apparent after comparing the considerably higher serum concentrations obtainable with amikacin with the concentrations achieved with gentamicin or tobramycin. The kill ratio, or the ratio of the peak serum concentration to the minimum inhibitory concentration (MIC) of the organism for which the drug is being considered, is the most persuasive evidence reported to date relating the influence of a pharmacokinetic index to effectiveness of antibiotic therapy. A few investigators have addressed the issue of antibacterial efficacy, relating the peak serum levels to the MIC of the organism (13–15). They found that a kill ratio of 4 to 8:1 resulted in significant antibacterial effectiveness and, in the in vivo studies, that the clinical success rate was 67 to >80% when this ratio was achieved.

In a study involving 2,741 clinical isolates, amikacin was the most active aminoglycoside tested, with 94% of the bacterial strains susceptible, as compared with 79 and 76%, respectively, for tobramycin and gentamicin (16). A breakdown by species tested showed that of 827 isolates of *P. aeruginosa*, 92% were susceptible to amikacin, whereas 83 and 78%, respectively, were susceptible to tobramycin and gentamicin. Of 182 isolates of *Serratia marcescens* tested, 91% were susceptible to amikacin, whereas 35 and 42%, respectively, were susceptible to tobramycin and gentamicin.

The activity of amikacin against some of the commonly encountered gram-negative organisms is comparable to the activity of gentamicin and tobramycin. Table 1 lists the mean MICs of the aminoglycosides to gentamicin-sensitive gram-negative rods. An important difference is the degree of activity of the aminoglycosides against *Pseudomonas* strains at clinically achievable concentrations. Table 2 summarizes data on activity of gentamicin, tobramycin, and amikacin against *Pseudomonas*. Amikacin is especially effective against many gentamicin- and tobramycin-resistant isolates of Enterobacteriaceae and *Pseudomonas* (Table 3) (6,8,9,11,17,18). Cross-resistance of gentamicin-resistant strains is observed much more frequently with tobramycin than with amikacin (19).

Although some activity has been shown against gram-positive organisms, the therapeutic usefulness of amikacin, like gentamicin and tobramycin, is limited to synergistic combinations with other agents when considered in the treatment of staphylococcal or enterococcal infections. Among the gram-positive organisms, amikacin is active against *Staphylococcus aureus* and *Staphylococcus epidermidis* (20–22). Amikacin exhibits weak activity against group A streptococci and *Streptococcus viridans* (23,24). Pneumococci are generally resistant and amikacin is active against the enterococcus only when combined with a penicillin (20,23,25). Although synergy has been shown when amikacin is combined with a penicillin against isolates of *Streptococcus faecalis*, gentamicin has much greater activity and remains the aminoglycoside of choice when used in combination to treat enterococcal infection (26,27).

TABLE 1. *Mean MIC of gentamicin, tobramycin, and amikacin for gentamicin-sensitive gram-negative rods*[a]

Organism	No. of strains	Mean MIC (μg/ml) Gentamicin	Tobramycin	Amikacin
Escherichia coli	52	0.5	1.0	2.0
Enterobacter spp.	18	0.5	0.5	1.0
Citrobacter spp.	14	0.5	0.5	1.0
Proteus mirabilis	32	0.5	1.0	2.0
Indole-positive *Proteus*	23	0.5	0.5	1.0
Klebsiella spp.	16	0.5	0.5	1.0
Pseudomonas aeruginosa	17	1.0	0.25	1.0
Serratia spp.	7	0.5	2.0	2.0

MIC, minimum inhibitory concentration.
[a]Data from ref. 132.

Amikacin has some activity against *Bacteroides urealyticus*, but in general is clinically ineffective against anaerobic bacteria, including *Bacteroides fragilis*, fusobacteria, clostridia, peptostreptococci, and other anaerobic cocci (24,28,29).

Although amikacin exhibits moderate in vitro activity against *Listeria monocytogenes, H. influenzae*, and *Mycobacterium pneumoniae*, other agents are preferable, and amikacin is not used for treatment of infections caused by these organisms (30–34). Amikacin exhibits in vitro and in vivo activity against *Nocardia asteroides* (35–37).

Amikacin is active in vitro against *Legionella pneumophilia*, but is not effective therapy for Legionnaires' pneumonia since treatment failures have been reported (38–41).

Amikacin has activity against some strains of *Mycobacterium tuberculosis* (42). *Mycobacterium chelonei* and *Mycobacterium fortuitum* are quite susceptible in vitro and amikacin has been clinically successful

TABLE 2. *Comparative activity of the aminoglycoside antibiotics at clinically achievable concentrations against* Pseudomonas *strains*

Reference	No. of *Pseudomonas* strains	Percent inhibited by: Gentamicin (4 μg/ml)	Tobramycin (4 μg/ml)	Amikacin (16 μg/ml)
Stewart and Bodey (7)	100	97	97	98
Young and Hewitt (4)	50	76	98	89
Price et al. (23)	110	67	—	93
Kluge et al. (55)	130	60	88	94
Dhawan et al. (133)	632	54	94	91
Braveny et al. (134)	228	89	90	99
Kelly and Matsen (56)	22	77	81	92

in the treatment of infections caused by these mycobacteria (43–45).

The major advantage of amikacin is its effectiveness against many gentamicin- and tobramycin-resistant gram-negative isolates. This has been proven clinically by successful treatment both of patients infected with resistant organisms and of patients who had previously failed aminoglycoside therapy (5,9,18,46).

RESISTANCE

The usefulness of the aminoglycosides is often limited by the emergence of bacterial resistance. Geographic variations in the number of resistant organisms sometimes result in strikingly different susceptibility patterns from one institution to another. Three mechanisms of bacterial resistance have been identified. First, alteration of the cellular transport system which effectively blocks the drug transport into the cell, resulting in decreased intracellular accumulation of the aminoglycoside. Second, alteration in the ribosomal target site of aminoglycoside attachment results in the inability of the drug to bind to the ribosome. The third mechanism is the elaboration of enzymes which inactivate the aminoglycoside (47).

TABLE 3. *Susceptibility of gentamicin-resistant gram-negative rods to tobramycin and amikacin*[a]

Organism	No. of strains	Percent susceptible at clinically achievable concentrations[b]: Tobramycin	Amikacin
Pseudomonas aeruginosa	32	75	85
Klebsiella aerogenes	13	15	92
Escherichia coli	7	0	72
Enterobacter spp.	25	0	100
Providencia spp.	35	14	92
Indole-positive *Proteus*	11	0	100
Acinetobacter spp.	27	30	33

[a]Data from ref. 132.
[b]Clinically achievable concentrations for tobramycin = 4 μg/ml, and for amikacin = 16 μg/ml.

Primary concern is focused on the mechanism involving enzymatic transformation. Since this mechanism is plasmid-mediated, the ability of bacteria to produce these enzymes may be passed to sensitive strains during bacterial conjugation. These plasmids, or R-factors, are capable of being transferred among gram-negative organisms, creating the potential for serious problems. Most resistance encountered clinically is attributable to the mechanism involving aminoglycoside-inactivating enzymes (48,49). There are currently 11 aminoglycoside-inactivating bacterial enzymes that have been identified. These enzymes will either adenylate or phosphorylate hydroxyl groups, or acetylate amino groups on the aminoglycoside molecule.

The structure of gentamicin or tobramycin is vulnerable to inactivation by eight of the aminoglycoside-inactivating enzymes, whereas amikacin is only inactivated by two of these enzymes. This structural difference gives amikacin a great advantage over gentamicin or tobramycin, and makes it quite useful against many of the gentamicin- or tobramycin-resistant bacterial strains. The decreased susceptibility of amikacin to enzyme degradation explains its high degree of activity against gentamicin- or tobramycin-resistant bacterial strains. In an in vitro study comparing aminoglycoside activity against clinical gram-negative isolates highly resistant to gentamicin (MIC $\geq$ 80 μg/ml), amikacin proved extremely effective in inhibiting all strains at clinically achievable concentrations (Table 4). To date, the majority of resistance encountered to amikacin appears to be due to the mechanism involving decreased penetration of

TABLE 4. *Activity of tobramycin and amikacin against clinical isolates highly resistant to gentamicin[a]*

Organism	No. of isolates	Mean MIC (μg/ml) Gentamicin	Tobramycin	Amikacin
Klebsiella pneumoniae	22	498	90	0.54
Enterobacter aerogenes	4	>1,360	160	1.25
Enterobacter cloacae	16	>1,700	162	0.99
Escherichia coli	8	1,240	126	1.25
Citrobacter freundii	1	1,280	160	1.25
Proteus mirabilis	1	640	5	2.5
Proteus morganii	3	>1,387	82	2.5
Proteus rettgeri	1	2,560	160	2.5
Proteus vulgaris	1	1,280	160	1.25

MIC, minimum inhibitory concentration.
[a]Data from ref. 135.

the drug into the bacterial cell. This type of resistance appears to be nonspecific and the vulnerability is shared by all other aminoglycosides. Little or no intracellular accumulation of the drug occurs because the organisms are severely impaired in their ability to transport the drug into the cell. This type of resistance is not plasmid mediated (50). Although strains resistant to gentamicin or tobramycin involving the inactivating enzymatic mechanism are sensitive to amikacin, strains resistant by this nonenzymatic mechanism are generally completely cross-resistant to all three aminoglycosides (19,51).

SYNERGY

In terms of patient survival, synergistic combinations of antibiotics have been shown to be more effective than either agent used alone. Synergy between β-lactam antibiotics (penicillins and cephalosporins) and aminoglycosides has been shown in vitro and in vivo. The mechanism of this synergistic action has been hypothesized to be an increase in the porosity of the bacterial cell wall produced by penicillin damage, thereby allowing more effective ingress of the aminoglycoside into the cell to the ribosomal site of action (52). An easy and quite useful role for this phenomenon is in the treatment of enterococcal endocarditis by increasing the bactericidal action of penicillin on enterococci, which are almost always resistant, in vitro, to either antibiotic alone (53,54). The decrease of the MIC to both antibiotics used in synergistic combinations makes it possible to reach higher levels of antibacterial activity in the serum of the patient, which is associated with a more favorable outcome than therapy with single agents. The combination of amikacin and a semisynthetic penicillin is synergistic against *P. aeruginosa, S. marcescens, E. coli, Klebsiella* spp., and *Proteus mirabilis* (55–58). In one study, the necessary concentration of amikacin to inhibit 90% of *P. aeruginosa* isolates was reduced from 12 to 5 μg/ml (approximately 1/6 achievable serum concentration) when combined with carbenicillin (55). Klastersky et al. (58) demonstrated synergy of amikacin and carbenicillin in 93.6% of 48 strains of *P. aeruginosa*. In the treatment of patients with serious gram-negative infections, the combination of an aminoglycoside and a penicillin provides a broader spectrum of activity and is synergistic against *Pseudomonas* and various Enterobacteriaceae (59–62).

Synergistic combinations are superior in vivo to single drug therapy, especially in patients whose natural mechanisms of defense against infection are poor, as in the neutropenic cancer patient. Successful treatment of gram-negative bacillemia in neutropenic patients has been achieved with combinations of broad-spectrum penicillins plus an aminoglycoside, and cephalosporins plus an aminoglycoside (63–66).

Response rates have been high for amikacin combined with carbenicillin, ticarcillin, cefazolin, or cephalothin as empiric therapy in febrile, neutropenic, immunocompromised patients (67–69). Because of the importance of antibiotic-resistant gram-negative rods, especially *P. aeruginosa*, encountered in these patients, amikacin's greater activity against aminoglycoside-resistant strains makes it the drug of choice in this situation. Although the importance of the adjustment of doses or change in antibiotics based on culture and sensitivity reports is well appreciated, investigators have shown that favorable clinical outcome is directly related to initial selection of an appropriate combination in the granulocytopenic, immunocompromised host (64). Amikacin has proven to be currently the most broadly active aminoglycoside, especially in terms of resistant organisms. Therefore, amikacin is considered the preferred aminoglycoside component of the antibiotic combination used as initial empiric therapy for serious infection in seriously ill, compromised hosts. A new area of interest is the combination of amikacin and the newer extended-spectrum penicillins or a third-generation cephalosporin. These new agents have remarkably wide spectra and enhanced in vitro effectiveness against many organisms, including *E. coli, S. marcescens, Klebsiella* spp., *Proteus* spp., and especially strains of *P. aeru-*

ginosa resistant to carbenicillin, ticarcillin, and the aminoglycosides.

Table 5 shows the synergistic activity of amikacin combined with one of the newer agents against various organisms. In a study of the synergistic efficacy of amikacin plus the newer β-lactam antibiotics against multi-resistant gram-negative organisms, piperacillin or cefotaxime in combination with amikacin proved to be the most powerful synergistic combination by inhibiting 81 and 85%, respectively, of multidrug-resistant Enterobacteriaceae (70). The synergistic activity of gentamicin, tobramycin, or amikacin with azlocillin or ticarcillin against 100 strains of *P. aeruginosa* was studied. The combination of amikacin plus azlocillin proved superior to the others by exhibiting synergy for 66% of the strains, while tobramycin–azlocillin and gentamicin–azlocillin were synergistic for 64 and 57%, respectively, of the strains tested. Resistance to gentamicin or tobramycin was frequent and resulted in lack of synergy for the combinations with azlocillin or ticarcillin. The amikacin–azlocillin combination effectively reduced the MICs to clinically achievable levels for all strains exhibiting the synergistic effect (71).

An in vitro study of the synergistic activity of amikacin or piperacillin combined with moxalactam, cefoperazone, or cefotaxime against aminoglycoside-sensitive and -resistant isolates of *P. aeruginosa* and *S. marcescens* showed moxalactam or piperacillin plus amikacin to be the most frequently synergistic. Moxalactam–amikacin was synergistic for 79% of amikacin-sensitive *P. aeruginosa*, whereas piperacillin–amikacin was synergistic for 88% of amikacin-resistant *P. aeruginosa*. The combination of piperacillin and amikacin was synergistic for 100% of the amikacin-sensitive *S. marcescens* strains tested (72). A study of the susceptibility of 100 clinical isolates of *S. marcescens* to combinations of moxalactam or cefotaxime and gentamicin, tobramycin, or amikacin, showed that moxalactam or cefotaxime plus amikacin was the most active combination against the gentamicin-resistant or -sensitive strains. Twenty-two strains of *Serratia* were resistant to both gentamicin and cephalothin. Results of the combinations used against these strains showed only 6% synergy with gentamicin–moxalactam, 2% synergy with gentamicin–cefotaxime, 4% synergy with tobramycin–moxalactam, and 2% synergy with tobramycin–cefotaxime. The combination of amikacin and moxalactam was synergistic for 14% of the strains, and amikacin–cefotaxime was synergistic for 4% of the strains (73). Although the results of these in vitro synergy studies suggest very promising and exciting clinical applications of synergistic antimicrobial combinations in the treatment of serious infections, clinical significance must ultimately be determined by carefully conducted, comparative clinical trials.

In a prospective, randomized, double-blind study of piperacillin or ticarcillin plus amikacin as empiric therapy for febrile, granulocytopenic, cancer patients, the combination of piperacillin and amikacin provided

TABLE 5. *Comparative synergistic activity of amikacin with the newer β-lactam antibiotics*

Combination	Organism	No. of isolates	Percent isolates synergistically inhibited	MIC_{90} (μg/ml) for the combination
Amikacin				
+ Moxalactam (72)	*Pseudomonas aeruginosa*	42	79	2 + 16
+ Piperacillin (72)	*P. aeruginosa*[a]	8	88	0.12 + 4
+ Ceftazidime (136)	*P. aeruginosa*[a]	13	85	8 + 32
+ Cefoperzone (72)	*P. aeruginosa*	42	43	4 + 8
+ Azlocillin	*P. aeruginosa*	39	85	—
+ Piperacillin (72)	*Serratia marcescens*	10	100	2 + 128
+ Cefotaxime (73)	*S. marcescens*	100	100	—
+ Azlocillin or cefotaxime (137)	*Serratia* spp.	18	78	—
+ Cefotaxime (137)	*Escherichia coli*	26	85	—
+ Cefotaxime (137)	*Klebsiella* spp.	39	77	—
+ Azlocillin (137)	*Proteus mirabilis*	25	72	—

MIC_{90}, minimum inhibitory concentration for 90% of strains tested.
[a]Amikacin-resistant *P. aeruginosa* tested.

excellent efficacy and safety as compared with ticarcillin–amikacin. Fifty-eight percent of microbiologically and clinically documented infections treated with piperacillin–amikacin showed improvement, whereas 56% of patients receiving ticarcillin–amikacin improved. An important difference was noted in the recovery of resistant organisms. Patients receiving ticarcillin–amikacin became colonized with more resistant gram-negative bacilli much more frequently (50%) than did patients receiving piperacillin–amikacin (6%) (74).

A prospective, randomized, double-blind study of moxalactam or ticarcillin plus amikacin as empiric therapy for febrile, granulocytopenic, cancer patients showed that the combination of moxalactam plus amikacin was more often synergistic and as effective as the ticarcillin–amikacin combination. In the moxalactam–amikacin and ticarcillin–amikacin groups, 70% of the microbiologically documented infections improved, whereas 96 and 83%, respectively, of the clinically documented infections improved (75).

A word of caution concerning the problem of enterococcal superinfection encountered with moxalactam therapy. Moxalactam, as well as the other clinically used third-generation cephalosporins—cefotaxime, cefoperazone, and ceftizoxime—has no activity against the enterococcus. Enterococcal infection or colonization has been reported in patients after moxalactam therapy (76). All patients were compromised hosts and no patient had enterococci isolated in pretherapy cultures. The potential benefit of the synergistic combination of the third-generation cephalosporins with an aminoglycoside may pose a therapeutic dilemma for the clinician, since the aminoglycosides also have no activity against the enterococcus. The patients most likely to benefit from this combination, i.e., seriously ill, compromised hosts, are likely to have key predisposing factors for enterococcal superinfection.

INACTIVATION BY PENICILLIN

The semisynthetic penicillins carbenicillin and ticarcillin, as well as the newly developed penicillin derivatives azlocillin, piperacillin, and mezlocillin, have been shown to interact with and inactivate the aminoglycosides. This chemical inactivation has been seen in vitro when both drugs are mixed together and in vivo in patients with impaired renal function who are receiving both drugs and are accumulating the penicillin. The inactivation of the aminoglycosides by the semisynthetic penicillins has been shown to have a direct relationship to time and concentration of the penicillin. Inactivation is greater as the drugs are allowed to incubate longer (77–80). A significantly greater inactivation of gentamicin or tobramycin by carbenicillin, ticarcillin, azlocillin, mezlocillin, and piperacillin, than inactivation of amikacin has been reported (81). Amikacin has been reported to be the least inactivated even when incubated with very high concentrations of ticarcillin, carbenicillin, or piperacillin (77,82). Adam and Haneder (83), using the combination of amikacin plus mezlocillin or piperacillin, reported no in vitro inactivation of amikacin even with extremely high (3,000 μg/ml) concentrations of the penicillins. The resistance of amikacin to this inactivation appears to be due to its structure. The 4-amino-2-hydroxybutyric acid group at the C-1 amino group (Fig. 1) protects the amino group by stereochemical interference, thereby making the amino group inaccessible for chemical reaction or alteration of the configuration of the molecule.

The clinical implications of this interaction are important in patients with impaired renal function. Since the renal excretion of the drugs is delayed, higher levels of the drugs are present for prolonged periods, allowing greater time for the interaction to occur. If patients with impaired renal function are receiving both an aminoglycoside and a semisynthetic penicillin, and the clinician has failed to modify the penicillin dose according to the degree of renal dysfunction, accumulation with significant elevation of penicillin serum levels may occur. This will result in significant aminoglycoside inactivation, and unexpected shortening of the aminoglycoside half-life, with significant decrease in serum levels (84). This inactivation has not been demonstrated in patients with normal renal function, since the antibiotics are eliminated from the body at a rate faster than the interaction between them can occur. The in vitro inactivation is also of concern when processing serum samples for determination of aminoglycoside concentration. In patients concomitantly receiving a semisynthetic penicillin, the sample should be tested or frozen immediately to minimize the inactivation of the aminoglycoside.

Because of its stability in the presence of penicillins, amikacin is the drug of choice for the treatment of severely ill patients when the combination of a semisynthetic penicillin and aminoglycoside is indicated.

PHARMACOLOGY

Amikacin, like other aminoglycosides, is a polar cationic molecule that is relatively insoluble in lipids.

Absorption from the gastrointestinal tract is negligible, and penetration of the eye and central nervous system is very poor. Elimination is completely dependent on renal function since these drugs are removed from the body by glomerular filtration. The pharmacokinetic properties of gentamicin and tobramycin are very similar, whereas the properties of amikacin are almost identical to those of kanamycin.

Absorption

Generally, aminoglycosides are administered by the intramuscular or intravenous routes. Amikacin is rapidly and nearly completely absorbed when administered intramuscularly, producing peak serum concentration 60–90 min after administration (85,86). The intravenous route is preferred to intramuscular administration in seriously ill patients in whom complete absorption is critical. Following intravenous administration, the true serum peak will occur after a rapid distributive phase of the drug, approximately 30–45 min after the end of the infusion (87,88). Notable differences in the achievable peak serum concentrations of gentamicin, tobramycin, and amikacin are chiefly a function of dosage, with consideration of desirable therapeutic concentrations and toxic concentrations. Peak serum concentrations of gentamicin and tobramycin are almost identical when identical doses are used in the same patient (89). The peak serum concentration achieved with amikacin is four to five times higher than the concentration achieved with gentamicin or tobramycin. An intravenous infusion of 1.5 mg/kg gentamicin or tobramycin over 20–30 min will produce peak serum concentrations of 4–8 μg/ml at the end of the infusion, while infusion of 7.5 mg/kg amikacin over 20–30 min will produce peak serum concentrations of 25–30 μg/ml.

Several investigators have commented on the unpredictability of serum concentrations achieved using gentamicin or tobramycin (90–96). The reasons for this unpredictability are not completely understood but they include altered renal function, age, body temperature, lean body weight, and variability in distribution volume (97–99).

Wide interpatient variations are seen with the use of gentamicin or tobramycin, resulting in suboptimal serum concentrations even when recommended dosage regimens are employed (100). In the therapy of infections caused by gram-negative organisms, treatment failures have resulted from subtherapeutic doses of gentamicin (101). Conventional dosage regimens, such as 3–5 mg/kg/day, will often produce undesirably low peak serum levels, and many times will result in prolonged periods of subinhibitory serum concentrations, which increases the risk of resistance and breakthrough bacteremia (102). The emergence of gentamicin or tobramycin resistance has been attributed to the selection of a few colonies of resistant organisms encouraged to proliferate by subinhibitory concentrations (103,104).

Achievement of adequate serum levels has been associated with greater therapeutic response in the therapy of serious gram-negative sepsis. In a study of patients with gram-negative sepsis treated with gentamicin, an 84% response rate was found in those patients with adequate serum concentrations, whereas only a 23% response rate was found in those patients having subtherapeutic serum concentrations (105). Amikacin, when given in doses of 7.5 mg/kg, achieves peak serum concentrations that are approximately seven times the average MIC for most organisms (106,107). In contrast, one study using gentamicin or tobramycin in the treatment of serious gram-negative infection showed that the peak aminoglycoside serum concentration failed to exceed the MIC of the infecting organism in 17–33% of the cases (108). Baltch et al. (109) reported that following the administration of 1.5 mg/kg doses of gentamicin, peak serum concentrations failed to achieve the MIC for the microorganism in 22% of patients treated. Riff and Jackson (96) reported suboptimal serum concentrations in 30% of patients receiving the standard gentamicin dosage regimen. Cipolle et al. (98) reported that young patients with normal serum creatinine required significantly higher daily dosages of tobramycin to achieve optimal serum concentrations. Amikacin has the advantage of a more predictable pharmacokinetic behavior. In a crossover study comparing the pharmacokinetics of amikacin to gentamicin, amikacin was found to have less variability in achieving satisfactory serum concentrations, and was judged more predictable than gentamicin (110). Amikacin has the advantage of a greater therapeutic ratio than that seen with gentamicin or tobramycin. With amikacin, the ratio between the achieved peak serum concentration and the MIC for sensitive organisms is much greater. Therefore, if any minor variations in achievable peak concentration or excretion of amikacin occur, they are less likely to alter serum levels to a point close to or below the MIC or to exceed toxic levels (111).

Distribution

Since amikacin, like other aminoglycosides, is relatively insoluble in lipids, its distribution volume is similar to the extracellular space. Like kanamycin, it is minimally protein bound (12). It is distributed poorly throughout some tissue compartments, such as adipose tissue, ocular tissue, and the central nervous system. Therapy of bacterial endophthalmitis requires periocular injections, and therapy of meningitis requires intraventricular administration to ensure concentrations adequate to eradicate infecting organisms (86,112,113). Amikacin has been shown to penetrate gall bladder tissue, and gall bladder and common duct bile, even in the presence of obstruction, in concentrations exceeding the MICs of the most commonly encountered organisms in hepatobiliary tract infections (114–117). Amikacin penetrates into bronchial secretions in concentrations higher than the MICs for many gram-negative bacteria encountered in respiratory tract infections (118,119). Lung and heart tissue concentrations of amikacin were found to exceed the MICs for the gram-negative organisms isolated from patients in one study (120). Amikacin reaches high enough concentrations in synovial fluid that instillation into infected joints is unnecessary (121). Amikacin, like all aminoglycosides, has an affinity for renal cortical tissue and concentrates to levels 10–40 times those found in serum (122). Urine is the only body fluid in which the aminoglycosides are more concentrated than in serum.

Excretion

Amikacin is not metabolized and is excreted unchanged in the urine, filtered almost entirely by the glomerulus. In patients with normal renal function, approximately 95% of a dose can be recovered in the urine within 24 h after administration (110). Complete urine recovery can be accomplished when urine is collected for 20–30 days after administration of last dose. The half-life of the drug is significantly longer in patients with renal dysfunction and patients with decreased renal function will have decreased urinary concentrations of amikacin. As with all aminoglycosides, adjustment of dose is necessary in patients with renal insufficiency, due to major changes in the pharmacokinetics of the drug (88,123). Since elimination is solely via renal mechanisms, hepatobiliary disease has little or no effect on the rate of amikacin elimination.

DOSAGE

The initial or loading dose of amikacin is recommended in patients with serious infections. A loading dose is administered to saturate body tissue and fluids, and to quickly achieve concentrations within the therapeutic range. For amikacin, the loading dose is 7.5 mg/kg regardless of the patient's renal function. Since amikacin is poorly distributed to adipose tissue, the dose is based on lean body weight in obese patients. In patients with ascites, a shift in the distribution of amikacin from the plasma to the large fluid compartment results in lower serum concentrations, necessitating larger doses to achieve adequate concentrations. These patients should be dosed on total body weight rather than lean body weight. Subsequent maintenance doses are adjusted in patients with renal dysfunction and in patients with rapidly changing renal function, to assure that the peak concentrations are within the therapeutic range and trough concentrations are not excessive. The recommended maintenance dose for adults with normal renal function is 15 mg/kg/day, divided into two or three equal doses administered at equal intervals. The dose should be decreased in direct proportion to the measured creatinine clearance in patients with renal dysfunction (94,123). There are many methods available for the adjustment of dosage in patients with renal dysfunction. The same dose may be given at a decreased dosing frequency, or the dose may be decreased while maintaining the dosing frequency. In the treatment of serious infections, it is preferable to decrease the dose and maintain the dosing interval to prevent the serum concentrations from dropping below the MIC for the organism. There are several published methods that provide a means for adjusting dosage regimens in patients with decreased renal function. A dosing nomogram, which estimates creatinine clearance from serum creatinine and permits the clinician the choice of doses and dosing intervals dependent on the degree of renal function and the severity of the infection, is the best method available to estimate dosage at this time (124). Other methods include increasing the dosing interval based on the patient's serum creatinine (125), or increasing the dosing interval based on estimation of the drug's half-life (123), but these methods may result in substantial variations in serum concentrations or substantial error in the prediction of an adequate maintenance dose. Although nomograms provide the clinician with a tool to easily calculate initial dose, further dosage adjustments should be based on measured peak and trough concentrations.

In patients undergoing hemodialysis or peritoneal dialysis, amikacin half-life is decreased when compared with predialysis values. Investigators have reported a 90% decrease following hemodialysis, and only a 30% decrease following peritoneal dialysis.

However, amikacin clearance following dialysis is so variable that serum concentrations should be monitored to prevent toxicity (126,127).

ADVERSE EFFECTS

The most important adverse effects limiting the clinical use of all aminoglycosides are nephrotoxicity and ototoxicity. The frequency of these effects is difficult to assess, due to difficulty in interpreting data from toxicity studies. The problem with comparing the nephrotoxicity of gentamicin, tobramycin, and amikacin is that no well-designed, prospective, randomized study has compared all three agents. Other confounding factors include different underlying diseases of study patients, lack of definite criteria assessing toxicity, concurrent treatment with other nephrotoxic medications, and failure to establish a proper baseline in study patients. Animal studies are of limited value in extrapolation to humans, but serve as useful models. Most studies of the comparative nephrotoxicities of aminoglycosides have utilized large multiples of the human dose. Animal data should be viewed cautiously since the relationship to the clinical situation may not be applicable.

Aminoglycosides damage the proximal tubular cells of the kidney, sparing the glomeruli. Tissue accumulation studies have shown that aminoglycosides have an affinity for renal cortical tissue. The comparative extent of this accumulation has been examined in animals and studies have shown that gentamicin accumulates in the highest concentrations, followed by tobramycin and amikacin (128,129). Wold and coworkers (130) dosed amikacin seven times higher than tobramycin in rats and found amikacin less nephrotoxic. Hottendorf and Gordon (131) examined the dose-response relationship over a range of low multiples of the human dose in rats, and found gentamicin to be more nephrotoxic than tobramycin, which was more nephrotoxic than amikacin. Unlike amikacin, the mg/kg human dose equivalent of gentamicin and tobramycin was significantly nephrotoxic in rats. Other animal data indicate that the nephrotoxic liability of amikacin is no greater than that of tobramycin or gentamicin, and in some studies amikacin appears to be less nephrotoxic.

Table 6 summarizes published reports of comparative, prospective, and randomized studies on the nephrotoxicity of aminoglycosides. Careful examination of these studies shows that the three aminoglycosides are equally nephrotoxic; little evidence appears to support a consistent pattern favoring one aminoglycoside over the others.

Risk factors associated with the development of nephrotoxicity include preexisting renal disease, prolonged therapy, previous therapy with an aminoglycoside, and concurrent administration of other nephrotoxic substances. Nephrotoxicity appears to be dose related and more common in elderly debilitated patients, patients with a contracted intravascular volume, and those with preexisting renal disease. Nephrotoxicity is usually mild and reversible, with usual onset after 5–7 days of therapy, but could be clinically manifested after cessation of therapy. The best method of predicting and monitoring nephrotoxicity in patients receiving aminoglycosides is measurement of urinary cast excretion, which will increase before the serum creatinine becomes elevated. This is a much more sensitive indicator of aminoglycoside effect on the proximal tubule than other tests of renal function.

The ototoxic effects of the aminoglycosides result in permanent loss of inner ear function. The ototoxicity of amikacin, like kanamycin, is primarily cochlear (6,69). The spectrum includes tinnitus, mild high-frequency loss noted on audiograms, and conversational range loss. It is often bilateral and irreversible. Vestibular dysfunction with vertigo, ataxia or nystagmus may also occur. The overall incidence of clinically overt ototoxicity in patients given usual doses for not more than 2 weeks is approximately 2–5%. The ototoxic effects of the aminoglycosides are potentiated by concomitant administration of other ototoxic drugs. Patients receiving aminoglycosides should be carefully observed for signs and symptoms of ototoxicity. If long-term therapy is anticipated, baseline and sequential audiograms should be performed. Several risk factors may be associated with a greater potential for the development of nephrotoxicity or ototoxicity (Table 7). A large number of variables which may be interrelated seem to predispose patients to a higher risk of toxicity. The risk of nephrotoxicity and ototoxicity may be reduced by monitoring serum peak and trough concentrations. Increased risk of ototoxicity has been associated with consistently elevated peak serum concentrations (>12 μg/ml for gentamicin or tobramycin, >35 μg/ml for amikacin). Nephrotoxicity appears to be related to trough concentrations consistently >2 μg/ml for gentamicin or tobramycin, or >10 μg/ml for amikacin. A very low therapeutic ratio is seen with gentamicin and tobramycin, i.e., the therapeutic and toxic doses are very close. With amikacin, however, the ratio between the achievable serum concentrations and the MICs of sensitive organisms is much greater. Amikacin has the advantage of achieving higher peak serum concentrations, com-

TABLE 6. *Summary of studies examining aminoglycoside nephrotoxicity*

Reference	Nephrotoxic criteria	Concurrent drugs	Percent nephrotoxic: Gentamicin	Tobramycin	Amikacin	Comments
Love et al. (67)	↑ Cr(s) >0.4 mg/dl	Ticarcillin	8.6	NT	7.5	Cancer patients; no significant difference
Lau et al. (69)	>100% of baseline when Cr(s) ≤ 1.3 mg/dl	Carbenicillin	8.5	NT	8	Cancer patients; no significant difference[a]
Keating et al. (138)	↑ Cr(s) > 2.5 mg/dl	Carbenicillin	10	NT	7	Cancer patients; no significant difference[a]
Feld et al. (139)	↑ Cr(s) > 1.4 mg/dl		NT	21	15	Cancer patients
Plaut et al. (140)	↑ Cr(s) > 0.5 mg/dl	Cephalosporins	36	23	25	Surgical patients; critically ill patients, no significant difference
Wade et al. (141)	↑ Cr(s) > 0.4 mg/dl	Cephalothin Methicillin	30.4 10	20.8 4.3	NT NT	<10 days therapy; no significant difference[a]
Smith et al. (142)	↑ Cr(s) > 0.4 mg/dl	Penicillin G	11	NT	8	Amikacin, 24 mg/kg/day[a]
Smith et al. (143)	↑ Cr(s) > 0.5 mg/dl	Methicillin Nafcillin	26	12	NT	Nephrotoxicity significant, $p < 0.02$[a]
Lerner et al. (144)	↑ Cr(s) > 50% of baseline	—	15.4	NT	0	Amikacin, 15 mg/kg/day[a] Gentamicin, 5 mg/kg/day[a]

NT, not tested; ↑ Cr(s), increase in serum creatinine.
[a]Serum levels monitored, doses adjusted accordingly.

pared with gentamicin and tobramycin, thereby affording a greater range between therapeutic and toxic concentrations. Nonetheless, monitoring serum concentration and appropriate adjustment of dose, along with an effort to avoid other predisposing factors, will reduce the risk of toxicity due to amikacin.

SUMMARY

Amikacin, a semisynthetic analog of kanamycin, is very active against most gram-negative bacteria including gentamicin- and tobramycin-resistant strains.

TABLE 7. *Predisposing factors associated with increased risk of aminoglycoside ototoxicity or nephrotoxicity*

Elderly patients with preexisting renal disease
Patients with compromised renal function
Excessively high peak and/or trough concentrations
Total dose for course of therapy
Duration of therapy
Previous treatment with an aminoglycoside
Concurrent use of ototoxic or nephrotoxic drugs
Dehydration

The effectiveness of amikacin in the treatment of serious gram-negative bacillary infections is well documented. Due to its resistance to inactivating enzymes, it is the aminoglycoside of choice for the treatment of known or suspected serious gram-negative infections caused by organisms resistant to gentamicin or tobramycin. Amikacin should be part of an empiric antibiotic regimen for the therapy of suspected sepsis in febrile, leukopenic immunocompromised hosts since it exhibits enhanced activity against the organisms most frequently encountered in this patient population. High response rates have been reported with the use of amikacin combined with β-lactam antibiotics in immunocompromised or granulocytopenic patients. It exhibits impressive in vitro synergy against aminoglycoside-sensitive and -resistant organisms when used in combination with the new acylureidopenicillins and third-generation cephalosporins. Amikacin has the advantage of being the aminoglycoside least inactivated by the semisynthetic penicillins. Amikacin achieves high and predictable serum concentrations and has a favorable therapeutic index. Its potential for nephrotoxicity and ototoxicity is not significantly different than that encountered with gentamicin or tobramycin. Amikacin appears to be the preferred aminoglycoside for use at the present time because of its activity against gentamicin- and tobramycin-resistant organisms, its low resistance potential, its relative low degree of inactivation by the semisynthetic penicillins, and its superior pharmacokinetic profile.

REFERENCES

1. Kawaguchi H, Naito T, Nakagawa S, et al. BB-K8, a new semisynthetic aminoglycoside antibiotic. *J Antibiot* 1972;25:695–708.
2. Bryan LE, Van Den Elzen HM. Streptomycin accumulation in susceptible and resistant strains of *E. coli* and *P. aeruginosa*. *Antimicrob Agents Chemother* 1976;9:928–38.
3. Bryan LE, Kowland SK, Van Den Elzen HM. Mechanism of aminoglycoside antibiotic resistance in anaerobic bacteria: *Clostridium perfringens* and *Bacteroides fragilis*. *Antimicrob Agents Chemother* 1979;15:7–13.
4. Young LS, Hewitt WL. Activity of five aminoglycoside antibiotics in vitro against gram-negative bacilli and *Staphylococcus aureus*. *Antimicrob Agents Chemother* 1973;4:617–25.
5. Price KE, Pursiano TA, DeFuria MD, et al. Activity of BB-K8 (amikacin) against clinical isolates resistant to one or more aminoglycoside antibiotics. *Antimicrob Agents Chemother* 1974;5:143–52.
6. Meyer RD, Lewis RP, Carmalt ED, et al. Amikacin therapy for serious gram-negative bacillary infections. *Ann Intern Med* 1975;83:790–800.
7. Stewart D, Bodey GP. In vitro activity of sisomicin, an aminoglycoside antibiotic, against clinical isolates. *J Antibiot* 1975;28:149–55.
8. Rahal JJ, Simberkoff MS, Kagan K, et al. Bactericidal efficacy of Sch20569 and amikacin against gentamicin-sensitive and resistant organisms. *Antimicrob Agents Chemother* 1976;9:595–9.
9. Sharp PM, Saenz CA, Martin PR. Amikacin (BB-K8) treatment of multiple-drug-resistant *Proteus* infections. *Antimicrob Agents Chemother* 1974;5:435–8.
10. Knothe H. In vitro susceptibility of recently isolated gram-negative bacteria to gentamicin, sisomicin, tobramycin, amikacin. *J Infect Dis* 1976;134:S271–4.
11. Keane CT, English LF, Wise R. *Providencia stuartii* infections. *Lancet* 1975;1:1045.
12. Clark JT, Libke RD, Regamey C, et al. Comparative pharmacokinetics of amikacin and kanamycin. *Clin Pharmacol Ther* 1974;15:610–6.
13. Grasso S, Meinardi G, De Carneri I, et al. New in vitro model to study the effect of antibiotic concentration and rate of elimination of antibacterial activity. *Antimicrob Agents Chemother* 1978;13:570–6.
14. Merrickin D, Robinson GN. Antibiotic levels in experimentally infected mice in relation to therapeutic effect and antibacterial activity in vitro. *J Antimicrob Chemother* 1979;5:423–9.
15. Klastersky J, Daneau D, Swings G, et al. Antibacterial activity in serum and urine as a therapeutic guide in bacterial infections. *J Infect Dis* 1974;129:187–93.
16. Price KE, Casson K, De Regis RG, et al. Amikacin: antimicrobial properties and resistance mechanisms affecting its activity. *Am J Med* 1977;62:14–24.
17. Noriega ER, Leibowitz RE, Richmond AS, et al. Nosocomial infection caused by gentamicin-resistant, streptomycin-sensitive *Klebsiella*. *J Infect Dis* 1975;131:S45–50.
18. Tally FP, Louie TJ, Weinstein WM, et al. Amikacin therapy for severe gram-negative sepsis: emphasis on infection with gentamicin-resistant organisms. *Ann Intern Med* 1975;83:484–8.
19. Price KE, DeFuria LD, Pursiano TA. Amikacin, an aminoglycoside with marked activity against antibiotic-resistant clinical isolates. *J Infect Dis* 1976;134:S239–61.
20. Finland M, Garner C, Wilcox C, et al. Susceptibility of recently isolated bacteria to amikacin in vitro: comparison with four other aminoglycoside antibiotics. *J Infect Dis* 1976;134:S297–307.
21. Semel J, Trenholme G, Levin S. Gentamicin- and clindamycin-resistant *Staphylococcus aureus*. *Am J Med Sci* 1980;280:4–9.
22. Sabath LD, Garner C, Wilcox C, et al. Susceptibility of *Staphylococcus aureus* and *Staphylococcus epidermidis* to 65 antibiotics. *Antimicrob Agents Chemother* 1976;9:962–9.
23. Price KE, Chisholm DR, Misiek M, et al. Microbiological evaluation of BB-K8, a new semisynthetic aminoglycoside. *J Antibiot* 1972;25:709–31.
24. Finland M. Changing patterns of susceptibility of common bacterial pathogens to antimicrobial agents. *Ann Intern Med* 1972;76:1009–36.
25. Sapico FL, Keys TF, Hewitt WL. Experimental enterococcal endocarditis. II. Study of in vitro synergism of penicillin and streptomycin. *Am J Med Sci* 1972;263:128–35.
26. Gutschik E, Jepsen OB, Mortensen I. Effect of combinations of penicillin and aminoglycosides on *Streptococcus faecalis*: a comparative study of seven aminoglycoside antibiotics. *J Infect Dis* 1977;135:832–6.
27. Calderwood SA, Wennersten C, Moellering RC, et al. Resistance to six aminoglycoside aminocyclitol antibiotics among enterococci: prevalence, evolution, and relationship to synergism with penicillin. *Antimicrob Agents Chemother* 1979;12:401–5.
28. Finegold SM, Sutter VL. Susceptibility of gram-negative anaerobic bacilli to gentamicin and other aminoglycosides. *J Infect Dis* 1971;124:S56–8.
29. Gorbach SL, Bartlett JG. Anaerobic infections. *N Engl J Med* 1974;290:1289–94.
30. Moellering RC, Medoff G, Leech I, et al. Antibiotic synergism against *Listeria monocytogenes*. *Antimicrob Agents Chemother* 1972;1:30–4.
31. Hirsch HA, Finland M. Susceptibility of *Haemophilus influenzae* to 21 antibiotics in vitro. *Am J Med Sci* 1960;239:33–40.
32. Waitz JA, Moss EL, Dribe CG, et al. Comparative activity of sisomicin, gentamicin, kanamycin, and tobramycin. *Antimicrob Agents Chemother* 1972;2:431–7.
33. Yu PK, Washington JA. Comparative in vitro activity of 3 aminoglycosidic antibiotics: BB-K8, kanamycin, and gentamicin. *Antimicrob Agents Chemother* 1973;4:133–48.
34. Jao RL, Finland M. Susceptibility of *Mycoplasma pneumoniae* to 21 antibiotics in vitro. *Am J Med Sci* 1967;253:639–50.
35. Bach MC, Sabath LD, Finland M. Susceptibility of *Nocardia asteroides* to 45 antimicrobial agents in vitro. *Antimicrob Agents Chemother* 1973;3:1–8.
36. Dalovisio JR, Pankey GA. In vitro susceptibility of *Nocardia asteroides* to amikacin. *Antimicrob Agents Chemother* 1978;13:128–9.
37. Yogev R, Greenslade T, Firlit CF, et al. Successful treatment of *Nocardia asteroides* infection with amikacin. *J Pediatr* 1980;96:771–3.
38. Edelstein PH, Meyer RD. Susceptibility of *Legionella pneumophilia* to twenty antimicrobial agents. *Antimicrob Agents Chemother* 1980;18:403–8.
39. Thornsbury C, Baker CN, Kirven LA. In vitro activity of

antimicrobial agents on Legionnaires disease bacterium. *Antimicrob Agents Chemother* 1978;13:78–80.
40. Baird IM, Fay D, Thompson RL, et al. Clinical manifestations and treatment of Legionnaires' disease. *Am J Med Sci* 1979;277:223–32.
41. Legionnaires' disease—Medical staff conference, University of California, San Francisco. *West J Med* 1978;129:480–5.
42. Garcia-Rodriguez JA, Martin F, Sasney MC. Activity of amikacin against *Mycobacterium tuberculosis*. *J Antimicrob Chemother* 1978;4:293–4.
43. Dalovisio JR, Pankey GA. In vitro susceptibility of *M. fortuitum* and *M. chelonei* to amikacin. *J Infect Dis* 1978;137:318–21.
44. Booth JE, Jacobson JA, Kurrus TA, et al. Infection of prosthetic arthroplasty by *Mycobacterium fortuitum*. *J Bone Joint Surg [Am]* 1979;61:300–2.
45. Speert DP, Munson D, Mitchell C, et al. *Mycobacterium chelonei* septicemia in a premature infant. *J Pediatr* 1980;96:681–3.
46. Meyer RD, Kraus LL, Pasiecznik KA. In vitro susceptibility of gentamicin-resistant Enterobacteriaceae and *Pseudomonas aeruginosa* to netilmicin and selected aminoglycoside antibiotics. *Antimicrob Agents Chemother* 1976;10:677–81.
47. Davies J, Smith DI. Plasmid-determined resistance to antimicrobial agents. *Annu Rev Microbiol* 1978;32:496–518.
48. Bryan LE, Shahrabada MS, Van den Elzen HM. Gentamicin resistance in *Pseudomonas aeruginosa*: R-factor mediated resistance. *Antimicrob Agents Chemother* 1974;6:191–9.
49. Davis J. Bacterial resistance to aminoglycoside antibiotics. *J Infect Dis* 1971;124:S7–10.
50. Bryan LE, Haraphongse R, Van den Elzen HM. Gentamicin resistance in clinical isolates of *Pseudomonas aeruginosa* associated with diminished gentamicin accumulation and no detectable enzymatic modification. *J Antibiot* 1976;29:743–5.
51. Davies J, Courvalin P. Mechanisms of resistance to aminoglycosides. *Am J Med* 1977;62:868–72.
52. Moellering RC Jr, Weinberg AN. Studies on antibiotic synergism against enterococci, II: effect of various antibiotics on the uptake of C^{14} labeled streptomycin by enterococci. *J Clin Invest* 1971;50:2580–4.
53. Moellering RC Jr, Wennersten C, Weinstein AJ. Penicillin-tobramycin synergism against enterococci: a comparison with penicillin and gentamicin. *Antimicrob Agents Chemother* 1973;3:526–9.
54. Moellering RC Jr, Wennersten C, Weinberg AN. Synergy of penicillin and gentamicin against enterococci. *J Infect Dis* 1971;124:S207–9.
55. Kluge RM, Standiford HC, Tatem B, et al. Comparative activity of tobramycin, amikacin, and gentamicin alone and with carbenicillin against *Pseudomonas aeruginosa*. *Antimicrob Agents Chemother* 1974;6:442–6.
56. Kelly MT, Matsen JM. In vitro activity, synergism, and testing parameters of amikacin, with comparisons to other aminoglycoside antibiotics. *Antimicrob Agents Chemother* 1976;9:440–7.
57. Weinstein RJ, Young LS, Hewitt WL. Comparison of methods for assessing in vitro antibiotic synergism against *Pseudomonas* and *Serratia*. *J Lab Clin Med* 1975;86:853–62.
58. Klastersky J, Nyamubeya B, Vandenborre L. Antimicrobial effectiveness of kanamycin, aminosidin, BB-K8, sisomicin, gentamicin and tobramycin combined with carbenicillin or cephalothin against gram-negative rods. *J Med Microbiol* 1974;7:465–72.
59. Comber KR, Basker MJ, Osborne CD, et al. Synergy between ticarcillin and tobramycin against *Pseudomonas aeruginosa* and Enterobacteriaceae in vitro and in vivo. *Antimicrob Agents Chemother* 1977;11:956–64.
60. European Organization for Research on Treatment of Cancer: The EORTC International Antimicrobial Therapy Project Group. Three antibiotic regimens in the treatment of infection in febrile granulocytopenic patients with cancer. *J Infect Dis* 1976;137:14–29.
61. Hoecker JL, Pickering LK, Groschel D, et al. Current concepts of bacteremia in children with malignancies. *Cancer* 1979;44:1939–44.
62. Schimpff S, Satterlee W, Young VM, et al. Empiric therapy with carbenicillin and gentamicin for febrile patients with cancer and granulocytopenia. *N Engl J Med* 1971;284:1061–5.
63. Anderson ET, Young LS, Hewitt WL. Antimicrobial synergism in therapy of gram-negative rod bacteremia. *Chemotherapy* 1978;24:45–54.
64. Love LJ, Schimpff SC, Schiffer CA, et al. Improved prognosis for granulocytopenic patients with gram-negative bacteremia. *Am J Med* 1980;68:643–8.
65. Keating MJ, Bodey GP, Valdivieso M, et al. A randomized comparative trial of three aminoglycosides. Comparison of continuous infusion of gentamicin, amikacin, and sisomicin combined with carbenicillin in the treatment of infections in neutropenic patients with malignancies. *Medicine* 1979; 58:159–70.
66. Klastersky J, Meunier-Carpentier F, Prevost JM. Significance of antimicrobial synergism for the outcome of gram-negative sepsis. *Am J Med Sci* 1977;173:157–67.
67. Love LJ, Schimpff SC, Hahn DM, et al. Randomized trial of empiric antibiotic therapy with ticarcillin in combination with gentamicin, amikacin, or netilmicin in febrile patients with granulocytopenia and cancer. *Am J Med* 1979;66:603–10.
68. Hahn DM, Schimpff SC, Young VM, et al. Amikacin and cephalothin: empiric regimen for granulocytopenic cancer patients. *Antimicrob Agents Chemother* 1977;12:618–24.
69. Lau WK, Young LS, Black RE, et al. Comparative efficacy and toxicity of amikacin/carbenicillin versus gentamicin/carbenicillin in leukopenic patients. *Am J Med* 1977;62:959–66.
70. Glew P, Pavuk R. Synergistic efficacy of new beta lactam antibiotics plus amikacin versus drug resistant enteric gram-negative bacteria. 12th International Congress of Chemotherapy, Florence, Italy, July 1981. Abstract 846.
71. Smith RP, Sutphen NT, Matzkowitz A, et al. Synergistic activity of cyclocillin and ticarcillin with aminoglycosides against *Pseudomonas aeruginosa*. Proceedings of the 21st Interscience Conference on Antimicrobial Agents and Chemotherapy, Chicago, Illinois, November 1981.
72. Kurtz TO, Winston DJ, Bruckner DA, et al. Comparative in vitro synergistic activity of new beta-lactam antimicrobial agents and amikacin against *P. aeruginosa* and *S. marcescens*. *Antimicrob Agents Chemother* 1981;20:239–43.
73. Markowitz SM, Sibilla DJ. Comparative susceptibilities of clinical isolates of *Serratia marcescens* to newer cephalosporins, alone and in combination with various aminoglycosides. *Antimicrob Agents Chemother* 1980;18:651–5.
74. Wade JC, Schimpff SC, Neuman KA, et al. Piperacillin or ticarcillin plus amikacin: a double-blind prospective comparison of empiric antibiotic therapy for febrile granulocytopenic cancer patients. *Am J Med* 1981;71:983–90.
75. de Jongh C, Wade J, Schimpff SC, et al. Moxalactam plus amikacin or ticarcillin plus amikacin: double blind comparison of empiric antibiotic therapy for febrile granulocytopenic cancer patients. Proceedings of the 72nd Annual Meeting of American Association for Cancer Research, April, 1981. Abstract C-332.
76. Yu VL. Enterococcal superinfection and colonization after therapy with moxalactam, a new broad-spectrum antibiotic. *Ann Intern Med* 1981;94:784–5.
77. Pickering LK, Gearhart P. Effect of time and concentration

upon interaction between gentamicin, tobramycin, netilmicin, or amikacin and carbenicillin or ticarcillin. *Antimicrob Agents Chemother* 1979;15:592–6.
78. Flournoy DJ. Factors influencing the inactivation of aminoglycosides by beta-lactams. *Methods Find Exp Clin Pharmacol* 1979;1:233–8.
79. Riff LJ, Jackson GG. Laboratory and clinical conditions for gentamicin inactivation by carbenicillin. *Arch Intern Med* 1972;138:887–91.
80. Davies M, Morgan JR, Anand C. Interaction of carbenicillin and ticarcillin with gentamicin. *Antimicrob Agents Chemother* 1975;7:431–4.
81. Pickering LK, Rutherford I. Effect of concentration and time upon inactivation of tobramycin, gentamicin, netilmicin and amikacin by azlocillin, carbenicillin, mecillinam, mezlocillin and piperacillin. *J Pharmacol Exp Ther* 1981;217:345–9.
82. Hale DC, Jenkins R, Matsen JM. In-vitro inactivation of aminoglycoside antibiotics by piperacillin and carbenicillin. *Am J Clin Pathol* 1980;74:316–9.
83. Adam D, Haneder J. Studies on the inactivation of aminoglycoside antibiotics by acylureidopenicillins and piperacillin. *Infection* 1981;9:182–5.
84. Parry MF, Neu HC. Pharmacokinetics of ticarcillin in patients with abnormal renal function. *J Infect Dis* 1976;133:46–9.
85. Bodey GP, Valdivieso M, Feld R, et al. Pharmacology of amikacin in humans. *Antimicrob Agents Chemother* 1974;5:508–12.
86. Cabana BE, Taggart JG. Comparative pharmacokinetics of BB-K8 and kanamycin in dogs and humans. *Antimicrob Agents Chemother* 1973;3:478–83.
87. Lode H, Grunert K, Koeppe P, et al. Pharmacokinetic and clinical studies with amikacin, a new aminoglycoside antibiotic. *J Infect Dis* 1976;134:S316–22.
88. Plantier J, Farrey AW, O'Neill MA, et al. Pharmacokinetics of amikacin in patients with normal or impaired renal function. *J Infect Dis* 1976;134:S323–30.
89. LeRoy A, Humbert G, Oksenhendler G, et al. Pharmacokinetics of aminoglycosides in subjects with normal and impaired renal function. *Antibiot Chemother* 1978;25:163–80.
90. Anderson AC, Hodges GR, Barnes WG. Determination of serum gentamicin sulfate levels. *Arch Intern Med* 1976;136:785–7.
91. Regamey C, Gordon RC, Kirby WM. Comparative pharmacokinetics of tobramycin and gentamicin. *Clin Pharmacol Ther* 1973;14:396–403.
92. Naba KG, Westenfelder SR, Madson PO. Pharmacokinetics of the aminoglycoside antibiotic tobramycin in humans. *Antimicrob Agents Chemother* 1973;3:469–73.
93. Simon VK, Mosinger EU, Malerczy V. Pharmacokinetic studies of tobramycin and gentamicin. *Antimicrob Agents Chemother* 1973;3:445–50.
94. Kaye D, Levison ME, Labovitz ED. The unpredictability of serum concentrations of gentamicin: pharmacokinetics of gentamicin in patients with normal and abnormal renal function. *J Infect Dis* 1974;130:150–4.
95. Barza M, Brown RB, Shen D, et al. Predictability of blood levels of gentamicin in man. *J Infect Dis* 1975;132:165–74.
96. Riff LJ, Jackson GG. Pharmacology of gentamicin in man. *J Infect Dis* 1971;124:S98–105.
97. Gyselynck AM, Forrey A, Cutler R. Pharmacokinetics of gentamicin: distribution and plasma and renal clearance. *J Infect Dis* 1971;124:S70–6.
98. Cipolle RJ, Seifert RD, Zaske DE, et al. Systematically individualizing tobramycin dosage regimens. *J Clin Pharmacol* 1980;20:570–80.
99. Sawchuk RJ, Zaske DE. Pharmacokinetics of dosing regimens which utilize multiple intravenous infusion. *J Pharmacokinet Biopharm* 1976;4:183–95.
100. Zaske DE, Cipolle RJ, Strata RG. Gentamicin dosage requirements: wide interpatient variations in 242 surgery patients with normal renal function. *Surgery* 1980;87:164–9.
101. Jackson GG, Riff LJ. *Pseudomonas* bacteremia: pharmacologic and other basis for failure of treatment with gentamicin. *J Infect Dis* 1971;124:S185–91.
102. Anderson ET, Young LS, Hewitt WL. Simultaneous antibiotic levels in "breakthrough" gram-negative rod bacteremia. *Am J Med* 1976;61:493–7.
103. Echeverria P, Lew MA, Smith AL. Apparent emergence of aminoglycoside resistant *Escherichia coli* during neonatal meningitis. *N Engl J Med* 1975;293:913–4.
104. Walker SH. Aminoglycoside-resistant *Escherichia coli*. *N Engl J Med* 1976;295:225–6.
105. Noone P, Parson TMC, Pattison JR, et al. Experience in monitoring gentamicin therapy during treatment of serious gram-negative sepsis. *Br Med J* 1974;1:477–81.
106. McHenry MC, Wagner JG, Hall PM, et al. Pharmacokinetics of amikacin in patients with impaired renal function. *J Infect Dis* 1976;134:S343–8.
107. Pollock AA, Berger SA, Richmond AS, et al. Amikacin therapy for serious gram-negative infection. *JAMA* 1977;237:562–4.
108. Reymann MT, Bradac JA, Cobbs CG, et al. Correlations of aminoglycoside dosages with serum concentrations during therapy of serious gram-negative bacillary disease. *Antimicrob Agents Chemother* 1979;16:353–61.
109. Baltch AL, Hammer M, Smith RP, et al. *Pseudomonas aeruginosa* bacteremia. *J Lab Clin Med* 1979;94:201–14.
110. Walker JM, Wise R, Mitchard M. The pharmacokinetics of amikacin and gentamicin in volunteers: a camparison of individual differences. *J Antimicrob Chemother* 1979;5:95–9.
111. Farchione LA, Chudzik GM. Serum concentrations and inhibitory ratios during amikacin therapy of gram-negative infections. *J Clin Pharmacol* 1978;18:432–8.
112. Wirt TC, McGee ZA, Oldfield EH, et al. Intraventricular administration of amikacin for complicated gram-negative meningitis and ventriculitis. *J Neurosurg* 1979;50:95–9.
113. Sklaver AR, Greenman RL, Hoffman TA. Amikacin therapy of gram-negative bacteremia and meningitis. *Arch Intern Med* 1978;138:713–6.
114. Hanebrough JF, Clark JE, Reimer LG. Concentrations of kanamycin and amikacin in human gallbladder bile and wall. *Antimicrob Agents Chemother* 1981;20:515–7.
115. Le Frock J, Schell R, Tillotson J, et al. Amikacin levels in the human biliary tract. 11th International Congress of Chemotherapy and 19th Interscience Conference on Antimicrobial Agents and Chemotherapy, October 1979, Boston, MA. Abstract 621.
116. Bermudez RH, Lugo A, Ramirez-Ronda CH, et al. Amikacin sulfate levels in human serum and bile. *Antimicrob Agents Chemother* 1981;19:352–4.
117. Rubinstein E, Beer-Gehler G, Dubner J, et al. Amikacin levels in the human biliary tract. *Proceedings of the 10th International Congress on Chemotherapy*, 1977;2:998.
118. Berthelot G, Bergogne-Berezin E, Ever P. Amikacin levels in human bronchial secretions. Proceedings of the 18th Interscience Conference on Antimicrobial Agents and Chemotherapy, Atlanta, GA, 1978. Abstract 388.
119. Dull WL, Alexander MR, Kasik JE. Bronchial secretion levels of amikacin. *Antimicrob Agents Chemother* 1979;16:767–71.
120. Farago E, Kiss J, Gomory A, et al. Amikacin: in vitro bacteriologic studies, levels in human serum, lung and heart tissue, and clinical results. *Int J Clin Pharmacol Biopharm* 1979;17:421–8.

121. Schurman DJ, Wheeler R. Bone and joint gram-negative infection and amikacin treatment. *Am J Med* 1977;S62:160–4.
122. Edwards CQ, Smith CR, Baughman KL, et al. Concentrations of gentamicin and amikacin in human kidneys. *Antimicrob Agents Chemother* 1976;9:925–7.
123. Pijck J, Hallynck T, Soep H, et al. Pharmacokinetics of amikacin in patients with renal insufficiency: relation of half-life and creatinine clearance. *J Infect Dis* 1976;S134:331–41.
124. Sarubbi FA, Hull JH. Amikacin serum concentrations: prediction of levels and dosage guidelines. *Ann Intern Med* 1978;89:612–8.
125. Levy J, Klastersky J. Correlation of serum creatinine concentrations and amikacin half-life. *J Clin Pharmacol* 1975;15:705–7.
126. Regeur L, Colding H, Jensen H, et al. Pharmacokinetics of amikacin during hemodialysis and peritoneal dialysis. *Antimicrob Agents Chemother* 1977;11:214–8.
127. Madhavan T, Yaremchuk K, Levin N, et al. Effect of renal failure and dialysis on the serum concentration of the aminoglycoside amikacin. *Antimicrob Agents Chemother* 1976;10:464–6.
128. Sairio E, Kasanen A, Kangas L, et al. The nephrotoxicity and renal accumulation of amikacin, tobramycin and gentamicin in rats, rabbits and guinea pigs. *Exp Path* 1978;15:370–5.
129. Nieminen L, Kasanen A, Kangas L, et al. Renal accumulation of amikacin, tobramycin and gentamicin in the rat. *Experientia* 1978;34:1135–6.
130. Wold JS, Robbins DO, Gries CL, et al. The comparative nephrotoxicity of aminoglycoside antibiotics in the rat. Society of Toxicology 18th Annual Meeting, March, 1979, New Orleans, Louisiana. Abstract 39.
131. Hottendorf GH, Gordon LL. Comparative low-dose nephrotoxicities of gentamicin, tobramycin and amikacin. *Antimicrob Agents Chemother* 1980;18:176–81.
132. Drasar FA, Farrell W, Maskell J, et al. Tobramycin, amikacin, sisomicin, and gentamicin resistant gram-negative rods. *Br Med J* 1976;2:1284–7.
133. Dhawan V, Marso E, Martin WJ, et al. In vitro studies with netilmicin compared with amikacin, gentamicin, and tobramycin. *Antimicrob Agents Chemother* 1977;11:64–73.
134. Braveny I, Voeckl J, Machka K. Antimicrobial activity of netilmicin in comparison with gentamicin, sisomicin, tobramycin, and amikacin, and their resistance patterns. *Drug Res* 1980;30:491–5.
135. Tselentis J, Legakis NJ, Nicolas KJ, et al. Comparative in vitro activity of netilmicin, amikacin, tobramycin and sisomicin against gentamicin highly-resistant Enterobacteriaceae. *Chemotherapy* 1980;26:409–17.
136. Stevens P, Hong D. Mechanisms of the synergy of amikacin and ceftazidime against amikacin resistant *Pseudomonas aeruginosa*. 8th International Congress of Pharmacology, Tokyo, Japan, July 1981.
137. Zinner SH, Klastersky J, Goya H. In vitro and in vivo studies of three antibiotic combinations against gram-negative bacteria and *Staphylococcus aureus*. *Antimicrob Agents Chemother* 1980;20:463–9.
138. Keating MJ, Bodey GP, Valdivieso M, et al. A randomized comparative trial of three aminoglycosides—comparison of continuous infusion of gentamicin, amikacin and sisomycin combined with carbenicillin in the treatment of infections in neutropenic patients with malignancies. *Medicine* 1979;58:159–70.
139. Feld R, Valdivieso M, Bodey GP, et al. Comparison of amikacin and tobramycin in the treatment of infections in patients with cancer. *J Infect Dis* 1977;135:61–6.
140. Plaut ME, Schentag JJ, Jusko WJ. Aminoglycoside nephrotoxicity: comparative assessment in critically ill patients. *J Med* 1979;10:257–66.
141. Wade JC, Smith CR, Petty BG, et al. Cephalothin plus an aminoglycoside is more nephrotoxic than methicillin plus an aminoglycoside. *Lancet* 1978;2:604–6.
142. Smith CR, Baughman KL, Edwards CQ, et al. Controlled comparison of amikacin and gentamicin. *N Engl J Med* 1977;296:349–53.
143. Smith CR, Lipsky JJ, Laskin OL, et al. Double-blind comparison of the nephrotoxicity and auditory toxicity of gentamicin and tobramycin. *N Engl J Med* 1980;302:1106–9.
144. Lerner S, Seligsohn R, Matz G. Comparative clinical studies of ototoxicity and nephrotoxicity of amikacin and gentamicin. *Am J Med* 1977;62:S113–8.

Therapeutic Drug Monitoring
7:26–35 © 1985 Raven Press, New York

Review

Oral Contraceptive Drug Interactions

Anne M. Baciewicz

Department of Clinical Pharmacy Practice, College of Pharmacy, St. John's University, Jamaica, New York, U.S.A.

Summary: Approximately 50 million women use oral contraceptives (OC). Studies and case reports demonstrate that OC failure may be caused by rifampin, anticonvulsant drugs, and possibly some antibiotics. Contraceptive steroids may interfere with the metabolism of the benzodiazepines, theophylline, and the glucocorticoids. Future investigation will document the clinical significance of other OC interactions as well as give rise to new interactions. **Key Words:** Oral contraceptives—Drug interactions.

An estimated 50 million women use oral contraceptives (OC) (1). With the widespread acceptance of the contraceptive steroids, they are frequently prescribed with other medications.

Evidence indicates that certain drugs may impair the efficacy of OC. The converse is also true: that contraceptive steroids may modify the action of various drugs.

These drug interactions may be caused by induction or inhibition of hepatic microsomal enzymes, interference with the enterohepatic circulation of steroid metabolites, competition between two drugs for a common metabolizing enzyme, or induction of an opposite physiological effect (2). Certain drugs such as rifampin and the anticonvulsants phenobarbital and phenytoin are known to be enzyme inducers of the cytochrome P-450 monooxygenase system (3–6). These agents have been reported to increase the metabolism of the OC (7–36). In contrast, contraceptive steroids may inhibit the mixed function oxidase system. Ethinylestradiol, 5 mg/kg/day given over 5 days, decreased cytochrome P-450 in the livers of male rats and was associated with a decreased turnover of the P-450 pool (37). However, these effects occurred at concentrations greater than those that follow usual doses in humans. OC are capable of inhibiting the oxidative pathways of certain drugs that are metabolized through the cytochrome P-450 and P-448 systems, thereby reducing their clearance. Those drugs affected by OC which are predominantly eliminated by the P-450 system include chlordiazepoxide (38,39), diazepam (40,41), antipyrine (42–49), and aminopyrine (50), whereas predominant metabolism by the P-448 system occurs for theophylline (51–54) and caffeine (55). The potential for clinically significant drug interactions exists between OC and other agents.

Address correspondence and reprint requests to Dr. A. M. Baciewicz at Department of Clinical Pharmacy Practice, College of Pharmacy, St. John's University, Jamaica, NY 11439, U.S.A.

ANTITUBERCULOUS DRUGS

Rifampin

Menstrual abnormalities and pregnancy have occurred in tuberculosis patients treated simultaneously with OC and rifampin. Reimers and Ježek (7) described an increased incidence of intermenstrual breakthrough bleeding in 38 of 51 women treated with concomitant OC and rifampin. Nocke-Finck et al. (8,9) reported that 5 of 88 women with tuberculosis became pregnant while taking rifampin and OC, while 62 experienced spotting, intermenstrual bleeding, or amenorrhea.

TABLE 1. *Oral contraceptives: antituberculous drug interactions*

Observation	Drugs	Reference
38 of 51 women: intermenstrual or breakthrough bleeding	RIF	Reimers and Ježek (7)
5 of 88 women: pregnant 62 of 88 women: intermenstrual or breakthrough bleeding, amenorrhea	RIF	Nocke-Finck et al. (8,9)
1 pregnancy	RIF	Hirsh (10)
1 pregnancy	RIF, INH, ETB	Kropp (11)
3 pregnancies: 2 women	RIF, INH, ETB	Hirsh et al. (12)
1 pregnancy	RIF	Piquet et al. (13)
2 pregnancies: 1 woman	RIF, INH, ETB	Skolnick et al. (14)
1 pregnancy	RIF, INH, ETB	Lafaix et al. (15)
3 pregnancies: 3 women	RIF, INH, ETB	Bessot et al. (16)
1 pregnancy	RIF, INH	Gupta and Ali (17)
1 woman: amenorrhea	RIF, INH	Altschuler and Valenteen (18)

RIF, rifampin; INH, isoniazid; ETB, ethambutol.

Case reports of pregnancies and alterations in the menstrual cycle have been described by other authors in regular OC users taking rifampin (10–18) (Table 1). The interaction of a low-dose combination OC with antitubercular drugs was studied by Joshi et al. (19). Nine women were treated with rifampin, 8–10 mg/kg. Three experienced menstrual irregularities, and two showed a premenstrual rise of plasma progesterone levels >4 ng/ml, suggesting an ovulatory cycle. Both plasma levels and the area under the curve were significantly reduced for norethisterone.

Bolt and associates (20) demonstrated a fourfold increase in the rate of hydroxylation of estradiol and ethinylestradiol paralleled by an increase of cytochrome P-450 liver content. This was observed in liver biopsies of patients treated for 6–10 days with 600 mg rifampin daily.

In 1977, Bolt et al. (21) assessed the pharmacokinetics and metabolism of ethinylestradiol in volunteers who received a 6-day course of rifampin, 600 mg. The half-life decreased from 7.5 $\pm$ 1.7 h to 3.3 $\pm$ 0.9 h in patients taking ethinylestradiol alone and ethinylestradiol and rifampin, respectively. Simultaneously with the decrease in half-life induced by rifampin, there was a twofold increase in the rate of hydroxylation of ethinylestradiol. Back et al. (22) found results similar to those of Bolt and associates (21).

Gelbke et al. (23) observed the influence of rifampin, 600 mg/day, on the metabolic fate of mestranol in several women. Both treated and untreated women had the same urinary excretion of mestranol and 2-hydroxy-ethinylestradiol. In contrast, the urinary excretion of ethinylestradiol was lower in the women treated with rifampin (3.5–4.9%) as compared with the control group (15–23%).

The progesterone component of the OC was studied by Back et al. (24). They assessed the effect of rifampin, 450–600 mg/day, on the pharmacokinetics of norethisterone, 1 mg, in eight women. Rifampin caused a significant reduction in the area under the curve for norethisterone from 37.8 $\pm$ 13.1 to 21.9 $\pm$ 5.9 ng/ml·h. The plasma β half-life of norethisterone was also reduced from 6.2 $\pm$ 1.7 h to 3.2 $\pm$ 1.0 h.

It is imperative to counsel women who will receive OC and rifampin simultaneously. The possible ineffectiveness of the OC, along with the suggestion to use other means of birth control, should be emphasized to the patient and documented in the chart.

ANTICONVULSANT DRUGS

Breakthrough bleeding and OC failure have been noted in women taking anticonvulsant drugs and contraceptive steroids concurrently. Table 2 summarizes the interactions of the various anticonvulsants—phenytoin, phenobarbital, carbamazepine, and primidone—that have been implicated in causing pregnancy (25–32). The British Committee on Safety of Medicines received 23 reports of pregnancies secondary to OC failure (33,34). John (35) noted an increased failure rate of OC in women taking anticonvulsant drugs.

Several studies addressed the influence of OC on anticonvulsants. Espir et al. (56) conducted a crossover trial of 20 epileptic women receiving various anticonvulsants with Norinyl-l (mestranol, 0.05 mg, and norethisterone, 1 mg; Syntex). They showed that a low-dose estrogen/progestogen contraceptive had no significant effect on the average frequency of seizures, in comparison with placebo. One patient developed symptoms of anticonvulsant toxicity shortly after beginning Norinyl-1.

Back et al. (36) investigated the interaction of various anticonvulsants and Ovran (ethinylestradiol, 50 μg, and levonorgestrel, 250 μg; Wyeth) in five women. The plasma levels of ethinylestradiol and norgestrel were at the lower limit of normal in women taking anticonvulsants, compared with control subjects. They

TABLE 2. *Oral contraceptives: anticonvulsant drug interactions*

No. of pregnancies	Drug(s)	Reference
1	Phenytoin	Kenyon (25)
6	Phenytoin, primidone, phenobarbital, or methylphenobarbital	Hempel et al. (26)
1	Phenytoin and phenobarbital	Janz and Schmidt (27)
1	Phenytoin, phenobarbital, and Ethosuximide	Janz and Schmidt (27)
1	Primidone	Janz and Schmidt (27)
1	Phenobarbital	Gagnaire et al. (28)
2	Butobarbital	Gagnaire et al. (28)
1	Phenytoin and carbamazepine	Janz and Schmidt (29)
1	Phenytoin, carbamazepine, and primidone	Janz and Schmidt (29)
1	Phenytoin and phenobarbital	Janz and Schmidt (29)
1	Phenytoin and primidone	Janz and Schmidt (29)
1	Primidone	Janz and Schmidt (29)
2	—[a]	Janz and Schmidt (30)
2	Primidone	Belaisch et al. (31)
1	Phenobarbital	Belaisch et al. (31)
1	Phenytoin	Coulam and Annegers (32)
1	Phenobarbital	Coulam and Annegers (32)
1	Phenytoin and phenobarbital	Coulam and Annegers (32)
1	Methylphenobarbital	Coulam and Annegers (32)

[a] Anticonvulsant drugs administered, type not specified.

also studied the interaction of *phenobarbital*, 30 mg twice daily, on OC therapy in four women. Their results showed no significant change in the plasma ethinylestradiol concentration for the group, but a marked variation in levels was noted in two women with breakthrough bleeding. No changes in plasma concentrations of northindrone, norgestrel, progesterone, or follicle-stimulating hormone were seen. There was a significant increase in the sex hormone binding globulin capacity, probably because of increased protein synthesis by phenobarbital. These changes are consistent with the interindividual variation in the microsomal enzyme inducing effect of phenobarbital in humans.

Hempel et al. (26) investigated the effect of *phenobarbital*, 0.05–0.1 g, for 7–10 d in 51 women who regularly used OC. Breakthrough bleeding or spotting occurred in 30 of the 51 women, and one pregnancy occurred.

Hooper et al. (57) studied the influence of plasma protein binding of *diphenylhydantoin* (DPH, phenytoin) in several groups of patients. They noted no significant differences among plasma protein binding of DPH in pregnant women, women taking OC, healthy women, or healthy men.

DeLeacy et al. (58) observed the effects of low-dose estrogen on plasma *phenytoin* levels. Their results showed higher plasma phenytoin levels relative to drug dose in OC users versus controls. There was no significant difference in plasma phenytoin levels and drug dose in women who did not use OC and men.

Bäckström (59) noted no definite correlation between changes in hormone concentrations and levels of phenytoin, phenobarbital, or carbamazepine after evaluating seven epileptic patients during six menstrual cycles.

In women taking both OC and various anticonvulsants, it would be advisable to counsel them to use additional forms of birth control, documentation being made in the patient's chart. The enzyme-inducing effect of the barbiturates, phenytoin, or other antiepileptic drugs might render the OC ineffective by increasing the hydroxylation of estrogen and progesterone. It would be advisable to monitor these women for clinical signs and symptoms of anticonvulsant toxicity, along with periodic measurement of anticonvulsant levels, as OC may influence the metabolism of antiepileptic drugs.

ANTIBIOTICS

The effect of ampicillin on OC effectiveness has been addressed in several studies. Friedman et al. (60) studied the effect of Demulen (ethinylestradiol, 50 μg, and ethynodiol diacetate, 1 mg; Searle) with placebo or ampicillin, 250 mg four times daily for 16 days, during two consecutive menstrual cycles in 11 volunteers. Serum estradiol, progesterone, luteinizing hormone, and follicle-stimulating hormone were suppressed in 10 of 11 patients during both study cycles. All cycles appeared to be anovulatory. Estrogen-dependent testosterone-binding globulin capacity was unaffected by ampicillin.

Joshi et al. (61) studied the interaction of a low dose combination OC (norethisterone acetate, 1 mg, and ethinylestradiol, 30 μg) with ampicillin, 500 mg twice daily for 5–7 days, in six women. Ampicillin did not alter the peak or 24-h plasma levels of the area under the curve for norethisterone or ethinylestradiol. Furthermore, the OC did not alter the peak level of ampicillin. Progesterone levels were in the anovulatory range in all ampicillin-treated cycles. Philipson (62) noted no significant difference in ampicillin plasma and urine levels produced by a single oral dose of ampicillin, 500 mg, administered to 10 women taking OC.

Back et al. (63) studied 13 women taking long-term OC therapy (ethinylestradiol, 30–50 μg, and levonorgestrel, 150–250 μg, or norethisterone acetate, 1 mg) and ampicillin, 500 mg three times daily for 8 days, compared with a control cycle without ampicillin. There was no significant change in the plasma concentrations of ethinylestradiol, levonorgesterol, follicle-stimulating hormone, or progesterone.

Dossetor (64) reported three patients who became pregnant while taking ampicillin and OC.

Ampicillin has been shown to decrease urinary estrogen excretion in pregnant and nonpregnant women (65–72). Ampicillin does not significantly lower the concentration of plasma unconjugated estrogens (65,69,72,73). Plasma and urinary progesterone levels did not manifest any consistent effect during concurrent ampicillin therapy (66,70,73,74).

Pulkkinen and Willman (75,76) reported the reduction of urinary estrogen excretion and plasma levels by both phenoxymethylpenicillin and neomycin for 3 days in pregnant women.

The possible explanation for the effect of antibiotics on endogenous steroid production strongly suggests that antibiotics, by reducing intestinal bacterial flora, inhibit steroid glucuronide conjugate hydrolysis in the gut. This inhibition could possibly cause fecal loss of steroid conjugates and by impairing normal steroid reabsorption would result in lower plasma and urine levels of certain steroid metabolites (77).

Studies or case reports regarding OC and other antibiotics have been described. Joshi et al. (61) studied the effect of a low-dose combination OC and metronidazole, 400 mg three times a day for 6–8 days, in 10 women. Metronidazole did not alter the peak or 24-h plasma levels and the area under the curve for norethisterone or ethinylestradiol. The peak level of metronidazole was unchanged. Progesterone levels were in the anovulatory range in 22 of 25 metronidazole treated cycles.

Grimmer et al. (78) described the concomitant administration of cotrimoxazole, 1 g twice daily for 7 days, in nine women taking a long-term OC with a control cycle. Cotrimoxazole significantly increased the plasma concentration of ethinylestradiol, while the follicle-stimulating hormone concentration was significantly suppressed. No significant changes were noted in the plasma concentration of levonorgestrel or progesterone. The rise in ethinylestradiol plasma levels during cotrimoxazole therapy is attributed to inhibition of ethinylestradiol metabolism by microsomal hydroxylation liver enzymes.

Swenson et al. (79) examined the effect of a 10-day course of oral tetracycline, 250 mg four times a day (four women), or ampicillin, 250 mg four times a day (one woman), on the urinary and fecal excretion of the OC ethinylestradiol. These antibiotics decreased the urinary excretion and increased the fecal excretion of ethinylestradiol. The mean half-life of ethinylestradiol decreased during antibiotic administration.

Reports of pregnancy have been attributed to interactions between OC and tetracycline (80,81), oxacillin (82), sulphamethoxypyridazine (26), and chloramphenicol (26). The British Committee on Safety of Medicines received 38 reports of pregnancies in women taking OC and antibiotics other than rifampin (33,34).

DeSano and Hurley (83) observed 16 pregnancies in women taking OC in conjunction with an antimicrobial (penicillin, ampicillin, tetracycline, sulfonamides, cephalexin) and antihistamines.

The Committee on the Safety of Medicines in the United Kingdom and the Netherlands Centre for the Monitoring of Adverse Reactions to Drugs reported 22 cases of possible interactions between griseofulvin, an antifungal agent, and OC (84). Twenty women experienced transient intermenstrual bleeding or amenorrhea when receiving concomitant long-term OC and griseofulvin, 500 to 1,000 mg daily. In four women reexposed to griseofulvin, the original reaction recurred. Unintended pregnancies occurred in two additional patients. However, both women were also receiving sulfonamides or cotrimoxazole.

Two hypotheses have been proposed to explain the failure of OC when antibiotics are prescribed (85,86). One theorizes that antibiotics change the intestinal flora affecting bacterial hydrolysis of steroid conjugates. This causes an interruption of the enterohepatic circulation of contraceptive steroids, leading to escape ovulation (85). The other hypothesis is that antibiotics induce liver microsomal enzymes, which accelerate estrogen metabolism resulting in subtherapeutic blood estrogen levels (86).

Ampicillin and other antibiotics appear unlikely to diminish the effectiveness of the OC, but further research is needed to delineate the significance of this interaction. However, it would be advisable to counsel the patient about this potential interaction and to document this action in the chart. Women should be encouraged to use an additional method of birth control when taking antibiotics, especially if they are taking ampicillin and OC simultaneously.

BENZODIAZEPINES

There is a variation in the effect of the OC on the benzodiazepines. Studies suggest that those benzodiazepines which are highly metabolized by oxidation, such as chlordiazepoxide, diazepam, and nitrazepam, have an impaired clearance and increased half-life in women receiving OC (38–41,87). In contrast, drugs metabolized primarily by glucuronide conjugation, such as oxazepam or lorazepam, have the same or an increased clearance in OC users (39,88). The reason for conflicting results in the benzodiazepines that are conjugated is unclear, but they may be due to a smaller sample in the Patwardhan et al. (39) study. Tables 3 and 4 summarize the studies of those benzodiazepines which are oxidized or glucuronidated, respectively.

OC users who are receiving long-term benzodiazepines that are highly oxidized should be monitored for potential increased clinical effects. A dosage reduction may be required. However, women using OC and glucuronidated benzodiazepines may have decreased steady-state plasma levels and require increased benzodiazepine doses. The clinical importance of these interactions requires further study.

THEOPHYLLINE

Four studies have addressed the effect of OC on theophylline disposition. Jusko et al. (51) studied the effect of OC on theophylline in eight patients. The use of OC was associated with a decreased total serum theophylline clearance in smokers only. Theophylline clearance diminished from 71 ± 30 ml/h/kg in smoking subjects not using OC to 55 ± 21 ml/h/kg in smoking subjects using OC.

Tornatore et al. (52) examined the usage of chronic OC on the disposition of a single oral dose of aminophylline, 4 ml/kg, in eight women versus a control group of eight women. The OC users had a significantly lower total plasma clearance of theophylline, 35.1 ± 5.6 ml/h/kg, versus that in women not using OC, 53.1 ± 14.5 ml/h/kg. The half-life of theophylline was also significantly prolonged in the OC group versus nonusers, being 9.79 ± 1.43 h and 7.34 ± 1.75

TABLE 3. *Oral contraceptives: oxidized benzodiazepines*

Drug	Subjects	Protein binding (%) [B or U]	Mean halflife (h)	Mean total clearance (ml/min/kg or ml/min*)	Mean unbound clearance (ml/min/kg or ml/min*)	Reference
CLDZ 0.6 mg/kg i.v.	11 M	97.0 (1.20) B	8.9 (2.50)	0.43 (0.12)	15.6 (5.3)	Roberts et al. (38)
	11 F	95.5 (1.40) B	14.8 (5.90)	0.35 (0.17)	8.7 (5.0)	
	7 F–OC	93.6 (1.50) B	24.3 (12.0)	0.34 (0.12)	5.7 (3.0)	
CLDZ 0.6 mg/kg i.v.	6 C	97.5 (0.24) B	11.6 (5.91)	33.2 (12.4)*		Patwardhan et al. (39)
	6 F–OC	96.1 (0.62) B	20.6 (8.08)	13.4 (4.69)*		
DZP 10 mg i.v.	6 M		34.9 (13.0)	25.2 (4.57)*		Giles et al. (40)
	5 F–OC		73.8 (49.3)	20.0 (7.09)*		
DZP 10 mg i.v.	11 M		36.0 (14.8)	27.9 (9.85)*		Giles et al. (40)
	10 F		40.3 (11.9)	28.7 (9.39)*		
DZP 10 mg i.v.	8 C	1.23 (0.07) U	47.0 (4.00)	0.45 (0.04)		Abernethy et al. (41)
	8 F–OC	1.23 (0.08) U	69.0 (9.00)	0.27 (0.02)		
NTZP 5 mg oral	6 M	11.4 (0.01) U	27.3 (1.30)	59.3 (2.70)*	530 (37)*	Jochemsen et al. (87)
	6 F	12.4 (0.50) U	28.7 (1.45)	57.0 (4.15)*	459 (40)*	
	6 F–OC	13.5 (0.04) U	30.9 (2.25)	46.1 (4.35)*	333 (30)*	

SD in parentheses. B, bound; U, unbound; CLDZ, chlordiazepoxide; DZP, diazepam; NTZP, nitrazepam; OC, oral contraceptives; C, controls; M, male; F, female.

TABLE 4. *Oral contraceptives: glucuronidated benzodiazepines*

Drug	Subjects	Protein binding (%) [B or U]	Mean halflife (h)	Mean total clearance (ml/min/kg or ml/min*)	Mean $V_{d\ ss}$ (L/kg or L*)	Reference
LRZP	15 C	10.3 (0.4) U	13.1 (0.8)	1.25 (0.1)	1.33 (0.07)	Abernethy et al. (88)
2 mg i.v.	15 F–OC	10.3 (0.3) U	12.2 (1.2)	1.50 (0.1)	1.45 (0.06)	
LRZP	8 C	92.5 (0.72) B	14.0 (6.2)	77.4 (32.9)*	75.7 (17.5)*	Patwardhan et al. (39)
2 mg i.v.	7 F–OC	92.9 (0.76) B	6.0 (3.1)	288.9 (165.9)*	113.5 (30.3)*	
OXZP	14 C	4.6 (0.3) U	7.6 (0.6)	1.60 (0.1)	1.05 (0.07)	Abernethy et al. (88)
30 mg oral	17 F–OC	4.9 (0.2) U	7.2 (0.6)	2.03 (0.2)	1.19 (0.14)	
OXZP	6 C	97.1 (1.22) B	12.1 (5.08)	97.9 (69.4)*		Patwardhan et al. (39)
45 mg oral	5 F–OC	97.3 (0.46) B	7.71 (3.23)	251.2 (106.9)*		

SD in parentheses. $V_{d\ ss}$, steady-state volume of distribution; LRZP, lorazepam; OXZP, oxazepam; B, bound; U, unbound; C, controls; F, females; OC, oral contraceptives.

h, respectively. The clearance of ethinylestradiol was approximately 30% lower in OC users. A significant positive correlation was noted between the plasma clearance of theophylline and the clearance of ethinylestradiol.

Roberts et al. (53) assessed the influence of OC on theophylline disposition in a control group of 13 women and 10 women using chronic OC. The elimination half-life of theophylline was increased in nonusers versus OC users from 386 ± 157 min to 523 ± 110 min, respectively. The plasma clearance of theophylline was decreased from 0.98 ± 0.32 ml/min/kg in nonusers to 0.70 ± 0.15 ml/min/kg in OC users.

Gardner et al. (54) investigated the effect of both acute and chronic OC use on a single oral dose of aminophylline, 4 mg/kg, in 49 women. OC caused a 28% decrease in theophylline clearance as well as a 19% increase in theophylline half-life. Single-dose exposure in OC nonusers did not significantly alter theophylline pharmacokinetics for the group. However, in a subgroup of smokers, significant decreases in clearance were evident. Analogous results were found for half-life. Areas under the serum concentration–time profiles of norgestral and ethinylestradiol were examined in 27 women as indices of OC exposure. The lowest values of theophylline clearance were noted in subjects with the largest area under the serum concentration–time curve of both steroids.

Gotz et al. (89) assessed the influence of the progestin medroxyprogesterone on theophylline disposition in a crossover blind study in 11 patients. Their data indicated that medroxyprogesterone, 20 mg three times daily for 4 weeks, had no significant effect on the pharmacokinetic parameters of theophylline in patients with moderate to severe obstructive pulmonary disease.

The effect of OC on theophylline disposition is probably due to decreased oxidation via the cytochrome P-448 system. Patients receiving concomitant OC and theophylline should be monitored for possible theophylline toxicity, both clinically and with periodic determinations of theophylline serum levels, as theophylline has a narrow therapeutic range.

GLUCOCORTICOIDS

The effect of OC use on glucocorticoid metabolism is significant. Spangler et al. (90) noted a 3- to 20-fold reduction in the corticosteroid dose for skin diseases with the concomitant administration of estrogens in nine females. The addition of estrogens to the corticosteroid therapy caused an average threefold rise in the concentration of unconjugated serum corticosteroids and cortisol-binding globulin.

Three studies address the alteration of prednisolone metabolism by OC. Kozower et al. (91) noted a significant increase in the half-life and a twofold decrease in the metabolic clearance rate of prednisolone in three women taking OC versus controls.

Legler and Benet (92) observed marked alterations in prednisolone pharmacokinetics in six OC users versus six controls receiving 0.53 mg/kg prednisolone intravenously. OC significantly increased the area under the prednisolone plasma concentration–time curve from 143 μg·ml/min to 858 μg·ml/min and the half-life from 115 ± 21 min to 279 ± 31 min, as well as significantly decreasing the average plasma clearance from 5.05 ± 1.99 ml/min/kg to 0.813 ± 0.158 ml/min/kg and the steady-state volume of distribution from 46.6 ± 8.5 L to 17.2 ± 2.8 L. Women receiving OC and prednisolone showed a dramatic increase in prednisolone plasma levels as a result of a greater than fivefold decrease in clearance along with a threefold decrease in distribution volume.

TABLE 5. *Clinically significant oral contraceptive drug interactions*

Drug (reference)	Comments
Rifampin (7–24)	Document counseling in the chart Use other forms of birth control
Anticonvulsants (25–36, 56–59) Barbiturates Phenytoin	Document counseling in the chart Use other forms of birth control Clinically monitor patients for symptoms of anticonvulsant toxicity Monitor serum anticonvulsant levels May need to adjust anticonvulsant dose
Theophylline (51–54)	Clinically monitor patients for symptoms of theophylline toxicity Monitor serum theophylline levels May need to decrease theophylline dose

TABLE 6. *Other oral contraceptive drug interactions*

Drug (reference)	Comments
Antibiotics (60–64,78–84) Ampicillin	Document counseling in the chart Encourage women to use an additional form of birth control
Benzodiazepines (38–41,87,88)	Clinically monitor patients for increase or decrease in benzodiazepine response May need to adjust benzodiazepine dose depending on the benzodiazepine
Glucocorticoids (90–93)	Clinically monitor patients for increased glucocorticoid side effects May need to decrease glucocorticoid dose
Acetaminophen (94–97)	Clinically monitor patients for optimal analgesic and antipyretic effect May need to increase acetaminophen dose
Anticoagulants (98,99)	Monitor prothrombin time May need to adjust anticoagulant dose
Other drugs (26,42–40,55,83, 100–114)	

Boekenoogan et al. (93) assessed the effects of 40 mg intravenous prednisolone in eight female OC users, and in eight men, and five women. Plasma clearance of total prednisolone in women receiving OC was 96 ± 9 ml/min/1.73 m^2, significantly lower than the clearance in male and female controls of 205 ± 46 ml/min/1.73 m^3 and 187 ± 22 ml/min/1.73 m^2, respectively. The prednisolone half-life and mean residence time were increased, while the steady-state volume of distribution was decreased, in OC users. Evaluation of free prednisolone parameters in women taking OC showed a significantly lower clearance and decreased volume of distribution along with a twofold increase in the area under the free concentration–time curve.

The addition of OC to the treatment regimen of patients receiving corticosteroids may result in potentiation of beneficial and adverse effects related to corticosteroids. Possibly this may be compensated for by reduction of the steroid dose.

ACETAMINOPHEN

Several studies have addressed the potential interaction between OC and acetaminophen. Abernethy et al. (94) studied the effect of chronic low-dose OC on the pharmacokinetics of intravenous acetaminophen (650 mg) in eight women and eight controls. OC users had a significantly increased total metabolic clearance of acetaminophen at 5.81 ± 0.48 ml/min/kg, versus 3.12 ± 0.38 ml/min/kg for controls. The contraceptive users also had a significantly decreased elimination half-life, 2.12 ± 0.13 h versus 2.71 ± 0.09 h for controls.

Mitchell et al. (95) noted similar results in seven OC users and seven controls who were given 1.5 g acetaminophen orally. Plasma acetaminophen clearance increased from 287 ± 13 ml/min to 470 ± 51 ml/min in OC users, whereas elimination half-life decreased from 2.40 ± 0.14 h to 1.67 ± 0.16 h. The increased clearance of acetaminophen in OC users resulted from increased glucuronidation on the drug.

Miners et al. (96) studied the influence of OC on paracetamol, 1,000 mg orally, in eight men, eight women, and eight women receiving OC. *Salivary* concentrations were used to determine paracetamol clearance. Paracetamol clearance in women using OC was 49% greater than in female controls and 22% higher than in men. The half-life of paracetamol was correspondingly decreased in the OC users compared with both men and women. Glucuronidation and oxidative metabolism of paracetamol were both induced in OC users by 78 and 36%, respectively. Mucklow et al. (97) observed a 30% increase in paracetamol clearance in women taking OC, using *saliva* samples.

As the metabolic clearance of acetaminophen is increased in women taking OC, acetaminophen dosage may have to be increased to obtain optimal analgesic and antipyretic response. The increased oxidative metabolism of the drug in OC users may be a risk factor in the development of acetaminophen-induced hepatotoxicity in women.

OTHER DRUGS

Potential interactions may exist between OC and other drugs. Studies have been done with anticoagulants (98,99), antidepressants (imipramine and clomipramine) (100–107), antipyrine (42–49), and phenylbutazone (43–45,108). Further investigation is warranted for vitamin D (45,109), antihistamines (83), butaperazine (110), aspirin (108), meperidine (111,112), other analgesics (26), metoprolol (113), aminopyrine (50), caffeine (55), and clofibric acid (114).

CONCLUSION

It is important for physicians to be cognizant of drugs that are influenced by OC, as concurrent drug administration is their responsibility. A summary of clinically significant drug interactions is listed in Table 5. Other potential OC drug interactions are listed in Table 6. Drugs that cause OC failure will require an increased OC estrogen dose and/or an alternative contraceptive modality. Most drugs that are modified by OC require a dosage decrease when administered concomitantly. Discontinuation of the OC will necessitate a dosage increase of the interacting agent. Anticipation of new OC drug interactions should be expected with further investigation.

Acknowledgment: The author acknowledges the assistance of the librarians at Queens Hospital Center and St. John's University and of Elaena Quattrocchi in obtaining the articles used for this work.

REFERENCES

1. Stokes B. *Filling the family planning gap* (Worldwatch paper 12). Washington, DC: Worldwatch Institute, 1977:17.
2. Roberton YR, Johnson ES. Interactions between oral contraceptives and other drugs: a review. *Curr Med Res Opin* 1976;3:647–61.
3. Miquet JP, Mavier P, Soussy CJ, Dhumequx D. Induction of hepatic microsomal enzymes after brief administration of rifampicin in man. *Gastroenterology* 1977;79:924–6.
4. Pessayre D, Mazel P. Induction and inhibition of hepatic drug metabolizing enzymes by rifampin. *Biochem Pharmacol* 1976;25:943–9.
5. Conney AH. Pharmacological implications of microsomal enzyme induction. *Pharmacol Rev* 1967;19:317–66.
6. Marshall WJ. Role of steroid hormones in hepatic microsomal enzyme induction. *Biochem Pharmacol* 1971;20:1723–5.
7. Reimers D, Ježel A. Rifampin und andre antituberkulotika bei gleichzeitiger oraler kontrazeption. *Prax Pneumol* 1971;25:255–62.
8. Nocke-Finck L, Breuer H, Reimers D. Wirkung von rifampicin auf den menstruationszyklus und die ostrongenausscheideidung bei einnahme oraler kontrazeptiva. *Dtsch Med Wochenschr* 1973;98:1521–3.
9. Nocke-Finck L, Breuer H, Reimers D. Effects of rifampin on menstrual cycle and on estrogen excretion in patients taking oral contraceptives [Abstract]. *JAMA* 1973;226:378.
10. Hirsch A. Pilules endormies. *Nouv Presse Med* 1983;2:2957.
11. Kropp R. Rifampicin und ovulationshemmer. *Prax Pneumol* 1974;28:270–2.
12. Hirsch A, Tillement JP, Chrétien J. Effets contrariants de la rifampicine sur les contraceptifs oraux: a propos de trois grossessess non désirées observées chez deux malades. *Rev Fr Mal Respir* 1975;3:174–82.
13. Piquet B, Muglioni JF, Chaline G. Contraception orale et rifampicine. *Nouv Presse Med* 1975;4:115–6.
14. Skolnick JL, Stoler BS, Katz DB, Anderson WH. Rifampin, oral contraceptives and pregnancy. *JAMA* 1976;236:1382.
15. Lafaix C, Cadoz M, Richard A, Patouillard P. L'effet "antipilule" de la rifampicine. *Med Hyg* 1976;1181:181–2.
16. Bessot JC, Petitjean R, Vandevenne A, Rempp M, Burghard G. Interference de la rifampicine sur les contraceptives oraux. *J Med Strasbourg* 1977;8:131–4.
17. Gupta KC, Ali MY. Failure of oral contraceptive with rifampicin. *Med J Zambia* 1980–1981;15:23.
18. Altschuler SL, Valenteen JW. Amenorrhea following rifampin administration during oral contraceptive use. *Obstet Gynecol* 1974;44:771–2.
19. Joshi JV, Joshi UM, Sankolli GM, et al. A study of interaction of a low-dose combination oral contraceptive with anti-tubercular drugs. *Contraception* 1980;21:617–29.
20. Bolt HM, Kappus H, Bolt M. Effect of rifampicin treatment on the metabolism of oestradiol and 17α-ethinyloestradiol by human liver microsomes. *Eur J Clin Pharmacol* 1975;8:301–7.
21. Bolt HM, Bolt M, Kappus H. Interaction of rifampicin treatment with pharmacokinetics and metabolism of ethinyloestradiol in man. *Acta Endocrinol* 1977;85:185–97.
22. Back DJ, Breckenridge AM, Crawford FE, et al. The effect of rifampicin on the pharmacokinetics of ethynylestradiol in women. *Contraception* 1980;21:135–43.
23. Gelbke HP, Gethman U, Knuppen R. Influence of rifampicin treatment on the metabolic fate of [4 – ^{14}C]mestranol in women. *Horm Metab Res* 1977;9:415–9.
24. Back DJ, Breckenridge AM, Crawford F, et al. The effect of rifampicin on norethisterone pharmacokinetics. *Eur J Clin Pharmacol* 1979;15:193–7.
25. Kenyon IE. Unplanned pregnancy in an epileptic [Letter]. *Br Med J* 1972;1:686–7.
26. Hempel von E, Bohm W, Carol W, Klinger G. Medikamentose enzyminduktion und hormonale kontrazeption. *Zentralbl Gynakol* 1973;95:1451–7.
27. Janz D, Schmidt D. Anti-epileptic drugs and failure of oral contraceptives [Letter]. *Lancet* 1974;1:1113.
28. Gagnaire JC, Tchertchian J, Revol A, Rochet Y. Grossessess sous contraceptifs oraux chez les patients recevant des barbituriques [Letter]. *Nouv Presse Med* 1975;4:3008.
29. Janz D, Schmidt D. Antiepileptika und die sicherheit oraler kontrazeptiva. *Bibl Psychiatr* 1975;151:82–4.
30. Janz S, Schmidt D. Sulla sicurezza dei contraccetivi orali in corso di trattamento antiepilettico. *Lega Italiano Contro L'Epilessia. Bollettino* 1976;15–6:113–5.

31. Belaisch J, Druguez P, Janaud A. Influence de certains médicaments sur l'action des pilules contraceptives. *Nouv Presse Med* 1976;5:1645–6.
32. Coulam CB, Annegers JF. Do anticonvulsants reduce the efficacy of oral contraceptives? *Epilepsia* 1979;20:519–26.
33. Anon. Drug interactions with oral contraceptive steroids. *Br Med J* 1980;281:93–4.
34. Back DJ, Breckenridge AM, Crawford FE, MacIver M, Orme MLE, Rowe PH. Interindividual variation and drug interactions with hormonal steroid contraceptives. *Drugs* 1981;21:46–61.
35. John A. Epilepsy and the pill [Letter]. *Br Med J* 1976;2:528.
36. Back DJ, Bates M, Bowden A, et al. The interaction of phenobarbital and other anticonvulsants with oral contraceptive steroid therapy. *Contraception* 1980;22:495–503.
37. MacKinnon M, Sutherland E, Simon FR. Effects of ethinyl estradiol on hepatic microsomal proteins and the turnover of cytochrome P-450. *J Lab Clin Med* 1977;90:1096–1106.
38. Roberts RK, Desmond PV, Wilkinson GR, Schenker S. Disposition of chlordiazepoxide: sex differences and effects of oral contraceptives. *Clin Pharmacol Ther* 1979;25:826–31.
39. Patwardhan RV, Mitchell MC, Johnson RF. Schenker S. Differential effects of oral contraceptives steroids on the metabolism of benzodiazepines. *Hepatology* 1983;3:248–53.
40. Giles HG, Sellers EM, Naranjo CA, Frecker RC, Greenblatt DJ. Disposition of intravenous diazepam in young men and women. *Eur J Clin Pharmacol* 1981;20:207–13.
41. Abernethy DR, Greenblatt DJ, Divoll M, Arendt R, Ochs HR, Shader RI. Impairment of diazepam metabolism by low-dose estrogen-containing oral-contraceptive steroids. *N Engl J Med* 1982;306:791–2.
42. O'Malley K, Stevenson IH, Alexander W. Increased antipyrine half-life in women taking oral contraceptives. *Scott Med J* 1970;15:454–6.
43. O'Malley K, Stevenson IH, Crooks J. Impairment of human drug metabolism by oral contraceptive steroids. *Clin Pharmacol Ther* 1972;13:552–7.
44. Carter DE, Goldman JE, Bressler R, Huxtable RJ, Christian CD, Heine MW. Effect of oral contraceptives on drug metabolism. *Clin Pharmacol Ther* 1974;15:22–31.
45. Carter DE, Bressler R, Hughes MR, Haussler MR, Christian CD, Heine MW. Effect of oral contraceptives on plasma clearance. *Clin Pharmacol Ther* 1975;18:700–7.
46. Homeida M, Halliwell M, Branch RA. Effects of an oral contraceptive on hepatic size and antipyrine metabolism in premenopausal women. *Clin Pharmacol Ther* 1978;24:228–32.
47. Abernethy DR, Greenblatt DJ. Impairment of antipyrine metabolism by low-dose oral contraceptive steroids. *Clin Pharmacol Ther* 1981;29:106–10.
48. Teunissen MWE, Srivastava AK, Breimer DD. Influence of sex and oral contraceptive steroids on antipyrine metabolite formation. *Clin Pharmacol Ther* 1982;32:240–6.
49. Fraser HS, Mucklow JC, Bulpitt CJ, Kahn C, Mould G, Dollery CT. Environmental factors affecting antipyrine metabolism in London factor and office workers. *Br J Clin Pharmacol* 1979;7:237–43.
50. Herz R, Koelz HR, Haemmerli UP, Benes I, Blum AL. Inhibition of hepatic demethylation of aminopyrine by oral contraceptive steroids in humans. *Eur J Clin Invest* 1978;8:27–30.
51. Jusko WJ, Gardner MJ, Mangione A, Schentag JJ, Koup JR, Vance JW. Factors affecting theophylline clearances: age, tobacco, marijuana, cirrhosis, congestive heart failure, obesity, oral contraceptives, benzodiazepines, barbiturates, and ethanol. *J Pharm Sci* 1979;68:1358–66.
52. Tornatore KM, Kanarkowski R, McCarthy TL, Gardner MJ, Yurchak AM, Jusko WJ. Effect of chronic oral contraceptive steroids on theophylline disposition. *Eur J Clin Pharmacol* 1982;23:129–34.
53. Roberts RK, Grice J, McGuffie C, Heilbronn L. Oral contraceptive steroids impair the elimination of theophylline. *J Lab Clin Med* 1983;101:821–5.
54. Gardner MJ, Tornatore KM, Jusko WJ, Kanarkowski R. Effects of tobacco smoking and oral contraceptive use on theophylline disposition. *Br J Clin Pharmacol* 1983;16:271–80.
55. Patwardhan RV, Desmond PV, Johnson RF, Schenker S. Impaired elimination of caffeine by oral contraceptive steroids. *J Lab Clin Med* 1980;95:603–8.
56. Espir M, Walker ME, Lawson JP. Epilepsy and oral contraception. *Br Med J* 1969;1:294–5.
57. Hooper WD, Bochner F, Eadie MJ, Tyrer JH. Plasma protein binding of diphenylhydantoin. Effects of sex hormones, renal and hepatic disease. *Clin Pharmacol Ther* 1974;15:276–82.
58. DeLeacy EA, McLeay CD, Eadie MJ, Tyrer JH. Effects of subjects' sex and intake of tobacco, alcohol and oral contraceptives on plasma phenytoin levels. *Br J Clin Pharmacol* 1979;8:33–6.
59. Bäckström T. Estrogen and progesterone in relation to different activities in the central nervous system. *Acta Obstet Gynecol Scand* 1977;66(suppl):1–17.
60. Friedman CI, Huneke AL, Kim MH, Powell J. The effect of ampicillin on oral contraceptive effectiveness. *Obstet Gynecol* 1980;55:33–7.
61. Joshi JV, Joshi UM, Sankholi GM, et al. A study of interaction of low-dose combination oral contraceptive with ampicillin and metronidazole. *Contraception* 1980;22:643–52.
62. Philipson A. Plasma and urine levels produced by an oral dose of ampicillin 0.5 g administered to women taking oral contraceptives. *Acta Obstet Gynecol Scand* 1979;58:69–71.
63. Back DJ, Breckenridge AM, MacIver M, et al. The effects of ampicillin on oral contraceptive steroids in women. *Br J Clin Pharmacol* 1982;14:43–8.
64. Dossetor J. Drug interactions with oral contraceptives. *Br Med J* 1975;4:467–8.
65. William K, Pulkkinen MO. Reduced maternal plasma and urinary estriol during ampicillin treatment. *Am J Obstet Gynecol* 1971;109:893–6.
66. Trybuchowski H. Effect of ampicillin on the urinary output of steroidal hormones in pregnant and non-pregnant women. *Clin Chim Acta* 1973;45:9–18.
67. Tikkanem MJ, Pulkkinen MO, Aldercreutz H. Effect of ampicillin treatment on the urinary excretion of estriol conjugates in pregnancy. *J Steroid Biochem* 1973;4:439–40.
68. Tikkanen MJ, Adlercreutz H, Pulkkinen MO. Effects of antibiotics on oestrogen metabolism [Letter]. *Br Med J* 1973;2:369.
69. Boehm FH, DiPietro DL, Goss DA. The effect of ampicillin administration on urinary estriol and serum estradiol in the normal pregnant patient. *Am J Obstet Gynecol* 1974;119:98–103.
70. Martin F, Peltonen J, Laatikai T, Pullinen M, Adlercreutz H. Excretion of progesterone metabolism and estriol in faeces from pregnant women during ampicillin administration. *J Steroid Biochem* 1975;6:1339–46.
71. Adlercreutz H, Martin F, Tikkanen MJ, Pulkkinen M. Effect of ampicillin administration on the excretion of twelve oestrogens in pregnancy urine. *Acta Endocrinol* 1975;80:551–7.
72. Sybulski S, Maughan GB. Effect of ampicillin administration on estradiol, estriol, and cortisol levels in maternal plasma and on estriol levels in urine. *Am J Obstet Gynecol* 1976;124:379–81.
73. Adlercreutz H, Martin F, Lehtinen T, Tikkanen MJ, Pulkkinen MO. Effect of ampicillin administration on plasma

conjugated and unconjugated estrogen and progesterone levels in pregnancy. *Am J Obstet Gynecol* 1977;128:266–71.

74. Martin F, Peltonen J, Laatikainen T, Tikkanen M, Pulkkinen M. Excretion of unconjugated and conjugated progesterone metabolites in pregnancy urine during ampicillin administration. *Clin Chim Acta* 1974;55:71–80.
75. Pulkkinen M, Willman K. Maternal oestrogen levels during penicillin treatment [Letter]. *Br Med J* 1971;4:48.
76. Pulkkinen MO, Willman K. Reduction of maternal estrogen excretion by neomycin. *Am J Obstet Gynecol* 1973;115:1153.
77. Orme ML, Back DJ. Therapy with oral contraceptive steroids and antibiotics. *J Antimicrob Chemother* 1979;5:124–6.
78. Grimmer SFM, Allen WL, Back DJ, Breckenridge AM, Orme M, Tjia J. The effect of cotrimoxazole on oral contraceptive steroids in women. *Contraception* 1983;28:53–9.
79. Swenson L, Goldin B, Gorbach SL. Effect of antibiotics on fecal/urinary excretion of ethinyl estradiol, an oral contraceptive [Abstract]. *Gastroenterology* 1980;78:1332.
80. Bacon JF, Shenfield GM. Pregnancy attributable to interaction between tetracycline and oral contraceptives. *Br Med J* 1980;280:293.
81. Lequeux A. Grossesse sous contraceptif oral après prise de tétracycline. *Louvain Med* 1980;99:413.
82. Silber TJ. Apparent oral contraceptive failure associated with antibiotic administration. *J Adolesc Health Care* 1983;4:287–9.
83. DeSano EA Jr, Hurley SC. Possible interactions of antihistamines and antibiotics with oral contraceptive effectiveness. *Fertil Steril* 1982;37:853–4.
84. van Dijke CPH, Weber JCP. Interaction between oral contraceptives and griseofulvin. *Br Med J* 1984;288:1125–6.
85. Rubin D. Antibiotics and oral contraceptives [Letter]. *Arch Dermatol* 1981;117:189.
86. Proudfit C. Concurrent oral contraceptive and antibiotic therapy. *JAMA* 1981;246:2076.
87. Jochemsen R, Van der Graff M, Boeijinga JK, Breimer DD. Influence of sex, menstrual cycle and oral contraception on the disposition of nitrazepam. *Br J Clin Pharmacol* 1982;13:319–24.
88. Abernethy DR, Greenblatt DJ, Ochs HR, et al. Lorazepam and oxazepam kinetics in women on low-dose oral contraceptives. *Clin Pharmacol Ther* 1983;33:628–32.
89. Gotz VP, Dolly FR, Block AJ. Influence of medroxyprogesterone on theophylline disposition. *J Clin Pharmacol* 1983;23:281–4.
90. Spangler AS, Antoniades HN, Sotman SL, Inderbitizin TM. Enhancement of the anti-inflammatory action of hydrocortisone by estrogen. *J Clin Endocrinol* 1969;29:650–5.
91. Kozower M, Veatch L, Kaplan MM. Decreased clearance of prednisolone, a factor in the development of corticosteroid side effects. *J Clin Endocrinol Metab* 1974;38:407–12.
92. Legler UF, Benet LZ. Marked alterations in prednisolone elimination for women taking oral contraceptives [Abstract]. *Clin Pharmacol Ther* 1982;31:243.
93. Boekenoogen SJ, Szefler SJ, Jusko WJ. Prednisolone disposition and protein binding in oral contraceptive users. *J Clin Endocrinol Metab* 1983;56:702–9.
94. Abernethy DR, Divoll M, Ochs HR, Ameer B, Greenblatt DJ. Increased metabolic clearance of acetaminophen with oral contraceptive use. *Obstet Gynecol* 1982;60:338–41.
95. Mitchell MC, Hanew T, Meredith CG, Schenker S. Effects of oral contraceptive steroids on acetaminophen metabolism and elimination. *Clin Pharmacol Ther* 1983;34:48–53.
96. Miners JO, Attwood J, Birkett DJ. Influence of sex and oral contraceptive steroids on paracetamol metabolism. *Br J Clin Pharmacol* 1983;16:503–9.
97. Mucklow JC, Fraser HS, Bulpitt CJ, Kahn C, Mould G, Dollery CT. Environmental factors affecting paracetamol metabolism in London factory and office workers. *Br J Clin Pharmacol* 1980;10:67–74.
98. Schrogie JJ, Solomon HM, Zieve PD. Effect of oral contraceptives on vitamin K–dependent clotting activity. *Clin Pharmacol Ther* 1967;8:670–5.
99. De Teresa E, Vera A, Ortigosa J, Alonso Pulpon L, Puente Arus A, De Artaza M. Interaction between anticoagulants and contraceptives: an unsuspected finding. *Br Med J* 1979;2:1260–1.
100. Prange AJ, Wilson IC. The effect of oestrogen on imipramine response in depressed women. *Proceedings of the fifth World Congress of Psychiatry.* Mexico City, 1971:477.
101. Prange AJ. Estrogen may well affect the response to antidepressants. *JAMA* 1972;219:143–4.
102. Khurana RC. Estrogen-imipramine interaction [Letter]. *JAMA* 1972:222:702–3.
103. Beaumont G. Drug interactions with clomipramine (Anafranil). *J Int Med Res* 1973;1:480–4.
104. Gringras M, Beaumont G, Grieve A. Clomipramine and oral contraceptives: an interaction study—clinical findings. *J Int Med Res* 1980;8(suppl 3):76–80.
105. John VA, Luscombe DK, Kemp H. Effects of age, cigarette smoking and the oral contraceptive on the pharmacokinetics of clomipramine and its desmethyl metabolite during chronic dosing. *J Int Med Res* 1980;8(suppl 3):88–95.
106. Luscombe DK, John V. Influence of age, cigarette smoking and the oral contraceptive on plasma concentrations of clomiparmine. *Postgrad Med J* 1980;56(suppl 1):99–102.
107. Luscombe DK, Jones RB. Effects of concomitantly administered drugs on plasma levels of clomipramine and desmethylclomipramine in depressive patients receiving clomipramine therapy [Abstract]. *Postgrad Med J* 1977;53(suppl 4):77–8.
108. Gupta KC, Joshi JV, Hazari K, Pohujani SM, Satoskar RS. Effect of low estrogen combination oral contraceptive on metabolism of aspirin and phenylbutazone. *Int J Clin Pharmacol Ther Toxicol* 1982;20:511–3.
109. Schreurs WHP, van Rijn HJM, Van den Berg H. Serum 25-hydroxycholecalciferol levels in women using oral contraceptives. *Contraception* 1981;23:399–406.
110. Khaled El-Yousef M, Manier DH. Estrogen effects on phenothiazine derivative blood levels [Letter]. *JAMA* 1974;228:827–8.
111. Crawford JS, Rudofsky S. Some alterations in the pattern of drug metabolism associated with pregnancy, oral contraceptives, and the newly-born. *Br J Anaesth* 1966;38:446–54.
112. Stambaugh JE Jr, Wainer IW. Drug interaction 1: meperidine and combination oral contraceptives. *J Clin Pharmacol* 1975;38:46–51.
113. Kendall MJ, Quarterman CP, Jack DB, Beeley L. Metoprolol pharmacokinetics and the oral contraceptive pill. *Br J Clin Pharmacol* 1982;14:120–2.
114. Miners JO, Robson RA, Birkett DJ. Gender and oral contraceptive steroids as determinants of drug glucuronidation: effects on clofibric acid elimination. *Br J Clin Pharmacol* 1984;18:240–3.

Therapeutic Drug Monitoring
7:36–40 © 1985 Raven Press, New York

Simultaneous Plasma Carbamazepine and Carbamazepine-Epoxide Concentrations in Pharmacokinetic and Bioavailability Studies

W. D. Hooper, A. R. King, M. Patterson, R. G. Dickinson, and M. J. Eadie

Department of Medicine, University of Queensland, Brisbane, Australia

Summary: A comparative bioavailability study of carbamazepine (CBZ) in tablets and a syrup preparation was carried out in six volunteers, using a crossover design. Plasma and saliva samples were collected at appropriate times, and the plasma specimens were analyzed by high performance liquid chromatography for concentrations of CBZ and its epoxide metabolite (CBZ-EP). Analysis of the data showed that the preparations were equally bioavailable, although absorption was faster from the syrup and gave higher maximum plasma levels of CBZ. In other respects the preparations were pharmacokinetically equivalent. Analysis of simultaneous plasma CBZ and CBZ-EP concentration–time data by iterative curve fitting to a one-compartment linear model permitted the calculation of elimination kinetic parameters of the CBZ-EP; the mean elimination half-life was 6.9 ± 2.7 h. Failure of the salivary CBZ concentrations soon after drug intake to correlate with simultaneous plasma CBZ levels rendered the salivary data useless for bioavailability comparison, but prompted a further study of salivary CBZ levels.
Key Words: Carbamazepine—Carbamazepine-epoxide—Bioavailability—Pharmacokinetics.

The bioavailability of the anticonvulsant carbamazepine (CBZ) has been the subject of several published reports. The lack of a parenteral formulation has prevented documentation of the absolute bioavailability of CBZ, but several workers have compared the availability from tablets with that from a variety of organic solutions (1–3). The finding of similar area under the concentration–time curve ($AUC_{0-\infty}$) values from tablets and solutions has been interpreted as indicating that bioavailability from tablets is fairly complete, although the recovery of 10–15% of an oral dose as CBZ in feces (4) and the wide variability seen in absorption half-life (5) suggest that this may not always be true.

Address correspondence and reprint requests to Dr. W. D. Hooper at Department of Medicine, Clinical Sciences Building, Royal Brisbane Hospital, Herston, Qld. 4029, Australia.

The lingering uncertainty of the bioavailability of CBZ necessitates a demonstration of bioequivalence with established products before a new formulation of CBZ can be released. In this context we have carried out a bioavailability comparison between CBZ tablets (Tegretol; Ciba-Geigy) and a thixotropic suspension of CBZ developed for pediatric use (Ciba-Geigy). The study was a conventional comparative bioavailability trial, similar in most respects to one previously reported from the United States (3). The time courses of the plasma concentrations of CBZ and its main metabolite carbamazepine-10,11-epoxide (CBZ-EP) were followed.

To avoid the inconvenience of blood sampling between 8 and 24 h, and to gain some additional data points during this interval in which the maximum drug concentration may well occur, saliva was collected for

TABLE 1. *Characteristics of subjects*

Subject	Age (yr)	Sex	Weight (kg)
A	21	F	54
B	20	M	65
C	20	M	70
D	27	M	69
E	27	M	67
F	30	M	76

CBZ assay at the same times as blood sampling and additionally at 10, 12, and 14 h from dosage. Saliva to plasma CBZ concentration ratios are reported to be reasonably constant over the range of values encountered in human therapeutics (6), and it has been shown that the salivary drug concentration corresponds with the non–protein bound CBZ concentration in plasma (7).

The pharmacokinetic and bioavailability data are reported here. The study revealed limitations in the interpretation of salivary CBZ measurements, which have been explored further and are reported separately (8).

MATERIALS AND METHODS

Protocol for Bioavailability Study

The bioavailability study was a comparison between CBZ tablets (Ciba-Geigy) and a thixotropic suspension of CBZ (also Ciba-Geigy). The study followed a standard crossover design in six intelligent, healthy adult volunteers who gave their informed consent. Personal details of the subjects are provided in Table 1. On day 1 all subjects took 600 mg CBZ orally following an overnight fast. The drug was taken with water and swallowed immediately. Three subjects received the drug as three 200-mg tablets, while the others took the drug as 30 ml of syrup (100 mg/5 ml). On day 15 the procedure was repeated, with each subject receiving the alternate formulation. After each CBZ administration, venous blood (5 ml) was collected at 0, 0.5, 1, 2, 3, 4, 6, 8, 24, 32, 48, 56, 72, 80, 96, and 108 h for measurement of plasma CBZ and CBZ-EP concentrations. Saliva samples (2–3 ml) were collected without stimulation at these times, and additionally at 1.5, 2.5, 5, 10, 12, and 14 h. Plasma and saliva samples were stored at −20°C until assayed.

Drug Assays

Plasma CBZ and CBZ-EP were assayed concurrently by a standard high performance liquid chromatography (HPLC) procedure similar to one previously described (9). Plasma (1 ml) was mixed with 0.1 ml hydrochloric acid (0.2 *M*) and extracted with chloroform (5 ml), in tubes containing 10 μg of internal standard (10-methoxy-CBZ). The chloroform extract was evaporated to dryness and the residue reconstituted in 50–100 μl methanol, of which 20 μl was injected into the HPLC. This consisted of a Tracor 950 HPLC pump, a Rheodyne 7125 RV injector, a Waters μBondapak C-18 column (10 μm), a Tracor 970A variable wavelength UV detector, and a Shimadzu R201 strip chart recorder. The detector was set at 215 nm, and the mobile phase was methanol-water (55% methanol, vol/vol) at 1 ml min^{-1} flow rate. Retention times were approximately 5.75, 8.25, and 10.25 min for CBZ-EP, CBZ, and 10-methoxy-CBZ, respectively. Concentrations were determined by measurement of peak height ratios and comparison with standards prepared from drug-free plasma.

Data Analysis

The data analysis for the bioavailability study was performed by fitting plasma CBZ and CBZ-EP concentration–time data to one- and two-compartment linear pharmacokinetic models with first-order absorption, using an iterative least-squares curve-fitting program MULTI (10) run on an Apple II plus microcomputer. The equations fitted were of the form

$$C_t = \Sigma a_i e^{-b_i t}$$

and provision was made for the calculation of an absorption lag time (T_{delay}) during the fittings.

The one-compartment linear model with first-order absorption was used for all bioavailability comparisons. AUC_{0-t} was calculated by trapezoidal rule integration, and $AUC_{0-\infty}$ by adding AUC_{0-t} to Ct/k (i.e., to $AUC_{t-\infty}$) for each set of concentration–time data. C_{max} and T_{max} values were read directly from the experimental data. Plasma half-life was calculated as $0.693/k$.

In a separate analysis of the plasma concentration–time data, plasma CBZ and CBZ-EP concentration–time values for each study were fitted simultaneously to linear equations for a one-compartment model with first-order absorption of CBZ and first-order CBZ-EP formation, to calculate in particular the elimination kinetics of the epoxide, again using the program MULTI. The data were fitted simultaneously to the

TABLE 2. *Bioavailability comparisons*

Parameter	Mean value			Paired	
	Solution	Tablets	*df*	*t* test	p value
k (h^{-1})	0.02203	0.0195	5	1.7049	NS
$AUC_{0-\infty}$ (mg h L^{-1})	416.2493	417.3278	5	0.342	NS
$AUC_{0-\infty}$ $\times k$ (mg L^{-1})	8.89914	8.40913	5	0.5507	NS
k_a (h^{-1})	1.88157	0.41853	5	2.5992	<0.05
T_{delay} (h)	0.14373	0.21028	5	0.4279	NS
T_{max} (h)	2.83	9.67	5	2.0815	NS
C_{max} (mg/L)	8.58	6.75	5	3.1421	<0.05

See text for description of parameters. NS, not significant.

following equations [cited by Wagner (11)] where the t values included a time delay:

$$C_{CBZ} = \frac{Dose}{V} \frac{k_a}{(k_a - k)} (e^{-kt} - e^{-k_a t})$$

and

$$C_{CBZ\text{-}EP} = \frac{k_a k_f D_m}{V_m} \left[\frac{e^{-kt}}{(k_a - k)(k_m - k)} - \frac{e^{-k_a t}}{(k_a - k)(k_m - k_a)} + \frac{e^{-k_m t}}{(k_m - k_a)(k_m - k)} \right]$$

where V is the apparent volume of distribution of CBZ, k_a is the absorption rate constant of CBZ, k is the elimination rate constant of CBZ, k_f is the CBZ-EP formation rate constant, D_m is the amount of CBZ-EP formed, V_m is the apparent volume of distribution of CBZ-EP, and k_m is the CBZ-EP elimination rate constant.

RESULTS

The mean plasma concentration–time data for CBZ and CBZ-EP are shown graphically in Fig. 1 for the tablets and in Fig. 2 for the syrup. The general similarities of the plasma CBZ and CBZ-EP concentration–time curves produced by the tablet and syrup preparations are obvious. At all times after 2–3 h there was parallelism between plasma and saliva CBZ concentrations for both tablets and syrup (not shown), the salivary levels being approximately 22% of the simultaneous plasma levels. Unfortunately, in the first 2–3 h after CBZ intake, there was a conspicuous lack of consistent relationship between plasma and salivary drug concentrations. Because of this, the salivary data could not be used further for the pharmacokinetic and bioavailability studies. However, the reason for the aberrant behaviour of the salivary CBZ levels relative to plasma levels in the first few hours after drug intake has been made the subject of a separate study (8).

Mean values for CBZ pharmacokinetic parameters relating to bioavailability are shown in Table 2. Mean $AUC_{0-\infty}$ values were virtually identical for the tablets (417.3 mg L h^{-1}) and syrup (416.2 mg L h^{-1}), as were the $AUC_{0-\infty} \times k$ values. Elimination rate constants, absorption delay times, and times to reach peak plasma CBZ concentrations did not show statistically significant differences between the two preparations. However, the mean absorption rate constant was greater to a statistically significant degree for the syrup (1.88157 h^{-1}) than for the tablet (0.41853 h^{-1}), and peak plasma CBZ level was statistically significantly higher for the syrup (8.58 as compared with 6.75 mg L^{-1}). This correlated with the observation that the volunteers tended to become drowsy in the first few hours after taking CBZ syrup, but not after taking the tablets.

Elimination pharmacokinetic parameters calculated from simultaneous fitting of plasma CBZ and CBZ-EP concentration–time data are given in Table 3. Also shown for comparison are the values for apparent elimination half-life of CBZ-EP derived when only the concentration–time data for this compound were fitted to a one-compartment model. Much lower values for the elimination half-life of CBZ-EP were found in every instance using the simultaneous fitting technique (mean 6.9 ± 2.7 h; range 4.0–10.3 h) than when CBZ-EP data alone were used for the calculation (mean 19.4 ± 3.4 h; range 15.8–24.1 h).

DISCUSSION

The present study shows that virtually identical amounts of CBZ are absorbed from tablets and from a syrup preparation of the drug. This equivalence in the extent of absorption of the drug occurred despite differences in the rates of absorption from the two preparations. The drug absorbed faster from the syrup than from tablets, and this led to higher peak plasma CBZ levels and a greater sedative effect soon after the dosage. Such a difference in the rate of drug entry can be of clinical importance. In the case of the CBZ syrup preparation studied, it might be wise to avoid undesirable sedation soon after drug intake by subdividing the daily dose more frequently than would be necessary if the tablets were used.

There have been several reports on the pharmacokinetics of CBZ-EP. Eichelbaum et al. (12) found that

TABLE 3. *Simultaneous fit of one-compartment model to drug and metabolite plasma level data*

Subject	Carbamazepine			Carbamazepine-epoxide		
	k_a (h^{-1})	k (h^{-1})	$t_{1/2}$ (h)	k (h^{-1})	$t_{1/2}$ (h)	$t_{1/2}{}^a$ (h)
A1	0.1799	0.02275	30.47	0.0856	8.09	21.33
A2	12.7490	0.02802	26.74	0.1075	6.45	15.78
B1	0.3081	0.2152	32.21	0.0677	10.25	21.85
B2	1.7536	0.02128	32.57	0.1748	3.97	18.35
C1	0.2761	0.02517	27.54	0.0865	8.01	18.70
C2	0.9219	0.02761	25.10	0.1057	6.56	16.49
D1	1.2599	0.02247	30.85	0.1351	5.13	15.47
D2	0.5230	0.02003	34.61	0.0867	7.99	19.35
E1	0.5106	0.01767	39.23	0.0703	9.86	18.93
E2	0.8480	0.01311	52.88	0.0703	9.87	24.08
F1	1.5313	0.01648	42.66	0.7707	0.98	45303.7
F2	0.2478	0.01976	35.08	0.1268	5.47	16.37
		Mean	33.95		6.89	19.40[b]
		SD	7.89		2.73	3.42

Subjects A1, B1, C1, D2, E2, and F2 received carbamazepine syrup. See text for description of parameters.

[a] $t_{1/2}$ calculated from fitting epoxide data only.

[b] Excluding F1.

the post–steady-state elimination half-life of CBZ-EP (16.7 ± 5.0 h) was similar to that of CBZ (20.9 ± 5.0 h). Westenberg et al. (13) reached the same conclusion, and interpreted this as implying that the CBZ concentration–time profile in these circumstances was actually reflecting its rate of formation. They sur-

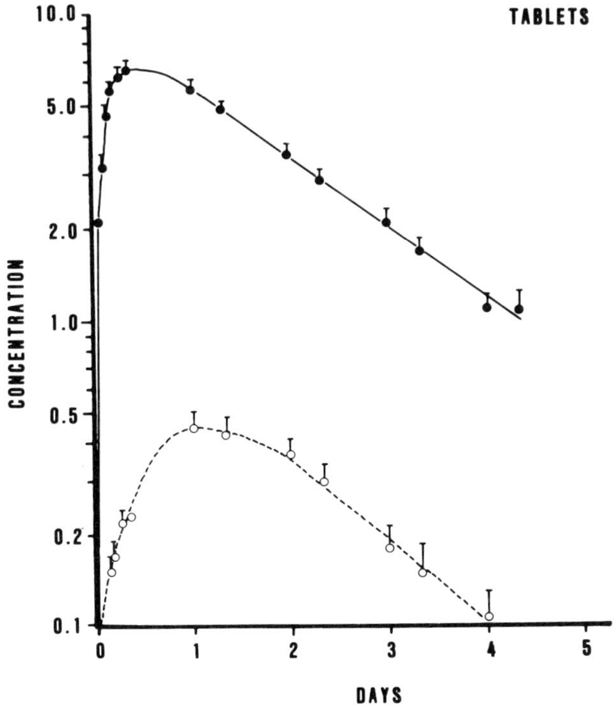

FIG. 1. Plasma concentrations (μg ml^{-1}) of carbamazepine (CBZ) (closed circles, solid line) and carbamazepine-10,11-epoxide (open circles, dashed line) following administration of 600 mg CBZ as tablets. Data points show mean values for six subjects, with one-half standard error indicated by the error bars.

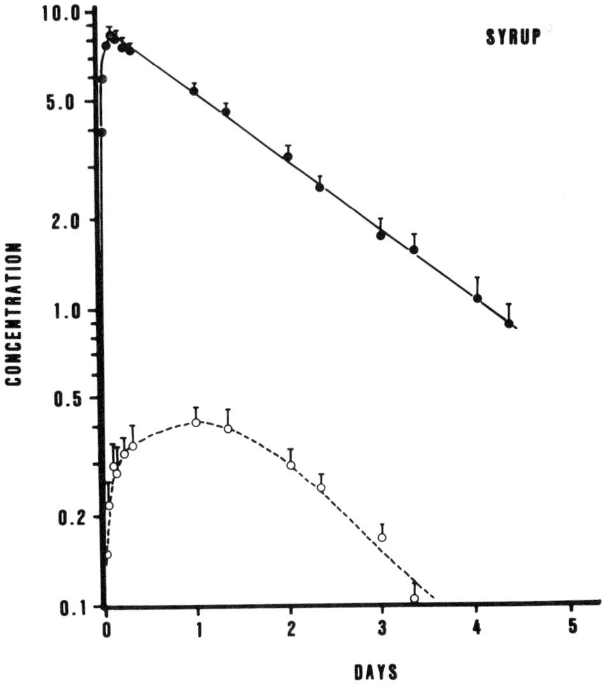

FIG. 2. Plasma concentrations (μg ml^{-1}) of carbamazepine (CBZ) (closed circles, solid line) and carbamazepine-10,11-epoxide (open circles, dashed line) following administration of 600 mg CBZ as syrup.

mised that the true elimination rate of CBZ-EP must be substantially greater than that of CBZ, and invoked several assumptions to calculate possible elimination half-lives of CBZ-EP in the range of 1–3 h. We are aware of only one study in which CBZ-EP itself has been administered to volunteers (14), and this gave plasma half-lives in the range of 4.6–6.9 h in four volunteers, by direct measurement.

We have analyzed our data by simultaneous iterative curve-fitting for CBZ and CBZ-EP, and have obtained a mean elimination half-life for CBZ-EP of 6.9 ± 2.7 h. This value is in good agreement with the directly measured values reported by Tomson et al. (14), and is substantially lower than that calculated by fitting the CBZ-EP data alone, using the same curve-fitting algorithm (19.4 ± 3.4 h; Table 3). The simultaneous fitting technique appears capable of yielding valid elimination rate data for a rapidly eliminated metabolite, whereas fitting to the metabolite data alone may yield erroneous elimination rate values that more nearly represent metabolite formation rate. CBZ-EP is reported to possess antiepileptic properties (15). If its elimination half-life were similar to that of CBZ, it could be worth developing as an independent anticonvulsant. However, its real elimination half-life suggests that it would have to be taken too frequently to be a convenient drug for long-term therapy.

The fact that the salivary CBZ data measured soon after drug intake did not correlate with the simultaneous plasma CBZ data invalidated the use of the salivary data for bioavailability assessment in the present study. This outcome was not fully expected, and it suggested the need for the further investigations reported in the accompanying article (8).

Acknowledgment: We thank Ciba-Geigy Australia Ltd. for the supply of CBZ, CBZ-EP, and 10-methoxy-CBZ, and for financial support of the study.

REFERENCES

1. Rawlins MD, Collste P, Bertilsson L, Palmer L. Distribution and elimination kinetics of carbamazepine in man. *Eur J Clin Pharmacol* 1975;8:91–6.
2. Levy RH, Pitlick WH, Troupin AS, Green JR, Neal JM. Pharmacokinetics of carbamazepine in normal man. *Clin Pharmacol Ther* 1975;17:657–68.
3. Wada JA, Troupin AS, Friel P, Remick R, Leal K, Pearmain J. Pharmacokinetic comparison of tablet and suspension dosage forms of carbamazepine. *Epilepsia* 1978;19:251–5.
4. Faigle JW, Feldman KF. Pharmacokinetic data of carbamazepine and its major metabolites in man. In: Schneider H, Janz D, Gardner-Thorpe C, Meinardi H, Sherwin AL, eds. *Clinical pharmacology of antiepileptic drugs.* Berlin: Springer, 1975:159–65.
5. Cotter LM, Smith GA, Hooper WD, Tyrer JH, Eadie MJ. The bioavailability of carbamazepine. *Proc Aust Assoc Neurol* 1975;12:123–8.
6. Kristensen O, Larsen HF. Value of saliva samples in monitoring carbamazepine concentrations in epileptic patients. *Acta Neurol Scand* 1980;61:344–50.
7. MacKichan JJ, Duffner PK, Cohen ME. Salivary concentrations and plasma protein binding of carbamazepine and carbamazepine-10,11-epoxide in epileptic patients. *Br J Clin Pharmacol* 1981;12:31–7.
8. Dickinson RG, Hooper WD, King AR, Eadie MJ. Fallacious results from measuring salivary carbamazepine concentrations. *Ther Drug Monit* 1985;7:41–5.
9. McKauge L, Tyrer JH, Eadie MJ. Factors influencing simultaneous concentrations of carbamazepine and its epoxide in plasma. *Ther Drug Monit* 1981;3:63–70.
10. Yamaoka K, Tanigawara Y, Nakagawa T, Uno T. A pharmacokinetic analysis program (Multi) for microcomputers. *J Pharm Dyn* 1981;4:879–85.
11. Wagner JG. Biopharmaceutics and relevant pharmacokinetics. Hamilton, Illinois: Drug Intelligence Publications, 1971:293–4.
12. Eichelbaum M, Ekbom K, Bertilsson L, Ringberger VA, Rane A. Plasma kinetics of carbamazepine and its epoxide metabolite in man after single and multiple doses. *Eur J Clin Pharmacol* 1975;8:337–41.
13. Westenberg HGM, van der Klein E, Oei TT, Zeeuw RA. Kinetics of carbamazepine and carbamazepine-epoxide, determined by use of plasma and saliva. *Clin Pharmacol Ther* 1978;23:320–8.
14. Tomson T, Tybring G, Bertilsson L. Pharmacokinetics of carbamazepine-10,11-epoxide in healthy volunteers. *Acta Neurol Scand* 1982;65(suppl 90):205–6.
15. Morselli PL, Bossi L, Gerna M. Pharmacokinetic studies with carbamazepine in epileptic patients. In: Birkmayer W, ed. *International symposium on epileptic seizures-behaviour-pain.* Berne:Huber, 1975:141–50.

Therapeutic Drug Monitoring
7:41–45

Fallacious Results from Measuring Salivary Carbamazepine Concentrations

R. G. Dickinson, W. D. Hooper, A. R. King, and M. J. Eadie

Department of Medicine, University of Queensland, Brisbane, Australia

Summary: During a carbamazepine (CBZ) relative bioavailability study involving tablets and a syrup preparation, salivary drug concentrations appeared disproportionately high relative to simultaneous plasma drug concentrations in the first 2–3 h after oral drug intake. This raised the suspicion of contamination of saliva by retention of drug in the mouth. In a separate study CBZ was retained in the mouth in tablet form (whole or crushed) or in syrup, for only 5 s before being spat out, and the mouth was carefully rinsed. Despite this, measurable salivary concentrations, sufficient to cause substantial error if extrapolated to simultaneous plasma drug concentrations, were present for at least 2 h after drug administration. CBZ in these studies disappeared from saliva with an apparent mean half-life of 21.0 ± 4.8 min. This experience suggests that, in therapeutic drug monitoring, salivary CBZ concentrations for at least 2 h after dosage may lead to invalid conclusions about simultaneous plasma CBZ concentrations. **Key Words:** Carbamazepine—Saliva concentrations—Pharmacokinetics.

Measurement of salivary drug concentrations has sometimes been advocated as an alternative to measuring plasma drug concentrations (1). Salivary measurement has the advantage of avoiding the discomforts of venipuncture, which is a particularly important consideration in children. Saliva-to-plasma carbamazepine (CBZ) concentration ratios are reported to be reasonably constant over the range of values encountered in human therapeutics (2). In the light of this knowledge, we carried out a CBZ bioavailability study utilizing simultaneous plasma and salivary drug concentration measurements at times when blood collection was convenient, but with salivary measurements only when venisection was difficult to organize. Simple precautions were taken to minimize CBZ retention in the mouth after ingestion (3). It was thought that such an experimental plan would enhance the accuracy of the study by providing an increased number of data points for analysis. Instead, it revealed a major source of error in the salivary CBZ concentrations soon after drug ingestion. This source of error would also be likely to apply in certain routine therapeutic drug monitoring situations during clinical practice.

The details of the bioavailability study have been reported separately (4). The salivary CBZ data that were obtained in that study, and further investigations to elucidate the problems that arose, are described here.

MATERIALS AND METHODS

CBZ Bioavailability Study

The bioavailability study was designed to assess the comparative bioavailabilities of CBZ from tablets and from a syrup preparation. The study protocol, details of the subjects investigated, the method employed for measuring plasma CBZ concentrations, and the methods of pharmacokinetic data analysis are all described in the accompanying article (4).

Address correspondence and reprint requests to Dr. R. G. Dickinson at Department of Medicine, Clinical Sciences Building, Royal Brisbane Hospital, Herston, Qld. 4029, Australia.

TABLE 1. *Characteristics of the four volunteers for the additional saliva studies*

Subject	Age (yr)	Sex	Weight (kg)
I	25	F	67
II	22	M	75
III	22	M	70
IV	21	M	64

Saliva Sampling and Assay

Saliva samples (approximately 5 ml) were collected from the subjects participating in the bioavailability study, without stimulation, at all of the times when blood samples were collected (0, 0.5, 1, 2, 3, 4, 6, 8, 24, 32, 48, 56, 72, 80, 96, and 108 h) as well as at 1.5, 2.5, 5, 10, 12, and 14 h. Urine samples were stored at −20°C until analyzed. After thawing, specimens were mixed on a vortex mixer, then centrifuged at 1,000 *g* to remove particulate matter. The clear supernatant was sampled for assay.

The high performance liquid chromatography assay technique was very similar to that used for plasma specimens (4). Aliquots of up to 2 ml were assayed, only one fifth of the quantity of internal standard was used (i.e., 2 μg 10-methoxy-CBZ), and standard curves were constructed using either drug-free saliva or water, which were found to be indistinguishable. In some instances a peak for the epoxide metabolite (CBZ-EP) was observed in the chromatograms, but the concentrations were so low in most samples that accurate quantitation was not possible and no further attempt was made to analyze those data.

Additional Salivary Studies

The results of the salivary CBZ determinations in the bioavailability study prompted additional studies of CBZ in saliva. These studies were carried out in another group of four adult volunteers, whose personal characteristics are given in Table 1. Each volunteer participated in three separate studies (A, B, and C). Procedure A required each subject to hold three 200-mg CBZ tablets on the tongue for 5 s, then to spit them out, rinse the mouth carefully with 50 ml water, spit that out, and subsequently provide approximately 3-ml saliva samples after 30, 60, and 120 min had passed. The tablets typically began to disintegrate after 5 s. Procedure B was similar, except that three crushed tablets were placed on the tongue for 5 s. In procedure C, 30 ml CBZ syrup was held in the mouth for 5 s before rinsing and providing the saliva samples. The subjects had no food or drink during the first 60 min after treatment. The order for the three procedures was randomized, and individual studies were separated by at least 1 day. CBZ concentrations in saliva were determined as above.

RESULTS

In the bioavailability study described in the accompanying article (4), it was pointed out that salivary and plasma CBZ concentrations declined in parallel once 2–3 h had elapsed after drug intake. Salivary CBZ levels after 3 h averaged 22% of the simultaneous plasma CBZ concentrations. The mean elimination half-life of CBZ, calculated from the salivary data from 3 h onward, was 29.39 h, whereas the mean half-life calculated from the plasma level data was 32.66 h. In contrast with this close relationship between salivary and plasma CBZ concentrations after 2–3 h, there was a gross disparity between the plasma and saliva CBZ profiles at the earlier points (Figs. 1 and 2). This disparity was more pronounced in the case of the syrup (Fig. 2), for which the early salivary CBZ concentrations were very much higher than would have been expected by comparison with the later values. Indeed, for the initial points after dosing, salivary levels were often higher than simultaneous plasma CBZ levels. This clearly suggested contamination of early saliva samples with unabsorbed drug, a suspicion that prompted further studies.

The results of the additional studies on CBZ in saliva are shown in Table 2. After 11 of the CBZ administrations, there was a substantial concentration of CBZ measurable in saliva over the 30–120 min period following a mere 5 s of drug contact with the mouth. The disappearance of CBZ from the mouth reasonably approximated first-order kinetics, with calculated half-times of 21.0 ± 4.8 min (range 13–32 min) in the 11 studies for which values were obtained. Although the bioavailability study had suggested a greater problem with contamination of saliva following administration of the syrup (Fig. 2), the crushed tablets gave the higher saliva CBZ levels for three of the four subjects in these studies (Table 2).

DISCUSSION

There have been several studies of CBZ concentrations in the saliva of patients treated with this drug, and these studies have been reviewed recently (1). Most authors have found an excellent correlation between saliva levels and unbound CBZ concentration in plasma (3,5), or between saliva levels and total

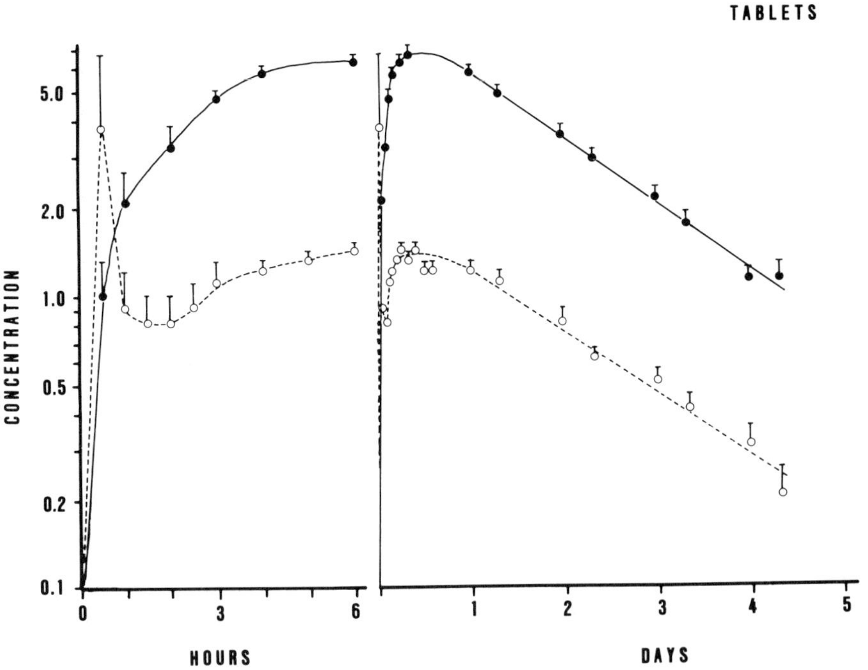

FIG. 1. Plasma (closed circles, solid line) and saliva (open circles, dashed line) carbamazepine (CBZ) concentrations (μg ml⁻¹) following administration of 600 mg CBZ as tablets. Data points show mean values for six subjects, with one-half standard error indicated by the error bars. The time scale has been expanded at left to illustrate clearly the early time points.

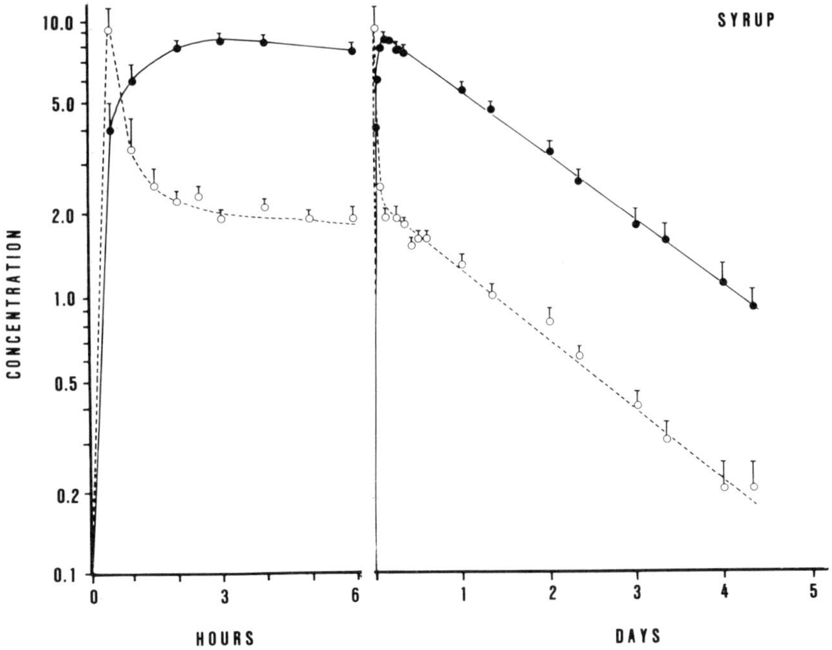

FIG. 2. Plasma and saliva carbamazepine (CBZ) concentrations (μg ml⁻¹) following administration of 600 mg CBZ in syrup preparation. Symbols as in Fig. 1.

plasma levels (2). There have, on the other hand, been occasional reports of aberrant results for salivary CBZ concentrations. Thus, Rylance et al. (6) reported generally good correlations between saliva and total plasma concentrations of CBZ in 15 children, but noted that in one instance, after administration of crushed tablets in orange juice to a 3.5-year-old child, contamination of saliva by the dose was detected for up to 1.5 h. Similarly, Goldsmith and Ouvrier (7) commented on contamination of saliva samples in the cases of children who chewed their tablets. Paxton et al. (8) noted substantial fluctuations in both salivary CBZ and CBZ-EP levels throughout the day, whether syrup or tablets were administered. They recommended that saliva samples for CBZ monitoring be taken just before administration for a trough level, and after 1–2 or 2–5

TABLE 2. *Salivary CBZ concentrations (mg L^{-1}) following 5 s of buccal contact with CBZ*

		Saliva CBZ concentration after various treatments		
Subject	Time (h)	Whole tablet	Crushed tablet	Syrup
I	0.5	0.24	0.40	0.62
	1	0.07	0.13	0.12
	1.5	0.05	0.04	0.06
	2	0.03	0.03	0.04
II	0.5	2.18	3.56	1.17
	1	0.36	0.33	0.17
	1.5	0.06	0.18	0.05
	2	0.02	0.15	0.04
III	0.5	0.04	1.59	0.61
	1	0.02	0.11	0.08
	1.5	ND[a]	0.03	0.03
	2	ND[a]	0.03	0.03
IV	0.5	9.06	10.44	3.73
	1	3.50	4.82	1.38
	1.5	1.74	1.42	0.50
	2	0.51	0.53	0.21

Administration of whole tablets usually resulted in the tablets being spat out, still recognizable as tablets.

[a]ND, nothing detected.

h for determination of peak concentration following syrup or tablet administration, respectively, seemingly without realising that their results may have been confounded by residual drug remaining in the mouth. Problems with contamination of saliva samples following drug administration have been reported for phenytoin (9), even when it is administered in capsules (10).

The results from our bioavailability study (4) suggested major problems with contamination of saliva by the CBZ dose, following administration of either tablets or syrup to adult volunteers, who neither chewed the tablets nor retained the dose for any appreciable time in the mouth. One published study has reported findings similar to ours (11). This contrasted with most previous reports of CBZ contamination in saliva assays, which related to observations in children, and identified chewing or crushing of tablets as the causative factor. For this reason we designed a simple additional study of the effects of exposing the oral cavity to CBZ in various dosage forms for 5 s. This time was selected as the minimum practicable and reproducible one to study, and also as a contact time with the mouth that might reasonably occur in the ordinary clinical situation. The finding of substantial concentrations of CBZ in saliva for up to 2 h after this brief exposure, with an apparently first-order disappearance of drug, was rather surprising. It is presumably a consequence of the high lipophilicity of CBZ, which may be rapidly taken up into the lipoidal cell membranes of the mucosa of the mouth, and only slowly leached out again into the saliva.

This finding has obvious significance for therapeutic drug monitoring of CBZ, and probably other lipophilic drugs, in saliva. Most of the articles on the topic cited by Mucklow (1) advocated the use of saliva for therapeutic drug monitoring, but only a few have identified this obvious pitfall as a serious concern, and then mainly in certain restricted circumstances (e.g., chewed tablets). It is disconcerting to find authors even speculating on the possible role of active transport mechanisms for drugs in the salivary glands to explain a higher saliva:plasma concentration ratio in the absorption phase than in the elimination phase in single dose studies (12). The case for using salivary estimations in therapeutic drug monitoring has been established repeatedly, but the need for caution in selecting sampling times must be stressed again, as has recently been done by Knott and Reynolds (3).

If salivary concentration levels were measured in the one subject receiving regular CBZ therapy on one occasion soon after drug intake, and on another occasion several hours later, a largely artifactual difference in salivary drug concentrations might mislead the clinician into believing that the patient was not complying with therapy, or that the drug had a much faster elimination than in reality. The latter conclusion could suggest the need for more frequent drug administration than was really necessary.

Awareness of this possible fallacy in measuring salivary concentrations of CBZ, and perhaps of other drugs, may enhance the reliability of measuring salivary drug concentrations as a guide to therapy, and may reduce the risk of inappropriate therapeutic decisions.

Acknowledgment: We thank Ciba-Geigy Australia Ltd. for the supply of CBZ, CBZ-EP, and 10-methoxy-CBZ, and for financial support of these studies.

REFERENCES

1. Mucklow JC. The use of saliva in therapeutic drug monitoring. *Ther Drug Monit* 1982;4:229–47.
2. Kristensen O, Larsen HF. Value of saliva samples in monitoring carbamazepine concentrations in epileptic patients. *Acta Neurol Scand* 1980;61:344–50.
3. Knott C, Reynolds F. The place of saliva in antiepileptic drug monitoring. *Ther Drug Monit* 1984;6:35–41.
4. Hooper WD, King AR, Patterson M, Dickinson RG, Eadie MJ. Simultaneous plasma carbamazepine and carbamazepine-epoxide concentrations in pharmacokinetic and bioavailability studies. *Ther Drug Monit* 1985;7:36–40.

5. MacKichan JJ, Duffner PK, Cohen ME. Salivary concentrations and plasma protein binding of carbamazepine and carbamazepine-10,11-epoxide in epileptic patients. *Br J Clin Pharmacol* 1981;12:31–7.
6. Rylance GW, Butcher GM, Moreland T. Saliva carbamazepine levels in children. *Br Med J* 1977;2:1481.
7. Goldsmith RF, Ouvrier RA. Salivary anticonvulsant levels in children: a comparison of methods. *Ther Drug Monit* 1981;3:151–7.
8. Paxton JW, Aman MG, Werry JS. Fluctuations in salivary carbamazepine and carbamazepine-10,11-epoxide concentrations during the day in epileptic children. *Epilepsia* 1983;24:716–24.
9. Ayers GJ, Burnett D. Drug formulation and salivary phenytoin measurements. *Lancet* 1977;1:656.
10. Paxton JW, Foote S. Aberrantly high phenytoin concentrations in saliva. Precaution in monitoring phenytoin concentrations in whole saliva. *Br J Clin Pharmacol* 1979;8:508–9.
11. Wada JA, Troupin AS, Friel P, Remick R, Leal K, Pearmain J. Pharmacokinetic comparison of tablet and suspension dosage forms of carbamazepine. *Epilepsia* 1978;19:251–5.
12. Danhof M, Breimer DD. Therapeutic drug monitoring in saliva. *Clin Pharmacokinet* 1978;3:39–57.

Therapeutic Drug Monitoring
7:46–50 © 1985 Raven Press, New York

Determination of Total and Free Plasma Carbamazepine Concentrations by Enzyme Multiplied Immunoassay: Interference with the 10,11-Epoxide Metabolite

Manuela Contin, Roberto Riva, Fiorenzo Albani, *Emilio Perucca, and Agostino Baruzzi

*Laboratory of Neuropharmacology, Institute of Neurology, University of Bologna, Bologna, and *Institute of Medical Pharmacology, University of Pavia, Pavia, Italy*

Summary: The performance of the enzyme multiplied immunoassay technique (EMIT) in the measurement of total and free plasma carbamazepine (CBZ) levels was assessed in 140 clinical specimens and compared with a reference high pressure liquid chromatography (HPLC) technique. Free drug was measured in plasma filtrates obtained by the Free Level system. Both total and free CBZ levels as determined by EMIT correlated strongly with corresponding HPLC values (r = 0.88 and 0.92, respectively). Plasma CBZ concentrations, however, were higher by EMIT than by HPLC. The degree of CBZ overestimation by EMIT was relatively small (about 14%) in whole plasma but quite considerable (35% on average) in the filtrates. As a result, estimated values of free CBZ fraction were also higher for EMIT than for HPLC. Separate experiments in vitro suggested that the discrepancies between the two methods were due to cross-reaction of the EMIT reagent with the 10,11-epoxide metabolite of CBZ. The greater degree of overestimation for the free drug can be explained by the higher proportion of less protein-bound metabolite in the filtrates. These results need to be taken into account in the interpretation of free CBZ level data from laboratories using different techniques. **Key Words:** Carbamazepine—Free fraction—Enzyme multiplied immunoassay technique—High pressure liquid chromatography—Interference.

Although several studies have shown good agreement between plasma antiepileptic drug levels determined by enzyme multiplied immunoassay technique (EMIT) and gas-liquid chromatography (GLC) or high pressure liquid chromatography (HPLC) (1–3), there is now evidence that for carbamazepine (CBZ) the EMIT reagent shows some cross-reactivity with the pharmacologically active 10,11-epoxide metabolite (CBZ-E), which can result in overestimation of the actual CBZ concentration (4,5).

Theoretically, the degree of interference should be greater when free rather than total drug concentration is being measured, because of the higher proportion of less protein-bound metabolite in plasma water (plasma filtrate). In a recent study, however, Levy et al. (5) were unable to find any difference between the magnitude of CBZ overestimation in whole plasma and in plasma filtrates; as a result, the free CBZ fraction was not overestimated by EMIT.

The present study was designed to reevaluate in a larger population of patients the discrepancies between EMIT and HPLC CBZ determinations in whole plasma and plasma filtrates and to assess the contribution of CBZ-E to such discrepancies. In contrast with the data reported by Levy et al. (5), we found that EMIT results in moderate overestimation of the free CBZ fraction.

Address correspondence and reprint requests to Dr. M. Contin at Institute of Neurology, Via Foscolo 7, I-40123 Bologna, Italy.

PATIENTS AND METHODS

Blood samples were collected into heparinized tubes (8–10 IU heparin/ml blood) from 140 epileptic patients receiving constant therapy (for at least 2 months) with CBZ, alone (n = 78) or in combination with phenobarbital (n = 62). Each sample was taken at 11 a.m., 3 h after the first daily dose. The plasma was separated immediately and stored at −20°C until analyzed within 2 weeks. This collection and storage procedure does not alter plasma CBZ binding (unpublished observations).

Plasma filtrates (300 μl) at 25°C were obtained in duplicate from 1 ml plasma aliquots by using the Free Level system (Syva, Palo Alto, CA) according to the procedure recommended by the manufacturer. The concentrations of CBZ in whole plasma and plasma filtrates were determined in each sample by both EMIT and an HPLC method that allowed the simultaneous measurement of CBZ-E. According to this method, modified from Mihaly et al. (1), 300 μl of whole plasma or plasma filtrate (both filtrates from the same specimen were pooled together) was extracted with 4 ml chloroform in alkaline medium (50 μl 6 N NaOH) and the dried extract redissolved in mobile phase (methanol:water, 55:45, vol/vol) prior to injection into a Perkin Elmer series 3 chromatograph equipped with a reversed-phase column (RP-18, 10 μm Lichrosorb, 25 cm long) and a spectrophotometric detector setting at 210 nm. The recoveries of CBZ and CBZ-E were 99 and 97%, respectively, over the concentration range examined (2.1–50.8 μmol/L for CBZ, and 1.2–11.9 μmol/L for CBZ-E). The coefficient of variation (CV) for EMIT CBZ analyses was 2.7% at a concentration of 7.4 μmol/L (n = 10). The CV of the HPLC procedure was 3.6% for CBZ (14.0 μmol/L, n = 10) and 5.6% for CBZ-E (6.7 μmol/L, n = 10). To evaluate the possible interference by CBZ-E, studies with patients' plasma were supplemented with separate sets of analyses performed on quality control samples containing CBZ without CBZ-E (Seronorm; Pharmacia AED) and normal human plasma spiked with CBZ and variable amounts of CBZ-E (Table 1). These specimens were processed exactly like the patients' samples.

RESULTS AND DISCUSSION

The relationship between total CBZ concentrations as determined by EMIT and HPLC, respectively, is shown in Fig. 1. Although EMIT appeared to overestimate slightly the total CBZ concentrations (HPLC taken as reference technique), the equation of the regression line ($y = 5.5 + 0.95\ x$; $r = 0.885$, *df* 138) indicated that the correlation between the two methods was good and that the difference in accuracy over the examined concentration range was too small to be clinically important (EMIT values were, on the average, 14% higher than HPLC values).

When free rather than total CBZ concentrations were considered, a different pattern emerged (Fig. 2). Although the correlation between the two methods was again quite strong ($r = 0.921$), free EMIT concentrations were considerably greater than corresponding HPLC values, the degree of overestimation averaging 35% over the examined concentration range (equation of the regression line: $y = 0.89 + 1.17\ x$; *df* 138). Because of the different degree of overestimation between free and total drug, estimates of free CBZ fraction were also significantly higher by EMIT than by HPLC (means ± SD 20.3 ± 2.7% vs. 17.1 ± 2.1%; $p < 0.001$, Student's *t* test) even though their distribution was similar with both methods (Fig. 3).

The concentration of total and free CBZ-E in the clinical specimens averaged 5.4 ± 2.1 μmol/L (range 1.6–13.2 μmol/L) and 2.0 ± 0.8 μmol/L (range 0.55–5.0 μmol/L), respectively. The CBZ-E/CBZ ratios averaged 0.18 ± 0.05 (range 0.09–0.40) for total levels and 0.38 ± 0.12 (range 0.16–0.95) for free levels. A positive correlation was found between degree of EMIT overestimation of free CBZ levels (difference between EMIT value and HPLC value divided by HPLC value) and free plasma CBZ-E concentration (slope 0.46; intercept 0.68; $r = 0.34$, *df* 138; $p < 0.001$): this correlation, however, was too weak to have any predictive value. More clear-cut evidence that the discrepancies between the two methods were caused by cross-reaction of the EMIT antibody with the epoxide metabolite was provided by the results of the in vitro studies. In a first experiment, a diluted quality control sample containing CBZ without CBZ-E was analyzed by both methods on seven consecutive runs using the calibrator sets employed for free drug determinations. In this sample, EMIT and HPLC gave identical results (15.3 ± 1.0 μmol/L vs. 15.3 ± 0.6 μmol/L, respectively; n = 7), thus excluding that the discrepancy observed in clinical samples was related to differences in the accuracy of the calibrators used in the two methods.

The interfering effect of CBZ-E was directly assessed by adding variable amounts of this metabolite to a sample of normal human plasma spiked with CBZ (33.9 μmol/L). As shown in Table 1, concentrations of CBZ-E yielding increasing CBZ-E/CBZ ratios within the clinical range induced only a slight overestimation

TABLE 1. *CBZ-E interference in the EMIT determination of total and free CBZ concentration: effect of adding increasing amounts of the metabolite to a sample of normal human plasma spiked with 33.9 μmol/L CBZ*

		Total plasma CBZ		Free plasma CBZ		
Added CBZ-E (μmol/L)	CBZ-E/CBZ ratio[a]	Estimated value (μmol/L)	Overestimation[a] (%)	Estimated value (μmol/L)	Overestimation[a] (%)	Estimated free CBZ fraction (%)
0	—	33.4	—	6.8	—	20.4
2.0	0.06	35.5	6.3	7.3	7.3	20.5
4.0	0.12	34.7	3.9	7.1	4.4	20.5
7.9	0.24	35.5	6.3	8.0	17.6	21.4
11.9	0.36	36.8	10.2	8.5	25.0	23.1
23.8	0.70	36.4	9.0	9.7	42.6	26.7

EMIT, enzyme multiplied immunoassay technique; CBZ, carbamazepine; CBZ-E, CBZ-10,11-epoxide.
[a]Estimated CBZ concentration in the absence of the epoxide taken as actual CBZ concentration.

of the total CBZ level but a progressive and appreciable increase of both free CBZ level and free CBZ fraction. At CBZ-E/CBZ ratios of 0.24 and 0.36 (the closest to the mean ratio observed in the clinical samples) the degrees of overestimation of free CBZ level were 18 and 25%, respectively.

In a recent study, Levy et al. (5) found plasma CBZ levels in 28 clinical specimens to be higher by EMIT than by a reference gas chromatography–mass spectrometry technique, with a mean overestimation of about 14% for total and 16% for free CBZ. These overestimations cancelled out each other in the calculation of free fraction so that no significant differences in free fractions between EMIT and GLC could be found. Our findings, based on a much larger number of specimens, disagree partly with these data. In fact, while the EMIT overestimation of total CBZ levels was virtually negligible and was identical with

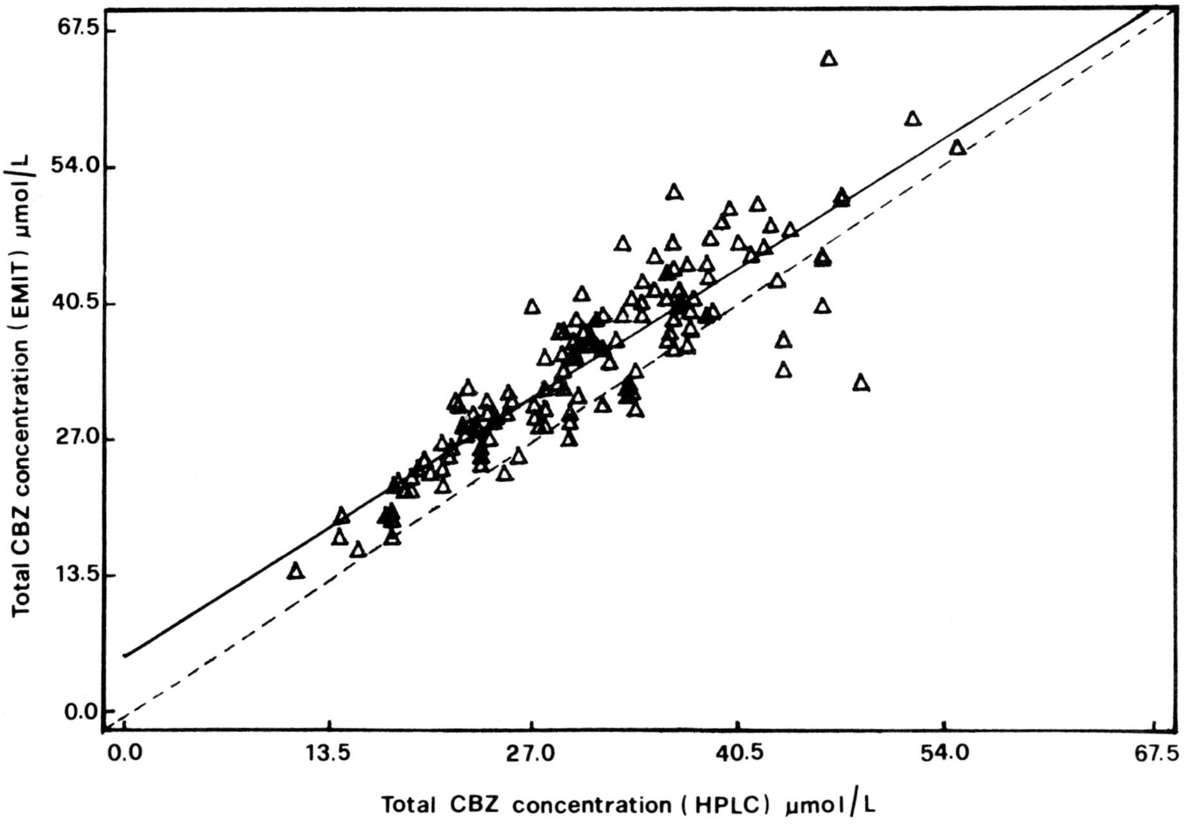

FIG. 1. Relationship between total carbamazepine (CBZ) concentrations determined by enzyme multiplied immunoassay technique (EMIT) and by high pressure liquid chromatography (HPLC); $r = 0.885$, intercept 5.5, $b = 0.95$, df 138.

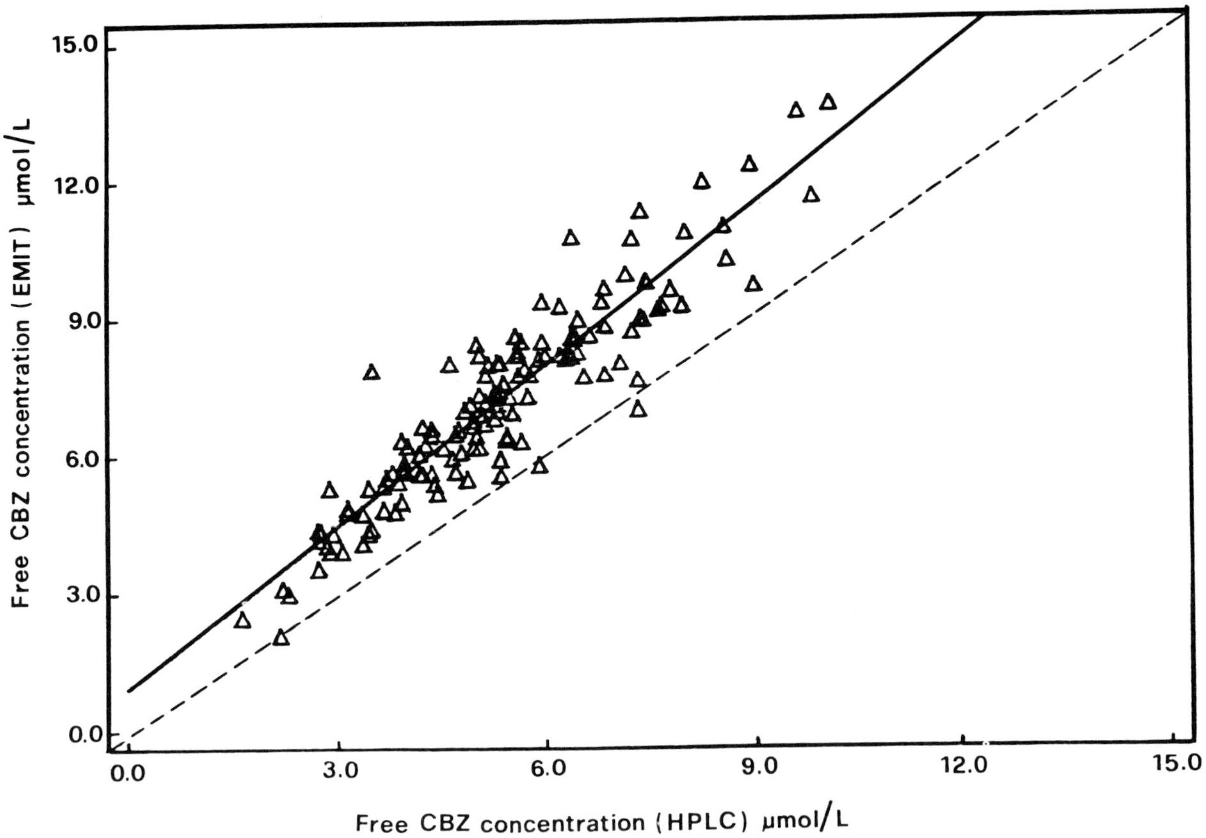

FIG. 2. Relationship between free carbamazepine (CBZ) concentrations determined by enzyme multiplied immunoassay technique (EMIT) and by high pressure liquid chromatography (HPLC); $r = 0.92$, intercept 0.89, $b = 1.17$, *df* 138.

that reported previously (14%), the overestimation of free CBZ levels was on average much greater (35 vs. 16%) so that the resulting free fraction values were also increased. These findings were theoretically expected in view of the lower protein binding of the cross-reacting CBZ-E (6) causing the metabolite/parent drug ratio (and the consequent interference) to be higher in plasma water than in whole plasma (6). The observation that the overestimation of free CBZ concentrations in our experiments was greater than that reported by Levy et al. (5) could be explained by differences in sampling time, which was not standardized in the latter study. In fact, the CBZ-E/CBZ ratio changes during the day in relation to drug intake and therefore the degree of analytical interference might fluctuate accordingly. This hypothesis, however, would not explain why the degree of overestimation of total CBZ concentration was identical in both studies.

In our experiments, no differences in degree of CBZ overestimation could be found between samples from patients undergoing polytherapy and samples from patients undergoing monotherapy, even though the CBZ-E/CBZ ratios were slightly increased in the first group (0.20 ± 0.07 vs. 0.16 ± 0.06 for total concentration, $p < 0.001$; 0.44 ± 0.17 vs. 0.34 ± 0.14 for free concentration, $p < 0.001$).

From the practical point of view, the fact that EMIT overestimates the concentration of CBZ (especially free CBZ) in patients' specimens does not necessarily affect the clinical usefulness of this method, which has clear advantages in terms of rapidity and simplicity. Indeed, the extremely good correlation between the two methods tested suggests that even for the free drug the observed differences in accuracy are of no serious consequence, provided that the same technique is consistently used in a given clinical setting and that the methodological discrepancies reported here are taken into account in the interpretation of drug monitoring data.

Moreover, at least for therapeutic drug monitoring purposes, the analytical interference due to the metabolite might result in a practical advantage, in view of the recent demonstration of the CBZ-E efficacy in trigeminal neuralgia (7). Further work, however, needs to be done on the clinical activity of the CBZ-E in epilepsy.

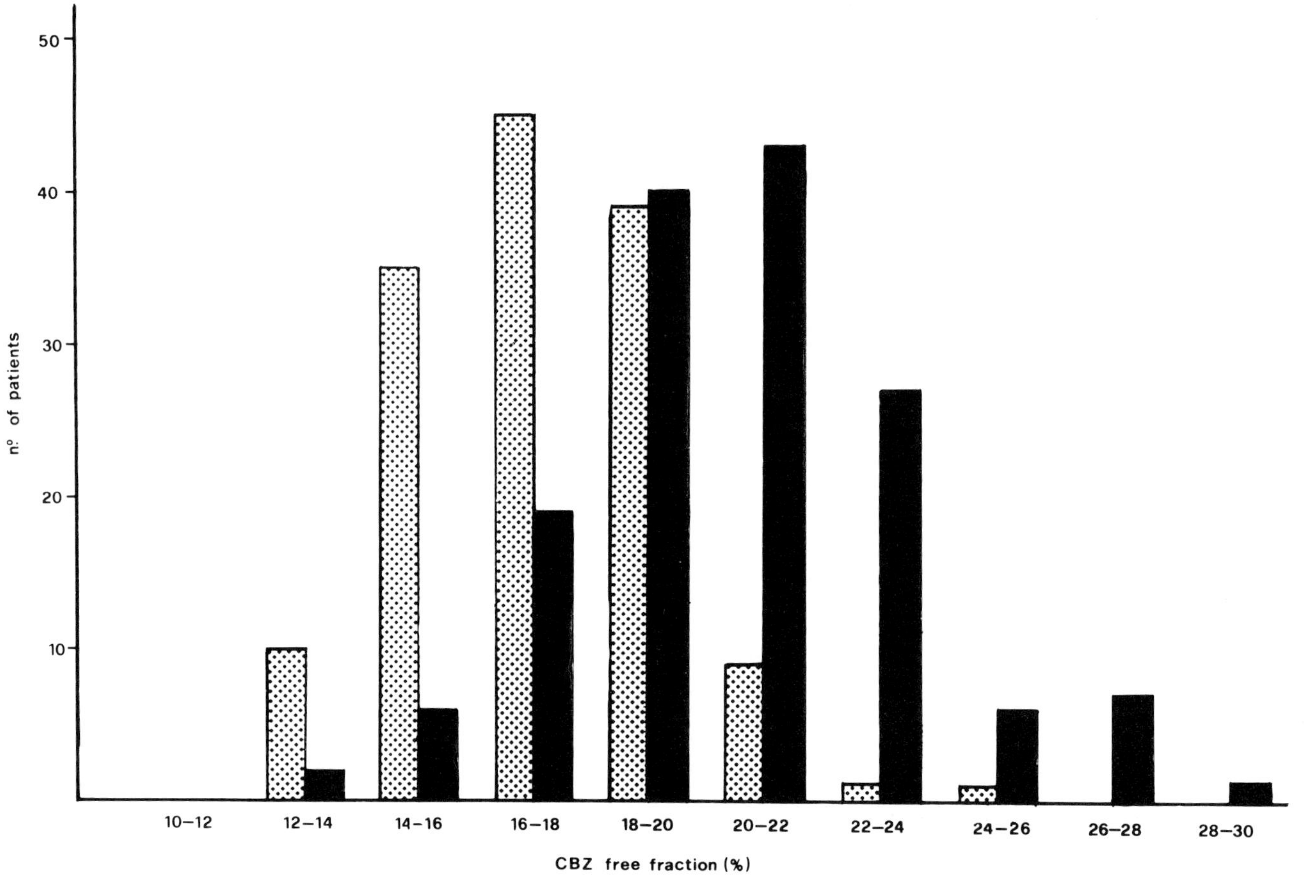

FIG. 3. Distribution of free carbamazepine (CBZ) fraction (%) in the 140 patients included in the study estimated by high pressure liquid chromatography (stippled bars) and enzyme multiplied immunoassay technique (solid bars).

Acknowledgment: This work was part of the "Progetto Finalizzato Medicina Preventiva e Riabilitativa" of the National Research Council of Italy, grant N.8302528. Carbamazepine and carbamazepine-10,11 epoxide were a gift of Ciba Geigy, Basel, Switzerland.

REFERENCES

1. Mihaly GW, Phillips JA, Louis WJ, Vajda FJ. Measurement of carbamazepine and its epoxide metabolite by high-performance liquid chromatography, and a comparison of assay techniques for the analyses of carbamazepine. *Clin Chem* 1977;23:2283–7.
2. Pesh-Imam M, Fretthold DW, Sunshine I, Kumar S, Terrentine S, Willis CE. High pressure liquid chromatography for simultaneous analysis of anticonvulsants: comparison with EMIT system. *Ther Drug Monit* 1979;1:289–99.
3. Meijer JWA, Rambeck B, Riedmann M. Antiepileptic drug monitoring by chromatographic methods and immunotechniques—comparison of analytical performance, practicability, and economy. *Ther Drug Monit* 1983;5:39–53.
4. Paxton JW, Donald RA. Concentrations and kinetics of carbamazepine in whole saliva, parotid saliva, serum ultrafiltrate, and serum. *Clin Pharmacol Ther* 1980;28:695–702.
5. Levy RH, Friel PN, Johno I, et al. Filtration for free drug level monitoring: carbamazepine and valproic acid. *Ther Drug Monit* 1984;6:67–76.
6. MacKichan JJ, Duffner PK, Cohen ME. Salivary concentrations and plasma protein binding of carbamazepine and carbamazepine-10,11-epoxide in epileptic patients. *Br J Clin Pharmacol* 1981;12:31–7.
7. Tomson T, Bertilsson L. Potent therapeutic effect of carbamazepine-10,11-epoxide in trigeminal neuralgia. *Arch Neurol* 1984;41:598–601.

Therapeutic Drug Monitoring
7:51–53 © 1985 Raven Press, New York

Carbamazepine–Phenytoin Interaction: Elevation of Plasma Phenytoin Concentrations Due to Carbamazepine Comedication

Janusz J. Zielinski, Dan Haidukewych, and Boris J. Leheta

Epilepsy Center of Michigan, Detroit, Michigan, U.S.A.

Summary: By intrapatient comparison at constant phenytoin (PHT) dose, the effect of carbamazepine (CBZ) comedication on PHT was studied in a group of 24 epileptic outpatients. In half of the patients with steady-state PHT plasma concentration, a significant increase of this concentration was noted after CBZ was added to their regimen. Twenty percent showed clinical manifestations of acute drug toxicity initially thought to be CBZ related. The mean PHT plasma concentration for the 12 patients (22.7 ± 5.64 μg/ml) as well as concentration/dose ratio for PHT (4.61 ± 1.65 μg/ml plasma per mg/kg/day dose) was significantly higher ($p < 0.001$) with concomitant administration of CBZ than when PHT was given alone: PHT concentration, 12.54 ± 3.93 μg/ml and PHT concentration/dose ratio, 2.52 ± 0.78 μg/ml plasma per mg/kg/day dose. Those patients with higher PHT plasma concentrations seem to be at higher risk of PHT toxicity due to CBZ comedication. **Key Words:** Phenytoin—Carbamazepine—TDx automated fluorescence polarization assay.

From a survey of the literature, the effect of carbamazepine (CBZ) on phenytoin (PHT) can be summarized as follows: The effect of CBZ comedication on plasma PHT concentration varies among patients and is generally not of great magnitude. Several authors have reported that CBZ caused a fall in plasma PHT concentration (1–3). Others have found no significant changes, whereas still others found that, if anything, there is a slight upward trend (4). The effect of CBZ on PHT in an individual patient is largely unpredictable (5). In contrast, the effect of PHT on CBZ is predictable. Numerous reports in the last decade (6–11) have demonstrated that CBZ metabolism is highly inducible by PHT, leading to significantly lower than expected CBZ concentrations.

Approximately 1 year ago, the senior author observed that some PHT-treated patients with steady-state plasma concentrations within the "therapeutic range" responded with clinical manifestations of drug toxicity after comedication with CBZ was started. Surprisingly, these cases presented with PHT concentrations above those previously noted on serial measurements. This early observation alerted us to the appearance of clinical or laboratory signs of PHT overdose in patients comedicated with CBZ. Since then, we have accumulated intrapatient data on serial observations of epileptic patients who were chronically medicated only with PHT and compared the data for the same patients after comedication with CBZ without a change of PHT dose. Here we report preliminary results on these retrospective observations.

Address correspondence and reprint requests to Dr. J. J. Zielinski at the Epilepsy Center of Michigan, 3800 Woodward Avenue, Detroit, MI 48201, U.S.A.

MATERIALS AND METHODS

Twenty-four epileptic outpatients with seizure disorder (11 female, 13 male; mean age 30.9 years, range 19–54 years) were involved in the study. All of them received only PHT. The daily dose remained un-

TABLE 1. *Intrapatient effects of CBZ on PHT in 24 patients after addition of CBZ to PHT-only regimens*[a]

Parameter[b]	PHT	PHT + CBZ	Percent difference
PHT dose	5.32 ± 1.28	5.32 ± 1.28	None
PHT L/D ratio	2.69 ± 0.80	3.78 ± 1.23	40.5[c]
PHT level	13.98 ± 4.68	19.00 ± 4.75	35.9[c]
CBZ dose		12.87 ± 3.78	
CBZ L/D ratio		0.36 ± 0.15	
CBZ level		4.31 ± 1.57	

CBZ, carbamazepine; PHT, phenytoin; L/D, level/dose.

[a]Data from serial observations over a 1-year period and presented as means ± SD.

[b]Dose = mg/kg/day; L/D ratio = μg/ml plasma per mg/kg/day dose; level = μg/ml plasma.

[c]$p < 0.001$.

TABLE 2. *Intrapatient effects of CBZ on PHT in Group A patients as compared with Group B patients*[a]

Parameter	PHT	PHT + CBZ	Percent difference
Group A: PHT elevated (n = 12)			
PHT dose	5.12 ± 1.19	5.12 ± 1.19	
PHT L/D ratio	2.52 ± 0.78	4.61 ± 1.65	82.9[b]
PHT level	12.54 ± 3.93	22.70 ± 5.64	81.3[b]
CBZ dose		12.94 ± 4.71	
CBZ L/D ratio		0.31 ± 0.13	
CBZ level		3.72 ± 1.17	
Group B: No change in PHT (n = 12)			
PHT dose	5.51 ± 1.37	5.51 ± 1.37	
PHT L/D ratio	2.86 ± 0.82	2.95 ± 0.81	3.1 (NS)
PHT level	15.42 ± 5.43	15.29 ± 4.79	−0.8 (NS)
CBZ dose		12.79 ± 2.84	
CBZ L/D ratio		0.40 ± 0.17	
CBZ level		4.89 ± 1.96	

CBZ, carbamazepine; PHT, phenytoin; L/D, level/dose; NS, not significant.

[a]No differences between Group A and B (see the text for description of Groups) for age, sex, or elapsed time (6 weeks) after initiation with CBZ and redetermination of anticonvulsant drug levels.

[b]$p < 0.001$.

changed for at least several months before CBZ was added to their regimen. Of the 24 studied, 18 were mentally retarded residents of group homes, and half of them showed various neurological deficits. Albumin, total bilirubin, and aminotransferases were within normal limits for all patients, and, clinically, no liver dysfunction was suspected. Trough, steady-state PHT and later CBZ plasma concentrations were measured as part of regular antiepileptic drug monitoring schedules. Abbott Diagnostics reagents and an Abbott TDx automated fluorescence polarization analyzer were used.

RESULTS AND DISCUSSION

Table 1 shows intrapatient data for the 24 patients medicated with only PHT, as compared with the same patients' data after CBZ comedication and without a change in PHT dose. The increase of PHT concentration (by 35.9%; $p < 0.001$) and of PHT concentration/dose ratio (by 40.5%; $p < 0.001$) on comedication with CBZ is evident. This finding was unexpected, and no precedent could be found for this in the literature.

The data for the 24 PHT patients comedicated with CBZ were divided into two groups. Group A (n = 12) consisted of patients who showed an elevation in their PHT concentration, which caused the attending epileptologist to order a repeat determination on the same specimens (elevation was confirmed). Group B (n = 12) consisted of those patients in whom PHT concentrations did not change on CBZ comedication. Table 2 shows the intrapatient data on the effect (Group A) and no effect (Group B) of CBZ on PHT concentration. For Group A, the large increase of PHT concentration/dose ratio (by 82.9%; $p < 0.001$) and PHT concentration (by 81.3%; $p < 0.001$) on comedication with CBZ is clearly evident. This effect is clinically significant because five cases responded to CBZ comedication with symptoms of acute drug toxicity. These symptoms were initially thought to be due to CBZ until PHT concentrations were determined.

Considering the mechanisms responsible, we can speculate that the lower CBZ concentration and CBZ concentration/dose ratio in Group A patients are due to an increased rate of CBZ metabolism. At the same time, the metabolism of PHT seems to slow down with the consequent accumulation of PHT in plasma. A careful search through the patients' neurological files produced no clinical features that could possibly be associated with the different CBZ effect between Groups A and B (sex, age, neurological findings, degree of mental retardation; there were no cases of liver or renal insufficiency). Moreover, as most of the patients were residents of selected group homes, their medications were administered by trained staff members, and therefore medical noncompliance could be ruled out.

CONCLUSIONS

CBZ added to the regimens of patients with steady-state PHT concentrations may result in a significant increase in plasma concentration of PHT. This may happen with or without manifestations of acute or subacute PHT toxicity. These findings were unexpected and occurred during adjustment of antiepileptic medication in a group of outpatients.

The undesired results of CBZ–PHT interaction may occur in clinical practice more often than expected, and may go unnoticed and unrecognized if the plasma concentration of PHT is not being monitored during the addition of CBZ. Monitoring plasma concentration of PHT is especially important in patients with epilepsy and concomitant mental retardation and/or neurologic handicap in whom clinical signs of PHT toxicity may easily be overlooked. Those patients in whom PHT plasma concentration is close to the upper limit of "therapeutic" range before they are comedicated with CBZ seem to be under higher risk of PHT toxicity.

As a matter of practical approach and to avoid probable intoxication with PHT in at-risk patients, plasma concentration of their medication is now carefully assessed in scheduled intervals after CBZ is added to their PHT regimen. Assessment is continued over a period of increasing CBZ dosage until a steady-state of both medications is achieved and maintained over a 3-month period.

REFERENCES

1. Hansen JM, Siersback-Nielsen K, Skovsted L. Carbamazepine-induced acceleration of diphenylhydantoin and warfarin metabolism in man. *Clin Pharmacol Ther* 1971;12:539–43.
2. Windorfer A Jr, Sauer W. Drug interactions during anticonvulsant therapy in childhood: diphenylhydantoin, primidone, phenobarbitone, clonazepam, nitrazepam, carbamazepine, and dipropylacetate. *Neuropadiatrie* 1979;8:29–41.
3. Perucca E. Clinical pharmacology and medical treatment. Part III: drug interactions. In: Laidlaw J, Richens A, eds. *A textbook of epilepsy*. New York: Churchill Livingstone, 1982:358–71.
4. Lander CM, Eadie MJ, Tyrer JH. Interactions between anticonvulsants. *Proc Aust Assoc Neurol* 1975;12:111–6.
5. Kutt H. Phenytoin interactions with other drugs. In: Woodbury DM, Penry JK, Pippenger CE, eds. *Antiepileptic drugs*. New York: Raven Press, 1982:227–40.
6. Hvidberg EF, Dam M. Clinical pharmacokinetics of anticonvulsants. *Clin Pharmakokinet* 1976;1:161–88.
7. Christiansen J, Dam M. Influence of phenobarbital and diphenylhydantoin on plasma carbamazepine levels in patients with epilepsy. *Acta Neurol Scand* 1973;49:543–6.
8. Christiansen J, Dam M. Drug interactions in epileptic patients. In: Schneider H, Janz D, Gardner-Thorpe C, Meinardi H, Sherwin AL, eds. *Clinical pharmacology of anti-epileptic drugs*. New York: Springer-Verlag, 1975:197–200.
9. Schneider H. Carbamazepine: the influence of other antiepileptic drugs on its serum level. In: Schneider H, Janz D, Gardner-Thorpe C, Meinardi H, Sherwin AL, eds. *Clinical pharmacology of anti-epileptic drugs*. New York: Springer-Verlag, 1975:189–96.
10. Johannessen SI, Standjord RE. The influence of phenobarbitone and phenytoin on carbamazepine serum levels. In Schneider H, Janz D, Gardner-Thorpe C, Meinardi H, Sherwin AL, eds. *Clinical pharmacology of anti-epileptic drugs*. New York: Springer-Verlag, 1975:201–5.
11. Rane A, Hojer B, Wilson JT. Kinetics of carbamazepine and 10,11-epoxide metabolite in children. *Clin Pharmacol Ther* 1976;19:276–83.

Therapeutic Drug Monitoring
7:54–60 © 1985 Raven Press, New York

Investigations of Long-Term Treatment with Perhexiline Maleate Using Therapeutic Monitoring and Electromyography

J. Pilcher, J. D. H. Cooper, D. C. Turnell, J. Matenga, R. Paul, and *J. D. F. Lockhart

*Coventry and Warwickshire Hospital, Coventry, and *Merrell Dow Research Institute, Merrell Dow Pharmaceuticals Limited, Egham, Surrey, England*

Summary: Experience is reported with 41 patients taking perhexiline maleate for angina pectoris for periods of up to 70 months, while serum concentrations of the drug were monitored, and liver function tests and electromyographic tests were made before and during treatment. Severe side effects did not occur unless serum perhexiline levels were greater than 1.5 mg/L. The drug seems effective for prolonged dosage, and the monitoring of weight, liver function test results, and serum concentrations should prevent or reduce toxicity. A starting dose of 100 mg daily is recommended. The drug is not recommended for routine use in angina pectoris. **Key Words:** Perhexiline—Angina pectoris—Serum concentrations—Liver function tests—Electromyography.

Perhexiline maleate (Px) is an effective antianginal agent (1,2) and has been shown to be superior to beta blockers (3) in this regard. The therapeutic use of Px is limited by serious side effects, and it is now reserved for the treatment of severe angina in patients who have failed to respond to, or who are unsuitable for, treatment with other antianginal drugs or surgery. Peripheral neuropathy (4,5) and hepatotoxicity (6,7) are the most important of the side effects and may occur from within a few weeks to up to 3 years from commencement of treatment.

In 1978, Singlas and colleagues (8) investigated the pharmacokinetics of Px in patients and found that those developing peripheral neuropathy had plasma Px concentrations greater than 2 mg/L. They concluded that the neuropathy was a direct toxic effect of Px due to its accumulation, which, in turn, was the result of slow hepatic metabolism in the affected individuals, possibly genetically determined. Px is metabolised by microsomal oxidation to more polar mono- and dihydroxy metabolites, and recently it has been shown that several similar drug oxidations in humans are under genetic control. The ability of an individual to metabolise debrisoquine has been used as a test to determine some pathways of oxidative capacity; this has been done by Shah et al. (9) in two groups of patients treated with Px, one group with neuropathy and the other without. Many more of the group with neuropathy were slow debrisoquine metabolisers, thus providing further confirmation that neuropathy is probably the result of accumulation of Px because of poor metabolism.

While a knowledge of the ability of an individual to metabolise debrisoquine may prove helpful in identifying patients at potential risk of developing neuropathy with Px, the test itself is time-consuming and may not be available in many areas; it may also show both false-positives and false-negatives in relation to observed Px toxicity. The development of a rapid and precise gas-liquid chromatographic technique for the measurement of Px in serum (10) has now made fea-

Address correspondence and reprint requests to J. Pilcher at Coventry and Warwickshire Hospital, Stoney Stanton Road, Coventry, CV1 4FH, England.

sible the monitoring of Px therapy by a district hospital service laboratory.

The main purpose of the study was to ascertain whether toxicity from Px therapy could be avoided by regular monitoring of serum Px concentrations and other indices of toxicity, such as abnormal liver function test results and weight loss. The possible development of subclinical electromyographic (EMG) abnormalities during Px treatment was also investigated in the same patients.

PATIENTS AND METHODS

A total of 41 patients were studied, divided into those who had not received Px previously (group 1) and those who were already receiving Px (group 2). All patients had angina pectoris due to coronary artery disease, confirmed by abnormal resting or exercise electrocardiograms and without evidence of other heart disease, diabetes mellitus, or neurological disorders. Patients continued to receive their previous medications, which included calcium antagonists, beta blockers (atenolol, metoprolol, propranolol), nitrites, and diuretics.

On each visit to the Cardiology Clinic, patients were examined, their weight and symptoms recorded, and a blood sample obtained for routine biochemical tests and for estimation of serum Px levels, which were done according to the procedure described by Cooper and Turnell (10). This comprises a single ether extraction of the drug from serum, followed by gas chromatographic separation of the analytes. The within-batch precision of this technique was obtained by analysing two pooled sera spiked with different levels of Px 20 times. When the method was optimised for monitoring Px therapy, the coefficients of variation of 9.1 and 3.2% at serum Px levels of 0.5 and 2.0 mg/L, respectively, were found, and the limit of detection was 0.09 mg/L. The between-batch precision was calculated by analysing the same two sera 20 times on different days. The sera had been aliquoted and deep-frozen. Coefficients of variation of 13.1 and 5.2% were obtained for the same serum Px concentrations. A mean recovery of 104% was calculated on the between-batch estimations. Assays performed on Px-free sera showed no endogenous peaks on the chromatogram. No interference from the Px metabolites or from the beta-blocking agents (acebutolol, metoprolol, oxprenolol, propranolol, timolol) was observed at the chromatographic peak elution times of the internal standard and Px.

Blood samples were, as far as possible, obtained at the same time of the day on each occasion and at a similar interval after the last dose of Px. However, this is not critical, as serum concentrations of the drug vary very little throughout 24 h in patients who have achieved steady-state (unpublished observation).

TABLE 1. *Characteristics of two groups of patients receiving perhexiline maleate (Px)*

	Group 1	Group 2
Number of patients	19 men	12 men 2 women
Age at first visit (yr)[a]	54 (43–73)	59 (50–76)
Time studied (mo)[a]	26 (5–34)	19 (7–33)
Previous myocardial infarction	5	6
Poor left ventricular function	3	3
Failed treatment with:		
beta blockers	9	6
coronary artery bypass graft	4	1
At termination of study:		
Total time of Px treatment (mo)[a]	26 (5–34)	42 (5–70)
Number still receiving Px	14	8
Number deceased	3	2
Number withdrawn	2	4

[a]Mean, with range in parentheses.

No formal assessment of anginal severity was made in any patients. Most had failed to respond to conventional treatments (Table 1), and consequently it was not thought ethical to subject them to a placebo intervention in order to obtain a drug-free baseline. Hence, assessments were open and based on a four-point scale, as follows: grade 0 indicated no improvement; grade 1 (+), slight improvement, but with patients not satisfied with their response; grades 2 and 3 (+ + and + + +) represented increasing improvement, satisfactory to the patients. In patients with a grade 3 response, angina was either completely suppressed or provoked only by heavy exertion. At no time during these assessments were the clinical staff aware of the serum Px levels.

Before patients in group 1 commenced Px therapy, blood was collected on 2 separate days to establish baseline biochemical measurements. Group 1 patients were given a starting dose of 100 mg Px daily. This dose was increased to 200 mg daily after 2 weeks unless good clinical response had been achieved or side effects had occurred. Patients were seen 2 to 8 weeks later and the dose increased to 300 mg daily if indicated. Upward dose adjustments were generally made without knowledge of serum Px levels. Thereafter, the patients were seen every 3 months, or more frequently when further dose adjustments might be made. Group 2 patients continued to receive the dose on which their conditions had been stabilised prior to the availability of serum concentrations of Px. Dosage was tailored to clinical response and the results of liver function tests. Dose reductions were made when serum Px concentrations greater than 2 mg/L were observed.

EMG studies were performed on both group 1 and group 2 patients and also on other patients receiving long-term Px treatment who did not undergo full biochemical tests. Group 1 patients were examined before commencing Px and then after 6 months and 2 years. Group 2 and other patients were examined at presentation and after 2 years whenever possible.

Antidromic sural sensory action potentials were obtained, latency, amplitude, and duration being noted. This nerve is not usually affected by extraneous pathological processes (11) and has well-established normal values and very little retrial variability (12). At the same time, posterior tibial nerve direct motor (M) and late (F) wave responses to the abductor hallucis were recorded. The F wave response rather than the Hoffmann (H) wave was chosen, as the latter often reflects upper motor neuron hyperexcitability, and the F wave is technically more satisfactorily obtained (13–15).

RESULTS

Of the 41 patients examined, only 33 underwent biochemical investigations (Table 1), and 40 had EMG studies. Fourteen patients of group 1 and eight of group 2 were still taking Px at the completion of the study.

Clinical Response and Serum Px Concentrations

Figure 1 shows the degree of improvement of angina pectoris and the corresponding serum Px concentrations.

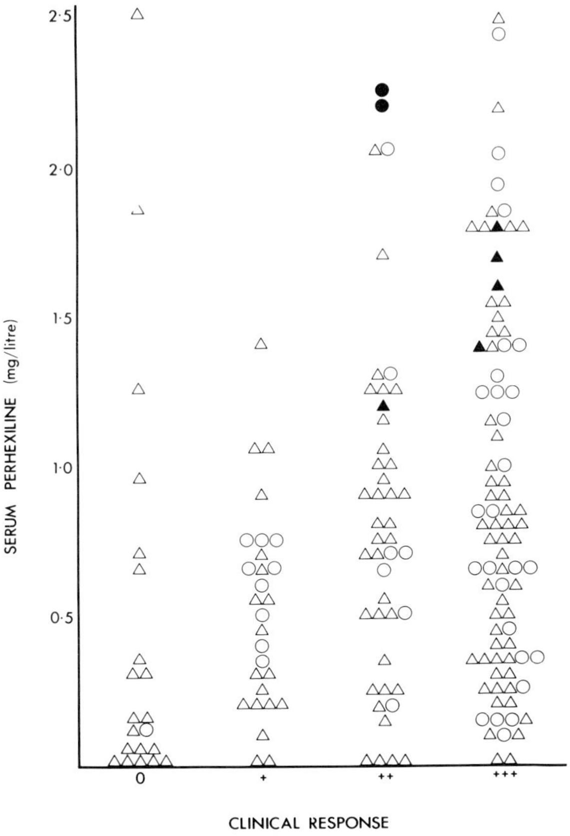

FIG. 1. Subjective response and serum perhexiline concentrations found on each patient visit during the study: patients with no subjective side effects (open triangles, group 1); patients with subjective side effects (filled triangles, group 1); patients with no subjective side effects (open circles, group 2); patients with subjective side effects (filled circles, group 2). Clinical response: 0, no improvement; +, some improvement; + +, good improvement; + + +, very good improvement—patients almost free of angina.

Group 1 Patients

The median serum Px concentrations for those showing no, some, good, and very good improvement were 0.14, 0.30, 0.75, and 0.79 mg/L, respectively. The 19 patients were examined on 136 occasions, and overall 13 showed good improvement, four were slightly improved, and two did not respond, one being withdrawn from treatment. Another patient was withdrawn later, following the observation of marginally abnormal EMG findings.

One patient died suddenly after the study commenced, having previously experienced good symptom relief. One patient with a good clinical response achieved serum Px concentrations of only 0.1 mg/L but was suspected of poor compliance; another sustained a myocardial infarction, after which his previously poor anginal control improved. Two others achieved fair anginal control after dose increases raised their serum Px concentrations. One other patient sustained a myocardial infarction, and two others died suddenly before their 2-year EMG visits.

Group 2 Patients

The median serum Px concentrations for those patients showing some, good, and very good improvement were 0.61, 0.70, and 0.84 mg/L, respectively. Patients were examined on 50 occasions, and all showed some improvement at some time during the study.

Relief of symptoms was maintained over the study period in eight patients, and two were well until their deaths of reinfarction. One patient was well for nearly

TABLE 2. *Range of serum perhexiline maleate (Px) concentrations (mg/L) in both group 1 and group 2 patients for different doses of the drug*

	Serum Px (mg/L)			
	Group 1		Group 2	
Dose Px/day	n	Range	n	Range
100	24	0–1.15	3[a]	1.02–1.86
200	55	0–1.44	16	0.14–2.43
300	42	0–2.50	20	0.10–2.19
400	7	0–2.60	11	0.61–4.50
600	8[a]	0.49–1.25	—	—

[a]Represents only one patient.

4 years, until his angina deteriorated and he required coronary artery surgery; one other had only a moderate response until he survived a myocardial infarction at 23 months and then became asymptomatic. The conditions of two patients were difficult to assess, and symptom relief was not maintained despite the achievement of serum Px concentrations greater than 2.0 mg/L; however, symptom relief deteriorated with reduced dosage and lower serum Px concentrations.

Among the other patients not undergoing full biochemical monitoring, two were admitted to hospital with high serum Px concentrations (3.23 and 4.5 mg/L), one showing definite clinical evidence of peripheral neuropathy. Following withdrawal of treatment, the serum Px concentrations were measured once a week for 7 weeks, and the half-lives of Px elimination were calculated as 10 and 14 days.

Dose and Serum Px Concentrations

Table 2 shows the range of serum Px concentrations obtained for both group 1 and group 2 patients at different doses.

Most group 1 patients experienced control of symptoms while receiving doses ranging from 100 to 400 mg of Px daily. One patient had no symptom relief while receiving Px up to and including the manufacturer's maximum recommended dosage of 400 mg daily. At that dose serum, Px concentrations ranged from 0 to 0.14 mg/L. The dose was increased to 600 mg daily, when good clinical improvement was obtained with a mean serum Px concentration of 0.90 mg/L, which may represent dose-dependent kinetics.

The 14 patients in group 2 achieved control with doses of 100 to 400 mg daily. Four patients receiving 400 mg daily had their doses reduced or withdrawn because of high serum Px concentrations.

Biochemical Measurements

Baseline Values

Seventeen patients from group 1 demonstrated no renal or liver dysfunction. One patient had a raised γ-glutamyl transferase (γ-GT), which was attributed to a high alcohol intake, and one other patient had unexplained elevated γ-GT activity, which remained high during the study. AST and ALT activities in serum for all the patients were within the laboratory's reference range.

Liver Function Tests

Values greater than twice the upper limit of normal were considered to represent a significant rise in enzyme activity.

In group 1, no abnormalities were seen in nine patients, and abnormally high serum enzyme levels in two patients were associated with myocardial infarction. Transient increases in AST, ALT, and γ-GT levels occurred in one patient with unchanged Px dosage. Another patient displayed transient enzyme rises with an increased dose. The Px dosage was actually reduced in four patients (one of them later developing EMG abnormalities, and one other having previously had abnormal values attributed to alcohol, as above). Enzyme levels returned to normal or pretreatment levels in all. Serum levels of Px in those whose dose was reduced ranged from 0.0 to 2.0 mg/L (mean 1.2 mg/L).

Only one of the group 2 patients showed elevated enzyme activity when his dose was increased; the activity returned to normal with dose reduction. The two patients admitted to the hospital with Px levels greater than 2 mg/L also showed elevated enzyme levels. These returned to normal 1 month after the drug was withdrawn. No other biochemical abnormalities were observed in either group 1 or group 2 patients.

EMG Studies

Group 1 Patients

Of the total 19 patients, 15 completed the EMG programme, 3 died before their 2-year visit, and 1 failed to attend. The patients who completed the 2-year period and who, at no time, reported any symptoms suggestive of neuropathy likewise showed no EMG abnormality. No statistically significant differences ($p > 0.05$, paired *t* test) were detected between pretreatment and treatment values of any of the tests performed.

One patient in this group who had no clinical evidence of neuropathy but did show marginal sensory EMG changes had a serum Px concentration of 2.23 mg/L. These EMG changes reverted to normal after cessation of Px.

Group 2 and Other Patients on Long-Term Treatment

Of 22 patients total, 3 patients who had been receiving Px for between 2 and 6 years had serum Px concentrations ranging from 2.2 to more than 4 mg/L, but no neurological or EMG abnormalities were found. One patient had a serum Px concentration of 3.6 mg/L and abnormal EMG findings. Unfortunately, sural nerve biopsy was inconclusive, but the EMG suggested a demyelinating neuropathy. However, as there was clinical neuropathy confirmed by EMG at his first presentation, it cannot be certain that Px was necessarily implicated, although this was assumed at the time, and his treatment was discontinued. Unlike the group 1 patient, his EMG did not subsequently revert to normal. No other patients in group 2 had elevated serum concentrations of Px or abnormal EMG findings.

Side Effects

Side effects were classified into two categories: first, those occurring in the initial dosing period of 3 months (for group 1 patients only when equilibration of the drug would not have been achieved), and second, those occurring during long-term therapy (all patients). Side effects were either subjective (volunteered by patient on direct questioning) or objective (from blood and EMG tests).

During the initial dosing period, three patients from group 1 complained of either visual blurring, headaches, or dizziness. However, these symptoms abated on continued therapy without dose reduction. Figure 1 also shows the serum Px concentrations observed when side effects occurred during long-term therapy. Of the group 1 patients, two complained of lethargy; one of these responded to a dose reduction producing a fall in serum Px from 1.69 to 0.73 mg/L, whereas the other received a maintenance dose of 600 mg daily to achieve anginal control and did not complain of malaise on further visits to the clinic. One patient was withdrawn from the study after 5 months of treatment because of tiredness and lethargy with little therapeutic response. A patient with a serum Px concentration of 1.81 mg/L complained of dizziness, which improved with dose reduction. Finally, in group 1, one patient complained of dizziness and blurred vision with a serum Px level of 1.88 mg/L. The side effects abated with a reduced dose, but the angina became worse.

In group 2, one patient with serum Px concentrations of 2.19 mg/L complained of dizziness, which disappeared with a lower dose and reduced serum Px concentrations. No other long-term side effects were observed in patients from group 2.

Weight Loss

Fifteen of the 19 patients in group 1 showed some weight loss over the period of the study. The mean weight for these patients at the beginning of the study was 82.1 kg, and the mean weight loss was 2.3 kg. The other four patients showed a slight gain in weight.

DISCUSSION

This study was primarily designed to evaluate the side effects of Px and to determine how they might be eliminated or reduced. Side effects of Px are of two main types: first, subjective effects without objective findings, and second, the more serious objective side effects, which may produce no subjective symptoms until after neurological or hepatic damage has already been sustained.

In a study of Px involving 363 patients (16), 220 subjective side effects were reported by 173 patients; the most common were dizziness, nausea, gastrointestinal symptoms, depression, tiredness, and headache—in that order. Most (64%) were reported during the first month of treatment, but in only 49 patients was the drug withdrawn, and the majority of the effects were transient. It was also noted that a significantly higher incidence of side effects was observed with a starting dose of 400 mg of Px daily than with 200 mg daily.

During the early clinical evaluation of Px, a starting dose of 400 mg daily was recommended, but this has now been amended in the manufacturer's data sheet to 100–200 mg daily. Horgan et al. (17) reported no side effects in 15 patients who had commenced treatment with 200 mg Px daily for 2 weeks. The results we report here certainly confirm the lower incidence of subjective side effects with a smaller starting dose, and we would suggest 100 mg daily.

Of the severe objective side effects that can arise during Px therapy, hepatotoxicity may, in rare cases, progress to hepatic cirrhosis with histological changes similar to those of alcoholic cirrhosis (6). However, raised liver enzyme levels due to the drug are common (16,18). Our results confirm this observation and suggest that serum ALT was the most useful assay to detect potential hepatotoxicity. While abnormal serum ALT results did occur early with Px treatment and tended to accompany a rise in serum Px concentrations, the serum Px level cannot properly be used to forecast hepatotoxicity. What is relevant is that with prompt dose reduction, abnormal enzyme levels return to normal. It is therefore mandatory that liver function tests be conducted on patients receiving Px, and the dose reduced, or even stopped, in response to abnormal results.

Symptomatic neurotoxicity with EMG abnormalities seems to be a late side effect. Thirteen patients with peripheral neuropathy studied by Singlas et al. (8) had been exposed to the drug for between 3 and 24 months (mean 12.4 months), and 10 patients studied by Fraser and Miller (19) had similarly been exposed for between 3 and 18 months (mean 10.3 months). EMG abnormalities in asymptomatic patients receiving Px have been reported by Maben et al. (20), who found that 17 of 22 patients had EMG changes, and Sebille (21), who found statistically significant EMG changes in 36 patients receiving Px. With the exception of one abnormality, the results in this study support those of Bouche et al. (22), who found no clinical or EMG disturbances in 20 asymptomatic patients who had taken Px for up to 2 years. The differences in these reports may be due to choice of population sample or, possibly, to undue reliance on H wave measurements in the former studies. Our own observations should be compared with the suggested incidence of 0.2% by the Intensified Adverse Drug Reporting Scheme in New Zealand (23). What seems certain is that peripheral neuropathy is associated with high levels of Px in serum, as was originally suggested by Singlas et al. (8). Indeed, in all confirmed cases to date in which the serum Px level has been measured, it has been greater than 2 mg/L. Rapid clinical recovery from neuropathy is the usual outcome when the drug is discontinued, but the return to normal EMG values may be prolonged, and in our experience (unpublished observations) of seven patients (collected over 7 years), six became asymptomatic, but only three of the six had EMGs that had reverted completely to normal within 18 months.

The results of monitoring serum Px concentrations demonstrate the wide variation of Px levels obtained in patients receiving the same dose, suggesting substantial differences in Px metabolism in the patients sampled (Table 2). Extreme examples of this are the one patient requiring a daily dose of 600 mg to achieve serum Px concentrations of around 1.0 mg/L, who can be recognised as a fast metaboliser of the drug, while two patients with high Px concentrations, in whom the elimination half-lives were measured at 10 and 14 days, are clearly slow metabolisers. These slow metabolisers probably represent the group of patients most likely at risk from accumulation of Px with the possibility of subsequent toxicity.

The results also demonstrate the apparent therapeutic range (Fig. 1), which lies between 0.1 and 1.5 mg/L, although a carefully controlled study is necessary to define this range more precisely. There was evidence to suggest that therapeutic response is positively related to serum concentration (Fig. 1), although some patients had a good antianginal response even when Px was not detected. This could be either because the concentration was below the limits of detection of the assay or because tissue levels of the bound drug may be higher than serum levels. However, in an open evaluation of this kind, a placebo effect or natural remission of symptoms seems more probable. The availability of an analytical method to measure serum concentrations of Px should now offer a means to prevent the development of peripheral neuropathy as a complication of treatment and to aid therapeutic response in fast metabolisers who might have poor response to treatment with normal recommended doses. Serum levels of Px above 2.0 mg/L are toxic, and levels above 1.5 mg/L should be regarded with suspicion, even in the absence of objective or subjective signs or symptoms.

Our conclusion is that it seems possible to avoid potentially dangerous accumulation of Px by routine monitoring of serum concentrations. Other criteria of good patient management, particularly that of administering the lowest effective dose, should continue to be observed. Regular liver function tests are mandatory, and any abnormalities of these tests or of EMG findings, side effects, or significant weight loss should prompt the clinician to ascertain the serum Px concentration and adjust the dose accordingly. Estimation of serum Px levels is certainly practicable, but it may be time-consuming. Ideally, one should like to be able to predict which patients are at risk, i.e., the slow metabolisers, before treatment. The debrisoquine test (9) may be helpful in this regard, and single-dose kinetic studies (24,25), including measurement of Px metabolites, will certainly identify slow metabolisers. However, the techniques are laborious, and neither is likely to be of value in the routine management of patients.

Finally, it should be stressed that, despite all these problems, Px may often succeed where other drugs have failed and thereby improve the quality of life in a group of patients whose prognosis is usually poor.

REFERENCES

1. Pilcher J, Chandrasekhar KP, Russell Rees J, Boyce MJ, Pierce TH, Ikram H. Long-term assessment of perhexiline maleate in angina pectoris. *Postgrad Med J* (Suppl) 1973;115–8.
2. Burns-Cox CJ, Chandrasekhar KP, Ikram H, et al. Clinical evaluation of perhexiline maleate in patients with angina pectoris. *Br Med J* 197i;4:586–8.
3. Mir MA, Kafetzakis EM. Assessment of perhexiline maleate in angiographically proven intractable angina: a double-blind trial. *Am Heart J* 1978;96:350–4.
4. L'Hermitte F, Fardeau M, Chedru F, Mallecourt J. Polyneuropathy after perhexiline maleate therapy. *Br Med J* 1976;1:1256.
5. Bousser MG, Bouche P, Brochard C, Herreman G. Peripheral neuropathies due to perhexiline maleate: seven case histories. *Cour et Medecine Interne* 1976;15:181–8.
6. Beaugrand M, Poupon R, Levy VG, et al. Hepatic lesions due to perhexiline maleate. *Gastroenterol Clin Biol* 1978;2:579–88.
7. Forbes GB, Rake MO, Taylor DJE. Liver damage due to perhexiline maleate. *J Clin Pathol* 1979;32:1282–5.
8. Singlas E, Goujet MA, Simon P. Pharmacokinetics of perhexiline maleate in anginal patients with and without peripheral neuropathy. *Eur J Clin Pharmacol* 1978;14:195–201.
9. Shah RR, Oates NS, Idle JR, Smith RL, Lockhart JDF. Impaired oxidation of debrisoquine in patients with perhexiline neuropathy. *Br Med J* 1982;284:295–9.
10. Cooper JDH, Turnell DC. A rapid method for the determination of perhexiline in serum using gas-liquid chromatography. *Ann Clin Biochem* 1980;17:155–8.
11. Burke D, Skuse NF, Lethlean AK. Sensory conduction of the sural nerve in polyneuropathy. *J Neurol Neurosurg Psychiatry* 1974;37:647–52.
12. Rosenfalk P. Electromyography—sensory and motor conduction findings in normal subjects. Laboratory of Clinical Neurophysiology. Copenhagen: Rigshospitalet, 1975;20–39.
13. McLeod JG, Wray SH. An experimental study of the F wave in the baboon. *J Neurol Neurosurg Psychiatry* 1966;29:196–200.
14. Magladery JW, Teasdale RD, Park AM, Languth HW. Electrophysiologic studies of reflex activity in patients with lesions of the nervous system. *Bull Johns Hopkins Hosp* 1952;91:219–44.
15. Shahani BT, Sumner AJ. Electrophysiological studies in peripheral neuropathy: early detection and monitoring. In: Stalberg E, Young RR, eds. *Clinical Neurophysiology*. Medical Reviews Neurology I. London: Butterworth, 1981:117–44.
16. Lockhart JDF, Masheter HC. Report of a multicentre monitored release study of perhexiline maleate in the prevention of angina pectoris. *Br J Clin Pract* 1976;30(a):172.
17. Horgan JH, O'Callaghan WG, Teo KK. Therapy of angina pectoris with low-dose perhexiline. *J Cardiovasc Pharmacol* 1981;3:566–72.
18. Howard DJ, Russell Rees J. Long term perhexiline maleate and liver function. *Br Med J* 1976;1:133.
19. Fraser DM, Miller HC. Perhexiline-induced neuropathy. *Br Med J* 1978;1:858.
20. Mabin D, Penther Ph, Blanc JJ. Electromyelogramme et vitesse de condition nerveuse au cours des traitement prolonges par la maleate de perhexiline. *Ann Cardiol Angeiol* 1977;26:401–6.
21. Sebille A. Etude electrophysiologique des neuropathies latentes indvite par la perhexiline. *EEG Clin Neurophysiol* 1978;45:666–70.
22. Bouche P, Bousser MG, Peytour MA, Cathala HP. Perhexiline maleate and peripheral neuropathy. *Neurology* 1979;29:739–43.
23. Coulter DM. Study of reasons for cessation of therapy with perhexiline maleate, sodium valproate, and labetalol in the intensified adverse reaction reporting scheme. *NZ Med J* 1981;93:81–4.
24. Amoah AGB, Gould BJ, Parke DV. Single dose pharmacokinetics of perhexiline administered orally to humans. *J Chromatogr* 1984;305:401–9.
25. Cooper RG, Evans DAP, Whibley EJ. Polymorphic hydroxylation of perhexiline maleate in man. *J Med Genetics* 1984;21:27–33.

Therapeutic Drug Monitoring
7:61–65 © 1985 Raven Press, New York

Assessment of Cyclosporin A in Whole Blood and Plasma in Five Patients with Different Hematocrits

R. P. Agarwal, R. A. McPherson, and G. A. Threatte

Clinical Laboratories, Georgetown University Hospital and Department of Pathology, Georgetown University School of Medicine, Washington, D.C., U.S.A.

Summary: Measurement of whole blood and plasma levels of cyclosporin A (CsA) by radioimmunoassay in kidney transplant recipients receiving the drug showed that CsA concentrations in plasma increased nonlinearly when whole blood levels of the drug exceeded 1,000 ng/ml. At low plasma levels (<200 ng/ml), most of the CsA in blood was in the nonplasma component, indicating that cellular elements have high affinity for CsA. Comparison of nonplasma CsA concentrations in two patients with hematocrit values of 32.5 and 35% showed that in the patient with a hematocrit of 35% the cellular associated drug was twice as great as that in the other patient, indicating that there may be significant differences in the cellular affinity of CsA in patients with similar hematocrits. Linear regression analysis of the cellular associated CsA versus plasma levels of the drug in a double-reciprocal plot showed a drug saturation capacity of 6,060 ng/ml in the nonplasma component of blood in the patient with a hematocrit of 35%. Similar analyses in the other patients indicated saturation capacities ranging from 4,750 to 10,400 ng/ml. **Key Words:** Cyclosporin A—Whole blood concentration—Plasma concentration—Cellular bound concentration—Cellular saturation.

Cyclosporin A (CsA), an immunosuppressive agent, is used in the prevention of graft rejection after kidney, liver, and heart transplantation and in the prevention of graft-versus-host disease after allogeneic bone marrow transplantation. The major side effects of CsA are nephrotoxicity, hypertension, hirsutism, tremor, and mild hepatic dysfunction. The enhancement of graft survival as well as a reduction in some of these adverse effects should be facilitated by the careful monitoring of serum, plasma, or whole blood concentrations of this drug. Cellular components of the blood have a high affinity for CsA (1,2). The distribution of the drug between plasma and cellular components of blood also depends on factors such as temperature and the time of incubation before separation of serum or plasma (3–7). Therefore, blood collection and plasma separation procedures must be carried out under standardized conditions to obtain clinically useful serum or plasma measurements.

There is controversy in the literature on the correlation of CsA concentrations in plasma and whole blood. Sandoz Ltd., the manufacturer of CsA, reported a good correlation (r = 0.87, n = 15) between the drug concentrations in plasma and whole blood (8). More recently, Bennett et al. (9) showed that there is poor correlation (r = 0.58, n = 34) between plasma and whole blood CsA concentrations. It is unclear whether values for whole blood or plasma will be more useful for monitoring clinical efficacy and undesired effects of the drug.

The present investigation was undertaken to estimate by radioimmunoassay (RIA) the uptake of CsA by cellular components of blood in five kidney trans-

Address correspondence and reprint requests to Dr. R. P. Agarwal at Clinical Laboratories, Georgetown University Hospital, 3800 Reservoir Road, Washington, DC 20007, U.S.A.

plant recipients and to determine to what extent distribution of the drug in blood depended on the hematocrit and total drug concentrations in serial specimens from individual patients. From the whole blood and plasma levels of CsA, we also estimated the cellular saturation capacity for the drug.

METHODS

We measured both peak and trough levels of CsA in plasma and whole blood of five renal transplant patients receiving the drug orally. Trough levels were obtained just prior to administration of the next dose, and peak levels were obtained approximately 3 h later. There was no restriction of food intake prior to the drug administration, since food apparently has no effect on either peak concentration or elimination of the drug (10).

Whole blood was drawn in Vacutainers containing ethylenediaminetetraacetic acid (EDTA) as an anticoagulant. Samples were allowed to stand at 4°C for 2 h, mixed by inverting for 5 min at 4°C, and aliquots removed and frozen at −20°C for at least 1 h to achieve hemolysis. Plasma from the remaining blood was removed by centrifugation at 4°C. CsA concentrations in plasma and hemolyzed blood were measured by RIA using a kit supplied by Sandoz Ltd. (Basel, Switzerland). Hematocrit (Hct) was determined by Coulter Counter.

The concentrations *(C)* of CsA (ng/ml) in the nonplasma component of whole blood were calculated from the following relationship:

$$C = \frac{A - B(1 - \text{Hct})}{\text{Hct}} \quad (1)$$

where *A* and *B* are the concentrations of CsA (ng/ml) in whole blood and plasma, respectively.

RESULTS

Sandoz recommends the use of heparinized blood in the test protocol for the RIA of CsA. To investigate the effect of EDTA (anticoagulant used in the present study) on the assay, samples of whole blood drawn from a kidney transplant recipient receiving the drug were divided equally into two Vacutainers containing EDTA and heparin. Samples were then treated for plasma separation and hemolysis as described in Methods. RIA of the plasma and whole blood samples containing the two anticoagulants yielded essentially identical results, showing that specimens containing EDTA could be used in place of heparinized samples.

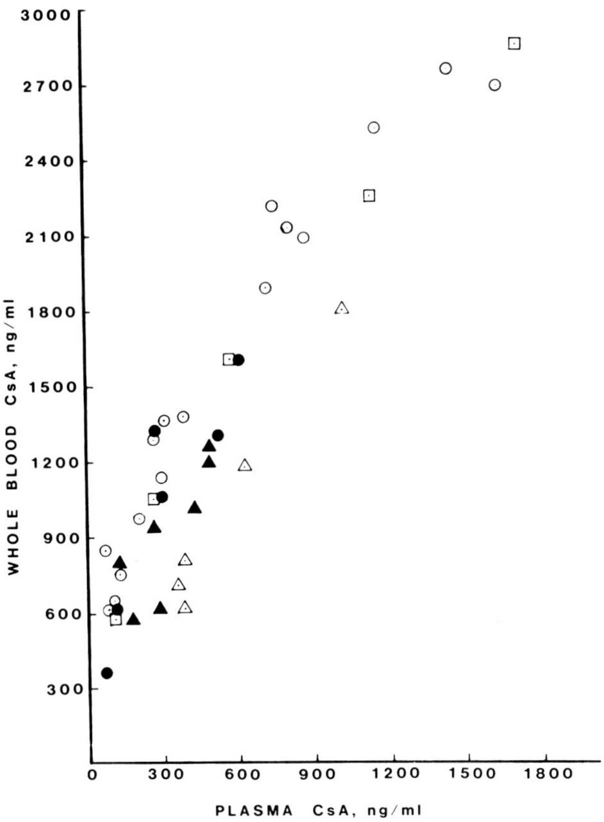

FIG. 1. Comparison of whole blood and plasma cyclosporin A (CsA) concentrations in five kidney transplant recipients with hematocrits ranging from 20 to 35.5%. Each symbol represents an individual patient.

The interassay coefficient of variation of CsA analyses in whole blood and plasma was ±5%. Mean values of CsA concentrations in the two quality control blood samples analyzed on 8 different days were 287 ± 18 (SD) and 1,614 ± 63 ng/ml, respectively.

In Fig. 1, whole blood CsA concentrations are plotted against the drug concentrations found in plasma of five kidney transplant recipients. Unweighted linear regression analysis of the data yielded the following equation: $y = 1.48x + 552$, with a correlation coefficient of 0.93. The Hct in these patients ranged from 20 to 35.5%. In four of the five patients with Hct of 20–32.5%, trough levels of whole blood CsA were within the therapeutic range (250–1,000 ng/ml) (11). In the case of the fifth patient with Hct of 35%, trough levels of CsA in blood reached 1,400 ng/ml. None of these patients experienced adverse effects of the drug.

A plot of whole blood versus plasma CsA concentrations in multiple specimens from one individual whose Hct varied only between 34.5 and 35.5% is shown in Fig. 2. Although plasma CsA concentrations

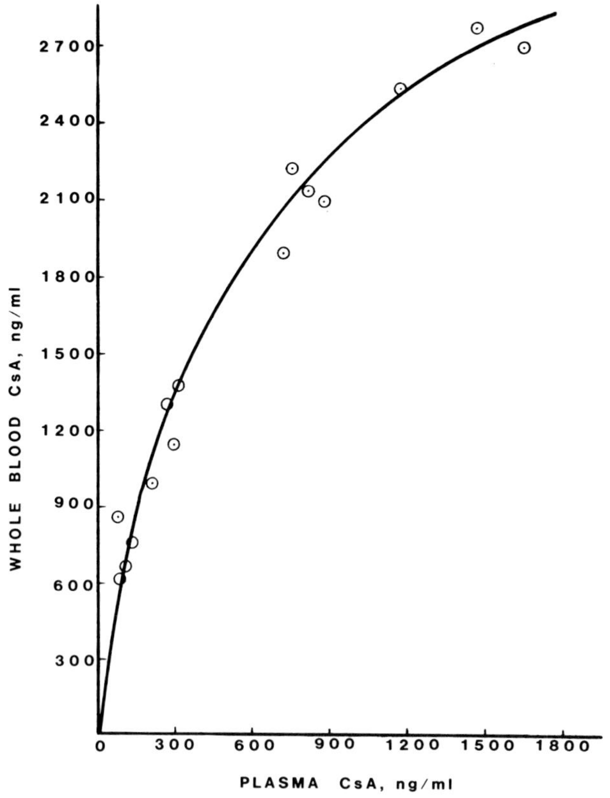

FIG. 2. Comparison of whole blood and plasma cyclosporin A (CsA) concentrations in a kidney transplant recipient with stable cell counts (hematocrit = 34.5–35.5%).

in these specimens appeared to increase linearly with whole blood concentrations up to about 1,000 ng/ml in whole blood, at higher concentrations of the drug, the relationship was nonlinear.

In Fig. 3 CsA concentrations (calculated from Eq. 1) in the nonplasma component of whole blood are plotted against those found in plasma of two patients with modal Hct values of 32.5 and 35%. These results indicate that the cellular affinity for CsA in the patient with Hct of 35% was almost twice as great as that in the patient with Hct of 32.5% at corresponding plasma levels of the drug.

Figure 4 illustrates the variation of the ratio of nonplasma CsA to plasma CsA (cellular/plasma concentration gradient) as a function of the plasma CsA concentrations found in the five patients studied. At low levels (<200 ng/ml) of plasma CsA, this ratio ranged from 12 to 28. At higher concentrations of the drug, values of the cellular/plasma concentration gradient of CsA gradually decreased to about 3 in the peak specimens. The CsA concentration in the nonplasma component is referred to as the cellular associated drug, since it has been shown by in vitro study (1,2) that most of the nonplasma CsA in blood is associated with erythrocytes and lymphocytes.

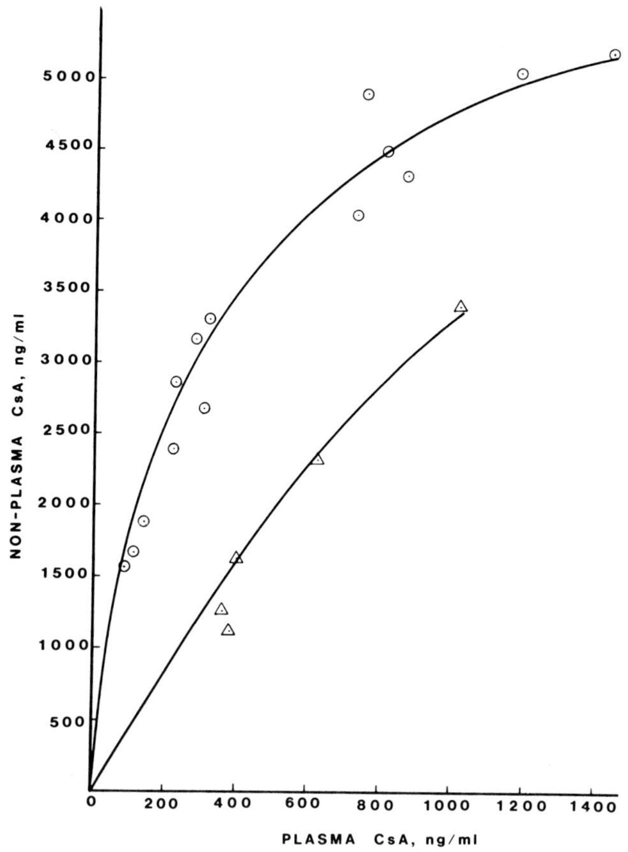

FIG. 3. Comparison of nonplasma versus plasma levels of cyclosporin A (CsA) in the blood of two patients with hematocrits of 32.5% (triangles) and 35% (circles).

Figure 5 shows a double-reciprocal plot of nonplasma CsA concentrations against plasma levels of the drug in the patient with Hct of 35% (Fig. 6) from whom the greatest number of samples were analyzed. Unweighted linear regression analysis of the data yielded the following equation: $y = 0.05x + 1.65 \times 10^{-4}$, with a correlation coefficient of 0.98.

DISCUSSION

When heparin was used as the anticoagulant, problems were sometimes encountered when the specimen clotted after refrigeration and freezing. EDTA proved to be the more effective anticoagulant, and samples could be used directly for Hct measurements by Coulter Counter as well. Since EDTA had no effect on the RIA of CsA, as shown in Results, we used blood

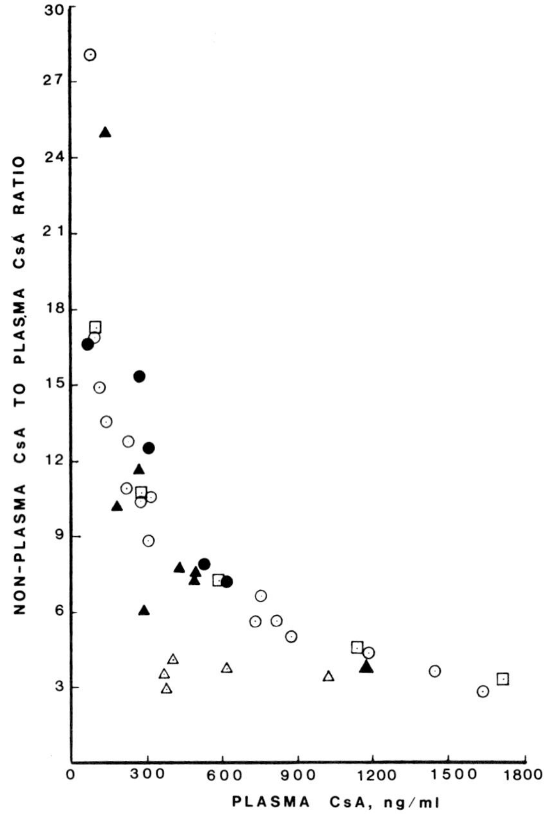

FIG. 4. Variation of cellular/plasma concentration gradient of cyclosporin A (CsA) as a function of plasma CsA levels. Each symbol represents an individual patient.

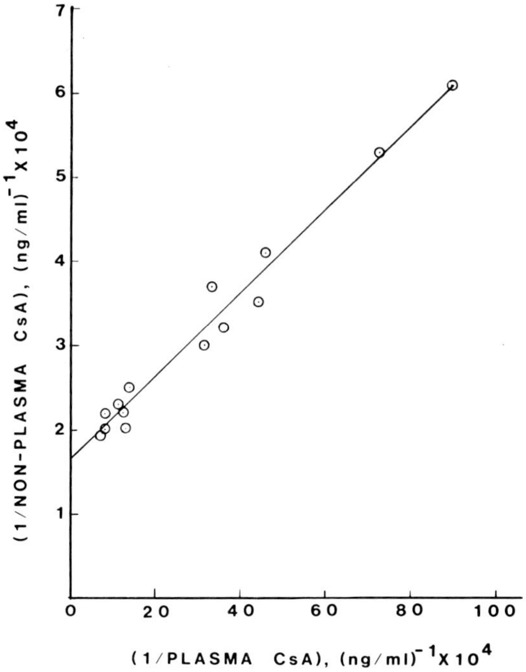

FIG. 5. Double-reciprocal plot of nonplasma cyclosporin A (CsA) concentrations versus plasma levels of CsA for patient with hematocrit of 35%. The line is drawn from an unweighted least-squares linear regression analysis of the data (shown by circles in Fig. 4) in the double-reciprocal form.

samples collected in the Vacutainers containing EDTA for the drug analysis.

There is disagreement in the literature on the correlation of CsA levels between whole blood and plasma. By linear regression analysis of whole blood and plasma concentrations of CsA in one patient, Wenk et al. (8) obtained the following equation: $y = 0.292x - 35.7$ (where y = values for plasma and x = values for whole blood), with a correlation coefficient of 0.87. Bennett et al. (9), on the other hand, showed that there was a poor correlation ($r = 0.58$, n = 34) between CsA concentrations in the two matrices. Although our results (Fig. 1) are in agreement with those reported by Wenk et al. (8) that there is a good correlation between whole blood and plasma CsA concentrations ($r = 0.93$, n = 39), linear regression analysis of these data is inappropriate, since it has been shown (2) in vitro that the uptake of CsA by erythrocytes is linear over only a narrow range of whole blood concentration (25–500 ng/ml). Saturation of cellular components at higher concentrations of the drug would lead to a nonlinear relationship. The results in Fig. 2 show that this is indeed true in vivo, and a nonlinear relationship was prominent at whole blood CsA levels of greater than 1,000 ng/ml. Because erythrocyte content after saturation would vary with Hct, curves comparing whole blood and plasma CsA levels would be different for different patients. Thus, linear regression analysis of the above data is of little clinical value.

The distribution of CsA between plasma and nonplasma components of the blood of two patients with Hct values of 32.5 and 35% is shown in Fig. 3. These data indicate that in the case of the patient with Hct of 35% (circles), the uptake of CsA by nonplasma components was almost twice as great as that in the other patient at corresponding plasma levels of the drug. Thus, among patients with similar Hct values, there may be significant differences in the cellular affinity for the drug.

Estimation of the cellular/plasma concentration gradient [ratio of nonplasma CsA to plasma CsA (Fig. 4)] of CsA reveals that at low plasma levels of the drug (<100 ng/ml) the cellular associated drug may be as much as 28-fold greater than that present in plasma, indicating that the cellular fractions in blood

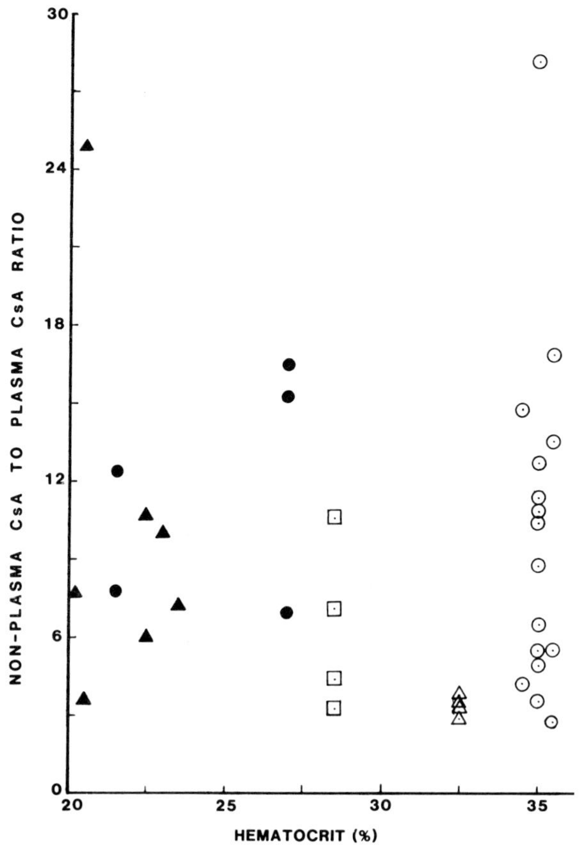

FIG. 6. Comparison of cellular/plasma concentration gradients of cyclosporin A (CsA) and hematocrits, showing variability in the cellular affinity between patients.

have a high affinity for CsA. At higher levels of plasma CsA, the cellular/plasma concentration gradient of the drug gradually dropped to about 3 as cellular components approached saturation. Among the five patients studied, the patient with lower cellular associated CsA (Fig. 3) had the lowest cellular/plasma concentration gradient of the drug (triangles, Fig. 4).

Figure 5 shows that there is a linear relationship when reciprocals of nonplasma CsA concentrations are plotted against the reciprocals of the plasma levels of the drug found in the patient with Hct of 35%. This plot shows that the limit of the reciprocals of nonplasma CsA concentrations would be 1.65×10^{-4} (ng/ml)$^{-1}$ as the reciprocal of the plasma level approaches zero. This leads to the conclusion that the saturation capacity of RIA-measured CsA in the nonplasma component for this patient is 6,060 ng/ml (reciprocal of 1.65×10^{-4}). Although fewer data were available for such analysis of other patients, estimates by linear regression showed that the slopes varied from 0.017 to 0.204, with a standard deviation of 0.074. The intercepts on the ordinate ranged from 0.96×10^{-4} to 2.10×10^{-4} (ng/ml)$^{-1}$, with a standard deviation of 0.47×10^{-4} (ng/ml)$^{-1}$. The saturation capacity (reciprocal of intercept) thus ranged from 4,750 to 10,400 ng/ml.

The distribution of CsA in blood is known to depend on temperature (1,3–7). At plasma CsA levels of less than 200 ng/ml, concentrations of the drug in plasma separated at 4°C may be as low as one-half of those in plasma separated at 37°C (1,4). At higher concentrations, however, as cellular components approach saturation, temperature had little effect on the drug distribution (1). Thus, at low CsA plasma levels, cellular/plasma ratios of the drug would be significantly higher at 4°C than at 37°C, while at levels approaching saturation, the temperature effects would be minimal, and our findings in vitro at 4°C are likely to reflect the in vivo distribution as well.

The results in Fig. 6 show that within the five patients, the maximum cellular/plasma ratio of CsA varied independently of the Hct. Since the affinity of cells for CsA, the Hct, and perhaps the saturation capacity of cells for CsA are probably independent variables, the distribution of CsA in blood can be seen as a complex function and therefore cannot be predicted directly from the RIA measurement of either whole blood or plasma CsA levels alone.

REFERENCES

1. Niederberger W, Lemaire M, Maurer G, Nussbaumer K, Wagner O. Distribution of cyclosporin in blood components and tissues. *Transplant Proc* 1983;15:2419–21.
2. Lemaire M, Tillement JP. Role of lipoproteins and erythrocytes in the in vivo binding and distribution of cyclosporin A in blood. *J Pharm Pharmacol* 1983;34:715–8.
3. Smith JM, Hows JM, Gordon-Smith EC. Stability of cyclosporin A in serum. *J Clin Pathol* 1983;36:41–3.
4. Hows JM, Smith JM. In vitro stability of cyclosporin A [Letter]. *J Clin Pathol* 1983;36:720–1.
5. Robinson CA, Ketchum CH. Monitoring of cyclosporin A: is it possible? *Ther Drug Monit* 1983;5:371–2.
6. Dieperink H. Temperature dependency of cyclosporin plasma levels. *Lancet* 1983;1:416.
7. Bandini G, Ricci P, Visani G, Tura S, Boschi S. Measuring cyclosporin in plasma. *Lancet* 1983;1:762.
8. Wenk M, Follath F, Abisch E. Temperature dependency of apparent cyclosporin A concentrations in plasma. *Clin Chem* 1983;29:1865.
9. Bennett MJ, Carpenter KH, Worthy E, Lilleyman JS. Cyclosporin concentrations in whole blood and plasma. *Clin Chem* 1984;30:817.
10. Keown PA, Stiller NR, Sinclair G, et al. The clinical relevance of cyclosporin blood levels as measured by RIA. *Transplant Proc* 1983;15:2438–41.
11. Beveridge T, Krupp P, McKibbin C. Lymphomas and lymphoproliferative lesions developing under cyclosporin therapy. *Lancet* 1984;1:788.

Therapeutic Drug Monitoring
7:66–73 © 1985 Raven Press, New York

Computer-Assisted Drug Assay Interpretation Based on Bayesian Estimation of Individual Pharmacokinetics: Application to Lidocaine

S. Vozeh, *R. Hillman, †M. Wandell, ‡T. Ludden, and §L. Sheiner

*Division of Clinical Pharmacology, Department of Internal Medicine, Kantonsspital, Basel, Switzerland; *Biotrack, Inc., Sunnyvale, California; †Clinical and Medical Affairs, Genetic Systems Corporation, Seattle, Washington; ‡University of Texas Health Sciences Center, San Antonio, Texas; and §Department of Laboratory Medicine, University of California, San Francisco, California, U.S.A.*

Summary: A microcomputer program for individualized drug level prediction based on Bayesian forecasting is presented. It is written so that the clinician can integrate patient demographics and drug levels to design a new dosage regimen tailored to an individual patient. The program's great flexibility and robustness make it appropriate for realistic clinical settings. A validation with a data set of lidocaine concentrations measured in 18 patients revealed that the program can predict serum lidocaine levels accurately enough to enhance individual patient dosage adjustment within a few hours after a dosage regimen is started. **Key Words:** Bayesian forecasting—Dose prediction—Lidocaine.

Recent advances in drug assay technology (1) allow the determination of serum drug concentrations with high precision (<10% error) within a few minutes. As a result, clinicians have become increasingly interested in how to estimate individual pharmacokinetics and predict future dosage regimens using measured drug levels. Although for some drugs the use of patient characteristics alone (e.g., body weight or creatinine clearance) has been helpful in individualizing drug dosage, for others the additional use of a few serum drug concentrations markedly improves pharmacokinetic parameter estimates and blood level predictability (2,3).

Several methods have been proposed for the estimation of individual pharmacokinetic parameters on the basis of one or more drug level determinations (4–6). Most of them, however, were developed with a particular drug in mind and are either drug or dosing regimen dependent, in the latter case requiring fixed schedules for sampling drug levels. A general method, first proposed by Sheiner et al. (7) and recently described in more detail by Sheiner et al. (8) uses an empirical Bayes approach. Apart from its general applicability, the most important difference between Bayesian and other approaches is that Bayesian methods use not only the information contained in the drug levels but also prior knowledge of the pharmacokinetic characteristics of the drug within a specific population. Although this approach has been shown to provide more accurate predictions (9,10), a nonlinear regression program is required to implement it. Programs using Bayesian forecasting have been described for micro- (11,12) and minicomputers (13). However, reports on the clinical utility of these programs are limited because of the difficulty of using them in a realistic clinical setting. As a result, to the extent that clinicians use aids, they still largely use nomograms

Address correspondence and reprint requests to Dr. M. Wandell at Genetic Systems Corporation, 3005 First Avenue, Seattle, WA 98121, U.S.A.

TABLE 1. *Estimates of population pharmacokinetic parameters for lidocaine*

Fixed effects		Random effects[a]	
Clearance *(CL)*	0.58 L/h/kg	$\sigma\eta_{CL}$	60%
V_1	0.64 L/kg	$\sigma\eta_{V_1}$	37%
K_{12}	1.35 h^{-1}	σ_{ϵ}[b]	21%
K_{21}	0.53 h^{-1}		
θ_5 (% decrease in *CL* with CHF)	46%		
θ_6 (% decrease in V_1 with CHF)	24%		

CHF, congestive heart failure. See text for description of parameters.
[a]Expressed as coefficient of variation.
[b]Intraindividual residual error between predicted and observed drug level.

or simple graphical methods for individual dose adjustment. The software package described herein was developed so that the clinical use of the Bayesian forecasting method could be furthered by a software package that is "user-friendly," generally applicable, and robust enough to be implemented in a routine clinical setting. The software was written to run on a Syva LP6500 (HP 85B) microcomputer system.

Although the package includes several drugs (lidocaine, theophylline, and aminoglycosides) the software and its validation for lidocaine are described here. Although distinct pharmacokinetic and statistical models are used for each drug, the general features of the program apply to all.

PHARMACOKINETIC AND STATISTICAL MODEL

The pharmacokinetics of lidocaine are described by a two-compartment open body model with elimination from the central compartment. The model is defined by four parameters: total body clearance *(CL)*, volume of distribution of the central compartment (V_1), and two microconstants (K_{12} and K_{21}).

The Bayesian approach requires estimates of the population mean and the interindividual variability for each parameter. These estimates were derived from more than 300 serum concentration measurements collected in 42 patients treated for arrhythmias after myocardial infarction (14). Alternative statistical models for describing the distribution of the pharmacokinetic parameters in the patient population were compared, and the effect of various factors (e.g., sex and weight) on lidocaine pharmacokinetics was tested using the Nonlinear Mixed Effects Model (NONMEM) (15). The model describing the interindividual variability of *CL* and V_1 in the population assumes a normal distribution for the logarithmic transformation of the parameters. Any remaining variability (residual error) between the drug assay result(s) and the concentration(s) predicted by the model is also assumed to be log-normally distributed. Both these assumptions are based on results of NONMEM analysis, which clearly indicated that log-additive error models were superior to simple additive ones. No distinct components of interindividual variability could be assigned to the microconstants K_{12} and K_{21}. The population parameters values are shown in Table 1.

Both *CL* and V_1 are normalized for body weight and are influenced by congestive heart failure (CHF). A fractional decrease in *CL* (additive under a log transformation) of 45% is assumed in patients with moderate CHF or liver function impairment. In patients with mild or moderate CHF, the predicted mean V_1 is decreased by 24%. For more detailed discussion of the NONMEM analysis see refs. 16 and 17.

Lidocaine is assumed to be administered by either an intravenous infusion or an intravenous bolus (modeled as a short infusion over 2 min). In a routine clinical setting, dosage information is frequently uncertain or incomplete. To accommodate such situations, the program allows the user to input a dose even if the actual amount of drug administered during a specified period of time cannot be ascertained. The degrees of uncertainty can be indicated by the user as small (e.g., irregular infusion rate), moderate (error more than 30%), large (e.g., line disconnected), or dose completely unknown. This option is implemented by defining an additional parameter, δ, for each uncertain dosing period. It is estimated along with *CL* and V_1 and represents the fraction of the dose actually administered. Each uncertain dose is multiplied by its corresponding δ. The "population value" for each δ is set to 1, and the "interindividual" variability (σ_{δ}) depends on the degree of uncertainty: 65% for small, 120% for moderate, 350% for large, and

640% for completely unknown dosage (δ is also assumed to be log-normally distributed; variability is here expressed as a coefficient of variation for convenience only). The greater the value of σ_δ (i.e., the greater the uncertainty) the more δ is allowed to differ from its initial value. For drugs administered on an outpatient basis (e.g., theophylline), the same approach is used to model compliance. A data check, included at the end of the dosage input, warns the user if the uncertainty in dosage is too high to obtain reliable parameter estimates.

The complete pharmacokinetic model relating serum concentration to V_1, CL, and δ can be written as follows:

$$C = \sum_{j=1}^{n} \frac{D_j \cdot \delta_j}{V_1 \cdot BW}\left[\frac{(k_{21} - \alpha)(1 - e^{\alpha T_j})}{\alpha(\alpha - \beta)} e^{-\alpha t_j} + \frac{(\beta - k_{21})(1 - e^{\beta T_j})}{\beta(\alpha - \beta)} e^{-\beta t_j}\right] \quad (1)$$

where

$$\alpha = \frac{1}{2}\left[K_{10} + K_{12} + K_{21} + \sqrt{(K_{10} + K_{12} + K_{21})^2 - 4K_{21}K_{10}}\right]$$

$$\beta = \frac{1}{2}\left[K_{10} + K_{12} + K_{21} - \sqrt{(K_{10} + K_{12} + K_{21})^2 - 4K_{21}K_{10}}\right]$$

and

$$K_{10} = \frac{CL}{V_1}$$

V_1 and CL are both adjusted depending on the degree of heart failure and liver disease (see above); BW is the body weight in kilograms; D_j is the jth infusion rate, δ_j is the parameter associated with uncertain doses; and t_j is the time between the start of the infusion and the time of the serum concentration measurement. T_j is equal to t_j if the jth infusion is still running and to the duration of the jth infusion otherwise.

The theoretical basis for the objective function (i.e., the function that has to be minimized with respect to the estimated parameters) used in Bayesian forecasting has been described in detail elsewhere (10). For lidocaine, it takes the following form:

$$\sum_{i=1}^{N} \frac{(\log C_i - \log \hat{C}_i)^2}{\sigma_\epsilon \cdot q^{r_i}} + \sum_{k=1}^{m} \frac{(\log \theta_k - \log \hat{\theta}_k)^2}{\sigma_{\eta k}} \quad (2)$$

where $\log C_i$ and $\log \hat{C}_i$ are the observed and calculated serum concentrations (log-transformed), respectively; θ_1 is CL, θ_2 is V_1, and θ_3 through θ_7 are the optional parameters; $\delta \cdot \sigma_\epsilon$ is the population parameter estimate of the standard deviation of the log residual error (Table 1). The expression q^{r_i} is a weighting function that acts to weight the impact of levels taken in the past less than recently obtained measurements. Decreasing weighting of old data in adaptive control systems was first proposed by Kalman (18) and applied in a similar form as herein by Peck et al. (11). r_i is the absolute difference between the sampling time of the most recent serum concentration and the ith measurement. q takes the value 1.005 for patients without either acute myocardial infarction (MI) or signs of CHF, 1.010 for patients with either MI or CHF, and 1.015 for patients with both MI and CHF. As q increases, the impact of past serum concentration measurement decreases more rapidly with time. The weighting function thus reflects clinical experience indicating that the lidocaine pharmacokinetic parameters may change more rapidly with time in patients with MI or CHF, without specifying the direction of the change. The upper bound on $\sigma_\epsilon \cdot q^{r_i}$ has been arbitrarily set at 0.5, approximately corresponding to the interindividual variability in lidocaine total body clearance.

PROGRAM DESCRIPTION

The general layout of the program is shown in Fig. 1 and consists of four main sections: data entry, editing, storage, and prediction. The user is taken through either a menu-driven "beginner's" version or an advanced version. Both versions include several safeguards against inappropriate data entry, such as "locking-out" unused keys during data entry and computation modes.

Data Entry

The data entry section allows input of patient identification and demographic data (e.g., name, birth date, height), drug level history, and dosage history.

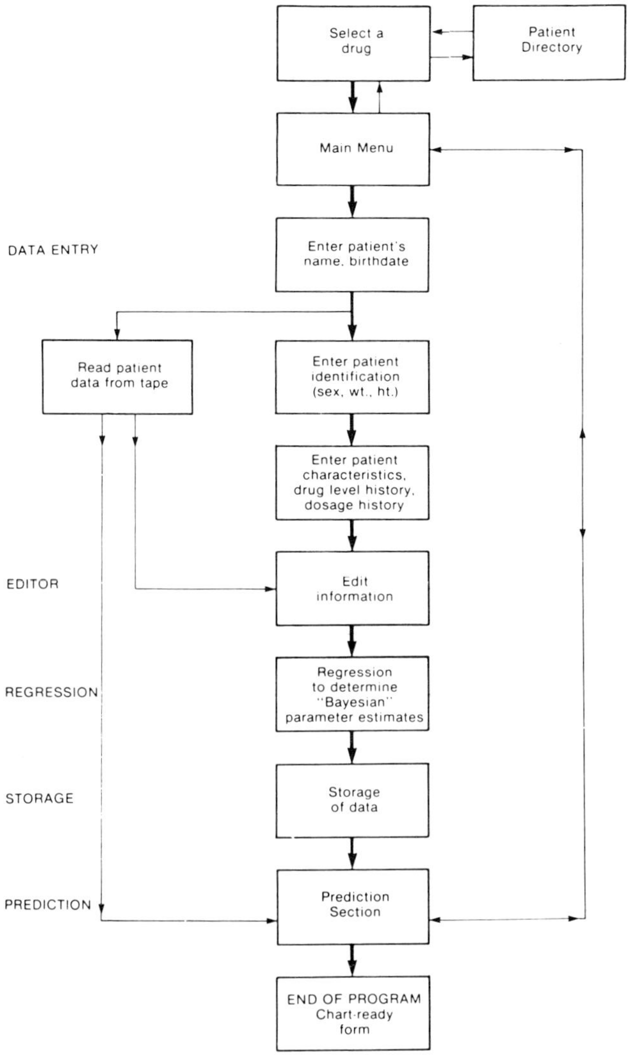

FIG. 1. Flow chart showing organization of the program.

Any information not available to the user can be entered as unknown, and default population values are used (although the data remains coded as unknown).

The patient characteristics are entered via a menu that is tailored specifically to each drug and the factors known to affect its pharmacokinetics. For lidocaine, the user is asked about degree of heart failure, presence or absence of liver disease, and occurrence of acute MI. Times of changes in disease severity (up to four per patient) can also be entered for heart failure and liver disease.

As many as 10 drug levels may be entered at any time after the first dose for a given patient. The dosage history, also entered via a menu, allows the user to specify unknown or uncertain dosage, and allows con-

```
********************************
    Lidocaine Predictor
JOHNSON,L
01,02,04(M,D,Y)
Sex:      Male
Weight:  60 kg
Height:  Unknown (170 cm assumed)
Smoker:  Yes
Acute M.I.:      Yes
Heart Failure:  Moderate
Liver Disease:  Absent
================================
        *Dosage History*
    PERIOD        Mode  Dose   Compl
No  from    to          (mg)
--------------------------------
1   20:00         i.v.  100    Inpt
    16Jun         bolus
2   20:00  00:00  i.v.  120/h  Inpt
    16Jun  17Jun  inf.
3   23:00         i.v.  50     Inpt
    16Jun         bolus
================================
```

FIG. 2. Chart-ready report form: summary of patient identification, characteristics, and dosage history.

venient entry of various rates of administration. Each patient file can accommodate up to 20 dosage "periods" (a period is defined as a single dose, a constant infusion rate, or multiple doses administered at regular intervals).

Throughout the process, the program makes plausibility checks to guard against errors in data entry. For example, the user is warned if drug levels are outside the range of the particular enzyme multiplied immunoassay technique (EMIT); if dosages exceed package insert recommendations; or if dosage schedules have gaps or overlaps in time. A warning is issued if the uncertainty in dosage could result in unreliable parameter estimates (see above). In all cases, the user is allowed to proceed without corrections if that is desired. In addition, the user is given frequent opportunities to change information while entering data. This feature includes an "error" option that sends the program back to the previous input. Once all information has been entered, the user can edit all data with a full-function editor and then obtain a chart-ready copy (Fig. 2) of the data entered, if that is desired.

Regression

The regression section is automatically called on completion of data entry and first displays the population parameters adjusted for the patient factors (e.g., weight, heart failure) known to affect the parameters. The program then iterates until the Bayesian Objective Function (Eq. 2) is minimized, at which time the

```
        *Concentrations*

No      Time        Measured  Predicted
                     (mg/l)     (mg/l)
-----------------------------------------
1   22:00/16Jun      1.5        1.7
2   00:00/17Jun      1.9        2.1
=========================================

**     Estimates of Patient's      **
** Pharmacokinetic Parameters **

Parameter    Mean    Conf.Int.(68%)
-----------------------------------------
Clearance
 (l/h)         50.4     40.9  -   62.1
Vc (l)         36.2     26.9  -   48.7
k12 (l/h)     1.35         constant
k21 (l/h)      .53         constant
 Terminal half life:     2.8 hours
=========================================
```

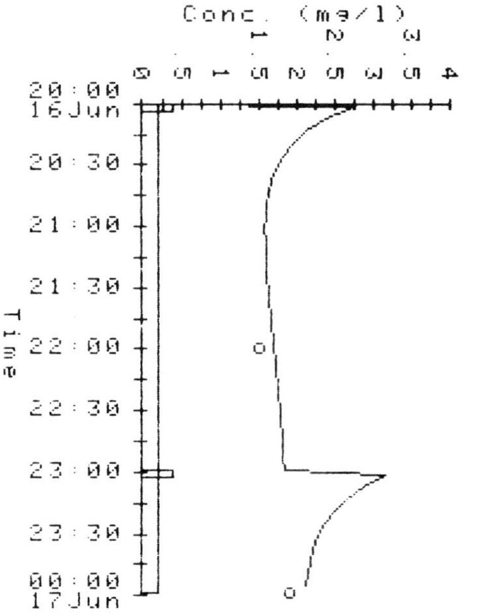

FIG. 3. Measured and predicted drug levels: individualized pharmacokinetic parameters and graph reported by regression section. l, liters; l/h, liters per hour; conf. int., confidence interval (which represents ±1 SD or approximately 68%).

individual predicted pharmacokinetic parameters *CL* and V_1 and their confidence interval (±1 SD) are printed. The two microconstants, K_{12} and K_{21}, assumed constant over the entire population are also incorporated in the output (Fig. 3). The user is informed if the parameter estimates of *CL* and V_1 are more than 2 SD from the population values. In addition, a graph showing the historical measured drug concentration(s) and estimated future concentration-versus-time profile is displayed and printed on request.

Data Storage

Following the regression section, the user is given the opportunity to store the patient data for later use. The program provides a directory of all stored patient information and allows for retrieval of either all previously entered information or the last parameter estimates.

Prediction

The prediction section can be used to forecast future serum drug concentration profiles. It is divided into two parts, as follows:

1. The "steady-state" section, which provides tables showing typical dosage regimens (e.g., constant infusion of lidocaine) required to maintain a desired steady-state level within the therapeutic range, including confidence intervals, as shown in Fig. 4. Alternatively, the user can construct an individual table of dosages, and the program will provide the steady-state levels and their respective confidence intervals. The disease state of the patient can then be changed and new tables generated.
2. The "non–steady-state" section allows the user to enter any additional dosage regimen(s) and/or disease changes and obtain a graph as well as point estimates (with confidence intervals) of future drug concentrations, as shown in Fig. 5.

Thus, the prediction section is designed to aid the clinician and does not prescribe any rigid schedule or fixed dosage regimen. It can be used with either population "estimates" or individualized parameters (Fig. 1). A hypothetical case can be simulated, or expected drug dosage requirements can be obtained before any drug levels have actually been taken.

The average time for an experienced user to enter a realistic case and obtain a forecast is 5–10 min. This includes the time necessary for the regression calculations, which require 1–5 min depending on the complexity of the case.

VALIDATION

Additional data from the same hospital (Kantonsspital, Basel, Switzerland), which was the source of the data yielding population parameter estimates, demonstrated excellent performance of the Bayesian algorithm when predicting serum concentrations on the basis of one or two lidocaine drug levels (14). To further validate the approach, data obtained in a different setting (University of Texas Health Science

```
********** PREDICTION **********

Infusion Rate      Css        Conf.Int.
  (mg/h)          (mg/l)        (68%)
---------------------------------------
    90              1.8       1.3 - 2.4
   135              2.7       2.0 - 3.6
   180              3.6       2.7 - 4.7
   225              4.5       3.4 - 5.9
---------------------------------------
Heart Failure:Moderate
Liver Disease:Absent
=======================================
```

FIG. 4. Table of predicted steady-state concentrations.

Center, San Antonio, TX, U.S.A.) were used. Serum lidocaine concentrations were measured using EMIT in 18 patients, 7 with heart failure, receiving lidocaine for ventricular ectopic beats. Blood samples were taken at 2–4 h after initiation of therapy and provided to the program as feedback for forecasting 10–14 h later (forecast 1) and 20–30 h later (forecast 2).

As a measure of accuracy and precision, the mean prediction error (measured minus predicted drug level) and its standard deviation are reported, respectively. A *t* test was used to detect statistically significant bias, i.e., whether the mean prediction error was different from zero. No significant bias was found. To test for differences in precision, the variances of the prediction error were compared using an *F* test. The results are summarized in Table 2. The precision and accuracy obtained when using only population pharmacokinetic parameters (i.e., no drug levels feedback) are also shown. A marked improvement in precision can be observed even when only one drug level is used, in agreement with previous findings (14).

TABLE 2. *Accuracy and precision of drug level forecasts*

	Individualized pharmacokinetic parameters (n = 18)		Population pharmacokinetic parameters (n = 17)	
	FC1	FC2	FC1	FC2
Mean prediction error (mg/L)	−0.10	−0.09	−0.084	0.082
Standard deviation	0.20	0.29	0.36	0.61
Coefficient of variation	11%	23%	32%	100%
t value[a]	NS (0.087)	NS (0.021)	NS (0.085)	NS (0.020)
F value[b]	3.24[c]	4.30[d]		

FC1 and FC2, forecasts 1 and 2, respectively (see the text); NS, not significant ($p > 0.05$).

[a]Mean error vs. 0.

[b]Error standard deviation, feedback predictions vs. population-based predictions.

[c]Significant ($p < 0.05$).

[d]Significant ($p < 0.01$).

DISCUSSION

A program for individualized drug level prediction based on Bayesian forecasting has been presented. It is written so that the clinician can integrate patient demographics and drug levels to design a new dosage regimen tailored to an individual patient. The program's great flexibility and robustness make it appropriate for realistic clinical settings. The program can predict serum lidocaine levels [as shown here and in a previous report (14)] accurately enough to enhance individual patient dosage adjustment within a few hours after a dosage regimen is begun.

Two alternative methods for the estimation of individual lidocaine pharmacokinetics have been proposed in the literature. Zito et al. (19) reported the use of indocyanine green clearance to estimate individual lidocaine clearance values. Although their data showed excellent correlation, the method required 10 blood samples for determination of indocyanine green concentrations, which limits its applicability under clinical circumstances. In addition, their prediction accuracy could not be reproduced by Bax et al. (20). Apart from being simpler and therefore more suitable for clinical use, the Bayesian method has two additional advantages. First, it yields individual estimates of both the volume of distribution and the total body clearance, allowing prediction of non–steady-state levels. Second, the samples used for feedback provide additional information as to whether the lidocaine serum concentration was in the therapeutic range at the time of sampling. Routledge et al. (6) recently described a close correlation between lidocaine concentration 1 h after a fixed loading dose and total body clearance in 33 subjects. They suggested the use of this relationship for individual dose adjustment. However, this method is applicable only to one particular dose and time of sampling, and has been tested in only six subjects to date.

Our results and the experience gathered in the last few years (9,10,14) indicate that Bayesian forecasting is superior to alternative nonstochastic methods with respect to both general applicability and prediction accuracy. However, the clinical application of the former method is still limited because of the lack of appropriate computer software. The development of a user-friendly and robust program package that can be implemented on an inexpensive microcomputer

PERIOD No	from	to	Mode	Dose (mg)	Compl
1	00:01 17Jun	18:00 17Jun	i.v. inf.	180/h	Inpt

Concentrations

No	Time	Predicted (mg/l)	Conf. Int. (68%)
1	07:00/17Jun	3.4	2.6- 4.4
2	16:00/17Jun	3.6	2.7- 4.7

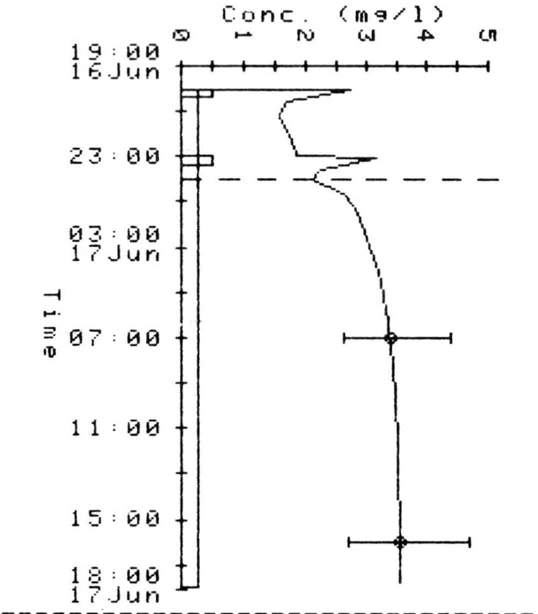

FIG. 5. Graphic display of predicted serum drug concentrations in response to a user-specific dosage regimen.

system should help bridge the gap between the theoretical advantages of this sophisticated forecasting method and its practical application.

In addition to improving patient care, rapid prediction methods represent an important tool for investigation of the serum concentration–effect relationships in controlled clinical trials. Further, such predictions can suggest future optimal sampling strategies, thereby aiding the clinician in determining when to take a sample for determining the next serum drug level. For many drugs, the clinical significance of achieving an optimum serum concentration in routinely treated patients can only be determined if the serum concentration can be prospectively adjusted within a narrow range (21). The development of sophisticated forecasting devices thus helps to define the clinical situations in which routine use of serum concentration measurements is warranted.

Acknowledgment: This work was supported by the Prof. Max Cloëtta Foundation. Dr. Vozeh was a visiting scientist at Syva Co. during the development of the computer software described in this article.

REFERENCES

1. Oellerich M. Enzyme immunoassays in clinical chemistry: present status and trends. *J Clin Chem Clin Biochem* 1980;18:197–208.
2. Sheiner LB, Halkin H, Peck C, Rosenberg B, Melmon KL. Improved computer assisted digoxin therapy. *Ann Intern Med* 1975;82:619–62.
3. Vozeh S, Koelz A, Martin E, Magun H, Scollo-Lavizzari G, Follath F. Predictability of phenytoin serum levels by nomograms and clinicians. *Eur Neurol* 1980;19:345–52.
4. Chiou WL, Gadalla MAF, Peng GW. Method for the rapid estimation of the total body clearance and adjustment of dosage regimens in patients during a constant rate intravenous infusion. *J Pharmacokinet Biopharm* 1978;6:135–51.
5. Anderson G, Koup J, Slaughter R, Drew Edwards W, Resman B, Hook E. Evaluation of two methods for estimating theophylline clearance prior to achieving steady state. *Ther Drug Monit* 1981;3:325–32.
6. Routledge PA, Stargel WW, Barchowsky A, Wagner GS, Shand DG. Control of lidocaine therapy: new perspectives. *Ther Drug Monit* 1982;4:265–70.
7. Sheiner LB, Rosenberg B, Melmon KL. Modelling of individual pharmacokinetics for computer aided drug dosage. *Computer Biomed Res* 1972;5:441–59.
8. Sheiner LB, Beal SB, Rosenberg B, Marathe VV. Forecasting individual pharmacokinetics. *Clin Pharmacol Ther* 1979;26:294–305.
9. Vozeh S, Muir KT, Follath F, Sheiner LB. Predicting individual phenytoin dosage. *J Pharmacokinet Biopharm* 1981;9:131.
10. Sheiner LB, Beal SB. Bayesian individualization of pharmacokinetics: simple implementation and comparison with non-Bayesian methods. *J Pharm Sci* 1982;71:1344–8.
11. Peck CC, Brown WD, Sheiner LB, Schuster BG. A microcomputer drug (theophylline) dosing program which assists and teaches physicians. In: *Proceedings of the Fourth Annual Symposium on Computer Applications in Medical Care*, 1980;994–8.
12. Sheiner LB. *Advise: user's manual.* A technical report of the Division of Clinical Pharmacology, University of California, San Francisco, California, 1981.
13. Kelman AW, Whiting B, Bryson SM. OPT: a package of computer programs for parameter optimization in clinical pharmacokinetics. *Br J Clin Pharmacol* 1982;14:247–56.
14. Vozeh S, Berger M, Wenk M, Ritz R, Follath F. Rapid prediction of individual dosage requirements for lidocaine. *Clin Pharmacokinet* 1984;9:354–63.
15. Beal SB, Sheiner LB. *NONMEM user's guide.* A technical report of the Division of Clinical Pharmacology, University of California, San Francisco, California, 1979.
16. Vozeh S, Katz G, Steiner V, Follath F. Population pharmacokinetic parameters in patients treated with oral mexiletine. *Eur J Clin Pharmacol* 1982;23:445–51.
17. Vozeh S, Wenk M, Follath F. Experience with NONMEM. *Drug Metab Rev* 1984;15:305–15.

18. Kalman RE. Design of self-optimizing control system. *Trans Am Soc Mech Engrs* 1958;80:468.
19. Zito RA, Reid PR, Longstretch JA. Variability of early lidocaine levels in patients. *Am Heart J* 1977;94:292–6.
20. Bax NDS, Tucker GT, Woods HF. Lidocaine and indocyanine green kinetics in patients following myocardial infarction. *Br J Clin Pharmacol* 1980;10:356–61.
21. Vozeh S, Kewitz G, Perruchoud A, et al. Theophylline serum concentration and therapeutic effect in severe acute bronchial obstruction: the optimal use of intravenous aminophylline. *Am Rev Resp Dis* 1982;125:181–4.

Therapeutic Drug Monitoring
7:74–80

Comparison of Eight Phenytoin Dosing Methods in Institutionalized Patients

Nora Flint, Larry M. Lopez, J. Daniel Robinson, Charles Williams, and Ronald B. Salem

Departments of Pharmacy Practice and Pediatrics, University of Florida Colleges of Pharmacy and Medicine, Gainesville, Florida, U.S.A.

Summary: Until now, no evaluation of phenytoin dosing methods has been undertaken in a large group of patients, to our knowledge. The goal of this study was to determine which of eight different dosing methods most accurately predicts a phenytoin steady-state concentration. Seventy-six patients were chosen, retrospectively, from a state-funded institution for the mentally retarded. Eligibility criteria included two or more different doses of phenytoin and corresponding plasma concentrations. Relative predictive performance was determined by comparing results of simple linear regression. Also, relative bias and precision were determined by comparing mean prediction errors, root mean squared errors, and respective 95% confidence intervals. Of the methods requiring one dose–concentration pair, Rambeck's nomogram was the best predictor of phenytoin concentrations. The methods requiring two known doses and plasma concentrations were more accurate. Their predictive performance was equivalent, although use of the Tozer equation might be preferred for its convenience. None of the methods tested were sufficiently precise to substitute for confirmatory serum phenytoin concentrations. **Key Words:** Phenytoin—Phenytoin dosing.

There is little dispute that optimal seizure control with phenytoin is attainable in patients with normal renal function when plasma concentration is maintained within the therapeutic range of 10–20 μg/ml (1–7). However, it can be difficult to achieve this range with standard dosage regimens because of the presence of nonlinearity of phenytoin pharmacokinetics and large intersubject differences in kinetic parameters (8–15). Consequently, alteration of a phenytoin dosage regimen may cause a disproportionately large change in plasma concentration. Numerous dosing methods (10,16–18) based on individual pharmacokinetic parameters have been developed to facilitate attainment of an optimal phenytoin plasma concentration.

Address correspondence and reprint requests to Dr. L. M. Lopez at University of Florida College of Pharmacy, Box J-4, JHMHC, Gainesville, FL 32610, U.S.A.

In general, the relationship between mean steady-state plasma concentration (C_{ss}), daily dose *(D)*, fraction absorbed *(F)*, and drug clearance *(CL)* is represented by the following equation:

$$F \times D = CL \times C_{ss} \quad (1)$$

For drugs following linear pharmacokinetic characteristics, *CL* is constant and independent of C_{ss}, provided renal, metabolic, and other clearance processes remain unchanged. In this situation, doubling of dose would result in doubling of steady-state plasma concentrations.

However, in the case of drugs following nonlinear pharmacokinetics, e.g., phenytoin, *CL* varies with C_{ss} as shown in the following equation:

$$CL = \frac{V_{max}}{K_m + C_{ss}} \quad (2)$$

where V_{max} is the maximum rate at which the drug

TABLE 1. *Summary of phenytoin dosing methods evaluated*

Method	Operational synopsis	Reference
1	Equation requiring only body surface area to predict a phenytoin dose	19
2A	Equation requiring one dose–plasma concentration to predict a second plasma concentration	20
2B	Equation requiring two dose–plasma concentrations to predict a third plasma concentration	20
3	Nomogram requiring one dose–plasma concentration to predict a dose that will achieve either 15 or 20 mg/ml	9
4	Nomogram requiring one dose–plasma concentration to predict a second plasma concentration	21
5	Nomogram requiring one dose–plasma concentration to predict a second plasma concentration	15
6	Graph requiring one dose–plasma concentration to predict a second plasma concentration	20
7	Graph requiring two dose–plasma concentrations to predict a third plasma concentration	16
8	Graph requiring two dose–plasma concentrations to predict a third plasma concentration	14
9	Graph requiring two dose–plasma concentrations to predict a third plasma concentration	15

can be metabolized and K_m is the plasma concentration when half-V_{max} is achieved. The relationship between D and C_{ss} is no longer proportional and is illustrated in the following equations:

$$D = \frac{V_{max} \times C_{ss}}{K_m + C_{ss}} \quad (3)$$

$$C_{ss} = \frac{D \times K_m}{V_{max} - D} \quad (4)$$

Equations 3 and 4 constitute the foundation upon which all methods for altering phenytoin dosage regimens rest. The common goal of these methods is to acquire an accurate estimate of an individual's V_{max} and K_m values for purposes of solving either Eq. 3 or 4.

Several studies have evaluated specific methods of predicting steady-state concentrations of phenytoin (Table 1). Some utilize one known plasma concentration and corresponding dose to predict another concentration with a new chosen dose. Other graphic methods require at least two steady-state plasma concentrations with corresponding doses to achieve a predicted concentration from a subsequent dose. Richens and Dunlop (9) proposed use of a nomogram utilizing a single known steady-state concentration and corresponding dose to predict a dose required to achieve a plasma concentration of either 15 or 20 μg/ml. However, this nomogram assumes an average K_m value of 3.8 μg/ml and does not allow for interpatient variation. Such variation can be secondary to differences in age, sex, height, weight, genetics, disease states, and duration of phenytoin intake (22). Despite this flaw, its use by others was found to be safe, since its predictions resulted in plasma concentrations that were either therapeutic or subtherapeutic most of the time. The greatest potential for toxicity with this method apparently occurs when an initial dose of 300 mg or more produces a steady-state plasma concentration of less than 5 μg/ml (18).

Rambeck et al. (21) reportedly developed an improved version of the Richens and Dunlop nomogram. It requires a single steady-state plasma concentration and corresponding dose, but does not limit itself to predicting doses required for plasma levels of 15 or 20 μg/ml. Any desired plasma level could be used to determine the needed dose. The authors concluded that the revised nomogram was superior, since it gave more accurate predictions of the change in plasma level after a dose change had occurred (21).

A third nomogram available for prediction of phenytoin doses and steady-state concentrations is that reported by Martin et al. (15). As with the other two nomograms, its use is also based on only a single, accurate steady-state plasma concentration and corresponding daily dose. This method determines how different the concentration for an individual patient is from the expected concentration. In addition, it can also predict a dose needed to attain a desired steady-state concentration. When Murphy et al. (18) evaluated this method, they found it to produce the greatest percentage of high or potentially toxic predictions.

There are four graphical methods available for obtaining assessments of individual K_m and V_{max} values (14–16,20). Three of the four methods require two or more accurate steady-state concentrations (14–16). The fourth method (20), requires only one steady-state concentration and utilizes orbits in the graph to predict a K_m and V_{max} for the individual patient. These graphs have not been tested extensively in a clinical setting.

Schumacher (23) evaluated those graphical methods requiring multiple C_{ss} values and concluded that the direct linear plot developed by Mullen (16) was the easiest and most rapid. However, this method appeared to be least accurate when steady-state concentrations used to construct the plot were much lower than those concentrations desired by the clinician. Other investigators (18,21) also found the direct linear plot safe and accurate.

Until now, as far as we are aware, no simultaneous evaluation of these dosing methods has been undertaken in a large group of patients. Also, previous evaluations of phenytoin dosing methods have compared no more than six different methods. Consequently, the goal of this study was to determine which of eight different dosing methods most accurately predicts phenytoin steady-state concentrations in a large group of institutionalized patients.

METHODS

Patient Selection

Patients were chosen from the clients residing at a state-funded institution for the mentally retarded (Sunland Center, Gainesville, FL, U.S.A.). This institution currently accommodates approximately 920 patients, and all age groups are represented. Nearly 40% of the clients in this institution have a known seizure disorder, and most of these receive phenytoin as part of their antiseizure therapy. Eligibility criteria for this study include two or more different doses of phenytoin and corresponding plasma concentrations obtained at least 4 weeks after initiating the dose or dosage change.

Patient eligibility was dependent on history of phenytoin use and observed steady-state plasma concentrations. Patients were excluded from the study if a demonstrated change in hepatic or renal function was found during the period of analysis. These changes were defined as either a rise in laboratory test results [e.g., serum glutamic-oxaloacetic transaminase (SGOT), serum glutamic-pyruvic transaminase (SGPT), serum creatinine] into abnormal range or a return to normal limits. In addition, a patient was excluded if his or her body weight changed more than 10% over the period of analysis.

Design

This study was conducted as a retrospective review of medical records of each patient with a history of phenytoin intake. Pharmacy records were reviewed to determine the dose of phenytoin received and the corresponding time period each patient received that particular dose.

TABLE 2. *Dilantin Kapseal Equivalent (DKE) values*

Dose/dosage form	DKE (mg)
100 mg = 1 capsule	100
130 mg = 1 capsule (100 mg) + 1 capsule (30 mg)	130
150 mg = 1 capsule (100 mg) + 1 tablet (50 mg)	154
250 mg = 2 capsules + 1 tablet	254
300 mg = 3 capsules	300
375 mg = 15 ml suspension (125 mg/5 ml)	408

An individual's dose and corresponding known plasma concentration were then utilized to predict a second concentration. This predicted concentration was compared with that recorded in the patient's chart.

Data Collection

Additional information tabulated from the charts of eligible patients included demographic data (e.g., age, weight, height, sex), dominant seizure type, and seizure frequency.

Each patient's complete drug regimen was noted over the period of time bordered by the chosen phenytoin concentrations. Any change in drug therapy was carefully dated, particular attention being given to drugs known to influence the disposition of phenytoin (e.g., other anticonvulsants, isoniazid, phenylbutazone, disulfiram, and cimetidine).

The specific phenytoin product was noted so that differences in bioavailability could be considered. All products of phenytoin were included in the study and transformed into a "Dilantin Kapseal Equivalent" (DKE) value. For example, a 100-mg capsule of Dilantin (phenytoin sodium) was equivalent to 100 mg DKE, and a 30-mg capsule of Dilantin was equivalent to 30 mg DKE, whereas a 50-mg tablet of Dilantin (phenytoic acid) was equivalent to 54 mg DKE, and a 125-mg Dilantin suspension was equivalent to 136 mg DKE (24). Other examples are summarized in Table 2.

Since several concentrations were often available from the same dose, criteria for determining the appropriate concentration to use in data analysis were developed. These criteria are summarized in Table 3. Reported plasma values were utilized in chronological order, i.e., the first level was used to predict the second level, and the first and second levels were used to predict the third level. To control potential bias in solving for predicted drug concentrations, all predic-

TABLE 3. *Inclusion and exclusion criteria for phenytoin concentrations*

Dosing methods	Inclusion	Exclusion
2A, 4, 5, 6 (only one prior phenytoin concentration needed)	1. Use the most recent value. 2. Concomitant drug therapy will be unchanged for the interval between obtaining levels.	1. An increased dose which results in a concentration that does not increase.
2B, 7, 8, 9 (all require at least two prior phenytoin concentrations)	1. Use the two most recent levels. 2. If more than two levels are available, use the two that are closest to the therapeutic range. 3. If more than two levels are available, use those which are nonlinear in relation to one another.	1. Same as entry no. 1 above. 2. Difference between two phenytoin concentrations is proportional to corresponding dose change.

tions were performed and tabulated before subsequent actual values were obtained.

Analysis of Phenytoin

Phenytoin was assayed by a gas-liquid chromatographic procedure previously described (25). This method has been used by the same laboratory for the past 10 years. The coefficient of variation of the assay has been determined from past quality control studies to be 5%.

Data Analysis

Mean actual and predicted phenytoin concentrations were compared using Student's t statistic for paired data. Individual actual and predicted values were further compared using simple linear regression. Multiplicative and additive biases were evaluated respectively by comparing observed slope with unity and the observed y-intercept with zero using Student's t statistic. Bias and precision were further evaluated by constricting a 95% confidence interval about the mean prediction error (MPE) and root mean squared prediction error (RMSE) for each method (26). In all instances, observed differences in data were considered significant if the corresponding p value was less than 0.05.

RESULTS

Charts of 360 patients receiving phenytoin were screened for inclusion and exclusion criteria. Plasma phenytoin concentrations from a total of 76 patients (21.1%) (53 male, 23 female) were eventually accepted for analysis. The patients' ages ranged from 13 to 65 years (mean ± SD, 32 ± 10 years).

Table 4 summarizes the various comparisons of actual and predicted phenytoin concentrations. Data are divided between those methods requiring a single known phenytoin concentration and those requiring at least two known phenytoin concentrations.

Mean predicted values for methods requiring at least two prior phenytoin concentrations were, without exception, lower than their corresponding actual values. In contrast, three of four mean predicted values from methods needing only one prior phenytoin concentration were higher than their actual counterparts. All of these differences, however, failed to achieve statistical significance.

For those methods requiring a single known phenytoin level, correlation between actual and predicted values was greatest with method 4. The observed correlation coefficient from method 2A was similar, and both were considerably greater than those associated with methods 5 and 6. The y-intercept and slope for method 4 were also closer to zero and unity, respectively, than those of any of the other methods. Use of method 5 only was associated with a y-intercept and slope significantly different from zero and unity, respectively. For these methods, MPEs were similar in magnitude, and the confidence interval for each included zero and overlapped with each other. The RMSEs for these methods were also similar, although no corresponding confidence interval contained zero.

Correlations between actual and predicted phenytoin concentrations resulting from use of methods requiring two known levels were similar for three of the

TABLE 4. *Comparison of phenytoin dosing methods*

Methods	Phenytoin concn. (μg/ml) Actual	Phenytoin concn. (μg/ml) Predicted	Correlation coefficient (*r*)	*y*-intercept (μg/ml)	Slope	MPE (μg/ml)	MPE—95% confidence interval (μg/ml)	RMSE (μg/ml)	RMSE—95% confidence interval (μg/ml)
Requiring one prior phenytoin concn.									
2A	12.7	13.9	0.60	−2.23	1.27	−1.19	−4.18 to 1.80	9.05	6.03 to 12.07
4	14.0	14.5	0.61	0.93	0.96	−0.44	−2.40 to 1.52	6.93	4.11 to 9.74
5	14.5	14.4	0.46	7.40[a]	0.48[a]	0.34	−1.33 to 2.01	5.64	3.58 to 7.69
6	13.3	14.0	0.41	5.32	0.66	−0.89	−3.26 to 1.48	8.22	4.48 to 11.96
Requiring two prior phenytoin concns.									
2B	13.2	11.8	0.86	1.56	0.78	1.40	−0.45 to 3.25	3.11	−0.63 to 6.85
7	12.9	10.7	0.87	0.92	0.76	2.20	−2.10 to 6.40	3.80	−1.46 to 9.06
8	12.9	10.9	0.84	0.82	0.78	1.97	−2.80 to 6.74	3.96	−1.22 to 9.14
9	12.5	12.0	0.63	4.8	0.57	0.57	−3.85 to 4.99	4.46	−0.41 to 9.32

MPE, mean prediction error; RMSE, root mean squared error.
[a] $p < 0.05$.

four methods tested. Use of method 9 was associated with the smallest correlation coefficient as well as the lowest slope and highest *y*-intercept value. None of the values obtained for slope and *y*-intercept, however, were significantly different from unity and zero, respectively. Use of method 9 resulted in the lowest MPE although all these values were comparable. Similarly, values for RMSE did not vary considerably between methods, and all confidence intervals for MPE and RMSE contained zero.

None of the methods tested demonstrated a clear superiority with respect to predicting therapeutic or nontherapeutic phenytoin concentrations. Further comparisons of data from patients receiving only phenytoin with those receiving additional antiseizure medications failed to significantly change results of previous analyses. The average K_m and V_{max} were calculated for this sample of patients using equations from method 2B. These data are summarized in Table 5. All values for these constants are consistent with previously reported values (20).

DISCUSSION

These data clearly demonstrate that two previous phenytoin levels and doses are far superior to one in the prediction of subsequent plasma concentrations. Such a finding is not surprising in view of the considerable variability associated with clearance of phenytoin and the need for a minimum of two concentrations for estimates of K_m and V_{max}. Intragroup analyses of data, however, fail to clearly distinguish one dosing method from another.

When the methods requiring a single known phenytoin dose and concentration were considered, the Martin nomogram (method 5) distinguished itself as perhaps the worst predictor of phenytoin levels. Its use resulted in a poor correlation between actual and predicted phenytoin concentrations and unacceptably high multiplicative and additive biases. In spite of these drawbacks, use of method 5 was least biased and most precise as evidenced by MPE, RMSE, and their respective confidence intervals. Of the remaining dose methods, the Rambeck nomogram (method 4) appeared to be the best predictor of phenytoin levels. Its use was associated with the best correlation between actual and predicted concentrations as well as the smallest multiplicative and additive biases. Also, it was associated with minimal bias, and its precision was comparable to the other methods. There is, how-

TABLE 5. *Michaelis-Menten constant (K_m) and maximal rate of phenytoin metabolism (V_{max})*

	K_m (μg/ml)	V_{max} (mg/kg/day)
All patients	7.80 ± 5.79[a]	6.95 ± 2.67
Patients receiving phenytoin alone	6.84 ± 5.82	6.17 ± 1.43
Patients receiving phenytoin plus other antiseizure medication	8.51 ± 5.97	7.53 ± 3.29

[a] All values are means ± SD. Literature averages for K_m = 6.6 μg/ml, and for V_{max} = 7.3 mg/kg/day.

ever, considerable overlap among confidence intervals for MPE and RMSE for all these methods. These similarities in data, together with overlapping confidence intervals, indicate that predictive performances of these methods are indistinguishable.

When data from methods requiring two known phenytoin doses and concentrations were evaluated, similarities in predictive performances were again noted. Correlation coefficients were similar, and multiplicative and additive biases were minimal and comparable. Bias and precision were similar and minimal as assessed by MPE and RMSE and the overlapping confidence intervals. The reason for the relatively poor performance of the Martin graph (method 9) is unclear and puzzling in view of its common derivation with the other methods (27,28). As before, similarities in regression data and overlapping confidence intervals suggest that these dosing methods are interchangeable.

These findings are similar to those reported by previous investigations. Murphy et al. (18), in a well-designed but smaller study, found that use of method 5 resulted in high predictions approximately 33% of the time. Vozeh et al. (27) reported that method 4 predicted phenytoin dosing requirements with comparable bias and precision to four other methods tested. The ability of method 4 to predict phenytoin concentrations, however, was not evaluated. Numerous investigators (17,18,21,23,29) have recommended routine use of the Mullen graph (method 7) because of its accuracy and ease of use. With the availability of hand-held programmable calculators and the equivalency of method 7 and method 2B, the latter method may be preferred for its relative convenience.

Measuring predictive performance using simple linear regression as a sole evaluative tool has been recently criticized (26). Instead, precision and bias should be evaluated by consideration of RMSE and MPE. Data from this study suggest that neither method used alone is sufficient for analyzing the comparative predictive performance of dosing methods. Consideration of data from methods requiring only one phenytoin dose and concentration will serve as a reasonable example of this point. If only RMSE and MPE were analyzed, the Martin nomogram (method 5) would be chosen as the best predictor of phenytoin levels. Its use was associated with the smallest MPE and RMSE. Further, its confidence interval for MPE encompassed zero. Yet, when these data were analyzed by linear regression, this same method was found to be inadequate because of unacceptable multiplicative and additive biases. On the basis of these findings, it is apparent that predictive performance of drug dosing methods preferably should be analyzed by both procedures.

Conclusions from these data may be restricted because of two important inherent limitations. First, the retrospective design assumed that all patient records were accurate and complete with respect to all variables considered. There was no direct way of confirming such a broad assumption. We noted, however, that observed K_m and V_{max} values were similar to those reported previously (20,27). It is apparent that this assumption was reasonable and that inaccuracies in charted information caused minimal variations in data. Second, predictive performance may have been affected by the time within a dosing interval when plasma was obtained for measurement of phenytoin content. Each method based its predictive capability on plasma samples obtained near the median of a dosing interval. It is likely that very few of these actual phenytoin concentrations met this criterion. Previous investigators (24) have examined differences in phenytoin concentrations between once- and thrice-daily dosing schedules. These differences failed to achieve statistical significance. It is reasonable to conclude, therefore, that variable time within a dosing interval had a similarly minimal effect on results of this study.

In conclusion, we recommend use of the Rambeck nomogram (method 4) to predict subsequent phenytoin levels when only one dose and one concentration are available. If two or more doses and concentrations of phenytoin are available, use of any of the methods assessed will yield equivalent and accurate predictions. Because of the overall lack of precision observed for all these dosing methods, all predictions should be confirmed with actual measurement of phenytoin concentrations.

REFERENCES

1. Buchthal F, Svensmark O, Schiller PJ. Clinical and electroencephalographic correlations with serum levels of diphenylhydantoin. *Arch Neurol* 1960;2:624–30.
2. Kutt H, McDowell F. Management of epilepsy with diphenylhydantoin sodium. *JAMA* 1968;203:969–72.
3. Borofsky LG, Louis S, Kutt H, Roginsky M. Diphenylhydantoin: efficacy, toxicity, and dose-serum level relationships in children. *J Pediatr* 1972;81:995–1002.
4. Dawson KP, Jamieson A. Value of blood phenytoin estimation in management of childhood epilepsy. *Arch Dis Child* 1971;46:386–8.
5. Houghton GW, Richens A, Toseland PA, Davidson S, et al. Brain concentrations of phenytoin, phenobarbitone, and primidone in epileptic patients. *Eur J Clin Pharmacol* 1975;9:73–8.
6. Kutt H, Winters W, Kokenge R, McDowell F. Diphenylhydantoin metabolism, blood levels, and toxicity. *Arch Neurol* 1964;11:642–8.

7. Lund L. Anticonvulsant effect of diphenylhydantoin relative to plasma levels: a prospective 3 year study in ambulant patients with generalized epileptic seizures. *Arch Neurol* 1974;31:289–94.
8. Bochner F, Hooper WD, Tyrer JH, Eadie MJ. Effect of dosage increments on blood phenytoin concentrations. *J Neurol Neurosurg Psychiatry* 1972;35:873–6.
9. Richens A, Dunlop A. Serum-phenytoin levels in management of epilepsy. *Lancet* 1975;2:247–8.
10. Atkinson AJ, Shaw JM. Pharmacokinetic study of a patient with diphenylhydantoin toxicity. *Clin Pharmacol Ther* 1973;4:521–8.
11. Koch-Weser J. The serum level approach to individualization of drug dosage. *Eur J Clin Pharmacol* 1975;9:1–8.
12. Kutt H, Brennan R, Dehejia H, Verebely K. Diphenylhydantoin intoxication. *Am Rev Resp Dis* 1970;101:377–94.
13. Gerber N, Wagner JG. Explanation of dose-dependent decline of diphenylhydantoin plasma levels by fitting to the integrated form of Michaelis-Menten equation. *Res Commun Chem Pathol Pharmacol* 1972;3:455–66.
14. Ludden TM, Hawkins DW, Allen JP, Hoffman SF. Optimum phenytoin-dosage regimens. *Lancet* 1976;1:307–8.
15. Martin E, Tozer T, Sheiner LB, Riegelman S. The clinical pharmacokinetics of phenytoin. *J Pharmacokinet Biopharm* 1977;5:579–96.
16. Mullen PW. Optimal phenytoin therapy: a new technique for individualizing dosage. *Clin Pharmacol Ther* 1978;23:228–32.
17. Mullen PW, Foster RW. Comparative evaluation of six techniques for determining the Michaelis-Menten parameters relating phenytoin dose and steady-state serum concentrations. *J Pharm Pharmacol* 1979;31:100–4.
18. Murphy JE, Bruni J, Stewart RB. Clinical utility of six methods of predicting phenytoin doses and plasma concentrations. *Am J Hosp Pharm* 1981;38:348–54.
19. Barot MH, Grant RHE, Maheendran KK, et al. Individual variation in daily dosage requirements for phenytoin sodium in patients with epilepsy. *Br J Clin Pharmacol* 1978;6:267–71.
20. Tozer TN, Winter ME. Phenytoin. In: Evans WE, Schentag JJ, Jusko WJ, eds. *Applied pharmacokinetics*. San Francisco: Applied Therapeutics, Inc, 1980:275–314.
21. Rambeck B, Beonigk HE, Dunlop A, Mullen PW, et al. Predicting phenytoin dose—a revised nomogram. *Ther Drug Monit* 1979;1:325–33.
22. Phillips PJ, Rain RW, Duncan BM. Serum phenytoin levels. *Lancet* 1975;2:926.
23. Schumacher GE. Using pharmacokinetics in drug therapy. VI: comparing methods for dealing with nonlinear drugs like phenytoin. *Am J Hosp Pharm* 1980;37:128–32.
24. Buchanan RA, Kinkel AW, Goulet JR, et al. The metabolism of diphenylhydantoin (Dilantin) following once-daily administration. *Neurology* 1972;22:126–30.
25. MacGee J. Rapid determination of diphenylhydantoin in blood plasma by gas-liquid chromatography. *Anal Chem* 1970;42:421–2.
26. Beal SI, Sheiner LB. Scientific commentary. Some suggestions for measuring predictive performance. *J Pharmacokinet Biopharm* 1981;9:503–12.
27. Vozeh S, Muir KT, Sheiner LB, Follath F. Predicting individual phenytoin dosage. *J Pharmacokinetic Biopharm* 1981;9:131–46.
28. Ludden TM. Individualization of phenytoin therapy [Letter]. *J Pharm Pharmacol* 1980;32:152.
29. Reidenberg MM, Odar-Cederlof I, vanBohr C, et al. Protein binding of diphenylhydantoin and desmethylimipramine in plasma from patients with poor renal function. *N Engl J Med* 1981;285:264–7.

Therapeutic Drug Monitoring
7:81–82 © 1985 Raven Press, New York

Therapeutic Blood Levels of Phenytoin in Treatment of Paroxysmal Choreoathetosis

Bor-Jeng Wang and *Yang-Chyuan Chang

*Section of Neurology, Department of Internal Medicine, Chung-Shan Medical College Hospital, Taichung, and *Department of Neurology, National Taiwan University Hospital, Taipei, Taiwan, Republic of China*

Summary: Eight patients with paroxysmal choreoathetosis received phenytoin therapy, starting from 50 mg of oral phenytoin with a gradual increment of the dose. After successful control of the paroxysmal attacks, blood levels of phenytoin in these patients were measured by enzyme immunoassay. The mean phenytoin blood level was 5.2 ± 3.2 μg/ml, with a range of 1.1–10.9 μg/ml. It is proposed that phenytoin can be maintained at a lower level in the treatment of paroxysmal choreoathetosis than in seizure control. **Key Words:** Paroxysmal choreoathetosis—Phenytoin—Therapeutic blood level.

Phenytoin has been reported to be effective for the treatment of paroxysmal choreoathetosis (1,2). The therapeutic blood level of phenytoin for this purpose has not been clarified. Clinically, it seems that a low phenytoin dose was sufficient to obtain a satisfactory result. It is the purpose of this study to establish the therapeutic phenytoin blood level for adequate treatment of paroxysmal choreoathetosis.

METHODS

Between 1980 and 1982, eight patients with paroxysmal choreoathetosis were included in the study. All patients had brief episodes of involuntary athetoid, ballistic, or dystonic movements of the extremities precipitated by voluntary movement. There were four patients with the familial and four with the nonfamilial disorder. The average age was 20.8 years (range 16–25 years). The age of onset of paroxysmal choreoathetosis was 12–19 years (average 14.9 years). Thus, the duration of illness before phenytoin therapy was about 6 years. The patients had never received anticonvulsant treatment before enrolling in this study.

Treatment was started with 50 mg of oral phenytoin, followed by an increase in dose of 50 mg every month. If the patient was free of attacks in the previous month, the daily dose was left unchanged. No other anticonvulsant drugs were used concomitantly. Successful treatment was defined as treatment with no more attacks within 6 months.

After the patients were successfully treated, blood samples taken before the morning dose of phenytoin were sent for determination of the phenytoin levels by enzyme immunoassay (Syva Co.).

RESULTS

Table 1 shows the therapeutic blood phenytoin levels in the eight patients with paroxysmal choreoathetosis. The mean therapeutic level was 5.2 μg/ml, with a standard deviation of 3.2 μg/ml and range of 1.1–10.9 μg/ml. The dose needed for successful treatment varied from 50 to 200 mg/day. There was no significant difference in the mean therapeutic levels between familial and nonfamilial cases. The mean therapeutic blood level in the patients with involvement of limbs on both sides during attacks was higher than that in the patients with only unilateral involvement (7.4 ± 3.2

Address correspondence and reprint requests to Dr. B.-J. Wang at Section of Neurology, Department of Internal Medicine, Chung-Shan Medical College Hospital 23, Section 1, Taichung Kang Rd., Taichung, Taiwan 400, Republic of China.

TABLE 1. *Phenytoin treatment in patients with paroxysmal choreoathetosis*

Patient	Age of onset (yr)	Duration of illness (yr)	Family history of the disorder	Involved limbs	Daily dose (mg)	Therapeutic level (μg/ml)
1	19	6	No	Left	150	6.0
2	15	3	Yes	Right	50	1.1
3	15	5	No	Left	100	3.1
4	16	5	No	Right	100	3.2
5	12	13	Yes	Both	200	9.0
6	13	3	Yes	Both	150	4.9
7	17	7	No	Both	200	10.5
8	12	5	Yes	Both	150	3.7

μg/ml versus 3.1 ± 1.6 μg/ml, $t = 2.44$ and $p < 0.05$).

There was a linear relationship (Fig. 1) between the therapeutic phenytoin blood level and the duration of illness before treatment ($r = 0.70$, $t = 2.40$ and $p = 0.05$); i.e., the longer the duration of illness before treatment, the higher was the therapeutic drug level.

DISCUSSION

After Merritt and Putnam introduced phenytoin for epilepsy in 1938 (3), the drug was widely studied and also applied in other neurological and even nonneurological diseases. In 1945, Michaux and Granier (4) published a report of a case of unilateral paroxysmal choreoathetosis that was responsive to phenytoin treatment. Stevens (1) in 1966 and Kertesz (2) in 1967 reported cases of paroxysmal kinesiogenic choreoathetosis, and several of their patients were satisfactorily treated with phenytoin at a daily dose of 200–300 mg.

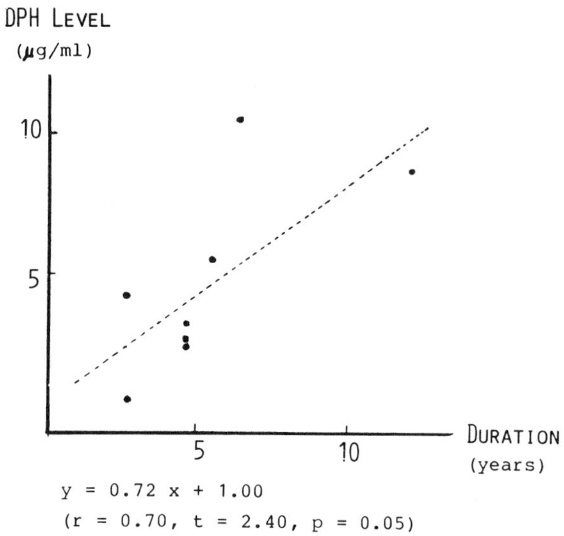

FIG. 1. Relationship between therapeutic phenytoin (DPH) level and duration of illness before DPH therapy.

Phenytoin, when used for seizure control, has been recommended at a daily maintenance dose of 150–600 mg for a therapeutic blood level of 10–20 μg/ml. In 1968, Bigger et al. (5) reported that the therapeutic phenytoin level for a cardiac antiarrhythmic effect ranged from 10 to 18 μg/ml. These findings might lead clinicians to use these data in phenytoin therapy for other neurological or nonneurological diseases. However, Lockman et al. (6) in 1973 noted that a blood phenytoin level above 4 μg/ml was effective in eliminating the pain associated with Fabry's disease.

In this study, the mean therapeutic phenytoin level for successful treatment of paroxysmal choreoathetosis was 5.2 μg/ml, and the daily dose ranged from 50 to 200 mg. In patients with shorter durations of illness before treatment, the required blood level and daily dose were even lower. Therefore, we conclude that to obtain satisfactory therapeutic effects with phenytoin in neurological disorders other than epilepsy, with minimization of possible side effects due to long-term treatment, adequate therapeutic levels of phenytoin should be individually evaluated for each disorder.

REFERENCES

1. Stevens H. Paroxysmal choreo-athetosis. *Arch Neurol* 1966;14:415–20.
2. Kertesz A. Paroxysmal kinesigenic choreoathetosis. *Neurology* 1967;17:680–90.
3. Merritt HH, Putnam TJ. Sodium diphenyl hydantoinate in treatment of convulsive disorders. *JAMA* 1938:111:1068–73.
4. Michaux L, Granier M. Epilepsie bravais-jacksonienne reflexe. *Ann Med Psychol* 1945;103:172.
5. Bigger JT, Schimidt D, Kutt H. Relationship between the plasma level of diphenylhydantoin sodium and its cardiac antiarrhythmic effects. *Circulation* 1968;38:363–74.
6. Lockman LA, Hunninghake DB, Krivit W, Desnick RJ. Relief of pain of Fabry's disease by diphenylhydantoin. *Neurology* 1973;23:872–5.

Therapeutic Drug Monitoring
7:83–86 © 1985 Raven Press, New York

Steady-State Serum Levels of Anticonvulsant Drugs in Chinese Epileptic Patients Living in Taiwan

Ming-Liang Lai

Department of Neurology, National Taiwan University, Taipei, Taiwan

Summary: Steady-state serum concentrations of phenytoin and phenobarbital were obtained in 70 epileptic patients in Taiwan and evaluated with respect to age, sex, and body weight. As demonstrated, the steady-state serum level of phenytoin is not affected by the age and sex of the patients or by phenobarbital used as a comedication. Thus, the main contributing factor influencing the steady-state serum concentration of phenytoin is the drug dosage. Among Chinese epileptic patients, the saturation of phenytoin metabolism occurs at the dosage of 4 mg/kg/day. **Key Words:** Epilepsy—Chinese—Phenytoin—Phenobarbital.

Regarding the genetic influence of drug metabolism (1–3), there have been studies (4,5) indicating that the disposition of phenytoin varies among ethnic groups. The following report is one part of an international combined study that was designed to investigate the pharmacogenetic variability in the distribution of anticonvulsants among the Asiatic peoples. It is concerned with the disposition of phenytoin and phenobarbital in Chinese epileptic patients living in Taiwan.

MATERIALS AND METHODS

From December 1, 1982, to March 31, 1983, 70 patients were evaluated for this study. Patients came from the clinics of the Department of Neurology, National Taiwan University Hospital. Their age, sex, body weight, and drug regimen were recorded.

Of the 21 patients receiving one drug, 18 used phenytoin only. Of 39 patients receiving two drugs concomitantly, 32 took phenytoin and phenobarbital. Because of the frequent interactions between anticonvulsant drugs and also because a few patients received other types of treatment, the patients who took phenytoin (acid form, 100 mg phenytoin per tablet; Dai-Nippon Pharmaceutical Company) and those who received phenytoin and phenobarbital simultaneously (LA tablet, 50 mg phenytoin and 20 mg phenobarbital per tablet; Department of Pharmacy, National Taiwan University Hospital) were used for further evaluation of the effects of patient characteristics on the disposition of phenytoin and phenobarbital. The sex ratio for the patients was 41 male/29 female in the whole group and 29 male/21 female in the evaluated group. The distributions for age, sex, and body weight are shown in Table 1.

Each patient placed in the normal range for blood albumin, globulin, bilirubin (both direct and indirect), glutamic-oxaloacetic transaminase (GOT), glutamic-pyruvic transaminase (GPT), zinc turbidity, urea nitrogen, and creatinine. After 2 weeks of a fixed dose of anticonvulsants, morning fasting serum was obtained from every patient to check the steady-state serum levels of the drugs. The measurement was performed by enzyme multiplied immunoassay technique (EMIT), a commercially available kit (Syva Corp., Palo Alto, CA, U.S.A.). Each measurement was duplicated using daily calibration of the standard curve. The *t* test and linear correlation were then statistically evaluated.

Address correspondence and reprint requests to Dr. M.-L. Lai at Department of Neurology, National Taiwan University, Taipei, Taiwan, R.O.C.

TABLE 1. *Age, sex, and body weight distribution of Chinese epileptic patients*

	Sex		Age (yr)						Body weight (kg)						
Treatment	M	F	≤9	10–19	20–29	30–39	40–49	≥50	≤29	30–39	40–49	50–59	60–69	70–79	80–89
DPH only (n = 18)	11	7	1	2	8	5	2	0	1	0	1	9	6	1	0
DPH + PB (n = 32)	18	14	1	5	13	6	6	1	0	1	4	15	9	2	1
PB only (n = 2)	2	0	0	2	0	0	0	0	0	1	0	1	0	0	0

DPH, diphenylhydantoin (or phenytoin); PB, phenobarbital.

RESULTS

Phenytoin

Age did not affect the disposition of phenytoin. This was true both in the patients who received phenytoin monotherapy and in those who received combination treatment with phenytoin and phenobarbital. Although the male patients had a lower mean phenytoin steady-state level (9.8 μg/ml) than that of the female patients (10.7 μg/ml), the difference was not significant (Table 2). The patients who received combination drug therapy had a phenytoin concentration comparable with that of those who received only phenytoin (9.9 μg/ml vs. 10.9 μg/ml). However, the patients who received 300 mg phenytoin/day did have a statistically higher steady-state phenytoin level than did those who received 200 mg/day.

The saturable metabolism of phenytoin is suggested by the steady-state phenytoin levels of 6.9 μg/ml (for 200 mg/day) and 12.7 μg/ml (for 300 mg/day), in which a 50% increase in the dosage level elevated the concentration to nearly twice the original value. This factor is better illustrated by the plot of the relationship between the steady-state serum phenytoin concentration versus daily phenytoin dose (Fig. 1), in which the relationship appears to be a hyperbolic curve with an upward turning of the curve at 250 mg/day or 4 mg/kg/day. For simplicity, linear correlation was used to predict the daily dose of phenytoin needed to obtain a therapeutic blood level (i.e., between 10 and 20 μg/ml). The two equations derived were $y = 3.1570x + 2.2659$ (monotherapy, $r = 0.32$, $p > 0.1$) and $y = 8.2683x - 7.9536$ (combined treatment, $r = 0.69$, $p < 0.01$), where y represents the steady-state serum phenytoin level in μg/ml and x represents the daily dose of phenytoin in 100 mg. From these equations, the daily dose of phenytoin was calculated to be between 245 and 562 mg/day for phenytoin mon-

TABLE 2. *Effects of age, sex, dose, and treatment on phenytoin levels*

	Sex		Age (yr)		Dose (mg/day)		
Treatment	M	F	<30	≥30	200	300	Total
DPH only							
n	11	7	11	7	5	10	18
Mean[a]	11.4	9.7	10.7	11.0	7.4	11.2	10.9
SD	4.8	4.8	5.2	4.3	2.4	4.1	4.8
DPH + PB							
n	18	14	19	13	11	7	32
Mean[a]	8.6	11.2	8.3	12.2[a]	6.7[b]	14.6[a]	9.9
SD	8.4	11.3	7.6	12.0	3.3	12.6	9.7
Total							
n	29	21	30	20	14	17	
Mean[a]	9.7[a]	10.7	9.2	11.7	7.1[a]	12.9[a]	
SD	7.3	9.5	6.9	9.8	3.0	8.5	

DPH, diphenylhydantoin (or phenytoin); PB, phenobarbital.
[a]DPH concentration in μg/ml.
[b]$t = 4.12$, $p < 0.01$.
[c]$t = 2.42$, $0.01 < p < 0.02$.

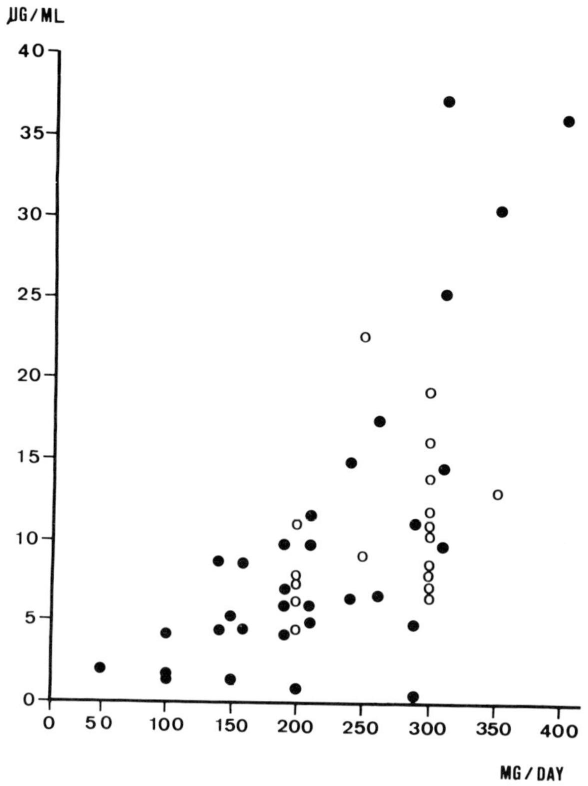

FIG. 1. Saturation kinetics of phenytoin: Data from patients who were treated with phenytoin and phenobarbital concomitantly (solid circles) and data from patients treated with phenytoin only (open circles).

otherapy and between 217 and 338 mg/day for phenytoin/phenobarbital combination therapy.

PHENOBARBITAL

The female epileptic patients had a larger daily dose of phenobarbital on the basis of body weight than did male patients. However, the serum steady-state phenobarbital level of the female patients was only slightly higher, and therefore the concentration/dose ratio was smaller than that of the male patients (Table 3). The difference, however, was not significant. These parameters were not affected by the age of the patients. While increasing the dose of phenobarbital, the daily dose per body weight increased and the steady-state serum level of phenobarbital increased, yet the concentration/dose ratio varied and no constant trend was observed.

DISCUSSION

In addition to genetic influence (1–3), age, sex, and body weight have been shown to be important determinants of the serum concentration–dose relationship for phenytoin in the Western countries (6–9). In this report, however, many trials using different age ranges were used, yet no significant association between serum steady-state level of phenytoin and age was revealed. The steady-state serum phenytoin concentration in adult Chinese epileptic patients seems to not be affected by age. This is in contrast to the studies of Grasela et al. (5), in which many Japanese pediatric patients were included. It was shown that patients who were less than 15 years old did have greater metabolic activity than did older patients. Because there were only three patients who were less than 15 years old in this study, it is possible that their small number biased the statistical significance of this report. Indeed, there also may be a difference between Chinese and Japanese peoples in phenytoin metabolism among patients in different age categories.

The slightly higher steady-state phenytoin level in the female patients in this study may be due to a higher daily phenytoin dosage (per body weight) in the female patients (5.09 mg/kg in female patients, 3.72 mg/kg in male patients). However, this minor difference is not significant. The results of this study, therefore, are consistent with other reports (6,8) from around the world and show that sex does not affect the phenytoin disposition in Chinese adult epileptic patients.

The exact nature of the interaction between phenobarbital and phenytoin is not fully understood. Phenobarbital induces liver microsomal enzymes for the metabolism of phenytoin, which at the same time competes with the phenytoin for the binding sites. The net effect may be an increase, decrease, or no change in phenytoin levels (10). The results of this study show that the steady-state concentration of phenytoin in adult Chinese epileptics who received only phenytoin did not vary much from the results obtained for those patients who received phenobarbital and phenytoin simultaneously.

The Michaelis-Menten equation is the best method for predicting the dosage needed to obtain therapeutic levels in epileptic patients (11–13). The major drawbacks are that the equation needs at least two estimates of steady-state phenytoin levels at different dosages, is time consuming, and sometimes is not practical in clinical situations. Because the equation's requirement regarding steady-state estimates was not fulfilled in this study and because the author thus wanted to avoid the pitfall of fitting the Michaelis-Menten equation to inappropriate data, the naive pooled data approach

TABLE 3. *Effects of age, sex, and daily dose on phenobarbital levels*

	Sex		Age (yr)		Dose (mg/day)					
	M (n = 18)	F (n = 13)	<30 (n = 19)	≥30 (n = 12)	40 (n = 3)	60 (n = 5)	80 (n = 9)	90 (n = 2)	100 (n = 5)	120 (n = 6)
D	1.22 (0.46)	1.90 (0.56)	1.50 (0.48)	1.52 (0.78)	0.69 (0.08)	1.14 (0.16)	1.41 (0.27)	1.52 (0.13)	1.81 (0.35)	2.30 (0.48)
C	16.7[a] (12.9)	13.4[a] (8.1)	15.7 (12.0)	17.5[a] (9.5)	8.2 (0.5)	10.4 (2.2)	13.5 (7.1)	17.8 (3.7)	23.8 (20.6)	20.3 (9.7)
C/D	11.54 (6.49)	8.52 (3.18)	10.70 (6.49)	9.60 (3.54)	11.94 (0.64)	9.16 (1.86)	9.44 (4.79)	11.65 (1.44)	13.53 (11.35)	9.06 (4.23)

All values are means, with SD in parentheses. D, daily dose of phenobarbital on body weight basis, mg/kg/day; C, phenobarbital concentration in μg/ml; C/D, concentration/dose ratio.
[a]Patients treated with phenytoin and phenobarbital.

was used (i.e., fitting all individuals' data together as though there were no individual kinetic difference) (14). From those data a simple linear regression was tried, and the equations listed previously were obtained. Clinically, these equations are more convenient for practical use. For an adult Chinese epileptic patient, the daily dosage for maintaining a steady-state serum phenytoin concentration between 10 and 20 μg/ml would be in the range of 245–562 mg if phenytoin only were being used. Therefore, a 200 mg daily dose may be used first; then later, with the help of drug monitoring, the dosage can be adjusted to maintain good seizure control.

The characteristic linear concentration–dose relationship of phenobarbital is well known (15,16). Since in this study there were two patients who used only phenobarbital to control their seizures, further work needs to be done to understand in more detail the kinetic patterns of phenobarbital among Chinese epileptic patients.

REFERENCES

1. Vasko MR, Bell RD, Daly DD, Pippenger CE. Inheritance of phenytoin hypometabolism: a kinetic study of one family. *Clin Pharmacol Ther* 1980;27:96–103.
2. Sloan TP, Idle JR, Smith RL. Influence of DH/DL alles regulating debrisoquine oxidation on phenytoin hydroxylation. *Clin Pharmacol Ther* 1981;29:493–7.
3. Eichelbaum M. Defective oxidation of the drugs. *Clin Pharmacokinet* 1982;7:1–22.
4. Chiba K, Ishizaki T, Miirua H, Minagawa K. Michaelis-Menten pharmacokinetics of diphenylhydantoin and application in the pediatric age patients. *J Pediatr* 1980;96:479–89.
5. Grasela TH, Sheiner LB, Rambeck B, et al. Steady-state pharmacokinetics of phenytoin from routinely collected patient data. *Clin Pharmacokinet* 1983;8:355–64.
6. Travers R, Reynolds EH, Gallagher B. Variation in response to anticonvulsants in a group of epileptic patients. *Arch Neurol* 1972;27:29–33.
7. Sherwin AL, Loynd JS, Bock GW, Sokolowski CD. Effects of age, sex, obesity and pregnancy on plasma diphenylhydantoin levels. *Epilepsia* 1974;15:507–21.
8. Houghton GW, Richens A, Leighton M. Effect of age, height, weight and sex on serum phenytoin concentration in epileptic patients. *Br J Clin Pharmacol* 1975;2:251–6.
9. Richens A. Clinical pharmacokinetics of phenytoin. *Clin Pharmacokinet* 1979;4:153–69.
10. Saunders GH, Penry JK. Phenobarbital/primidone: therapeutic use and serum concentration monitoring. In: Taylor WJ, Finn AL, eds. *Individualizing drug therapy*. New York: Gross, 1981:50–62.
11. Wagner JG. Properties of the Michaelis-Menten equation and its integrated form which are useful in pharmacokinetics. *J Pharmacokinet Biopharm* 1973;1:103–21.
12. Lundovist F, Wolthers H. The kinetics of alcohol elimination in man. *Arch Pharmacol Toxicol* 1958;14:265–89.
13. Mullen PW, Foster RW. Comparative evaluation of six techniques for determining the Michaelis-Menten parameters relating phenytoin dose and steady-state serum concentrations. *J Pharm Pharmacol* 1979;31:100–4.
14. Scheiner LB, Beal SL. Evaluation of methods for estimating population pharmacokinetic parameters. I. Michaelis-Menten model: routine clinical pharmacokinetic data. *J Pharmacokinet Biopharm* 1980;8:553–71.
15. Laidlaw J, Richens A. *A textbook of epilepsy*. Edinburgh: Churchill-Livingston, 1976:194.
16. Buchthal F, Lennox Buchthal MA. Phenobarbital: regulation of serum concentration to control of seizures. In: Woodbury DM, Penry JK, Schmidt RP, eds. *Antiepileptic drugs*. New York: Raven Press, 1972:335–41.

Therapeutic Drug Monitoring
7:87–91 © 1985 Raven Press, New York

Monitoring Drug Noncompliance in Epileptic Patients: Assessing Phenobarbital Plasma Levels

Seiichiro Takaki, Toru Kurokawa, and *Toshinobu Aoyama

*Departments of Pediatrics and *Pharmacy, Faculty of Medicine, Kyushu University, Fukuoka, Japan*

Summary: In an attempt to detect drug noncompliance in epileptic patients, we assessed phenobarbital plasma concentrations and examined the determinants of noncompliance in 252 outpatients, with 22 inpatients as controls. The plasma level of phenobarbital was measured at least twice, at mean intervals of 4.8 months. The percent difference (PD) between the minimum and maximum levels was calculated in each case. A PD of more than 35% was associated with noncompliance. The frequency of noncompliance was 19% in the outpatient group. The medication period, seizure-free period, and, secondarily, number of drugs and drug forms were found to be correlated with noncompliance. Noncompliance was not influenced by the age of the patient, sex, psychomotor development, or seizure type or frequency. The mean period until complete control of seizures was significantly shorter in compliant than in noncompliant patients.
Key Words: Epilepsy—Phenobarbital—Blood level—Compliance—Drug monitoring.

Compliance has been studied using questionnaires (1), verbal reports (2,3), interview (1,3), pill or bottle count (1–4), prescription rate (5,6), daily dispenser (7–9), or appointment keeping (6). Blood concentrations such as serum level/dose ratio (10) have also been used to confirm compliance. Data on compliance in children with epilepsy have rarely been reported (11). We assessed noncompliance by determining the levels of phenobarbital in plasma samples (12,13); the factors influencing compliance in epileptic children were also analyzed.

SUBJECTS

The subjects were 252 ambulatory epileptic outpatients. They ranged in age from 10 months to 25 years and 11 months (mean 10 years and 10 months). There were 129 males and 123 females. Patients or their parents were required to visit the clinic once or more a month, according to Japan's health insurance system rules. An estimation of the plasma level was made at least twice during the administration of the same prescription, including phenobarbital, and without prediction of the measurements of the plasma levels at steady state 1 month or more after the initiation or change in the prescription. Two blood samples were obtained, at a mean interval of 4.8 months. As a control group, 22 inpatients with epilepsy were also studied. The ages of the control group ranged from 5 years and 8 months to 22 years and 1 month (mean 15 years and 5 months). Because these patients were severely retarded and bedridden, the nursing staff administered the drugs directly, and blood samples were obtained in the morning, 3 h after the last dose.

Address correspondence and reprint requests to Dr. T. Kurokawa at Department of Pediatrics, Faculty of Medicine, Kyushu University 60, Fukuoka 812, Japan.

METHODS

Assessment of Noncompliance

Three methods were used to assess noncompliance: percent difference (PD) between minimum and max-

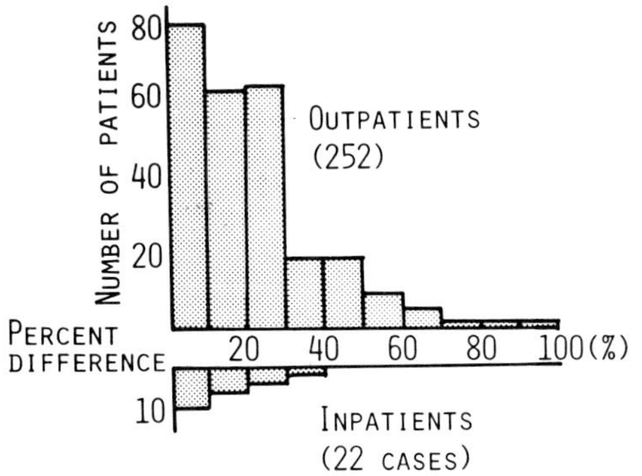

FIG. 1. Distribution of percent difference (between minimum and maximum plasma phenobarbital levels) among epileptic inpatients and outpatients.

imum plasma phenobarbital levels, prescription rate, and questionnaires. The plasma level was determined using the EMIT (enzyme multiplied immunoassay technique; Syva) method. The PD was calculated for each patient as follows:

$$\frac{\text{maximum plasma level} - \text{minimum plasma level}}{\text{maximum plasma level}} \times 100$$

The prescription rate is the percentage of the days of actual drug refill during 365 days or equivalent days if less than 1 year:

$$\frac{\text{no. of days actually refilled/yr}}{\text{365 days}} \times 100$$

Evaluation of PD

The PD in the outpatients ranged from nil to 100% (mean 20.8 ± 1.1%). The PD in the inpatients ranged from nil to 39.3% (mean 13.3 ± 2.3%), significantly less than that in the outpatients ($p < 0.05$; Fig. 1).

As a result of evaluation of the PD in the outpatients, the use of the rejection limit test of Thompson proved to be reliable in 199 patients (79.0% of the 252 outpatients), with a PD of less than 31.5%.

As for the correlation between PD *(x)* and prescription rate *(y)*, the equation of the regression line was $y = 0.13x + 101.1$, with $r = -0.315$. The correlation coefficient was significant ($p < 0.01$). When the limit was set at 35% for PD and at 95% for prescription rate, the correlation was highest ($\chi^2 = 34.85$) (Table 1). The coincidence rate at which PD and prescription rate were both normal (178 patients) or both abnormal (25 patients) was 80.6%.

TABLE 1. *Correlations (χ^2) between PD and prescription rate*

	PD		
Prescription rate (%)	30%	35%	40%
90	25.81	30.41	24.98
95	28.08	34.85	26.79
98	18.65	21.41	15.23

PD, percent difference between the minimum and maximum levels of plasma phenobarbital levels.

Interval Between Blood Samplings

The interval between the two blood samplings was 1–3 months in 89 cases, 4–6 months in 75, 7–9 months in 61, and 10–12 months in 27. The PD was 23.1 ± 3.2, 17.9 ± 1.7, 20.9 ± 2.0, and 20.9 ± 3.2%, respectively, in the four groups; these differences were not statistically significant.

RESULTS

Frequency of Noncompliance

Forty-eight (19.0%) of 252 patients were considered noncompliant because the PD was more than 35%. In 51 (20.2%), the prescription rate was less than 95%. The frequency of noncompliance as indicated by PD and by prescription rate was much the same (Fig. 2).

Factors Influencing Noncompliance

Factors Related to the Patients

Noncompliance was observed in 26 (20.2%) of 129 male and in 22 (17.9%) of 123 female patients. There was no significant correlation between the ages of the patients and the frequency of noncompliance, although the noncompliance rate tended to be high in those aged 15–19 years (Table 2). As to psychomotor

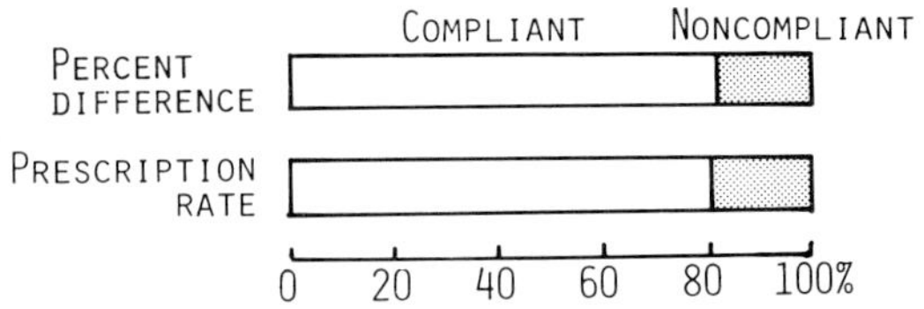

FIG. 2. Frequency of noncompliance in epileptic patients when data were analyzed by percent difference (PD) between minimum and maximum plasma phenobarbital levels and by prescription rate (see the text for details). The frequency was 19.0 and 20.2%, by PD and prescription rate, respectively.

TABLE 2. *Correlation between ages and noncompliance*

Ages (yr)	No. of patients	No. of noncompliant patients (%)
0–4	42	6 (14%)
5–9	74	10 (14%)
10–14	75	16 (21%)
15–19	40	12 (30%)
⩾20	21	4 (19%)

development, the noncompliant patients numbered 35 (21%) of 165 with normal development, 4 (24%) of 17 with borderline development, and 9 (13%) of 70 with delayed development; thus, development was not a determinant of compliance. The period from initial drug administration until the first blood sampling in 252 cases ranged from 1 month to 22 years and 2 months (mean 6 years and 8 months). The percentage of noncompliance was significantly lower in the group on drugs for 0–4 years than in the group on drugs for 5 years or longer ($p < 0.05$) (Fig. 3).

Factors Related to Epileptic Seizures

There were no significant correlations between type or frequency of seizures at the beginning of the illness and noncompliance, although the correlation with generalized seizures tended to be low, according to the percentage of noncompliant patients (Tables 3 and 4). With regard to the control of seizures, 31 (21%) of the 154 patients with uncontrolled seizures were noncompliant (i.e., occurrence of one or more seizures in the last 1 year) (Fig. 4). In the group in which the seizures were controlled, the percentage of noncompliant patients increased as the duration of seizure control lengthened.

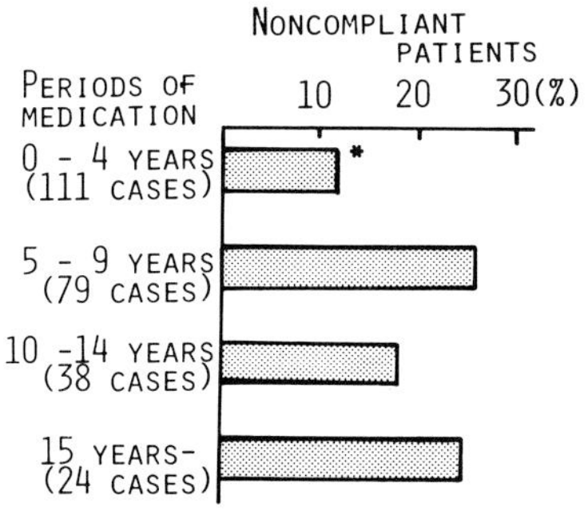

FIG. 3. Percentage of noncompliant epileptic patients in the various medication groups (by duration of medication). *$p < 0.05$.

TABLE 3. *Correlation between seizure type and noncompliance*

Type of seizure	No. of cases	No. of noncompliant patients (%)
Partial		
Simple partial	30	6 (20%)
Complex partial	17	6 (35%)
With secondary generalization	66	14 (21%)
Generalized		
Primary (convulsive)	82	14 (17%)
Primary (nonconvulsive)	18	2 (11%)
Secondarily generalized	37	5 (13%)
Unclassified	2	1 (50%)

Drug Factors

The number of drugs taken correlated with the percentage of noncompliant patients. Noncompliance amounted to 18% in the group prescribed phenobarbital only. As the number of drugs ingested increased, the noncompliance percentage decreased significantly, from 28% in the group on two drugs to 4% in those on five drugs or more ($p < 0.05$). Noncompliance was significantly lower in the group given a mixed drug form than in the group given a powder alone or a tablet alone (Table 5; $p < 0.01$).

Family Factors

The frequency of noncompliance was lowest in the group given drugs directly by parents, and was highest in the self-medicated group (Fig. 5).

Noncompliance and Prognosis

Analyzing the 96 patients with seizure control, 31 (39%) of 79 compliant patients and 6 (35%) of 17 noncompliant patients attained seizure control within 1 year after beginning anticonvulsant therapy; there

TABLE 4. *Correlation between seizure frequency and noncompliance*

Seizure frequency	No. of cases	No. of noncompliant patients (%)
One episode	6	1 (17%)
Less than one per year	42	12 (29%)
Yearly	89	14 (16%)
Monthly	48	8 (17%)
Weekly	30	6 (20%)
Daily	37	7 (19%)

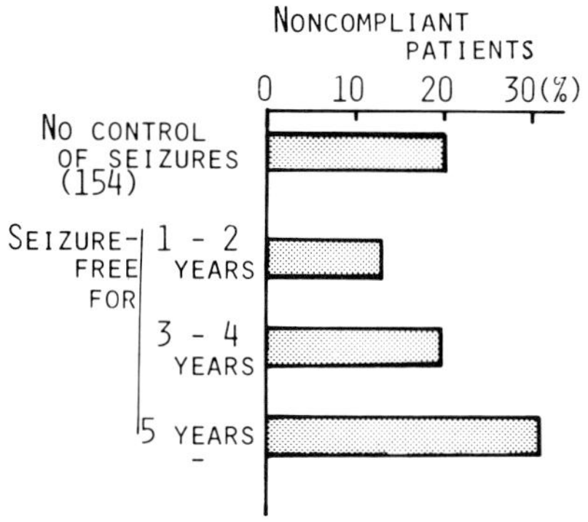

FIG. 4. Relationship between seizure control and percentage of noncompliant patients.

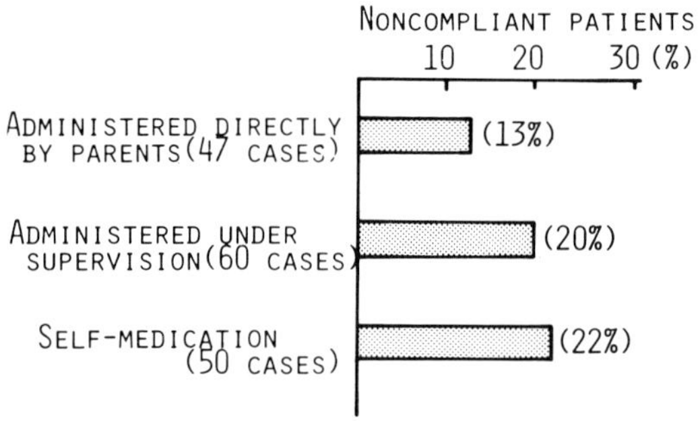

FIG. 5. Relationship between family factors affecting drug administration and percentage of noncompliant patients.

were no differences between the compliant and noncompliant groups. Twenty-two patients with seizure control after drug administration for 1 year or more have been seizure free for more than 3 years. The periods from the beginning of drug therapy to the last seizure were 70.3 ± 13.2 months in 17 of 22 compliant patients and 126.0 ± 21.9 months in the remaining 5 noncompliant patients (Fig. 6). The period from the beginning of therapy to the last seizure was significantly longer in the noncompliant group ($p < 0.05$).

DISCUSSION

Blood levels (3,6) or serum level/dose ratios (10) are indications of adequate drug intake; however, the levels do not necessarily reflect compliance. Although the serum level/dose ratio is a rather direct method to check compliance, it varies within the individual, as well as with the age of the patient (14,15), and in relation to interactions with other drugs (16,17).

Phenobarbital has a long half-life (13), and there are only slight daily variations when the drug is ingested regularly. The blood level of phenobarbital is little influenced by drug form (18,19) or food intake (20), compared with findings for sodium valproate or phenytoin (21). Other investigators have monitored

TABLE 5. *Drug forms and noncompliance*

Drug form	No. of patients	No. of noncompliant patients (%)
Powder	150	35 (23%)
Tablet	47	10 (21%)
Elixir	2	0 (0%)
Mixed	53	4 (8%)[a]

[a]Significantly lower in mixed form than in powder or tablet form ($p < 0.01$).

compliance using the protocol of two or more measurements of blood levels of anticonvulsant drugs (22–25). However, statistical analyses of the variability of these levels have been unsatisfactory, except in the study by Leppik et al. (24,25), in which noncompliance was associated with a coefficient of variation of more than 20% in the plasma concentration of phenytoin, in several measurements. In our study, a 35% PD for phenobarbital blood concentration was a reasonable limit of compliance.

The frequency of noncompliance in epileptic children has been reported to be 46.2% (6 of 13, as assessed by drug concentration in urine or saliva) (11). Noncompliance was less frequent in the present series, probably because the interval between clinical visits was relatively short (1 month or less). Wannamaker et al. (26) reported improvement in blood levels of antiepileptic drugs following the reduction of intervals from a mean of 3.4 months to 1.1 months. There were no correlations between type or frequency of seizures and percentage of noncompliance in our study. Generalized major (tonic-clonic) seizures were found to be related to compliance in adults (6).

We found compliance to be good when the duration of drug intake was less than 5 years. This is consistent with Lund's findings (27) that compliance was good shortly after the beginning of therapy. Compliance in epileptic children is better than in adults, probably because of parental supervision and a relatively short duration of drug ingestion.

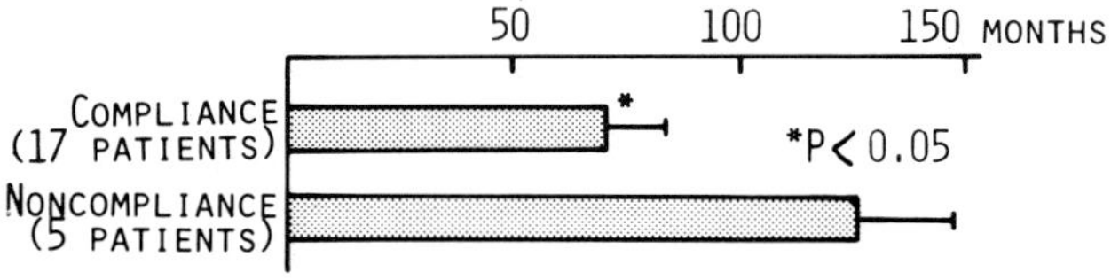

FIG. 6. Comparison of the periods from beginning of therapy to control of seizures in compliant and noncompliant patients.

There are no available data concerning compliance and prognosis. Our study revealed that the period until control of seizures in epileptic patients with disease of a moderately difficult degree, i.e., for whom 1 year or more is required to achieve control, was shorter in the compliant patients than in the noncompliant patients.

Acknowledgment: We thank Professors N. Goya (Department of Pediatrics) and M. Horioka (Department of Pharmacy) for their support and M. Ohara for comments on the manuscript.

REFERENCES

1. Bergman AB, Werner RJ. Failure of children to receive penicillin by mouth. *N Engl J Med* 1963:268;1334–8.
2. Park LC, Lipman RS. A comparison of patient dosage deviation reports with pill counts. *Psychopharmacologia* 1964;6:299–302.
3. Fletcher SW, Pappius EM, Harper SJ. Measurement of medication compliance in a clinical setting: comparison of three methods in patients prescribed digoxin. *Arch Intern Med* 1979;139:635–8.
4. Roth HP, Caron HS, Hsi BP. Measuring intake of a prescribed medication: a bottle count and a tracer technique compared. *Clin Pharmacol Ther* 1970;11:228–37.
5. Kugou T, Hirata J, Hosokawa K. Compliance in epilepsy. *Rinsho Seishin Igaku* 1978;9:731–7.
6. Peterson GM, McLean S, Millingen KS. Determinants of patient compliance with anticonvulsant therapy. *Epilepsia* 1982;23:607–13.
7. Lund M. Failure to observe dosage instructions in patients with epilepsy: the short-term effect of a daily dispenser. *Acta Neurol Scand* 1973;49:295–306.
8. Moulding TS, Onstad GD, Sbarboro JA. Supervision of outpatient drug therapy with the medication monitor. *Ann Intern Med* 1970;73:559–64.
9. Moulding TS. The unrealized potential of the medication monitor. *Clin Pharmacol Ther* 1979;25:131–6.
10. Buchthal F, Lennox-Buchthal MA. Relation of serum concentration to control of seizure. In: Woodbury DM, Penry JK, Schmidt RP, eds. *Antiepileptic drugs*. New York: Raven Press, 1972;335–43.
11. Zysset T, Rudeberg A, Vassella F, Kupfer A, Bircher J. Phenytoin therapy for epileptic children: evaluation of salivary and plasma concentrations and of methods of assessing compliance. *Dev Med Child Neurol* 1981;23:66–75.
12. Kugou T, Takahashi S, Hirata J, Hosokawa K. Repeated measurement of antiepileptic drug level in the same patients. *Nou to Hattatsu* 1979;11:531–8.
13. Woodbury DM, Fingel E. Drugs effective in the therapy of the epilepsies. In: Goodman LS, Gilman A, eds. *The pharmacological basis of therapeutics*. New York: Macmillan, 1975;201–26.
14. Heimann G, Gladtke E. Pharmacokinetics of phenobarbital in childhood. *Eur J Clin Pharmacol* 1977;12:305–10.
15. Kitahara H. Blood level of anticonvulsant drugs in children. II: Dose and blood level relationships. *Nou to Hattatsu* 1979;11:417–28.
16. Patel IH, Levy RH, Cutler RE. Phenobarbital–valproic acid interaction. *Clin Pharmacol Ther* 1980;27:515–521.
17. Wilder BJ, Willmore LG, Bruni J, Villarreal HJ. Valproic acid: interaction with other anticonvulsant drugs. *Neurology* 1978;28:892–6.
18. Lund L. Clinical significance of genetic inequivalence of three different pharmaceutical preparations of phenytoin. *Eur J Clin Pharmacol* 1974;119–124.
19. Takaki S, Kurokawa T, Hanai T, Nakao Y, Aoyama T. Blood concentration of antiepileptic drugs—differences with individuals and drug forms. *Nou to Hattatsu* 1979;11:548–53.
20. Windorfer A, Stunkel S, Weinmann HM. Influences on the absorption of diphenylhydantoin preparations. *Neuropediatrics* 1978;9:120–26.
21. Maynert EW. Phenobarbital, mephobarbital and metharbital: absorption, distribution and excretion. In: Woodbury DM, Penry JK, Schmidt RP, eds. *Antiepileptic drugs*. New York: Raven Press, 1972;303–10.
22. Bryant SG, Ereshefsky L. Determinants of compliance in epileptic outpatients. *Drug Intell Clin Pharm* 1981:15:572–7.
23. Driessen O, Hoppener R. Plasma levels of phenobarbital and phenytoin in epileptic outpatients. *Eur Neurol* 1977;15:135–42.
24. Leppik IE, Cloyd JC, Sawchuk RJ. Coefficient of variation as measure of compliance. *Lancet* 1978;i:849.
25. Leppik IE, Cloyd JC, Sawchuk RJ, Pepin SM. Compliance and variability of plasma phenytoin levels in epileptic patients. *Ther Drug Monit* 1979;1:475–83.
26. Wannamaker BB, Morton WA Jr, Gross AJ, Saunders S. Improvement in antiepileptic drug levels following reduction of intervals between clinic visits. *Epilepsia* 1980;21:155–62.
27. Lund L. Clinical significance of genetic inequivalence of three different pharmaceutical preparations of phenytoin. *Eur J Clin Pharmacol* 1974;7:119–24.

Therapeutic Drug Monitoring
7:92–94 © 1985 Raven Press, New York

No Influence of Doxycycline on Theophylline Pharmacokinetics

*†J. H. G. Jonkman, *W. J. V. van der Boon, *R. Schoenmaker, *A. Holtkamp, and *J. Hempenius

**Laboratory for Drug Analysis, Departments of Biopharmaceutics and Clinical Pharmacokinetics, Assen, and †Department of Pharmaceutical and Analytical Chemistry, State University, Groningen, The Netherlands*

Summary: The influence of the antibiotic drug doxycycline on steady-state pharmacokinetics of theophylline was studied in nine healthy adults by comparing the pharmacokinetic parameters measured during a 9-day course of theophylline alone and during comedication with doxycycline. Theophylline plasma concentrations were measured by means of high performance liquid chromatography analysis. Trough theophylline plasma concentrations were measured on days 1–8. On day 9 of each of the two periods of drug administration, a plasma concentration–time curve was evaluated. No influence of doxycycline on absorption, elimination, and volume of distribution of theophylline was found. Mean steady-state plasma concentrations were not significantly different during the two treatments. It is concluded that the drugs can be given concomitantly without any dosage adjustment of theophylline. **Key Words:** Doxycycline—Theophylline—High performance liquid chromatography.

Theophylline is widely used as a bronchodilator in patients with chronic obstructive lung disease. Because the drug has a short half-life of elimination (~7–8 h) and a rather narrow therapeutic window (~7.5–20 mg L^{-1}), individualized dosage schedules are desirable. Since up to 90% of a theophylline dose is biotransformed, drugs influencing the liver function may affect the elimination of theophylline, e.g., enzyme inducers such as phenytoin and phenobarbital increase theophylline clearance, while some other drugs such as allopurinol, propranolol, cimetidine, and the antibiotics erythromycin and troleandomycin decrease theophylline clearance (1).

Recently, Mathis et al. (2) reported a study in which theophylline pharmacokinetic parameters were determined before and after a 7-day tetracycline course of 1 g daily in eight healthy volunteers. The total body clearance was reduced by 9.4% and the half-life of elimination was increased by 9.7%; however, these differences were not statistically significant.

We studied the effect of doxycycline on theophylline clearance. Doxycycline, a semisynthetic tetracycline-type antibiotic, is frequently used together with theophylline during acute exacerbations of bronchitis and infections of the upper and lower respiratory tract. Doxycycline is partially metabolized in the liver, and no information is available on its influence on theophylline pharmacokinetics.

MATERIALS AND METHODS

The study had an open, randomized crossover design with controlled intake of the medications during two periods of 10 days (long enough to reach steady state and to show possible interactions), with a washout period of at least 4 days.

Address correspondence and reprint requests to Dr. J. H. G. Jonkman at Laboratory for Drug Analysis, Departments of Biopharmaceutics and Clinical Pharmacokinetics, P.O. Box 147, 9400 AC Assen, The Netherlands.

Nine healthy, nonsmoking human volunteers (three female and six male; aged 24.3 ± 6.1 years; weighing 69.2 ± 8.2 kg) participated in this trial (Table 1). All subjects had cardiac, renal, and hepatic function within the normal range, as judged by physical examination and from the usual laboratory tests. They were informed orally and in written form about the purpose, procedures, and risks of the study, and were asked to give written consent (in compliance with the Signed Informed Consent Recommendations of the U.S. Food and Drug Administration). All participants had an extensive medical (physical) examination before and after completion of the study, and they were observed and questioned for any side effects during the study. No other drugs were taken for 2 weeks prior to and during the study.

A dose of 350 mg theophylline [as one capsule containing 100 mg theophylline and one capsule containing 250 mg theophylline (Somophyllin CRT; Fisons)] was given on an empty stomach at 7:30 a.m. and at 7:30 p.m. on days 1–8. On day 9, a last dose was given at 7:30 a.m.

A dose of 100 mg doxycycline [as one tablet of 100 mg Vibramycin (Pfizer)] was given at 7:30 a.m. and at 7:30 p.m. on day 1 and at 7:30 a.m. on days 2–9.

Blood samples were taken just before dosing on days 1–9 and during a period of 33 h after the dose on day 9.

Theophylline plasma concentrations were measured by means of a selective high performance liquid chromatography method in which other xanthines do not interfere (3).

The difference between individual pharmacokinetic parameters, as obtained after the two different treatments, was analyzed by using the *t* test for paired observations.

RESULTS AND DISCUSSION

Table 1 shows the characteristics of eight of the nine subjects (nos. 2–9) as well as pharmacokinetic parameters obtained on day 9 during both drug courses. Because subject 1 had high theophylline plasma concentrations and substantial side effects, including vomiting, a loss of medication by vomiting cannot be excluded. It was therefore decided not to use the data for subject 1 in the statistical analysis.

In general, the sustained-release theophylline capsules were well tolerated by the subjects. Only a slight headache was reported on day 1 by subjects 1 and 4,

TABLE 1. *Subject characteristics and pharmacokinetic parameters obtained after the last dose of 350 mg theophylline on day 9*

		Subject									Significance
		2	3	4	5	6	7	8	9	Mean ± SD	(n = 8)
Sex		M	M	M	M	M	M	F	F		
Age (yr)		23	21	23	25	25	21	21	40	24.9 ± 6.3	
Weight (kg)		82	71	66	75	74	73	63	65	71.1 ± 6.3	
Pharmacokinetic parameters											
Dose ($mg\ kg^{-1}$)		4.27	4.93	5.30	4.67	4.73	4.79	5.56	5.38	4.95 ± 0.43	—
C_{min} ($mg\ L^{-1}$)	A	4.2	9.2	5.8	5.1	5.5	5.1	7.8	4.4	5.9 ± 1.7	NS
	B	3.7	7.3	8.1	6.2	4.4	5.7	8.1	3.8	5.9 ± 1.8	
C_{max} ($mg\ L^{-1}$)	A	7.0	13.8	11.8	8.5	8.1	8.8	12.5	7.3	9.7 ± 2.6	NS
	B	6.0	10.4	12.8	7.8	6.5	8.6	11.1	8.5	9.0 ± 2.3	
C_{ss} ($mg\ L^{-1}$)	A	5.3	10.9	8.4	6.5	6.0	6.5	9.2	6.0	7.4 ± 1.9	NS
	B	4.8	8.7	8.6	6.3	5.2	7.0	9.4	6.2	7.0 ± 1.7	
t_{max} (h)	A	3.5	3.0	3.0	3.0	3.0	3.0	4.0	3.0	3.2 ± 0.4	NS
	B	5.0	4.0	2.8	6.0	3.5	3.1	4.2	3.0	4.0 ± 1.1	
$(t_{1/2})_{el}$ (h)	A	6.3	9.9	6.0	7.1	6.5	7.1	5.8	4.2	6.6 ± 1.6	NS
	B	7.4	8.9	7.3	6.0	6.5	6.9	11.4	5.1	7.4 ± 2.0	
CL^a ($L\ h^{-1}$)	A	5.51	2.67	3.47	4.50	4.88	4.52	3.17	4.83	4.19 ± 0.98	NS
	B	6.09	3.34	3.40	4.64	5.57	4.17	3.11	4.70	4.38 ± 1.08	
$V_d{}^b$ (L)	A	50.0	38.1	30.2	45.9	45.7	46.3	26.7	29.3	39.0 ± 9.2	NS
	B	65.3	42.8	36.0	40.4	52.5	41.8	51.2	34.4	45.6 ± 10.2	
$AUC^{0\rightarrow 33}$ ($mg\ L^{-1}\ h$)	A	93.20	221.54	147.08	118.56	104.16	118.42	153.98	103.37	132.54 ± 41.73	NS
	B	88.95	171.35	146.11	111.59	94.10	124.44	185.18	100.72	127.81 ± 36.21	

A, results obtained during the period of administration of theophylline (Somophyllin CRT) alone; B, results obtained during the period of administration of theophylline in combination with doxycycline (Vibramycin); AUC, area under the plasma concentration–time curves; NS, not significant ($p > 0.05$).

[a] Overall total body clearance, $CL = V_d \times k_{el}$.

[b] Overall volume of distribution, V_d = Dose/(AUC $\times\ k_{el}$).

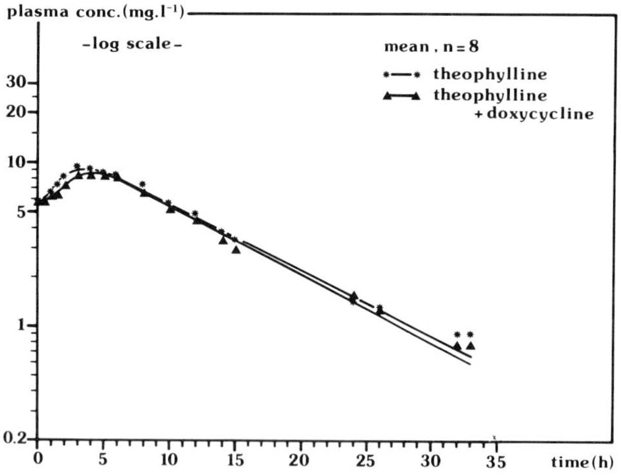

FIG. 1. Mean theophylline plasma concentration–time curves as observed on days 9 and 10 during both studies (semilogarithmic scale).

and a slight tremor was experienced on day 1 and day 2 by subjects 8 and 9.

During comedication with doxycycline, the frequency and severity of side effects were much more pronounced; only subject 7 did not report any side effects. Severe nausea was reported by subject 1 (with vomiting on days 1, 2, 8, and 9) and subject 9 (with vomiting on day 1). Nausea was also reported by subjects 3, 4, and 8, while slight nausea was experienced by subjects 2 and 6. Diarrhea was reported by subject 3 (days 1 and 3) and some dizziness by subject 4 (day 4). These symptoms (mainly gastrointestinal) are well known side effects of doxycycline and may be caused by the fact that the doxycycline tablets were taken on an empty stomach; food might have diminished the gastric upset.

In both treatments steady state was established on day 3. Mean values of minimum theophylline plasma concentrations (C_{min}) in the morning on days 3–9 were all close to 6 mg L^{-1}.

Figure 1 shows the mean theophylline plasma concentration–time curves, as observed on days 9 and 10 during both studies, on a semilogarithmic scale.

The rate of absorption of theophylline on day 9 was normal, with minor variation among the subjects (t_{max} = time to peak, 3.2 ± 0.4 h, and C_{max} = peak concentration, 9.7 ± 2.6 mg L^{-1}). Cotreatment with doxycycline tended to result in a somewhat slower absorption (time to peak, 4.0 ± 1.1 h), with lower peak concentration (9.0 ± 2.3 mg L^{-1}), but the difference was not statistically significant ($p > 0.05$). Also, the values for the areas under the plasma concentration–time curves were not significantly different after the addition of doxycycline, indicating that no important interaction is present at the absorption level.

Values observed for half-life of elimination ($t_{1/2}$), volume of distribution (V_d), and clearance *(CL)* are well within the range reported in healthy volunteers (Table 1). Addition of doxycycline did not significantly change mean values of these pharmacokinetic parameters. Thus, mean steady-state theophylline plasma concentrations (C_{ss}) were not significantly different during the two treatments. It is probable that no adjustment of theophylline dosage is required when the drug is given together with doxycycline.

REFERENCES

1. Jonkman JHG, Upton RA. Pharmacokinetic drug interactions with theophylline; a review. *Clin Pharmacokinet* 1984;9:309–34.
2. Mathis JW, Prince RA, Weinberger MM, Mc Elnay JC. Effect of tetracycline hydrochloride on theophylline kinetics. *Clin Pharmacy* 1982;1:446–8.
3. Jonkman JHG, Schoenmaker R, Greving JE, De Zeeuw RA. Rapid and selective theophylline serum and saliva assay by means of high pressure liquid chromatography. *Pharm Weekbl [Sci]* 1980;2:49–53.

Therapeutic Drug Monitoring
7:95–100

Evaluation of the Du Pont Theophylline Assay Adapted to a Centrifugal Analyzer

*†Roger L. Boeckx and *Sara T. Munson

**Department of Laboratory Medicine, Childrens' Hospital National Medical Center, and †Department of Child Health and Development, The George Washington University School of Medicine and Health Sciences, Washington, D.C., U.S.A.*

Summary: We evaluated the Du Pont Theophylline Assay, a particle-enhanced turbidimetric inhibition immunoassay (PETINIA) for the measurement of theophylline in human serum. The procedure was applied to the Cobas-Bio centrifugal analyzer, and was compared to an enzyme immunoassay (EMIT) method and a high performance liquid chromatographic (HPLC) procedure. Day-to-day precision was 3.7% (1 SD coefficient of variation) at 7.1 mg/L, 3.3% at 17.7 mg/L, and 3.9% at 27.8 mg/L. The assay was linear up to 40 mg/L, and the correlation between the PETINIA, EMIT, and HPLC methods was good [PETINIA/EMIT: $y = 0.94x + 0.63$, $r = 0.98$, $S_{yx} = 1.13$; PETINIA/HPLC: $y = 1.00x - 0.89$, $r = 0.99$, $S_{yx} = 0.66$, where S_{yx} is the standard deviation of the residual error of regression], when evaluated using specimens from 135 patients receiving theophylline. No interference from hemolysis, lipemia, icterus, or other methylxanthines was observed. Of the major metabolites of theophylline, only 1,3-dimethyluric acid showed any significant cross-reactivity (2.1 mg/L apparent theophylline at 20 mg/L 1,3-dimethyluric acid). The method is reliable and cost-effective for the measurement of theophylline in serum. **Key Words:** Particle-enhanced turbidimetric inhibition immunoassay (PETINIA)—Enzyme multiplied immunoassay technique (EMIT)—High performance liquid chromatography (HPLC)—Theophylline assay.

The monitoring of serum theophylline concentration is a necessary component of the treatment of asthma and neonatal apnea (1–4). Various methods have been described for the measurement of theophylline concentration in body fluids. These include high performance liquid chromatography (HPLC) (5), enzyme immunoassay (6), fluorescence polarization immunoassay (7), substrate-labeled fluorescent immunoassay (8), and gas-liquid chromatography (9).

We report here the evaluation of the Du Pont Theophylline Assay, a novel analytical approach for the measurement of theophylline in serum. The particle-enhanced turbidimetric inhibition immunoassay (PETINIA) is a homogeneous immunoassay technique that employs a latex particle–theophylline conjugate and a theophylline-specific monoclonal antibody (10,11). The reaction between the anti-theophylline antibody and the latex–theophylline conjugate results in the formation of light-scattering particles that cause an increase in the turbidity of the reaction mixture. Unlabeled theophylline, when added to the system, occupies theophylline sites on the antibody and inhibits the rate of increase in turbidity. The rate of particle aggregation is monitored by measuring the absorbance at 340 nm, and this rate of increase of the absorbance of the reaction mixture is inversely proportional to the concentration of theophylline. The development of

Address correspondence and reprint requests to Dr. R. L. Boeckx at Department of Laboratory Medicine, Childrens' Hospital National Medical Center, 111 Michigan Avenue NW, Washington, DC 20010, U.S.A.

latex particles, specifically designed for use in PETINIA, has recently been described (12), and a PETINIA for theophylline is commercially available, but only for use on the aca analyzer manufactured by E. I. du Pont de Nemours and Co. (Wilmington, DE, U.S.A.) (11). We used PETINIA reagents that had been specifically formulated for use with spectrophotometers other than the Du Pont aca and compared the performance of the assay with an enzyme immunoassay and an HPLC method.

MATERIALS AND METHODS

Instrumentation

We used the Cobas Bio centrifugal analyzer (Roche Analytical Instruments, Inc., Nutley, NJ, U.S.A.), equipped with the DENS option, for the PETINIA and EIA procedures. The DENS option allows automatic calculation of results using a nonlinear standard curve derived by means of a four-parameter logit function.

For HPLC we used an M-45 solvent delivery system (Waters Associates, Inc., Milford, MA, U.S.A.), a model 7125 6-port rotary injector fitted with a 20-μl loop (Rheodyne Inc., Cotati, CA, U.S.A.), an LC-6 UV absorbance detector (Bioanalytical Systems, Inc., West Lafayette, IN, U.S.A.), and a C-18 reversed-phase column (Biophase ODS 4.6 × 250 mm, 5-μm particle size; Bioanalytical Systems). The mobile phase was pumped at a rate of 1.6 ml/min at ambient temperature. The absorbance of the column eluent was monitored at 273 nm.

Reagents

PETINIA reagents and calibrators were supplied by Du Pont. Each reagent kit consists of a vial of theophylline–particle reagent, a vial of theophylline–specific monoclonal (mouse) antibody reagent, a bottle of phosphate buffer, and a set of six calibrators (0, 2, 5, 10, 20, and 40 mg/L). A working particle solution was prepared as recommended by the manufacturer, by mixing 1 part of theophylline–particle reagent and 15 parts phosphate buffer. The other reagents were used as supplied.

Enzyme immunoassay reagents [enzyme multiplied immunoassay technique (EMIT)] and calibrators were purchased from Syva Co. (Palo Alto, CA, U.S.A.). EMIT reagents were reconstituted as recommended by Syva. A working solution of reagent A was prepared by mixing 1 part reconstituted reagent A with 11 parts EMIT theophylline buffer solution. Reagent B was used as reconstituted.

Anhydrous theophylline, β-hydroxyethyltheophylline, caffeine, theobromine, 8-chlorotheophylline, 3-methylxanthine, 1-methyluric acid, and 1,3-dimethyluric acid were obtained from Sigma Chemical Co. (St. Louis, MO, U.S.A.). HPLC-grade acetonitrile, methanol, chloroform, 2-propanol, sodium acetate, and glacial acetic acid were purchased from Scientific Products (Columbia, MD, U.S.A.).

A stock solution of 50 mg theophylline in 100 ml deionized water was prepared. Dilutions of this stock solution with drug-free serum were made to provide working standards containing theophylline at concentrations of 5, 10, 20, and 50 mg/L. These solutions were divided into 100-μl aliquots and frozen at −50°C until used. The internal standard solution was prepared by diluting a stock solution of β-hydroxyethyltheophylline (1 g/L in acetonitrile) in acetonitrile to a final concentration of 15 mg/L. A 0.01 *M* acetate buffer was prepared by adjusting the pH of a 0.01 *M* solution of sodium acetate to 4.0 with a 0.01 *M* solution of acetic acid. The mobile phase consisted of 100 ml of acetonitrile added to 900 ml of the acetate buffer.

Procedures

The HPLC procedure is a modification of the method of Ou and Frawley (5). To 100 μl of sample (standard, serum, or control) was added 100 μl of working internal standard solution and 2.0 ml of chloroform:2-propanol (95:5, vol/vol). The mixture was vortex-mixed for 30 s and centrifuged (5 min at 3,000 *g*). The lower layer was transferred to a clean test tube and evaporated under a stream of air at 40°C. The residue was dissolved in 75 μl methanol, and 20 μl was injected onto the column. Results were calculated using the peak height ratio method.

For the PETINIA procedure, the primary reagent well was filled with 8 ml of the working particle solution, and the secondary reagent well was filled with 1.0 ml of antibody reagent.

For the EMIT procedure, the primary reagent well was filled with 7 ml of working reagent A solution, and the secondary reagent well was filled with 1 ml of reagent B.

The settings used on the Cobas Bio for the PETINIA and EMIT are shown in Table 1.

RESULTS

The within-run precision of the PETINIA was evaluated by analyzing 10 aliquots of three different con-

TABLE 1. *Cobas Bio settings for the PETINIA and EMIT methods*

Parameter	PETINIA	EMIT
Calculation factor	1,000	1,000
Standard 1 conc. (μg/ml)	0	0
Standard 2 conc. (μg/ml)	2.0	2.5
Standard 3 conc. (μg/ml)	5.0	5.0
Standard 4 conc. (μg/ml)	10.0	10.0
Standard 5 conc. (μg/ml)	20.0	20.0
Standard 6 conc. (μg/ml)	40.0	40.0
Limit	0	20
Temperature (°C)	37.0	30.0
Type of analysis	7.3	7.3
Wavelength (nm)	340	340
Sample volume (μl)	3	3
Diluent volume (μl)	20	70
Reagent volume (μl)	300	215
Incubation time (s)	30	20
Start reagent volume (μl)	20	18
Time of first reading (s)	0.5	5.0
Time interval (s)	10	10
Number of readings	4	4
Blanking mode	0	0
Printout mode	0	0

PETINIA, particle-enhanced turbidimetric inhibition immunoassay; EMIT, enzyme multiplied immunoassay technique.

centrations of quality control material (TheraChem anticonvulsant/theophylline control; Fisher Diagnostics, Orangeburg, NY, U.S.A.) in the same analytical run. The "low" and "high" materials were analyzed as reconstituted, following the manufacturer's instructions, and a "mid-level" material was prepared by mixing equal volumes of the "low" and "high" materials. In addition, the same within-run analysis was performed for each of the six PETINIA calibrator materials. The results of the within-run precision study are shown in Table 2.

Day-to-day precision was evaluated by analyzing aliquots of the same three quality control materials (low, mid, high) on 20 consecutive days, by each of the three methods (PETINIA, EMIT, HPLC). The results of the day-to-day precision study are shown in Table 3.

We determined the stability of the PETINIA standard curve. The Cobas Bio was calibrated, and each of the six calibrators were assayed on subsequent days. A single lot of working particle solution (see Materials and Methods) was used throughout the study. The solution was stored at 4°C. We found that the calibration curve was stable for at least 35 days.

The linearity of the PETINIA was evaluated by analyzing a number of specimens specifically prepared by combining quality control materials and calibrators to cover a range of theophylline concentrations from 0 to

TABLE 2. *Within-run precision of the PETINIA for theophylline*

	Mean (mg/L)	SD (mg/L)	CV (%)
Low	7.1	0.1	1.8
Mid	17.3	0.5	2.9
High	27.4	0.7	2.6
0.0 calibrator	0.0	0.0	—
2.0 calibrator	2.0	0.1	3.1
5.0 calibrator	4.9	0.1	2.3
10.0 calibrator	9.8	0.2	2.2
20.0 calibrator	20.3	0.3	1.6
40.0 calibrator	36.6	0.6	1.7

Ten samples at each concentration were analyzed in each case. SD, standard deviation; CV, 1 SD coefficient of variation expressed as a percentage; PETINIA, particle-enhanced turbidimetric inhibition immunoassay.

40 mg/L. All measurements were made in duplicate. The results of this study are shown in Fig. 1.

A split-sample correlation study, using specimens from 135 patients receiving theophylline, was performed to compare the performance of the PETINIA with the EMIT and HPLC methods. The results are

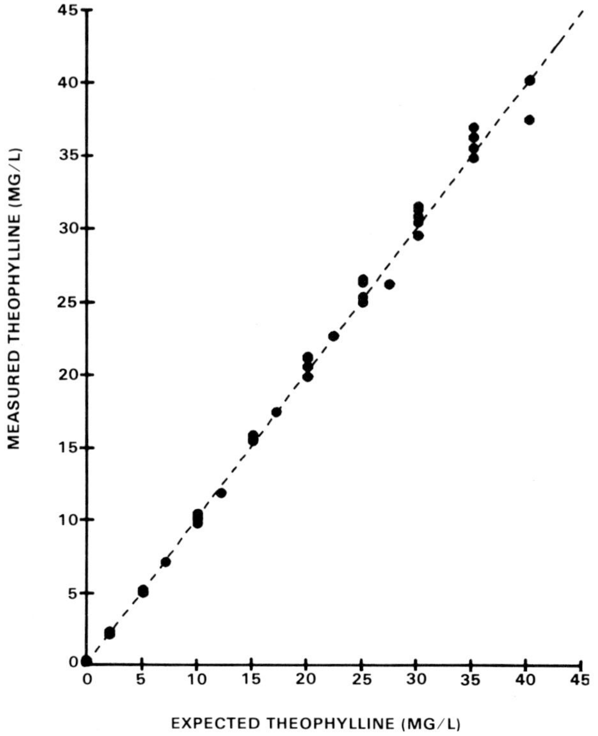

FIG. 1. Linearity of the particle-enhanced turbidimetric inhibition immunoassay (PETINIA). Each point is the mean of duplicate analyses. Linear regression analysis yielded the following straight line through the 50 data points: $y = 1.00x + 0.6$; r = 0.99; $S_{yx} = 0.706$. The dashed line is the line of identity.

TABLE 3. *Day-to-day precision of the theophylline assays*

Assay	Low	Mid	High
EMIT			
Mean (mg/L)	7.3	17.8	27.6
SD	0.3	0.8	1.5
CV (%)	4.1	4.5	5.4
HPLC			
Mean (mg/L)	8.0	18.6	29.0
SD	0.2	0.4	0.8
CV (%)	2.5	1.9	2.6
PETINIA			
Mean (mg/L)	7.1	17.7	27.8
SD	0.3	0.6	1.1
CV (%)	3.7	3.3	3.9

Each material was analyzed on 20 consecutive days. SD, standard deviation; CV, 1 SD coefficient of variation expressed as a percentage; EMIT, enzyme multiplied immunoassay technique; HPLC, high performance liquid chromatography; PETINIA, particle-enhanced turbidimetric inhibition immunoassay.

presented in Fig. 2. Regression analysis (13) of the results obtained when comparing PETINIA *(y)* with EMIT *(x)* gave the following equation for the best-fitting straight line: $y = 0.94x + 0.63$, $r = 0.98$, $S_{yx} = 1.13$, where S_{yx} is the standard deviation of the residual error of regression. The equation of the best-fitting straight line through the data obtained when comparing PETINIA *(y)* with HPLC *(x)* was $y = 1.00x - 0.89$, $r = 0.99$, $S_{yx} = 0.66$.

We evaluated the effect of hemolysis, lipemia, and icterus on the PETINIA. Samples were prepared by adding theophylline to a drug-free serum pool, to a concentration of 15.0 mg/L. Samples were treated with hemoglobin (prepared by hemolyzing packed red cells), triglycerides [by adding various amounts of Intralipid, 20% (Cutter Biological, Emeryville, CA, U.S.A.)], and bilirubin (prepared as a 20 g/L solution in 0.1 *M* NaOH–0.1 *M* Na_2CO_3). No interference was observed from hemoglobin concentrations up to 4,530 mg/L, triglyceride concentrations up to 5,700 mg/L, or bilirubin concentrations up to 342 mg/L.

The potential interference of a number of other methylxanthines, related drugs, and theophylline metabolites

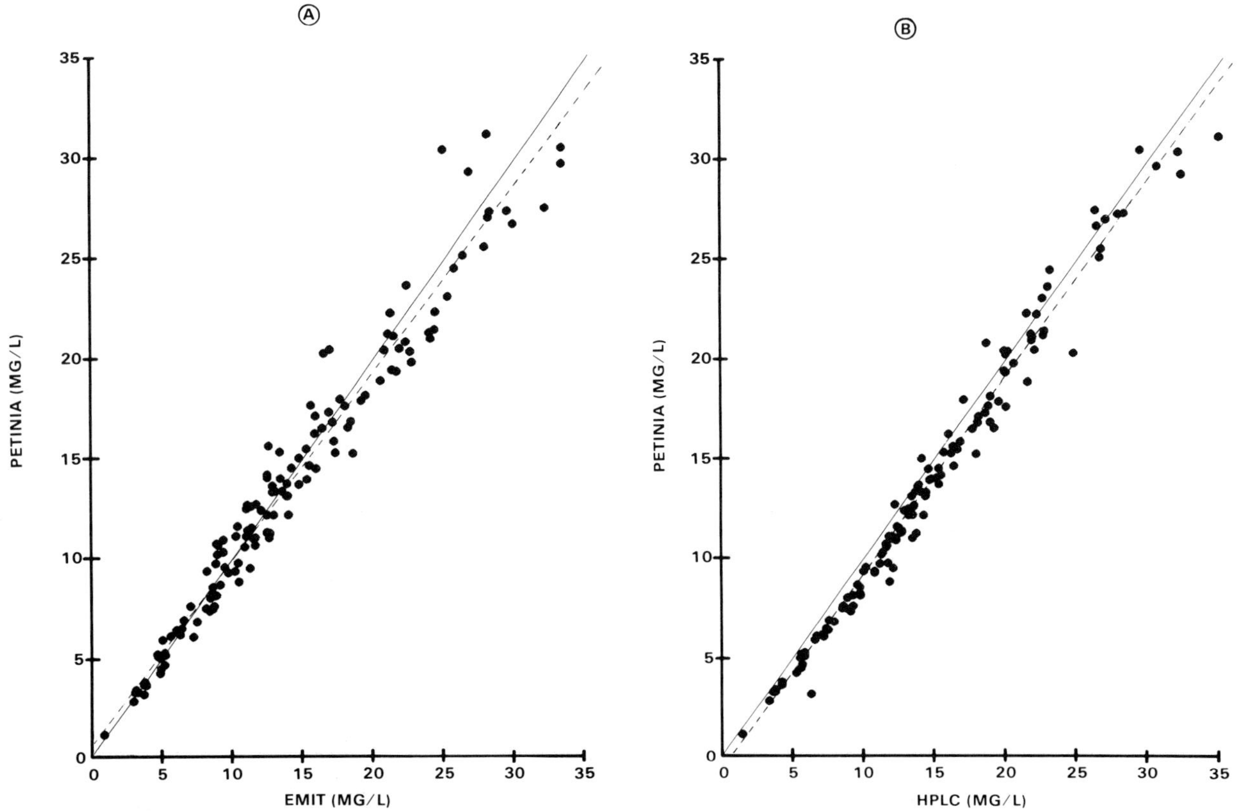

FIG. 2. Comparison of the three methods using samples from 135 patients receiving theophylline. **A:** Comparison of particle-enhanced turbidimetric inhibition immunoassay (PETINIA) and enzyme multiplied immunoassay technique (EMIT). **B:** Comparison of PETINIA and high performance liquid chromatography (HPLC). The dashed line is the best-fitting straight line determined using the Deming method (13). The solid line is the line of identity.

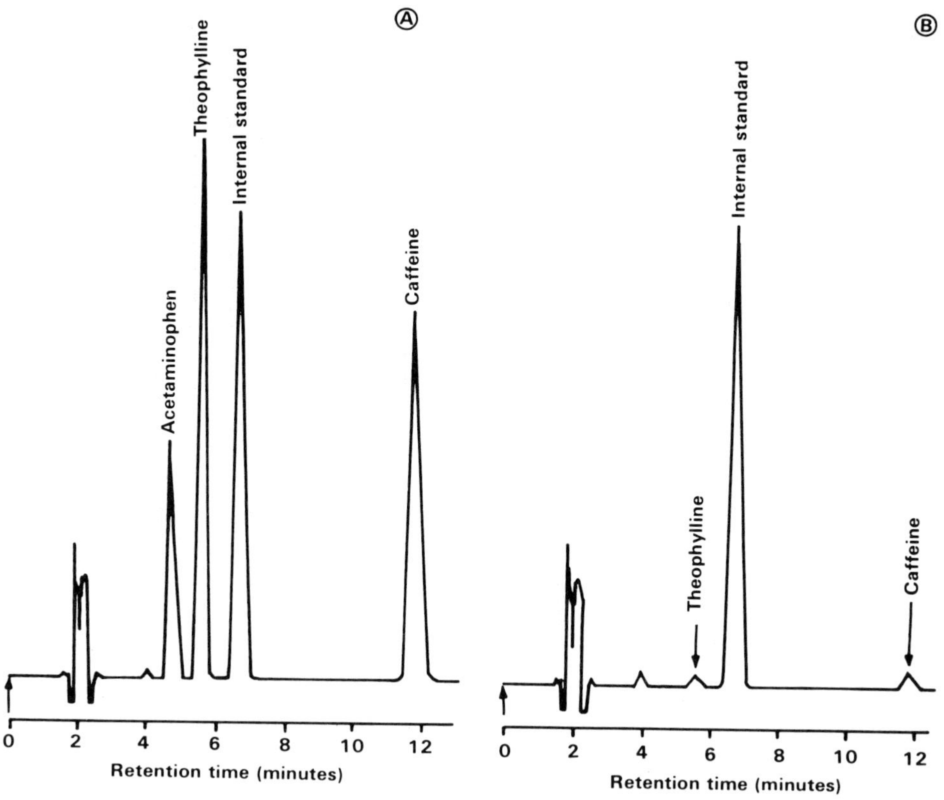

FIG. 3. Chromatogram of high performance liquid chromatography standard containing 20 mg/L each of acetaminophen, theophylline, and caffeine **(A)** and the particle-enhanced turbidimetric inhibition immunoassay (PETINIA) zero calibrator **(B)**, showing the presence of small amounts of theophylline and caffeine.

was evaluated. Each interfering compound was added to drug-free serum at final concentrations of 20 mg/L and 100 mg/L, and the treated serum samples were analyzed for theophylline using the PETINIA. Results of the interference study are shown in Table 4.

DISCUSSION

The Du Pont PETINIA for theophylline is a stable, accurate, and precise method for the measurement of theophylline in serum. When used with a centrifugal analyzer, such as the Cobas Bio, this procedure will provide rapid turnaround of theophylline analyses.

The precision of the method ranged from 3.3 to 3.9%, and exceeded the performance of the enzyme immunoassay method. HPLC did, however, provide somewhat better precision.

The method was linear to 40 mg/L. An evaluation of sample dilution procedures showed that samples in which the theophylline concentration exceeded 40 mg/L could be adequately diluted with water, normal saline, "zero" calibrator, or drug-free serum, but dilution with drug-free serum gave the best results.

TABLE 4. *Measured theophylline concentrations resulting from potential interferents in the PETINIA*

Potential interferent	Concentration (mg/L)	Theophylline measured (mg/L)
Caffeine	20	<0.1
	100	0.2
Theobromine	20	0.2
	100	0.9
8-Chlorotheophylline	20	0.9
	100	4.4
3-Methylxanthine	20	0.3
	100	1.4
1,3-Dimethyluric acid	20	2.1
	100	10.5
1-Methyluric acid	20	<0.1
	100	0.1

Each value is the mean of duplicate determinations. PETINIA, particle-enhanced turbidimetric inhibition immunoassay.

In a study of 135 patients, the PETINIA method, demonstrated good correlation with EMIT and HPLC, the two most commonly used methods for the determination of theophylline. Correlation with HPLC was better, as demonstrated by the higher correlation coefficient (r = 0.99) and lower standard error of the estimate (S_{yx} = 0.66). The correlation between the PETINIA and HPLC methods shows the existence of a small constant error. Analysis of the PETINIA calibrators by HPLC (Fig. 3) shows the presence of small amounts of theophylline (0.5 mg/L) and caffeine (1.0 mg/L) in the zero calibrator. This might account for the constant error that is observed. Correlation of PETINIA with EMIT was not as good as with HPLC, and showed significant scatter at higher theophylline concentrations. Correlation of EMIT *(y)* and HPLC *(x)* yielded the following equation: $y = 1.03x - 1.12$ (r = 0.97, S_{yx} = 1.76), and showed the same scatter at higher theophylline concentrations. This would suggest that the scatter that is observed in the PETINIA/EMIT correlation may be due to the EMIT method rather than to the PETINIA method.

No interference was observed from hemolysis, lipemia, or icterus, and no significant cross-reaction was noted with a number of other methylxanthines. 8-Chlorotheophylline at a concentration of 100 mg/L gave an apparent theophylline concentration of 4.4 mg/L. This compound is a component of a popular nonprescription medication for motion sickness (Dramamine, the 8-chlorotheophylline salt of diphenhydramine). Serum concentrations of 100 mg/L are never achieved from the administration of this agent.

Of the metabolites of theophylline (14), only 1,3-dimethyluric acid showed any significant cross-reactivity. At a concentration of 20 mg/L, 1,3-dimethyluric acid gave an apparent theophylline concentration of 2.1 mg/L. Although it is a major urinary metabolite of theophylline, this compound does not usually reach significant concentrations in the serum of patients receiving theophylline. Approximately 40% of a dose of theophylline is excreted in the urine as 1,3-dimethyluric acid (15). Presumably, this compound might accumulate in patients with renal failure.

The calibration curve of the PETINIA was stable for at least 35 days. This will allow some cost-saving to be realized, since the procedure will not need to be calibrated as frequently as other methods.

The performance of the PETINIA on the Cobas Bio analyzer was comparable to results obtained on the Du Pont aca analyzer (10,11). The PETINIA for theophylline should prove to be a widely applicable, reliable, cost-effective alternative for the measurement of serum theophylline concentration.

REFERENCES

1. Simons FER. Asthma. In: Moyer TP, Boeckx RL, eds. *Applied therapeutic drug monitoring*, vol 2. Washington, D.C.: American Association for Clinical Chemistry, 1984:207–11.
2. Hendeles L, Weinberger M. Theophylline. Therapeutic use and serum concentration monitoring. In: Taylor WJ, Finn AL, eds. *Individualizing drug therapy*, vol 1. New York: Gross, Townsend, Frank, Inc., 1981:31–65.
3. Aranda JV, Turmen T. Methylxanthines in apnea of prematurity. *Clin Perinatol* 1979;6:87–108.
4. Ogilvie RI. Monitoring plasma theophylline concentrations. *Ther Drug Monit* 1980;2:111–7.
5. Ou CN, Frawley VL. Concurrent measurement of theophylline and caffeine in neonates by an interference-free liquid-chromatographic method. *Clin Chem* 1983;29:1934–6.
6. Rubenstein KE, Schneider RS, Ullman EF. Homogeneous enzyme immunoassay. A new biochemical technique. *Biochem Biophys Res Commun* 1972;47:846–51.
7. Hill HD, Jolley ME, Wang CHJ, et al. Fluorescence polarization immunoassay (FPIA) for theophylline: clinical correlation and reagent stability. *Clin Chem* 1981;27:1086.
8. Messenger LJ, Li TM, Benovic JL, Burd JF. STAT assay for theophylline concentrations in human serum using a modified substrate labeled fluorescent immunoassay. *J Allergy Clin Immunol* 1980;65:175.
9. Least CJ, Johnson GF, Soloman HM. Gas-chromatographic microscale procedure for theophylline, with use of a nitrogen-sensitive detector. *Clin Chem* 1976;22:765–8.
10. Powell LM, Frey WA, Simons DM, Riabov DK, Jurga PA, Miller WK. A very precise measurement for theophylline on the Du Pont aca analyzer. *Clin Chem* 1983;29:1156.
11. Opheim KE, Glick MR, Ou C-N, et al. Particle-enhanced turbidimetric inhibition immunoassay for theophylline evaluated with the Du Pont aca. *Clin Chem* 1984;30:1870–4.
12. Litchfield WJ, Craig AR, Frey WA, Leflar CC. Novel shell/core particles for automated turbidimetric immunoassays. *Clin Chem* 1984;30:1489–93.
13. Cornbleet PJ, Gochman N. Incorrect least-squares regression coefficients in method-comparison analysis. *Clin Chem* 1979;25:432–8.
14. Baselt RC. *Disposition of toxic drugs and chemicals in man*. 2nd ed. Davis, California: Biomedical Publications, 1982:723–7.
15. Jenne JW, Nagasawa HT, Thompson RD. Relationship of urinary metabolites of theophylline to serum theophylline levels. *Clin Pharmacol Ther* 1976;19:375–81.

Therapeutic Drug Monitoring
7:101–107 © 1985 Raven Press, New York

Dual-Label Fluoroimmunoassay for Simultaneous Determination of Primidone and Phenobarbital

A. M. Sidki, D. S. Smith, and J. Landon

Department of Chemical Pathology, St. Bartholomew's Hospital, London, England

Summary: A dual-label magnetizable solid-phase fluoroimmunoassay for direct determination of serum levels of primidone and its main metabolite, phenobarbital, in a single tube was developed and optimized. Fluorescein isothiocyanate was used to label phenobarbital and a rhodamine 101 derivative (XRITC) to label primidone; these could be independently quantitated with no fluorimetric "cross-talk." The dual-label assay employs mixed immunochemical reagents but is otherwise similar in performance to conventional, single-drug, magnetizable solid-phase fluoroimmunoassays. The ability to measure simultaneously two related analytes, such as a drug and its metabolite, represents a useful extension of immunoassay. This was illustrated in the present work by assay of sera from patients on primidone therapy. Dual-label assay results correlated well with those by a conventional enzymoimmunoassay (for primidone) and by a polarization fluoroimmunoassay (for phenobarbital). **Key Words:** Primidone—Phenobarbital—Antiepileptic drugs—Fluoroimmunoassay—Drug assay—Monitoring therapy—Dual assay.

Monitoring circulating levels of drugs used for prophylactic treatment of epilepsy is useful in determining the proper dosage (1). When a drug (such as primidone) produces an active metabolite (phenobarbital), measurement of both species may be clinically useful in the management of therapy (2). We have already reported single-drug assays for primidone (3) and phenobarbital (4) using fluorescein-labeled drug and antibody coupled to magnetizable solid-phase particles.

Various methods have been devised for measuring combinations of drugs or hormones simultaneously. These include liquid and gas-liquid chromatographic systems to measure combinations of antiepileptics (5,6). Various dual-label radioimmunoassays (RIA) have been described, for example, the determination of triiodothyronine (T_3) and thyroxine (T_4) (7) or of T_4 and thyrotrophin (8) with ^{125}I and ^{131}I as labels. Weerasekera and colleagues (9) described a combined RIA/nonisotopic immunoassay for two steroid glucuronides in urine, employing tritium and a chemiluminescent label as tracers. Dual-label enzymoimmunoassay of T_4 and T_3 has also been reported (10), but the endpoint determinations were somewhat tedious and complicated because of the different incubation conditions required for the two enzymes employed (alkaline phosphatase and β-galactosidase). A sol particle immunoassay for simultaneous measurement of human placental lactogen and human chorionic gonadotrophin (11) utilized specific antibodies conjugated to silver and gold particles, respectively, with detection by atomic absorption spectroscopy.

Fluoroimmunoassay (FIA) is well suited to dual-label applications because of the simplicity, speed, and versatility of fluorescence measurement. Recently, a 4-methylcoumarin derivative of phenytoin and a β-galactosylcoumarin derivative of phenobarbital were employed in a nonseparation substrate-la-

Address correspondence and reprint requests to Dr. A. M. Sidki, Department of Chemical Pathology, St. Bartholomew's Hospital, 51 Bartholomew Close, London EC1A 7HL, England.

beled FIA for the simultaneous determination of phenytoin and phenobarbital (12). Labeling with fluorescein (green-emitting) and various rhodamines (orange- to red-emitting) has a long history in immunofluorescence, and quantitative applications with labeled antibodies have been reported (13,14). Established two-colour labeling pairs such as fluorescein isothiocyanate (FITC) and tetramethyl- or tetraethylrhodamine isothiocyanate are not ideal because of partial overlap of their fluorescence spectra, which must be compensated for electronically to obtain optimum accuracy (13,14). Superior red-emitting labels, based on the rhodamine 101 fluorophore, have recently been introduced (15). These have a comparatively high quantum yield in water and offer the important advantage that the excitation and emission spectra are red-shifted relative to those of the commoner rhodamine derivatives. XRITC is the isothiocyanate derivative of rhodamine 101, while "Texas Red" is sulforhodamine 101 with an active sulfonyl chloride function (16). Materials labeled with FITC and with either XRITC or Texas Red may be independently quantitated in mixtures because of their nonoverlapping emission and excitation spectra (16).

The present report gives a detailed description of the development of a dual-label, magnetizable solid-phase FIA for the simultaneous direct determination of primidone and phenobarbital. FITC and XRITC were employed for labeling phenobarbital and primidone derivatives, respectively.

MATERIALS AND METHODS

Reagents

Primidone was obtained from ICI (Macclesfield, Cheshire, U.K.); phenobarbital from Winthrop (Surbiton, Surrey, U.K.); XRITC from Research Organics (Cleveland, OH, U.S.A.); Triton X-100 and all organic solvents (Analar grade) from BDH (Poole, Dorset, U.K.); keyhole limpet hemocyanin (KLH) from Calbiochem-Behring Corp. (La Jolla, CA, U.S.A.); silica gel thin-layer chromatography sheets (DC-Alufolien Kieselgel 60 F_{254}, Art. 5554) from E. Merck (Darmstadt, F.R.G.); and pooled normal human serum from ILS (London, U.K.). Other drugs employed in the specificity studies were gifts from their respective distributors in the United Kingdom. Fluorescein-labeled phenobarbital (PB-FTC) was prepared as described previously (4). Sheep antiprimidone serum was obtained as reported elsewhere (3). Sheep antiphenobarbital serum was obtained by immunizing with 5-ethyl-5(4-aminophenyl)barbituric acid coupled to KLH by diazotization, employing procedures similar to those described previously (4). Each antiserum (2 ml) was covalently coupled by the cyanogen bromide method (3) to 1 g of magnetizable cellulose/iron oxide particles. The products were suspended in 20 ml of sodium phosphate buffer (100 mmol/L, pH 7.5) and stored at 4°C when they remained stable for at least 1 year.

Preparation of XRITC-Labeled Primidone

The 4-aminophenyl derivative of primidone (3 mg), prepared as described previously (3), was reacted with XRITC (8 mg) in 500 μl dimethylformamide for 3 h at room temperature. The reaction mixture was applied to silica gel sheets (70 μl per sheet) which were developed with chloroform:methanol:acetic acid (85:12:3, by volume). The major product (R_f 0.2) was removed and extracted into ethanol (2 ml per sheet), and the solution was stored at −20°C. The concentration of XRITC-labeled primidone (PR-XRTC) was estimated spectrophotometrically on the assumption that it has the same absorptivity as XRITC itself, with a peak extinction coefficient of 8.4×10^4 L mol^{-1} cm^{-1} (16). The PR-XRTC was found to be stable for more than 1 year when stored at −20°C and tested in the present assay.

Assay Standards

Primidone and phenobarbital were dissolved together in methanol at 1 g/L concentrations of each drug, and this stock solution was added to drug-free pooled normal human serum to obtain the required standard concentrations. Standards were stored at −20°C.

Patients' Specimens

Serum specimens from patients receiving primidone therapy were obtained from the Department of Chemical Pathology, The National Hospital for Nervous Diseases (Queen Square, London, U.K.). They were assayed for primidone by an enzymoimmunoassay (EMIT; Syva) and for phenobarbital by a polarization fluoroimmunoassay (PIA) (4).

Fluorimetry

Fluorescence was measured directly in disposable test tubes using a Perkin-Elmer model LS-5 Luminescence Spectrometer fitted with a cuvette adaptor (17). The excitation and emission wavelengths used for fluorescein were 492 and 517 nm, and for rhodamine 101, 577 and 607 nm, respectively (corresponding to the spectral peaks in each case). Excitation and emission monochromator slit widths were 5 nm in all cases. A red-sensitive photomultiplier was used throughout this work to ensure adequate response at the high wavelengths characteristic of rhodamine 101 fluorescence.

Dual-Label Fluoroimmunoassay Procedures

The assay tubes were disposable polystyrene test tubes (no. 55.484, 55 × 12 mm; Sarstedt, Leicester, Leicestershire, U.K.). Sodium borate (200 mmol/L, pH 10.0) containing Triton X-100 (1 ml/L) and sodium azide (1 g/L) was the diluent buffer. The elution reagent was a mixture of methanol and sodium bicarbonate buffer (50 mmol/L, pH 9.0, containing 10 ml/L Triton X-100) in the proportion of 4:1, by volume. The magnet used was a multipolar ferrite block magnet, with a flat surface of approximately 15 × 20 cm (Magnet Applications, London, U.K.).

Assay protocol. Assays were performed at room temperature, in duplicate. Into test tubes were pipetted 10 μl of standard or sample, followed by 100 μl of a mixture of the two tracers (PR-XRTC 400 nmol/L and PB-FTC 580 nmol/L) and, finally, 200 μl of a mixture of the two solid-phase coupled antisera (antiprimidone solid phase, 7.5 g/L, and antiphenobarbital solid phase, 5 g/L). After 30 min incubation with continuous mixing on a mechanical shaker, 1 ml of diluent buffer was added, the particles were sedimented to the bottom of the tubes on a magnet, and the supernates were aspirated to waste. Elution reagent (1.5 ml) was then added, the tubes were vortex-mixed, and the particles were sedimented again on the magnet. Finally, the fluorescence of the supernates (containing the eluted bound fractions of the tracers) was measured for each tracer at its optimal excitation and emission wavelengths. Two standard curves, one for primidone and the other for phenobarbital, were constructed by plotting the percentage of total fluorescence of each tracer bound against the serum standard concentration of the corresponding drug (Fig. 1).

RESULTS

Assay Optimization

Effect of pH

The use of an assay diluent buffer with pH 10.0 prevented serum protein interference with binding of the PR-XRTC tracer and, at pH 10.0, superimposable dual-label assay standard curves were obtained using standards prepared in buffer and in serum.

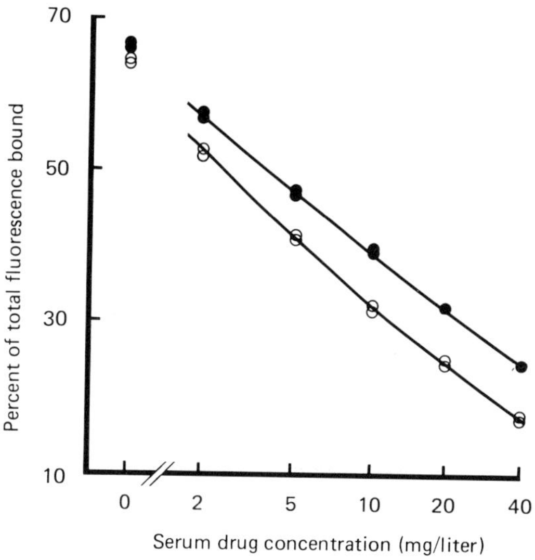

FIG. 1. Calibration curves for dual-label simultaneous fluoroimmunoassay of primidone and phenobarbital in serum. Measurement of rhodamine 101 fluorescence gives the primidone standard curve (closed circles) and measurement of fluorescein fluorescence gives the phenobarbital standard curve (open circles).

Choice of Elution Reagent

In preliminary experiments it was necessary to find an elution reagent that could elute both antibody-bound tracers from the solid phase efficiently and also yield a good fluorescence signal. A mixture of methanol:sodium bicarbonate buffer (50 mmol/L, pH 9.0, containing 10 ml/L Triton X-100) in the proportion of 4:1 by volume was suitable and proved easy to dispense with a repeating dispenser.

Antiserum Dilution Curves

Figure 2 shows the binding of PR-XRTC with double dilutions of antiprimidone magnetizable solid-phase particles. An amount of 1.5 mg per tube of these particles, which gave about 70% binding in the absence of primidone (zero concentration standard), was chosen for use in the dual-label system. A similar antibody dilution curve was obtained for phenobarbital, from which 1 mg per tube of the particles was chosen. Nonspecific binding for both tracers was less than 4%, as determined using magnetizable particles covalently linked to nonimmunized sheep serum (Fig. 2).

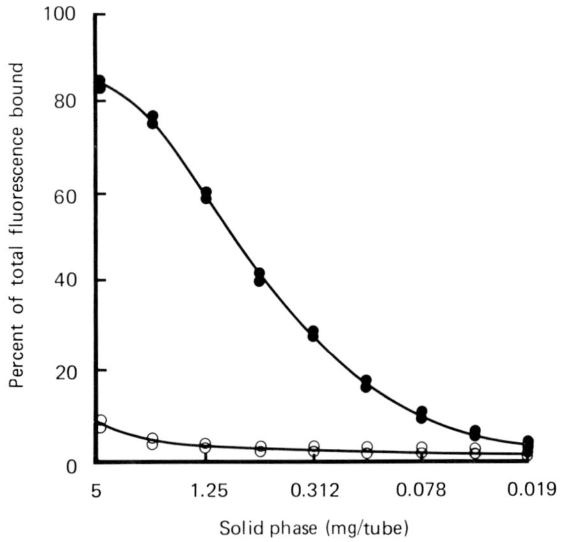

FIG. 2. Antibody dilution curves constructed with antiprimidone solid phase (closed circles) or nonspecific sheep solid phase (open circles), XRITC-labeled primidone being used as tracer.

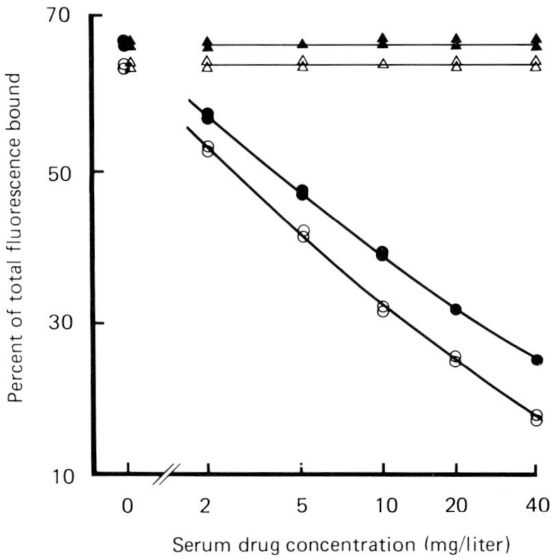

FIG. 4. Specificity of the dual-label fluoroimmunoassay system with mixed tracer and solid-phase reagents. With use of serum standards containing phenobarbital alone, fluorescein (open circles) or rhodamine 101 (closed triangles) fluorescence was measured. With serum standards containing primidone alone, rhodamine 101 (closed circles) or fluorescein (open triangles) fluorescence was measured.

Nonoverlapping Fluorescence Spectra of PR-XRTC and PB-FTC

Excitation and emission spectra for both PR-XRTC and PB-FTC in elution reagent are shown in Fig. 3. There is wide separation between the excitation and emission bands of the two fluorophores. By use of the excitation and emission wavelengths optimal for fluorescein, PR-XRTC at the concentration employed in the FIA gave a signal equivalent to that obtained from assay buffer alone (background signal). The same result was obtained with PB-FTC at excitation and emission wavelengths optimal for XRITC. Thus, there was no overlapping of spectra, and the two fluorophores could be quantitated independently of each other.

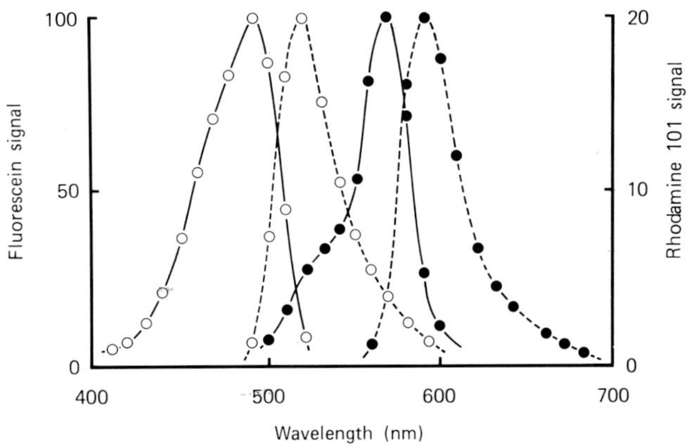

FIG. 3. Fluorescence excitation (solid lines) and emission (dotted lines) spectra of fluorescein-labeled phenobarbital (open circles) and rhodamine 101-labeled primidone (closed circles) in assay elution reagent.

Specificity of the Combined Immunochemical Systems

Three assays were performed simultaneously, the same assay protocol as described earlier being used, with the exception that only single-drug standards were used (i.e., primidone standards or phenobarbital standards prepared in pooled normal human serum) for running two of the assays while the third assay was performed as usual. Figure 4 shows the results, which indicate that there was no immunochemical interference of one assay with the other, and the mixed-drug standards gave curves that were superimposable with those of the corresponding individual specific drug standard curves.

Standard Curves

Figure 1 shows typical standard curves for dual-label FIA for primidone and phenobarbital. These cover the clinically important subtherapeutic, therapeutic, and toxic concentration ranges for primidone therapy (18).

Assay Validation

Precision and Accuracy

Primidone and phenobarbital were added at three different concentrations (low, medium, and high) to pooled normal human serum and assayed by dual-label FIA. Mean results for primidone were 4.9, 9.9, and 29.5 mg/L, with analytical recovery of 98.3, 99.5, and 98.5%, respectively. Mean phenobarbital results were 5.1, 9.9, and 30.6 mg/L, with analytical recovery of 101.0, 99.0, and 102.0%, respectively. Measurement of the same specimens 10 times in one assay gave within-assay coefficients of variation of 4.5, 3.0, and 3.5%, respectively, for primidone and 3.2, 2.5, and 4.0%, respectively, for phenobarbital.

Linearity

Three clinical samples containing high levels of primidone (22.0, 20.4, and 18.6 mg/L) and phenobarbital (60.0, 56.6, and 48.0 mg/L) were diluted 2-, 5-, and 10-fold with normal human serum and assayed in duplicate. The recoveries were calculated for each drug, and the average results for primidone were 99.0, 98.5, and 97.0%, and for phenobarbital 102.0, 101.0, and 98.0%, respectively.

Specificity

Phenobarbital did not cross-react at a level of 1 g/L with the antiprimidone serum, and the same result was obtained for primidone with the antiphenobarbital serum. The results of specificity studies of the two antisera against various compounds were similar to those obtained previously (3,4); there was no interference from any other antiepileptic drugs or their metabolites.

Correlations with Established Assay Methods

Results of the assay of primidone in 25 patients' specimens by the present method *(x)* and by enzymoimmunoassay *(y)* were related by the regression equation $y = 0.99x - 0.2$, with $r = 0.99$ (Fig. 5). The results of phenobarbital assay of the same specimens by this assay *(x)* and by PIA *(y)* gave a regression line $y = x - 0.6$, with $r = 0.99$ (Fig. 5). Both regression equations were calculated on the assumption that the two methods have equal precision characteristics (19).

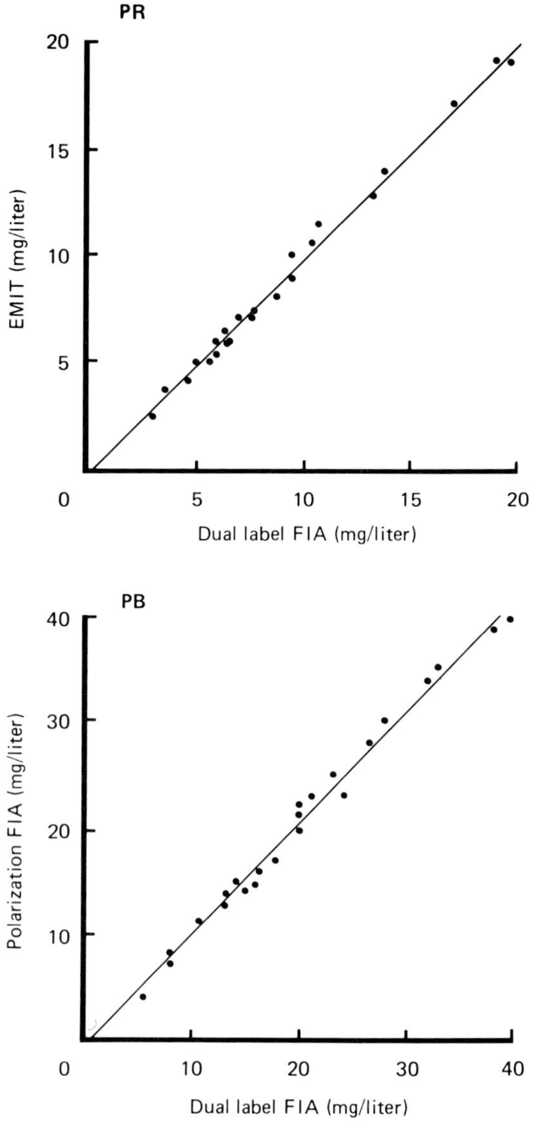

FIG. 5. Top: Correlation between concentrations of primidone (PR) in 25 patients' serum specimens as determined by dual-label fluoroimmunoassay (FIA) and by enzymoimmunoassay (EMIT). **Bottom:** Correlation between concentrations of phenobarbital (PB) in the same specimens as determined by dual-label FIA and by polarization FIA.

Phenobarbital/Primidone Ratio and Correlation

The mean serum primidone level for the 25 random patients' specimens was 9.7 mg/L (range 5–19 mg/L) and the mean phenobarbital level was 21.4 mg/L (range 4–40 mg/L). The mean serum phenobarbital/primidone ratio was 2.3 (range 1.3–4.2) with an SD of 0.95.

Linear regression analysis relating phenobarbital and primidone levels in the above specimens gave the equation (phenobarbital level) = 1.5 (primidone level) + 7.3, with $r = 0.65$.

DISCUSSION

The method presented here illustrates the use of FIA for the simultaneous measurement of a drug and its major metabolite. In attempts to develop dual-label RIA systems, the two iodine isotopes ^{125}I and ^{131}I have been used (7,8). However, the short half-life of ^{131}I (8.1 days) and the less than ideal distinction between the energies of the gamma emission from the two isotopes prevented further development of this approach.

Dual-label FIA has the advantages of technical simplicity, the greater stability of reagents, and the ease of end-point determination. Because the excitation and emission spectra of rhodamine 101 do not overlap with those of fluorescein (Fig. 3), XRITC was chosen together with FITC (16). The excitation maxima of fluorescein and rhodamine 101 are separated by 85 nm; in contrast, the two fluorophores involved in the substrate-labeled FIA (12) have maxima separated by only 35 nm, and this necessitated the use of nonoptimal excitation wavelengths to minimise mutual measurement interferences. Labeling at amino groups with XRITC is achieved in a manner similar to that with FITC. PR-XRTC was stable for more than 1 year when stored at −20°C.

There appears to be no reason why the method presented here could not be extended so that three or even more components could be measured simultaneously. This would increase the savings in time, reagent cost, and sample volume as compared with individually performed assays, with the last consideration being particularly important when the sample volume is limited, as in pediatric investigations.

The separation step in the present assay, which is simple and rapidly achieved by magnetic sedimentation, also serves to remove endogeneous fluorophores and other potential interfering substances present in the sample that may interfere in fluorescence end-point detection (3).

The precision and accuracy of the dual assay are similar to those for the primidone and phenobarbital FIAs reported previously (3,4), and the results for patients' specimens correlate well with those by the corresponding PIA for phenobarbital and enzymoimmunoassay for primidone.

In the limited number of serum specimens studied, the average phenobarbital/primidone ratio of 2.3 and the linear regression relationship between the levels of the two drugs were in close agreement with those reported previously (2). This report demonstrates the development and application of a novel dual-label FIA for simultaneous measurement of a drug and its major pharmacologically active metabolite in a single test tube. Other applications of interest for the dual-label assays would be the simultaneous measurement of concomitantly administered drugs and detection of two or more antibodies.

REFERENCES

1. Perucca E, Richens A. Antiepileptic drugs: clinical aspects. In: Richens A, Marks V, eds. *Therapeutic drug monitoring*. Edinburgh: Churchill Livingstone, 1981:320–48.
2. Fincham RW, Schottelius DD. Primidone: interactions with other drugs. In: Woodbury DM, Penry JK, Pippenger CE, eds. *Antiepileptic drugs*. New York: Raven Press, 1982:421–7.
3. Sidki AM, Rowell FJ, Landon J. Direct determination of primidone in serum or plasma by a magnetizable solid-phase fluoroimmunoassay. *Ann Clin Biochem* 1983;20:227–32.
4. Sidki AM, Pourfarzaneh M, Rowell FJ, Smith DS. Direct determination of phenobarbital in serum or plasma by polarization fluoroimmunoassay. *Ther Drug Monit* 1982;4:397–403.
5. Pesh-Imam M, Fretthold DW, Sunshine I, et al. High pressure liquid chromatography for simultaneous analysis of anticonvulsants: comparison with EMIT system. *Ther Drug Monit* 1979;1:289–99.
6. Meijer JWA. Antiepileptic drugs: analytical techniques. In: Richens A, Marks V, eds. *Therapeutic drug monitoring*. Edinburgh: Churchill Livingstone, 1981:349–69.
7. Denning CE, Schick LA, Boguslaski RC. The combined radioimmunoassay of triiodothyronine and thyroxine. *Clin Chim Acta* 1979;98:5–18.
8. Bluett MK, Reiter EO, Duckett GE, Root AW. Simultaneous radioimmunoassay of thyrotropin and thyroxine in human serum. *Clin Chem* 1977;23:1644–7.
9. Weerasekera DA, Kim JB, Barnard GJ, Collins WP. Multiple immunoassay: the simultaneous measurement of two urinary steroid glucuronides as an index of ovarian function. *J Steroid Biochem* 1983;18:465–70.
10. Blake C, Al-Bassam MN, Gould BJ, Marks V, Bridges JW, Riley C. Simultaneous enzyme immunoassay of two thyroid hormones. *Clin Chem* 1982;28:1469–73.
11. Leuvering JHW, Thal PJHM, van der Waart M, Schuurs AHWM. Sol particle immunoassay (SPIA). *J Immunoassay* 1980;1:77–91.
12. Dean KJ, Thompson SG, Burd JF, Buckler RT. Simultaneous determination of phenytoin and phenobarbital in serum or plasma by substrate-labeled fluorescent immunoassay. *Clin Chem* 1983;29:1051–6.
13. Loken MR, Parks DR, Herzenberg LA. Two-color immunofluorescence using a fluorescence-activated cell sorter. *J Histochem Cytochem* 1977;25:899–907.
14. Gillis TP, Thompson JJ. Double-label fluorescence immunoassay of bacteria. *J Clin Microbiol* 1978;8:351–3.
15. Ullman EF, Khanna PL. Fluorescence excitation transfer immunoassay (FETI). In: Langone JJ, Van Vunakis H, eds. *Methods in enzymology*, vol 74 (Immunochemical techniques, Part C). New York: Academic Press, 1981:28–60.
16. Titus JA, Haugland R, Sharrow SO, Segal DM. Texas Red, a hydrophilic, red-emitting fluorophore for use with fluorescein in dual parameter flow microfluorometric and fluorescence microscopic studies. *J Immunol Methods* 1982;50:193–204.

17. Kamel RS, Landon J, Smith DS. Magnetizable solid-phase fluoroimmunoassay of phenytoin in disposable test tubes. *Clin Chem* 1980;26:1281–4.
18. Fincham RW, Schottelius DD. Relation of plasma concentration to seizure control. In: Woodbury DM, Penry JK, Pippenger CE, eds. *Antiepileptic drugs*. New York: Raven Press, 1982:429–40.
19. Smith DS, Pourfarzaneh M, Kamel RS. Linear regression analysis by Deming's method. *Clin Chem* 1980;26:1105–6.

Therapeutic Drug Monitoring
7:108–114

Evaluation of an Automated System (Optimate) for Substrate-Labeled Fluorescent Immunoassays

Michael Sheehan and Geoffrey Caron

Good Samaritan Hospital and Medical Center, Portland, Oregon, U.S.A.

Summary: Performance characteristics of substrate-labeled fluorescent immunoassays for the drugs phenytoin, phenobarbital, primidone, carbamazepine, theophylline, gentamicin, tobramycin, amikacin, and quinidine run on an Optimate automated fluorometric analyzer were compared with those of automated enzyme multiplied immunoassays (EMIT) for the same drugs performed on a Cobas centrifugal analyzer for patient samples and controls. For 100 patient samples assayed by both systems for each drug, excellent correlations were obtained, with correlation coefficients ranging from 0.96 to 0.99. Likewise, very good within-run (n = 10) and between-run (n = 30) precision was obtained by both methods. Values for controls and clinical specimens by the Optimate methods calculated using the same-day calibration curves were not significantly different from those calculated from calibration curves stored 14 days, indicating at least 14-day curve stability for all assays. **Key Words:** Phenytoin—Phenobarbital—Primidone— Carbamazepine—Theophylline— Gentamicin—Tobramycin—Amikacin—Quinidine—Automated substrate-labeled fluorescent immunoassay— Optimate analyzer—Automated EMIT assays—Cobas centrifugal analyzer.

Substrate-labeled fluorescent immunoassays (SLFIAs) have been developed and reported (1–8) for a variety of therapeutic drugs. In these assays an antibody to the drug is raised and a fluorogenic derivative of the drug, β-D-galactosyl-umbelliferone-drug (GUD) is synthesized. The fluorogenic derivative, nonfluorescent under the conditions of the assay, is enzymatically hydrolyzed by β-galactosidase to yield a fluorescent product (UD). Binding of the drug antibody (AB) to GUD inhibits the enzymatic hydrolysis of the substrate. Competitive binding reactions are set up with a fixed amount of GUD and a limiting amount of AB in such a mannner that the drug in the serum sample competes with the GUD for the antibody binding sites. The fluorescence produced is thus proportional to the level of drug in the serum sample.

$$\begin{array}{c} \mathrm{GUD} + \mathrm{AB} + \mathrm{D} \\ \downarrow\uparrow \\ \mathrm{GUD}\cdot\mathrm{AB} + \mathrm{D}\cdot\mathrm{AB} \end{array} \quad \xrightarrow{\beta\text{-galactosidase}} \mathrm{G} + \mathrm{UD}$$

Although an automated SLFIA has been reported on for theophylline (9), the other reports have dealt with manual or semiautomated SLFIAs. Recently, a totally automated fluorometric analyzer, the Optimate (Ames Division, Miles Laboratories, Inc., Elkhart, IN, U.S.A.), specifically designed for performing SLFIAs, was introduced to the clinical market. It was the purpose of this study to compare the performance of SLFIAs for phenytoin, phenobarbital, primidone, carbamazepine, theophylline, gentamicin, tobramycin, amikacin, and quinidine on the Optimate with the performance of automated enzyme multiplied immunoassays (EMIT) for these same drugs.

Address correspondence and reprint requests to Dr. M. Sheehan at Good Samaritan Hospital and Medical Center, Portland, OR 97210, U.S.A.

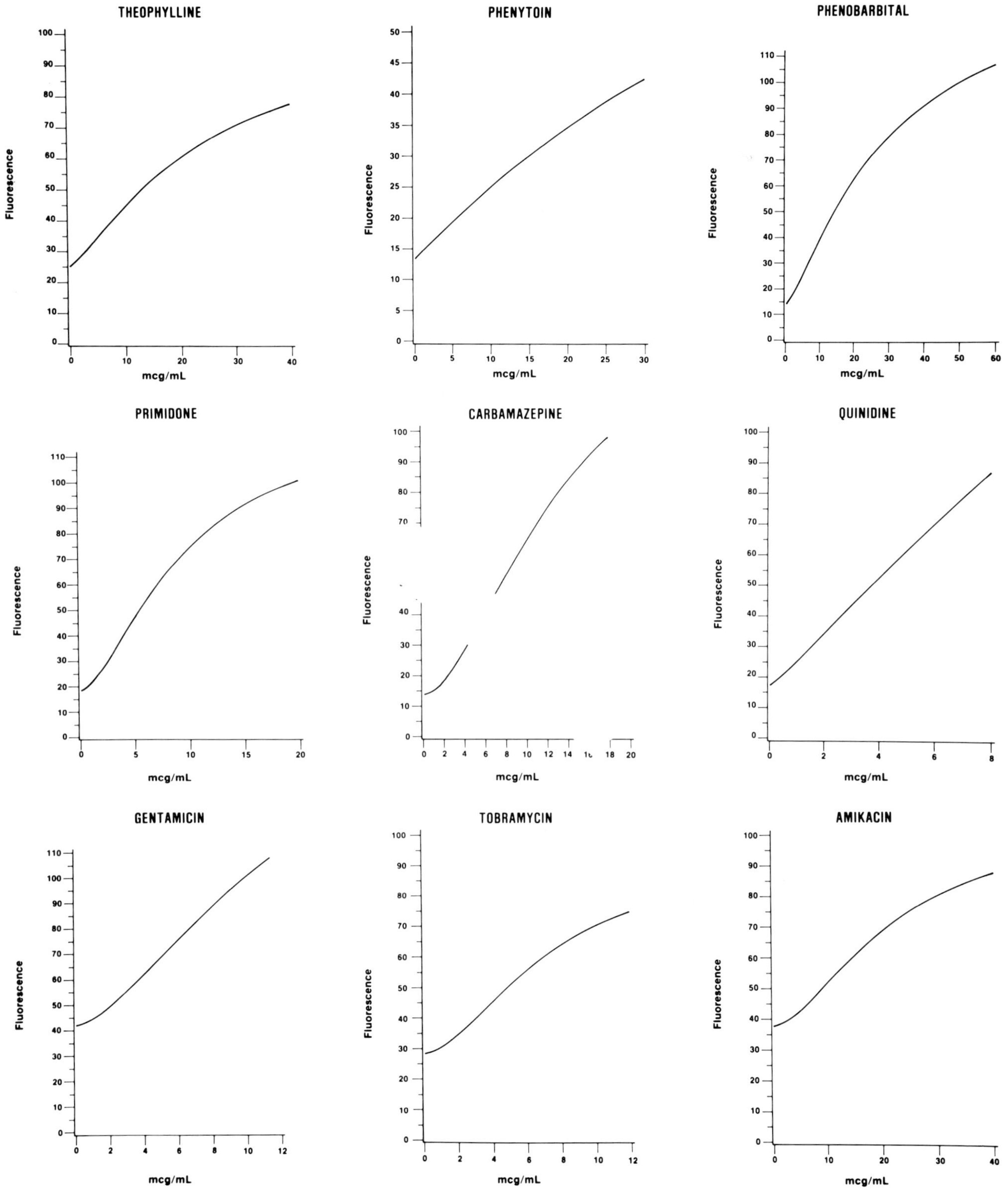

FIG. 1. Typical Optimate/substrate-labeled fluorescent immunoassay calibration curves, fitted using a four-parameter log-logit calculation.

TABLE 1. *Within-run precision comparisons*

Drug	Mean (μg/ml)	SD (μg/ml)	CV (%)
Quinidine			
Optimate/SLFIA[a]	3.1	0.12	3.9
Cobas Bio/EMIT[a]	2.9	0.08	2.8
Gentamicin			
Optimate/SLFIA	6.4	0.16	2.5
Cobas Bio/EMIT	6.7	0.20	3.0
Theophylline			
Optimate/SLFIA	14.6	0.30	2.1
Cobas Bio/EMIT	15.3	0.50	3.3
Tobramycin			
Optimate/SLFIA	5.7	0.30	4.6
Cobas Bio/EMIT	5.9	0.10	2.4
Phenytoin			
Optimate/SLFIA	13.9	0.40	2.9
Cobas Bio/EMIT	13.1	0.50	3.8
Phenobarbital			
Optimate/SLFIA	19.3	0.90	4.5
Cobas Bio/EMIT	20.4	1.0	4.8
Primidone			
Optimate/SLFIA	9.9	0.30	3.2
Cobas Bio/EMIT	9.9	0.30	3.2
Carbamazepine			
Optimate/SLFIA	10.3	0.30	3.1
Cobas Bio/EMIT	8.5	0.50	5.8
Amikacin			
Optimate/SLFIA	16.5	0.80	0.60
Cobas Bio/EMIT	15.3	5.1	3.8

n = 10. SLFIA, substrate-labeled fluorescent immunoassay; EMIT, enzyme multiplied immunoassay technique; CV, coefficient of variation.
[a]Midtherapeutic control.

MATERIALS AND METHODS

Apparatus

The SLFIAs were performed on the Optimate fluorometric analyzer. This system comprises five separable modules, each having several individual components. The components are housed in a single benchtop cabinet and consist of the optical components (fluorescence assays use a quartz-halogen lamp with 405 nm excitation and 450 nm emission filters), a carousel transport component (60 sample positions), computer (12K RAM + 96K PROM) and communications (keyboard + 20 character/s printer) components, pipettor/dilutor module, and digital dilutor module. The optical system contains a flow-through thermocuvet, temperature range 25–37°C, with ±0.2°C accuracy. All assays were performed at 37°C.

The EMIT assays (Syva Corporation, Palo Alto, CA, U.S.A.) were performed at 30°C on a Cobas centrifugal analyzer (Roche, Nutley, NJ, U.S.A.) interfaced for data reduction to an HP-85 (Hewlett-Packard, Corvallis, OR, U.S.A.) desk-top calculator.

Reagents and Samples

The TDA SLFIA reagents used on the Optimate were obtained from Ames. Directions for each assay were supplied by the manufacturer and followed without modification. Likewise, the EMIT reagents were obtained from Syva, and all assays were performed according to the Roche/Syva protocol, with the exceptions of gentamicin plus tobramycin (type 6 analysis used instead of type 3 with incubation time = 20 s, time of first reading 15 s, time interval = 30 s, and number of readings = 2) and theophylline (type 6 analysis instead of type 3, sample volume = 2 μl, reagent volume = 100 μl, start reagent volume = 10 μl, number of readings = 4, and printout mode = 2).

Liquid controls in the low (A), medium (B), and high (C) therapeutic range for each assay were obtained from Ames and stored at 4°C. Fresh controls were opened and used for each day's run. Clinical specimens (100 for each assay) were obtained from hospitalized patients and stored at −20°C until analysis. For each specimen, SLFIA and EMIT were performed on the same day for each of the nine drugs. Each specimen was also assayed on 2 consecutive days by both systems to minimize between-run analytic variation.

Procedures

For the SLFIAs, 8 μl of sample was diluted with 400 μl of buffer, and 20 μl of this mixture was combined with 20 μl of the appropriate AB/enzyme reagent and an additional 600 μl of buffer in the reaction cup. After 20 s, 20 μl of the GUD reagent and another 300 μl of buffer were added to the reaction cup and allowed to react with the sample for 240 s. The reaction mixture was then aspirated into the photometer and a fluorescence reading was taken. Drug concentrations for each sample were calculated by comparison of the fluorescence intensity of the sample with fluorescence produced by the appropriate standards on a logit-log plot.

For EMIT performed on the Cobas analyzer, generally (see above for exceptions) 3 μl of sample was mixed with a 150 μl aliquot of a 10:1 dilution of the AB/substrate reagent and incubated for 20 s. After 15 μl of the appropriate enzyme reagent was added and the resulting mixture underwent spinning for 5 s, absorbance readings were taken every 10 s over 70 s. Unknown drug concentrations were then determined

TABLE 2. *Between-run precision comparisons*

Drug	Control (μg/ml)	Optimate/SLFIA mean (μg/ml)	Cobas Bio/EMIT mean (μg/ml)	Optimate/SLFIA 0–1[a] (CV%)	Optimate/SLFIA 0–14[b] (CV%)	Cobas Bio/EMIT (CV%)
Quinidine	2	2.0	2.0	4.6	5.3	7.3
	4	4.0	3.9	2.6	3.6	3.5
	6	6.0	5.8	2.7	5.1	5.6
Gentamicin	2	2.1	2.1	8.6	7.3	2.9
	6	6.0	6.4	2.4	4.8	1.9
	10	10.5	9.1	2.6	7.9	5.2
Theophylline	5	5.0	5.0	7.9	7.8	4.0
	15	15.3	15.3	2.8	2.5	5.7
	25	25.2	24.7	2.1	2.2	5.3
Tobramycin	2	2.2	2.1	5.2	11.4	4.6
	6	6.2	6.0	3.9	7.2	1.9
	10	10.2	9.5	5.1	16.5	8.9
Phenytoin	7.5	8.4	7.0	5.7	5.7	3.9
	15	16.0	13.9	3.0	5.3	4.0
	25	26.3	23.0	2.7	6.5	4.5
Phenobarbital	15	16.1	14.8	2.7	2.8	2.2
	30	30.7	28.8	2.8	3.1	3.1
	50	51.1	47.3	3.5	5.3	3.5
Primidone	4	4.1	4.0	3.5	4.6	3.8
	12	12.6	11.6	3.2	3.5	3.0
	16	16.7	15.1	3.7	5.2	2.4
Carbamazepine	4	3.9	4.1	3.9	5.9	3.2
	12	12.3	11.4	2.7	3.0	4.7
	16	16.4	15.3	2.7	3.8	7.1
Amikacin	10	9.8	10.2	4.0	4.1	3.0
	20	19.7	19.7	2.7	3.7	4.5
	30	30.9	29.3	3.4	5.9	5.3

n = 22. Abbreviations as in Table 1.
[a]Same-day calibration curve.
[b]14-day stored calibration curve.

by comparison of the rate of absorbance change of the sample with absorbance rates produced by the appropriate standards on a logit-log plot.

RESULTS

Each system was calibrated daily to eliminate curve stability as a variable in the precision and correlation studies. Figure 1 illustrates typical calibration curves for the SLFIAs on the Optimate. Within-run precision was determined on both systems for the nine drugs by assaying 10 replicates of control B on 3 separate days. Table 1 lists the average of the three runs for each drug. Between-run precision was compared at low, medium, and high therapeutic levels (controls A, B, and C, respectively) over 30 runs. SLFIA results were calculated from calibration curves run on the same day as well as from calibration curves that had been stored for 14 days. Table 2 compares these results with the EMIT results.

The 100 clinical specimens were assayed on both systems on two consecutive days for the nine drugs. Mean values for the SLFIAs were plotted against the corresponding mean values for the EMIT assays for each drug. Regression lines for these plots are shown in Fig. 2. Results for these samples were also recalculated from 14-day stored calibration curves for the SLFIAs and correlated to the original EMIT results. Table 3 summarizes the day 1 and day 14 regression statistics for these assays.

DISCUSSION

Tables 1 and 2 reveal that overall precision of the SLFIAs on the Optimate is slightly better than that of EMIT performed on the Cobas analyzer. However, if the precision acceptability level is set at $\leq 10\%$ for the between-run coefficient of variation, both systems exhibited good to excellent precision, and the precision differences would not be considered clinically

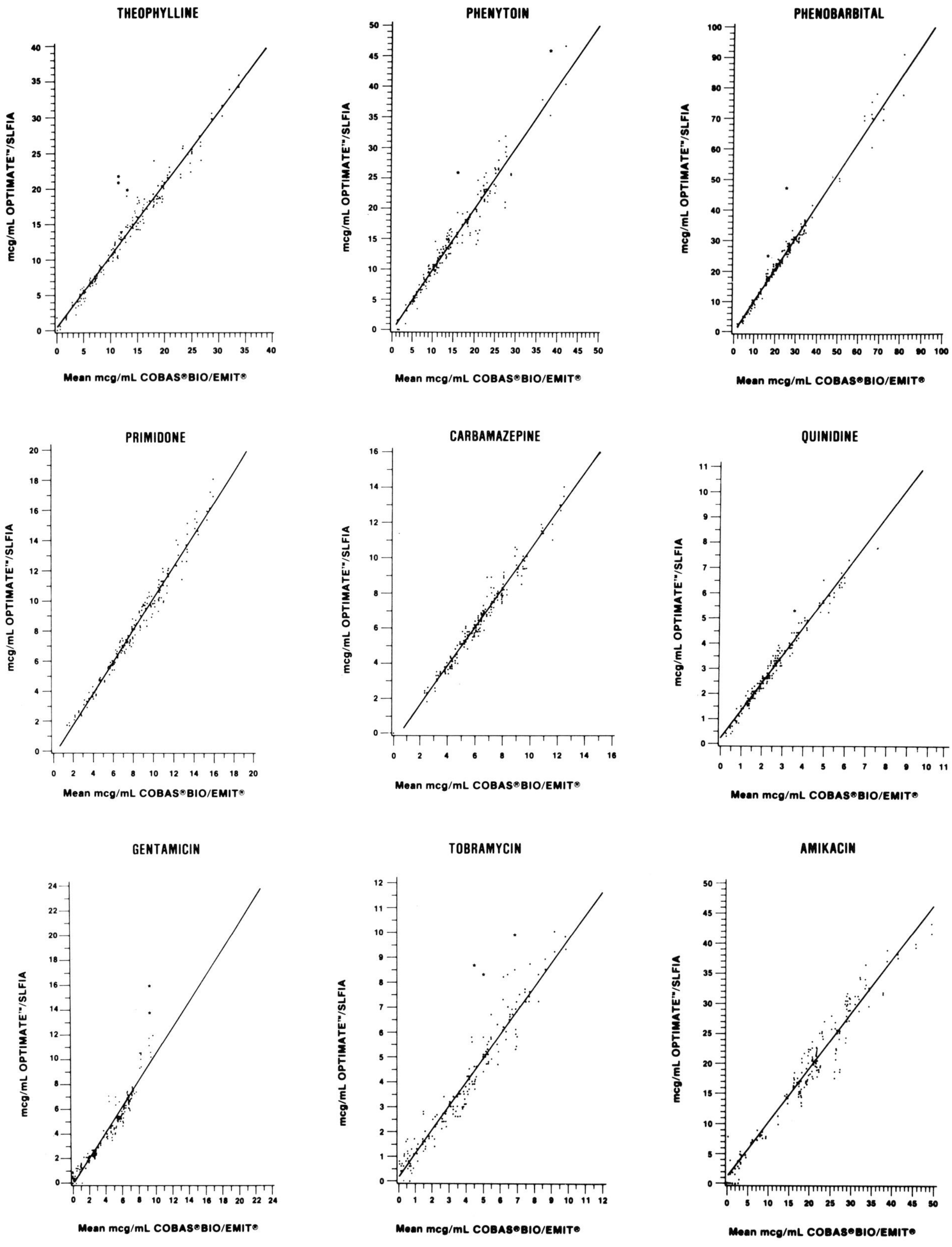

FIG. 2. Regression lines: Optimate/substrate-labeled fluorescent immunoassay (SLFIA) versus Cobas Bio/enzyme multiplied immunoassay technique (EMIT).

TABLE 3. *Regression statistics*

Drug	Regression line	Correlation coefficient
Quinidine		
Same-day calibration	$y = 1.10x + 0.19$	0.99
2-week-stored calibration	$y = 1.10x + 0.22$	0.98
Gentamicin		
Same-day calibration	$y = 1.05x - 0.20$	0.96
2-week-stored calibration	$y = 1.10x - 0.26$	0.94
Theophylline		
Same-day calibration	$y = 1.02x + 0.32$	0.99
2-week-stored calibration	$y = 1.01x + 0.35$	0.99
Tobramycin		
Same-day calibration	$y = 0.96x + 0.11$	0.97
2-week-stored calibration	$y = 0.94x + 0.20$	0.95
Phenytoin		
Same-day calibration	$y = 1.01x - 0.29$	0.98
2-week-stored calibration	$y = 1.02x - 0.50$	0.98
Phenobarbital		
Same-day calibration	$y = 1.05x - 0.55$	0.99
2-week-stored calibration	$y = 1.02x - 0.42$	0.99
Primidone		
Same-day calibration	$y = 1.05x - 0.41$	0.99
2-week-stored calibration	$y = 1.02x - 0.31$	0.99
Carbamazepine		
Same-day calibration	$y = 1.10x - 0.51$	0.98
2-week-stored calibration	$y = 1.08x - 0.51$	0.98
Amikacin		
Same-day calibration	$y = 0.91x + 0.73$	0.97
2-week-stored calibration	$y = 0.95x + 0.69$	0.97

significant. The EMIT procedures were generally more precise in the low therapeutic ranges, whereas the SLFIAs showed better precision in the medium and high therapeutic ranges. These trends are not unexpected, since the SLFIA calibration curves (Fig. 1) are flatter at the low end and steeper with less fall-off at the high end, compared with the EMIT calibration curves. It is of note, also, that with the exception of the gentamicin and tobramicin assays, no significant differences in precision were seen regardless of whether the 14-day stored calibration curves or the same-day curves were used to calculate the results.

Figure 2 and Table 3 demonstrate the good (tobramycin, gentamicin, and amikacin) to excellent (remaining drugs) correlations between the SLFIAs and EMIT procedures.

These results confirm that SLFIAs performed on the Optimate analyzer are clinically acceptable in terms of precision and accuracy. Table 3 also demonstrates that no significant differences in correlations were observed when 14-day-stored versus same-day calibration curves were used for the SLFIAs, indicating at least a 14-day curve stability for all nine assays on the Optimate. Four drug assays (theophylline, tobramycin, gentamicin, and phenytoin) were investigated further, and we established that their calibration curves were stable for at least 30 days. Although we did not systematically investigate the calibration curve stability of the Cobas/EMIT assays, it has been our experience that these curves are stable for less than 14 days; we generally recalibrate these assays at least every 3 days.

Both systems were easy to operate, little special training or expertise being required by the operator. Thus, with either system stat drug level monitoring can be provided on a 24-h basis without the necessity of having a toxicologist or specially trained person present or on call at all times. For any one particular drug on a specimen and the control, stat results are available from either system in about 10 min (assuming the Optimate has been precalibrated, which with the 14-day curve stability for this system would be the normal operating mode). Sample throughput for the Cobas/EMIT system (approximately 97 per hour) is slightly higher than for the Optimate (approximately 90 per hour). The total costs (including expendables) for performing these assays were comparable for both instrument–reagent combinations. Including the price of the instruments (plus service contracts) amortized over a 5-year period, we estimated the cost per test for 3,000 tests run at 100 tests per day over a 30-day period to be \$1.35 on the Optimate versus \$1.39 on the Cobas/EMIT system.

We found the Optimate to be extremely reliable (less than 1 day of down-time in more than 8 months of daily operation), and we believe that SLFIAs performed on the Optimate provide a precise, accurate, expedient, and economical mode of drug level monitoring.

Acknowledgment: This work was supported in part by a grant from the Ames Division of Miles Laboratories, Inc., Elkhart, IN, U.S.A., and we gratefully acknowledge the assistance of Mr. Lawrence Crowley, a Senior Clinical Research Associate with Ames, for his help in facilitating this study.

REFERENCES

1. Burd JF, Wong RC, Feeney JE, Carrico RJ, Boguslaski RC. Homogeneous reactant-labeled fluorescent immunoassay for therapeutic drugs exemplified by gentamicin determination in human serum. *Clin Chem* 1977;23:1402–8.
2. Wong RC, Burd JF, Carrico RJ, Buckler RT, Thoma JT, Boguslaski RC. Substrate-labeled fluorescent immunoassay for phenytoin in human serum. *Clin Chem* 1979;25:686–91.
3. Krausz LM, Hitz JB, Buckler RT, Burd JF. Substrate-labeled fluorescent immunoassay for phenobarbital. *Ther Dug Monit* 1980;2:261–72.
4. Li TM, Berovic JL, Buckler RT, Burd JF. Homogeneous substrate-labeled fluorescent immunoassay for theophylline in serum. *Clin Chem* 1981;27:22–6.
5. Thompson SG, Burd JF. Substrate-labeled fluorescent immu-

noassay for amikacin in human serum. *Antimicrob Agents Chemother* 1980;18:264–8.
6. Acton WJ, Van Duyn OM, Allen LV, Flournoy DJ. Evaluation of four assay methods for determination of tobramycin in human serum. *Clin Chem* 1982;28:177–80.
7. Miller JE, Li TM, Krausz LM, Wong RC, Burd JF. Substrate-labeled fluorescent immunoassay (SLFIA) for carbamazepine in serum [Abstract]. *Clin Chem* 1980;26:1002.
8. Sheehan M, Caron G. Evaluation of a fluorescent enzyme immunoassay for quinidine [Abstract]. *Clin Chem* 1982;28:1667.
9. Fingerhut B, Costanzo R, Chandri Z, Rizvi S. Automation of the homogeneous substrate-labeled fluorescent immunoassay for theophylline in serum: application to the determination of phenytoin and phenobarbital in serum. *Ther Drug Monit* 1982;4:419–25.

Therapeutic Drug Monitoring
7:115–120 © 1985 Raven Press, New York

Determination of Free Valproic Acid Concentrations Using the Amicon Micropartition MPS-1 Ultrafiltration System

Clark March and Robert V. Blanke

Department of Pathology, Medical College of Virginia, Virginia Commonwealth University, Richmond, Virginia, U.S.A.

Summary: Free valproic acid concentrations were determined using the MPS-1 ultrafiltration device marketed by Amicon with one YMB membrane per device. Valproic acid binding to the membrane was 5.6% of the free valproic acid concentration. The free valproic acid concentration increased as serial ultrafiltrate volumes were collected, suggesting that only small ultrafiltrate volumes should be collected from a large initial sample. The protein content of the ultrafiltrate was acceptable and was within the tolerances stated by Amicon. There was no significant difference between free valproic acid concentrations determined within 3 h of sample collection and those determined after storage at 4°C or − 20°C for 1 week. There was no significant difference between free valproic acid concentrations in serum and heparinized plasma samples collected simultaneously. **Key Words:** Free drug concentration—Valproic acid—Ultrafiltration.

This study was performed to determine the usefulness of measuring free valproic acid (VPA) concentrations using the ultrafiltration device made by Amicon, the Micropartition System MPS-1 (Amicon Corp., Danvers, MA, U.S.A.) with one YMB membrane. Others have used ultrafiltration devices to study free VPA concentrations (1). Cramer et al. (2) used both the Amicon (CF50) Centriflo cones and the FreeLevel System I (Syva, Palo Alto, CA, U.S.A.) to measure free VPA concentrations in plasma and serum. They found the methods to be comparable. It was noted that the FreeLevel device utilized two YMB membranes during ultrafiltration to decrease the probability of protein leakage. Haidukewych and Rodin (3) used the Ultrafree ultrafiltration device (Worthington Diagnostics, Millipore Corp., Freehold, NJ, U.S.A.) to measure free VPA concentrations in plasma. Godolphin et al. (4) used the FreeLevel device to measure free anticonvulsant concentrations in serum and plasma in an effort to determine which sample types were appropriate for a particular anticonvulsant drug.

Bachmann et al. (5) used the Amicon YMT membrane to measure free phenytoin levels in plasma and compared these results favorably with saliva phenytoin concentrations. Judd and Pesce (6) used the MPS-1 system to demonstrate the stability of free phenytoin concentrations over successive collections of ultrafiltrate after the initial ultrafiltrate was discarded.

It was the intent of this study to investigate those parameters that affect the determination of free VPA concentrations in an effort to validate the method for use in a routine laboratory setting. Specifically, the question of volume of the original sample collected as ultrafiltrate, as investigated by Judd and Pesce (6) for phenytoin, was examined in detail.

Address correspondence and reprint requests to C. March at Box 597, MCV Station, Richmond, VA 23298, U.S.A.

This work was performed as partial fulfillment of the requirements for the degree of Master of Science at the Medical College of Virginia, Virginia Commonwealth University (C.M.).

METHODS

Assays

The procedures for measuring free and total VPA concentrations were modifications of the gas chromatographic technique presented by Kupferburg (7). The internal standard (cyclohexanecarboxylic acid) concentrations were 349 and 174.5 μg/ml for the total and free VPA assays, respectively. The 6-ft stainless steel column was packed with 10% DEGS-PS on 80/100 Supelcoport (Supelco, Inc., Bellefonte, PA, U.S.A.). The oven temperature was maintained at 140°C for the total VPA assay and immediately ramped from 140 to 150°C at 8°C/min for the free VPA assay.

The total VPA extraction was performed by placing in a small test tube 200 μl of internal standard, 200 μl of serum or plasma, 100 μl of 1 N HCl, and 200 μl of chloroform. The tube was vortex-mixed, and centrifuged, and 1.5 μl of the chloroform layer was injected. The free VPA extraction was similar, 20 μl of internal standard, 100 μl of ultrafiltrate, 100 μl of 1 N HCl, and 50 μl of chloroform being used.

Linearity of the total VPA assay was determined over the range of 25 to 200 μg/ml by spiking blank serum with a methanolic solution of sodium valproate (Abbott Laboratories, North Chicago, IL, U.S.A.). The free VPA assay was checked over the range of 1 to 20 μg/ml, using water standards. Day-to-day precision of the total assay was assessed by use of a 65 μg/ml serum standard. The free assay precision was tested by use of a 10 μg/ml water standard.

Ultrafiltration

Either 0.5 or 1.0 ml of sample was introduced into the reservoir of the MPS-1 device with a 9-in pasteur pipet. One YMB membrane was used. The device was centrifuged in a fixed, tilted head centrifuge at 1,100 *g* until 100 μl of ultrafiltrate was collected. All ultrafiltrations were performed at 25°C.

VPA Binding to the Ultrafiltration Device

Eight YMB membranes were added to 3 ml of a 5 μg/ml VPA standard made in normal saline. The solution was mixed by swirling for 30 s every 5 min. Samples were withdrawn at 30, 60, and 90 min and assayed for free VPA.

Three complete support assemblies (reservoir, support base, O-ring, and collection cup) were placed in beaker containing 45 ml of a 6 μg/ml VPA standard made in normal saline. The solution was mixed by swirling for 30 s every 5 min. Samples were withdrawn at 30, 60, 90, and 120 min and assayed for free VPA.

Four normal saline standards of VPA (5, 10, 15, and 20 μg/ml) were assayed for free VPA before and after ultrafiltration through the YMB membrane.

Volume of Ultrafiltrate

(a) One milliliter of pooled serum from patients receiving VPA was ultrafiltered until 100 μl of ultrafiltrate was collected and removed for free VPA analysis. Ultrafiltration was continued until five sequential 100 μl fractions were collected. The experiment was done at total VPA concentrations of 74 and 40 μg/ml.

(b) Experiment (a) was repeated except that the reservoir was capped between each ultrafiltrate collection and the sample mixed by inversion five times. The total VPA concentrations were 67 and 40 μg/ml.

(c) Experiment (a) was repeated except that after each fraction was collected, an equal volume of ultrafiltrate from VPA free serum or distilled water was added back to the reservoir and mixed. The total VPA concentration was 60 μg/ml.

Protein Content of Ultrafiltrate

Experiment (a) was repeated (total VPA = 74 μg/ml). Protein concentration measured as albumin in the ultrafiltrate was determined by use of the Coomassie blue dye binding assay as described by Bradford (8). The assay was standardized by use of human serum albumin (Hyland Diagnostics, Deerfield, IL, U.S.A.).

Serum and heparin anticoagulated plasma samples were divided into 0.5 and 1.0 ml aliquots and ultrafiltered to collect 100 μl of ultrafiltrate. This corresponded to a 10% collection for the 1.0 ml sample and a 20% collection for the 0.5 ml sample. The protein content of the filtrate was determined as described above.

Storage

Serum samples were assayed within 3 h of collection for free and total VPA using a 0.5 ml sample. The remaining sample was aliquoted and stored at −20 and 4°C for 1 week. The aliquots were thawed at 25°C for 1 h while rotating at 10 r/min. Free and total VPA concentrations were again determined.

Serum Versus Plasma

Paired serum and heparinized plasma samples were drawn from patients receiving VPA. The samples were analyzed for free and total VPA within 3 h of collection by use of a 0.5 ml sample for ultrafiltration.

RESULTS

Linearity and Precision

The linearity data for the total VPA assay were as follows: slope = 6.88×10^{-3}, intercept = -0.048, and $r^2 = 0.997$, with a day-to-day (n = 10) coefficient of variation of 5.9%. The free VPA assay linearity data were as follows: slope = 2.25×10^{-1}, intercept = -0.027, and $r^2 = 0.998$, with a day-to-day (n = 10) coefficient of variation of 6.3%.

VPA Binding to the Ultrafiltration Device

The solution in which the membranes were soaked showed a decrease in VPA concentration of 7.0% at 30 min, 2.7% at 60 min, and 7.0% at 90 min (average 5.6%). The solution in which the support assemblies were soaked showed no decrease in VPA concentration over the 2-h period.

The peak height ratios calculated for the filtered and unfiltered standards showed a difference of 5.7, 6.8, 3.5, and 6.3% (average 5.6%) at concentrations of 5, 10, 15, and 20 μg/ml, respectively. In all cases, the unfiltered standards gave higher peak height ratios.

Volume of Ultrafiltrate

Figures 1 and 2 show the results of the sequential collection of 100-μl ultrafiltrates from 1.0 ml samples. In each case it can be observed that the free VPA concentration increased. In each case, the difference between the first fraction and the fifth fraction was found to be significant (Fig. 1: $p < 0.0005$ without mixing, $p < 0.005$ with mixing; Fig. 2: $p < 0.0005$ without mixing, $p < 0.01$ with mixing). In Fig. 1 (without mixing) the increase in mean free VPA concentration from the first fraction to the fifth fraction was 2.1 μg/ml. Since the total VPA concentration in that sample was 74 μg/ml, this increase represents 2.8% of the total VPA concentration in the original sample.

Figures 3 and 4 show how the results for the sequential collection of 100-μl ultrafiltrates are altered when VPA free ultrafiltrate solution or water is returned to the sample reservoir after the collection of the ultrafiltrate. The slope of the lines is the reverse of the case in Figs. 1 and 2. The only effect of mixing between fractions was to decrease the amount of centrifugation time required (5.5, 7, 9, 13, and 22 min for the unmixed samples vs. 5.5, 5.5, 6, 7.5, and 11.5 min for the mixed samples).

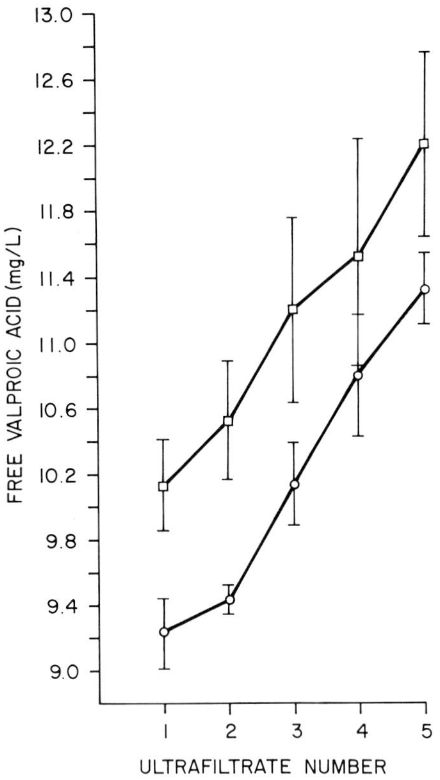

FIG. 1. Plot (mean and SD; n = 5) of free valproic acid concentration in five sequential 100-μl ultrafiltrates collected from a 1-ml sample with (squares) and without (circles) mixing between fractions. Total valproic acid concentrations were 67 mg/L for mixed sample and 74 mg/L for unmixed sample.

Protein Content of Ultrafiltrate

The same pooled serum used to perform the experiment in Fig. 1 (without mixing) was used in this experiment. The total albumin concentration of the pooled serum was 41 g/L. The highest concentration of protein measured in the ultrafiltrate in this series was 50 mg/L, or 0.12% of the total albumin concentration in the original sample. The difference between the mean protein content of the first fraction and that of the last fraction was 34.2 mg/L, or 0.08% of the total albumin concentration in the original sample.

In the 10 and 20% sample collection study, the average protein concentration in serum was 16.7 mg/L (range: none detected to 127) for the 10% collection, and 34.1 mg/L (range: none detected to 110) for the 20% collection. In plasma, the average protein con-

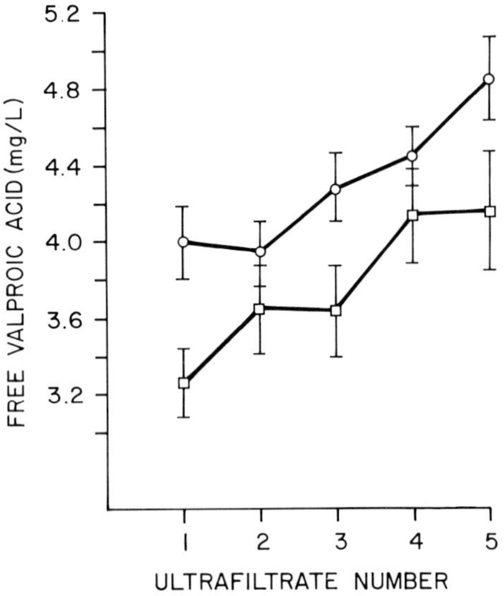

FIG. 2. Plot (mean and SD; n = 5) of free valproic acid concentration in five sequential 100-μl ultrafiltrates collected from a 1-ml sample with (squares) and without (circles) mixing between fractions. Total valproic acid concentration was 40 mg/L for both samples.

centration was 8.8 mg/L (range: none detected to 54) for the 10% collection, and 9.7 mg/L (range: none detected to 32) for the 20% collection.

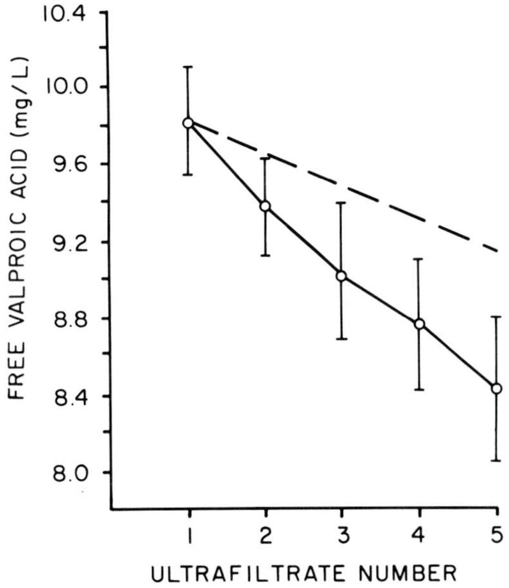

FIG. 3. Plot (mean and SD; n = 5) of free valproic acid concentration in five sequential 100-μl ultrafiltrates collected from a 1-ml sample. One hundred microliters of ultrafiltrate from valproic acid free serum was added to the sample reservoir after each fraction was collected. Dashed line represents expected decrease in free valproic acid concentration, assuming a constant free fraction as determined by the first collection.

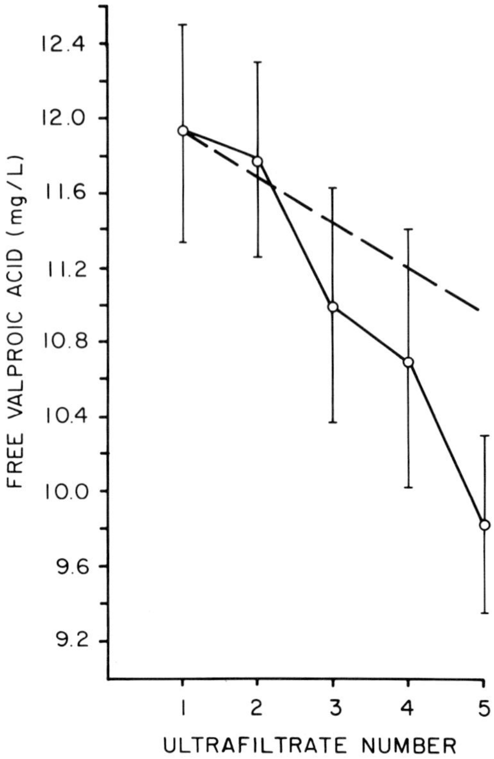

FIG. 4. Plot (mean and SD; n = 5) of free valproic acid concentration in five sequential 100-μl ultrafiltrates collected from a 1-ml sample. One hundred microliters of distilled water was added to the sample reservoir after each fraction was collected. Dashed line represents expected decrease in free valproic acid concentration, assuming a constant free fraction as determined by the first collection.

Storage

There was no significant difference ($p < 0.05$) in total VPA concentration between serum samples (n = 20) assayed within 3 h of collection and the same samples stored for 1 week at 4 or −20°C. Storage of serum samples (n = 19) for 1 week at 4 and −20°C resulted in no significant difference ($p < 0.05$) in free VPA concentrations when compared with values obtained when samples were assayed within 3 h of collection.

Serum Versus Plasma

The paired serum and heparinized plasma samples (n = 20) showed no significant difference ($p < 0.05$) in free VPA concentration when assayed within 3 h of collection.

DISCUSSION

The linearity and precision of the free and total VPA assays are adequate for use in a routine therapeutic drug monitoring laboratory.

Both tests for binding of VPA to the YMB membrane showed the same loss of VPA. This loss occurred within 30 min and did not seem to be concentration dependent. The standard solutions filtered through the membranes were in contact with the membranes for less than 10 min. The support apparatus and the collection cup did not bind a measurable amount of VPA. The value of 5.6% loss of VPA to the YMB membrane is close to the value of 7% that Judd and Pesce (6) demonstrated for phenytoin for the first 12.5% of the sample collected as ultrafiltrate. Cramer et al. (2) state that the YMB membrane used in the FreeLevel device had a low, nonspecific binding of VPA.

Several authors (6,9,10,11) have presented theoretical arguments to demonstrate that the volume of ultrafiltrate collected from the original sample has no effect on the free drug concentration as measured in the ultrafiltrate. Judd and Pesce (6) have shown this to be true for phenytoin when the MPS-1 device is used. The present study does not affirm theoretical predictions. There was a steady and significant increase in free VPA concentration from the first 100 μl of ultrafiltrate to the fifth. This was true at two total VPA concentrations and was independent of mixing to redistribute the protein gradient that develops during centrifugation. Haidukewych and Rodin (3) used the Ultrafree system to show an increase in free VPA between successive ultrafiltrates representing the first and second 10% of the original plasma sample. For their two patients, there were increases of 39 and 37% in free VPA concentration. The increases shown in Figs. 1 and 2 are not this large.

Judd and Pesce (6) cite the work of others to list four assumptions made in the theoretical arguments that suggest that free drug concentration is independent of the volume of ultrafiltrate collected. These assumptions are as follows: (a) The membrane does not significantly bind drug. (b) The protein leakage through the membrane is insignificant. (c) The equilibrium constant for the drug binding to the protein does not alter as protein concentration increases. (d) The drug and water are passed equally well by the membrane. Judd and Pesce state that each assumption needs to be validated for each drug and ultrafiltration system.

The first two assumptions were tested directly in this study. There is some binding of VPA to the YMB membrane. If this binding is saturable, one would expect to see results like those Judd and Pesce presented for phenytoin. Figures 1 and 2 show that this does not occur in this study. Membrane binding of VPA may be only part of the problem with this technique.

There is some protein leakage into the ultrafiltrate. In the protein content experiment and the experiment used to generate Fig. 1 (without mixing), the free VPA concentration rose by 2.8% of the total VPA concentration, whereas the protein concentration rose by only 0.08% of the total albumin concentration. Since VPA binds to albumin, it can be assumed that increased protein leakage can cause increased free VPA concentrations. However, the modest increase in protein in the ultrafiltrate cannot entirely explain the larger increase in VPA in the ultrafiltrate. The values for protein content in the ultrafiltrates are in agreement with values Joern (12) found for plasma using the Ultrafree system.

The last two assumptions listed by Judd and Pesce were not directly tested by this study. In the experiments that resulted in Figs. 3 and 4, the protein concentration in the sample reservoir is kept constant by the addition of VPA free serum ultrafiltrate or water. It was supposed that this technique would result in a constant free fraction for VPA. However, the figures show that free VPA concentrations decrease at a rate greater than would be expected for a constant free fraction and that the rate of decline is relatively constant. All the causes of this inconsistent binding of VPA to albumin are not known, but since VPA binding to YMB membranes and protein leakage are of insufficient magnitude to explain this inconsistency, the binding of VPA to albumin in a perturbed system becomes suspect.

The molecular weight of VPA is 144.2 daltons, and the stated performance of the YMB membrane is that it passes 95% of a solute with a molecular weight of 776 daltons (13). It is probably safe to assume that the YMB membrane passes water as easily as VPA.

Freezing and refrigeration of serum did not alter free VPA concentrations. Cramer and Mattson (14) used the Amicon Centriflo cones in an ultrafiltration technique to show that refrigeration and freezing did not alter VPA binding.

The free VPA concentrations of paired serum and plasma samples showed no significant difference. This is in agreement with results Cramer and Mattson (14) and Cramer et al. (15) published, although they used the Amicon Centriflo cone for ultrafiltration.

We conclude from this study that if the MPS-1 system is used with one YMB membrane to determine free VPA concentrations, a large initial sample volume must be used from which as small an ultrafiltrate volume as possible should be collected. This should minimize any disruption of the binding equilibrium that ultrafiltration may cause.

Acknowledgment: The authors wish to thank William R. Garnett, Pharm. D., for his help in obtaining patient samples appropriate for use in this study.

REFERENCES

1. Cramer JA, Mattson RH. Valproic acid: *in vivo* plasma protein binding and interaction with phenytoin. *Ther Drug Monit* 1979;1:105–16.
2. Cramer JA, Bennett DM, Mattson RH. Free and bound valproic acid separated by two methods of ultrafiltration. *Clin Chem* 1983;29:1441–2.
3. Haidukewych D, Rodin EA. Variable in vivo binding of valproic acid in epilepsy patients being medicated with other anticonvulsants. *Clin Chem* 1980;26:1634–5.
4. Godolphin W, Trepanier J, Farrell K. Serum and plasma for total and free anticonvulsant drug analysis: effects on EMIT assays and ultrafiltration devices. *Ther Drug Monit* 1983;5:319–23.
5. Bachmann K, Forney RB, Voeller K. Monitoring phenytoin in salivary and plasma ultrafiltrates of pediatric patients. *Ther Drug Monit* 1983;5:325–9.
6. Judd RL, Pesce AJ. Free drug concentrations are constant in serial fractions of plasma ultrafiltrate. *Clin Chem* 1982;28:1726–7.
7. Kupferburg HJ. Gas-liquid chromatographic quantitation of valproic acid. In: Pippenger CE, Penry JJ, Kutt H, eds. *Antiepileptic drugs.* New York: Raven Press, 1978: chapter 13.
8. Bradford MM. A rapid and sensitive method for quantitation of microgram quantities of protein utilizing the principle of protein-dye binding. *Anal Chem* 1976;72:248–54.
9. Whitlam JB, Brown KF. Ultrafiltration in serum protein binding determinations. *J Pharm Sci* 1981;70:146–50.
10. Sophianopoulos JA, Durham SJ, Sophianopoulos AJ, Ragsdale HL, Cropper WP. Ultrafiltration is theoretically equivalent to equilibrium dialysis but much simpler to carry out. *Arch Biochem Biophys* 1978;187:132–7.
11. Bowers WF, Fulton S, Thompson J. Ultrafiltration vs equilibrium dialysis for determination of free fraction. *Clin Pharmacokinetics* 1984;9(suppl 1):49–60.
12. Joern WA. Gas-chromatographic assay of free phenytoin in ultrafiltrates of plasma: test of a new filtration apparatus and specimen stability. *Clin Chem* 1981;27:417–21.
13. Package insert. Micropartition system MPS 1. Amicon Corporation, Danvers, MA, 11–80.
14. Cramer JA, Mattson RH. A simple method to obtain unbound antiepileptic drugs in blood. *Ther Drug Monit* 1982;4:107–8.
15. Cramer JA, McCarthy KA, Mattson RH. Free fraction of valproic acid is the same in serum and plasma. *Clin Chem* 1983;29:1449.

Therapeutic Drug Monitoring
7:121–122 © 1985 Raven Press, New York

Interference with High Performance Liquid Chromatographic Chloramphenicol Assay in a Patient Receiving Dobutamine

M. Beth Powel, C. Andrew Robinson, and Raymond L. Furner

Department of Pathology, University of Alabama in Birmingham, Birmingham, Alabama, U.S.A.

Summary: We report potential interference by dobutamine with our high performance liquid chromatography (HPLC) procedure for assaying chloramphenicol succinate and chloramphenicol. Interference was discovered in a 1-year-old boy receiving chloramphenicol succinate and dobutamine. The identity of the interfering substance was confirmed by HPLC and gas chromatography. **Key Words:** Chloramphenicol—High performance liquid chromatography—Dobutamine—Therapeutic drug monitoring.

CASE HISTORY

A 1-year-old boy with congenital heart disease was admitted to our institution for repair of a left pulmonary aneurysm and truncus arteriosis. He was transferred after 2 days to the Children's Hospital, where he appeared to be doing well. Ten days postoperatively he developed a low-grade fever in the early morning and evening. A spinal tap was performed, and a specimen for culture grew *Staphylococcus aureus*, which was treated with vancomycin and chloramphenicol succinate intravenously. Other medications given included furosemide, phenobarbital, spironolactone, aminophylline, methylprednisolone sodium succinate, and cimetidine. By 17 days postoperatively the child was in metabolic acidosis and renal failure, and was undergoing maximum life support, with a systolic blood pressure of less than 40 mm Hg. Twenty-four days postoperatively he was given dobutamine hydrochloride and steroids. Chloramphenicol succinate was discontinued on the 25th day.

Our laboratory began determining the patient's serum chloramphenicol levels on day 23, quantitating chloramphenicol and noting the presence or absence of the succinate ester. The therapeutic range is 0.7–2.3 mg/dl, with levels of more than 2.5 mg/dl considered toxic. The results are shown in Table 1. The continued detection of a peak coinciding with chloramphenicol succinate long after the disappearance of the metabolite caused the child's clinician and our laboratory to investigate possible interfering substances.

TABLE 1. *Serum chloramphenicol levels in a 1-year-old child*

Postoperative day	Hour of measurement	Chloramphenicol level (mg/dl)	Succinate
23	1948	5.2[a]	present
23	2145	5.4[a]	present
27	0500	0.09	present
30	0525	Nondetectable	present

[a]Toxic result. Chloramphenicol succinate was discontinued on day 25 postoperatively.

METHODS

For chloramphenicol analysis we used the method of Aravind et al. (1,2). The analysis is performed on a Waters 6000 high performance liquid chromatography (HPLC) system, using a Supelco C-18 column.

Address correspondence and reprint requests to Dr. C. A. Robinson at Department of Pathology, University of Alabama in Birmingham, University Station, Birmingham, AL 35294, U.S.A.

To investigate the interference we used the same HPLC system with a Hewlett-Packard model 1040A Diode Array Detector. Gas chromatography (GC) was performed on a Hewlett-Packard 5840A on an SP2250 column with a column temperature beginning at 180°C and rising 30°/min to 270°C. Prior to injection into the GC, both the extracted patient sample and dobutamine hydrochloride were treated with TriSil (Pierce), a silylating agent.

RESULTS

Since the spurious results were found just after the initiation of dobutamine HCl treatment, we elected to test it first for interference with our chloramphenicol assay.

Injection of a 1-μg/mL dobutamine hydrochloride standard through the HPLC column showed a retention time of 4.4 min, matching that of the chloramphenicol succinate standard. A sample from another patient known to be receiving dobutamine was extracted using the chloramphenicol procedure and showed a peak at the same retention time.

Analysis of the unknown substance was performed with a Hewlett-Packard model 1040A Diode Array Detector along with similar scans of chloramphenicol, chloramphenicol succinate, and dobutamine hydrochloride. This analysis showed that the unknown substance was definitely not chloramphenicol or chloramphenicol succinate, that only one substance was contained in the peak on the HPLC, and that the substance was suggestive of dobutamine hydrochloride.

For additional confirmation, the extracted patient serum sample and dobutamine hydrochloride were silylated and run through GC. Both dobutamine hydrochloride and the patient sample presented a peak at 8.3 min.

DISCUSSION

The succinate ester of chloramphenicol must be hydrolyzed to chloramphenicol for its antibacteriologic properties to be active. About 30% of the ester is excreted unchanged in the urine, the remainder being hydrolyzed to chloramphenicol and distributed widely to tissues and body fluids. The elimination half-life of chloramphenicol is approximately 4 h and is not changed significantly by renal dysfunction. Most of the drug is metabolized in the liver to the inactive glucuronide conjugate (3). The rapid hydrolysis of the succinate ester and relatively short half-life of chloramphenicol make it highly improbable that either would be detected in serum 4 days after the drug had been discontinued.

Dobutamine hydrochloride is a synthetic catecholamine used to improve ventricular contractility and is usually given by continuous infusion. It has a mean plasma half-life of about 2 min, metabolizing to dobutamine glucuronide and 3-*O*-methyldobutamine glucuronide. Both are inactive and are eliminated through the kidney (4).

Laboratories should be aware of the continuing possibility of interferences even in documented, well-established procedures as new drugs become available. Any unusual or unexpected results should be thoroughly researched by the laboratory and clinician.

REFERENCES

1. Aravind MK, Miceli JN. Chloramphenicol and chloramphenicol succinate. In: Sunshine I, ed. *Methodology for analytical toxicology*. Boca Raton: CRC Press, 1982.
2. Aravind MK, Miceli JN, Kauffman RE, Strebel L, Done AK. Simultaneous measurement of chloramphenicol and chloramphenicol succinate by high performance liquid chromatography. *J Chromatogr* 1980;221:176–81.
3. Ambrose PJ. Clinical pharmacokinetics of chloramphenicol and chloramphenicol succinate. *Clin Pharmacokinet* 1984;9:222–38.
4. Leier CV, Unverferth DV. Drugs five years later: dobutamine. *Ann Intern Med* 1983;99:490–6.

Therapeutic Drug Monitoring
7:123–126 © 1985 Raven Press, New York

Letters to the Editor

On the Interaction Between Phenytoin and Antineoplastic Agents

To the Editor: In their interesting article (1) on the interaction between phenytoin and antineoplastic agents, Sylvester and co-workers stated that only one other case report (2) in the literature has suggested that cisplatinum, vinblastine, and bleomycin therapy may adversely affect phenytoin absorption. Although this statement is essentially correct, another case report dealing with pharmacokinetic interaction between phenytoin and antineoplastic treatment (vinblastine, methotrexate, and carmustine) was published in 1983 (3). This work has been quoted in a comprehensive review on pharmacokinetic interactions of antiepileptic drugs (4).

The patient described in our report showed a marked decrease of plasma phenytoin concentrations and a subsequent reappearance of seizures after the beginning of an antineoplastic therapy cycle. The association of the clinical problems with the sudden large drop in phenytoin concentrations 24 h after vinblastine administration suggested a cause–effect relationship. As in the other cases (1,2), a substantial impairment of phenytoin absorption seemed to be the most obvious explanation of the observed phenomena. Given the fact that three case reports suggest that there is a clinically important interaction between antineoplastic drugs and phenytoin, we think that controlled studies of this interaction are required to optimize phenytoin treatment in patients concurrently receiving antineoplastic drug therapy.

Roberto Riva
Fiorenzo Albani
Agostino Baruzzi
Laboratory of Neuropharmacology
Institute of Neurology
University of Bologna
Bologna, Italy

References

1. Sylvester RK, Lewis FB, Caldwell KC, Lobell M, Perri R, Sawchuk RA. Impaired phenytoin bioavailability secondary to cisplatinum, vinblastine, and bleomycin. *Ther Drug Monit* 1984;6:302–5.
2. Fincham RW, Schottelius DD. Decreased phenytoin levels in antineoplastic therapy. *Ther Drug Monit* 1979;1:277–83.
3. Bollini P, Riva R, Albani F, et al. Decreased phenytoin level during antineoplastic therapy: a case report. *Epilepsia* 1983;24:75–8.
4. Perucca E. Pharmacokinetic interaction with antiepileptic drugs. *Clin Pharmacokinet* 1982;7:57–84.

Measurement of Cyclosporine: A Challenge to the Professional Laboratory Organizations

To the Editor: During the past year there has been a series of letters to the editor in this journal regarding the ability of clinical laboratories to monitor cyclosporine. This series started with a letter from Robinson and Ketchum (1) and continued with the letters of Schran and Abisch (2) and Paull et al. (3). Each proposes a different method for analysis of cyclosporine, each method yielding a different numerical result. We (4) have recently published our own opinion on this matter, which yields yet another analytically correct but different result of the concentration of cyclosporine. These differences are based on choice of specimen type, temperature of separation (if serum analysis is proposed), and analytical procedure [radioimmunoassay (RIA) vs. high performance liquid chromatography (HPLC)]. Briefly, the RIA procedure yields results approximately twofold higher than HPLC in identical specimens, the blood concentration of cyclosporine is approximately twofold that of plasma separated at 37°C, and plasma separated at 37°C is approximately twofold higher in concentration than plasma separated at 20°C (room temperature). Merging analytical procedures that differ by a predictable degree (because of cross-reactivity in the immunochemical method) with significant differences in specimen, whether it is serum separated at 20°C or 37°C, or whole blood, makes six distinctly different results possible.

This situation causes a great deal of confusion among transplant surgeons who wish to use cyclosporine concentration to guide them in making therapeutic decisions. There are effectively six different "therapeutic ranges" that must be considered, each of them dependent upon decisions made within the clinical laboratory regarding specimen handling and analytical procedures. As outlined in refs. 1 through 4, there are arguments that favor all six options, and each set of results is clinically useful within its own context. Physicians performing transplants are understandably confused and annoyed by the discrepancy that they see between laboratories and in the peer-reviewed literature. These annoyances are laboratory induced, and therefore it is up to the laboratories to resolve them.

Since reasonable arguments can be made in favor of any one of the six options available, I doubt that a consensus will be reached through individual efforts. Only the professional laboratory organizations active in the field of therapeutic drug monitoring can bring a broad enough spectrum of experience and understanding to bear on the problem to render an opinion that will be accepted by the majority of laboratories regarding the most clinically useful combination of specimen and procedure. The deliberations of these groups should consider that clinical utility is of paramount importance, and limitations of any particular technique should not influence the outcome of the final decision. I therefore challenge the College of American Pathologists Therapeutic Drug Monitoring Resource Committee and the American Association for Clinical Chemistry Therapeutic Drug Monitoring Subcommittee to study the problem of appropriate specimen and procedure for analysis of cyclosporine and render a *timely* opinion that could set the standard for laboratory practice in this field. Until such happens, I agree with the conclusions of Robinson and Ketchum (1): it is not a question of whether cyclosporine monitoring is necessary, but whether it is *uniformly* possible.

Thomas P. Moyer
Department of Laboratory Medicine
Mayo Clinic
Rochester, Minnesota, U.S.A.

References

1. Robinson CA, Ketchum CH. Monitoring of cyclosporin A: is it possible [Letter]? *Ther Drug Monit* 1983;5:371.
2. Schran H, Abisch E. Monitoring of cyclosporine: a status report [Letter]. *Ther Drug Monit* 1984;6:371.
3. Paull P, Britton K, Atkinson K, Biggs J. On the measurement of cyclosporine in plasma [Letter]. *Ther Drug Monit* 1984;6:373.
4. Faynor SM, Moyer TP, Sterioff S, McDonald MW. Therapeutic drug monitoring of cyclosporine. *Mayo Clin Proc* 1984;59:571–2.

Extraction of Interfering Substance from the Sera of Uremic Subjects Prior to Homogeneous Enzyme Immunoassay

To the Editor: The homogeneous enzyme immunoassay (EMIT, Syva Corp., Palo Alto, CA, U.S.A.) test has been shown to give artificially high results for serum phenytoin in some patients with renal disease (1). This report describes a method for removal of the interfering substance(s) using the PREP I (E. I. Du Pont de Nemours, Wilmington, DE, U.S.A.) automated sample processing system. This interference may be caused by the glucuronide conjugate of 5-(*p*-hydroxyphenyl)-5-phenylhydantoin (HPPH-glucuronide) (2,3). Syva (4) states that cross-reactivity with unconjugated HPPH is significant at concentrations greater than 8 μg/ml. The cross-reactivity to conjugated HPPH is reported to be significant at 20 μg/ml for some reagent lots (3). We observed the interference in phenytoin assays performed on the Du Pont ACA which uses EMIT reagents from Syva and is subject to the same interferences. It appears that this simple procedure can be used to prepare uremic specimens for analysis by EMIT on the Du Pont ACA.

Materials

Samples. Specimens were collected by venipuncture into 10-ml Vacutainer tubes (Becton Dickinson, Rutherford, NJ, U.S.A.) with no preservative. Serum was separated by centrifugation within 30 min and frozen until analysis.

Chemicals. Anhydrous sodium acetate, AR-grade, was purchased from Mallincrodt (Paris, KY, U.S.A.). The water used in all steps was double-distilled in glass and passed through a Barnstead D0809 Ultrapure (mixed bed) column (Barnstead Company of Sybron Corp., Boston, MA, U.S.A.). Chloroform and methanol, HPLC-grade, and acetic acid, ACS reagent-grade, were purchased from Fisher Scientific (Fairlawn, NJ, U.S.A.). For the gas-liquid chromatography (GLC), hydrogen was generated by a model 15EHG generator (General Electric, Wilmington, MA, U.S.A.), and 99.998% pure nitrogen and instrument grade air (<2 ppm H_2O, <0.1 ppm hydrocarbon) were purchased (Liquid Carbonic Corp., Chicago, IL, U.S.A.).

Standards. Internal standard 5-(*p*-methylphenyl)-5-phenyl-hydantoin (*p*-tolylphenytoin MPPH) and phenytoin metabolite DL-5-(*p*-hydroxyphenyl)-5-phenylhydantoin (5-HPPH) were purchased from Aldrich Chemical Co. (Milwaukee, WI, U.S.A.), and 5,5-

diphenylhydantoin (Dilantin) was purchased from Supelco (Bellefonte, PA, U.S.A.).

Reagents. A 1.0-mg/ml stock solution of phenytoin, MPPH internal standard, and 5-HPPH was prepared by dissolving 0.1 g of material in 100 ml methanol. Sodium acetate buffer, 1 mol/L, containing 410 ml of 1 N acetic acid and 590 ml of 1 mol/L sodium acetate, was adjusted to pH 4.8 with 1 N acetic acid. The GLC extraction reagent was prepared by diluting 2 ml of stock internal standard solution to 1 L with chloroform. The working standard of 10 mg/L was prepared by diluting 1 ml of stock standard to 100 ml with water.

Apparatus. A model 2100 chromatograph (Varian Instrument Division, Palo Alto, CA, U.S.A.) coupled with a Model 3380 recorder integrator (Hewlett-Packard, Avondale, PA, U.S.A.) was used for the GLC determinations. The GLC 6-ft glass column (Supelco) was packed with 2% SP-2110/1% SP-2510-DA on 100/120 Supelcoport. Extraction of specimens for enzyme immunoassay was carried out on a PREP I automated sample processor with type W extraction columns, and these analyses were performed on an ACA III. The instruments, columns, and reagent packs were from Du Pont (Phenytoin reagent pack lot Nos. C3139A and C3207A).

Procedures

GLC with manual extraction. The extraction procedure is that of Savory et al. (5).

One milliliter of sera buffered with 1 ml of sodium acetate buffer is extracted with 10 ml of extraction reagent. The extraction tube is mixed and then centrifuged for 2 min at moderate speed. The aqueous layer is discarded, and the chloroform layer is transferred to a clean tube and evaporated to dryness at 65°C under an air stream. Chloroform, 25 μl, is used to reconstitute the extract, and 3 μl is injected onto the column, the oven temperature being programmed from 160–260°C at 15°/min.

Quantification is based on peak area ratios of phenytoin to MPPH internal standard.

Enzyme immunoassay with automated extraction. Empty all fluid from the top of the type W cartridge and introduce 0.5 ml of sample and 0.5 ml of buffer. Use program No. 1 on the PREP I automated sample processor with 9.6 ml of water as solvent 1 and 9.6 ml chloroform as solvent 2. This program causes the column to be successively drained, washed with water, and eluted with chloroform. The chloroform solution is collected and evaporated under an air stream. Dissolve the residue by adding 0.1 ml of methanol and vortex-mixing. Reconstitute to volume by adding 0.4 ml of drug-free sera.

TABLE 1. *Serum phenytoin concentrations (μg/ml)*

Patient	Gas-liquid chromatography	ACA analyzer	ACA w/ extraction
WD[a]	2.7	10.2	3.1
DC[a]	6.5	19.6	7.4
SE[a]	6.8	14.4	5.9
MB[a]	10.6	33.9	10.6
EF[a]	11.5	17.5	11.3
DJ[a]	20.3	31.4	19.7
SF[b]	7.4	9.7	8.6
TO[b]	8.2	14.5	8.0
HF[b]	10.4	14.0	10.3
ON[b]	11.2	15.0	12.8
FS[b]	13.3	23.8	15.8
RP[b]	9.4	10.5	—
RP[b] (spiked[c])	9.4	22.6	8.2
Control	19.0	19.3	19.4
Control (spiked[c])	19.0	34.3	19.6

[a]Known uremic patient.
[b]Nonuremic patient (serum urea nitrogen = <21 mg/dl, creatinine = <1.4 mg/dl).
[c]Spiked with stock 5-(*p*-hydroxyphenyl)-5-phenylhydantoin (5-HPPH) to yield a 50 μg/ml 5-HPPH concentration.

Results

Table 1 gives the results of assays on the sera of several patients and a control material. Some of the patients where known to be uremic. After extraction of these sera with the PREP I, the ACA results were substantially in agreement with those from the GLC method. Sera and controls spiked with 5-HPPH at a concentration of 50 μg/ml gave increased enzyme immunoassay values similar to those seen in uremic patients (HPPH-glucuronide was unavailable). PREP extraction of these spiked sera also gave nearly quantitative recovery of phenytoin. Reference sera or water spiked with 5-HPPH gave only a small increase in the enzyme immunoassay value. The average phenytoin concentration for 24 patients was 103% of that found using the GLC reference method. This comparison study included the 12 patients indicated in Table 1 plus groups of three drug-free pool seras spiked at 10, 20, 30, and 40 μg/ml concentrations. The results of precision studies were as follows. Within run: n = 9, patient specimen; mean = 13.3 mg/L; coefficient of variation = 5.6%. Day to day: n = 15, quality control sera; mean = 19.4 mg/L; coefficient of variation = 7.9%.

Reconstitution with methanol and sera assures better recovery on samples with a phenytoin concentration above 40.0 μg/ml. ACA enzymatic diluent gives good recovery on samples with concentrations less than 40.0 μg/ml.

Discussion

The effect of artificially increased enzyme immunoassay phenytoin results in uremic patients has been previously observed by us and reported by others (1–3). It was inconvenient to perform the GLC analysis for all renal patients (especially the stat requests). Our goal was to develop a simple extraction procedure that would enable reliable phenytoin determinations by enzyme immunoassay in uremic patients. We found that the manual extraction used for GLC also worked. Chloroform, 10 ml, was used as the extraction reagent and then a 1 5.0-ml aliquot was evaporated down. The dried extract was then reconstituted with 0.1 ml methanol and 0.4 ml drug-free sera. Because of automation and ease of use we chose to work with PREP I. Our experiments indicated that the recoveries were close to 100% and that the interfering metabolite(s) extraction was complete.

Clark A. Rundell
Sue Ellen Tupper
Department of Pathology
Maine Medical Center
Portland, Maine, U.S.A.

References

1. Flacks H, Rasmussen JM. Renal disease may increase apparent phenytoin in serum as measured by enzyme-multiplied immunoassay. *Clin Chem* 1980;26:361–62.
2. Green PJ, Vlasses PH, Frauenhoffer SM, Hennessey KM. Phenytoin can be measured reliably in uremic patients by immunoassay. *Clin Chem* 1983;29:737.
3. Aldwin L, Kabakoff DS. Metabolite interference in homogeneous enzyme immunoassay of phenytoin. *Clin Chem* 1981;27:770–1.
4. Syva Corp., Palo Alto, CA. Package insert for the EMIT-aed, May 1982.
5. Savory J, Shipe JR. A comprehensive gas chromatographic procedure for measurement of drugs in biological material. *Ann Clin Lab* 1975;5:57–64.

Therapeutic Drug Monitoring
7:127–128 © 1985 Raven Press, New York

Book Reviews

Practical Immunoassay. The State of the Art. *Butt, W. R. (ed.).* Marcel Dekker, New York, 1984. 318 pp., $55.00.

This 14th volume of the Dekker series on clinical and biochemical analysis is devoted entirely to the immunological techniques currently in use at most clinical and research laboratories. The book is fairly comprehensive, with chapters on radioimmunoassays, enzyme immunoassays (EIA), fluoroimmunoassays, chemiluminescence assays, nephelometric assays, labeled antibody assays, and free hormone assays. In addition, one chapter is dedicated to the production and use of monoclonal antibodies, and another to data analysis and quality control.

Most sections were written with endocrinology assays in mind and may not be relevant to workers engaged in therapeutic drug monitoring and clinical pharmacology. The exception is the chapter on EIA that deals with competitive EIA for methotrexate as a detailed example of the technique. However, the basic principles of the techniques covered in all chapters could be equally applicable to most drugs and their metabolite immunoassays. The emphasis of the book is on basic principles, and detailed procedures for a given substance may not be found. However, example protocols are given for various procedures.

The book opens with a discussion of antibody preparation (the basic requirement of all immunoassays including drugs) using conventional animal immunization protocols, and the various methods used to separate antibody-bound ligands from free ligands. There is a brief introduction to each chapter. The author comments on the trend toward utilization of nonisotopic assays, especially employing two antibody immunometric assays. The technical advances and increasing use of nonisotopic assays are evident as one peruses the book.

The procedures for iodination are discussed in the second chapter. The most commonly used procedure, the chloramine-T method, is described in detail, and readers will also find a typical protocol for the iodination of 30,000 MW protein. A sample calculation of specific activity after iodination is included. Also discussed are problems associated with storage and disposal of isotopes and the disadvantages associated with their use.

The third chapter is concerned with the principles and practices of EIA in general. Earlier work in the field is reviewed, and recent developments are described. Principles of EIA, e.g., competitive, immunoenzymometric (IRMA), and enzyme-linked immunoassays (ELISA), as well as homogeneous EIAs based on enzyme ligand conjugates (enzyme multiplied immunoassay technique used widely for drug analysis), hapten substrate conjugates, or ligand modulator conjugates, are discussed. The merits of EIA are critically evaluated, and both advantages and disadvantages of using enzymes as ligands are listed. The criteria for choosing enzyme labels are outlined, and a procedure for preparation of enzyme labels is discussed in detail. The chapter is complete and provides an excellent bibliography.

Fluorescent probes have found wide application as labels in immunoassays: chapters 4 and 5 are concerned mainly with recent trends in their use. Time-resolved fluorescent measurements, using lanthanide series chelates, may some day develop assays of greater sensitivity than conventional fluorescent systems. The theoretical aspects of these assays are well covered in chapter 4; but few practical applications are discussed, suggesting that these techniques are still in their infancy. The material on chemiluminescence labels in immunoassays in chapter 5 documents the extreme sensitivity that can be obtained by these ligands if they are used in two-site immunometric assays.

Chapter 6 discusses the measurement of antibody-antigen complexes by their ability to scatter light (nephelometer). The kinetics of antigen-antibody reactions are thoroughly covered. As applications of these techniques are mainly restricted to larger proteins, this chapter has little to offer in terms of drug assays. The same is true of chapter 9, on the measurement of free hormones in the blood.

With the advent of monoclonal antibodies, the trend is to use antibodies as label ligands (both isotopic or nonisotopic). Chapter 7 describes the theoretical aspects of label antibody assays and their clinical use. The extreme sensitivity and precision of these assays are well documented.

The last chapter gives a broad review of some of the important aspects of data processing and quality control.

As each chapter is written by a different author, there is repetition of immunoassay principles in various chapters. Immunological techniques (competitive RIA, ELISA, IRMA, etc.) could have been described in one chapter at the beginning of the book. Despite this weakness, the book provides comprehensive coverage of the rapidly growing field of immunoassays. As these techniques are being vigorously applied for therapeutic drug monitoring, this book will be equally valuable to pharmacologists and toxicologists, as well as to clinical chemists. It is a valuable addition to the field of immunoassays.

Manjula K. Gupta

Marihuana in Science and Medicine. *Nahas, G.* Raven Press, New York, 1984. 324 pp., $48.00.

With the aid of three associates, the author presents a comprehensive review of the botanical and chemical properties of marihuana. Complementing this is a current assessment of its toxicology, pharmacology, clinical applications, and relationship to mental illness. Each chapter is extremely well documented and compared objectively. The text reads easily, provides excellent detailed information, is well indexed, and can be an effective reference source. It is worth the attention of all those concerned with the problems marihuana brings.

Irving Sunshine

Applications of Optimal Control Therapy in Biomedicine. *Swan, G. W.* Marcel Dekker, New York, 1984. 285 pp., $55.00.

Mathematical models of human physiological systems have been particularly valuable in the design of certain bioengineering systems. This book introduces the reader to basic concepts of optimal control theory and provides five major examples of applications of this theory. These examples include models of control of diabetes, management of thyroid disease, administration of drugs, control of cancer therapy, and control of problems of the circulatory system. For readers of *Therapeutic Drug Monitoring*, the chapter on the optimal administration of drugs is of particular interest and includes the development of the one-, two-, and three-compartmental models of pharmacological drug distribution. The chapter describes and derives the mathematics of a number of workers in this field, including the one-compartmental model of Bellman and the two-compartmental model of Buell and coworkers.

The orientation of the book is quite mathematical, and the models that are discussed probably have their prime utility in bioengineering. For example, the models on diabetes might be useful in the design of a feedback-controlled infusion insulin pump. In addition, these models are useful in designing simulation models for teaching. Unfortunately, this book is so mathematical that most readers will find the models difficult to follow. The drug models, for example, are too complex to use as simple pharmacokinetics simulations. Most of the models covered in this book, however, are sufficiently realistic that they can be rather useful in helping users understand the limitations and assumptions of some common modeling systems.

David Chou

Therapeutic Drug Monitoring
7:129 © 1985 Raven Press, New York

Editorial

Cyclosporine Quality Control Program is a Reality

As all of our readers are aware, there is major concern throughout the scientific community with respect to the interlaboratory reproducibility and reliability of the analytical radioimmunoassay (RIA) and high pressure liquid chromatographic (HPLC) assay techniques employed to determine cyclosporine drug concentrations. Many laboratories have modified the original RIA and HPLC assays in order to adapt them to their environment. Yet, there often were no interlaboratory studies carried out to verify that these modifications were indeed valid. It is with great pleasure that we print the following announcement from the Department of Pathology of the University of Pittsburgh:

A CYCLOSPORINE QUALITY CONTROL SURVEY PROGRAM, CALLED PITTSBURGH CYCLOSPORINE SURVEY, IS BEING INITIATED BY THE CLINICAL CHEMISTRY LABORATORY, DEPARTMENT OF PATHOLOGY, UNIVERSITY OF PITTSBURGH SCHOOL OF MEDICINE. THOSE LABORATORIES UNDERTAKING THE MEASUREMENT OF CYCLOSPORINE, EITHER BY RIA OR HPLC, ARE ENCOURAGED TO PARTICIPATE. SIX TIMES PER YEAR, EACH PARTICIPANT WILL RECEIVE TWO 1-ML WHOLE BLOOD SPECIMENS CONTAINING KNOWN AMOUNTS OF CYCLOSPORINE AT TWO DIFFERENT LEVELS. THE RESULTS OF THESE ANALYSES FROM EACH PARTICIPANT WILL BE ANALYZED STATISTICALLY FOLLOWING THE FORMAT OF THERAPEUTIC DRUG MONITORING PROGRAM AND/OR COLLEGE OF AMERICAN PATHOLOGISTS' SURVEY, AND WILL BE CONVEYED BACK TO THE PARTICIPANTS. THE COST OF THE SURVEY IS $200/YEAR. CHECKS MUST BE MADE PAYABLE TO PITTSBURGH CYCLOSPORINE SURVEY.

FOR ADDITIONAL INFORMATION PLEASE CONTACT ROSEMARIE BALOH, SUPERVISOR, AT CLINICAL CHEMISTRY LABORATORY 203 DESOTO STREET, PITTSBURGH, PA 15261. TELEPHONE, (412) 647–3765

We would strongly urge every laboratory in the world engaged in the monitoring of cyclosporine, regardless of technique, to enroll in this quality control program. It is essential that all of us actively participate together in order that we can exchange information and standardize cyclosporine monitoring throughout the world. It is obvious that through participation in this program, each of us will be assured that our assays are performing in an appropriate manner, and even more importantly, we will be able to identify the differences in the various methodologies and make the appropriate adjustments to improve the assays.

We gratefully acknowledge and express our thanks to Dr. Ajit Sanghvi and Ms. Rosemarie Baloh for their willingness to institute and sponsor this program. With our support, the program will be a success and ultimately result in better patient care.

C. E. Pippenger
Cleveland, Ohio

Therapeutic Drug Monitoring
7:130–147 © 1985 Raven Press, New York

Review

Clinical Pharmacokinetics of Sulfonamides in Children: Relationship Between Maturing Kidney Function and Renal Clearance of Sulfonamides

Tom B. Vree, Yechiel A. Hekster, and *Rob J. J. Lippens

*Departments of Clinical Pharmacy and *Paediatrics, Sint Radboud Hospital, University of Nijmegen, Nijmegen, The Netherlands*

The pharmacokinetic properties of sulfonamides in adults are well described (1–7). It has been shown that in most cases elimination is governed by metabolism of the parent compound at the *p*-aminophenyl group at the N_4 atom, leading to formation of N_4-acetylsulfonamides possessing no antibacterial activity (Fig. 1). Sulfonamides are, to varying extents, excreted by the kidneys in characteristic ways. Depending on the structure and the substituent at the N_1 atom, the parent drugs are excreted either by glomerular filtration or by active tubular secretion followed by reabsorption (7). The N_4-acetylsulfonamide metabolites are excreted predominantly by active tubular secretion independent of the N_1 substituent (7).

Overall elimination of sulfonamides in adults depends on renal function. Whether elimination processes in general are age dependent has yet to be determined. However, this determination is especially important for assessing dosage regimens of sulfonamides in children undergoing supportive antiinfectious care during the treatment of neoplastic diseases. When the mechanism by which the elimination process of (particular) sulfonamides occurs in relation to age is clear, it may become possible to predict how sulfonamide kinetics will vary with age. Anticipation of decreased elimination requires the physician to change dosage regimens to reduce the risks of accumulation and severely adverse, toxic, effects. However, data on pharmacokinetic characteristics of sulfonamides in young children are relatively scarce, mainly due to the fear of administering sulfonamides to children under the age of 1 year, due to the expected and observed side effects and the uncertainty about the kinetics and preferable dosage regimens.

KIDNEY FUNCTION

The functional capacity of the kidney in young infants is lower than in older children and adults. Although glomeruli and tubules are present at the time of birth, they are not of full proportion or capacity (8–12).

Glomerular Function

The creatinine clearance in preterm infants at birth is extremely low, with the level dependent on the number of gestational weeks. At 28 weeks, the creatinine clearance is only 0.35 ml/min, which increases to ~3 ml/min at 40 weeks (13).

The glomerular filtration rate (GFR) at birth is ~2.5 ml/min (20 ml/min/1.73 m^2) and increases gradually over 12 months to 28 ml/min (115 ml/min/1.73 m^2), the average increase being ~2 ml/min/month (10%) (9,10,13–27). The increase in the GFR is due to increased renal blood flow, a gradual shift from juxtamedullar nephrons to cortical nephrons, and

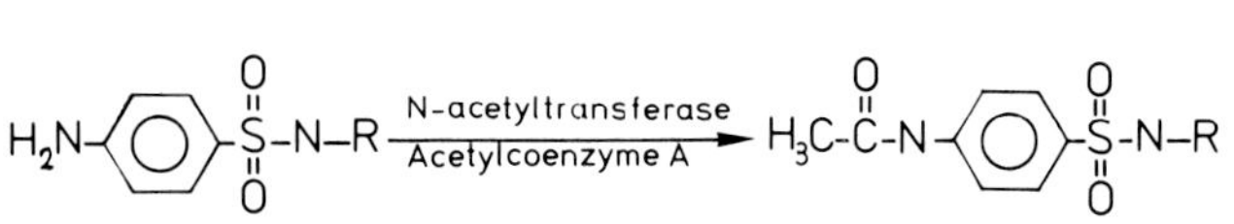

FIG. 1. Metabolism of sulfonamides.

Address correspondence and reprint requests to T. B. Vree at Department of Clinical Pharmacy, Sint Radboud Hospital, University of Nijmegen, Geert Grooteplein Zuid 8, Nijmegen, The Netherlands.

changes in the glomerular capillary surface and permeability (15,16,18,21,28–32,82).

Tubular Function

The tubular secretory capacity for *p*-aminohippuric acid (PAH), a parameter for active tubular secretion, also correlates strongly with age (12,17,21,23,30). Infants under 1 year of age show an extremely variable capacity for excretion of PAH (23,33), ranging from 12 ml/min (25 ml/min/1.73 m^2) at the time of birth to 200–300 ml/min at 1 year of age (9,34,35).

Another parameter for tubular functioning is the active reabsorption of glucose and β-2-microglobulin (36). As the kidney matures, the reabsorption of β-2-microglobulin by the tubule increases and the overall renal excretion rate and apparent renal clearance diminish (37,38). Reabsorption of β-2-microglobulin decreases when kidney function is impaired (38).

Tubuloglomerular Balance

The tubuloglomerular balance in the kidney shows a constant and maximum ratio of 5:1 between their respective clearance capacities from 1 to 50 years of age (29,39). From the data of Rubin et al. (23) and West et al. (26) it can be derived that in premature neonates the tubuloglomerular ratio is 3.5:1.

Reabsorption

When the tubule has to excrete compounds via active transport (40), these compounds are eligible for active reabsorption, as demonstrated for glucose and PAH (41–43). Active tubular reabsorption seems to be the last process to develop in the immature kidney, consequently there may be periods earlier in life when the sum of glomerular and tubular secretion exceeds tubular reabsorption, resulting in a temporarily higher renal clearance than found at older ages (12). The high glomerular rate of filtration, an heritage from our aquatic ancestors, continuously filters the entire circulating plasma volume twice an hour (44). At birth the glomerular surface is disproportionately large in comparison with the tubular surface (26). Thus the overall excretion–reabsorption processes are dependent on the number, age, and capacity of the tubules.

Whether tubule capacity increases by functional changes in the transport mechanism or has to be stimulated by endogenous waste products such as PAH, glucuronides, or sulfates is still an open question, the question being whether the active transport mechanism has to be trained to excrete these products.

The active tubular system can be stimulated by repetitive administration of compounds that have to be excreted predominantly by the active transport system, such as penicillins (16,40,45–50). The system is also gradually stimulated by the changing composition of the child's food over the year.

Urine Production

Urine production is already occurring in preterm life, and ranges from ~10 ml/h (0.167 ml/min) at 30 gestational weeks to 27 ml/h (0.45 ml/min) at 40 weeks (18,14,51,52). The concentration ability of the kidney and the urinary flow are less in young than in older infants (20).

In comparison with that of the adult, the kidney functioning of young infants must be considered "impaired." This impairment, due mainly to the immaturity of the glomeruli and tubules and their correspondingly limited functions, differs from that observed in adults, which usually results from the adverse effects of drugs, decreased cardiac output, nephropathy, pathophysiologic or other circumstances. Knowing that glomerular and tubular functions, the tubuloglomerular balance, and urine flow are less in young infants than in older children and adults, we can examine the effects of the kidney on the renal excretion of sulfonamides and overall elimination in young children.

CLINICAL PHARMACOKINETICS OF SULFONAMIDES

Sulfonamides are eliminated from the human body by metabolism, via acetylation, and by renal excretion. Each member of the large series of available sulfonamides shows its own kinetic parameters depending on its chemical structure and corresponding enzyme–drug structure interactions.

Kinetics of Acetylation

All sulfonamides become acetylated when metabolized, the yield of acetylation depending strongly on the structure of the sulfonamide, i.e, the N_1 substituent. How the N_1 substituent influences the acetylation reaction that takes place at the "opposite site" of the molecule, the N_4 atom, is as yet unclear.

It has recently been determined (33,53) that acetylation is a part of, or the result of, an acetylation–deacetylation equilibrium. The position of the equilibrium depends strongly on the N_1 substituent and the acetylating enzyme package in humans, slow–fast acetylation phenotype or fast–slow deacetylation phenotype, and in dogs, in which deacetylation dominates acetylation with the net outcome being a zero yield of acetylation. The impact of the position of the acetylation–deacetylation equilibrium is best illustrated by the facts that whereas sulfaethidole is not at all acetylated in humans, due to its high rate of deacetylation, and sulfamethizole is acetylated only 3%, sulfamethoxazole and sulfametrole are extensively acetylated due to their very low deacetylation rates (6). The rates of deacetylation of N_4-acetylsulfamethoxazole and N_4-acetylsulfametrole in humans are so low that in patients with normal kidney function no "metabolite" sulfamethoxazole and sulfametrole can be detected when the N_4-acetyl derivatives are administered (2,4).

Deacetylation of these two N_4-acetylsulfonamide derivatives was detected in patients with end-stage renal function and in beagle dogs, which deacetylate very rapidly (2,6,7). The deacetylation of N_4-acetylsulfonamide derivatives to sulfonamides contributes to the plasma concentration of the originally administered sulfonamide, thus influencing the observed or apparent half-life. All of these observations however, were made in adults.

In young children, the position of the acetylation–deacetylation equilibrium may differ from that in adults, if we extrapolate from results for the glucuronidation–deglucuronidation equilibrium (35). But as yet, no clear-cut mechanistic studies have been carried out on young volunteer children.

It is questionable whether a shift in the positions of these equilibria must be attributed to a lack of the conjugation reactions or to the impaired renal excretion, which makes the deconjugation visible and measureable (6,33,53). Because it is unlikely that such vital metabolic reactions as acetylation and glucuronidation are dependent on age, it is difficult to ascribe a decreased yield of acetylation to the metabolic reaction only and not to a secondary effect of impaired renal function (54–57). Furthermore, when the renal excretion of the formed glucuronide is impaired, alternative sulfate conjugation reactions may become relatively more important (58–61).

Cerebrospinal Fluid Passage of Sulfonamides

Sulfonamides pass through the blood–brain barrier. In clinical practice, sulfonamides can be used in the treatment of infections of susceptible strains of microorganisms in the brain ventricles, in the meninges, and in other brain regions (62). When the physician requests the determination of the concentration of sulfonamides in the aqueous humor or in the cerebrospinal fluid (CSF), the laboratory should ask for accompanying blood and urine samples to make the scarce and isolated CSF results more meaningful and to increase the number of blood samples from young children, which is indispensable for rational treatment of infection with sulfonamides in young children. Table 1 gives the values of the plasma concentrations, protein-binding levels, CSF concentrations, and CSF/plasma ratios of sulfamethoxazole and its N_4-acetyl derivative for several patients of various ages.

Renal Excretion of Sulfonamides and Their Metabolites

Based on their observed renal clearances and underlying mechanisms of renal excretion, the sulfonamides can be classified in three categories: (a) those

TABLE 1. *Ratio between cerebrospinal fluid (CSF) concentration (% total plasma concentration) and free (unbound) plasma concentration of sulfamethoxazole (S) and its metabolite* N_4*-acetylsulfamethoxazole* (N_4) *during co-trimoxazole therapy*

Subject	Age days (years)	Protein binding		CSF concentration (% of plasma conc.)		Concentration ratio (CSF/free plasma)		Sample source	Remarks
		S (%)	N_4 (%)	S	N_4	S	N_4		
1	15 (0.041)			73.4	59.1			Ventricle	
	35 (0.096)	53.5	74.6	30.2	11.1	0.65	0.44	Ventricle	
				30.8	11.7	0.66	0.46	Lumbar	
2	30 (0.082)	42.6	57.2	16.8 ± 4.9	39.5 ± 4.2	0.61	0.27		
3	(8.7)			36.9	54.5				
4	(12)			43.6	74.4				
5	(50)	57.8	78.2	27.5	9.7	0.65	0.45		Kidney impairment

excreted predominantly by active tubular secretion, (b) those excreted by glomerular filtration and tubular reabsorption, and (c) those excreted by active tubular secretion and tubular reabsorption.

Sulfonamides

Renal excretion predominantly by active tubular secretion. Compounds with a "free" sulfur atom in their N_1-substituted group, such as sulfamethizole and sulfathiazole, are excreted actively. The renal clearance values of these sulfonamides are high, usually higher than those of the corresponding metabolites (2). Probenecid comedication reduces the renal clearance until it equals the net remaining clearance of glomerular filtration and tubular reabsorption (7).

Renal excretion by glomerular filtration and tubular reabsorption. Sulfonamides that are excreted by glomerular filtration and tubular reabsorption invariably show low renal clearance values. Their renal clearance values are low in comparison with the renal clearance values of their metabolites. The renal clearance is dependent on such parameters of the tubular reabsorption as urinary pH and urinary flow. Members of this group are sulfamethoxazole, sulfametrole, sulfadiazine, sulfamerazine, and sulfadimidine.

Renal excretion by active tubular secretion and tubular reabsorption. The overall measured renal clearances of these drugs are low (~10 ml/min) and of the same magnitude as those of the corresponding N_4-acetylsulfonamide metabolites. Comedication with probenecid lowers the renal clearance value of the parent drug. Members of this group are sulfisomidine, sulfafurazole, and sulfaethidole.

N_4-*Acetylsulfonamide Derivatives*

The metabolite N_4-acetylsulfonamide is excreted predominantly by active tubular secretion. Probenecid

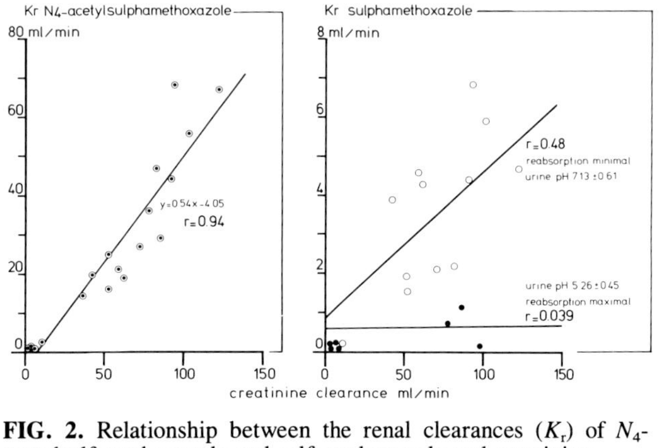

FIG. 2. Relationship between the renal clearances (K_r) of N_4-acetylsulfamethoxazole and sulfamethoxazole and creatinine.

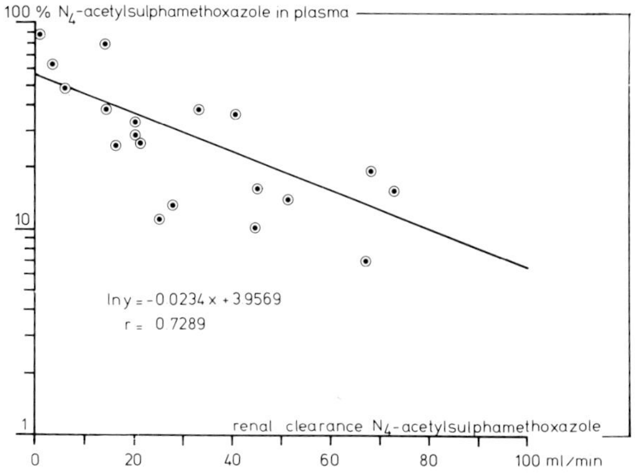

FIG. 3. Relationship between the renal clearance of N_4-acetylsulfamethoxazole and its concentration in plasma (% total concentration of parent drug plus metabolite).

comedication lowers the renal clearance to the level of the remaining glomerular filtration and tubular reabsorption processes. The intrinsic half-lives for the majority of these N_4-acetylsulfonamide derivatives (when administered as parent drugs) are 3.5–5 h, while the same compounds of group (c) above have half-lives from 10 to 22 h (7).

The tubular secretion of the metabolites is governed by the presence of the CH_3-CO-NH group and is independent of the N_1 substituent (7). The plasma concentration–time curve of the metabolite N_4-acetylsulfonamide, when administered as the parent drug, is biphasic, with an initial half-life of 3.5–5 h followed by one half-life identical to the intrinsic half-life of the formed sulfonamide metabolite. This biphasic behavior can be explained by the deacetylation of the N_4-acetyl derivative, and is not caused by alterations in the renal clearance of the compounds by the kidney (33,53).

Tubular Reabsorption and Sulfonamides

The process of tubular reabsorption can be measured in terms of its parameters, urine pH, and urinary flow. The urinary pH and the pK_a of the compound determine the fraction of the total concentration that is un-ionized according to the equation: $TPC = APC(1 - 10^{(pK_a\text{-}pH)})$ where TPC is true partition coefficient and APC is the apparent partition coefficient. The un-ionized fraction is eligible for reabsorption. Sulfonamides with an acidic pK_a of 5 to 6 are subject to tubular reabsorption due to the difference between urinary pH of 5 to 8 and pK_a value. The renal clearances of sulfamethoxazole (pK_a 5.70) and sulfametrole (pK_a 4.70) are dependent on urinary pH, whereas those of sulfadiazine (pK_a 6.40) and sulfadimidine (pK_a 7.40) are much less dependent on urinary pH.

When the major mechanism of renal excretion is active tubular secretion, the correlation between the renal clearance of the sulfonamide and urinary pH is very low, i.e., reabsorption and the resulting variations in the measured renal clearance values are relatively small in comparison with the active secretion process, which governs the total renal clearance of these particular sulfonamides (4).

Tubular reabsorption seems to be increased with low urinary flow rates. Low urinary flow means extensive water reabsorption and concentration processes occur in which the ionized sulfonamide is readily reabsorbed passively. When no active tubular secretion of the sulfonamide takes place, differences in the renal clearance values can be observed when the urinary pH is constant, whether acidic or alkaline (2,3,5). The influence of urinary flow on renal clearance then becomes visible.

Acidic urine, caused either by metabolic acidosis in neonate or adult patients or by immaturity of the kidney, causes extensive and measureable reabsorption of those sulphonamides that are excreted by the mechanisms glomerular filtration and tubular reabsorption.

Many sulfonamides inhibit the urge to micturate and thus reduce urinary flow (2). The risk of crystallization of the less soluble sulfonamide in the kidney nephrons increases with reduced flow and more acidic urine. This is a real risk with the long-term treatment and high dosages commonly used in the "era of the sulfonamides" (1940–1960) (63–65).

The occurrence of crystalluria results in the appearance of crystals of the sulfonamide and its metabolite in the urine and in mechanical obstruction of the nephron (66). This obstruction is manifested as a reduction in the measured renal clearance values of the particular sulfonamide. The reduced clearances return to normal values when (a) the dosage regimen is terminated; (b) the urinary pH changes from an acidic to an alkaline value, thus increasing solubilities; and (c) urinary flow increases (63,64,67).

Impaired Kidney Function and Sulfonamides

Sulfonamides

Kidney impairment logically affects the renal clearances and related overall elimination rate constants and half-lives of those compounds that are eliminated predominantly by renal excretion. Of the sulfonamides, impaired kidney function can affect the kinetics of sulfamethizole, sulfathiazole, sulfaethidole, sulfisomidine, and sulfafurazole.

The elimination characteristics of the group of compounds that are excreted by glomerular filtration and tubular reabsorption, and thus have low overall renal clearances, i.e., sulfametrole, sulfamethoxazole, sulfadiazine, sulfapyridine, sulfamerazine, and sulfadimidine, are relatively unaffected by impairment of kidney function. The overall elimination of these compounds proceeds predominantly by acetylation.

N_4-*Acetylsulfonamide Derivatives*

The elimination and related half-lives of N_4-acetylsulfonamide derivatives depend primarily on kidney function. There is a linear relationship between the measured creatinine clearance and the renal clearance of the N_4-acetylsulfonamide derivative, as has been shown for N_4-acetylsulfamethoxazole (6) in adult patients with various degrees of kidney impairment (Fig. 2).

Deteriorating kidney function interferes with the excretion of N_4-acetylsulfonamides. If the rate of conversion of sulfonamides to N_4-acetylsulfonamides remains constant, the plasma concentration of the N_4-acetylsulfonamide metabolite will increase to a steady-state concentration if dosage regimen is not changed. The steady-state concentration will depend on the rate of acetylation and the actual half-life of the parent drug.

The plasma concentration of the metabolite can be expressed as the percentage of total (parent drug + metabolite) sulfonamide concentration: $(N_4/N_4 + S) \times 100\%$ where N_4 is the metabolite and $N_4 + S$ is the parent drug plus the metabolite. With kidney impairment and growing inability to excrete the metabolite, the percentage of the metabolite in the plasma will increase over time (5,67). Figure 3 shows the increase in the percentage of metabolite in the plasma with deteriorating kidney function, as illustrated by decreasing values of renal clearance of N_4-acetylsulfamethoxazole which is in turn related to decreasing renal clearance values of creatinine (demonstrated in Fig. 2). In a steady-state situation with normal kidney function the percentage of N_4-acetylsulfamethoxazole in plasma will be ~10% (5).

Thus it may be concluded that in adult patients the percentage of metabolite in the blood can be used as a predictor of kidney function. Decreased renal clearance value of the metabolite or increased percentage of the metabolite in plasma indicates that the renal clearance of the compound, and thus the overall kidney function, is impaired.

A summary of the current state of knowledge reveals that (a) the rates of acetylation and deacetylation are independent of kidney function and presumably not age dependent, (b) elimination of sulfonamides from which overall elimination proceeds mainly by renal excretion depends strongly on kidney function, and (c) the molecular structure of the sulfonamide derivative automatically determines the mechanism of elimination.

Now the two basic elements of maturation of kidney function and pharmacokinetics of the sulfonamide molecule can be coupled.

KIDNEY MATURATION VERSUS KIDNEY IMPAIRMENT

Before one understands the relationship between the kinetics of a particular sulfonamide and the age of the recipient, one has to precisely define the functional behavior or status of the kidney. The following functional states of the kidney can be distinguished: (a) immature with normal function, (b) immature with impaired function, (c) mature with normal function, (d) mature with impaired function, (e) aged with normal function, and (f) aged with impaired function.

Nomograms have been constructed to distinguish between immature kidney function and impaired immature kidney function by correcting for body height, weight, and surface area. Such methods have determined that an observed creatinine clearance of 25 ml/min in a 50-cm-tall, 3 week old child corresponds to the nomogram for an adult clearance of 100 ml/min, which is considered to be normal (27). Thus, this creatinine clearance of the child, 25 ml/min, is considered to be normal in respect to age and the state of development of the child's kidney. But this creatinine clearance limitation to 25 ml/min must still be considered reduced or impaired compared with creatinine clearance values in adults of 100–150 ml/min and the kinetic parameters of the drugs based thereupon.

Thus, a dualistic situation exists in young children in that although their kidney function is normal for their age and development, in comparison with values obtained in adults it is relatively reduced or impaired. For understanding the kinetic behavior of a drug in a child, the actual, never the corrected, creatinine clearance should be used. The corrected creatine clearance must be used only in determining whether the measured creatinine clearance value is normal for the actual age.

Immature Kidney Functioning and Resulting Half-lives of Sulfonamides

Research has been conducted which has determined that longer half-lives of sulfonamides are found in young infants and neonates than in older children and adults (23,26). The half-life of the parent drug, however, was the only parameter that could be obtained. The renal clearance values were not measured, although the concept of immature kidney function was

TABLE 2. *Half-life (h) of sulfonamides in children of different ages*

Compound	Age						Reference
	1–7 days	1–4 wk	1–12 m	2–7 yr	7–15 yr	Adults	
Sulfathiazole					10	4	(2,64)
Sulfamoxole			7.4			8	(2)
	19.5	11.5	10.5				(68)
Sulfisomidine	22	10	7.6			8	(2,69)
	18	10	8	8	8	8	(70)
Sulfisoxazole (furazole)	17.7	12.5	8.3			6 + 9	(2,69)
	18	10	8	8	8	8	(70)
Sulfadiazine	40					10–15	(71)
	20–10		10				(5,64,72)
Sulfaethidole			5.8			12	(2)
Sulfamerazine			24–60	10	18	21	(24,73)
						11;22	(2)
Sulfaperine			11.7			33	(2,63)
Sulfadimethoxine	120	88	44				(69)
			20				(68)
Sulfamethoxypyridazine	280	140	50	50	50	50	(74)
	200–100	70	50	50	50	50	(75)
Sulfaclomide					43	84	(24)
Sulfadoxine	14 days	140–70				110	(2,57)

known. Table 2 summarizes the observed half-lives of several sulfonamides at different stages of kidney development. These investigations were mainly carried out in the era of the sulfonamides, and no sulfamethoxazole or sulfametrole kinetic data were obtained in children. Sulfonamide therapy became of interest again with the introduction of the combination of sulfamethoxazole and trimethoprim in the fixed dosage ratio (5:1), which has since been followed by sulfametrole and sulfadiazine combined with trimethoprim. For the treatment of uncomplicated infections of the lower urinary tract, the use of trimethoprim alone receives and deserves greater attention (76,77).

Kinetics of Sulfonamides with Immature Kidney Function

As discussed in Immature Kidney Functioning and Resulting Half-Lives of Sulfonamides, the renal excretion of some sulfonamides may be dependent on the kidney function as expressed by the creatinine clearance. Because the creatinine clearance, a glomerular functional parameter, is age dependent, the renal clearance of the sulfonamides will also be age dependent. The fixed relationship in Fig. 2 is based on the constant ratio (5:1) between the maximum tubular secretion of PAH and the maximum glomerular filtration (capacity) of inulin and/or creatinine (39). The intact-nephron theory and the deterioration of the whole nephron proposed by Bricker (28) imply a linear relationship between the renal clearances of creatinine (glomerular filtration) and N_4-acetylsulfamethoxazole (active tubular secretion), as shown in Fig. 2.

In the young, immature kidney, there exists a tubuloglomerular imbalance (21,78) that may change the 5:1 ratio. In young children, for instance, the relationship between the clearance of N_4-acetylsulfamethoxazole (reflecting tubular function) and that of creatinine (reflecting glomerular function) may differ from the relationship found in adults (Fig. 2).

Figure 4 shows the relationship between the renal clearances of N_4-acetylsulfamethoxazole and creatinine in a group of children (ranging in age from 3 weeks to 19 years) who were treated with co-trimoxazole (Bactrim). The data are summarized in Tables 3 and 4.

Figure 4 also shows a similar relationship between the renal clearances of N_4-acetylsulfametrole and creatinine in a group of children of the same age range who were treated with Lidatrim (sulfametrole plus trimethoprim). These data are summarized in Tables 5 and 6. N_4-Acetylsulfamethoxazole and N_4-acetylsulfametrole respond in similar ways to the increase and maturation of kidney function. When the renal clearance of both compounds are taken together, which is possible because both compounds are excreted by the same mechanism (active tubular secretion), the relationship with the creatinine clearance reads: $K_rN_4 = 0.42(K_{r,creat}) + 4.81$ ($r = 0.81$), where K_r is the renal constant. The renal clearance values were calculated from urine samples and corresponding plasma samples over 2 to 4 months of treatment with either Bactrim or Lidatrim therapy for an infection during the treatment of acute lymphoblastic leukemia.

An example of a plasma concentration and renal excretion rate time profile over three periods of treatment with Lidatrim (start of treatment, steady state,

TABLE 3. *Pharmacokinetic parameters of sulfamethoxazole/trimethoprim[a] in children*

Subject	Age (yr)	Height (cm)	Weight (kg)	Dose (mg)	Percentage protein binding S (%)	N_4 (%)	TMP (%)	Half-life (h) S	N_4	TMP	N_4 (%)
1	0.041	47	2.6	40/8 b.i.d.	53.4	74.6	—	—	—	—	31
2	0.080	56	2.1	100/20 b.i.d.	42.6	57.2	29.5	—	—	—	46
3	0.58	63	5	80/16 s.d.d.	39.1	59.4	48.1	16	40	16	49
4	0.75	66	7.3	200/40 b.i.d.	—	—	—	—	—	—	39
5	3.6	89	12.5	200/40 b.i.d.	18.6	15.1	87.3	7	8	10.5	41
6	6.7	119	16	400/80 b.i.d.	—	—	—	8	8	8	22
7	8.7	134	26	800/160 b.i.d.	—	—	—	—	—	—	54
8	10	157	31	800/160 q.i.d.	—	—	—	10	10	10	11
9	11	155	30	800/160 q.i.d.	45.8	64.9	57.9	—	—	—	10
10	12	—	—	400/80 b.i.d.	—	—	—	—	—	—	19
11	13	147	32	400/80 s.d.d.	—	—	—	6	6	4.5	26
12	19	—	—	Steady state	—	—	—	6	6	—	11

Dashes indicate quantities not measured. S, sulfamethoxazole; N_4, N_4-acetylsulfamethoxazole; TMP, trimethoprim; N_4 (%), $(N_4/N_4 + S) \times 100\%$ in plasma. b.i.d., 2 × day; t.i.d., 3 × day; q.i.d., 4 × day; s.d.d., single daily dose.
[a]Bactrim 400/80.

TABLE 4. *Pharmacokinetic parameters of the urinary excretion of sulfamethoxazole/trimethoprim[a] in children*

Subject	Urinary flow (ml/min)	Urinary pH	Renal clearance (ml/min)						
			S_t	N_{4t}	TMP_t	S_f	N_{4f}	TMP_f	Creatinine
1	—	—	—	—	—	—	—	—	—
2	—	—	—	—	—	—	—	—	—
3	0.22 ± 0.16	6.80 ± 0.57	0.022 ± 0.020	0.84 ± 0.43	4.2 ± 2.08	0.038 ± 0.035	1.93 ± 1.04	7.04 ± 1.04	3.18 ± 1.43
4	—	—	—	—	—	—	—	—	—
5	0.27 ± 0.12	8.88 ± 0.23	0.094 ± 0.036	0.55 ± 0.23	0.34 ± 0.15	0.156 ± 0.073	0.63 ± 0.27	—	1.17 ± 0.49
6	0.84 ± 0.55	7.81 ± 0.40	2.15 ± 0.77	19.98 ± 2.63	—	—	—	—	—
7	0.92	5.66	0.95	22.0	—	—	—	—	—
8	0.44 ± 0.20	—	1.17 ± 0.82	22.92 ± 16.9	—	—	—	—	—
9	—	—	—	—	—	—	—	—	—
10	—	—	—	—	—	—	—	—	—
11	0.62 ± 0.16	7.28 ± 0.50	4.60 ± 2.27	21.52 ± 12.5	76.6 ± 57.2	—	—	—	59.0 ± 17.0
12	1.79 ± 0.81	7.31 ± 0.57	5.88 ± 1.03	56.34 ± 6.81	—	—	—	—	103 ± 35.1

Dashes indicate quantities not measured. S, sulfamethoxazole; S_t, total plasma concentration, S_f, unbound or free plasma concentration; N_4, N_4-acetylsulfamethoxazole; N_{4t}, total plasma concentration; N_{4f}, unbound or free concentration; TMP, trimethoprim; TMP_t, total plasma concentration; TMP_f, unbound or free plasma concentration.

[a]Bactrim 400/80.

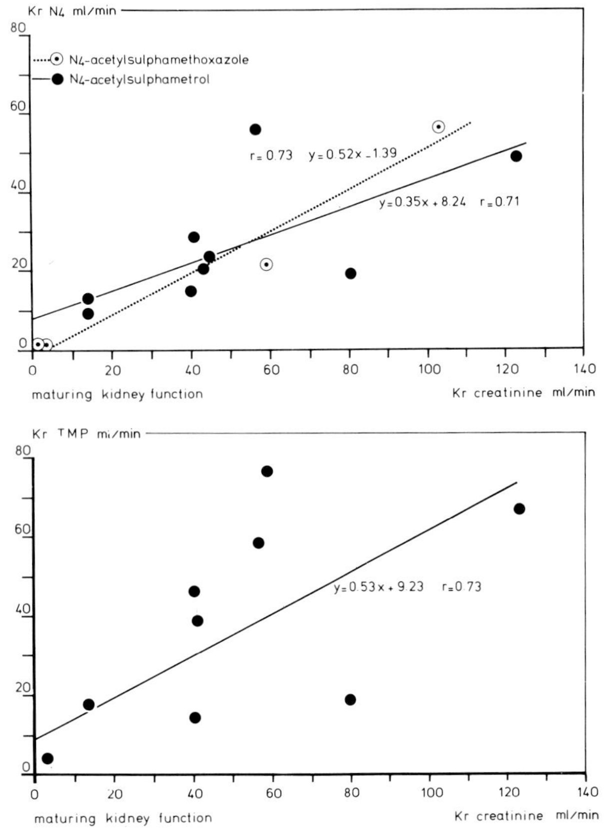

FIG. 4. Relationship between the renal clearances (K_r) of N_4-acetylsulfamethoxazole, N_4-acetylsulfametrole, and trimethoprim (TMP) and the creatinine clearance in children.

and final elimination after discontinuation of the dosage regimen) is shown in Fig. 5.

Figure 6 shows a steady-state plasma concentration–time profile of co-trimoxazole in a 6-month-old child with an impaired, immature kidney function, as expressed by a creatinine clearance of 3 ml/min. N_4-Acetylsulfamethoxazole has accumulated in the plasma, and the half-life of sulfamethoxazole is slightly increased due to deacetylation of the metabolite. Trimethoprim shows a half-life similar to that of sulfamethoxazole, which is also considered to be slightly increased.

Because of the known age dependency of tubular functioning, the renal clearance of both N_4-acetylsulfamethoxazole and N_4-acetylsulfametrole are age dependent, as is shown in Fig. 7. Even the renal clearance of trimethoprim, the comedication or coproduct of the sulfonamides in Bactrim and Lidatrim, is dependent on age (Fig. 8).

Trimethoprim is eliminated mainly (80%) by renal excretion via glomerular filtration, and therefore its kinetics depend on maturation of glomerular filtration (76,77) (Fig. 8).

If the renal clearance values of N_4-acetylsulfonamides and trimethoprim are age dependent and linearly related to the creatinine clearance, the creatinine clearance itself must also be age dependent. This relationship, as obtained from the data of the children participating in this investigation, is shown in Fig. 9.

The renal clearances of the parent sulfonamide drugs, sulfamethoxazole and sulfametrole, are age dependent (r = 0.90). The masking effect of tubular reabsorption and the influence of its parameters, urinary pH and urinary flow, is shown in Fig. 10. As in Fig. 2, two relationships can be distinguished for each drug.

TABLE 5. *Pharmacokinetic parameters of sulfametrole/trimethoprim[a] in children*

Subject	Age (yr)	Height (cm)	Weight (kg)	Dose (mg)	Percentage protein binding			Half-life (h)			N_4
					S	N_4	TMP	S	N_4	TMP	(%)
1	1.33	74	7.3	200/40 t.i.d.	79.5	90.0	69.7	—	—	—	12
2	1.75	84	10.8	1000/200 s.d.d.	—	—	—	—	—	—	11
											16
3	4.25	98	13.3	250/50 q.i.d.	75.0	87.7	56.5	5	5		11
4	4.58	108	17.3	200/40 s.d.d.	—	—	—	11	11	11	13
5	5.70	112	19.5	300/60 t.i.d.	—	—	—	8	8		10
6	6.70	117	19.2	400/80 q.i.d.	71.6	78.5	66.1	—	—	—	13
7	6.75	119	16	400/80 q.i.d.	—	—	—	8	8	8	17
8	9.20	138	36.5	800/160 q.i.d.	68.2	60.0	61.7	11	11	8	5
9	12.3	162	43.1	400/80 q.i.d.	57.4	64.2	59.4	6	6	5	21
10	12.5	126	20.2	200/20 t.i.d.	—	—	—	—	—	—	16
11	14.7	164	52.1	800/160 q.i.d.	80.2	89.5	71.7	13	18	10	10

S, sulfametrole; N_4, N_4-acetylsulfametrole; TMP, trimethoprim; N_4 (%), (N_4/N_4 + S) × 100% in plasma. See Table 3 for dosage abbreviations.

[a]Lidatrim, 400/80.

TABLE 6. *Pharmacokinetic parameters of the urinary excretion of sulfametrole/trimethoprim[a] in children*

Subject	Age (yr)	Urinary flow (ml/min)	Urinary pH	Renal clearance (ml/min)						
				S_t	N_{4t}	TMP_t	S_f	N_{4f}	TMP_f	Creatinine
1	1.33	0.35 ± 0.22	7.40 ± 0.61	0.96 ± 0.67	13.2 ± 4.9	18.1 ± 16.6	4.77 ± 3.03	132 ± 44	159 ± 62	13.6 ± 6.0
2	1.75	0.54 ± 0.28	6.85 ± 0.39	1.18 ± 0.45	14.8 ± 6.3	46.1 ± 27.5	—	—	—	40.1 ± 24.7
		0.12 ± 0.03	6.61 ± 0.64	0.45 ± 0.28	9.4 ± 0.28	9.4 ± 4.1	—	—	—	13.9 ± 6.2
3	4.25	0.33 ± 0.22	7.90 ± 0.23	3.89 ± 1.79	20.9 ± 3.2	—	23.5 ± 4.30	92.4 ± 25.6	—	43.0 ± 16.9
4	4.58	0.39 ± 0.24	6.55 ± 0.68	1.49 ± 0.87	23.8 ± 14.4	—	—	—	—	44.5 ± 25.4
5	5.70	0.86 ± 0.54	6.53 ± 0.54	4.06 ± 2.48	56.5 ± 18.5	—	—	—	—	—
6	6.70	0.51 ± 0.17	6.14 ± 0.30	0.14 ± 0.11	24.6 ± 7.5	14.1 ± 2.6	—	—	—	13.3 ± 1.9
		1.63 ± 0.72	8.44 ± 0.50	4.24 ± 1.90	32.9 ± 10.5	38.8 ± 15.6	—	—	—	13.3 ± 1.9
7	6.75	0.99 ± 0.49	7.63 ± 0.40	2.93 ± 1.75	31.0 ± 13.1	32.7 ± 13.9	—	—	—	—
8	9.20	1.65 ± 1.24	7.18 ± 0.78	1.39 ± 0.74	55.8 ± 24.6	58.3 ± 26.7	3.78 ± 2.07	220 ± 130	187 ± 102	56.6 ± 16.2
9	12.3	0.83 ± 0.73	5.50 ± 0.09	0.08 ± 0.08	37.0 ± 1.8	53.6 ± 9.2	0.27 ± 0.18	200 ± 71	107 ± 26	20.7 ± 4.7
		1.43 ± 0.18	7.10 ± 0.93	5.85 ± 2.87	66.6 ± 33.0	40.8 ± 8.8	14.4 ± 7.0	167 ± 17	89 ± 33	20.7 ± 4.7
10	12.5	0.46 ± 0.14	7.10 ± 0.10	1.08 ± 0.80	18.9 ± 6.3	18.7 ± 6.3	—	—	—	18.6 ± 5.5
11	14.7	1.42 ± 0.94	6.13 ± 0.39	0.65 ± 0.73	48.6 ± 8.1	67.1 ± 23.1	0.66 ± 0.44	—	142 ± 13	123 ± 39.5

S, sulfametrole; S_t, total plasma concentration; S_f, unbound or free plasma concentration; N_4, N_4-acetylsulfametrole; N_{4t}, total plasma concentration; N_{4f}, unbound or free plasma concentration; TMP, trimethoprim; TMP_t, total plasma concentration; TMP_f, unbound or free plasma concentration.

[a]Lidatrim, 400/80.

Unlike the creatinine clearance shown in Fig. 2, the low-renal-clearance line cannot be attributed solely to acidic urinary pH and low urinary flow. There must exist more parameters that determine the renal clearances of both sulfametrole and sulfamethoxazole in young children. The percentage of N_4-acetylsulfonamide metabolite in plasma is increased in impaired kidney function (6,67) and also in young children (Figs. 3 and 11).

An interesting discrepancy between the behaviors of N_4-acetylsulfamethoxazole and N_4-acetylsulfametrole can be observed. N_4-Acetylsulfamethoxazole accumulates in plasma when its renal clearance is reduced due to impaired kidney function (Fig. 2) or immaturity (Fig. 11). N_4-Acetylsulfametrole shows a constant percentage in plasma of ~10%. This should mean that the kidney function is maximal for this compound. Figure 7 shows that even the renal clearance of N_4-acetylsulfametrole is age and capacity dependent. One explanation may be that due to the lower water solubility of N_4-acetylsulfamethoxazole in comparison with that of N_4-acetylsulfametrole, crystalluria of N_4-acetylsulfamethoxazole inhibits renal excretion and causes the accumulation (66,67). The higher solubility of N_4-acetylsulfametrole and available kidney function results, then, in a low percentage of N_4-acetylsulfametrole in children, which is fully comparable to the situation in adults (1,5,79,80). Additional evidence of crystalluria of N_4-acetylsulfamethoxazole in young children is the fact that, as shown in Fig. 7, the renal clearance of N_4-acetylsulfamethoxazole is systematically lower than that of N_4-acetylsulfametrole. This situation is reversed in adults (1,3,5).

Immature Kidney Function and the Use of Sulfonamide–Trimethoprim Combinations

In a study conducted by the Department of Paediatrics at Sint Radboud Hospital, some children were treated with sulfamethoxazole–trimethoprim (co-trimoxazole) and other chilren with sulfametrole–trimethoprim. The characteristics of these children, dosages, and kinetic parameters such as age, sex, protein binding, half-life, renal clearance, and penetration in CSF are summarized in Tables 1 and 3–6, and examples of the plasma concentration–time curves are given in Figs. 5 and 6.

It can be noticed from Table 1 that the protein binding of sulfamethoxazole varies between 40 and 50%, and that of its metabolite, between 57 and 75%. These values do not differ from values obtained in adults (2). The same observation can be made for sulfametrole and its metabolite N_4-acetylsulfametrole.

The measured half-lives of sulfamethoxazole and N_4-acetylsulfamethoxazole in children are similar and identical, respectively, to adult values (Table 3). The same observation is made for sulfametrole and N_4-acetylsulfametrole (Table 5).

The renal clearance values of sulfamethoxazole and sulfametrole are low (~5 ml/min, based on total plasma concentration), and depend on urinary flow and urinary pH and only minimally on age (1,2,5).

This means that the main metabolic pathway of sulfamethoxazole and sulfametrole in infants is acetylation. As in adults, deacetylation reactions must be extremely slow. In children with a starting kidney function and creatinine clearance of 25 ml/min deacetylation is not reflected in the half-life of elimination of the parent sulfonamide.

The renal clearances of the metabolites N_4-acetylsulfamethoxazole and N_4-acetylsulfametrole are clearly age dependent, i.e., dependent on tubular functioning and creatinine clearance, and thus on the tubuloglomerular capacity ratio, in analogy to data observed in adults (Fig. 7).

THE EFFICIENCY PRINCIPLE

From the kinetic viewpoint, infections in adult patients with normal kidney function can be treated with sulfamethoxazole–trimethoprim, sulfametrole–trimethoprim, or sulfadiazine–trimethoprim. Preference for one of these three combinations depends in part on the susceptibility of the pathogen and the experience of the clinician. Loss of the active parent sulfonamide by acetylation can be compensated for with a subsequent dose.

The possibility that one compound may be acetylated at either a fast or a slow rate and that its elimination kinetics depend on the genetic enzyme package of the patient must be avoided unless the population of patients for which the sulfonamide is meant to be prescribed is a uniformly "fast" or "slow" acetylator population. To avoid the problem of fast versus slow acetylation and resulting different half-lives and kinetic behaviors of the administered sulfonamide, the ideal sulfonamide has to be acetylated in a unimodel way or administered to a unimodal group of humans (i.e., in Eskimos, sulfadimidine acetylation is fast, 100%) or animals (i.e., in dogs, no acetylation occurs, due to extremely fast deacetylation). The selection of sulfadiazine by the World Health Organization as the essential drug for developing countries (81) reduces the question of the main acetylator phenotype of the country.

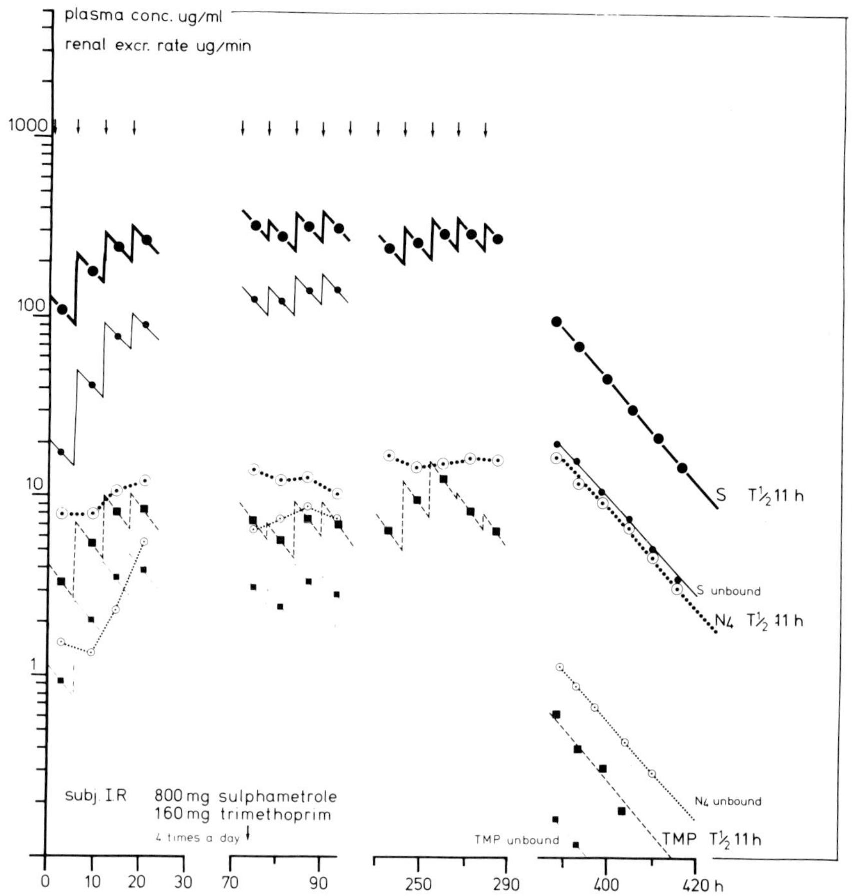

FIG. 5. Plasma concentration–time profiles of sulfametrole (S), its metabolite N_4-acetylsulfametrole (N_4), and trimethoprim (TMP) in a child over a period of 18 days. $T_{1/2}$, half-life.

The inactive metabolite N_4-acetylsulfonamide will be excreted by healthy, normal kidneys without any problem when the dosage regimen does not exceed 1,200–2,400 mg sulfonamide/day both in children over 2 years of age and in adults. The ranking of the positions of the acetylation–deacetylation equilibria of sulfadiazine, sulfamethoxazole, and sulfametrole is then relatively trivial.

In patients with impaired renal function, acetylation proceeds at normal rate, but since elimination by renal excretion is more or less impaired the metabolite will accumulate in the body. To avoid side effects due to the accumulating metabolite, the dosages of the parent drug must be reduced to obtain a lower steady-state concentration of the active sulfonamide. This may, however, result in undertreatment or less effective treatment (6,33,53). Thus changing the choice of sulfonamide to a derivative that is less acetylated is preferable to dosage reduction of the sulfonamide–trimethoprim combination.

The ideal sulfonamide–trimethoprim combination for patients with impaired kidney function is the one in which both compounds are eliminated mainly by renal excretion and have identical half-lives (i.e., both sulfaethidole and trimethoprim have half-lives of 9 h). It can be expected that dosage reduction as a consequence of reduced kidney function in this drug combination can be based on the same mechanism of elimination, i.e, renal excretion.

This principle and prerequisite for drug combination, i.e., that the individual components be handled by the body in the same way, is very important for the administration of the drug to young infants. When the same drug combination for which kinetic parameters have been obtained in adults is administered to young children, drug elimination is reduced due to reduced or immature kidney function. Thus the same rules for establishing the dosage regimen are valid for adults and young children when kidney function is the principal parameter. Using information on clinical effects and kinetic behavior obtained in adults for treatment of neonates, infants, and children should be avoided when one is not yet certain about the kinetic mechanisms and the maturity of the eliminating organs.

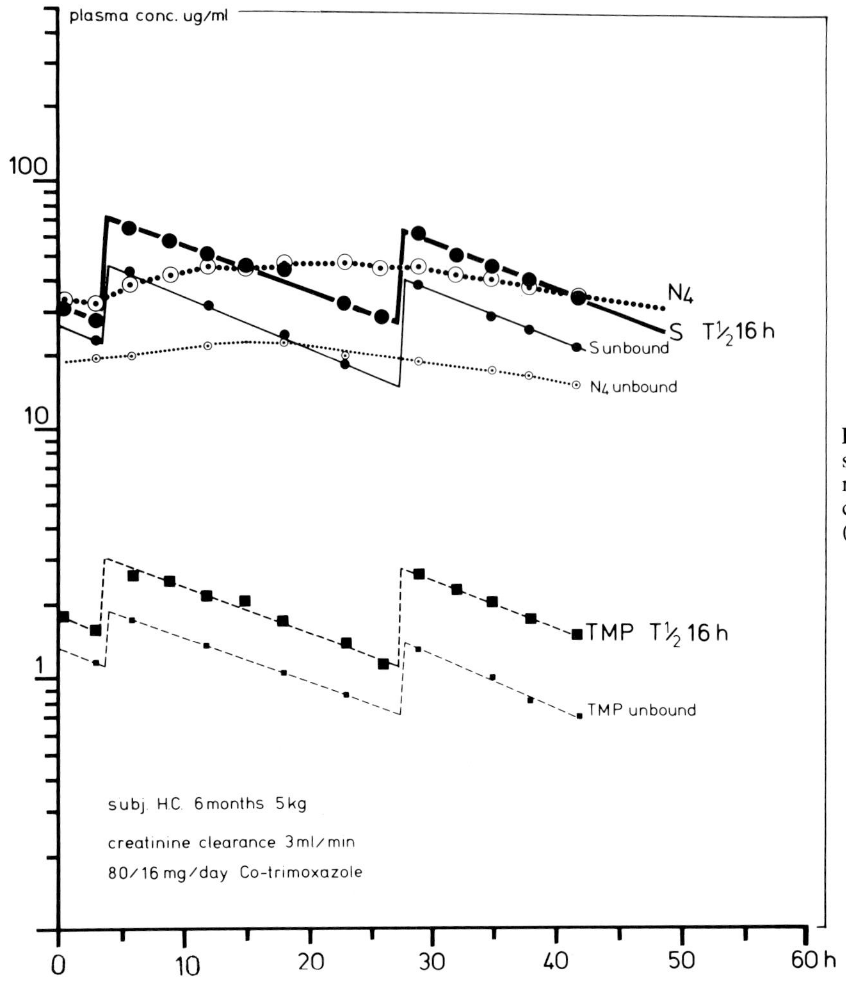

FIG. 6. Plasma concentration–time profiles of sulfamethoxazole, its metabolite N_4-acetylsulfamethoxazole (N_4), and trimethoprim (TMP) in a child with impaired, immature kidney function (creatinine clearance 3 ml/min). $T_{1/2}$, half-life.

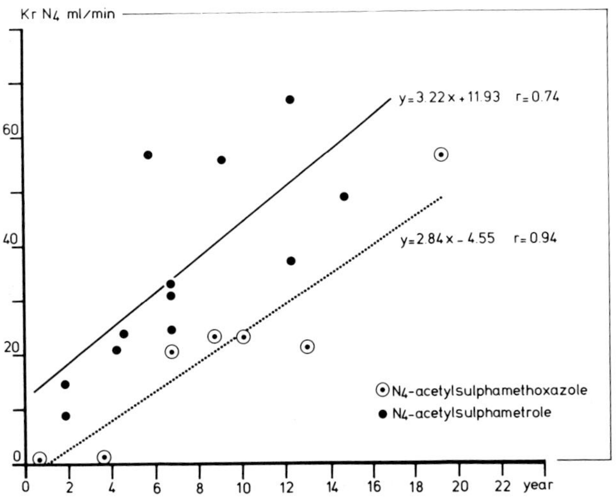

FIG. 7. Relationship between the renal clearances (K_r) of N_4-acetylsulfamethoxazole and N_4-acetylsulfametrole and age in children.

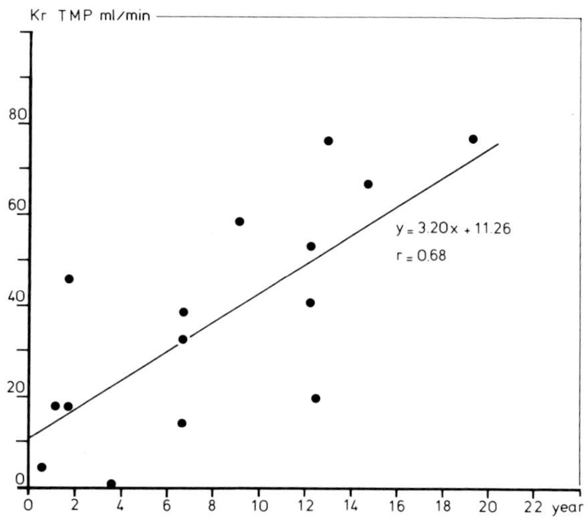

FIG. 8. Relationship between the renal clearance of trimethoprim (K_r TMP) and age in children.

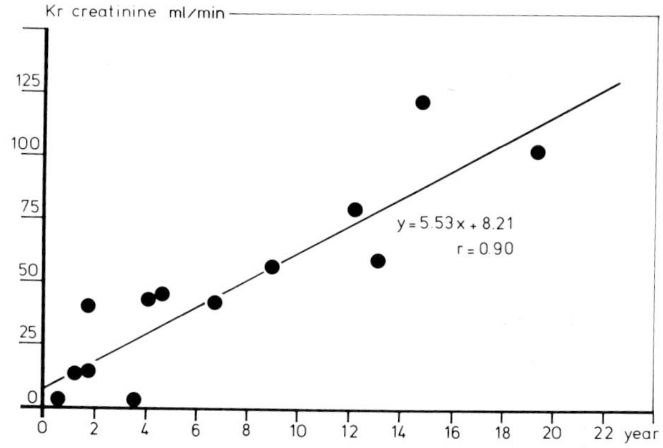

FIG. 9. Relationship between the renal clearance (K_r) of creatinine and age in children.

Adverse Effects of Sulfonamide–Trimethoprim Combinations

In 38 children with malignancies, elective decontamination of the digestive tract was carried out by oral administration of either trimethoprim–sulfamethoxazole (20/100 mg/kg/24 h divided in 2–4 h doses), or trimethoprim–sulfametrole, (20/100 mg/kg/24 h, divided in 3–4 h doses), colistin (6 mg/kg/24 h, 1 dose/day), or miconazole (15 mg/kg/24 h, 1 dose/day). In 27 children with malignancies, either trimethoprim–sulfamethoxazole or trimethoprim sulfametrole (both in doses of 100/20 mg/kg/24 h divided in 4 doses) was administered orally or i.v. during 37 periods of fever during aplastic bone marrow stages in cytostatic treatment. Various antibiotics were combined with co-trimoxazole. The adverse reactions that occurred during this treatment were difficult to interpret. Table 7 compares the adverse reactions with administration of trimethoprim–sulfamethoxazole to those with administration of trimethoprim–sulfametrole. In these groups of patients, no differences could be discerned. Disappearance of the adverse reactions after discontinuation of the co-trimoxazole may be considered an indication that the adverse reactions were due to the administration of that drug. Co-trimoxazole is a weak inhibitor of the enzyme dihydrofolate reductase, and to establish that the adverse reactions could be due to inhibition of this enzyme, leucovorin (citrovorum factor) was administered orally to 10 children prior to the administration of co-trimoxazole. In four of these children, vomiting occurred. However, no rash was observed in any of the 10 children.

It can be concluded then that no difference can be observed in the occurrence of side effects in children treated with high doses of either trimethoprim–sulfamethoxazole or trimethoprim–sulfametrole.

ETHICAL CONSIDERATIONS

The maturation of the kidney in children is shown by the increase in the functional capacity of the nephrons, as expressed by the renal clearance of a drug, drug metabolite, or endogenous compound. When a dosage regimen for a drug has to be calculated, ideally the reference renal clearance values and reference half-lives of the drug and its metabolites should be known. To obtain the required data, the drug should be administered to healthy young children or neonates in the same manner as they are administered to healthy adult volunteers, and samples should be taken. Because young children cannot volunteer to undergo a kinetic reference study, it is not ethical to carry out such experiments. Thus studies are limited to occasions when a sulfonamide is therapeutically indicated in treatment of a child and it is possible or desirable to take one or more small samples from that child. The problem with this approach is that, as in the present investigation, the data may deviate from the reference values because of the disease state of the children. Despite this interference by the diseases, the effect of maturation on kidney function can be demonstrated by the increase in renal clearance values of the drug with time.

DOSAGE TIME INTERVALS

When a steady-state plasma concentration obtained with intermittent dosing is desired and when in this plasma concentration, for instance, a variation of 20% is allowed, the following formula can be used:

$$\Delta t = t_{\max} + t_{0.8} \qquad (1)$$

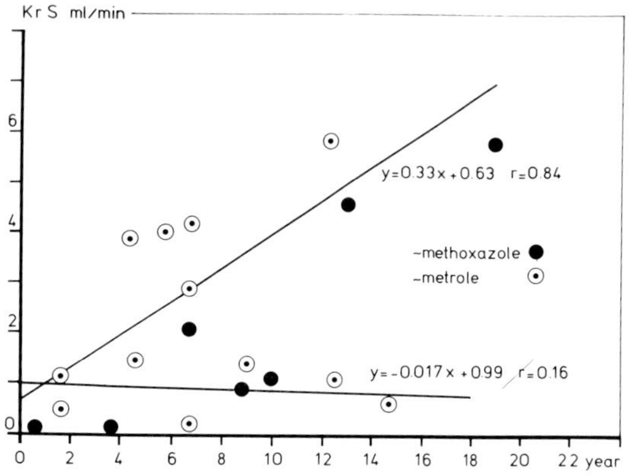

FIG. 10. Relationships between the renal clearances of sulfamethoxazole and sulfametrole (K_rS) and age in children.

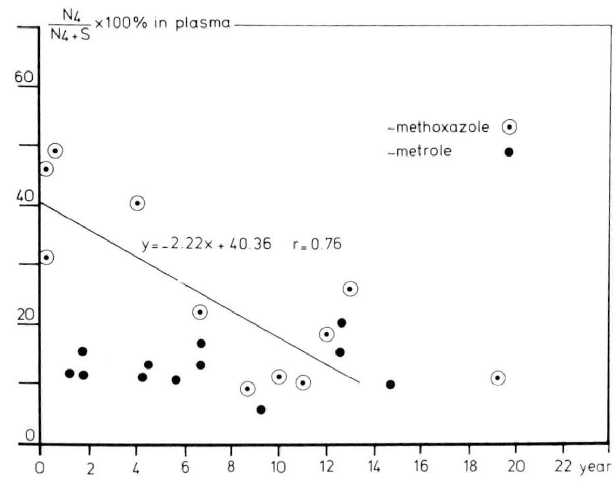

FIG. 11. Relationship between the concentrations of N_4-acetylsulfamethoxazole and N_4-acetylsulfametrole (% total concentration of parent drug plus metabolite in plasma) and age in children.

where Δt is the dosage time interval, t_{max} ($t_{100\%} = t_{1.0}$) is the time in hours that passes between the administration of the drug and attainment of the maximal plasma concentration ($C_{t\ max} = C_{t100\%} = C_{t1.0}$), $t_{max} = 0$ after an intravenous bolus injection and varies after an oral or intramuscular dose, and $t_{0.8}$ is the time (h) at which the plasma concentration has decreased by 20% ($C_{t80\%}$) from the maximal plasma concentration.

When $C_{t0.8} = C_{t1.0}\, e^{(-k_{el} \cdot t_{0.8})}$ and $k_{el} = (0.693\ t_{1/2})$ are substituted in Eq. 1, the following equation is derived:

$$\Delta t = \tfrac{1}{3} t_{1/2} + t_{max} \qquad (2)$$

The elimination constant k_{el} (the sum of the summations of the metabolic rate constants Σk_m and the renal rate constants Σk_r, consisting of glomerular filtration, tubular secretion, and reabsorption) can be expressed as $k_{el} = \Sigma k_m + \Sigma k_r$. The resulting steady-state plasma concentration is

TABLE 7. *Adverse reactions to sulfamethoxazole/trimethoprim (A) and sulfametrole/trimethoprim (B) combinations in children with malignancies*

Reaction	A (n = 39)	B (n = 26)
Anorexia + nausea + vomiting	15	26
Rash	4	7
Elevations of SGOT and SGPT levels	2	2

SGOT, serum glutamic–oxaloacetic transaminase; SGPT, serum glutamic–pyruvic transaminase.

$$C_{ss} = \frac{FD}{Vk_{el}\Delta t} \qquad (3)$$

where C_{ss} represents the steady state plasma concentration, D is the dosage, V is the volume of distribution, and F is the bioavailability. When k_{el} is substituted in Eq. 3, the equation for the C_{ss} becomes

$$C_{ss} = \frac{1.44\ FDt_{1/2}}{V\Delta t} \qquad (4)$$

The dosage regimen calculation in infants must be based on the functional state of the kidney, as characterized by the creatinine clearance. For the three following groups of sulfonamides, characterized by different mechanisms of renal excretion, individual dosage regimen calculations should be followed.

Renal Excretion by Glomerular Filtration and Tubular Reabsorption

For these compounds, the main route of elimination of the parent drug is by acetylation ($k_{el} = k_m$). Compounds include sulfamethoxazole, sulfametrole, sulfamoxole, sulfadiazine, and sulfamerazine. The N_4-acetylsulfonamide derivatives are excreted predominantly by active tubular secretion. The half-life of elimination is independent of kidney function, but depends on the acetylation–deacetylation equilibrium. Less acetylated compounds, such as sulfadiazine with its high rate of deacetylation which increases its half-life from 15 to 30 h at a creatinine clearance of <25 ml/min (2) should be preferred.

Sulfamethoxazole and sulfametrole show identical half-lives of 9–12 h and very low rates of deacetylation. Sulfamethoxazole is less acetylated than sulfametrole and may be preferred. The metabolite N_4-acetylsulfamethoxazole, however, is much less soluble than N_4-acetylsulfametrole (1,2), may crystallyze earlier in the nephron, and subsequently may inhibit its renal excretion (67), resulting in accumulation of N_4-acetylsulfamethoxazole in plasma (Fig. 2). The percentage of N_4-acetylsulfamethoxazole in plasma should be ~10%, but in young children is 40% (Fig. 11). This accumulation is not seen with sulfametrole and N_4-acetylsulfametrole. Thus sulfametrole (or sulfametrole–trimethoprim) is preferred over sulfamethoxazole (or sulfamethoxazole–trimethoprim) in children with reduced or immature kidney function.

Renal Excretion by Active Tubular Secretion

Administration of sulfonamides that are eliminated predominantly by active tubular secretion must be based on the creatinine clearance. The half-life of elimination is governed by the renal clearance constant k_r and is proportional to the kidney function and creatinine clearance. The compounds are sulfamethizole ($t_{1/2}$ = 2 h), sulfathiazole ($t_{1/2}$ 3 h), and sulphathiourea ($t_{1/2}$ 3 h).

Renal Excretion by Active Tubular Secretion and Tubular Reabsorption

The overall low renal clearance of these compounds makes extensive acetylation possible. Sulfisoxazole (furazole) is highly acetylated (30–60%) and should be avoided. Sulfisomidine is slightly acetylated (~10%) and shows a mediate half-life of 9 h. Sulfaethidole is not acetylated and shows a half-life of 12 h. Sulfadoxine is very slightly acetylated (~3%) but shows the longest half-life, 110 h.

CLINICAL IMPLICATIONS

For the selection and administration of sulfonamides and combinations of sulfonamides with trimethoprim, allowance should be made for the following factors: (a) The kidney function of the young child may be immature and reduced in comparison with that of adults. (b) Dosage regimens and kinetic parameters of drugs are obtained mainly from adults. (c) The mechanisms of elimination of the drug to be administered to a young child must be known. (d) Sulfonamides that are unimodally acetylated are preferred over those that show a fast–slow acetylation phenotype. (e) Sulfonamides that are not or are only slightly acetylated are preferred over ones that are extensively acetylated. The combination of a sulfonamide and trimethoprim must be based on similar routes of elimination, i.e., renal excretion. Adjustment of the dosage regimen of sulfonamides that are eliminated mainly by renal excretion can be guided by the renal clearance of creatinine, and for the calculation of the dosage regimen in young children, the actual, not the corrected, creatinine clearance must be used.

Acknowledgment: Ita Baars, Margriet Baakman, Tom Janssen, Emiel Termond, and Marian Tijhuis are thanked for skillful analyses of the sulfonamides in many samples; Marijn Oosterbaan and Dr. L. Monnens, for discussions; Dr. J. C. M. Hafkenscheid and co-workers, for determinations of creatinine concentrations; Marijcke Schoots van de Siepkamp, for typing the manuscript; and the nurses of the Department of Paediatrics, Sint Radboud Hospital, for careful collection of the blood and urine samples.

REFERENCES

1. Hekster YA, Vree TB, Damsma JE, Friesen WT. Pharmacokinetics of sulphametrole and its metabolite N_4-acetylsulphametrole in man. *J Antimicrob Chemother* 1981;8:133–44.
2. Hekster YA, Vree TB. Clinical pharmacokinetics of sulphonamides and their N_4-acetyl derivatives. *Antibiot Chemother* 1982;31:22–118.
3. Vree TB, Hekster YA, Baars AM, Damsma JE, van der Kleijn E. Pharmacokinetics of sulphamethoxazole in man. Effects of urinary pH and urine flow on metabolism and renal excretion of sulphamethoxazole and its metabolite N_4-acetylsulphamethoxazole. *Clin Pharmacokinet* 1978;3:319–29.
4. Vree TB, Hekster YA, Damsma JE, van der Kleijn E, O'Reilly WJ. Pharmacokinetics of N_1-acetyl- and N_4-acetylsulphamethoxazole in man. *Clin Pharmacokinet* 1979;4:310–9.
5. Vree TB, O'Reilly WJ, Hekster YA, Damsma JE, van der Kleijn E. Determination of the acetylator phenotype and pharmacokinetics of some sulphonamides in man. *Clin Pharmacokinet* 1980;5:274–94.
6. Vree TB, Hekster YA, Damsma JE, van Dalen R, Hafkenscheid JCM, Friesen WT. Renal excretion of sulphamethoxazole and its metabolite N_4-acetylsulphamethoxazole in patients with impaired kidney function. *Ther Drug Monit* 1981;3:129–35.
7. Vree TB, Hekster YA, Damsma JE, Tijhuis M, Friesen WT. Pharmacokinetics and mechanism of renal excretion of short acting sulphonamides and N_4-acetylsulphonamides in man. Structural requirements of sulphonamides for active tubular secretion. *Eur J Clin Pharmacol* 1981;20:283–92.
8. Barne HI, Hare WK, McNamara N, Hare RS. Influence of postnatal age on kidney function of premature infants. *Proc Soc Exp Biol Med* 1948;69:55–67.
9. Guignard JP, Torrado A, Da Cunha O, Gautier E. Glomerular filtration rate in the first three weeks of life. *J Pediatr* 1975;87:268–72.
10. Guignard JP, Torrado A, Feldman H, Gautier E. Assessment of glomerular filtration rate in children. *Helv Paediatr Acta* 1980;35:437–47.
11. Leake RD, Trygstad CW. Glomerular filtration rate during the period of adaptation to extrauterine life. *Pediatr Res* 1977;11:959–62.
12. Schreiter G. Neuere physiologische und klinische Aspekte der Nierenfunktion bei Frühgeborenen. *Dtsch Gesundheitswes* 1966;21:433–41.
13. Arant BS. Developmental patterns of renal functional maturation compared in the human neonate. *J Pediatr* 1978;92:705–12.
14. Arant BS. Adaptation of the infant to an external milieu. In: Gruskin AB, Norman ME, eds. *Pediatric nephrology.* The Hague, Boston, London: Martinus Nijhoff Publishers, 1981:265–72.
15. Bräunlich H, Splinter FK. Renale Ausscheidung von Langzeitsulfonamiden bei Flüssigkeitsbelastung und Änderung des pH-Werten des Harns. *Acta Biol Med Ger* 1976;35:793–8.
16. Bräunlich H. Excretion of drugs during postnatal development. *Pharmacol Ther* 1981;12:299–320.
17. Calcagno PL, Rubin MI. Renal excretion of para-aminohippurate in infants and children. *J Clin Invest* 1963;42:1632–9.
18. Chantler C. The kidney. In: Godfrey S, Baum JD, eds. *Clinical paediatric physiology.* Oxford, London: Blackwell Scientific Publications, 1980:356–98.
19. Houston IB, Oetliker O. The growth and the development of

the kidneys. In: Davies JA, Dobbing J, eds. *Scientific foundation of pediatrics*. London: Heineman, 1974:297–307.
20. Lindeman RD. Age changes in renal function. In: Goldman R, Rockstein M, eds. *The physiology and pathology of human aging*. New York: Academic Press, 1975:19–38.
21. Morselli PL, Franco-Morselli R, Bossi L. Clinical pharmacokinetics in newborns and infants. Age-related differences and therapeutic implications. *Clin Pharmacokinet* 1980;5:485–527.
22. Rowe JW, Andres R, Tobin JD, Norris AH, Shock NW. The effect of age on creatinine clearance in men: a cross-sectional and longitudinal study. *J Gerontol* 1976;31:155–63.
23. Rubin MI, Bruck E, Rapoport M. Maturation of renal function in childhood: clearance studies. *J Clin Invest* 1949;28:1144–62.
24. Traeger A. Der Altersgang der renalen Elimination von Arzneimitteln beim Menschen. *Zentralbl Pharm* 1977;116:591–9.
25. Weil WB. The evaluation of renal function in infancy and childhood. *Am J Med Sci* 1955;229:678–92.
26. West JR, Smith HW, Chasis H. Glomerular filtration rate, effective renal blood flow, and maximal tubular excretory capacity in infancy. *J Pediatr* 1948;32:10–8.
27. Winberg J. The 24-hour true endogenous creatinine clearance in infants and children without renal disease. *Acta Paediatr* 1959;48:443–52.
28. Bricker NS, Morrin PAF, Kime SW. The pathologic physiology of chronic Bright's Disease. *Am J Med* 1960;28:77–98.
29. Edelmann CM. Developmental renal physiology. In: Gruskin AB, Norman ME, eds. *Pediatric nephrology*. London: Martinus Nijhoff Publishers, 1981:15–27.
30. Loggie JMH, Kleinman LI, van Maanen EF. Renal function and diuretic therapy in infants and children. *J Pediatr* 1975;86:485–96.
31. Schnermann J, Levine DZ. Tubular control of glomerular filtration rate in single nephrons. *Can J Physiol Pharmacol* 1975;53:326–9.
32. Tisher CC. Functionele anatomie van de nier. *Tempo Med Nederland* 1981;7:9–24.
33. Vree TB, Hekster YA, van der Kleijn E. Significance of apparent half-lives of a metabolite with a higher elimination rate than its parent drug. *Drug Intell Clin Pharm* 1982;16:124–31.
34. Fawer C-L, Torrado A, Guignard J-P. Maturation of renal function in full-term and premature neonates. *Helv Paediatr Acta* 1979;34:11–21.
35. Neims AH. Renal elimination of drugs at various ages. In: Turner P, Padgham C, Hedges A, eds. *Clinical pharmacology and therapeutics*. London: MacMillan, 1980:117–23.
36. Aperia A, Broberger O, Elinder G, Herin P, Zetterström R. Postnatal development of renal function in pre-term and full-term infants. *Acta Paediatr Scand* 1981;70:183–7.
37. van Oort A, Monnens L, van Munster P. Beta-2-microglobulin clearance, an indicator of renal tubular maturation. *Int J Pediatr Nephrol* 1980;1:80–4.
38. Vree TB, Guelen PJM, Jongman-Nix B, Walenkamp GHIM. The relationship between the renal clearance of creatinine and the apparent renal clearance of beta-2-microglobulin in patients with normal and impaired kidney function. *Clin Chim Acta* 1981;114:93–9.
39. Baethke R, Golde G, Gahl G. Sulphamethoxazole/trimethoprim: pharmacokinetic studies in patients with chronic renal failure. *Eur J Clin Pharmacol* 1972;4:233–40.
40. Peters L. Urinary excretion of drugs. In: Brodie BB, Erdös EG, Maickel RP, Lindgren P, eds. *Metabolic factors controlling duration of drug action*. London: Pergamon Press, 1961:179–91.
41. Cho KC, Cafruny EJ. Renal tubular reabsorption of *p*-aminohippuric acid (PAH) in the dog. *J Pharmacol Exp Ther* 1970;173:1–12.
42. Rennick BR. Renal excretion of drugs: tubular transport and metabolism. *Annu Rev Pharmacol* 1972;12:141–57.
43. Rennick BR. Renal tubule transport of organic cations. *Am J Physiol* 1981;240:F83–9.
44. Thurau K, Boylan JW. Acute renal success. The unexpected logic of oliguria in acute renal failure. *Am J Med* 1976;61:308–15.
45. Frenzel J, Bräunlich H, Schramm D, Kersten I, Zwacka G. Effect on maturation of kidney function in newborn infants of repeated administration of water and electrolytes. *Eur J Clin Pharmacol* 1977;11:317–20.
46. Hewitt WR, Hook JB. Identification of renal anion transport systems with substrate stimulation and transport ontogeny. *Pharmacologist* 1976;18:232.
47. Hook JB, Hewitt WR. Development of mechanisms for drug excretion. *Am J Med* 1977;62:497–506.
48. Hook JB, Bailie MD. Perinatal renal pharmacology. *Annu Rev Pharmacol Toxicol* 1979;19:491–509.
49. Rind H, Gladtke E. Pharmacokinetische Untersuchungen zur Sulfonamidtherapie bei Trimenonkindern. *Monatsschr Kinderheilkd* 1964;112:239–40.
50. Taggart JV. Mechanisms of renal tubular transport. *Am J Med* 1958;24:774–84.
51. Campbell S, Wladimiroff JW, Dewhurst CJ. The antenatal measurement of fetal urine production. *J Obstet Gynaecol Br Cwlth* 1973;80:680–6.
52. Wladimiroff JW, Campbell S. Fetal urine-production rates in normal and complicated pregnancy. *Lancet* 1974;i:151–3.
53. Vree TB, Hekster YA, van der Kleijn E. De betekenis van halfwaardetijden van geneesmiddelenmetabolieten. *J Drug Res* 1981;6:1029–35.
54. Vest M. Insufficient glucuronide formation in the newborn and its relationship to the pathogenesis of icterus neonatorum. *Arch Dis Child* 1958;33:473–6.
55. Vest MF, Streiff RR. Studies on glucuronide formation in newborn infants and older children. *J Dis Child* 1959;98:688–93.
56. Vest MF, Rossier R. Detoxification in the newborn: the ability of the newborn infant to form conjugates with glucuronic acid, glycine acetate and glutathione. *Ann NY Acad Sci* 1963;111:183–97.
57. Vest M. Stoffwechsel und therapeutischer Effekt des Langzeitsulfonamids 4-Sulfanilamido-5,6-dimethoxypyrimidin (Fanasil) beim Säugling und Kind. *Schweiz Med Wochenschr* 1966;96:920–8.
58. Levy G, Khanna NN, Soda DM, Tsuzuki O, Stern L. Pharmacokinetics of acetaminophen in the human neonate: formation of acetaminophen glucuronide and sulfate in relation to plasma bilirubin concentration and D-glucaric acid excretion. *Pediatrics* 1975;55:818–25.
59. Miller RP, Roberts RJ, Fisher LJ. Acetaminophen elimination kinetics in neonates, children and adults. *Clin Pharmacol Ther* 1976;19:284–94.
60. Rane A, Tomson G. Prenatal and neonatal drug metabolism in man. *Eur J Clin Pharmacol* 1980;18:9–15.
61. Rane A. Drug metabolism at various ages—young. In: Turner P, Padgham C, Hedges A, eds. *Clinical pharmacology and therapeutics*. London: MacMillan, 1980:98–107.
62. Friedrich H, Hänsel G. Liqourspiegel-untersuchungen einer Trimethoprim–sulfamethoxazole-kombination im Ventrikelliquor bei neurochirurgischen Patienten. *Acta Neurochir (Wien)* 1977;37:271–80.
63. Lehr D, Slobody L, Greenberg W. The use of a sulfadiazeine–sulfathiazole mixture in the treatment of children. *J Pediatr* 1946;29:275–85.
64. Lehr D. Clinical toxicity of sulfonamides. *Ann NY Acad Sci* 1957;69:417–47.

65. Prien EL. The mechanism of renal complications in sulfonamide therapy. *N Engl J Med* 1945;232:63–8.
66. Woolley JL, Ragouzeous A, Brent DA, Sigel CW. Sulfonamide crystalluria: isolation and identification of sulfamethoxazole and four metabolites in urinary calculi. In: Nelson JD, Grassi C, eds. *Current chemotherapy and infectious disease*. American Society for Microbiology, Washington. 1980:552–4.
67. Vree TB, Hekster YA, van Dalen R. Het meten van de concentratie van sulfonamiden in bloed en urine van patienten met gestoorde nierfunktie. *Folia Chemother (Roche)* 1981;1–30.
68. Schönfeld H. Resorption, Verteilung und Ausscheidung neuerer Sulfonamide beim Säugling. *Chemotherapy* 1962;4:8–30.
69. Rind H, Gladtke E. Die Aktivierung der Sulfonamidelimination bei reifen und unreifen Neugeborenen durch Complamin. *Klin Wochenschr* 1965;43:904–5.
70. Krauer B, Spring P, Dettli L. Zur Pharmacokinetik der Sulfonamide im ersten Lebensjahr. *Pharmacol Clin* 1968;1:47–53.
71. Fichter EG, Curtis JA. Sulfonamide administration in newborn and premature infants. *Pediatrics* 1956;18:50–8.
72. Richmond JB, Kravitz H, Segar WE. Sulfonamide dosage in early infancy. *J Pediatr* 1950;36:539–49.
73. Forbes GB, Perley A, Dehlinger J. The use of sulfamerazine in infants and children. *J Pediatr* 1946;28:24–36.
74. Dost FH, Gladtke E. Pharmacokinetik des 2-Sulfanilamido-3-methoxy-pyrazin beim Kind (Elimination, enterale Absorption, Verteilung und Dosierung). *Arzneimittelforsch* 1969;19:1304–7.
75. Sereni F, Perletti L, Marubini E, Mars G. Pharmacokinetic studies with a long-acting sulfonamide in subjects of different ages. *Pediatr Res* 1968;2:29–37.
76. Friesen WT, Hekster YA, Vree TB. Trimethoprim: clinical use and pharmacokinetics. *Drug Intell Clin Pharm* 1981;15:325–30.
77. Friesen WT, Hekster YA, Boerema JBJ, Vree TB, Nieste HLG, van der Kleijn E. Recent developments in the treatment of acute urinary infections. *J Clin Hosp Pharm* 1981;6:1–11.
78. Lott RS, Hayton WL. Estimation of creatinine clearance from serum creatinine concentration. *Drug Intell Clin Pharm* 1978;12:140–50.
79. Fowle ASE, Bye A, Hariri F, Middlemiss D, Naficy K. The dosage of co-trimoxazole in childhood. *Eur J Clin Pharmacol* 1975;8:217–22.
80. Marks MI, Kazemi M, Hales B, Neims AH. Pharmacokinetic studies of trimethoprim–sulfamethoxazole in children with gastroenteritis. *J Infect Dis* 1973;128(suppl):622–5.
81. World Health Organization. *The selection of essential drugs*. World Health Organization, Geneva. Second report Rep. Series. 1979;641.
82. Schwartz GJ, Haycock GB, Spitzer A. Plasma creatinine and urea concentration in children: normal values for age and sex. *J Pediatr* 1976;88:828–35.

Therapeutic Drug Monitoring
7:148–158 © 1985 Raven Press, New York

Review

Therapeutic Drug Monitoring in Pediatric Acute Drug Intoxications

*†Kent E. Opheim and †Vidmantas A. Raisys

**Department of Laboratories, Children's Orthopedic Hospital and Medical Center, and †Department of Laboratory Medicine, University of Washington School of Medicine, Seattle, Washington, U.S.A.*

Diagnosis and treatment of acute intoxication resulting from drug ingestion remain frequent and formidable problems for the pediatrician. Traditionally, the physician has relied on the use of supportive therapy, based on established and clearly understood physiological principles, as the first and primary mode of treatment. With the current greater availability of serum drug assays, the use of drug concentration data and the application of pharmacokinetic principles would appear to offer rational and attractive advantages in the medical management of the poisoned patient. Plasma drug levels may be used in the treatment of overdose to (a) confirm diagnosis, (b) assess the severity of intoxication, (c) predict the time course of toxic effects, (d) allow for decisions to treat the patient prophylactically for delayed toxicity, (e) facilitate the choice of treatment in order to accelerate the removal of drug from the body, and (f) assure adequate drug elimination.

Compared with blood level measurements for routine therapeutic drug monitoring, correlations between drug concentrations during overdose and clinical effects are sometimes poor. Poor documentation of the size of dose, time of ingestion, drawing of blood samples during a prolonged absorptive phase, sampling over too short a time interval to obtain accurate elimination parameters, drug interactions with other unknown ingested drugs, and a high degree of interindividual variation all contribute to this lack of correlation. Finally, the general lack of data on drug disposition during human development and during acute intoxication has severely limited the clinical application of pharmacokinetic principles in the pediatric patient.

Address correspondence and reprint requests to Dr. K. E. Opheim at Clinical Laboratories, Children's Orthopedic Hospital and Medical Center, P.O. Box C-5371, Seattle, WA 98105, U.S.A.

INCIDENCE OF POISONING IN CHILDREN

Data compiled by the National Clearinghouse for Poison Control Centers (1) show that in 1978, 60% of the 150,000 reported cases of poisonings involving liquids and solids occurred in children under 5 years of age. Because it is estimated that only 1 in 10 cases of poisoning is reported, the real incidence is probably much higher. For this same age group, these data show that one half of the cases resulted from the ingestion of a therapeutic drug, obtained either by prescription or over the counter. There has been a general decrease in the incidence of poisonings in children under 5 years of age in the United States since the 1960s. This decline has been attributed to both the introduction of child-resistant packaging of medications and household products and increased consumer awareness of potential poisons. For aspirin alone, only 13 deaths were reported for children under 5 years of age in 1979, compared with an average of 140 per year in the early 1960s. Table 1 lists the number of deaths associated with drug ingestion during 1979 for various age groups. Although children under 5 years of age account for nearly 25% of reported drug ingestions, they represent only 4% of drug-related mortality. The relatively high incidence of drug ingestion by toddlers (peaking between 1.5 and 4 years of age) (2) and their relatively low mortality rate correlates with their active exploration of the environment and the resulting ingestion of either small amounts of toxic drugs or compounds of low toxicity. The higher incidence of drug-related mortality in adults and adolescents re-

TABLE 1. *Number of deaths from poisoning in the United States during 1978, grouped by age*[a]

Drug	Age (yr)				
	<5	5–9	10–14	15–19	20–65 +
Antibiotics and other antimicrobials	—	—	—	—	15
Hormones and synthetic substitutes	1	—	—	—	16
Hematological agents (including antihistamines)	8	2	1	1	46
Analgesics and antipyretics	18	1	4	28	401
Sedatives and hypnotics	1	—	2	16	212
Autonomic nervous system and psychotherapeutic drugs (including antidepressants)	10	3	2	12	141
Central nervous system stimulants and depressants	2	1	—	9	33
Cardiovascular drugs (primarily cardiac glycosides)	—	—	—	—	172
Gastrointestinal drugs	1	—	—	—	3
Other and unspecified drugs	7	3	6	51	677
Alcohol	—	—	1	8	354
Total	48	10	16	125	2,070

[a]Data obtained from the National Clearinghouse for Poison Control Centers (1).

flects intentional drug ingestion (true accidental poisoning being rare) (1).

PEDIATRIC PHARMACOKINETICS

For monitoring acute intoxication, knowledge of the time course of serum drug concentrations may be useful if such levels can be related to the magnitude or duration of intoxication. However, well-documented information providing these relationships for children is lacking, limiting the usefulness of blood-level monitoring in these acute situations. This comparative lack of pharmacokinetic data limits or excludes the therapeutic use of many drugs in children [Shirkey (3) has termed such children therapeutic orphans]. Frequently, and often incorrectly, estimates of drug disposition in children must be made using pharmacokinetic parameters derived from the study of adults. Several monographs and reviews have recently been written that begin to address the need for basic pediatric pharmacokinetic information (4–7).

Continuous and rapid physiologic changes are associated with the basic stages of human development: (a) neonates (birth to 1 month); (b) infants (1 month to 5 years); (c) prepubescent children (6–10 years); (d) pubescent children (10–14 years); and (e) children over 15 years of age, who exhibit adult patterns of drug utilization. Although physiologic functions that determine pharmacokinetic parameters are numerous and evolve at different rates, some general statements concerning drug disposition at various ages can be made.

In the neonatal period, drug clearance is usually much lower than in children and adults, primarily as a result of immature renal and hepatic function. Interestingly, the lack of some of the enzymes required for drug metabolism that are acquired in later development can result in qualitatively different pathways for drug elimination; for example, theophylline is partially converted to caffeine in neonates (8). From infancy through early childhood, drug elimination usually occurs at a significantly higher rate than in adults, as maturing organ function contributes to a greater effect per unit of body weight than in the adult. At puberty, the child's patterns for handling drugs rapidly approach those of adults.

PHARMACOKINETICS IN DRUG OVERDOSE

Pharmacokinetic parameters applicable to therapeutic doses of certain drugs may change as a result of dose-dependent and pathophysiologic consequences of an overdose (9), a phenomenon known as toxicokinetics (10). An overdose commonly delays drug absorption, due to delay in gastric emptying or in dissolution of the larger mass, i.e., in a therapeutic dose aspirin absorption is usually completed within 1 h, but after ingestion of a large dose may be delayed for more than 6 h.

The extent of absorption, bioavailability, may be increased due to saturation of presystemic or first-pass metabolism. Similarly as plasma protein-binding sites become saturated, the free, unbound, fraction of drug increases resulting in an increased volume of distribution for the drug. In overdose, for example, the volume of distribution of salicylate may increase sharply as a result of the increase of the free fraction of drug in the serum (11). Increases in the free level of drug may then lead to a greater clinical or toxic effect than would be expected from the drug's total level, as free concentrations generally correlate more closely with clinical effect.

Elimination is, for most drugs, a first-order process (i.e., the amount eliminated per unit of time is directly proportional to the plasma concentration). If a rate-determining enzymatic process becomes saturated, drug elimination becomes zero order (ie., a constant amount is eliminated per unit of time) and an increase in the drug's half-life, as seen for high doses of theophylline (12), salicylate (11), phenytoin (13), and acetaminophen (14), may be observed.

Certain pathophysiologic changes induced by drug overdose may affect pharmacokinetic parameters, often resulting in delay of drug absorption or elimination. These include changes in gastrointestinal motility (15), cardiovascular and pulmonary function (16), acid–base balance (17), hepatic function (18), renal function (19), and temperature regulation (20).

TREATMENT OF DRUG OVERDOSE

Diagnosis of drug intoxication is often difficult; symptoms may mimic those of disease, and the patient history may be unreliable or unobtainable, especially for children. The use of drug screening tests to determine whether drug ingestion occurred has proven useful in many hospital centers. The cost effectiveness of such testing and the extent to which the results affect medical decision making are sparsely documented and subject to controversy. Even when the source of intoxication is identified, the information is often not used in patient management, since for the majority of drugs and other toxic agents there are no specific treatments or antidotes. Supportive therapy to maintain circulation and respiration may be the only approach; the adage, "treat the patient, not the poison," applies in a vast majority of the cases (21–23).

Once the patient has been stabilized by means of supportive care, procedures may need to be initiated to remove unabsorbed drug from the gastrointestinal tract and to increase the rate of drug elimination from the blood. Traditionally, emesis and gastric lavage have been used to remove unabsorbed drug from the stomach. Emesis is often initiated using syrup of ipecac since the use of apomorphine to induce vomiting in children is not recommended due to its narcotic depressant effect. Gastric lavage may be used to empty the stomach when emesis is contraindicated, as in a comatose patient, but may have limited use when large, solid dosage forms have been ingested.

For the drug not removed by emesis or lavage, the use of activated charcoal to bind unabsorbed drug has proven safe and effective. Concomitant administration of activated charcoal with syrup of ipecac or a specific antidote will render both agents less effective. Cathartics (i.e., solutions of magnesium sulfate) are useful for hastening the passage of toxin through the gastrointestinal tract in some situations (i.e., ingestion of enteric drug formulations), but have not been well studied.

In some cases of toxicity, diuresis may be used to enhance the elimination of the drug from the blood. Resorption of drugs that are weak acids or weak bases may be inhibited in the kidney when they are converted to their ionized forms (ion trapping). If the pH of the patient's urine can safely be adjusted by infusion of sodium bicarbonate, weak acids such as salicylate or phenobarbital may be more efficiently eliminated in the urine. Similarly weak bases such as amphetamines may be better eliminated if one acidifies the urine by administration of an agent such as ascorbic acid or ammonium chloride.

The use of dialysis, peritoneal or hemodialysis, is most effective for the removal of drugs that are of low molecular weight, highly water soluble, not highly bound to plasma proteins, and have low volumes of distribution. Hemoperfusion, passing the patient's blood through a column filled with activated charcoal or other drug-absorbent material, is a newer technique that is sometimes more effective than dialysis, but is still limited to drugs with low volumes of distribution. Since dialysis and hemoperfusion are not benign procedures for the patient, they should be used only in cases of severe toxicity when a substantial increase in drug clearance, above endogenous clearance, can be achieved (24,25).

Measuring drug concentrations to monitor the effectiveness of the above procedures for enhancing drug elimination may be very useful. For example, if the drug concentration in the serum continues to rise after emesis or lavage, there may be considerable unabsorbed drug still in the gastrointestinal tract and further treatment, i.e., administration of charcoal, may be called for. Measurement of serum levels before and after dialysis or hemoperfusion should be used to monitor the effectiveness of treatment.

Information on poisons (10,26–28) and overdose treatment (29,30) may be found in numerous sources, though some may be out of date and should be used cautiously. Currently, *Poisindex* (31), a computer-generated microfiche compendium, updated and distributed on a quarterly basis, is the largest source of such data for drugs as well as for toxic plants, snakes, and household products. Overdose treatment protocols given in *Poisindex* have become the treatment standards for the nation's network of 500 Poison Control Centers.

SALICYLATE

Salicylate (in the form of aspirin, acetylsalicylic acid) is a widely used therapeutic agent possessing analgesic, antipyretic, and antiinflammatory properties. Salicylate ingestion remains a frequent cause of drug intoxication for both children and adults; in 1978 there were 3,300 cases reported for children under 5 years of age and 1,200 cases in older individuals (1). Two extensive journal supplements discuss the therapeutic merits and toxic aspects of aspirin and acetaminophen usage (32,33).

Aspirin has a systemic half-life of 15–20 min and is hydrolyzed to salicylic acid, primarily in the liver. Peak salicylate serum concentrations usually occur within 1 h after a therapeutic dose; after ingestion of larger doses peak levels may be delayed and may not occur until after 6 h (or >24 h, with enteric coated tablets) due to delayed dissolution and gastric emptying (11).

In both therapeutic and toxic doses, salicylate shows dose-dependent elimination. Quantitatively, the two most important metabolic pathways for salicylate (conjugation with glycine and conjugation with glucuronic acid) become saturated even at therapeutic concentrations. The apparent half-life may extend up to 15 to 30 h in overdose, as compared with 3 to 6 h after therapeutic intake (11,34). An increase in salicylate plasma concentration or a decrease in albumin concentration or blood pH may result in an enlarged volume of distribution. This may potentiate toxicity by increasing the level of salicylate in the brain (9). The symptoms of acute salicylate intoxication (which include nausea; vomiting; tinnitus; hypernea; disorientation; and in severe cases, convulsions or coma) are nonspecific and complicate diagnosis. In older children and adults, respiratory alkalosis is common, whereas in younger children a mixed respiratory alkalosis and predominating metabolic acidosis are frequently seen.

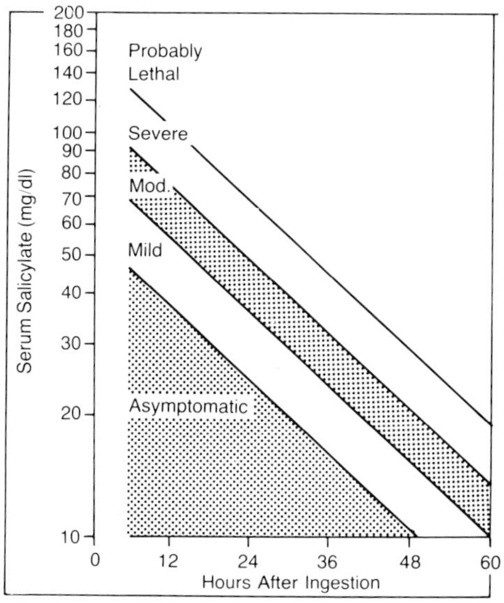

FIG. 1. Nomogram relating serum salicylate concentration to expected severity of intoxication at varying times following the ingestion of a single dose of salicylate. [From Done (37). Copyright 1960, American Academy of Pediatrics.]

Treatment is usually directed first toward correcting serious acid–base and electrolyte imbalances and then toward removing unabsorbed drug through emesis or lavage. This is usually followed by administration of activated charcoal and a cathartic. Sodium bicarbonate solution may be administered parenterally to correct severe acidosis and is also indicated for alkalinization of the urine. Alkaline diuresis (pH > 8) is highly effective in increasing the elimination of salicylate by ion trapping the anionic form in the urine and preventing its resorption by the kidney. In severe poisoning, hemodialysis may be necessary and is considered superior to either peritoneal dialysis or hemoperfusion (31,35,36).

Serum-level determinations for salicylate are only occasionally used for monitoring antiinflammatory treatment (therapeutic range, 10–20 mg/dl). However, serum levels are good prognostic indicators for acute ingestion. An initial blood level should be obtained at least 6 h after ingestion; levels obtained prior to this may still reflect absorption–distribution kinetics and must be interpreted with caution. Serial levels should be used to confirm that drug absorption has ceased. The initial level can be evaluated using the Done nomogram (Fig. 1) (37) to estimate the probable severity of the ingestion. This nomogram should be used only to assess acute overdose, not chronic intoxication. In severely toxic patients (those with >130 mg/dl salicylate at 6 h or with clinical deterioration and lack of response to other measures) hemodialysis may be required.

The most frequently used procedure for the determination of salicylate concentrations in serum remains the venerable colorimetric procedure of Trinder (38) or a modification thereof. Assays employing chromatographic methods, including high performance liquid chromatography (HPLC), are also available (39).

ACETAMINOPHEN

Acetaminophen (*N*-acetyl-*p*-aminophenol) was introduced in the United States in the mid-1950s. The drug has analgesic and antipyretic actions similar to those of aspirin (40,41). In the United States, acetaminophen is sold under ~50 brand names and in almost 200 preparations with other drugs (42). Because acetaminophen has fewer gastrointestinal side effects than aspirin, it is widely promoted to the public as a safe alternative. With the increased use of the drug has come an increase in deliberate and accidental poisoning, which can be life threatening or fatal.

Acetaminophen is rapidly absorbed from the gastrointestinal tract after oral administration of therapeutic doses, with peak levels usually occurring within 2 h (43). However when the dose is increased, absorption is prolonged and peak serum levels may not occur until after 4 h. Once absorbed, acetaminophen is metabolized mainly by glucuronidation and sulfation in the liver (44,45). The conjugation pattern changes with age. The urinary glucuronide/sulfate ratio is 0.34 in neonates and 0.75 in children 3–9 years of age, significantly lower than that seen in adolescents and adults (1.61 and 1.80, respectively) (46). A small fraction of acetaminophen is excreted unchanged, and ~4% is oxidized to a reactive metabolite that is conjugated with glutathione to yield a mercapturic acid derivative (47). When hepatic glutathione is depleted by ≥70%, as it is after ingestion of large amounts of acetaminophen, the reactive metabolite binds covalently to liver macromolecules, causing hepatic necrosis (48). Individual susceptibility to acetaminophen toxicity depends on the level of hepatic glutathione and the amount of the reactive metabolite generated. Microsomal enzyme inducers, such as phenobarbital, enhance the production of the potentially toxic metabolite (49). The plasma half-life of acetaminophen after therapeutic doses is ~2 h, but may increase severalfold after ingestion of large amounts of the drug. This increased plasma half-life is considered a good indicator of potential hepatotoxicity (50).

The clinical course of acetaminophen overdose has four stages (51). Stage I occurs in the first 24 h after drug ingestion. The patient may have nausea, vomiting, diaphoresis, and general malaise. The onset of these symptoms occurs ~6 h after ingestion of large amounts of acetaminophen. By 14 h after ingestion, all patients show these symptoms. Stage II occurs 24 to 48 h after ingestion. In this stage, the patient begins to feel better, but laboratory tests will show liver involvement. At this time aspartate aminotransferase, alanine aminotransferase, and bilirubin levels become elevated, and prothrombin time increases. Stage III occurs 3 to 4 days after ingestion, with liver function tests reaching their highest values. In less severe poisoning, recovery occurs at Stage IV, 7–8 days after drug ingestion, with liver function returning to normal. In untreated severe cases, death may occur from hepatic failure.

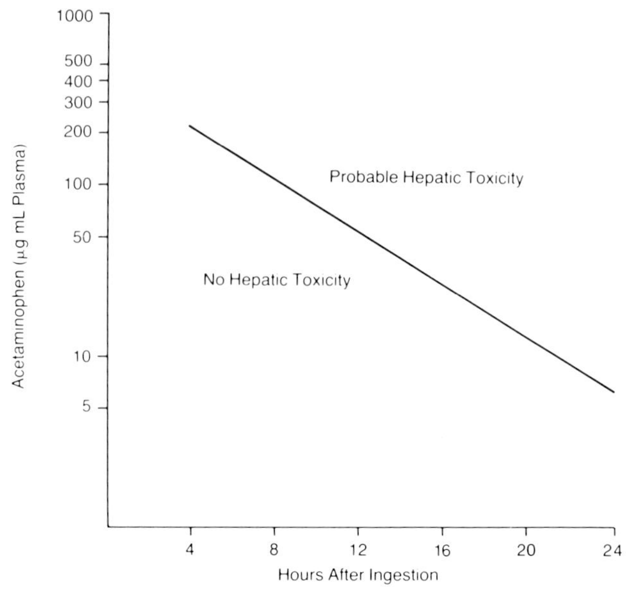

FIG. 2. Nomogram relating plasma acetaminophen concentration to expected severity of intoxication at varying times following the ingestion of a single dose of acetaminophen. [From Rumack and Matthew (52). Copyright 1975, American Academy of Pediatrics.]

The initial treatment of an overdosed patient should consist of emesis or gastric lavage to remove unabsorbed acetaminophen. Activated charcoal or saline cathartics should not be used, since they can inhibit absorption of the antidote, *N*-acetylcysteine (Mucomyst). Blood should be drawn for plasma acetaminophen determination at least 4 h after ingestion of the drug. Blood drawn earlier than 4 h may not show the peak plasma drug concentration (31). The plasma acetaminophen concentration should then be plotted on the Rumack–Matthew nomogram (Fig. 2) (52); if the acetaminophen concentration is in the toxic region,

N-acetylcysteine treatment should be instituted as suggested by Rumack (31).

The incidence of severe liver toxicity after acetaminophen overdose in children under 6 years of age is low; in the United States only one fatal case, involving a 3-year-old child, has been reported (53). Peterson and Rumack (54) reported five cases of children under 6 years of age who had toxic plasma acetaminophen levels and whose treatment with *N*-acetylcysteine was delayed up to 20 h postingestion; none showed hepatotoxicity. In the same report, another group of eight children who had ingested large amounts of acetaminophen and vomited had plasma acetaminophen levels close to zero, indicating that emesis was effective for drug removal. In prepubescent children (7–12 years old) who had toxic plasma acetaminophen levels, the liver toxicity correlated with the time of initiation of *N*-acetylcysteine therapy. The limited information available suggests that young children may metabolize acetaminophen differently than adults. It is possible that in children the potentially toxic metabolite is not formed, which would explain the lack of hepatotoxicity. However, until more information is obtained from clinical studies, children who ingest toxic amounts of acetaminophen should receive the same therapeutic treatment as adults (54).

An accurate and precise method should be used for serum acetaminophen determination. A specific colorimetric method can be used for plasma acetaminophen determination (55). Chromatographic procedures such as HPLC or gas–liquid chromatography (GLC) can be used. An HPLC procedure using protein precipitation with acetonitrile and reverse-phase chromatography (56) is less time consuming than gas–liquid chromatography. A urine screening test for *p*-aminophenol is an adequate test for phenacetin ingestion, but it should not be used for acetaminophen ingestion. *p*-Aminophenol is not produced in significant amounts in the metabolism of acetaminophen.

ALCOHOLS

Alcoholic beverages are readily accessible in most households. Consequently, accidental and intentional ethanol intoxication is common in children who are trying to imitate adults.

Ethanol, a sedative that affects the central nervous system, is rapidly absorbed from the gastrointestinal tract and reaches peak blood levels in 30 min to 3 h (57). The presence of food and ingestion of large amounts of alcoholic beverages will slow down the rate of absorption. Once alcohol is absorbed into the blood, it is distributed throughout the body water. The volume of distribution is 0.58–0.70 L/kg (57). Ninety percent of the ingested alcohol is metabolized by oxidation by the liver alcohol dehydrogenase, and only 5–10% is lost in urine and in the exhaled breath. Generally elimination appears to follow zero order kinetics at a rate of 15 mg/dl/h (58). Some evidence suggests that at high concentrations of alcohol other mechanisms, including metabolism by microsomal oxidizing enzymes and increased renal excretion, contribute to enhanced ethanol elimination (59,60). Clinical manifestations of intoxication, as well as legally defined intoxication, usually occur at blood alcohol levels >100 mg/dl. Fatalities in alcohol-intolerant individuals may occur at levels as low as 350 mg/dl.

Treatment of acute alcohol intoxication is directed first toward prevention of further absorption of alcohol. Emesis or gastric lavage is recommended, followed by administration of activated charcoal to reduce alcohol absorption (31). Hemodialysis can eliminate ethanol faster than hepatic oxidation; however, it is usually not indicated unless the toxicity is severe or hepatic elimination is impaired. Hypoglycemia is a common complication of acute alcohol intoxication and should be treated accordingly (61).

Methanol is a common ingredient in household and industrial products. Although methanol poisonings are not as common as ethanol poisonings, they are more severe. Methanol is rapidly absorbed from the gastrointestinal tract and metabolized by liver alcohol dehydrogenase (62) first to formaldehyde and then to formic acid, which may cause severe metabolic acidosis and permanent blindness (63). Initial treatment consists of emesis or gastric lavage to remove unabsorbed methanol (31). Because methanol is oxidized by alcohol dehydrogenase, which favors ethanol, methanol oxidation can be competitively inhibited by ethanol administration (64). To achieve saturation of alcohol dehydrogenase with ethanol, a blood ethanol concentration of 100 mg/dl or higher should be maintained. In a patient with a blood methanol concentration of 20 mg/dl or higher, ethanol administration should be instituted and continued until the blood methanol concentration decreases to below 20 mg/dl or until no acidosis is present. When acidosis is severe and unresponsive to therapy or when the blood methanol concentration is higher than 50 mg/dl, hemodialysis should be performed (31).

Isopropyl alcohol (isopropanol or rubbing alcohol) is sometimes accidentally ingested by children. Intoxication has also been reported following excessive sponging with isopropyl alcohol probably due to the child's inhalation of isopropanol vapors (65).

Isopropyl alcohol is readily absorbed from the gastrointestinal tract and reaches peak levels within 1 h after ingestion. Isopropanol is metabolized in the body to acetone; and both acetone and isopropanol are excreted in the urine. The rate of isopropanol elimination is lower than that for ethanol. Toxic effects are noted at plasma levels of 50 mg/dl or higher, and fatalities have been reported at 150 mg/dl (31).

Initial treatment after oral ingestion of isopropanol should be directed toward decreasing absorption from the stomach through emesis or gastric lavage, followed then by administration of activated charcoal and a cathartic. Hemodialysis is an effective treatment for severe intoxication (31). Measurement of isopropanol and acetone in the blood may be used to monitor treatment.

Gas–liquid chromatographic (GLC) methods are available that can measure all three of these alcohols (66). Commercially available kits employing enzymatic (alcohol dehydrogenase) methods can also be used for ethanol determination (67).

IRON

Iron, in the form of ferrous salts or chelates, is widely available for therapeutic or nutritional purposes. Iron poisoning in children is relatively frequent, with over 300 cases reported in 1979 (1). Attractive iron dosage forms, brightly colored and sugar coated, have contributed to this problem. Toxic effects from ingestion of these compounds correlate best with their content of elemental iron. Minimal toxic symptoms are likely to occur at dosage levels of 20–60 mg iron/kg; the average lethal dose is estimated to be 200–250 mg iron/kg (68). Elemental iron content of the many available dosage forms varies widely and is listed in a recent publication by Krenzelok and Hoff (69). The Food and Drug Administration requires that products containing over 250 mg iron per container be packaged in child-resistant containers.

Initial clinical manifestations of iron overdose include vomiting, upper abdominal pain, and diarrhea. The corrosive nature of large amounts of iron compounds on the gastrointestinal mucosa may cause significant intestinal irritation and severe blood loss resulting in shock. This may be followed by a transient phase, lasting for up to 12 h, during which initial symptoms abate. In severe toxicity, death may result from profound shock, acidosis, and gastrointestinal and hepatic necrosis (31).

Treatment of iron overdose is directed first toward the removal of unabsorbed iron by emesis or lavage. Iron not removed through this treatment may be converted to less absorbable salts by administration of sodium bicarbonate by lavage. Unabsorbed tablets are radiopaque and can be observed with abdominal x-ray. To increase elimination of iron from the blood, the chelating agent deferoxamine can be given parenterally. The pink- to orange-colored iron–deferoxamine complex is rapidly excreted in the urine; deferoxamine treatment may be discontinued when the color of the urine returns to normal.

Serum iron levels are important in the management of iron ingestion. Absorption for most iron preparations is not complete before 2–3 h after ingestion, and distribution may continue for up to 6 h (70). Serial monitoring is appropriate to determine this time course. Rumack has recommended that both serum iron level and total iron-binding capacity (TIBC) be measured (31); when the total iron concentration exceeds the binding capacity of the serum, free serum iron is present and the patient should be considered toxic. Concentrations of iron greater than 350 μg/dl generally exceed the TIBC of normal serum (the reference value for TIBC is <400 μg/dl). Reference values for serum iron concentration for children range from 60 to 150 μg/dl and show considerable diurnal variation within this range.

Colorimetric procedures are available for the determination of serum iron concentration and TIBC (71).

THEOPHYLLINE

Theophylline (1,3-dimethylxanthine) is used as a bronchodilator for the treatment of asthma and as a respiratory stimulant for the treatment of neonatal apnea. The therapeutic range suggested for control of asthma is 10–20 μg/ml; a lower range (6–11 μg/ml) is recommended for treating apnea in premature newborns. Interpretation of theophylline levels in newborns is complicated by the fact that newborns are uniquely able to metabolize a significant portion of a theophylline dose to caffeine (1,3,7-trimethylxanthine), also a potent respiratory system stimulant (8). The elimination half-life of theophylline is age dependent, with that of premature infants ranging from 14 to 58 h; young children, from 2 to 6 h; and older children and adults, from 4 to 12 h (72,73). Additionally, dose-dependent elimination kinetics, with a prolonged half-life, have been suggested for high doses of theophylline (12).

Intoxication with theophylline due to disease-induced alterations in kinetics or to accidental or suicidal ingestion is not uncommon among children taking the drug (9). Toxic symptoms correlate well with theophylline serum concentrations: Minor adverse effects such as nausea and vomiting occur at concentrations >25 μg/ml, and serious toxic effects, including seizures and cardiac arrhythmias, become more frequent at levels of >50 μg/ml (72).

Treatment of theophylline overdose begins with removal of unabsorbed drug, through emesis (with syrup of ipecac) or gastric lavage. This is followed by oral administration of activated charcoal and a cathartic such as magnesium sulfate. Serum levels of theophylline should be monitored until concentrations return to the therapeutic range (<20 μg/ml) to verify that elimination is satisfactory (31). For patients with very high levels (>50 μg/ml) and severe clinical toxicity, charcoal hemoperfusion has been used successfully to hasten theophylline clearance (74,75).

Theophylline is most frequently monitored using an enzyme multiplied immunoassay technique (EMIT) (76) or HPLC (77).

PHENYTOIN

Phenytoin (Dilantin) is an anticonvulsant drug frequently prescribed for children. Intoxication with phenytoin is not uncommon because of the well-documented dose dependency of its elimination (and its greatly increased half-life), which may result in phenytoin accumulation even with therapeutic doses. Phenytoin absorption may be prolonged after an overdose, with the peak level occurring between 24 and 48 h after ingestion (compared with 3–12 h for a therapeutic dose); the delay is due to phenytoin's poor water solubility and its effect in reducing gastrointestinal motility. Phenytoin is highly protein bound (usually >90%); whether this amount of binding decreases as a result of phenytoin overdose is not known (13,78).

Toxic symptoms correlate with serum concentrations. At 20–30 μg/ml nystagmus is noted, at 30–40 μg/ml ataxia appears, and at concentrations of >40 μg/ml drowsiness and disorientation occur (79). Paradoxical intoxication with increased seizure frequency has been reported for patients with chronically high phenytoin levels (80).

Treatment of phenytoin overdose begins with removal of unabsorbed drug through emesis or gastric lavage, followed by administration of activated charcoal and a cathartic (31). Dialysis, diuresis, and charcoal hemoperfusion have proven to be of no value.

Serum levels of phenytoin allow severity assessment and elimination monitoring. Phenytoin serum concentrations are frequently monitored using EMIT (81); chromatographic procedures employing GLC (82) and, more recently, HPLC (83) are available. Techniques for monitoring free unbound concentrations of phenytoin are becoming more widely available; free levels correlate better with clinical condition for those patients with protein-binding abnormalities such as uremia and hypoalbuminemia (84).

PHENOBARBITAL

Phenobarbital continues to be widely prescribed as an anticonvulsant and sedative drug for children and adults, and accidental poisoning in children is not uncommon. Absorption of even therapeutic doses of phenobarbital is slow and peak levels may not occur until 6–18 h after ingestion (85). The absorption of therapeutic doses of sedative barbiturates, such as amobarbital, pentobarbital, and secobarbital, is more rapid with peak levels occurring within 2 h but may be delayed when overdose amounts are ingested. The elimination half-life of phenobarbital in infants and children is 40–70 h, which is shorter than that in adolescents and adults (86).

Initial treatment of phenobarbital overdose is directed toward prevention of further absorption of the drug. Emesis or gastric lavage should be initiated, followed by administration of activated charcoal and a cathartic. Alkaline diuresis, to achieve a urinary pH of 7–8, is somewhat effective in the treatment of phenobarbital intoxication (31). However, this mode is ineffective for treating intoxication with most other barbiturates, such as pentobarbital or secobarbital, since their pK_a values are higher and the ionized forms cannot be trapped in the urine (87). Hemodialysis or charcoal perfusion may be used in patients who do not respond to forced alkaline diuresis.

Toxic symptoms correlate with plasma concentration levels of phenobarbital of >65 μg/ml, usually associated with lethargy, stupor, and possible coma (88). Individuals who have become tolerant to the drug through chronic administration may not show these effects until higher concentrations are reached. Measurement of serum phenobarbital levels can aid in monitoring the progress of drug elimination. Phenobarbital serum levels can be monitored using EMIT (81), HPLC (83), or GLC (82).

TRICYCLIC ANTIDEPRESSANTS

Tricyclic antidepressant drugs comprise a relatively new and large class of therapeutic agents and include amitriptyline, desipramine, doxepin, imipramine, nortritptyline, and protriptyline. The increasing availability of these drugs to suicide-prone, depressed patients and to children treated for nocturnal enuresis has resulted in a dramatic increase in their involvement in acute intoxication. In 1978 as many as 10 deaths in children under 5 years of age resulted from ingestion of these drugs (1).

After ingestion of large amounts of tricyclic antidepressants, peak plasma levels could be delayed because the anticholinergic action of the drugs may reduce gastrointestinal motility. As for most other drug overdoses, the initial treatment should be directed toward removal of unabsorbed drug by emesis or gastric lavage, followed by administration of activated charcoal and a cathartic (31). Dialysis and hemoperfusion are ineffective in removing tricyclic antidepressants because of the large volumes of distribution and high degrees of protein binding associated with the drugs. Signs of serious toxicity are associated with plasma levels of 1 μg/ml (89). The elimination half-lives for these drugs are long (90) and cardiac complications, which may be fatal, can occur days after ingestion if plasma concentrations of tricyclic antidepressant remain elevated (91).

Measuring plasma levels of tricyclic antidepressants (and their active metabolites, if present) may be useful for confirming acute intoxication (92). However, correlations with clinical toxicity or with treatment outcome, which might warrant continued serial monitoring, have not been established.

Reliable methods are now available that measure the plasma levels of a tricyclic antidepressant and its active metabolites; the use of HPLC is particularly attractive (93).

CONCLUSION

Insufficient information is available to fully describe drug disposition following drug overdose; this lack of potentially useful information is an especially acute problem in the pediatric age group. What little information does exist is often derived from poorly documented case reports, frequently involving a single adult individual. All too often, data are obtained by extrapolation of pharmacokinetic data derived from studies using therapeutic doses of drug.

The clinical laboratory, working with the pharmacy and medical services, is in an excellent position to study the pharmacokinetics of drug overdose and to evaluate the effectiveness of treatment modalities. In their review of overdose pharmacokinetics, Rosenberg et al. (9) have suggested guidelines for acquiring these data in a rational manner. Appropriately timed blood sampling and measurement during the course of recovery would provide a better understanding of drug absorption and elimination. Drug measurement should include measurement of levels of active metabolites and of free levels when appropriate. Similarly, data are needed to define the effects on drug–protein binding resulting from high drug concentration, drug-induced physiological changes, and the interactions of multiple drug ingestion. Finally, treatment protocols for enhancing drug elimination, such as charcoal administration or hemoperfusion, should be preceded with and followed by drug-level determinations to assess the treatment's effectiveness and to provide insight into future therapeutic procedures.

Note added in proof: Subsequent to the submission of this manuscript an enzyme multiplied immunoassay for acetaminophen has become available. In addition, fluorescence polarization immunoassays for use with the Abbott TDx (Abbott Laboratories, North Chicago, IL, U.S.A.) automated drug assay system are now available for the measurement of acetaminophen, theophylline, phenobarbital, and phenytoin.

Acknowledgment: We gratefully acknowledge the help of Dr. William O. Robertson, Seattle Poison Center, Children's Orthopedic Hospital and Medical Center, for his constructive suggestions; and Ms. Lois McAnally, Department of Laboratory Medicine, for her help in the preparation of this article.

REFERENCES

1. *National Clearinghouse for Poison Control Centers Bulletin* Rockville, Maryland: United States Department of Health and Human Sciences, Bureau of Drugs, Division of Poison Control. 1981;25:1–15.
2. Deeths TM. Poisoning in children: a statistical study of 1057 cases. *J Pediatr* 1971;78:299–305.
3. Shirkey H. Infants and children are becoming therapeutic orphans. *J Pediatr* 1968;72:119–20.
4. Mirkin BL, ed. *Clinical pharmacology and therapeutics: a pediatric perspective*. Chicago: Year Book Medical Publishers, 1978.
5. Morselli PL, ed. *Drug disposition during development*. New York: Spectrum Publications, 1977.
6. Rane A, Wilson JR. Clinical pharmacokinetics in infants and children. *Clin Pharmacokinet* 1976;1:2–24.
7. Yaffe SJ, Sjögvist F, Alvan G. Pharmacological principles in the management of accidental poisoning. *Pediatr Clin North Am* 1970;17:495–507.
8. Bory C, Baltassat P, Porthault M, Bethenod M, Frederich A, Aranda JV. Biotransformation of theophylline to caffeine in premature newborn. *Lancet* 1978;2:1204–5.
9. Rosenberg J, Benowitz NL, Pond S. Pharmacokinetics of drug overdose. *Clin Pharmacokinet* 1981;6:161–92.
10. Rumack BH, Peterson RG. Clinical toxicology. In: Doull J, Klassen CD, Amdur MO, eds. *Casarett and Doull's toxicol-*

ogy: the basic science of poisons, 2nd ed. New York: Macmillan, 1980:677–98.
11. Levy G. Clinical pharmacokinetics of aspirin. *Pediatrics* 1978;62(suppl):867–72.
12. Weinberger M, Genchansky E. Dose-dependent kinetics of theophylline disposition in asthmatic children. *J Pediatr* 1977;91:820–4.
13. Richens A. Clinical pharmacokinetics of phenytoin. *Clin Pharmacokinet* 1979;4:153–69.
14. Slattery JT, Levy G. Acetaminophen kinetics in acutely poisoned patients. *Clin Pharmacol Ther* 1979;25:184–95.
15. Nimmo WS. Drugs, diseases and altered gastric emptying. *Clin Pharmacokinet* 1976;1:189–203.
16. Benowitz NL, Rosenberg J, Becker CE. Cardiopulmonary catastrophes in drug-overdosed patients. *Med Clin North Am* 1979;63:267–96.
17. Gabow PA, Anderson RJ, Potts DE, Schrier RW. Acid–base disturbances in salicylate-intoxicated adult. *Arch Intern Med* 1978;138:1481–4.
18. Mitchell JR, Jollow DJ, Gillette JR, Brodie BB. Drug metabolism as a cause of drug toxicity. *Drug Metab Dispos* 1973;1:418–23.
19. Mitchell JR, McMurty RJ, Statham CN, Nelson S. Molecular basis for several drug-induced nephropathies. *Am J Med* 1977;62:518–26.
20. Popovic V, Popovic P. *Hypothermia in biology and medicine*. New York: Grune & Stratton, 1974.
21. Curry AS, ed. *The poisoned patient: the role of the laboratory*. Amsterdam: Elsevier, 1974.
22. Walberg CB, McCarron MM. Role of therapeutic monitoring in drug overdosage. In: *Therapeutic Drug Monitoring Continuing Education and Quality Control Program, vol. 1*. Washington, D.C.: American Association of Clinical Chemistry 1980:1–7.
23. Wiltbank TB, Sine HE, Brody BB, et al. Are emergency toxicology measurements really used? *Clin Chem* 1974;20:116–20.
24. Gibson TP, Nelson HA. Drug kinetics and artificial kidneys. *Clin Pharmacokinet* 1977;2:403–26.
25. Takki S, Gambertoglio JG, Honda DH, Tozer TN. Pharmacokinetic evaluation of hemodialysis in acute drug overdose. *J Pharmacokinet Biopharm* 1978;3:181–92.
26. Baselt RC. *Disposition of toxic drugs and chemicals in man. vol. 1: Centrally-acting drugs*. Canton, Connecticut: Biomedical Publications, 1978.
27. Baselt RC. *Disposition of toxic drugs and chemicals in man. vol. 2: Peripherally-acting drugs and common toxic chemicals*. Canton, Connecticut: Biomedical Publications, 1978.
28. Klaassen CD. Toxicology. In: Gilman AG, Goodman LS, Gilman A, eds. *The pharmacological basis of therapeutics*, 6th ed. New York: Macmillan, 1980;1602–14.
29. Arena JM. *Poisoning: toxicology, symptoms, treatments*, 4th ed. Springfield, Illinois: Charles C Thomas, 1979.
30. Dreisbach RH. *Handbook of poisoning: diagnosis & treatment*, 9th ed. Los Altos, California: Lange Medical Publications, 1977.
31. Rumack BH, ed. *Poisindex*. Denver: Micromedex, 1982.
32. Winchester, JF, ed. Aspirin and acetaminophen. *Arch Intern Med* 1981;141 (Special Issue):273–404.
33. Rumack BH, ed. Aspirin and acetaminophen: a comparative view for the pediatric patient, with particular regard to toxicity, both in therapeutic and in overdose. *Pediatrics* 1978;62(suppl):865–946.
34. Levy G. Pharmacokinetics of salicylate elimination in man. *J Pharm Sci* 1965;54:959–67.
35. Temple AR. Acute and chronic effects of aspirin toxicity and their treatment. *Arch Intern Med* 1981;141:364–9.
36. Winchester JF, Gelfand MC, Helliwell M, Vale JA, Goulding R, Schreiner GE. Extracorporeal treatment of salicylate or acetaminophen poisoning—is there a role? *Arch Intern Med* 1981;141:370–4.
37. Done AK. Salicylate intoxication: significance of measurements of salicylate in blood in cases of acute ingestion. *Pediatrics* 1960;26:800–7.
38. Trinder P. Rapid determination of salicylate in biological materials. *Biochem J* 1954;57:301–3.
39. Cham BE, Johns D, Bochner F, Imhoff DM, Rowland M. Simultaneous liquid-chromatographic quantitation of salicylic acid, salicyluric acid, and gentisic acid in plasma. *Clin Chem* 1979;25:1420–5.
40. Beaver WT. Mild analgesics: a review of their clinical pharmacology. *Am J Med Sci* 1965;250:577–604.
41. Beaver WT. Mild analgesics: a review of their clinical pharmacology. *Am J Med Sci* 1966;251:576–99.
42. Koch-Weser J. Acetaminophen. *N Engl J Med* 1976;295:1297–300.
43. Rawlins MD, Henderson DB, Hijab AR. Pharmacokinetics of paracetamol (acetaminophen) after intravenous and oral administration. *Eur J Clin Pharmacol* 1972;11:283–6.
44. Cummings AJ, King ML, Martin BK. A kinetic study of drug elimination: the excretion of paracetamol and its metabolites in man. *Br J Pharmacol Chemother* 1967;29:150–7.
45. Nelson E, Morioka T. Kinetics of the metabolism of acetaminophen by humans. *J Pharm Sci* 1963;52:864–8.
46. Miller RP, Roberts RJ, Fischer LJ. Acetaminophen elimination kinetics in neonates, children, and adults. *Clin Pharmacol Ther* 1975;19:284–94.
47. Mitchell JR, Thorgeirsson SS, Potter WZ, Jollow DJ, Keiser H. Acetaminophen-induced hepatic injury: protective role of glutathione in man and rationale for therapy. *Clin Pharmacol Ther* 1974;16:676–84.
48. Mitchell JR, Jollow DJ, Potter WZ, Gillette JR, Brodie BB. Acetaminophen-induced hepatic necrosis. IV. Protective role of glutathione. *J Pharmacol Exp Ther* 1973;187:211–7.
49. Jollow DJ, Mitchell JR, Potter WZ, Davis DC, Gillette JR, Brodie BB. Acetaminophen-induced hepatic necrosis. II. Role of covalent binding in vivo. *J Pharmacol Exp Ther* 1973;187:195–202.
50. Prescott LF, Wright N, Roscoe P, Brown SS. Plasma-paracetamol half-life and hepatic necrosis in patients with paracetamol overdosage. *Lancet* 1971;1:519–22.
51. Rumack BH, Peterson RC, Koch GG, Amara JA. Acetaminophen overdose: 662 cases with evaluation of oral acetylcysteine treatment. *Arch Intern Med* 1981;141:380–5.
52. Rumack BH, Matthew H. Acetaminophen poisoning and toxicity. *Pediatrics* 1975;55:871–6.
53. Nogen AG, Bremmer JE. Fatal acetaminophen overdosage in a young child. *J Pediatr* 1978;92:832–3.
54. Peterson RG, Rumack BH. Age as a variable in acetaminophen overdose. *Arch Intern Med* 1981;141:390–3.
55. Walberg CB. Determination of acetaminophen in serum. *Anal Toxicol* 1977;1:79–80.
56. Black M, Sprague K. Rapid micromethod for acetaminophen determination. *Clin Chem* 1978;24:1288–9.
57. Redetzki HM. Treatment of ethanol intoxication. *Hosp Formul* 1979;14:934–6.
58. Wallgren H, Barry H III. *Actions of alcohol. Biochemical, physiological and psychological aspects*, vol 1. New York: Elsevier, 1970:17–73.
59. Feinman L, Baraona E, Matsuzaki S, Korsten M, Lieber CS. Concentration dependence of ethanol metabolism in vivo in rats and man. *Alcohol Clin Exp Res* 1978;2:381–5.
60. Hammond KB, Rumack BH, Rodgerson DO. Blood ethanol: a report of unusually high levels in a living patient. *JAMA* 1973;226:63–4.
61. Tolis AD. Hypoglycemic convulsions in children after alcohol ingestion. *Pediatr Clin North Am* 1965;12:423–5.
62. Mani JC, Pietruszko R, Theorell H. Methanol activity of

alcohol dehydrogenases from human liver, horse liver, and yeast. *Arch Biochem Biophys* 1970;140:52–9.
63. McMartin KE, Ambre JJ, Tephly TR. Methanol poisoning in human subjects: role for formic acid accumulation in the metabolic acidosis. *Am J Med* 1980;68:414–8.
64. McCoy HG, Cipolle RJ, Ehlers SM, Sawchuk RJ, Zaske DE. Severe methanol poisoning: application of a pharamcokinetic model for ethanol therapy and hemodialysis. *Am J Med* 1979;67:804–7.
65. Senz EH, Goldfarb DL. Coma in a child following use of isopropyl alcohol in sponging. *J Pediatr* 1958;53:322–3.
66. Baselt RC. *Analytical procedures for therapeutic drug monitoring and emergency toxicology*. Davis, California: Biomedical Publications, 1980:298–9.
67. Redetzki HM, Dees WL. Comparison of four kits for enzymatic determination of ethanol in blood. *Clin Chem* 1976;22:83–6.
68. Stein M, Blayney D, Feit T, Goergen TG, Micik S, Nyhan WL. Acute iron poisoning in children. *West J Med* 1976;125:289–97.
69. Krenzelok EP, Hoff JV. Accidental childhood iron poisoning: a problem of marketing and labeling. *Pediatrics* 1979;63:591–6.
70. Robertson WO. Iron poisoning: a problem of childhood. *Top Emerg Med* 1979;1:57–63.
71. Tietz NW. Electrolytes. In: Tietz NW, ed. *Fundamentals of clinical chemistry*. Philadelphia: WB Saunders, 1976:873–944.
72. Hendeles L, Weinberger M, Johnson G. Monitoring serum theophylline levels. *Clin Pharmacokinet* 1978;3:294–312.
73. Ogilvie RI. Clinical pharmacokinetics of theophylline. *Clin Pharmacokinet* 1978;3:267–93.
74. Russo ME. Management of theophylline intoxication with charcoal-column hemoperfusion. *N Engl J Med* 1979;300:24–6.
75. Ehlers SM, Zaske DE, Sawchuk RJ. Massive theophylline overdose: rapid elimination by charcoal hemoperfusion. *JAMA* 1978;240:474–5.
76. Koup JR, Brodsky B. Comparison of homogeneous enzyme immunoassay and high pressure liquid chromatography for the determination of theophylline concentration in serum. *Am Rev Respir Dis* 1978;117:1135–8.
77. Butrimovitz GP, Raisys VA. An improved micromethod for theophylline determination by reverse-phase liquid chromatography. *Clin Chem* 1979;25:1461–4.
78. Morselli PL. Antiepileptic drugs. In: Morselli PL, ed. *Drug disposition during development*. New York: Spectrum Publications, 1977:311–60.
79. Kutt H, McDowell F. Management of epilepsy with diphenylhydantoin sodium. *JAMA* 1968;203:167–70.
80. Troupin AS, Ojemann LM. Paradoxical intoxication: a complication of anticonvulsant administration. *Epilepsia* 1975;16:753–8.
81. Legaz M, Raisys VA. Correlation of the "EMIT" antiepileptic drug assay with a gas liquid chromatographic method. *Clin Biochem* 1976;9:35–8.
82. Kupferberg HJ. Quantitative estimation of diphenylhydantoin, primidone and phenobarbital in plasma by gas–liquid chromatography. *Clin Chim Acta* 1970;29:283–8.
83. Kabra PM, McDonald DM, Marton LJ. A simultaneous high-performance liquid chromatographic analysis of the most common anticonvulsants and their metabolites in the serum. *J Anal Toxicol* 1978;2:127–33.
84. Booker HE, Darcey B. Serum concentrations of free diphenylhydantoin and their relationship to clinical intoxication. *Epilepsia* 1973;14:177–84.
85. Leal KW, Troupin AS. Clinical pharmacology of antiepileptic drugs: a summary of current information. *Clin Chem* 1977;23:1964–8.
86. Saunders GH, Penry JK. Phenobarbital/primidone: therapeutic use and serum concentration monitoring. In: Taylor WJ, Finn AL, eds. *Individualizing drug therapy: practical applications of drug monitoring*. New York: Gross, Townsend, Frank, 1981:49–62.
87. Hadden J, Johnson K, Price L, Giardina E. Acute barbiturate intoxication: concepts of management. *JAMA* 1969;209:893–900.
88. Buchthal F, Lennox-Buchthal MA. Phenobarbital: relation of serum concentration to control of seizures. In: Woodbury DM, Penry JK, Schmidt RP, eds. *Antiepileptic drugs*. New York: Raven Press, 1972:335–43.
89. Petit JM, Spiker DG, Ruwitch JF, Ziegler VE, Weiss AN, Biggs JT. Tricyclic antidepressant plasma levels and adverse effects after overdose. *Clin Pharmacol Ther* 1976;21:47–51.
90. Spiker DG, Biggs JT. Tricyclic antidepressants: prolonged plasma levels after overdose. *JAMA* 1976;236:1711–2.
91. Callaham M. Tricyclic antidepressant overdose. *JACEP* 1979;8:413–25.
92. Bailey DN, Van Dyke C, Langov RA, Jatlow PI. Tricyclic antidepressants: plasma levels and clinical findings in overdose. *Am J Psychiatry* 1978;135:1325–8.
93. Kabra PM, Mar NA, Marton LJ. Simultaneous liquid chromatographic analysis of amitriptyline, nortriptyline, imipramine, desipramine, doxepin, and nordoxepin. *Clin Chim Acta* 1981;111:123–32.

Therapeutic Drug Monitoring
7:159–167 © 1985 Raven Press, New York

Review

Chloramphenicol: Clinical Pharmacology in Pediatrics

Angela M. Ristuccia

Clinical Pharmacokinetic Services, Infectious Disease Division, Department of Medicine, Nassau Hospital, Mineola, and State University of New York at Stony Brook School of Medicine, Stony Brook, New York, U.S.A.

Chloramphenicol, initially identified as a natural product of *Streptomyces venezuelae* in 1947 (1), was the first recognized broad-spectrum antibiotic. Its structure and a method for its chemical synthesis were elucidated in 1948, and large-scale production and clinical trials began shortly thereafter. Chloramphenicol quickly gained acceptance after proving clinically effective against serious infections caused by a great variety of bacterial and rickettsial agents. Reports of its serious hematopoietic toxicity began to appear by 1950 (2,3). As a result, the indications for the use of chloramphenicol narrowed and its use declined. Recently, there has been a resurgence in the use of chloramphenicol. Major contributing factors to its increased use include the emergence of organisms, particularly *Streptococcus pneumoniae* and *Hemophilus influenzae* type b, resistant to less toxic agents; the reliable penetration and the excellent levels achieved in body tissues and fluids, coupled with its broad antimicrobial spectrum; and the development of rapid and accurate methods for determination of chloramphenicol blood levels. Chloramphenicol has thus reassumed a major role in the chemotherapy of infection.

CHEMISTRY

Chloramphenicol occurs as fine, needle-like crystals with an extremely bitter taste. It is freely soluble in ethanol (400 mg/ml), but only slightly soluble in water (2.5 mg/ml). Its molecular weight is 323.14 and its melting point 151°C. Aqueous solutions have a pH of 5.5 and are very stable (4). Although four possible diastereoisomers, only one is microbiologically active.

Address correspondence and reprint requests to Dr. A. M. Ristuccia at Clinical Pharmacokinetic Services, Infectious Disease Division, Nassau Hospital, Mineola, NY 11501, U.S.A.

MECHANISM OF ACTION

Chloramphenicol is primarily a bacteriostatic agent, blocking protein synthesis by reversible inhibition of the peptidyl transferase reaction at the 50S ribosomal subunit of bacteria (5). Peptide chains whose synthesis was interrupted by chloramphenicol can be completed when the drug is removed (6). Chloramphenicol has been shown to exert a bactericidal effect on *Hemophilus influenzae, Neisseria meningitidis*, and *Streptococcus pneumoniae* (7–9); hence its use for treatment of meningitis caused by these organisms. The bactericidal effect is dependent on the growth phase of the bacterial cells. Actively dividing cells die rapidly, whereas resting cells remain viable for long periods (10,11). The site of action of chloramphenicol is the single ribosomal protein receptor that also serves as that of erythromycin, oleandomycin, troleandomycin, clindamycin, and lincomycin (12,13).

It is generally accepted that chloramphenicol does not inhibit ribosomal protein synthesis in mammalian cells by the same mechanism as in bacterial cells (14). Protein synthesis in mammalian ribosomes, unlike that in bacterial ribosomes, is apparently unaffected by chloramphenicol (14). The effect of chloramphenicol on mitochondria appears to explain the dose-related hematopoietic toxicity of the drug.

SPECTRUM

The spectrum of activity of chloramphenicol is shown in Table 1. The drug is active against a wide variety of gram-positive and gram-negative bacteria, rickettsia, chlamydia, and mycoplasma. Organisms are considered highly susceptible to chloramphenicol if inhibited by 4 μg/ml, and moderately susceptible if inhibited by 16 μg/ml. Organisms almost universally sensitive include *Streptococcus pneumoniae*, group A

TABLE 1. *In vitro susceptibility of bacterial isolates to chloramphenicol*[a]

Organism	No. of strains	MIC range (μg/ ml)	Cumulative percentage inhibited[b]
Gram-positive			
Staphylococcus aureus	36	3.1–12.5	98 (12.5)
Staphylococcus epidermidis	35	1.6–25	95 (3.2)
Streptococcus pneumoniae	199	1.4–4.0	90 (3.8)
Group D Streptococcus			
Non-enterococcus	74	<1.9–16	97 (7.8)
Enterococcus	332	6.3–>100	56 (100)
Listeria	10	4–16	—
Gram-negative			
Escherichia coli	1,114	5–>20	87 (25)
Hemophilus sp.	122	0.1–3.1	95 (0.8)
Hemophilus influenzae	68	0.1–5.0	96 (1.0)
Klebsiella pneumoniae	132	1–>20	77 (20)
Neisseria gonorrhoeae	172	0.5–1.5	100 (<5)
Neisseria meningitidis	56	0.5–2	100 (2)
Salmonella sp.	17	5–10	100 (10)
Anaerobes			
Bacteroides sp.	72	0.25–12.5	100 (12.5)
Bacteroides fragilis	83	0.8–12.5	100 (12.5)
Clostridium perfringens	77	1.6–6.2	99 (3.2)
Fusobacterium sp.	18	0.1–6.2	100 (6.2)
Peptococcus	145	0.1–>25	97 (3.1)
Peptostreptococcus	72	0.2–6.2	96 (3.1)

MIC, minimum inhibitory concentration.
[a]See reference (15).
[b]Value in parentheses is concentration (μg/ml) at which inhibition occurs.

beta-hemolytic streptococci, viridans streptococci, enterococci, *Neisseria* species, *Hemophilus* species, corynebacteria, *Aeromonas hydrophila, Pasteurella multocida, Bacillus, Brucella, Bartonella, Listeria,* and virtually all obligately anaerobic bacteria. Chloramphenicol is also frequently active against *Salmonella* and *Shigella*. Its activity against *Enterobacteriaceae* is variable. Chloramphenicol is not active against *Pseudomonas aeruginosa*, fungi, or mycobacteria.

Although natural and acquired resistance to chloramphenicol has been demonstrated in some organisms, and has slowly increased over the years, it is relatively uncommon in a number of the life-threatening infections for which chloramphenicol is considered a first-line antibiotic. These infections include typhoid fever and the invasive salmonella infections, some anaerobic infections, rickettsial infections, and bacterial meningitis. Resistance to chloramphenicol was noted within a few years of its introduction. In 1955 epidemic strains of shigella resistant to many drugs, including chloramphenicol, appeared, leading investigators to recognize the phenomenon of transferable drug resistance mediated by R plasmids (16). Although chloramphenicol plasmid-mediated resistance was first observed in gram-negative bacteria (17), it also occurs in gram-positive organisms such as streptococci and *Staphylococcus aureus* (18). In vitro resistance to chloramphenicol has been shown to be induced in a stepwise manner. Plasmid-borne chloramphenicol resistance is due to the presence in resistant organisms of the enzyme chloramphenicol-acetyltransferase, which catalyzes acetylation of the molecule rendering the molecule unable to bind to the bacterial ribosome and thus microbiologically inactive. An excellent review of this topic has recently been published (19).

Resistance to chloramphenicol and the presence of the acetyltransferase enzyme have been documented in *Hemophilus influenzae* type b, but the incidence of resistance among clinical isolates of *Hemophilus influenzae* and *Streptococcus pneumoniae* remains very low in most countries (20,21). Since chloramphenicol achieves concentrations that are bactericidal against *Hemophilus influenzae* type b in the cerebrospinal fluid (CSF), it remains the drug of choice for the treatment of meningitis caused by this organism, especially if the organism is a β-lactamase producer (22,23). The vast majority of clinical isolates of *Bacteroides fragilis* remain sensitive to chloramphenicol, and the usefulness of the drug for infections involving this organism remains unchallenged.

PHARMACOKINETICS

Chloramphenicol is available as chloramphenicol base (in capsules) and palmitate ester (in liquid suspension) for oral administration. The parent compound, chloramphenicol base, is reserved for oral administration in capsule form because of its extreme bitterness; it cannot be given parenterally, because it is insoluble. Esters such as the palmitate form are used in liquid preparations for oral use. There are problems with the bioavailability of orally administered chloramphenicol. Absorption of the different preparations varies with particle size. Glazko et al. (24) reported a twofold difference in the peak serum concentrations achieved following oral administration of various preparations. These differences in bioavailability were due to differences in the in vitro solubility of the capsules.

The esters of chloramphenicol are biologically inactive and must be hydrolyzed to active chloramphenicol (25,26). The orally administered palmitate ester must be hydrolyzed in the duodenum by pancreatic lipases to allow complete absorption of active chloramphenicol (25,27). The absorption of the oral preparations is complete (24,28). Although liquid suspensions are especially useful in treating children who cannot swallow capsules, these suspensions are sometimes poorly absorbed from the gastrointestinal (GI) tract (27), possibly due to the poor aqueous solubility of the ester used in the preparation. One study in neonates (29) showed that the palmitate ester produced peak concentrations that were as much as 30% lower than those achieved in older children given equivalent doses. Also, the time to peak concentration in these newborns was delayed, occurring 12 h after administration. This decreased absorption may have been due to the newborns having less GI esterase activity. Absorption from the GI tract may not be reliable in this age group and therefore should not be used to treat serious infection. Numerous other studies comparing orally and parenterally administered chloramphenicol in infants and older children have recently been published (30–34). These studies report that higher serum concentrations of active chloramphenicol were achieved with orally administered chloramphenicol than after intravenous (i.v.) administration. One must conclude that in spite of the decreased bioavailability of orally administered chloramphenicol palmitate in comparison with chloramphenicol base, it is superior than that of the succinate ester given i.v. Oral administration of chloramphenicol palmitate appears to offer significant therapeutic advantages in the pediatric patient who can tolerate the oral route.

The esters of chloramphenicol that are freely water soluble, and therefore suitable for parenteral administration, are the sodium succinate and glycinate forms. Again, these esters must be hydrolyzed in the body to release the active drug (25,26). The hydrolysis of chloramphenicol succinate occurs in the liver; however, the rate at which this occurs is unpredictable and extremely variable in pediatric patients. Studies in newborns have shown a large variability in both serum concentration achieved and the half-life of chloramphenicol after i.v. administration of recommended doses (35–37). Half-lives extending to >48 h or even infinity (i.e., no decrease in serum concentration during the study period) have been reported. A close look at the recent literature shows that ~5% of the patients in any series will have no detectable change in chloramphenicol concentration during a dosing interval (35,38). One recent study of the pharmacokinetics of chloramphenicol in low-birth-weight infants showed peak serum concentrations ranging from 11 to 36 μg/ml and half-lives ranging from 10 to >48 h in infants 1–8 days old. In infants 11 days to 8 weeks old, peak serum concentrations ranged from 10 to 36 μg/ml and half-lives from 5 to 16 h (36).

On the basis of these data showing great variation in serum concentrations and half-life values in neonates, especially low-birth-weight and preterm babies, the following dosages are recommended during the neonatal period. Premature and full-term infants <2 weeks of age should receive 25 mg/kg/day i.v. All infants >2 weeks of age should receive 50 mg/kg/day i.v. in two divided doses. Infants 2–4 weeks old should receive 50 mg/kg/day i.v. divided into four doses. Infants >4 weeks old and children should receive 50–100 mg/kg/day in four divided doses.

In infants <4 weeks of age chloramphenicol serum concentrations are most unpredictable (39,40). One of the greatest concerns of the pediatrician treating infants with chloramphenicol is toxic accumulation of the drug leading to fatal cardiovascular collapse (the "gray syndrome"), which is usually seen when chloramphenicol concentrations are >40 μg/ml (28,41,42). The clinician should closely monitor serum levels to ensure concentrations within the therapeutic range; susceptible organisms are defined as having minimum inhibitory concentrations (MICs) of ≤16 μg/ml of chloramphenicol. Serum concentrations exceeding 25 μg/ml are considered potentially toxic in terms of reversible bone marrow suppression (43,44). With these limitations in mind, the clinician should optimally dose the patient so that concentrations of 10–20 μg/ml are achieved.

The intramuscular route of administration should not be used because absorption is very poor and several reports of clinical failure due to subtherapeutic serum concentrations of active drug have appeared.

There is wide interpatient variation in the metabolism and excretion of chloramphenicol in the pediatric population. Once absorbed and hydrolyzed, the unesterified free form of the drug is in turn metabolized in the liver to the biologically inactive chloramphenicol glucuronide (47). The glucuronide is excreted mainly by renal tubular secretion. Approximately 10%

of circulating free chloramphenicol is not conjugated, but is directly excreted, unchanged, in the urine by glomerular filtration (47). Various authors have reported that in infants and children anywhere from 2 to 82% of an i.v. dose is excreted unchanged in the urine (30,31,38,48,49). This variable metabolism and variable excretion of chloramphenicol means that a significant amount of an administered dose will never be converted to the microbiologically active form (31,48). In premature infants and neonates, the rate of metabolism of chloramphenicol is decreased due to immature liver function. Renal tubular mechanisms are also considerably immature in the first weeks of life. For these reasons, doses of chloramphenicol that are satisfactory in older infants may produce high and prolonged serum concentrations in neonates.

Chloramphenicol is widely distributed in body fluids and tissues. Pleural, peritoneal, and synovial fluid concentrations have been reported as 30–50% of simultaneously observed serum concentrations. Consistently high concentrations are achieved in the central nervous system in either the presence or absence of inflammation. In lumbar CSF and ventricular fluid, concentrations of 50–90% of serum levels have been reported (35,50). Brain tissue levels 9 × the serum concentration and brain abscess concentrations of 25% of the serum level have been reported (51,52). Chloramphenicol has the unique ability to penetrate well into the aqueous humor and vitreous humor (53). Levels in lung, myocardium, and spleen generally range from 5 to 20 μg/ml (54). Joint fluid levels of ≥50% of serum concentration have been reported in patients with septic arthritis (55,56).

Levels of free chloramphenicol can be measured by use of microbiologic (57), radioenzymatic (58,59), and high pressure liquid chromatographic (60) techniques.

TOXICITY

The most important adverse effect of chloramphenicol is on the hematologic system; serious and fatal blood dyscrasias have occurred following its administration (Table 2). Chloramphenicol is associated with two different types of effects on the bone marrow: (a) a predictable, dose-related, reversible depression that can be prevented or modified by monitoring serum concentrations, and (b) an idiosyncratic reaction resulting in aplastic anemia, which cannot be predicted or prevented in susceptible patients. The dose-related form is considered an extension of the pharmacologic effect of chloramphenicol (61–63). It is postulated that chloramphenicol affects mammalian mitochondrial enzymes in much the same way that it affects organisms. In addition to its effect on other mitochondrial enzymes, chloramphenicol inhibits synthesis of ferrochelatase, the enzyme responsible for the final step in heme synthesis (64). This inhibition is responsible for the selective effect of chloramphenicol on erythropoiesis. Peripherally, there is decreased iron utilization and increased serum iron. The dose-related toxicity is characterized by anemia, with or without thrombocytopenia or leukopenia, increased serum iron, vacuolization, and maturation arrest of erythroid and myeloid precursors (44). This effect is related to dose and duration of therapy and associated with serum concentrations >25 μg/ml. As expected, toxicity has been observed most frequently in premature infants in whom hepatic enzyme systems and other physiologic processes are immature resulting in higher serum levels for prolonged periods of time.

TABLE 2. *Features of chloramphenicol-induced bone marrow toxicity*

	Type of toxicity	
Feature	Dose-related	Idiosyncratic
Incidence	In all patients receiving high doses and prolonged therapy	1:25,000–1:41,000 courses
Mechanism	Extension of pharmacologic effect	Unknown
Predisposing factors	Liver dysfunction, inappropriate dosing, serum concentrations >25 μg/ml	Genetic (?)
Onset	Usually day 5 of therapy	From 2 weeks to 12 months after discontinuation
Outcome	Returns to normal after drug is discontinued	Often fatal
Monitoring parameters	Complete blood cell count with differential and platelet counts and measurements of serum iron level and iron-binding capacity	None

Contrary to what is seen in studies of normal volunteers, this dose-related toxicity is usually clinically seen as early as day 5 of therapy. This early onset is probably due to increased myeloproliferation secondary to infection. Recovery usually occurs within 1 to

3 weeks after discontinuation of the drug. Anemia and decreased reticulocyte counts do not necessarily contraindicate the continued use of the drug. Patients should be monitored with complete blood cell counts, including differential and platelet counts, and serum iron determinations every 4–5 days during therapy (65). In addition, serum iron level and iron-binding capacity should be determined at the onset of therapy for use as a baseline.

The second type of blood dyscrasia, aplastic anemia, is idiosyncratic, irreversible, and fatal in ≥50% of affected patients. In one study, 70% of the patients were 2–9 years old (66). The pathogenesis of the aplastic anemia is unclear. It is characterized by bone marrow hypoplasia or aplasia. Peripherally, it is most often manifested by pancytopenia, but in a few cases one, two, or all major cell types (erythrocytes, leukocytes, and thrombocytes) may be depressed. Onset has been reported to be from 2 weeks to 12 months following discontinuation of the chloramphenicol (66–69). This toxicity cannot be predicted by monitoring blood counts, because the irreversible stage occurs before changes are seen.

The relative risk of developing aplastic anemia following oral or parenteral therapy is the subject of some controversy. It has been suggested that development of aplastic anemia is associated only with the oral use of chloramphenicol (70,71), but this should be critically reviewed. No valid scientific data are available to support this conclusion. This association may be due in part to the fact that a very large number of patients have received the drug orally. Data are not available comparing the incidence of bone marrow aplasia following oral and parenteral therapy. Unfortunately, most studies examining the incidence of aplastic anemia have failed to document any route of administration (66,69). The suggestion that it is the oral use of the drug that causes the toxicity has been based on the false conclusion that only a very few cases of aplastic anemia have developed following parenteral administration (72). The vast difference in the number of courses of therapy given by one route versus the other prevents the issue from being settled on epidemiologic grounds. Also lacking is a definite mechanism for the fatal aplasia, although many hypotheses exist (71,73–76). One must conclude that the available data are inadequate to support the belief that the exclusive use of i.v. chloramphenicol will result in greater safety.

A very serious nonhematopoietic toxicity given considerable attention is the "gray syndrome." In 1959, a report of unexplained peripheral vascular collapse occurred in infants given high doses of chloramphenicol (28). Other reports described a high mortality rate following respiratory distress syndrome and circulatory collapse in premature infants treated with the drug (77). This clinical picture in infants treated with chloramphenicol became characteristic and was termed the "gray syndrome." In most cases, therapy had been instituted within the first 48 h of life. Symptoms first appeared after 3–4 days of continued treatment with high doses of chloramphenicol (100 mg/kg/day) (29). Symptoms appear in the following order: (a) abdominal distention, with or without emesis; (b) progressive pallid cyanosis; (c) vasomotor collapse, frequently accompanied by irregular respiration; and (d) death within a few hours of the onset of symptoms (29). Serum chloramphenicol levels were unusually high (>90 μg/ml) in these patients, but the gray syndrome has been reported at levels of 75 μg/ml (77). The neonate is especially predisposed to this toxicity since immaturity of the hepatic glucuronyl transferase system results in impaired metabolism of chloramphenicol and elevated, prolonged serum concentrations (78). This toxicity is due to the free drug rather than its metabolite (29). The gray syndrome is seen most frequently in premature and full-term infants during the first week after birth, but has been reported in older infants and toddlers (79,80); the oldest infant with gray syndrome reported to date was 25 months old (81).

Management of overdosed infants is complex and often unsuccessful. Hemodialysis and peritoneal dialysis remove only minimal concentrations of chloramphenicol (82,83). Exchange transfusion has yielded variable results (84,85). Charcoal hemoperfusion seems to be quite promising, since it is effective in decreasing chloramphenicol concentrations by ~60% (86,87).

Other adverse effects associated with chloramphenicol use are very rare. Optic neuritis and peripheral neuritis have been associated with long-term therapy (88,89).

INTERACTIONS

Chloramphenicol competes with other compounds metabolized by the hepatic microsomal enzyme system. Phenytoin metabolism has been reported to be inhibited by chloramphenicol (90–94). Since phenytoin is often administered to control seizure activity in patients with meningitis, phenytoin concentrations should be monitored and dosages appropriately altered to prevent toxicity in these patients. A brief report on the enhancement of chloramphenicol metabolism by concomitantly administered phenytoin in a

7-year-old child has recently been published (95). The peak concentration of chloramphenicol was reduced by ~46% with concomitant phenytoin. Following the addition of phenobarbital therapy, the chloramphenicol peak concentration declined further, to 63% of its already reduced level. Interestingly enough, both the phenytoin and the phenobarbital concentration remained within their therapeutic ranges. The obvious consequences of subtherapeutic chloramphenicol concentrations, especially in patients with central nervous system infections, emphasized the need for close monitoring of chloramphenicol levels in such cases.

Phenobarbital increases chloramphenicol metabolism resulting in subtherapeutic concentrations (95–97). In one report, a child receiving 100 mg/kg/day of chloramphenicol, with resultant peak concentrations of 31 μg/ml, was started on phenobarbital therapy, and after 5 days the chloramphenicol peak concentration decreased to 5 μg/ml (96).

Chloramphenicol decreases the metabolism of other drugs such as dicumarol and tricyclic antidepressants, with resultant increases in their respective adverse effects (98). A report on the interaction between chloramphenicol and acetaminophen resulting in decreased chloramphenicol metabolism and increased chloramphenicol half-life has recently been published (99). However, due to several inherent faults in the study, the results should be viewed very cautiously until they can be confirmed.

Patients receiving phenytoin and/or phenobarbital while on chloramphenicol therapy should have serum concentrations of all three medications measured at least one time during the course of therapy. If this is not done, special effort should be made to monitor these patients closely for signs and symptoms of toxicity or therapeutic failure.

THERAPEUTIC USAGE

Chloramphenicol should be reserved for treatment of selected, serious infections caused by susceptible organisms when potentially less toxic antibiotics are ineffective or contraindicated. Chlorampenicol is considered the drug of choice for typhoid fever and enteric fevers caused by susceptible organisms (70, 100,101). Chloramphenicol appears superior to trimethoprim–sulfamethoxazole for the treatment of typhoid fever (102). Amoxicillin has proven superior to ampicillin and may be as effective as chloramphenicol for treatment of this disease (103). Strains of chloramphenicol-resistant *Salmonella typhi* and other salmonella have been reported in Southeast Asia (104). Those strains of chloramphenicol-resistant *Salmonella typhi* that caused the typhoid epidemic in Mexico in the early 1970s returned to their original sensitivity after the epidemic subsided (105). Chloramphenicol is considered the drug of choice in penicillin-allergic patients with meningitis caused by *Hemophilus influenzae, Streptococcus pneumoniae*, or *Neisseria meningitidis* (106). Over the years, the percentage of *Hemophilus influenzae* type b strains resistant to ampicillin has steadily increased to the current level of 15–30% of clinical isolates. Consequently, ampicillin, once regarded as equally effective to chloramphenicol for *Hemophilus influenzae* type b meningitis, is no longer dependable (107,108). Chloramphenicol may be preferable for treatment of other invasive *Hemophilus influenzae* infections, including pneumonia, cellulitis, bacteremia, arthritis, and epiglottitis.

Because chloramphenicol has the unique ability to cross the blood–brain barrier and is active against most organisms causing brain abscess, it is considered a drug of choice for empirical treatment of brain abscess prior to culture and sensitivity results (109–111). Chloramphenicol is especially useful for temporal lobe abscess of otic origin, usually caused by a mixed bacterial flora, including anaerobes such as *Bacteroides fragilis* (112). Although tetracycline may be preferred in treating older patients, chloramphenicol is preferred in treating young children with rickettsial diseases and melioidosis (113,114). There is renewed interest in using chloramphenicol for the treatment of gram-negative anaerobic infections. Although clindamycin, metronidazole, cefoxitin, and ticarcillin or mezlocillin are also effective against the anaerobes, including *Bacteroides fragilis*, clinicians seem to prefer chloramphenicol for serious infection, especially of the central nervous system.

Chloramphenicol clearly remains a valuable and lifesaving agent in today's clinical practice, even with the introduction of newer antibiotics. Its unique pharmacokinetic characteristics, coupled with its antimicrobial spectrum, make it an ideal agent for the treatment of many life-threatening infections. The use of this drug must be combined with a full understanding of its limitations. Careful patient monitoring will allow the pediatrician to maximize its therapeutic efficacy and minimize the risk of drug-related toxicity.

REFERENCES

1. Ehrlich J, Gottlieb D, Burkholder PR, et al. *Streptomyces venezuelae*, the source of Chloromycetin. *J Bacteriol* 1948;56:567.
2. Rich ML, Ritterhoff RJ, Hoffman RJ. A fatal case of aplastic

anemia following chloramphenicol therapy. *Ann Intern Med* 1950;33:1459–67.
3. Volini IF, Greenspan I, Ehrlich L, et al. Hemopoietic changes during administration of chloramphenicol. *JAMA* 1950;142:1333–5.
4. Weiss PJ, Andrew ML, Wright WW. Solubility of antibiotics in twenty-four solvents: use in analysis. *Antibiot Chemother* 1957;7:374–6.
5. Cundliffe E, McQuillen K. Bacterial protein synthesis: the effects of antibiotics. *J Mol Biol* 1967;30:137–46.
6. Green CE, Cameron HJ, Julian GR. Recovery of polysome function of T4-infected *E. coli* after brief treatment with chloramphenicol and rifampin. *Antimicrob Agents Chemother* 1975;7:549–54.
7. Overturf GD, Wilkins J, Leedom JM, et al. Susceptibility of *Hemophilus influenzae*, type b, to ampicillin at Los Angeles County/University of Southern California Medical Center. *J Pediatr* 1975;87:297–300.
8. Rahal JJ Jr, Simberkoff MS. Bactericidal and bacteriostatic action of chloramphenicol against meningeal pathogens. *Antimicrob Agents Chemother* 1979;16:13–8.
9. Wehrle PF, Mathies AW, Leedom JM, et al. Bacterial meningitis. *Ann NY Acad Sci* 1967;145:488–98.
10. Bacchus AN, Javor GT. Stability of *Escherichia coli* membrane proteins during chloramphenicol treatment. *Antimicrob Agents Chemother* 1975;8:387–9.
11. Gupta RS. Killing and lysis of *E. coli* in the presence of chloramphenicol: relation to cellular magnesium. *Antimicrob Agents Chemother* 1975;7:748.
12. Pongs O, Bald R, Erdman VA. Identification of chloramphenicol binding protein in *E. coli* ribosome by affinity labeling. *Proc Natl Acad Sci USA* 1973;70:2229–33.
13. Vazguez D. Binding of chloramphenicol to ribosomes. The effect of a number of antibiotics. *Biochim Biophys Acta* 1966;114:277–88.
14. Yunis AA. Concluding remarks. International Symposium on Chloramphenicol–thiamphenicol. *Postgrad Med J* 50(suppl 5):1974;149.
15. Lorian V. Species incidence and trends in susceptibility. In: Lorian V, ed. *Antibiotics in laboratory medicine*. Baltimore: Williams & Wilkins, 1980:653–5.
16. Watanale T. Infective heredity of multiple drug resistance in bacteria. *Bacteriol Rev* 1963;27:87–115.
17. Shaw WV. The enzymatic acetylation of chloramphenicol by extracts of R factor-resistant *E. coli*. *J Biol Chem* 1967;242:687–93.
18. Miyamura S, Ochiai H, Nitahara Y, et al. Resistance mechanism of chloramphenicol in *Streptococcus haemolyticus, Streptococcus pneumoniae*, and *Streptococcus faecalis*. *Microbiol Immunol* 1977;21:69–97.
19. Shaw WV. Bacterial resistance to chloramphenicol. *Br Med Bull* 1984;40:36–41.
20. Jahn G, Laufs R, Kaulfers PM, et al. Molecular nature of two *Haemophilus influenzae* R factors containing resistances and the multiple integration of drug resistance transposons. *J Bacteriol* 1979;138:584–97.
21. Roberts M, Corney A, Shaw WV. Molecular characterization of three chloramphenicol acetyltransferases isolated from *Haemophilus influenzae*. *J Bacteriol* 1982;151:737–41.
22. Feldman WE, Manning NS. Effect of growth phase on the bactericidal action of chloramphenicol against *Haemophilus influenzae* type b and *Escherichia coli* K-1. *Antimicrob Agents Chemother* 1983;23:551–4.
23. Turk DC. A comparison of chloramphenicol and ampicillin as bactericidal agents for *Haemophilus influenzae* type b. *J Med Microbiol* 1977;10:127–31.
24. Glazko AJ, Kinkel AW, Alegnani WC, et al. An evaluation of the absorption characteristics of different chloramphenicol preparations in normal human subjects. *Clin Pharmacol Ther* 1968;9:472–83.
25. Glazko AJ, Edgerton WH, Dill WA, et al. Chloromycetin Palmitate—a synthetic ester of Chloromycetin. *Antibiot Chemother* 1952;2:234–42.
26. Ross S, Burke FG, Rice EC. The use of Chloromycetin Palmitate in infants and children: a preliminary report. *Antibiot Chemother* 1952;2:199–207.
27. Glazko AJ, Dill WA, Kazenko A, et al. Physical factors affecting the rate of absorption of chloramphenicol ester. *Antibiot Chemother* 1958;8:516–27.
28. Sutherland JM. Fatal cardiovascular collapse of infants receiving large amounts of chloramphenicol. *Am J Dis Child* 1959;97:761–7.
29. Weiss CF, Glazko AJ, Weston JK. Chloramphenicol in the newborn infant. A physiological explanation of its toxicity when given in excessive doses. *N Engl J Med* 1960;262:787–94.
30. Kauffman RE, Miceli JN, Strebel L, et al. Pharmacokinetics of chloramphenicol and chloramphenicol succinate in infants and children. *J Pediatr* 1981;98:315–20.
31. Kauffman RE, Thirumoorthi MC, Buckley JA, et al. Relative bioavailability of intravenous chloramphenicol succinate and oral chloramphenicol palmitate in infants and children. *J Pediatr* 1981;99:963–7.
32. Pickering LK, Hoecker JL, Kramer WG, et al. Clinical pharmacology of two chloramphenicol preparations in children: sodium succinate (IV) and palmitate (oral) esters. *J Pediatr* 1980;96:757–61.
33. Tuomanen E, Smith A, Powell K, et al. Oral chloramphenicol pharmacokinetics in *H. influenzae* b meningitis [Abstract]. *Twentieth interscience conference on antimicrobial agents and chemotherapy*. New Orleans: 1980:[abstract]186.
34. Yogev R, Kolling WM, Williams T. Pharmacokinetic comparison of intravenous and oral chloramphenicol in patients with *Haemophilus influenzae* meningitis. *Pediatrics* 1981;67:656–60.
35. Friedman CA, Lovejoy FC, Smith AL. Chloramphenicol disposition in infants and children. *J Pediatr* 1979;95:1071–7.
36. Glazer JP, Danish MA, Plotkin SA, et al. Disposition of chloramphenicol in low birth weight infants. *Pediatrics* 1980;66:573–8.
37. Rajchgot P, Prober CG, Soldin S, et al. Initiation of therapy in the newborn infant. *J Pediatr* 1982;101:1018–21.
38. Sack CM, Korys JR, Opheim KE, et al. Chloramphenicol succinate kinetics in infants and young children. *Pediatr Pharmacol* 1982;2:93.
39. Black SB, Levine P, Shinefield HR. The necessity for monitoring chloramphenicol levels when treating neonatal meningitis. *J Pediatr* 1978;92:235–6.
40. Hodgman JE, Burns LE. Safe and effective chloramphenicol dosage for premature infants. *Am J Dis Child* 1961;101:140–8.
41. Lietman PS. Chloramphenicol and the neonate—1979 view. *Clin Perinatol* 1979;6:151–62.
42. Thompson WL, Anderson SE, Lipsky JJ, et al. Overdose of chloramphenicol. *JAMA* 1975;234:149–50.
43. McCurdy PR. Plasma concentration of chloramphenicol and bone marrow suppression. *Blood* 1963;21:263–72.
44. Scott JL, Finegold SM, Belkin GA, et al. A controlled double blind study of the hematologic toxicity of chloramphenicol. *N Engl J Med* 1965;272:1137–42.
45. DuPont HL, Hornick RB, Weiss CF, et al. Evaluation of chloramphenicol acid succinate therapy of induced typhoid fever and Rocky Mountain spotted fever. *N Engl J Med* 1970;282:53–7.
46. Shah PN, D'Souza J, Dattani KK. Absorption of chloram-

phenicol by various routes of administration. *India J Med Res* 1977;65:549–53.
47. Glazko AJ, Wolf LM, Dill WA, et al. Biochemical studies on chloramphenicol. *J Pharmacol Exp Ther* 1949;96:445–59.
48. Sack CM, Korys J, Opheim K, et al. Pharmacokinetics of chloramphenicol-succinate after intravenous administration. *Pediatr Res* 1980;14:472.
49. Slaughter RL, Pieper JA, Cerra FB, et al. Chloramphenicol sodium succinate kinetics in critically-ill patients. *Pharmacol Ther* 1980;28:69–77.
50. Dunkle LM. Central nervous system chloramphenicol concentration in premature infants. *Antimicrob Agents Chemother* 1978;13:427–9.
51. Kramer PW, Griffith RS, Campbell RL. Antibiotic penetration of the brain. A comparative study. *J Neurosurg* 1969;31:295–302.
52. Black P, Graybill JP, Charache P. Penetration of brain abscess by systemically administered antibiotics. *Neurosurgery* 1973;38:705–9.
53. Leopold IH, Nichols AC. Penetration of chloramphenicol into the eye. *Arch Ophthalmol* 1950;44:22.
54. Gray JG. The concentration of chloramphenicol in human tissue. *Clin Lab Notes* 1955;72:778.
55. Joeson CT. The diffusion of antibiotics through the synovial membrane. *J Bone Joint Surg* 1955;37A:107.
56. Rapp GE, Griffith RS, Hebble WM. The permeability of traumatically inflamed synovial membrane to commonly used antibiotics. *J Bone Joint Surg* 1966;48:1534–40.
57. Bannatyne RM, Cheung R. Chloramphenicol bioassay. *Antimicrob Agents Chemother* 1979;16:43–5.
58. Lietman PS, White TJ, Shaw WV. Chloramphenicol: an enzymological microassay. *Antimicrob Agents Chemother* 1976;10:347–53.
59. Smith AL, Rosenberg IR, Smith DH, et al. Enzymatic microassay of chloramphenicol. *Pediatr Res* 1975;9:345.
60. Sample RHB, Glick MR, Kleiman MB, et al. High-pressure liquid chromatographic assay of chloramphenicol in biologic fluids. *Antimicrob Agents Chemother* 1979;15:491–3.
61. Freeman KB. Inhibition of mitochondrial and bacterial protein synthesis by chloramphenicol. *Can J Biochem* 1970;48:479.
62. Martelo OJ, Manyan DR, Smith US, et al. Chloramphenicol and bone marrow mitochondria. *J Lab Clin Med* 1969;74:927.
63. Ratzan J, Moore MAS, Yunis AA. Effect of chloramphenicol and thiamphenicol in the in vitro colony-forming cell. *Blood* 1974;43:363–9.
64. McKay R, Druyan R, Getz GS. Intramitochondrial localization of delta aminolevulinic acid synthetase and ferrochelatase in rat liver. *Biochem J* 1969;114:45.
65. Oski F. Hematologic consequences of chloramphenicol therapy. *J Pediatr* 1979;94:515.
66. Best WR. Chloramphenicol-associated blood dyscrasias—a review of cases submitted to the AMA Registry. *JAMA* 1967;201:181–8.
67. Helbriegel KP, Gross R. Follow-up studies in chloramphenicol-induced aplastic anemia. *Postgrad Med J* 1974;50:S136.
68. Polak BC, Wesseling H, Schut D, et al. Blood dyscrasias attributed to chloramphenicol. A review of 576 published and unpublished cases. *Acta Med Scand* 1972;192:409–14.
69. Yunis AA, Bloomberg GR. Chloramphenicol toxicity: clinical features and pathogens. *Prog Hematol* 1967;4:138–59.
70. Gleckman RA. Warning—chloramphenicol may be good for your health. *Arch Intern Med* 1975;135:1125–6.
71. Holt R. The bacterial degradation of chloramphenicol. *Lancet* 1967;1:1259–60.
72. Wallerstein RO, Condit PK, Kasper CK, et al. Statewide study of chloramphenicol therapy and fatal aplastic anemia. *JAMA* 1969;208:2045–50.
73. Dameshek W. Chloramphenicol aplastic anemia in identical twins—a clue to pathogenesis. *N Engl J Med* 1969;281:42–3.
74. Morley A, Trainor K, Remes J. Residual marrow damage: possible explanation for idiosyncrasy to chloramphenicol. *Br J Haematol* 1976;32:525–31.
75. Nagao T, Mauer AM. Concordance for drug-induced aplastic anemia in identical twins. *N Engl J Med* 1969;281:7–11.
76. Yunis AA. Chloramphenicol-induced bone marrow suppression. *Semin Hematol* 1973;10:225–34.
77. Burns LE, Hodgman JE, Cass AB. Fatal circulatory collapse in premature infants receiving chloramphenicol. *N Engl J Med* 1959;261:1318–21.
78. Meissner HC, Smith AL. The current status of chloramphenicol. *Pediatrics* 1979;64:348–56.
79. Maddox RR, Reigart JR, Anastasio GA. Gray toddler syndrome at recommended chloramphenicol succinate dosage in a critically ill infant. *Drug Intell Clin Pharm* 1982;16:477–9.
80. Morton K. Chloramphenicol overdosage in a 6-week-old infant. *Am J Dis Child* 1961;102:430.
81. Craft AW, Brocklebank JT, Hey EN. The "gray toddler": chloramphenicol toxicity. *Arch Dis Child* 1974;49:235–237.
82. Greenberg PA, Randford JP. Removal and absorption of antibiotics in blood of patients with renal failure undergoing peritoneal dialysis. *Ann Intern Med* 1967;66:465.
83. Kunin CM, Glazco AJ, Finland M. Persistence of antibiotics in blood of patients with acute renal failure. II. Chloramphenicol and its metabolic products in the blood of patients with severe renal failure or hepatic cirrhosis. *J Clin Invest* 1959;38:1498–1508.
84. Kessler DL, Smith AL, Woodrum DR. Chloramphenicol toxicity in a neonate treated with exchange transfusion. *J Pediatr* 1980;96:140.
85. Stevens DC, Kleiman MB, Leitman PS, et al. Exchange transfusion in acute chlorotoxicity. *J Pediatr* 1981;99:651–3.
86. Freundlich M, Cynamon H, Tamer A, et al. Management of chloramphenicol intoxication in infancy by charcoal hemoperfusion. *J Pediatr* 1983;103:485–7.
87. Mauer SM, Chavers BM, Kjellstrand CM. Treatment of an infant with severe chloramphenicol intoxication using charcoal column hemoperfusion. *J Pediatr* 1980;96:136–9.
88. Huang NM, Harley RD, Promadhattavedi V, et al. Visual disturbances in cystic fibrotics following chloramphenicol administration. *J Pediatr* 1966;68:32–44.
89. Wallenstein L, Synder J. Neurotoxic reaction to Chloromycetin. *Ann Intern Med* 1952;36:1526–8.
90. Adams HR, Isaacson EL, Masters BS. Inhibition of hepatic microsomal enzymes by chloramphenicol. *J Pharmacol Exp Ther* 1977;203:388.
91. Boolek RE, Reidenberg MM, Orr L. Inhibition of diphenylhydantoin metabolism by chloramphenicol. *Lancet* 1973;1:150.
92. Koup J, Gibaldi M, McNamara P, et al. Interaction of chloramphenicol with phenytoin and phenobarbital. *Clin Pharmacol Ther* 1978;24:571.
93. Rose JQ, Choi HK, Schentag JJ, et al. Intoxication caused by the interaction of chloramphenicol and phenytoin. *JAMA* 1977;237:2630–1.
94. Vincent FM, Mills C, Sullivan JK. Chloramphenicol-induced phenytoin intoxication. *Ann Neurol* 1978;3:469.
95. Powell DA, Nahata MC, Durrell DC, et al. Interactions among chloramphenicol, phenytoin, and phenobarbital in a pediatric patient. *J Pediatr* 1981;98:1001–3.
96. Bloxham RA, Durbin GM, Johnson T, et al. Chloramphenicol and phenobarbitone: a drug interaction. *Arch Dis Child* 1979;54:76–7.

97. Krasinski K, Kusmiesz H, Nelson JD. Pharmacologic interactions among chloramphenicol, phenytoin and phenobarbital. *Pediatr Infect Dis* 1982;1:232.
98. Christensen LK, Skousted L. Inhibition of drug metabolism by chloramphenicol. *Lancet* 1969;2:1,397–9.
99. Buchanan N, Moodley GP. Interaction between chloramphenicol and paracetamol. *Br Med J* 1979;2:307–8.
100. Anderson ES, Smith HR. Chloramphenicol resistance in the typhoid bacillus. *Br Med J* 1972;3:329–31.
101. Robertson RP, Wahab MFA, Raasch FO. Evaluation of chloramphenicol and ampicillin in *Salmonella* enteric fever. *N Engl J Med* 1968;278:171–6.
102. Snyder MJ, Peroni J, Gonzalez O, et al. Comparative efficacy of chloramphenicol, ampicillin, and co-trimoxazole in the treatment of typhoid fever. *Lancet* 1976;2:1155–7.
103. Neu HC. Amoxicillin. *Ann Intern Med* 1979;90:356–60.
104. Sharma KB, Blum Bhat M, Pasrucha A, et al. Multiple antibiotic resistance among salmonellae in India. *J Antimicrob Chemother* 1979;5:15–21.
105. Ryder RW, Blake PA. Typhoid fever in the United States, 1975 and 1976. *J Infect Dis* 1979;139:124–6.
106. Westenfelder GO, Paterson YL. Life-threatening infection: choice of alternate drugs when penicillin cannot be given. *JAMA* 1969;210:845–8.
107. Barrett FF, Taber LH, Morris CR, et al. A 12 year review of antibiotic management of *Hemophilus influenzae* meningitis. *J Pediatr* 1972;81:370–7.
108. Feigin RD, Stechenberg BW, Chang MJ, et al. Prospective evaluation of treatment of *Hemophilus influenzae* meningitis. *J Pediatr* 1976;88:542–8.
109. Brewer NS, MacCarty CS, Wellman WE. Brain abscess: a review of recent experience. *Ann Intern Med* 1975;82:571–6.
110. Finegold SM, Bartlett JG, Chow AW, et al. Management of anaerobic infections. *Ann Intern Med* 1975;83:375–89.
111. Heineman HS, Braude AI. Anaerobic infection of the brain. *Am J Med* 1963;35:682–97.
112. deLouvois J. The bacteriology and chemotherapy of brain abscess. *J Antimicrob Chemother* 1978;4:395–413.
113. Haynes RE, Sanders DY, Cramblett HG. Rocky Mountain spotted fever in children. *J Pediatr* 1970;76:685–93.
114. Kelsey DS. Rocky Mountain spotted fever. *Pediatr Clin North Am* 1979;26:367–376.

Therapeutic Drug Monitoring
7:168–173 © 1985 Raven Press, New York

Theophylline Serum Concentrations in Ambulatory Patients with Chronic Obstructive Pulmonary Disease

James W. Bredon, *J. Lyle Bootman, *William N. Jones, *William F. McGhan, †Donald G. Perrier, and ‡Sammy C. Campbell

*United States Public Health Service, Pineridge, South Dakota; *Department of Pharmacy Practice, College of Pharmacy, and Department of Internal Medicine, College of Medicine, University of Arizona, and ‡Veterans Administration Medical Center, Tucson, Arizona, U.S.A.; and †College of Pharmacy, University of Otago, Dunedin, New Zealand*

Summary: A two-part study was designed to investigate the application of theophylline serum concentration data at a Veterans Administration Medical Center. The investigation was unique in its use of ambulatory patients instead of hospitalized patients as study subjects for assessing the use of laboratory tests. As has been found in other studies that examined different drugs and involved hospitalized subjects, this investigation discovered significant problems in the ordering, application, and documentation of these data when judged against established criteria. There was no significant difference in the appropriate use of these drugs between physicians specializing in pulmonary versus general medicine. Of clinical importance also are the findings that confirm a positive correlation between the proper use of these tests and improvement in patient outcome, and the demonstrated relationships between clinical symptoms and subtherapeutic and toxic serum concentrations of theophylline. **Key Words:** Theophylline—Serum concentration—Chronic obstructive pulmonary disease—Enzyme multiplied immunoassay technique.

A review by Ogilvie (1) reported on a variety of studies that have demonstrated the beneficial effects of theophylline and its analogs. However, a major concern among prescribers of these drugs has been the toxicity associated with their use in some patients (2). Adverse reactions ranging in severity from mild to fatal have been reported (3–5). Furthermore, a report by Zwillich et al. (6) demonstrated that serious toxicity in the form of generalized seizures can occur without being preceded by signs of less severe reactions. The 50% mortality rate and the seizures' resistance to anticonvulsant therapy made this form of theophylline toxicity of particular concern because it can be resistant to conventional methods of treatment.

Therapeutic effectiveness and toxicity have been shown to correlate closely with the concentration of theophylline in serum (7–9). Bronchodilation is thought to be minimal at 5 μg/ml, whereas concentrations in the therapeutic range of 10 to 20 μg/ml are considered to be most effective (10–12). Above 20 μg/ml, adverse reactions become a threat and are more prevalent and severe as concentrations increase past this point (13,14).

The achievement of serum concentrations within the relative narrow range necessary for safe and effective therapy with these drugs is made more difficult by the large variations in serum concentrations found among individuals equivalently dosed. Age, cardiovascular and pulmonary status, level of tocacco use, presence of liver disease or obesity, type of diet, and concurrent use of certain drugs are thought to effect theophylline disposition (15–21).

These factors point to the necessity for individualizing dosage regimens with these drugs. The availability of laboratory assays for theophylline in serum that are accurate, reasonable in cost, and rapidly done has made the use of these assays an important tool in efforts to provide optimum therapy (22,23). Trained clinical observation combined with the proper use of

Address correspondence and reprint requests to Dr. J. L. Bootman at Department of Pharmacy Practice, College of Pharmacy, University of Arizona, Tucson, AZ 85721, U.S.A.

theophylline serum concentration data has been shown to be effective in providing relief of bronchoconstriction while avoiding toxicity (24).

Studies concerned with the application of serum concentrations to make dosage recommendations have raised questions about the appropriate use of this technology. Examination of the sampling process and use of the data obtained from assays for gentamicin, digoxin, and phenytoin in four separate studies demonstrated significant problems in terms of the correct utilization of serum drug concentrations for making rational therapeutic decisions (25–28). Omission of information on the laboratory order, as well as inappropriate times for obtaining samples, resulted in data being unusable for many patients. The absence of indications that assay results were ever acknowledged in any way or used to effect therapy was also demonstrated as a frequent problem. Each of these studies, however, was done using hospitalized patients as study subjects.

PURPOSE

There are few available reports assessing the application of serum concentration data in ambulatory patients. Theophylline and its congeners are frequently used in outpatients to treat chronic obstructive pulmonary disease (COPD) over extended periods of time. This investigation was conducted to achieve the following objectives: (a) to assess the appropriateness of the use of theophylline serum concentration data in a series of ambulatory patients under treatment for COPD at a Veterans Administration medical center, (b) to compare physicians specializing in pulmonary medicine with physicians specializing in general medicine in terms of their use of theophylline serum concentration data, (c) to assess the ability of physicians practicing at the study hospital to determine which patients are at risk from subtherapeutic or toxic serum concentrations, as shown by the decision to request a laboratory determination, and (d) to determine whether the signs and symptoms noted by physicians in their assessments of the study subjects could be related to theophylline serum concentrations found in these patients.

METHODS

The first part of this investigation involved review of the medical records of 100 patients. This part was undertaken to accomplish objectives (a) and (b). For this purpose, patient numbers (corresponding to Social Security numbers) were obtained from the clinical laboratory files of patients for whom a theophylline serum concentration assay had been performed during the 8-month period prior to the beginning of this retrospective investigation. Only those assays reported as being ordered for outpatients were included. The medical records for these patients were requested and reviewed initially for diagnosis. Only those patients with a diagnosis of COPD and for whom an oral formulation of theophylline, aminophylline, or oxtriphylline had been prescribed were selected for inclusion in the first phase of the study. The records of the first 100 patients who met these criteria were then further reviewed and the following information recorded: age, sex, height, weight, diagnosis of other chronic or acute illnesses, other medications used, smoking history, theophylline product prescribed and directions for use, and the date and result of the laboratory report of the theophylline serum concentration assay in the patient's file.

The second part of this investigation was a prospective study lasting 4 months. This portion accomplished objectives (c) and (d). Patients who presented a prescription to the outpatient pharmacy at the hospital for an oral theophylline, aminophylline, or oxtriphylline product were interviewed by the investigator. Patients who had not been taking one of these drugs for at least the preceding 2 weeks were not considered for inclusion in the study. Patients who had been seen in the outpatient clinics and who had reported having a blood sample drawn for a theophylline serum concentration became part of the pool of subjects from which the "physicians' group" was selected. Those patients who had been seen in the outpatient clinic regarding their pulmonary condition and who had not had blood drawn for a theophylline assay on their most recent appointment were asked to participate in the study. These patients constituted the "investigator's group" in this study. There were no patients who refused to participate in the study. All assays were accomplished via the enzyme multiplied immunoassay technique (EMIT, Syva Corporation).

The medical records of patients for whom theophylline serum concentrations were ordered by the investigator (investigator's group) and those of the patients who had assays ordered by their physician (physicians' group) were reviewed for the following information: age, sex, height, weight, diagnosis of active chronic or acute illnesses, other medications used, smoking history, and the physician's assessment of the patient's pulmonary status at the most recent examination. Changes were recorded (as noted by the physician) that revealed improvement or deterioration in the patient in symptoms of dyspnea or shortness of breath, coughing, sputum production, wheezing, or exercise tolerance. The following was also noted for patients having theophylline assays ordered by the physician: reason the assay was ordered, theophylline product prescribed and directions for use, time of sampling and time of last dose for the assay, and results of the assay.

RESULTS AND DISCUSSION

In the first part of this study, the medical records of 50 patients from the pulmonary clinics and 50 patients from the general medicine clinics were evaluated. All patients were men, with ages ranging from 46 to 82 years (mean ± SD, 62.5 ± 8.2 years). Pulmonary patients' ages ranged from 47 to 82 years (mean ± SD, 62.3 ± 8.8 years). General medicine patients' ages ranged from 46 to 79 years (mean ± SD, 62.8 ± 7.5 years).

A review of medical records produced the results summarized here.

In 65% of the 100 medical records reviewed, there were no statements indicating the reason the theophylline assay had been ordered. Therefore, only 35 charts (35%) had documentation of the reason the theophylline serum concentration assay was requested.

All of the 100 laboratory reports recorded the time the blood was drawn for the assay. When patients reported to the outpatient phlebotomists, the time was stamped on each laboratory report by a time clock just prior to the actual drawing of the blood sample.

Twenty-six laboratory reports had no indication of the time the patient had taken his last dose of theophylline prior to the time blood was taken for the assay.

Sixty-four of the 100 records had no indication that the theophylline assay was acknowledged or interpreted, up to and including the time of the patient's next appointment after the assay was requested.

Of 61 patients who had theophylline serum concentrations outside of the 10 to 20 μg/ml range, 13 (21.3%) were above 20 μg/ml, 13 (21.3%) were below 5 μg/ml, and 35 (57.4%) were in the range of 5 to 9.9 μg/ml. Thirty-two (52.5%) of the 61 patients outside of the 10 to 20 μg/ml range had no changes ordered in their theophylline dosage in response to the report. Conversely, 39 patients had a serum theophylline concentration in the range of 10 to 20 μg/ml.

As for the direction of dosage changes made in response to reported theophylline serum concentrations, 41 dosage changes were made in the 100 patients observed. Of the dosage changes made, 25 (61%) were judged appropriate (dose increased when concentration was less than 10 μg/ml and decreased when concentration was greater than 20 μg/ml). The remaining 16 dosage changes (39%) were judged questionable, since no justification was found in these patients' medical records for the changes made. Chi-square analysis (Table 1) revealed no difference between pulmonary and general medicine physicians in making dosage changes judged to be appropriate or inappropriate.

TABLE 1. *Comparison of physician specialty in dosage adjustments judged appropriate and questionable*

Physician specialty	Dosage adjustment: No. of appropriate[a]	No. of questionable[a]	Total[a]
Pulmonary	13 (61.9)	8 (38.1)	21 (100.0)
General medicine	12 (60.0)	8 (40.0)	20 (100.0)
Total	25 (61.0)	16 (39.9)	41 (100.0)

$\chi^2 = 0.04$; $df = 1$; NS.
[a]Percentages in parentheses.

To assess the outcome of changes in dosage that were judged "appropriate" or "inappropriate," the physicians' assessment of the patient, classified as "improved," "unchanged," "deteriorated," or "no assessment" was compared with appropriate and inappropriate designations in the 41 patients who had dosage changes. These results are shown in Table 2. The categories designated as "deteriorated," "unchanged," and "no assessment" were combined to permit χ^2 analysis. This procedure showed a significant difference in the response of patients who had appropriate changes in dosage as compared with those who had inappropriate changes. This suggests that a change in

TABLE 2. *Physician's assessment of patient's condition after appropriate and questionable changes in theophylline dosage*

Classification of dosage change	Physician's assessment: No. of improved[a]	No. of deteriorated, unchanged, or no assessment[a]	Total[a]
Appropriate	16 (64.0)	9 (36.0)	25 (100.0)
Questionable	4 (25.0)	12 (75.0)	16 (100.0)
Total	20 (48.8)	21 (51.2)	41 (100.0)

$\chi^2 = 4.48$; $df = 1$; $p < 0.05$.
[a]Percentages in parentheses.

dosage classified as "appropriate" was more likely to result in the physicians' assessment of the patients' clinical state as improved when compared with dosage changes classified as "inappropriate."

In the second part of this study, data were collected and analyzed to evaluate whether theophylline serum concentrations were different in patients who had these assays requested by their physician as compared with those who did not have this laboratory test ordered.

Results were obtained from 77 physician-ordered theophylline plasma concentration assays in ambulatory patients. These values were compared with the values obtained in 102 outpatients who had theophylline serum concentrations ordered by the investigator after the physician who examined the patient made a decision not to request the assay.

The ages of patients whose assays were physician-ordered ranged from 29 to 85 years (mean ± SD, 61.0 ± 9.4 years). One of the 77 patients was a woman (1.3%). Ages of the investigator's subjects ranged from 33 to 83 years (mean ± SD, 61.3 ± 7.4 years). Two of the 102 subjects were women (1.9%).

Table 3 shows the number of patients from each group who had theophylline serum concentrations within the ranges indicated as <5 μg/ml, 5 to 9.9 μg/ml, 10 to 20 μg/ml, and >20 μg/ml. Chi-square analysis revealed no significant differences between the two groups in numbers of patients having serum concentrations in these ranges ($\chi^2 = 4.157$; $df = 3$; NS). Further statistical analysis using Student's t test to determine differences between the means of the theophylline serum concentrations found in the physicians' and investigator's patients also showed no significant differences ($t = 1.05$; $df = 177$; NS). The mean (± SD) theophylline serum concentrations were 11.0 ± 5.9 and 10.0 ± 6.0 μg/ml in the physicians' group and the investigator's group, respectively.

The physicians' progress notes were reviewed and data tabulated that revealed any complaint of increased difficulty in breathing or a report by patients of any symptom that could be the result of toxic serum concentrations of theophylline.

When physicians' assessments were examined to determine whether a report of increasing difficulty in breathing could be associated with theophylline serum concentrations that were different from those found in subjects without shortness of breath, a trend in the direction of subtherapeutic theophylline concentrations in subjects complaining of increasing dyspnea was found (Table 4). The differences were shown to be statistically significant by χ^2 analysis ($\chi^2 = 12.241$; $df = 2$; $p < 0.01$).

Patients' reports of symptoms that have been related to theophylline toxicity were also recorded. These symptoms included headache, irregular heart rhythms, nausea or emesis, dizziness, hypotension, precordial pain, agitation or restlessness, and evidence of seizures; they were tabulated and analyzed. Table 5 shows comparison of the theophylline serum concentrations in subjects reporting none of these symptoms and subjects who did complain of one or more of these symptoms that were possibly caused by theophylline toxicity. The results reveal a definite trend toward increasing symptoms of toxicity as serum concentrations increase. This is borne out by χ^2 analysis, which shows a statistically significant difference between the groups ($\chi^2 = 28.264$; $df = 2$; $p < 0.001$). Although there is a statistically significant relationship between toxic manifestations and theophylline concentration, these results may not reflect clinical importance for the toxic manifestations seen, since certain manifestations can appear at any concentration.

DISCUSSION AND RECOMMENDATIONS

Analysis of the results from the first part of the study reveal problems in both the way theophylline assays were ordered at the study hospital and in documentation and interpretation of the assays. These results are not markedly different from previous data

TABLE 3. *Number of theophylline serum concentrations within ranges from physicians' and investigator's groups*

	Serum concentration (μg/ml)[a]				
Subject group	<5	5–9.9	10–20	>20	Total no. (%)
Physicians' patients	10 (12.0)	25 (32.5)	35 (45.4)	7 (9.1)	77 (100.0)
Investigator's patients	23 (22.5)	36 (35.3)	38 (37.2)	5 (4.9)	102 (100.0)
Total	33 (18.4)	61 (34.1)	73 (40.8)	12 (6.7)	179 (100.0)

$\chi^2 = 4.16$; $df = 3$; NS.
[a]Percentages in parentheses.

TABLE 4. *Number of subjects assessed by physicians as having increased dyspnea with subtherapeutic, therapeutic, and potentially toxic theophylline serum concentrations*

Physicians' assessment	Serum concentration (μg/ml)[a]			
	<10	10–20	>20	Total
Increased dyspnea	60 (64.5)	30 (32.3)	3 (3.2)	93 (100.0)
No change or improved	34 (39.5)	43 (50.0)	9 (10.5)	86 (100.0)
Total	94 (52.5)	73 (40.8)	12 (6.7)	179 (100.0)

$\chi^2 = 12.24$; $df = 2$; $p < 0.01$.
[a]Percentages in parentheses.

from other authors examining different drugs (25–28). A reason for ordering the assay and a notation in the chart that an assay had been ordered were not indicated in 65% of the records reviewed. Ideally, the reason for obtaining theophylline levels and the response to the result should be noted in the progress notes. Interpretation of the laboratory test is made simpler if complete data are available. In an outpatient setting where the patient may not be seen shortly after a previous visit, not knowing why a level was obtained at the prior visit may make an assessment of the result more difficult. Not having a reason noted in 65% of the cases may reflect less-than-optimal charting habits or a questionable reason for obtaining a level. Considering also that 64% of the records revealed no evidence that the assay results were acknowledged or used to change therapy, it is reasonable to suspect that documentation of these laboratory test results is often forgotten, ignored, or lost. An alternative possibility is that the interpretation of a theophylline result may be less likely if the reason for ordering the test was unclear.

An interesting finding resulted when the physician's assessment of the patient, at the next examination after a change in dosage was made, was compared with the classification of the change as "appropriate" or "inappropriate." A statistically significant difference was found, indicating that a change in dosage classified as "appropriate" was more likely to result in a physician's assessment of the patient's clinical state as improved when compared with dosage changes classified as "inappropriate." A reasonable conclusion is that properly ordered, documented, and interpreted theophylline assays that provide accurate, usable results can have the direct result of improving the patient's clinical state.

When pulmonary clinic and general medicine clinic physicians were compared in terms of their ability to use theophylline assays properly, no significant differences were found. A conclusion supportable by this finding is that the observed increased frequency of use of these drugs and assays by physicians specializing in pulmonary medicine had no effect on improving the appropriateness of these assays.

Statistical analysis of the findings in the second part produced no evidence that physicians at the study hospital could determine whether ambulatory patients under treatment were at risk from theophylline serum concentrations above or below the therapeutic range of 10 to 20 μg/ml.

A significant relationship was found between patient complaints of an increasing difficulty in breathing or symptoms of toxicity and their serum theophylline concentrations. Theophylline serum concentrations outside the therapeutic range were related to signs and symptoms of inefficacy and toxicity. This concentra-

TABLE 5. *Number of subjects assessed by physicians as having symptoms of possible theophylline toxicity with subtherapeutic, therapeutic, and toxic theophylline serum concentrations*

Physicians' assessment	Serum concentration (μg/ml)[a]			
	<10	10–20	>20	Total
Symptoms of toxicity	10 (27.8)	17 (47.2)	9 (25.0)	36 (100.0)
No symptoms of toxicity	84 (58.7)	56 (39.2)	3 (2.1)	143 (100.0)
Total	94 (52.5)	73 (40.8)	12 (6.7)	179 (100.0)

$\chi^2 = 28.26$; $df = 2$; $p < 0.001$.
[a]Percentages in parentheses.

tion–efficacy/toxicity relationship suggests that a more extensive investigation involving patient-specific factors, possibly related to the serum theophylline concentration, may be useful in any attempt to utilize the assay in patient management more effectively.

Evidence presented here suggests that the physician's examination and clinical assessment of the patient may not reveal ineffective or excessive theophylline dosage. The judicious use of theophylline serum concentration data to achieve and maintain therapeutic doses could result in improvement in patients with a disabling disease while helping to avoid the serious consequences of a possible overdose.

A limitation of this study is that the results cannot be extrapolated to other populations. Much of the information was collected retrospectively, which brings forth another set of limitations. Despite some of these concerns, it is believed that certain recommendations can be made. They are as follows:

Guidelines should be developed with recommendations from the laboratory, pharmacy, and medical services and the pharmacy and therapeutic committee to advise those ordering or interpreting theophylline assays on their appropriate use. A sheet containing these instructions should be provided to each new physician. An abbreviated form might also be developed to include with the laboratory slip used in reporting results of the assay.

The clinical pharmacy service should become involved with the laboratory and medical services to improve theophylline therapy by reviewing theophylline level results and recording these data in the patient's medical record on a routine basis. Whenever exceedingly high concentrations are found, the physician should also be notified by telephone.

Additional studies should be conducted to examine more thoroughly the outcome of properly used theophylline serum concentration data in terms of clinical improvement of patients. Also, studies should be designed to examine the relationship between the use of theophylline serum concentration data and the frequency of hospitalizations and emergency room visits.

REFERENCES

1. Ogilvie RJ. Clinical pharmacokinetics of theophylline. *Clin Pharmacokinet* 1978;3:267–93.
2. Sheiner LB. Intelligent use of drug blood level data is helpful in managing patients. In: Lasagna L, ed. *Controversies in therapeutics*. Philadelphia: WB Saunders, 1980.
3. Yarnell PR, Chu NS. Focal seizures and aminophylline. *Neurology* 1975;25:819–22.
4. Jacobs MH, Senior RM, Kessler G. Clinical experience with theophylline: relationships between dosage, serum concentration and toxicity. *JAMA* 1976;235:1983–6.
5. Iberti TJ, Hammond RS. Massive oral theophylline poisoning. *South Med J* 1978;71:965–6.
6. Zwillich CW, Sutton FD, Neff TA, et al. Theophylline-induced seizures in adults; correlation with serum concentrations. *Ann Intern Med* 1975;82:784–7.
7. Jenne JW, Wyze E, Rood FS, et al. Pharmacokinetics of theophylline—application to adjustment of the clinical dose of aminophylline. *Clin Pharmacol Ther* 1972;13:349–60.
8. Jackson RH, McHenry JI, Moreland FB, et al. Clinical evaluation of elixophyllin with correlation of pulmonary function studies and theophylline serum levels in acute and chronic asthmatic patients. *Dis Chest* 1964;45:75–85.
9. Levy G, Koysooko R. Pharmacokinetic analysis of the effect of theophylline on pulmonary function in asthmatic children. *J Pediatr* 1975;86:789–93.
10. Mitenko PA, Ogilvie RI. Rational intravenous doses of theophylline. *N Engl J Med* 1973;289:600–3.
11. Mitenko PA, Ogilvie RI. Pharmacokinetics of intravenous theophylline. *Clin Pharmacol Ther* 1973;14:509–13.
12. Sheiner LB, Tozer TN. Clinical pharmacokinetics: the use of plasma concentrations of drugs. In: Melmen KL, Morrelli HF, eds. *Clinical pharmacology—basic principles in therapeutics*. New York: Macmillan, 1978.
13. Kordash TR, VanDellen RG, McCall JT. Theophylline concentrations in asthmatic patients after administration of aminophylline. *JAMA* 1977;238:139–41.
14. Weinberger MM, Matthay RA, Ginchansky EJ, et al. Intravenous aminophylline dosage: use of serum theophylline measurements for guidance. *JAMA* 1976;235:2110–3.
15. Powell JR, Vozeh S, Hopewell P, et al. Theophylline disposition in acutely ill hospitalized patients: the effect of smoking, heart failure, severe airways obstruction and pneumonia. *Am Rev Resp Dis* 1978;118:229–38.
16. Kappas A, Anderson KE, Conney AH, et al. Influence of dietary protein and carbohydrates on antipyrene and theophylline metabolism in man. *Clin Pharmacol Ther* 1976;20:643–53.
17. Weinberger M, Hudgel D, Spector S, et al. Inhibition of theophylline clearance by troleandomycin. *J Allergy Clin Immunol* 1977;59:228–31.
18. Cummins LH, Kozak PP, Gillman SA. Erythromycin's effect on theophylline blood levels. *Pediatrics* 1977;59:144–5.
19. Landay RA, Gonzales MA, Taylor JC. Effect of phenobarbital on theophylline disposition. *J Allergy Clin Immunol* 1978;62:27–9.
20. Neilsen-Kudsk F, Magnussen I, Jacobsen P. Pharmacokinetics of theophylline in ten elderly patients. *Acta Pharmacol Toxicol* 1978;42:226–34.
21. Gal P, Jusko WJ, Yurchak AM, et al. Theophylline disposition in obesity. *Clin Pharmacol Ther.* 1978;23:438–44.
22. Hendeles L, Weinberger M, Johnson G. Monitoring serum theophylline levels. *Clin Pharmacokinet* 1978;3:294–312.
23. Koch-Weser J. The serum level approach to individualization of drug dosage. *Eur J Clin Pharmacol* 1975;9:1–8.
24. Wyatt R, Weinberger M, Hendeles L. Oral theophylline dosage for the management of chronic asthma. *J Pediatr* 1978;92:125–30.
25. Wilson JT, Wilkinson GR. Delivery of anticonvulsant drug therapy in epileptic patients assessed by plasma level analysis. *Neurology* 1974;24:614–23.
26. Anderson AC, Hodges GR, Barnes WG. Determination of serum gentamicin sulfate levels: ordering patterns and use as a guide to therapy. *Arch Intern Med* 1976;136:785–7.
27. Flynn TW, Pevonka PM, Yost RL, et al. Use of serum gentamicin levels in hospitalized patients. *Am J Hosp Pharm* 1978;35:806–8.
28. Slaughter RL, Schneider PJ, Visconti JA. Appropriateness of use of serum digoxin and tigitoxin assays. *Am J Hosp Pharm* 1978;35:1376–9.

Therapeutic Drug Monitoring
7:174–180 © 1985 Raven Press, New York

Bayesian Pharmacokinetic/Pharmacodynamic Forecasting of Prothrombin Response to Warfarin Therapy: Preliminary Evaluation

Jennifer M. Svec, Robert W. Coleman, *Dennis R. Mungall, and †Thomas M. Ludden

*Pharmacy Service, Veterans Administration Medical Center, Palo Alto, *Biotrack Corporation, Sunnyvale, California, and †College of Pharmacy, University of Texas, Austin, Texas, U.S.A.*

Summary: The ability of a pharmacokinetic/pharmacodynamic Bayesian forecasting computer program to predict prothrombin response to warfarin therapy was investigated. The performance of the program was evaluated retrospectively in an inpatient study population of 45 subjects. Predictions of prothrombin response at discharge, based on zero to five serially measured prothrombin ratios, were compared. Precision of prediction was measured by root mean squared error (rmse), bias was measured by average prediction error, and significance ($p < 0.05$) was determined by 95% confidence intervals and correlation coefficients. Eleven (3.8%) predictions exceeded established limitations of the pharmacokinetic/pharmacodynamic model and were excluded from data analysis. Correlations between measured and predicted prothrombin ratios for all methods were significant. The five prothrombin ratio feedbacks provided the most accurate predictions (rmse 0.219). These predictions were significantly better than the population parameter (rmse 0.418), one (rmse 0.401), and two (rmse 0.459) prothrombin ratio feedback predictions. The predictions based on population parameters and one prothrombin ratio feedback were significantly biased. When provided with sufficient feedback, the bias was not apparent and the predictive performance improved with each additional prothrombin ratio. The predictive performance of the four and five prothrombin ratio feedbacks is sufficient to provide clinically useful dosage guidelines early in the course of warfarin therapy. The population parameter estimates require further delineation in order to improve the performance of limited prothrombin ratio feedback predictions. **Key Words:** Warfarin—Pharmacokinetics—Pharmacodynamics—Bayesian forecasting—Anticoagulation.

The pharmacokinetic and pharmacodynamic properties of warfarin vary widely among individuals (1–5). Because of this variation and the narrow therapeutic window between optimal anticoagulation and significant risk of hemorrhage, coagulation tests such as the prothrombin time are routinely used to determine dosage requirements. Ideally, coagulation test results could be used early in the course of therapy to determine individual warfarin dosage requirements. This would assure therapeutic efficacy and safety, and aid in decreasing the length of hospitalization. However, the complexity of warfarin's pharmacokinetic and pharmacodynamic effect makes achieving this ideal difficult.

Several methods have been proposed for facilitating individualization of warfarin therapy (6–13). These methods range from trial-and-error dose titration to computer-generated estimates of dose requirements.

Address correspondence and reprint requests to Dr. D. R. Mungall at Biotrack Corporation, 1234 Elko Drive, Sunnyvale, CA 94086, U.S.A.

Despite this variation in sophistication, proposed methods have not allowed for assessment of individual warfarin pharmacokinetic and pharmacodynamic variables based on measured prothrombin response and pharmacokinetic/pharmacodynamic population parameter estimates.

Sheiner et al. (14,15) have suggested methods for estimating population pharmacokinetic parameters and using the parameters to forecast individual pharmacokinetic variables. This Bayesian forecasting method has been applied to several commonly used drugs, including theophylline, phenytoin, lidocaine, and aminoglycoside antibiotics (16–18).

A study by Mungall et al. (5) recently assessed the population pharmacokinetics of warfarin in 163 subjects. These population pharmacokinetic parameters have subsequently been used, in part, in the development of a Bayesian forecasting computer program to predict warfarin pharmacokinetics, pharmacodynamics, and prothrombin response. [WARFDA. T. M. Ludden and D. R. Mungall. College of Pharmacy, University of Texas, Austin, TX (HP-85 computer, Hewlett-Packard Corporation, Palo Alto, CA, U.S.A.).]

The purpose of this study was to evaluate the predictive performance of the Bayesian forecasting program. The objectives of the study were as follows: (a) to compare the predictive performance of the program when given from zero to five measured prothrombin ratios, (b) to identify predictions based on data that exceed the bounds limitations of the pharmacokinetic/pharmacodynamic model, and (c) to evaluate the program's population parameter estimates.

METHODS

The study group consisted of 51 patients selected from anticoagulation clinic records at the Medical Center Hospital, San Antonio, TX, U.S.A., and the Veterans Administration Medical Center, Palo Alto, CA, U.S.A. During the study period, all patients were hospitalized for thromboembolic disorders, including deep vein thrombosis (66%), pulmonary embolism (12%), arterial graft occlusion (10%), and other indications (12%). There were 12 women and 38 men, most of whom received concurrent or prior heparinization (96%). The patients' ages ranged from 18 to 78 years (mean 58 years). Patients receiving concurrent therapy with drugs known to alter warfarin clearance were excluded.

Data collection was by retrospective chart review. Patients had daily prothrombin times obtained in the morning and received daily warfarin doses in the early evening. An average of 8.5 prothrombin times was obtained for each patient.

Pharmacokinetic Model

The pharmacokinetic model used in this program is a one-compartment open model for bolus administration. Warfarin absorption is assumed to be complete and instantaneous with plasma concentration described by the following equation for first-order elimination:

$$C_p(t) = C_{p0} \times e^{-krt} \quad (1)$$

where $C_p(t)$ is the plasma warfarin concentration at any time t during a dosing interval, C_{p0} is the initial post-"bolus" plasma concentration, and kr is the first-order warfarin elimination rate constant.

Pharmacokinetic/Pharmacodynamic Model

The model proposed by Theofanous and Barile (20) is used in this program to describe the pharmacodynamic response to warfarin. This model describes the time course of warfarin effect on coagulation after single or multiple doses, as follows:

$$\mathrm{PCA}(t) = P^0 e^{-k_d t} - [mk_r/(k_d)^2](1 - e^{-k_d t} - k_d t) - (m/k_d)(1 - e^{-k_d t})\ln(C_{p0}/C_p^{max}) \quad (2)$$

where PCA(t) is the prothrombin complex activity at time t (h); k_d is the first-order rate constant for PCA degradation; m is the constant relating the plasma warfarin concentration to clotting factor synthesis (slope of the log dose–response curve); C_{p0} is the warfarin plasma concentration at the beginning of a specified dosing interval; and C_p^{max} is the warfarin plasma concentration at which clotting factor synthesis rate approaches zero. At plasma concentrations where $C_p > C_p^{max}$, prothrombin synthesis is completely blocked and Eq. 2 no longer applies. During the time that $C_p > C_p^{max}$, the appropriate equation is

$$\mathrm{PCA}(t) = P^0\, e^{-k_d t} \quad (3)$$

where P^0 is the PCA at the time when C_p initially exceeds C_p^{max} and t is the length of time C_p remains greater than C_p^{max}. In addition, when C_p declines below the minimum effective concentration, C_p^{min}, there is no block of prothrombin synthesis, and PCA will increase back toward control values according to the equation

$$\mathrm{PCA}(t) = 100 - [(100 - P^0) - e^{-k_d t}] \quad (4)$$

where 100% is assumed to be the control PCA value, P^0 is the PCA at the time when C_p declines below

C_p^{min}, and t is the time that C_p remains below C_p^{min}. Note that C_p^{max} can be calculated from C_p^{min}, k_d, and m according to the following formula:

$$C_p^{max} = C_p^{min} e^{100k_d m} \quad (5)$$

Prothrombin complex activity was related to prothrombin time with the following relationship (12):

$$\text{PCA}(\%) = 100\%/[(3.636PR) - 2.636] \quad (6)$$

where PR is prothrombin ratio, which is defined as the measured prothrombin time divided by the control prothrombin time value.

The five pharmacokinetic/pharmacodynamic variables and the P^0 are estimated by Bayesian nonlinear regression analysis. These values are derived from population parameters *(P)* by finding the values of the individual kinetic/dynamic variables *(p)* that minimize the sums of the squared weighted residuals of parameter values, and observed [PCA_{ob}] and predicted [PCA_{pr}]. Parameter values are modified by a factor (CV) that represents the relative standard deviation for the P. Prothrombin response data are weighted by a factor (SD) that represents the standard deviation of measurement error attributable to both intraindividual variation and error in the PCA estimate. Thus, the following function is minimized:

$$\sum_1^n \{[\log(P) - \log(p)]/\text{CV}\}^2 + \sum_1^n [(\text{PCA}_{ob} - \text{PCA}_{pr}/\text{SD})^2] \quad (7)$$

where n is number of prothrombin ratios measured. An HP-85 microcomputer program originally developed for theophylline (18) was modified to accomplish warfarin data analysis.

Initial parameter values were estimated from data presented in previous studies. The pharmacokinetic parameter values (clearance and volume of distribution) were based on NONMEM [(nonlinear mixed effect model) Lewis B. Sheiner, B. Rosenberg, and V. V. Marathe. University of California, San Francisco, CA, U.S.A.] analysis of warfarin in 163 subjects (5). The pharmacodynamic parameter values (PCA degradation rate constant, slope of the log dose–response, and C_p^{min}) were average literature values (19,20). The population parameters are presented in Table 1.

The ability of the warfarin Bayesian forecasting program to predict prothrombin response at time of discharge, based on zero to five initial measured prothrombin ratios (feedbacks), was examined. The time periods between the fifth prothrombin ratio and the discharge prothrombin ratio ranged from 1 to 8 days (mean 3.8). Predictions less than 48 h into the future were excluded from analysis.

TABLE 1. *Population parameters*

NONMEM analysis
CL (clearance) = (3.5 − 0.026 × age) × (wt/70)^{21} L/day ± 0.1[a]
V_d (volume of distribution) = 0.11 L/kg ± 0.3[a]
Literature values
K_d (degradation rate constant) = 1.01 days^{-1} ± 0.3[a]
P_0 (initial prothrombin ratio) = 1
$C_{P\,min}$ (minimum effective concentration) = 0.4 mg/L ± 0.3[a]
m (slope of dose response curve) = 30% ± 0.3[a]
w (PCA weighting factor) = 0.2 + 0.1 × (PCA observed)

PCA, prothrombin complex activity.
[a]Relative standard deviation for parameters.

Comparison of relative predictive performance was evaluated by computing correlation coefficients *(r)* and root mean squared error (rmse) (21). Mean prediction error and 95% confidence intervals were used to determine bias. Predictions of PCA of <10% where the model is known to be inaccurate were "flagged" by the program and excluded from analysis. Significance is defined as $p < 0.05$ and was determined by correlation coefficients and the 95% confidence intervals of the rmse.

RESULTS

Six (6 of 51) subjects were excluded because of concurrent administration of drugs known to interact with warfarin (aspirin, trimethoprim-sulfamethoxazole). Five (5 of 45) predictions based on five prothrombin ratios, and two (2 of 45) predictions based on four prothrombin ratios were excluded because blood for discharge prothrombin times was drawn less than 48 h after the final prothrombin ratio. Ten (10 of 263) predictions were excluded from data analysis for violating the bounds limitation of the kinetic/dynamic model. Excluded predictions occurred as follows: using five prothrombin ratios, 1 of 40; four prothrombin ratios, 3 of 43; three prothrombin ratios, 4 of 45; and two prothrombin ratios, 2 of 45.

The correlations between measured prothrombin ratios and predicted prothrombin ratios for all methods were significant (Figs. 1–6). The five prothrombin ratio feedback provided the most accurate predictions (rmse 0.219). These predictions were significantly better than the population parameter (rmse 0.418), one (rmse, 0.401) and two (rmse 0.459) prothrombin ratio predictions (Fig. 7). Differences between the four prothrombin ratio predictions (rmse 0.283) and either the population parameter, or one or two prothrombin ratio predictions approached but did not achieve significance (Fig. 7).

The predictions based on population parameters and one prothrombin ratio feedback were significantly

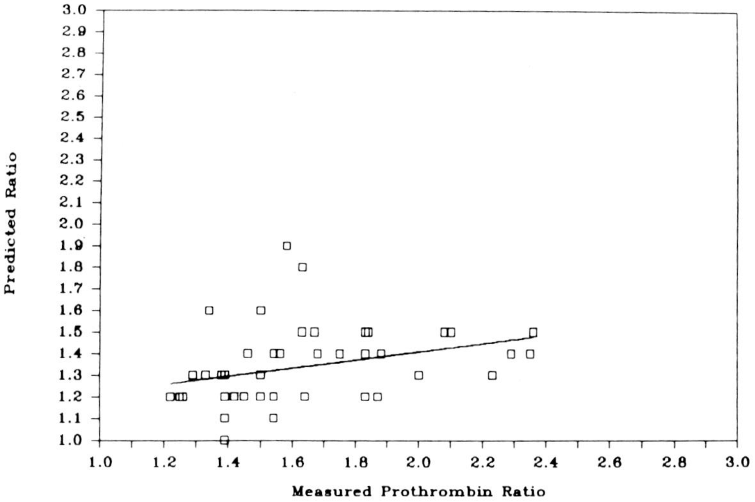

FIG. 1. Predicted versus measured prothrombin ratios based on population parameters. Solid line represents the regression line (n = 45; r = 0.32; r^2 = 0.10; y = 0.188x + 1.03).

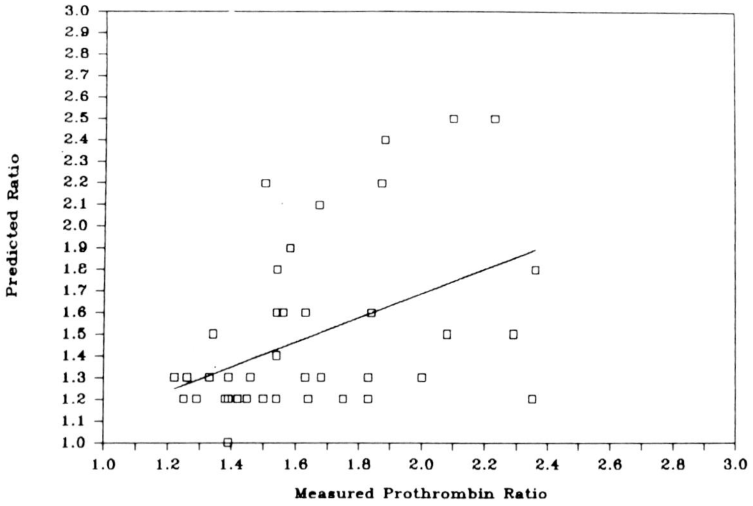

FIG. 2. Predicted versus measured prothrombin ratios based on one prothrombin ratio feedback. Solid line represents the regression line (n = 45; r = 0.44; r^2 = 0.19; y = 0.566x + 0.557).

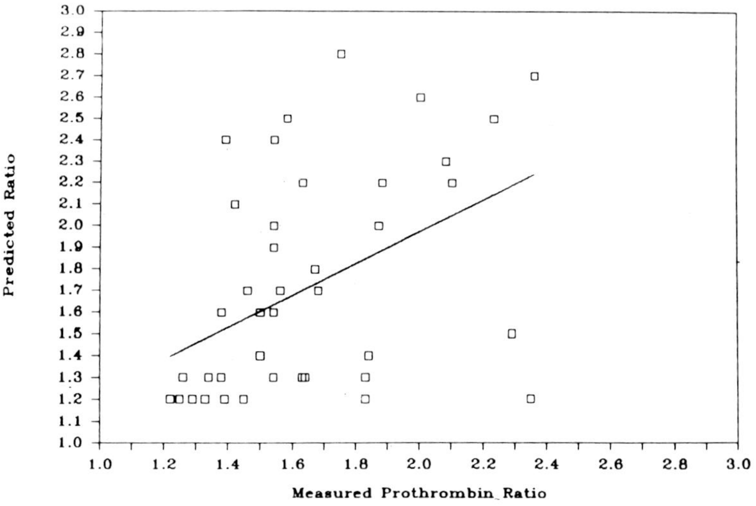

FIG. 3. Predicted versus measured prothrombin ratios based on two prothrombin ratio feedbacks. Solid line represents the regression line (n = 43; r = 0.45; r^2 = 0.20; y = 0.739x + 0.496).

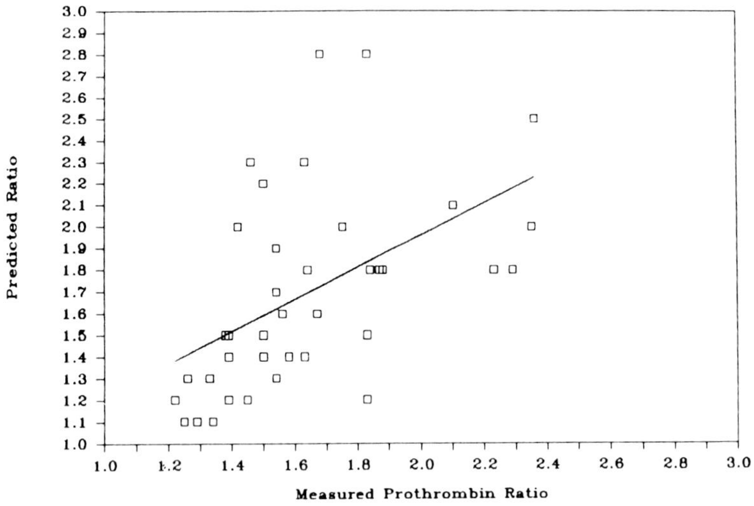

FIG. 4. Predicted versus measured prothrombin ratios based on three prothrombin ratio feedbacks. Solid line represents the regression line (n = 41; $r = 0.50$; $r^2 = 0.25$; $y = 0.742x + 0.478$).

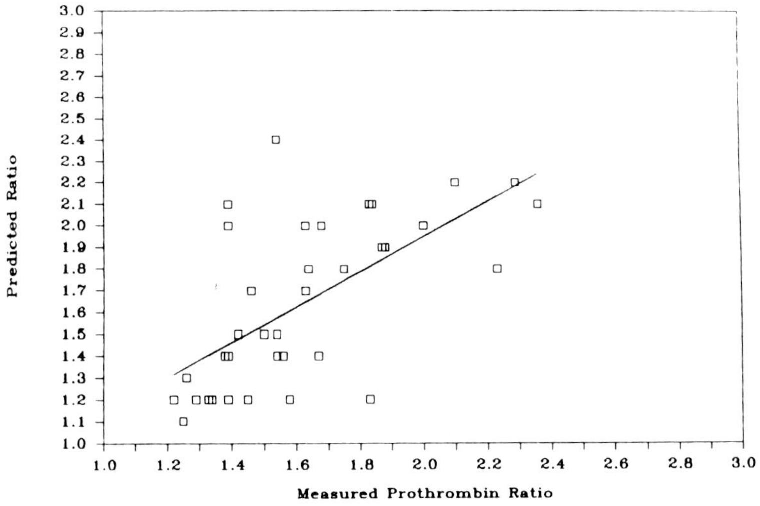

FIG. 5. Predicted versus measured prothrombin ratios based on four prothrombin ratio feedbacks. Solid line represents the regression line (n = 40; $r = 0.64$; $r^2 = 0.41$; $y = 0.812x + 0.326$).

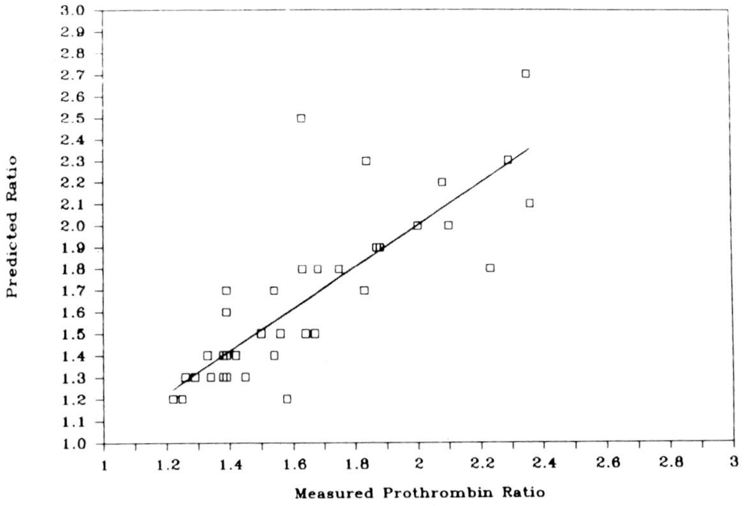

FIG. 6. Predicted versus measured prothrombin ratios based on five prothrombin ratio feedbacks. Solid line represents the regression line (n = 39; $r = 0.81$; $r^2 = 0.66$; $y = 0.972x + 0.058$).

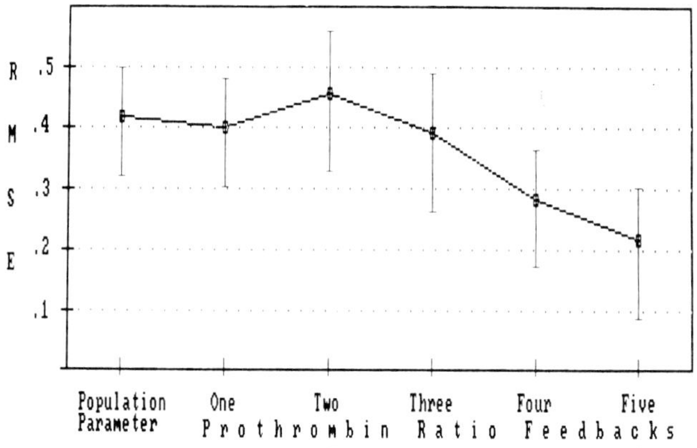

FIG. 7. Root mean squared error (rmse) with 95% confidence intervals for all predictions. Rectangular symbols represent rmse value. Ends of vertical lines represent high and low 95% confidence intervals.

biased, i.e., the 95% confidence interval of the prediction error did not include zero (Fig. 8). Predictions were biased toward underestimating the measured prothrombin ratio; therefore, dosages based on these parameters would routinely be excessive (Figs. 1, 2, and 8). When provided sufficient feedback (greater than two prothrombin ratios) the bias is not apparent and the predictive performance improves with each additional prothrombin ratio (Figs. 7 and 8).

DISCUSSION

The Theophanous and Barile model is valid only when serum concentrations correspond to the linear portion of the dose response curve, i.e., response is >20 and <80% of maximal. This potential for model failure represents a possible limitation to the clinical application of the model. However, in the study population only 3.8% (11 of 263) of the program's predictions yielded highly questionable values. The majority (four) of these occurred after three prothrombin feedbacks, and only one questionable prediction was observed after 4 days of therapy.

The reliability of Bayesian forecasting is largely dependent on accurate initial population parameter estimates. Sheiner et al. (15) recommend determining parameters by sophisticated computer methodologies capable of identifying the influence of multiple factors on parameter distribution (NONMEM). Pharmacokinetic parameters utilized in the Bayesian forecaster were determined by NONMEM analysis (5); however, this analysis is not currently available for the pharmacodynamic parameters. These latter values were extracted from two studies, one with a small study population (19) and another with "normal" subjects (20). Significant bias in the population parameter and single prothrombin ratio predictions indicate that the parameter estimates did not accurately represent the study population. The excellent predictions of the four and five prothrombin ratios reflect the deemphasizing of the population parameters (least square fitting) and illustrate the performance ability of the model.

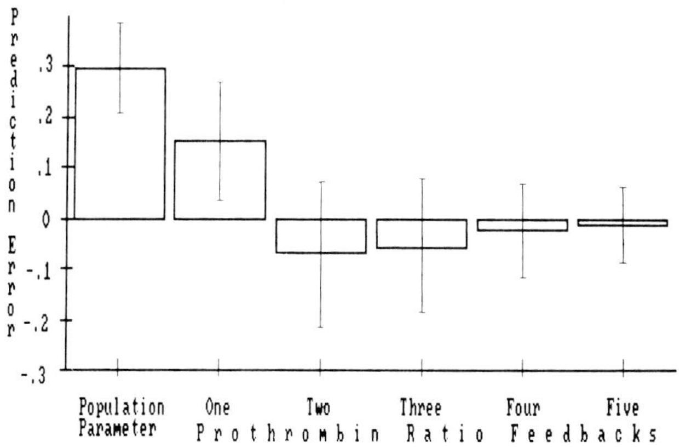

FIG. 8. Prediction error with 95% confidence intervals for all predictions. Horizontal top of bars greater than zero or bottom of bars less than zero represent prediction error value. Ends of vertical lines represent 95% confidence intervals.

CONCLUSIONS

The predictive performance of the four and five prothrombin ratio feedbacks is sufficient to provide clinically useful dosage guidelines early in the course of therapy. These guidelines could be utilized to reduce the average length of hospitalization and thus significantly reduce health care costs.

Further delineation of the true population parameter estimates for this model and the weighting factors for the response data should improve the performance of predictions based on limited prothrombin feedback (three or less). Studies to refine the population parameter estimates are currently ongoing.

REFERENCES

1. Routledge PA, Chapman PH, Davie DM, Rawlings MD. Factors affecting warfarin requirements. *Eur J Clin Pharmacol* 1979;15:319–22.
2. Coon WW, Willis PW. Some aspects of pharmacology of oral anticoagulants. *Clin Pharmacol Ther* 1970;11:312–6.
3. O'Reilly RA, Aggeler PM. Determinants of the response to oral anticoagulants in man. *Pharmacol Rev* 1970;22:33–93.
4. Kelly JG, O'Malley K. Clinical pharmacokinetics of oral anticoagulants. *Clin Pharmacokinet* 1979;4:1–15.
5. Mungall DA, Marshall J, Ludden TM, Hawkins DW, Crawford MH. Population kinetics of warfarin. Paper presented to Second world conference on clinical pharmacology, Washington, DC, August 9, 1983.
6. Routledge P, Bell J, Davies D, Cavonogh J, Rawlins M. Predicting warfarin requirements. *Lancet* 1977;2:854–5.

7. Miller D, Brown M. Predicting warfarin manintenance dosage based on initial response. *Am J Hosp Pharm* 1979;36:1351–5.
8. McGhee J, Evans R, Wolfson P, et al. Predictability of warfarin maintenance dosage based upon initial response. *JAOA* 1981;80:335–8.
9. Sawyer W. Predictability of warfarin dosage requirements: theoretical considerations. *J Pharm Sci* 1976;68:432–4.
10. Williams D. A simple technique for predicting daily maintenance dose of warfarin. *Am J Surg* 1968;137:572–6.
11. O'Reilly RA, Aggeler PM. Studies on coumarin anticoagulant drugs: initiation of warfarin therapy without a loading dose. *Circulation* 1968;38:169–77.
12. Sheiner LB. Computer aided long term anticoagulation therapy. *Comp Biomed Res* 1969;2:507–18.
13. Sawyer W, Finn AL. Digital computer assisted warfarin therapy; comparison of two models. *Comp Biomed Res* 1979;12:221–31.
14. Sheiner LB, Rosenberg B, Marathe VV. Estimation of population characteristics of pharmacokinetic parameters from routine clinical data. *J Pharmacokinet Biopharm* 1977;5:445–79.
15. Sheiner LB, Beal SL, Rosenberg B, Marathe VV. Forecasting individual pharmacokinetics. *Clin Pharmacol Ther* 1979;26:294–304.
16. Vozeh S, Muir KT, Sheiner LB, Follath F. Predicting individual phenytoin dosage. *J Pharmacokinet Biopharm* 1981;9:131–46.
17. Kelman AW, Whiting B, Bryson SM. Parameter optimization in clinical pharmacokinetics. *Comp Prog Biomed* 1982;14:239–48.
18. Peck CC, Brown WD, Sheiner LB, Schuster, BG. A microcomputer theophylline dosing program which assists and teaches physicians. *Proceedings 4th annual conference on computers in medical care.* 1980;2:988–91.
19. Theofanous TG, Barile RG. Multiple-dose kinetics of oral anticoagulants: methods of analysis and optimized dosing. *J Pharm Sci* 1973;62:261–6.
20. Nagashima R, O'Reilly RA, Levy G. Kinetics of pharmacologic effects in man: the anticoagulant action of warfarin. *Clin Pharmacol Ther* 1969;10:22–35.
21. Sheiner LB, Beal SL. Some suggestions for measuring predictive performance. *J Pharmacokinet Biopharm* 1981;9:503–12.

Therapeutic Drug Monitoring
7:181–184 © 1985 Raven Press, New York

Influence of High-Dose Pentobarbital on Theophylline Pharmacokinetics: A Case Report

*Gene A. Gibson, Robert A. Blouin, †Larry A. Bauer, Robert P. Rapp, and Phillip A. Tibbs

*College of Pharmacy and Department of Surgery, Division of Neurosurgery, College of Medicine, University of Kentucky Medical Center, Lexington, Kentucky; *Hospital of the University of Pennsylvania, Philadelphia, Pennsylvania; and †School of Pharmacy, University of Washington, Seattle, Washington, U.S.A.*

Summary: The effect of high dose pentobarbital coma therapy on the total body clearance of theophylline (CL_T) was evaluated in a neurosurgical patient. Preinduction and induction CL_T were 4.22 and 8.02 L/h, respectively, which represented a 95% increase in the CL_T as a consequence of pentobarbital therapy. Although barbiturates have been shown to induce hepatic microsomal enzymes, previous reports minimize their effect on CL_T in humans. This case report demonstrates remarkable alterations in the CL_T as a result of high doses of pentobarbital, necessitating the need for substantial dosage adjustments of theophylline. **Key Words:** Induction—Interaction—Pentobarbital—Theophylline.

Theophylline, which possesses a narrow therapeutic index, is used principally in the treatment of reversible airway obstruction (1). The drug is primarily metabolized by the mixed function oxidase system in hepatic microsomes, with less than 10% excreted unchanged in the urine (2). The disposition of theophylline has been shown to be accelerated by such factors as diet (3) and tobacco (4–7) or marijuana (6) smoking. Animal studies have suggested phenobarbital pretreatment induces the metabolism of theophylline, but studies in humans have produced conflicting results (8,9). Pentobarbital has been shown to stimulate the mixed function oxidase system in rats (10) and to increase the metabolism of various β-adrenergic blockers in humans (11–13). However, the influence of low or high doses of pentobarbital on the disposition of theophylline has not been evaluated. The following case report demonstrates an increase in the total body clearance of theophylline (CL_T) during a continuous intravenous infusion of high dose pentobarbital.

Address correspondence and reprint requests to Dr. R. A. Blouin at University of Kentucky, College of Pharmacy, Washington and Gladstone Streets, Lexington, KY 40536-0053, U.S.A.

CASE REPORT

J. T., a 47-year-old man (weight, 109 kg) with no history of smoking, was admitted to University Hospital with symptoms of an acute, severe headache accompanied by a loss of consciousness. At the time of admission the patient was awake and alert. A lumbar puncture, computerized axial tomography scan of the head, and angiogram confirmed a diagnosis of subarachnoid hemorrhage and revealed an aneurysm at the junction of the right cerebral and communicating arteries with no evidence of vasospasm. Further physical and laboratory data were remarkable only for a history of mild hypertension, which was untreated. Four days later he underwent surgery and the aneurysm was repaired. Postoperatively the patient's neurological status deteriorated and he became responsive only to pain bilaterally. Repeat cerebral angiography revealed vasospasm of the right artery. Infusions of isoproterenol and aminophylline were subsequently initiated to reverse the vasospasm, based on the recommendations of Flamm et al. (14). Eight hours later, the patient developed sinus tachycardia with a corresponding serum theophylline concentration of 20.6 μg/ml while on an aminophylline continuous infusion of 125 mg/h (1.15 mg/kg aminophylline). Aminophylline dosage was adjusted throughout the remainder of therapy to maintain serum concentrations within the therapeutic range (8–20 μg/ml). The patient's neurological function continued to deteriorate with an accompanied elevation in intracranial pressure (ICP), and therapy with mannitol, furosemide, and dexamethasone was initiated. Eventually, the ICP became refractory to therapy and a pentobarbital coma without hypothermia was initiated 8 h after surgery. The dosage of pentobarbital was titrated to maintain serum pentobarbital concentrations between 20 and 50 μg/ml. During pentobarbital therapy, theophylline serum concentrations became increasingly difficult to maintain, requiring several increases in the theophylline maintenance dose (Fig. 1). The cardiovascular function and ICP were stable and controlled for several days. However, therapy later became ineffective and the patient eventually died secondary to uncontrollable increased ICP.

METHODS

Aminophylline (85% anhydrous theophylline; Searle Laboratories) and pentobarbital (Nembutal; Abbott Laboratories) were administered by constant intravenous infusions, with dosage adjustments based on serum concentrations and clinical response. Medications administered prior to surgery consisted of phenytoin (500 mg, one dose only), propranolol, cimetidine, promethazine, hydralazine, aminocaproic acid, kanamycin, and reserpine. Medications administered postoperatively during theophylline and pentobarbital therapy consisted of isoproterenol, furosemide, mannitol, hydralazine, dexamethasone, cimetidine, gentamicin, cephalothin, kanamycin, and reserpine. Theophylline blood samples were obtained at 0, 10.0, and 19.0 h during the initial continuous infusion of aminophylline at 125 mg/h. At 19.0 h the aminophylline dose was decreased to 60 mg/h and additional blood samples were collected at 29.0 and 35.0 h. Serum theophylline versus time data were fitted by employing NONLIN, a least-squares linear regression program (15), according to the method described by Jusko et al. (16). The apparent volume of distribution was assumed to be 0.385 L/kg (total body mass) based on data by Gal et al. (17). Pentobarbital was started 8.0 h after the initiation of theophylline, with a 1.5 g loading dose given over 4 h followed by a constant infusion of 100 mg/h. It was assumed that the CL_T was unchanged during the first 35.0 h (regarded as the preinduction time period). CL_T was calculated during the pentobarbital induction period by taking the quotient of the theophylline dose (mg/h) and the steady-state serum concentration. Theophylline blood samples were collected at 129.0, 154.0, 176.0, and 203.0 h postinitiation of theophylline while on a continuous intravenous infusion of aminophylline (110 mg/h). The patient was considered to be at steady-state when two consecutive serum theophylline levels obtained at least 24.0 h apart were within a difference of 10% of one another. All blood samples were allowed to clot at room temperature and centrifuged. The serum was then collected and stored at −5°C until analysis, or stored at room temperature and analyzed within 6 h of collection. Serum theophylline concentrations were determined by high performance liquid chromatography using a method previously described (18). Between- and within-run coefficient of variation determinations were both within 5.0%.

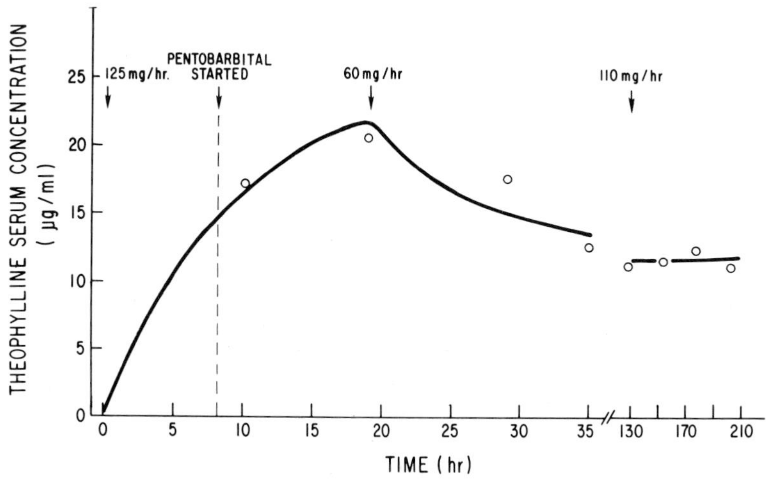

FIG. 1. Theophylline serum concentrations during the time of treatment for vasospasm. Open circles indicate observed theophylline concentrations during therapy. Solid line describes best-fit computer estimates of theophylline concentrations. Arrows indicate times of changes in rates of infusions of aminophylline.

RESULTS

The theophylline serum concentration versus time profile is shown in Fig. 1. The computer-fitted estimate of CL_T during the first 35.0 h of theophylline (preinduction period) was 4.22 L/h. The correlation coefficient between the observed and computer estimated concentrations was high ($r = 0.966$). In contrast, the mean estimate CL_T between days 5 and 8 of pentobarbital therapy was 8.02 L/h, a 95% increase in CL_T.

DISCUSSION

This report demonstrates the induction potential of high-dose pentobarbital on the CL_T. The induction appeared to occur rapidly and was of sufficient magnitude to warrant frequent theophylline dosage adjustments. Data analysis revealed a 95% increase in the CL_T during the pentobarbital induction period.

Theophylline has been shown to be primarily metabolized by the liver, with less than 10% of a dose being excreted unchanged in the urine (2). The influence of the enzyme-inducing agents contained in cigarette and marijuana smoke on the clearance of theophylline has been well described (4–6). However, the importance of barbiturates causing clinically significant alterations in the CL_T has not been substantiated. Lohmann et al. (19) reported an increase in the metabolism of theophylline as a result of pretreatment with the enzyme inducer 3-methylcholanthrene and phenobarbital using in vitro rat tissue. Mannering had previously reported that 3-methylcholanthrene produced an increase in the synthesis of a modified cytochrome, P-448, whereas phenobarbital promoted an increase in the liver microsome cytochrome P-450 (20). Therefore, it was concluded that the metabolism of the theophylline involved P-448 (primary) and P-450 (secondary) in its metabolic pathway (19). Stimulation of either cytochrome P-448 or P-450 pathways could theoretically influence the disposition of theophylline. Although animal studies support this contention (10), significant alterations in CL_T have only been demonstrated by inducers of P-448 in humans (4,6) while the effects of phenobarbital and other inducers of P-450 remain inconclusive (8,9).

The characteristics of pentobarbital induction on the P-450 enzyme system have been previously described. Valerino et al. (10) demonstrated a significant increase in the synthesis of cytochrome P-450 following repeated injection of pentobarbital. This increase was observed within a 24-h period and plateaued within 8 days. The autoinduction of pentobarbital in cats was also shown to have a rapid onset and was completed within 7 days (21). Additionally, pentobarbital in humans has been reported to increase the total body clearance of metoprolol and alprenolol by 30–40% within 10 days of therapy (11–13). Recently, Paladino et al. (22) reported a dramatic increase (33%) in the total body clearance of theophylline as a consequence of secobarbital therapy.

The enzyme induction ability of the barbiturates in animals has been related to the lipid solubility and plasma half-life of the compound (23,24). These results have been contradicted by studies of the induction of theophylline metabolism by phenobarbital (8,9) and pentobarbital (this report). The reason for these differences may be the result of other factors. The study by Valerino et al. (10) suggests pentobarbital stimulates hepatic enzymes and increases cytochrome P-450 content at a faster rate and to a greater extent during the first 48 h than do similar doses of phenobarbital. Later in the study phenobarbital would consistently stimulate hepatic enzymes and cytochrome P-450 content to a significantly greater degree, thus implying that the difference in the onset of induction is a result of the difference in lipid solubility between pentobarbital and phenobarbital. Furthermore, data published by Yamamato et al. (25) demonstrate that the constant release of pentobarbital from a pellet induces the metabolism of pentobarbital faster than do intermittent injections. These results imply that the onset of cytochrome P-450 induction may be related to the lipophilicity of the inducing agent, while the extent of induction is related to the length of time the enzymes are exposed to the inducing agent. Thus, in our case, the pronounced effect of pentobarbital on the induction of the metabolism of theophylline may be the result of the higher lipid solubility of pentobarbital as well as the constant maintenance of high serum levels during pentobarbital coma therapy.

Our observations indicate a clinically significant change in CL_T during a high-dose, continuous infusion of pentobarbital. This interaction most likely involves the induction of the hepatic cytochrome mixed-function oxidase microsomal enzymes. Theophylline serum concentrations should therefore be carefully monitored while patients are on this combination. Additionally, well-controlled studies are needed to further examine the enzyme induction potential of the barbiturates on the various forms (isozymes) of the cytochrome P-450 system and assess the clinical significance of such interactions.

REFERENCES

1. Piafsky KM, Ogilvie RI. Dosing of theophylline in bronchial asthma. *N Engl J Med* 1975;292:1212–22.
2. Thompson RD, Nagasawa HT, Jenne JW. Determination of theophylline and its metabolites in human urine and serum by high pressure liquid chromatography. *J Lab Clin Med* 1974;84:585–93.
3. Kappas A, Anderson KE, Conney AH, Alvares AP. Influence of dietary protein and carbohydrates on antipyrine and theophylline metabolism in man. *Clin Pharmacol Ther* 1976;20:643–53.
4. Hunt SN, Jusko WJ, Yurchak AM. Effect of smoking on theophylline disposition. *Clin Pharmacol Ther* 1976;19:546–51.
5. Jenne J, Nagasawa M, McHugh R, MacDonald F, Wyse E. Decreased theophylline half-life in cigarette smokers. *Life Sci* 1975;17:195–7.
6. Jusko WJ, Schentag JJ, Clark JK, Gardner M, Yurchak AM. Enhanced biotransformation of theophylline in marijuana and tobacco smokers. *Clin Pharmacol Ther* 1978;24:406–10.
7. Powell JR, Thiercelin J, Vozeh S, Sansom L, Riegelman S. The influence of cigarette smoking and sex on theophylline disposition. *Am Rev Respir Dis* 1977;116:17–23.
8. Landay RA, Gonzalez MA, Taylor JC. Effect of phenobarbital on theophylline disposition. *J Allergy Clin Immunol* 1978;62:27–9.
9. Piafsky KM, Sitar OS, Ogilvie RI. Effect of phenobarbital on the disposition of intravenous theophylline. *Clin Pharmacol Ther* 1977;22:336–9.
10. Valerino DM, Vesell ES, Aurori KC, Johnson AO. Effects of various barbiturates on hepatic microsomal enzymes. *Drug Metab Dispos* 1974;2:448–57.
11. Alvan G, Piafsky K, Lind M, vonBahr C. Effect of pentobarbital on the disposition of alprenol. *Clin Pharmacol Ther* 1977;22:316–22.
12. Collste P, Seideman P, Borg K, Haglund K, vonBahr C. Influence of pentobarbital on effect and plasma levels of alprenol and 4-hydroxy-alprenolol. *Clin Pharmacol Ther* 1979;25:423–7.
13. Haglund K, Seideman P, Collste P, Borg K, vonBahr C. Influence of pentobarbital on metoprolol plasma levels. *Clin Pharmacol Ther* 1979;26:326–9.
14. Flamm ES, Ransohoff J. Treatment of cerebral vasospasm by control of cyclic adenosine monophosphate. *Surg Neurol* 1976;6:223–6.
15. Metzler CM. NONLIN—a computer program for parameter estimation in nonlinear situations. Kalamazoo, Michigan: The Upjohn Co., 1969.
16. Jusko WJ, Garner MJ, Mangione A, Schentag JJ, Koup JR, Vance JW. Factors affecting theophylline clearances: age, tobacco, marijuana, cirrhosis, congestive heart failure, obesity, oral contraceptives, benzodiazepines, barbiturates, and ethanol. *J Pharm Sci* 1979;68:1358–66.
17. Gal P, Jusko WJ, Yurchak AM, Franklin BA. Theophylline disposition in obesity. *Clin Pharmacol Ther* 1978;23:438–44.
18. Blouin RA, Elgert JF, Bauer LA. Theophylline clearance: effect of marked obesity. *Clin Pharmacol Ther* 1980;28:619–26.
19. Lohmann SM, Miech RP. Theophylline metabolism by the rat liver microsomal system. *J Pharmacol Exp Ther* 1976;196:213–25.
20. Mannering GJ. Microsomal enzyme system which catalyze drug metabolism and drug disposition. Baltimore: Williams & Wilkens, 1971.
21. Okamoto M, Rosenberg HC, Boisse NR. Tolerance characteristics produced during the maximally tolerable chronic pentobarbital dosing in the cat. *J Pharmacol Exp Ther* 1975;192:555–64.
22. Paladino JA, Blumer NA, Maddox RR. Effect of secobarbital on theophylline clearance. *Ther Drug Monit* 1983;5:133–9.
23. Ioannides C, Parke DV. Mechanism of induction of hepatic microsomal drug metabolizing enzymes by a series of barbiturates. *Pharm Pharmac* 1975;27:739–46.
24. Pelkonen O, Karki NT. Effect of physicochemical and pharmacokinetic properties of barbiturates on the induction of drug metabolism. *Chem Biol Interact* 1973;7:93–9.
25. Yamamoto I, Ho IK, Loh HH. Acceleration of pentobarbital metabolism in tolerant mice induced by pentobarbital pellet implantation. *Life Sci* 1977;20:1353–63.

Therapeutic Drug Monitoring
7:185–190 © 1985 Raven Press, New York

Effect of Associated Antiepileptic Treatment on Valproate-Induced Hyperammonemia

G. Zaccara, M. Paganini, R. Campostrini, *F. Moroni, †T. Valenza, ‡A. Messori, M. Bartelli, G. Arnetoli, and R. Zappoli

*Centre for Epilepsy of the 2nd Neurological Institute and *Department of Pharmacology, University of Florence; and †Clinical Analysis Laboratory and ‡Hospital Pharmacy, Florence, Italy*

Summary: It has recently been shown that acute changes of venous blood ammonia (NH_3) may predict short-term adverse effects of valproic acid (VPA). In the present study, the time course of NH_3 concentration after a single oral dose of VPA (800 mg) was monitored in 68 epileptic patients. Patients were classified into four groups: previously untreated patients (group A, n = 21), patients under treatment with either phenobarbital (group B, n = 14) or phenytoin (group C, n = 13) or both (group D, n = 20). In each patient, venous blood for the NH_3 assay was taken before the VPA dose (predose level) and at 1, 2, 3, and 4 h after the dose (postdose levels). While in patients receiving only VPA the postdose NH_3 concentrations did not differ from the predose level, in each of groups B, C, and D the postdose concentrations appeared to be significantly higher than the predose concentration. The greatest increase was observed in group D. In the light of the data reported in the literature, those patients whose NH_3 concentration after the VPA dose exceeds 100 μg/dl should be considered at higher risk for short-term, VPA-induced adverse effects during long-term therapy. Thus, our data suggest that caution should be exercised in adding VPA to anticonvulsant treatments including phenobarbital or phenytoin or both. **Key Words:** Adverse effects—Anticonvulsants—Drug interactions—Hyperammonemia—Valproic acid.

Hyperammonemia is one of the most frequent adverse effects of therapy with valproic acid (VPA) (1–4). In patients receiving multiple anticonvulsants, the addition of VPA to the antiepileptic treatment may elicit a considerable increase in blood ammonia (NH_3) concentration as well as alterations of the patient's state of consciousness (5). The pathogenesis of such a modification of NH_3 metabolism is not yet understood. In healthy volunteers, VPA increases the release of NH_3 from the kidney (6); however, this fact is not sufficient to explain the VPA-induced increase in arterial blood NH_3 concentration that has been observed in patients receiving concurrent treatment with phenobarbital (PB) (7).

Address correspondence and reprint requests to Dr. G. Zaccara at 2nd Neurological Institute, University of Florence, viale Morgagni 85, 50134 Florence, Italy.

In a recent report we suggested that the time course of venous blood NH_3 concentrations after an oral loading dose of VPA may predict short-term adverse effects when the drug is added to the therapeutic regimen (8). In fact, monitoring the acute changes of NH_3 in venous blood seems to be of value for predicting the occurrence of drowsiness and obtundation.

In the present study, the measurement of venous blood NH_3 concentration at various times after a single oral VPA dose was extended to previously untreated epileptic patients and to patients receiving treatment with PB, phenytoin (PHT), or both.

METHODS

Patient Population

Sixty-eight epileptic patients who were scheduled for VPA therapy were studied. The patients were divided into four groups: 21 patients not previously treated with anticonvulsants (group A), 14 taking PB (group B), 13 taking PHT (group C), and 20 being treated with the combination of PB and PHT (group D). Patients' demographic data are given in Table 1. All patients of groups B, C, and D had begun treatment with PB, PHT, or both at least 3 months prior to inclusion in the study. No changes in the dosage regimen of PHT and PB had been made during the 4 weeks preceding the patients' inclusion in the study. The type and duration of the disease in the four groups are described in Table 2. The duration of the disease was much longer in groups B, C, and D.

Study Protocol

In each patient, after an overnight fast, venous blood for the assay of antiepileptic drugs and NH_3 was taken at 9 a.m. before the administration of a standard loading dose of VPA (800 mg in a 50 ml water solution) and at 1, 2, 3, and 4 h after the dose. (In groups B, C, and D, the plasma concentrations of PB and PHT were determined only from the predose blood sample.) The patients were not allowed to eat or to have physical exercise before the last venipuncture. However, each patient had a standard cup of coffee with milk and sugar a few minutes after the VPA dose.

In all patients, the occurrence of short-term adverse effects induced by VPA was assessed over the 4 weeks after the loading dose, as previously described (8).

Assays for NH_3 and Anticonvulsants

Blood NH_3 concentration was measured in duplicate within 10 min after each venipuncture (9). The plasma concentrations of antiepileptic drugs were measured by gas-liquid chromatography (GLC) (10,11).

Data Evaluation and Statistical Analysis

In each of the four study groups, the baseline NH_3 plasma levels and the four concentrations measured at 1, 2, 3, and 4 h after the VPA dose were compared by using the repeated-measurement analysis of variance (ANOVA) (12), the significance level being $p = 0.05$. To assess the magnitude of the variations of NH_3 relative to the baseline level, we used the parameter DX_{AV} defined as $DX_{AV} = NH_{3,AV} - NH_{3,BL}$ (where $NH_{3,AV}$ is the mean of the four NH_3 concentrations measured at 1, 2, 3, and 4 h after the VPA dose and $NH_{3,BL}$ is the baseline level). The DX_{AV} value was therefore calculated for each of the 68 patients. To compare the DX_{AV} values between the four patient groups, the one-way ANOVA was employed. [Simultaneous pairwise comparisons were performed by the Bonferroni procedure (12).]

The *t* test for unpaired samples and Pearson's correlation coefficient were also used, when appropriate.

RESULTS

The measured plasma concentrations of VPA, PHT, and PB are shown in Table 3.

Figure 1 shows the time course of venous NH_3 concentration after the loading dose of VPA in the four groups of patients.

In patients receiving only VPA, the four postdose NH_3 concentrations did not change significantly in comparison with the baseline level. Conversely, in each of the other three patient groups, the postdose NH_3 concentrations appeared to be, on the average, higher than the baseline level. As shown in Fig. 1, the

TABLE 1. *Patient data*

	Group A VPA (n = 21)	Group B VPA + PB (n = 14)	Group C VPA + PHT (n = 13)	Group D VPA + PB + PHT (n = 20)
Age (yr)	28.1 ± 3.9 (17–60)	31.0 ± 13.5 (17–53)	40.2 ± 14.3 (19–64)	35.2 ± 12.9 (17–58)
Weight (kg)	61.8 ± 17.5 (46–95)	67.3 ± 11.3 (51–82)	67.1 ± 10.4 (49–85)	69.0 ± 12.6 (50–92)
PB dosage (mg/day)[a]	—	143 (100–200)	—	146 (50–250)
PHT dosage (mg/day)[b]	—	—	308 (200–400)	282 (150–400)

Values are means ± SD; range in parentheses. VPA, valproic acid; PB, phenobarbital; PHT, phenytoin.

[a]PB was administered in a single daily dose at ~9 p.m.

[b]PHT was administered in two divided doses at ~9 a.m. and ~9 p.m.

TABLE 2. *Type and duration[a] of epilepsy in the four groups of patients*

	Type of epilepsy			
	Primary generalized (n)	Secondary generalized (n)	Partial (n)	Duration[b] (yr)
Group A	15	1	5	2.2 (0.08–20)
Group B	9	1	4	16.5 (1–33)
Group C	6	0	7	15.6 (1–40)
Group D	7	0	13	20.3 (1–38)

[a]Time elapsed since first seizure.
[b]Mean, with range in parentheses.

highest increase was observed in the group previously treated with PB and PHT.

As measured by the repeated ANOVA, the difference between the baseline NH_3 level and the postdose concentrations was significant in groups B, C, and D (group B, $F = 3.44$, $p = 0.014$; group C, $F = 2.72$, $p = 0.04$; group D, $F = 6.45$, $p = 0.0002$). No significant difference was observed in group A ($F = 0.71$, $p = 0.58$).

The DX_{AV} values are shown in Fig. 2. The values (mean ± SE) of this parameter measured in the four groups were as follows: 1.0 ± 2.2 (group A), 19.5 ± 6.7 (group B), 14.0 ± 4.5 (group C), and 38.2 ± 10.3 (group D).

The difference between the DX_{AV} values in the four groups was significant, as shown by the one-way ANOVA ($F = 5.68$, $p = 0.002$). As regards the simultaneous pairwise comparisons, only the difference between groups A and D reached the significance level.

In Fig. 2, those patients who experienced short-term adverse effects have been differentiated from symptom-free patients. Overall, short-term adverse effects were observed in nine patients, while the remaining 59 patients were symptom free. (Adverse affects were noted in zero, one, one, and seven patients of groups A through D, respectively.) The response in NH_3 levels to the VPA test dose, as measured by DX_{AV}, was significantly different between these two patient groups (mean DX_{AV} ± SE in symptomatic patients, 71.7 ± 17.4; mean DX_{AV} ± SE in symptom-free patients, 11.1 ± 2.2; $p = 0.001$ by the *t* test for unpaired samples).

No correlation was found between the DX_{AV} values and the 9 a.m. plasma levels of PB in groups B and D ($r = 0.22$, $n = 34$, $p = 0.20$). Conversely, a weak though significant correlation between the DX_{AV} values and the 9 a.m. plasma levels of PHT was observed in groups C and D ($r = 0.36$, $n = 33$, $p = 0.04$).

The VPA plasma levels measured after the test dose were consistently lower in groups B, C, and D than in group A (Table 3). At each of the four sampling times, the difference in VPA plasma concentration between the four groups was significant, as measured by the one-way ANOVA (1 h level: $F = 6.23$, $p < 0.001$; 2 h level: $F = 7.24$, $p < 0.001$; 3 h level: $F = 14.0$, $p < 0.001$; 4 h level: $F = 10.3$, $p < 0.001$).

DISCUSSION

Our study shows that a single oral dose of VPA (800 mg) administered to previously untreated adult epileptic patients does not change the venous blood NH_3 concentration, whereas the same dose administered to patients taking PB, PHT, or both elicits a significant increase in the NH_3 concentration. Our data are in agreement with previous observations suggesting that the VPA-induced increase in arterial blood NH_3 is more clear-cut in patients undergoing long-term treatment with PB than in untreated patients (7).

TABLE 3. *Measured plasma levels of VPA, PB, and PHT in the four patient groups*

	Group A VPA	Group B VPA + PB	Group C VPA + PHT	Group D VPA + PB + PHT
VPA plasma level (μmol/ml)				
1 h[a]	542 ± 137	462 ± 104	379 ± 59	445 ± 110
2 h[a]	475 ± 114	404 ± 68	326 ± 42	379 ± 112
3 h[a]	453 ± 85	377 ± 64	286 ± 46	336 ± 94
4 h[a]	404 ± 91	338 ± 52	268 ± 44	302 ± 87
PB plasma level (μmol/ml)[b]	—	110 ± 71	—	120 ± 57
PHT plasma level (μmol/ml)[b]	—	—	46 ± 34	51 ± 34

Values are means ± SD. VPA, valproic acid; PB, phenobarbital; PHT, phenytoin.
[a]Time elapsed since the VPA loading dose.
[b]Steady-state plasma level measured at 9 a.m. on the first day of the study.

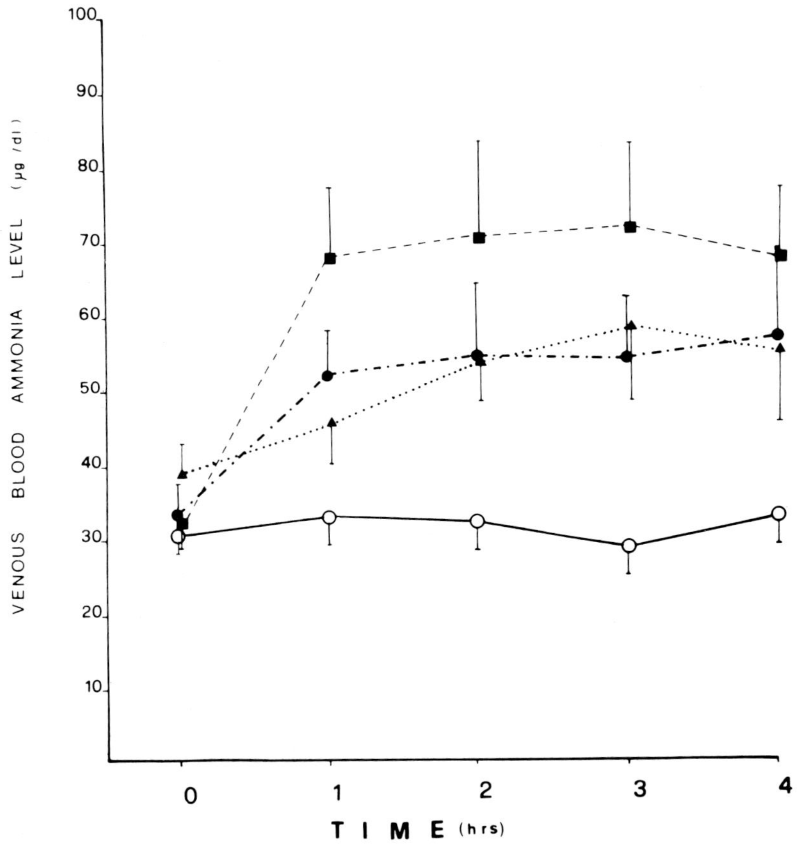

FIG. 1. Time course of venous blood ammonia concentration after the loading dose of valproic acid in the four groups of patients (group A, open circles; group B, filled circles; group C, triangles; group D, squares). Values are means ± SE.

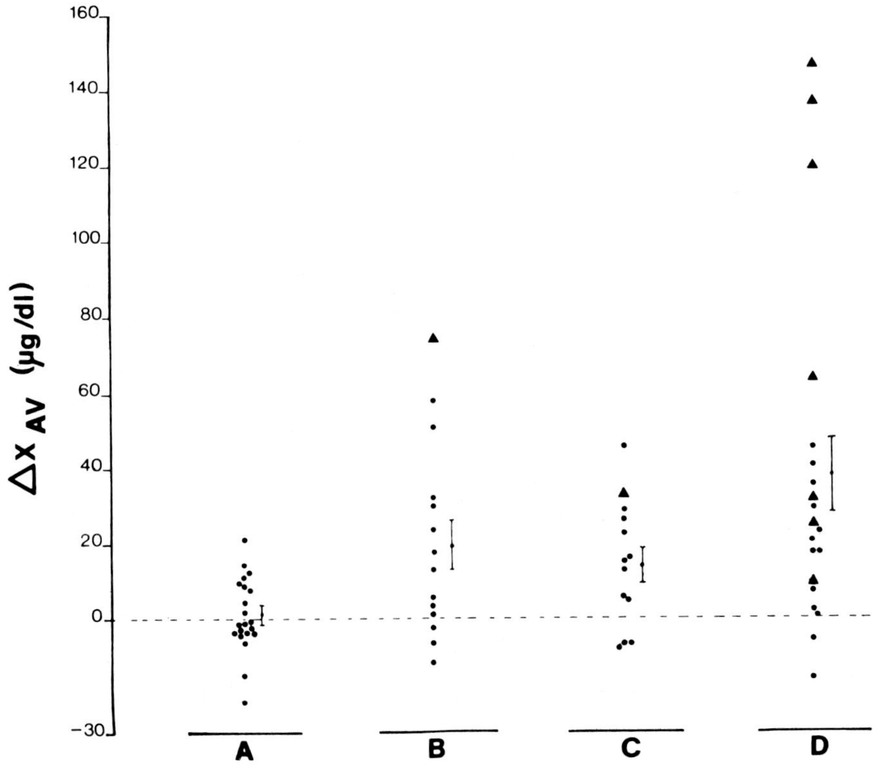

FIG. 2. Increase in venous blood ammonia concentration after the valproic acid (VPA) dose, as measured by the parameter DX_{AV} (circles, symptom-free patients; triangles, symptomatic patients, i.e., patients who complained of drowsiness or more serious alterations of the state of consciousness within the first month of VPA therapy).

Interestingly enough, the patients treated with combined PB and PHT had the greatest increase in NH_3 after the loading dose of VPA.

The pairwise comparisons of the DX_{AV} values between the four patient groups show that only the difference between group A and group D is significant. However, a trend was distinguishable in two additional pairwise comparisons, namely, group A versus group B and group A versus group C. In the latter two cases, failure to reach statistical significance can be explained by the small number of patients examined.

In the three groups of patients receiving long-term anticonvulsant therapy, there were subjects who did not show reproducible changes of NH_3 concentrations, possibly because genetic factors may be involved in determining the extent to which VPA alters the metabolism of NH_3 (R. Campostrini et al., unpublished observations in identical twins).

The results concerning the correlation between DX_{AV} and the plasma levels of PB or PHT cannot be easily interpreted, mainly because of the limited number of patients included in our study. A significant correlation, in fact, has only been found for PHT. As shown in Table 3, the VPA plasma levels were, on the average, higher in patients undergoing monotherapy than in patients undergoing polytherapy. This finding is consistent with the data reported in the literature (13).

With regard to the relation between the acute changes of NH_3 after the VPA dose and the occurrence of short-term adverse effects, the data from the present study confirm substantially the findings obtained in our previous investigation (8). In fact, the hyperammonemia observed after the VPA test dose was more evident in symptomatic patients than in symptom-free patients.

The reasons why the concurrent administration of some anticonvulsants potentiates the interference of VPA with NH_3 metabolism are unknown. It may be suspected that enzyme induction is involved. Both PB and PHT are in fact inducers of the enzyme systems capable of oxidizing VPA. It has recently been shown in experimental animals that PB pretreatment greatly increases the blood content of the ω- and ω-1 oxidation products of VPA (14). Indeed, one of these metabolites (4-en-VPA) has been found to be hepatotoxic in experimental animals (15).

One may therefore hypothesize that these products impair the urea cycle enzymes in human liver. Should this hypothesis be true, the same mechanism (production of toxic VPA metabolites) would be involved in VPA-induced liver injury (16) as well as in the alterations of NH_3 metabolism that are observed in patients undergoing polytherapy.

In conclusion, our data are of value in providing insight into the reasons why some VPA-induced adverse effects are almost exclusively observed in patients undergoing multiple drug therapy (5,8,17–23). Also, our findings suggest that caution should be exercised in adding VPA to anticonvulsant treatments including PB, PHT, or both. In fact, those patients whose NH_3 concentration after the loading VPA dose exceeds 100 μg/dl are at higher risk for short-term, VPA-induced adverse effects such as drowsiness, obtundation, or more serious alterations of the state of consciousness during long-term therapy (8). In our view, in those cases where addition of VPA to a previous anticonvulsant regimen is judged to be necessary, venous NH_3 concentrations should be monitored at the beginning of VPA therapy to select those subjects who are at higher risk for VPA-induced, short-term adverse effects (8).

Acknowledgment: This work was supported in part by grants from Consiglio Nazionale delle Ricerche (No. 83.02528.56) and from the University of Florence. The technical assistance of Mrs. Loriana Bendoni is gratefully acknowledged.

REFERENCES

1. Bathshaw ML, Brusilow SW. Valproate-induced hyperammonemia. *Ann Neurol* 1982;11:319–21.
2. Marescaux C, Warter JM, Laroye M, et al. Le valproate de sodium: una drogue hyperammonemiante. Etude chez l'epileptique et chez le volontaire sain. *J Neurol Sci* 1983;58:195–209.
3. Murphy JV, Marquardt K. Asymptomatic hyperammonemia in patients receiving valproic acid. *Arch Neurol* 1982;39:591–2.
4. Williams CA, Tiefenbach S, McReynolds JW. Valproic acid-induced hyperammonemia in mentally retarded adults. *Neurology (NY)* 1984;34:550–3.
5. Zaccara G, Paganini M, Campostrini R, Arnetoli G, Zappoli R, Moroni F. Hyperammonemia and valproate-induced alterations of the state of consciousness. A report of eight cases. *Eur Neurol* 1984;23:104–12.
6. Warter JM, Brandt C, Marescaux C, et al. The renal origin of sodium-valproate-induced hyperammonemia in fasting humans. *Neurology (NY)* 1983;33:1136–40.
7. Warter JM, Marescaux C, Brandt C, et al. Sodium valproate associated with phenobarbital: effects of ammonia metabolism in humans. *Epilepsia* 1983;24:628–33.
8. Zaccara G, Campostrini R, Paganini M, et al. Acute changes of blood ammonia may predict short-term effects of valproic acid. *Neurology (NY)* 1984;34:1519–21.
9. Tada K, Okuda K, Watanabe K, Yasuo I, Yamada S. A new method for screening for hyperammonemia. *Eur J Pediatr* 1979;130:105–10.
10. Riva R, Albani F, Baruzzi A. Rapid quantitative determination of underivatized carbamazepine, phenytoin, phenobarbital and p-hydroxyphenobarbital in biological fluids by packed column gas chromatography. *J Chromatogr* 1980;221:75–84.
11. Riva R, Albani F, Baruzzi A. Rapid and simple GLC deter-

mination of valproic acid and ethosuximide in plasma of epileptic patients. *J Pharm Sci* 1982;71:110–1.
12. Wallenstein S, Zucker CL, Fleiss JL. Some statistical methods useful in circulation research. *Circ Res* 1980;47:1–9.
13. Levy RH. Variability in level-dose ratio of valproate: monotherapy versus polytherapy. *Epilepsia* 1984;25(suppl):S10–13.
14. Heinemeyer G, Nau H, Hildebrandt A, Roots T. Oxidation and glucuronidation of valproic acid in male rats. Influence of phenobarbital, 3-methylcolantrene, beta-naphtoflavone and clofibrate. *Biochem Pharmacol* 1985;32:133–9.
15. Schafer H, Luhrs R. On the responsibility of the metabolite pattern for potential side effects in the rat being treated with valproic acid, 2-propylpenten-2-oic acid, and 2-propylpenten-4-oic acid. In: Levy RH, Pitlick WH, Eichenbaum M, Meijer J, eds. *Metatabolism of antiepileptic drugs*. New York: Raven Press, 1984:73–81.
16. Jeavons PM. Non–dose-related side effects of valproate. *Epilepsia* 1984;25(suppl):S50–5.
17. Coulter DL, Allen RJ. Secondary hyperammonemia: a possible mechanism for valproate encephalopathy. *Lancet* 1980;1:310–1.
18. Coulter DL, Allen RJ. Hyperammonemia with valproic acid therapy. *J Pediatr* 1981;99:317–9.
19. Jeavons PM. Valproate toxicity. In: Woodbury DM, Penry JK, Pippinger CE, eds. *Antiepileptic drugs*. New York: Raven Press, 1982:604–16.
20. Marescaux C, Warter JM, Micheletti G, Rumbach L, Coquillat G, Kurtz D. Stuporous episodes during treatment with sodium valproate: report of seven cases. *Epilepsia* 1982;23:297–305.
21. Rawat S, Borkowsky WJ, Swick HK. Valproic acid and secondary hyperammonemia. *Neurology (NY)* 1981;31:1173–4.
22. Sackellares JC, Lee SI, Dreifuss FE. Stupor following administration of valproic acid to patients receiving other antiepileptic drugs. *Epilepsia* 1979;20:697–703.
23. Zaret BS, Becker RR, Marini AM, Wagle N, Passarelli C. Sodium valproate-induced hyperammonemia without clinical hepatic dysfunction. *Neurology (NY)* 1982;32:206–8.

Therapeutic Drug Monitoring
7:191–196 © 1985 Raven Press, New York

Red Blood Cell Electrolytes for Monitoring Digoxin Therapy in Adults

C. J. van Boxtel, R. Koopmans, B. Oosterhuis, and *F. J. Hoek

*Clinical Pharmacology Section, Departments of Medicine and Pharmacology, Academical Medical Center, and *Clinical Chemistry Laboratory, Department of Medicine, University Hospital of Amsterdam, Amsterdam, The Netherlands*

Summary: Red blood cell (RBC) electrolyte concentrations were determined, with a method that can be applied easily in any clinical chemistry laboratory, in 18 patients not on digoxin therapy and 37 patients on maintenance digoxin therapy for various diagnoses. Of the digoxin-treated patients, 11 had electrocardiographic changes and other clinical evidence of digoxin toxicity. Mean RBC sodium was higher and mean RBC potassium was lower in patients on prolonged digoxin therapy than in controls, and these changes were more pronounced in patients with toxic symptoms. In the group of 11 patients with toxicity, a positive correlation was found between the ratio of RBC sodium to potassium and plasma digoxin levels ($r = 0.8234$, $p < 0.05$). Plasma digoxin concentrations did not clearly distinguish between toxic and nontoxic patients. The RBC sodium/potassium ratio, however, identified 35 of 37 patients correctly, with two patients from the toxic and two patients from the nontoxic group giving the same results. Changes in intracellular erythrocyte electrolytes in adults appear to correlate closely with clinical signs of digoxin toxicity. **Key Words:** Erythrocytes—Red blood cells—Sodium levels—Potassium levels—Digoxin.

Cardiac glycosides are commonly thought to exert their pharmacological effect by inhibiting the membrane-bound Na^+,K^+-adenosine triphosphatase (ATPase). This inhibition occurs in many tissues, including red blood cells (RBC). The predicted effect of that inhibition, a fall in the RBC potassium concentration and a rise in RBC sodium, has been described in many studies (1–7). Theoretically, these RBC electrolyte changes can be expected to reflect the clinical effect of cardiac glycosides better than the plasma digoxin level (3,8,9). The latter is a pharmacokinetic variable, while RBC electrolytes represent a pharmacodynamic effect.

There are some indications of a relationship between RBC electrolytes and the clinical response to digoxin. Loes et al. (2) found that RBC electrolytes discriminated between toxic and nontoxic digoxin-taking patients better than did the plasma digoxin level. On the other hand, Henion et al. (6), despite finding a significant relationship between plasma digoxin concentration and RBC electrolytes, found that the latter predicted digoxin toxicity more poorly than did the drug plasma concentration. The findings by Aronson et al. (10) indicate that the decrease in ventricular rate in patients with atrial fibrillation correlates better with RBC ^{86}Rb uptake than with the plasma digoxin level. Ford et al. (11) established a correlation of RBC sodium with the therapeutic effect of digoxin administered for cardiac failure (shortening of the electromechanical systole). They found no correlation between this therapeutic effect and the plasma digoxin level.

Several studies have tried to establish a temporal relationship between digoxin administration and RBC electrolytes. Ford et al. (11) found a rise in RBC sodium over the first few days of treatment. In chronically treated patients (>2 months) RBC sodium was not significantly different from that in the control group, unless toxicity was present. In agreement with these findings, Morgan et al. (4) found RBC sodium

Address correspondence and reprint requests to Dr. C. J. van Boxtel at Clinical Pharmacology Section, Departments of Medicine and Pharmacology, Academical Medical Center, Meibergdreef 9, 1105 AZ Amsterdam, The Netherlands.

in a large group of chronically treated nontoxic patients to be either slightly elevated or not elevated. Loes et al. (7) studied two pediatric cases. RBC electrolyte changes seemed to peak at about 24–48 h after digoxin administration during chronic treatment or a considerable overdose.

The aim of our study was to establish the usefulness of the ratio of RBC sodium to RBC potassium [as described by Loes et al. (2)] for the diagnosis of digoxin toxicity in adults, using methods that can easily be applied in any clinical chemistry laboratory. We further correlated plasma digoxin levels with RBC potassium, RBC sodium, and the ratio of RBC sodium to RBC potassium; and we studied the temporal changes in RBC electrolytes after administration of a single dose of digoxin.

MATERIALS AND METHODS

Patients

The patients for this study consisted of 18 controls not treated with digoxin and 37 patients on maintenance digoxin therapy for various diagnoses. The 55 subjects were either visiting the cardiology, internal medicine, or infectious diseases outpatient clinics of the university hospital of the University of Amsterdam, or were inpatients of the hospital. Two categories of patients were studied in addition to the 18 controls: 26 patients on maintenance digoxin therapy without signs of toxicity and 11 patients on maintenance digoxin therapy, who had electrocardiographic changes and other clinical evidence of digoxin toxicity. Diagnosis of digitalis toxicity was established by the cardiologist treating the patient. The ultimate criterion was an existing arrhythmia, one not seen before digitalis treatment in that particular patient and which disappeared within 48 h after digoxin withdrawal. Nontoxic subjects and controls were chosen at random from the outpatient and inpatient populations.

Temporal relationships between RBC electrolytes and plasma digoxin concentration were studied. After informed consent had been obtained, a single oral dose of 1 mg digoxin was given to one healthy volunteer, and 18 samples of blood were collected during the 55 h after dosage. Two groups of two rabbits were given doses of digoxin intravenously, 0.050 and 0.075 mg/kg, respectively, and 9–11 samples were taken during the 3 and 4.5 h after dosage.

Electrolyte Determinations

Blood from patients was taken at least 6 h after the last dose. All samples were centrifuged within 2 h after they were obtained. RBCs were washed twice with a 0.25 *M* sucrose solution and hemolyzed by dilution with distilled water. Sodium and potassium were determined by flame photometry. Per sample electrolyte concentrations were corrected for sucrose trapping. Sucrose trapping was determined by centrifuging a specimen of the packed erythrocytes after the last washing at high speed (12,000 *g*) in a microhematocrit centrifuge. The mean hematocrit of packed cells determined by this method was 0.83 ± 0.01 (mean ± SEM). The standard error of the mean of duplicate RBC sodium determinations was ± 0.2 mEq/L, and for the potassium determinations, ± 0.8 mEq/L.

Plasma Digoxin Analyses

Plasma digoxin concentrations were estimated by enzyme immunoassay (EMIT, Merck), this being the routine for digoxin monitoring in our hospital. RBC digoxin had to be determined by radioimmunoassay (RIA), as hemoglobin interferes with the enzyme assay. All samples were analyzed in duplicate. Ten plasma samples with digoxin concentrations ranging from 0.4 to 3.4 ng/ml were reanalyzed with RIA. The regression equation for the correlation graph of RIA (x) and EMIT (y) determinations was $y = 0.9977x + 0.2533$ $(r = 0.9789)$. Standard errors for EMIT digoxin analyses were 0.20 ng/ml (sample concentrations, >2 ng/ml), 0.04 (sample concentrations, 1–2 ng/ml), and 0.02 (sample concentrations, <1 ng/ml).

Statistical Analyses

For comparison of the means of plasma electrolytes, RBC electrolytes, and plasma digoxin obtained in each group, Student's *t* test was used. The values in this article represent two-tailed probabilities. Regression lines and correlation coefficients were calculated by the method of least squares.

RESULTS

Following administration of a single dose of digoxin to a healthy subject, no changes in RBC electrolyte concentrations were seen during 55 h after dosage. RBC digoxin uptake was very fast. The concentration–time curve of RBC digoxin was about the same as the curve for plasma digoxin (Fig. 1). Administration of considerably higher doses of digoxin to rabbits (comparable to 5–10 mg orally in a human) resulting in digoxin plasma levels of 25 ng/ml initially, which decreased in 4.5 h to 5 ng/ml, produced no changes in RBC electrolytes during the first 4.5 h after dosing.

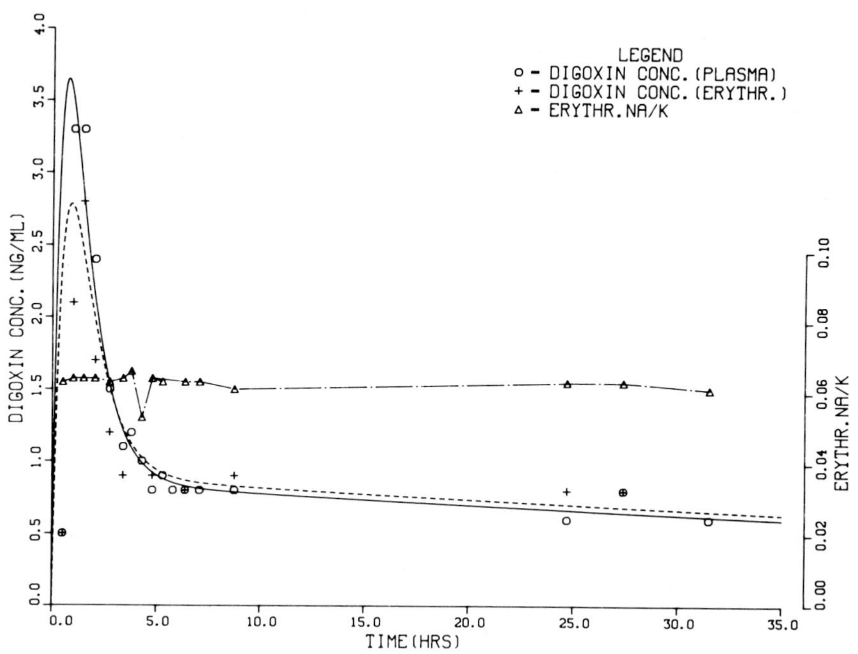

FIG. 1. Time course of drug concentration and red blood cell Na/K ratio in a healthy volunteer after administration of an oral dose of 1 mg digoxin.

Electrolyte and plasma digoxin concentrations obtained for the different groups of patients are given in Table 1. Mean plasma sodium and potassium concentration and mean RBC potassium concentration for the nontoxic digoxin-using group and the control group were not statistically significantly different. However, differences between RBC sodium and the ratio of RBC sodium to RBC potassium for these two groups were statistically significant ($p < 0.005$). For the toxic and the nontoxic digoxin-using groups, differences between plasma sodium and potassium concentrations were not statistically significant. The differences between these two groups for RBC sodium, RBC potassium, and the ratio of RBC sodium to RBC potassium were all significant at the $p < 0.001$ level, and also mean digoxin concentrations differed significantly ($p < 0.001$). Individual measurements of electrolyte ratios and digoxin levels in the toxic and nontoxic digoxin-taking patients are shown in Fig. 2.

RBC electrolyte concentrations were correlated with the plasma digoxin level. The ratio of RBC sodium to RBC potassium had a coefficient of correlation of 0.8307 ($p < 0.001$) with the plasma digoxin level for the whole group of patients on maintenance digoxin therapy ($n = 37$). This correlation was almost entirely due to the group of toxic patients ($n = 11$). If their ratios and plasma digoxin levels alone were correlated, the coefficient of correlation was 0.8234 ($p < 0.005$). The nontoxic group ($n = 26$) did not follow this correlation ($r = 0.095$). For the whole group ($n = 37$), RBC sodium correlated better ($r = 0.8113$) with the plasma digoxin level than did RBC potassium ($r = 0.6596$). The ratio of RBC sodium to RBC potassium correctly identified 95% of

TABLE 1. *Plasma and red blood cell electrolytes and plasma digoxin levels*

Group	No. of patients	RBC Na (mEq/L)	Plasma Na (mEq/L)	RBC K (mEq/L)	Plasma K (mEq/L)	RBC Na/K ratio	Plasma digoxin (ng/ml)
Control	18	6.1 ± 0.4	135.9 ± 0.6 (n = 9)	103.3 ± 2.4	3.9 ± 0.1 (n = 9)	0.06 ± 0.004	—
Nontoxic	26	8.0 ± 0.4[a]	135.2 ± 1.0 (n = 24)	101.1 ± 1.3	4.1 ± 0.1 (n = 24)	0.08 ± 0.004[a]	1.3 ± 0.1
Toxic	11	15.7 ± 1.3[b]	132.1 ± 1.6 (n = 9)	90.1 ± 2.6[b]	4.3 ± 0.2 (n = 9)	0.18 ± 0.01[b]	3.0 ± 0.5[b]

Values are means ± SEM. RBC, red blood cell.
[a] $p < 0.005$.
[b] $p < 0.001$.

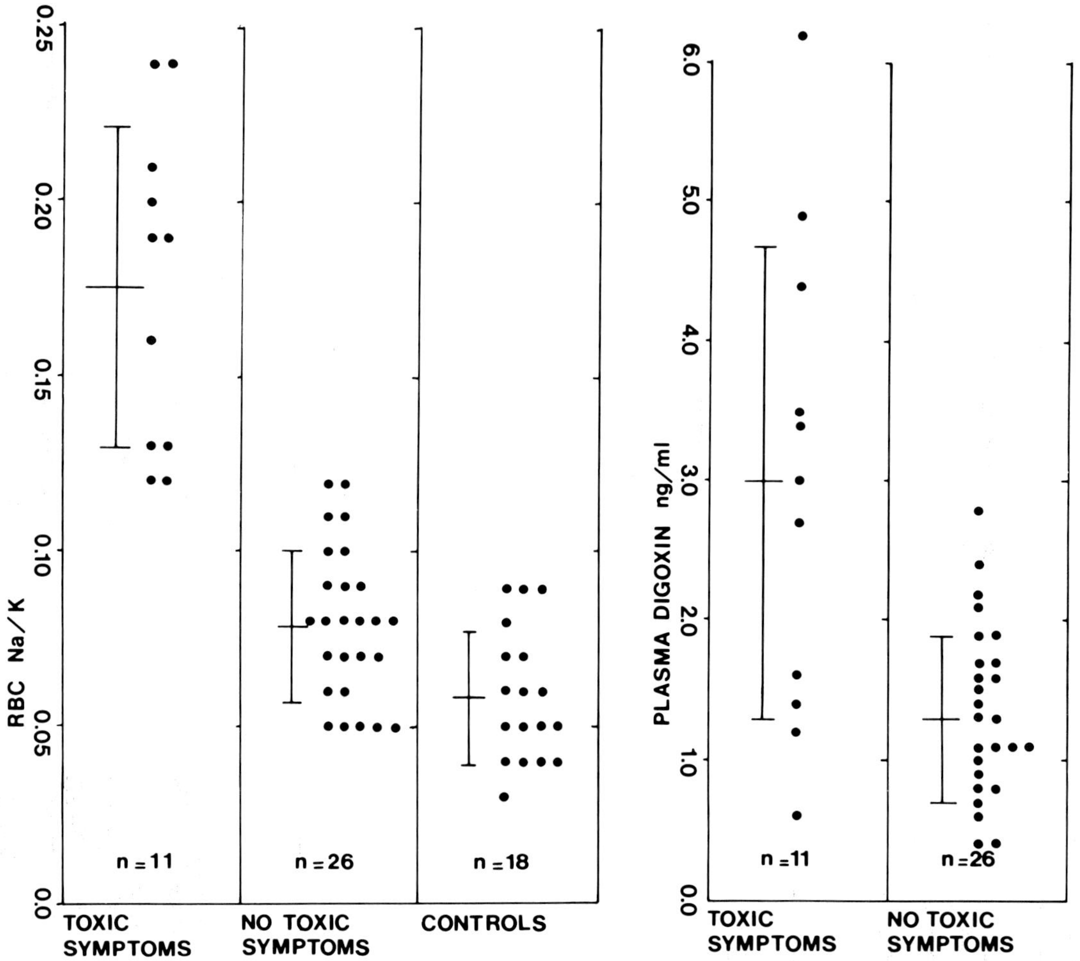

FIG. 2. Red blood cell electrolyte ratios and plasma digoxin levels and means ± SEM in patients and controls.

the patients in a group of 11 toxic and 26 nontoxic patients, while the plasma digoxin levels in the same group correctly identified 78% of the patients. RBC sodium or RBC potassium alone was less informative than the two combined (correctly identifying 89 and 84% of the patients, respectively). Sensitivity, specificity, and predictive value of both the RBC electrolyte ratio and the plasma digoxin concentration are shown in Table 2. A cutoff value for RBC Na/K ratio to diagnose toxicity has been put at 2 standard deviations above the mean ratio in the digoxin-treated patients with no clinical signs of toxicity.

TABLE 2. *Efficacy of pharmacodynamic versus pharmacokinetic monitoring of digoxin therapy*

	RBC Na/K > 0.12 (%)	Digoxin > 2 ng/ml (%)
Sensitivity TP/(TP + FN) × 100	82	64
Specificity TN/(TN + FP) × 100	100	85
Predictive value TP/(TP + FP) × 100	100	64

RBC, red blood cell; TP, true positive; TN, true negative; FN, false negative; FP, false positive.

DISCUSSION

Digoxin overdose is associated with considerable changes in RBC sodium and potassium. These changes can be useful for the diagnosis of digoxin toxicity. In this article, it is shown that the ratio of RBC sodium to RBC potassium is a better parameter for identifying toxic and nontoxic patients than the plasma digoxin concentration. Our findings are in agreement with those of Loes et al. (2). In contrast to their study, we made an at-random sampling of control patients, patients chronically using digoxin, and patients admitted to the hospital for possible digoxin toxicity. Although our results in adults are comparable with those obtained in children (2), they are not in accordance with those of Henion et al. (6), who also studied adults. They found less favorable figures for sensitivity, specificity, and predictive value of RBC electrolytes; but their values given for group means of RBC Na/K ratios were also different. In this respect, it is important that our method of RBC preparation is different from that in both the studies mentioned. Ours is very simple and easier to handle and could therefore be more reproducible.

RBC potassium concentrations are less well correlated with the plasma digoxin level than are sodium concentrations. Morgan et al. (4) comment on this and suggest that the rise in sodium and the fall in potassium are probably of the same magnitude in molar terms, but that the sodium changes are proportionally larger than potassium changes and therefore better correlated with the plasma digoxin level. Although RBC potassium concentrations are less well correlated with the plasma digoxin level, they are useful. The combination of sodium and potassium in a ratio of RBC sodium to RBC potassium discriminates better among toxic and nontoxic patients than RBC sodium alone.

After initiation of digoxin therapy, changes in RBC electrolytes become apparent only after a few days (7,11). We found in rabbits that even very high digoxin concentrations do not produce measurable changes in RBC electrolyte concentrations during the first few hours. Our data suggest, however, that receptor binding could occur very quickly, as the RBC digoxin concentration is nearly the same as the plasma digoxin concentration during the first 55 h after a single dose. The fact that digoxin does have rapid effects on ^{86}Rb uptake in erythrocytes (10) is not in contradiction with our observations. With radioactive Rb, small ion fluxes are measured in a very sensitive way, while we are observing the overall effects of changes in these ion fluxes on electrolyte pools. The delay in RBC electrolyte changes can be explained by a time-consuming electrolyte redistribution process, after blocking of the Na^+,K^+-ATPase by digoxin. Changes in myocardial cell electrolytes probably are much faster, as ions actively pass over the cell membrane with each depolarization. Ford et al. (11) found RBC sodium to be significantly altered in two groups of toxic and recently digitalized patients. They did not find significant changes in RBC sodium in a chronically (more than 2 months) digoxin-taking but nontoxic group. The cause of this change in electrolyte concentration with steady digoxin concentration possibly lies in a decreasing sensitivity of the receptor (the Na^+,K^+-ATPase). Alternatively, there may be an increased number of Na^+,K^+-ATPase receptor sites per RBC. This would mean that a more or less acute event has taken place in digoxin toxicity. Our findings indicate that differences of RBC electrolytes between controls and chronically digoxin-taking nontoxic patients are indeed very small as compared with differences between the latter group and the toxic group.

With regard to other factors, apart from digoxin, that can potentially influence RBC electrolytes, the following should be said. An influence of diuretics on RBC electrolytes has been shown (12). However, the two clinical studies of major importance thus far (2,6) have both found RBC cations to be comparable between patients that do and patients that do not take diuretics together with digitalis. Furthermore, a better correlation of signs of digoxin toxicity with RBC electrolytes in comparison with plasma digoxin levels is understandable in view of the fact that altered gradients of electrolytes with increased RBC sodium content are known to increase the risk of digitalis intoxication and arrhythmias (13). Whether diuretics have contributed to those electrolyte changes is thus of less importance, on the condition that RBC electrolyte changes mirror those in cardiac cells.

If, indeed, changes in RBC electrolytes after digoxin administration take a few days to occur, it can be inferred that by the same mechanism they will stay altered for some time after digoxin is withheld. Such a delay will have two consequences. First, determination of the ratio of RBC sodium to RBC potassium for diagnosing toxicity during the first few days of therapy may give false negative results. Second, and of more importance, during several days after digoxin has been withheld, one could still retrospectively diagnose an overdose with such pharmacodynamic monitoring of digitalis therapy.

REFERENCES

1. Kettlewell M, Nowers A, White R. Effect of digoxin on human red blood cell electrolytes. *Br J Pharmacol* 1972;44:165–7.
2. Loes MW, Singh S, Lock JE, Mirkin BL. Relation between plasma and red cell electrolyte concentrations and digoxin levels in children. *N Engl J Med* 1978;299:501–4.
3. Wessels F, Samizadeh A, Losse H. Diagnosis der Digitalis Intoxikation durch Bestimmung der Erythrocyten-electrolyte. *Klin Wochenschr* 1974;52:341–5.
4. Morgan DB, Cumberbatch M, Cohn S, et al. The erythrocyte sodium and potassium in patients treated with digoxin. *Br J Clin Pharmacol* 1980;10:127–33.

5. Clifford TC, Bentyman W. Changes in erythrocyte potassium in patients with cardiac failure treated with digitalis. *Clin Chem* 1958;4:311–5.
6. Henion WA, Montondo D, Hilal A, Bayer R, Cohen J. Changes in red blood cell electrolyte concentrations in digitalis intoxication. *Am Heart J* 1983;106:14–20.
7. Loes MW, Lock JE, Singh S, Mirkin BL. The kinetics of red blood cell electrolyte alterations following digoxin administration. *Dev Pharmacol Ther* 1981;3:50–4.
8. Wessels F, Samizadeh A, Heinze A, Tasche V. Erythrozytenelectrolyte als Parameter einer wirksamen Digitalisierung. *Verh Dtsch Ges Inn Med* 1975;81:1672–4.
9. Grahame-Smith DG. The foxglove. 1978: Some aspects of the clinical pharmacology of digoxin. Part V. In: Dickenson CJ, Morris J, eds. *Developments in cardiovascular medicine*. London: MTP Press Ltd, 1978.
10. Aronson JK, Grahame-Smith DG, Hallis KF, Hibble AF, Wigley F. Monitoring digoxin therapy: 1. Plasma concentrations and an in vitro assay of tissue response. *Br J Clin Pharmacol* 1977;4:213–21.
11. Ford AR, Aronson JK, Grahame-Smith DG, Carver JG. Changes in cardiac glycoside receptor sites, ^{86}rubidium uptake and intracellular sodium concentrations in the erythrocytes of patients receiving digoxin during the early phases of treatment of cardiac failure in regular rhythm and of atrial fibrillation. *Br J Clin Pharmacol* 1979;8:125–34.
12. Walter U. Red blood cell sodium and potassium after hydrochlorothiazide. *Clin Pharmacol Ther* 1981;30:373–7.
13. Mason DT, Zelis R, Lee G, Hughes JL, Spann JF, Amsterdam EA. Current concepts and treatment of digitalis toxicity. *Am J Cardiol* 1971;27:546–59.

Therapeutic Drug Monitoring
7:197–201

Influence of Body Fat on the Volume of Distribution of Theophylline

Peter J. Jewesson and Robin J. Ensom

Division of Clinical Pharmacy, Faculty of Pharmaceutical Sciences, University of British Columbia, Vancouver, British Columbia, Canada

Summary: Twenty-six acutely bronchospastic patients admitted to the emergency room of an acute care hospital were studied to determine the influence of body fat on the volume of distribution (V_d) of theophylline. Total body weight (TBW), height, skinfold thickness (at three sites), and theophylline levels around an intravenous aminophylline dose were measured. Ideal body weight (IBW), percentage of body fat, and absolute and relative V_d of theophylline were calculated. V_d of theophylline correlated better with IBW than TBW. No relationship was identified between V_d normalized to IBW and either percentage of body fat or the ratio of TBW to IBW. This indicates that in our sample (0.8 IBW < TBW < 1.4 IBW), distribution of theophylline into adipose tissue was not an important determinant of V_d. Theophylline's V_d was best estimated by the formula V_d (L) = 0.419(L/kg) × IBW(kg). **Key Words:** Body fat—Theophylline—Distribution.

The therapeutic range of serum theophylline for the treatment of bronchospastic disorders is narrow (10–20 μg/ml), and even within that range, concentration changes have been shown to result in a considerable variation in both efficacy and incidence of toxicity (1–4). Therefore, it is appropriate that the dosage requirements for theophylline be as accurate as possible. One important determinant of theophylline dosage requirements is volume of distribution (V_d).

The calculation of an appropriate loading dose of theophylline is dependent on an accurate estimation of a patient's V_d. A similar estimation is essential to the pharmacokinetic interpretation of a serum drug level during non–steady-state kinetics. The V_d of theophylline ranges between 0.3 and 0.7 L/kg (2). Acidemia, pregnancy, and hepatic cirrhosis have been demonstrated to cause an increase in this parameter, while sex, smoking history, asthma, and acute pulmonary edema reportedly have no effect (4,5).

Address correspondence and reprint requests to Dr. R. Ensom at Division of Clinical Pharmacy, Faculty of Pharmaceutical Sciences, 2146 East Mall, Vancouver, British Columbia, Canada, V6T 1W5.

The influence of obesity on the V_d of theophylline has been the subject of two previous studies (6,7). However, the results of these reports conflict. Gal et al. (6) conclude that theophylline readily distributes into fat and that loading dose is best calculated on the basis of total body weight (TBW), whereas Rohrbaugh et al. (7) state that theophylline is not extensively distributed into adipose tissue and loading dose calculations should be based on ideal body weight (IBW).

The objectives of this study were as follows: (a) to determine the V_d of theophylline in a sample of acutely bronchospastic patients; (b) to determine whether TBW or IBW is more strongly associated with the calculated V_d; and (c) to determine whether measures of adiposity are related to V_d.

METHODS

Patient Selection

The study population included 26 asthmatic patients (15 men and 11 women, aged 17 to 83 years) admitted to the emergency department of a 550 bed, general, acute care hospital. All patients were prescribed intravenous loading doses of aminophylline for the treatment of an acute bronchospastic attack. Informed consent was obtained from all participants. Participants with known factors affecting the disposition of theophylline, including liver disease, congestive heart failure, and pregnancy, were excluded. No attempt was made to exclude acidemic patients, as these patients were considered to be representative of the typical acutely bronchospastic population.

Drug Administration

The loading dose of aminophylline was determined by the casualty officer independent of this study and ranged from 1.75 to 7.0 mg/kg (Table 1). Each dose was administered in a 100 ml minibag solution of 5% dextrose in water or normal saline during ~30 min. In all cases, this was immediately followed by a continuous infusion of aminophylline at a rate ranging from 0.25 to 0.94 mg/kg/h.

Measurements

Within 30 min prior to the administration of intravenous aminophylline, ~10 ml of venous blood was drawn for theophylline assay. Thirty minutes after the completion of the loading dose infusion, a second blood sample was also drawn from the antecubital vein of the arm uninvolved in the aminophylline infusion. All blood specimens were collected in a red or red/gray tris(2-butoxyethyl phosphate (TBEP)-free evacuated blood specimen tube (Vacutainer, Becton Dickinson). Samples were allowed to clot. They were then centrifuged, and the serum was separated and frozen until analysis. All specimens were assayed for theophylline by homogeneous enzyme immunoassay (EMIT, Syva). Serum theophylline concentrations were calculated from daily calibration curves obtained with standards provided by the manufacturer. Within-run and day-to-day precision were determined; the data yielded a coefficient of variation (CV) of <10 and 4%, respectively.

Within 24 h of the aminophylline loading dose, height, weight, and skinfold thickness measurements

TABLE 1. *Summary of individual patient data*

Patient	Age (yr)	Sex	Smoke/ Drug[a]	Weight (kg) Total	Ideal	% > or < ideal	Height (cm)	Aminophylline dose (mg)	C_{pre} (μg/ml)	C_{post} (μg/ml)	V_d/TBW (L/kg)	V_d/IBW (L/kg)	K_e[b] (h^{-1})	Body fat (%)
1	57	M	—	51.2	63.4	−19	168.5	250	0	6.8	0.523	0.423	0.100	11.9
2	38	M	—	58.5	69.2	−15	176.5	200	2.5	7.8	0.471	0.398	0.079	10.1
3	62	M	1	53.4	61.9	−14	166.6	300	0	8.9	0.471	0.405	0.127	16.3
4	53	M	1	53.0	60.8	−13	165.0	250	0	5.6	0.588	0.512	0.165	10.0
5	22	M	—	62.0	70.8	−12	178.7	350	1.2	9.3	0.522	0.457	(0.091)	8.4
6	50	F	—	41.6	46.2	−10	148.6	150	10.8	19.7	0.261	0.235	0.132	22.9
7	63	F	—	55.5	60.7	−9	171.0	250	0	5.8	0.538	0.491	0.160	29.6
8	69	F	1	42.6	46.1	−8	148.4	300	0	12.3	0.433	0.401	0.076	—
9	83	M	—	51.6	55.9	−8	158.2	275	0	10.2	0.360	0.333	(0.091)	—
10	24	M	1	62.4	64.8	−4	170.5	400	0	12.1	0.378	0.363	(0.141)	15.7
11	61	F	—	42.1	43.9	−4	145.1	150	0	4.4	0.578	0.554	(0.091)	24.2
12	40	M	—	66.3	67.2	−1	173.7	200	8.1	11.0	0.354	0.349	0.158	14.7
13	17	M	1	71.4	67.2	+6	173.8	125	23.4	25.6	0.267	0.284	0.094	13.7
14	28	F	1	68.6	62.9	+9	174.3	300	1.2	7.8	0.446	0.486	0.152	24.6
15	62	M	—	74.6	67.8	+10	174.6	350	0	9.2	0.382	0.421	0.079	24.8
16	30	F	1	61.5	55.2	+11	162.5	350	1.8	12.1	0.413	0.460	0.073	29.8
17	52	F	—	62.3	55.7	+12	163.2	200	2.6	7.9	0.435	0.487	(0.091)	35.8
18	42	M	—	77.1	68.6	+12	175.7	250	0	6.2	0.396	0.445	(0.091)	23.3
19	39	F	—	52.6	46.3	+14	148.7	300	0	12.0	0.351	0.399	(0.091)	33.3
20	43	F	—	59.0	51.2	+15	156.3	150	5.3	11.4	0.245	0.283	0.222	30.0
21	50	M	1	66.5	57.3	+16	160.3	350	0	10.0	0.393	0.455	0.078	27.6
22	46	M	—	77.4	62.6	+24	167.5	500	0	12.0	0.390	0.482	0.088	27.3
23	47	F	—	69.6	52.4	+33	158.2	175	16.0	19.4	0.361	0.479	0.139	33.2
24	41	M	2	89.4	66.4	+35	172.6	400	0	12.4	0.269	0.362	(0.069)	28.4
25	46	M	—	107.6	77.1	+38	187.4	400	0	7.4	0.372	0.519	(0.091)	29.9
26	36	F	1	80.7	57.7	+41	166.3	150	6.4	10.4	0.301	0.421	0.130	34.5

C, serum theophylline concentration before (pre) and after (post) aminophylline loading dose; V_d, volume of distribution; TBW, total body weight; IBW, ideal body weight; K_e, elimination rate constant.

[a] 1 = smoker, 2 = concurrent cimetidine use.

[b] ( ) Literature estimates.

were obtained. Height was determined to the nearest 0.1 cm by use of a metric tape measure, with the barefoot patient standing erect, heels together, and arms hanging naturally by the sides. TBW was determined to the nearest 0.1 kg by use of a beam-balance scale, which was balanced prior to each measurement. Patients wore only a thin, hospital-issued cotton gown during this procedure.

Skinfold thickness measurements were obtained from right triceps, subscapular, and suprailiac sites by use of a set of skinfold calipers (Harpenden, British Indicators Inc.) according to accepted procedures (8–10). All measurements were made in triplicate by one investigator, and the median value to the nearest 0.1 mm was recorded. Body density was determined from the sum of these measurements by use of age-specific formulas determined by Durnin and Womersley (8). The resulting body density values were then converted to percentage of body fat by use of Siri's equation (11).

Calculations

IBW was estimated from sex and height by formulas derived from life insurance tables (12,13): IBW (men) = 51.65 kg + 1.85 kg/in of height > 5 ft; IBW (women) = 48.67 kg + 1.65 kg/in of height > 5 ft.

To permit specific comparisons with previous investigations of theophylline disposition relative to body fat, patients were categorized as lean if calculated IBW exceeded TBW, normal if TBW exceeded IBW but was less than 20% over IBW, and obese if TBW was at least 20% over IBW for both sexes (7).

V_d was calculated from the formula

$$V_d = \frac{K_0(1 - e^{-K_e(T_2 - T_1)})e^{-K_e(T_4 - T_2)} + K_{02}(1 - e^{-K_e(T_4 - T_3)})}{K_e(C_{post} - C_{pre}e^{-K_e(T_4)})}$$

where K_0 is the loading dose infusion rate constant (mg/h), K_{02} is the maintenance dose infusion rate constant (mg/h), T_1 is the time of the initiation of the loading dose infusion, T_2 is the end of the infusion, T_3 is the initiation time of the maintenance dose infusion, T_4 is the time of the second blood sample, and C_{pre} and C_{post} represent serum theophylline concentrations prior to and after administration of the loading dose, respectively. The elimination rate constant (K_e) was determined by the drug measurement service for 17 patients who were subsequently followed up by this service and subjected to further blood level determinations during their stay (14). The method of determining K_e involved a progressive iterative calculator program adjusting the estimated K_e in such a way that predicted serum concentrations were within 1% of the measured concentrations (15).

Specific elimination rate information was not available for nine patients. However, we chose not to exclude these patients. We justified their inclusion on the basis of the fact that preloading dose theophylline concentrations were 0 μg/ml in seven patients, with the remaining two patients having initial concentrations of <3 μg/ml. The interval between initiation of infusion (T_1) and the second blood sample (T_4) was <1.5 h for all nine patients, and minor inaccuracies in estimation of K_e would not be expected to influence our V_d determination. For these individuals, a history of smoking status and concurrent use of drugs known to influence the elimination of theophylline (cimetidine, erythromycin, anticonvulsants, and influenza vaccine) was established. Depending upon the presence or absence of these factors (two of the patients were smokers and one patient was currently taking oral cimetidine), K_e was estimated from average literature values and employed for the calculation of V_d (16–21).

Infusion set dead volume (~8%), infusion solution bag overfill (~5%) and drug volume (500 mg/10 ml) were accounted for in determination of actual theophylline loading and maintenance dosages administered to study patients. The aminophylline solution for injection contained 39.5 mg (79%) of theophylline per ml of solution (written communication, Abbott Laboratories).

Analysis

Statistical analysis was performed with the University of British Columbia Statistical Package for the Social Sciences (SPSS:9). A two-tailed Student's *t* test was used to compare mean V_d between lean, normal, and obese groups, and the Pearson correlation coefficient was used to examine the relationship between V_d, body fat, and weight. Statistical significance was set at $p < 0.05$.

RESULTS

Patient characteristics including sex, age, height, weight, percentage of body fat, and V_d are listed in Table 1. Percentage of body fat was not determined in two patients, as their ages exceeded the upper limits of the Durnin and Womersley formulas (8).

Figure 1 is a graph of V_d as a function of IBW. The positive association between V_d and IBW was stronger ($r = +0.69$, $p < 0.001$) than the relationship between V_d and TBW ($r = +0.56$, $p < 0.005$). The slope of the line represents average V_d of 0.419 L/kg IBW.

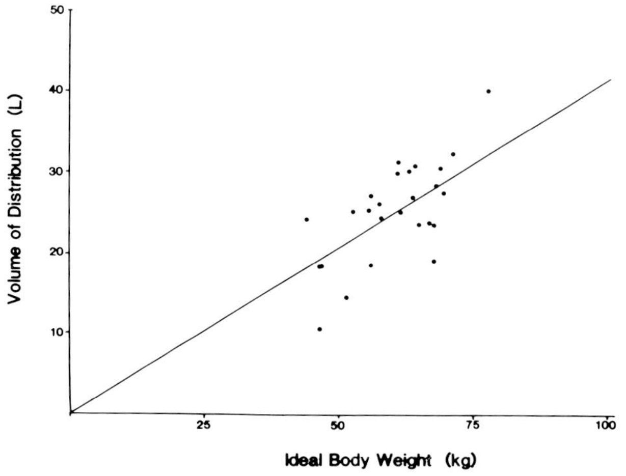

FIG. 1. Volume of distribution of theophylline in relation to ideal body weight.

Figure 2 is a graph of V_d as a function of IBW (V_d/I) and TBW (V_d/T) for patients categorized as lean (n = 12), normal (n = 9), or obese (n = 5). The V_d/I (mean ± SD) was 0.410 ± 0.087, 0.413 ± 0.079, and 0.453 ± 0.062 L/kg in lean, normal, and obese patients, respectively. This difference between groups was not significant. The V_d/T (mean ± SD) was 0.456 ± 0.10, 0.369 ± 0.070, and 0.338 ± 0.051 L/kg in lean, normal, and obese patients, respectively. When obese and lean patients were compared, this difference was significant ($p < 0.05$).

No significant relationship was found between V_d/I and percentage of body fat ($r = +0.187$) or between V_d/I and the ratio of TBW to IBW ($r = +0.160$).

DISCUSSION

An important aspect of this study is that the subjects represent an unselected sample of those patients admitted to the emergency room of this hospital for treatment of acute bronchospasm. Therefore, our sample is small and does not include as extreme a range of percentage of body fat as that present in the previously cited studies (6,7) in which obese subjects were specifically sought. The relationship of V_d to IBW and TBW that is identified in this study reflects that relationship which exists over a narrower range of total to ideal body weight ratios.

Another consideration is that our data were collected for patients receiving an intravenous aminophylline loading dose. Therefore, recommendations provided should be of particular relevance to this clinical situation.

The results of three of our analyses suggest that the distribution of theophylline into adipose tissue was not significant in our population. First, the strength of association for V_d versus IBW was greater than for V_d versus TBW. Second, neither V_d/I versus percentage of body fat nor V_d/I versus TBW/IBW (two indices of adiposity) resulted in a significant correlation. Finally, the mean V_d/I did not vary appreciably between the lean, normal, and obese groups (Fig. 2). However,

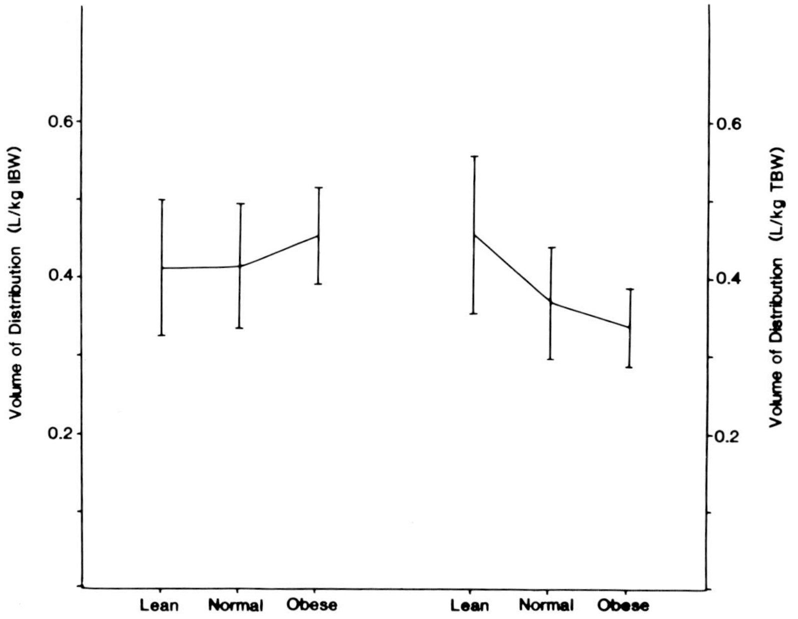

FIG. 2. Volume of distribution of theophylline normalized to ideal body weight (IBW) and total body weight (TBW) in lean, normal, and obese patients. Bars and vertical lines show mean ± 1 SD for data from 26 patients.

there was a significant difference between the mean V_d/T of the lean and obese groups. Our interpretation of the data is that IBW is preferable to TBW in determining V_d. Therefore, we would recommend that in the treatment of patients whose TBW is within 40% over and 20% under their IBW, the V_d of theophylline should be estimated by use of IBW. Specifically, our sample demonstrated an average V_d of 0.419 L/kg IBW.

The literature suggests that in the very obese patient a more complex relationship may exist. Both Gal et al. (6) and Rohrbaugh et al. (7) examined very obese patients whose TBW/IBW ratios were higher than in our sample. These studies confirm the trends identified in Fig. 2. In the sequence from lean patients to very obese patients, the mean V_d/I increases while the V_d/T decreases. Pharmacokinetic data obtained from a single 522.7 kg man as reported by Koup and Vawter (22) demonstrate this relationship in the extremely obese patient. The estimated V_d for this patient was 132.1 L, suggesting a V_d/I of 1.74 L/kg and a V_d/T of 0.25 L/kg.

These trends indicate that neither IBW nor TBW can be used alone to accurately predict V_d for all patients. We offer two possible theories to explain these findings: (a) although theophylline primarily distributes into lean tissue (as demonstrated by our sample) as the relative amount of adipose tissue increases, its contribution to the V_d of theophylline becomes significant; and/or (b) IBW based upon height may not be a good predictor of lean body mass in the very obese patient. We suspect that these individuals have a greater lean tissue mass to support their total mass than estimated by use of IBW formulas and therefore a larger V_d than their IBW would suggest.

In conclusion, our study supports the suggestion of Rohrbaugh et al. (7) that IBW be used to predict the V_d of theophylline. An average V_d of 0.419 L/kg of IBW was identified for patients whose actual weight is within 40% over and 20% under their ideal weight. Patients weighing >40% of their IBW should be considered separately, as there are indications that V_d cannot be accurately predicted from either IBW or TBW alone in this population.

Acknowledgment: This work was supported by University of British Columbia Research Grant 32-9606. We would like to acknowledge Dr. Chris Rumbal, Dr. Albert Scholtz, Dr. Francis Rosenberg, Sally Scotland, Richard Ward, and the staff of the emergency and pharmacy departments of St. Paul's Hospital for their contribution to this research.

REFERENCES

1. Ellis EF. Theophylline and derivatives. In: Middleton E Jr, Reed CE, Ellis EF, eds. *Allergy. Principles and Practice*. St. Louis: CV Mosby, 1978.
2. Hendeles L, Weinberger M, Johnson G. Theophylline. In: Evans WE, Schentag JJ, Jusko WJ, eds. *Applied pharmacokinetics. Principles of therapeutic drug monitoring*. San Francisco: Applied Therapeutics, 1980.
3. Jacobs MH, Senior RM, Kessler G. Clinical experience with theophylline: relationships between dosage, serum concentration and toxicity. *JAMA* 1976;235:1983–6.
4. Ogilvie RI. Clinical pharmacokinetics of theophylline. *Clin Pharmacokinet* 1978;3:267–93.
5. Van Dellen RG. Theophylline. Practical application of new knowledge. *Mayo Clin Proc* 1979;54:733–45.
6. Gal P, Jusko WJ, Yurchak AM, Franklin BA. Theophylline disposition in obesity. *Clin Pharmacol Ther* 1978;23:438–44.
7. Rohrbaugh TM, Danish M, Ragni MC, Yaffe SJ. The effect of obesity on apparent volume of distribution of theophylline. *Pediatr Pharmacol* 1982;2:75–83.
8. Durnin JV, Womersley J. Body fat assessed from total body density and its estimation from skinfold thickness: measurements on 481 men and women aged from 16 to 72 years. *Br J Nutr* 1974;32:77–97.
9. Lohman TG. Skinfolds and body density and their relation to body fatness: a review. *Hum Biol* 1981;53:181–225.
10. Mueller WH, Stallones L. Anatomical distribution of subcutaneous fat: skinfold site choice and construction of indices. *Hum Biol* 1981;53:321–35.
11. Siri WE. The gross composition of the body. *Adv Biol Med Phys* 1956;4:239–80.
12. Metropolitan Life Insurance Company. *Desirable weight in indoor clothing*. Statistical Bulletin No. 40, 1959.
13. Robinson JD, Lupkieqicz SM, Palenik L, Lopez LM, Arlet M. Determination of ideal body weight for drug dosage calculations. *Am J Hosp Pharm* 1983;40:1016–9.
14. Ensom RJ, Godwin CC, Nakagawa RS. The development of a drug measurement service at St. Paul's Hospital: a pharmacy perspective. *Can J Hosp Pharm* 1982;35:135–42.
15. Ensom RJ, Nakagawa RS. Calculator programs to deal with non-steady state, multiple dosage regimen clinical pharmacokinetics. *Int J Biomed Computing* 1983;14:287–309.
16. Jackson JE, Powell JR, Wandall M, Bentley J, Dorr R. Cimetidine decreases theophylline clearance. *Am Rev Respir Dis* 1981;123:615–7.
17. Roberts RK, Grice J, Wood L, Petroff V, McGuffie C. Cimetidine impairs the elimination of theophylline and antipyrine. *Gastroenterology* 1981;81:19–21.
18. Hunt SN, Jusko WJ, Yurchak AM. Effect of smoking on theophylline disposition. *Clin Pharmacol Ther* 1976;19:546–51.
19. Jenne J, Nagasawa H, McHugh R, MacDonald F, Wyse E. Decreased theophylline half-life in cigarette smokers. *Life Sci* 1975;17:195–8.
20. Jusko WJ, Schentag JJ, Clark JH, Gardner M, Yurchak AM. Enhanced biotransformation of theophylline in marihuana and tobacco smokers. *Clin Pharmacol Ther* 1978;24:406–10.
21. Powell RJ, Thiercelin JF, Vozeh S, Sansom L, Riegelman S. The influence of cigarette smoking and sex on theophylline disposition. *Am Rev Respir Dis* 1977;116:17–23.
22. Koup JR, Vawter TK. Theophylline pharmacokinetics in an extremely obese patient. *Clin Pharm* 1983;2:181–3.

Therapeutic Drug Monitoring
7:202–206 © 1985 Raven Press, New York

Falsely Elevated Digoxin Concentrations in Patients with Liver Disease

Bernd Rosenkranz and Jürgen C. Frölich

Institute of Clinical Pharmacology, Stuttgart, F.R.G.

Summary: Immunoreactive digoxin was determined in blood samples of 73 patients with liver disease who did not take any cardiac glycoside. Seventeen of these patients reproducibly showed false-positive results, as much as 3.6 ng/ml. Patients with concomitant renal disease had higher assay results (mean 1.9 ng/ml) than patients with normal renal function (mean 0.6 ng/ml). It is concluded that blood of a number of patients with liver disease of different causes contains a substance that interferes with digoxin radioimmunoassay. **Key Words:** Digoxin—Radioimmunoassay—Digoxin-like immunoreactivity—Liver disease.

Determination of digoxin plasma concentration is regarded as an important guide in digitalis therapy (1). Concentrations below 0.7 ng/ml are usually considered insufficient to exert a therapeutic effect, whereas patients with values of more than 2.0 ng/ml often show symptoms of toxicity (1). However, several recent reports cast some doubt on the reliability of measuring serum digoxin concentrations by radioimmunoassay (RIA) in certain patients. Thus, a so-called digitalis-like immunoreactive substance (DLIS) has been detected in sera of subjects not treated with any cardiac glycoside. False-positive digoxin levels have been observed in patients with renal (2,3) or combined renal and hepatic (4) failure as well as during the last trimester of pregnancy (5,6) and in premature or full-term infants (3,7–10). These findings make earlier studies on pharmacokinetics of digoxin during pregnancy and infancy questionable (11,12). More importantly, erroneous determinations of digoxin plasma concentrations may lead to inappropriate therapeutic decisions. We also report here that in patients with liver disease a circulating substance that causes false-positive RIA results can be detected.

Address correspondence and reprint requests to Dr. B. Rosenkranz at Institute of Clinical Pharmacology, Auerbachstr. 112, 7000 Stuttgart 50, F.R.G.

Dr. Frölich's present address is Medical School Hannover, Institute of Clinical Pharmacology, Konstanty-Gutschow-Str. 8, 3000-Hannover 61, F.R.G.

MATERIAL AND METHODS

Plasma or sera samples were obtained from 73 randomly selected patients with hyperbilirubinemia (serum bilirubin >2.4 mg/dl) due to different liver diseases such as fibrosis; cirrhosis; fatty liver; hepatitis; neoplasia of pancreas, bile duct, or liver, with or without metastases or acute liver failure following pituitary infarction (Sheehan syndrome). None of the patients were treated with digoxin, digitoxin, or any other cardiac glycoside. Ten patients received treatment with spironolactone, which is known to interfere with digoxin assays (13). Treatment with 200 mg spironolactone results in false-positive "digoxin" concentrations in the range of 0.2–0.4 ng/ml in patients with normal renal function.

The samples were analyzed by RIA using an antibody (antibody A) provided by Prof. Dr. G. Bodem (Bad Homburg, F.R.G.) (14). Iodinated and unlabeled digoxin were obtained from Becton Dickinson (Heidelberg, F.R.G.). Plasma or serum was added directly to the assay mixture; separation of antibody-bound and free digoxin was performed by adding charcoal and subsequent centrifugation. Assays were done in duplicates; accuracy of this procedure was verified by analysis of two spiked serum samples and by external quality control (Prof. Alan Richens, London, England).

Some of the samples were reanalyzed by a commercially available digoxin kit using antibody-coated tubes (Becton Dickinson) (antibody B) as well as by the TDx system using an automated fluorescence polarization immunoassay (FPIA) (Abbott Laboratories, Diagnostic Division, North Chicago, IL, U.S.A.) (antibody C). The lower limit of detection of all three assays is 0.2 ng/ml.

RESULTS

Seventeen of the 73 patients (23.3%) showed a false-positive digoxin level by RIA using antibody A. Clinical diagnoses, chemistry, concomitant drug therapy, and DLIS levels of these patients are shown in Table 1. Eleven patients had normal renal function (serum creatinine concentration of ≤1.4 mg/dl); 3 of the 17 patients concomitantly received spironolactone. When 10 of the 17 samples containing DLIS as determined by antibody A were reanalyzed by antibody B, false-positive digoxin levels were obtained in 9 of these patients (Table 1). There was a significant correlation between both assay results ($r^2 = 0.972$, $p < 0.05$) with antibody B giving about 50% of the values obtained by antibody A ($B = 0.534 \cdot A - 0.023$). Analysis of six samples by the TDx system (antibody C) gave values of ≤0.3 ng/ml, which were not significantly correlated with the results obtained with antibody A ($r^2 = 0.505$). Longitudinal observations in three patients (patients 2,3, and 11 in Table 1) for as long as 19 days showed only minimal changes (≤0.2 ng/ml) of the DLIS values.

To determine whether the cross-reacting material could be discerned by nonparallel shift in binding, four plasma samples were diluted two- and fourfold with blank plasma. Mean DLIS values (antibody A) of the undiluted samples and the two different dilutions were 3.3, 1.5, and 0.7 ng/ml.

DISCUSSION

The present data clearly show that blood of a number of patients with liver disease, irrespective of its cause, contains a substance that interferes with immunological digoxin determinations. This finding extends previous observations in patients with renal disease (2,3) and pregnancy (5,6). In our present study, false-positive values as great as 3.6 ng/ml have been detected in patients with concomitant hepatic and renal failure, numbers that sometimes even exceeded the therapeutic range of digoxin plasma concentrations (1) and were thus higher than those reported for renal disease alone (2). Patients without renal failure had lower false positive digoxin concentrations, which were often still close to the therapeutic range.

The observed divergent results obtained by use of three different antibodies clearly show that the measured "digoxin" concentrations were not caused by surreptitious digoxin intake. Similarly, other groups found different DLIS values when using several different assays in patients with renal disease or during pregnancy, or in newborns (2,6,8). In accordance with previous observations (3,4,9), determination of digoxin concentrations by the automated FPIA was the method least susceptible to the artifacts observed in patients with liver disease.

As in the other studies (2–10), the identity of the material interfering with the immunoassays is not clear. It might be argued that, because of the largely heterogeneous patient population (Table 1), different endogenous substances might be responsible for the false-positive digoxin assay results in our patients. However, the good correlation between the values obtained by the two antibodies A and B suggests that the material probably was identical in all patients and that it had a lower affinity to antibody B than to antibody A. Moreover, the parallel shift in binding caused by sample dilution indicates that the binding curve of the interfering substance to antibody A paralleled the binding curve of digoxin. Altogether, these results demonstrate that the false-positive digoxin values most probably were not the result of an unspecific interference with the assays used, but instead were caused by an endogenous circulating material with affinity to the anti-digoxin antibodies.

This substance might either be excessively produced in patients with liver disease and/or renal failure, or its concentration might increase by an impairment of either its degradation or its excretion. Recently DLIS has been detected in concentrated plasma of healthy volunteers (15,16). Besides binding to digoxin antibodies, this factor inhibits Na,K-adenosine triphosphatase (17) and seems to play a role in sodium homeostasis (16–18). Although reported values did not exceed 0.2 ng/ml of digoxin equivalents in these studies, it is possible that this factor might be elevated in patients with liver disease. Furthermore, catecholamines and glucocorticoids in animal experiments have been shown to induce formation of a factor interfering with digoxin immunoassays (19). On the other hand, it is also possible that a structurally related hormone

TABLE 1. *Clinical diagnoses, blood chemistry, and concomitant drug therapy of patients with false positive digoxin levels*

Patient No.	Age (yr)	Sex	Diseases	Bilirubin (mg/dl)	SGPT (U/ml)	AP (U/ml)	Albumin (g/dl)	Creatinine (mg/dl)	Concomitant medication	Digitalis-like immunoreactive substance (ng/ml)		
										Antibody A	Antibody B	Antibody C
Patients with serum creatinine ≤ 1.4 mg/dl												
Without spironolactone treatment												
1	62	M	Liver cell carcinoma	27.3	25	1,020	2.3	0.7	Oxazepam Vitamin K Lactulose	0.4	ND	0.3
2	54	M	Alcoholic liver cirrhosis	4.4	36	147	2.4	0.6	Oxazepam Clomethiazol Vitamin B	0.5	0.3	ND
3	47	F	Alcoholic liver cirrhosis with coma Miliary tuberculosis	14.9	9	672	3.7	1.4	Lactulose Vitamins B Furosemide Amoxicillin Diazepam	0.7	0.3	0.1
4	69	F	Hepatitis	11.1	430	250	4.6	0.7	Lactulose	0.3	ND	0.2
5	37	M	Fatty liver Alcoholism Diabetes mellitus II	5.4	59	713	4.4	0.8	Insulin	0.3	0	ND
6	39	M	Alcoholic liver cirrhosis	7.5	30	360	2.9	0.9	Vitamins B Ranitidine Paromomycin Lactulose	0.6	ND	ND
7	53	M	Liver cirrhosis with coma	19.3	29	388	2.4	0.7	Tilidin	0.3	0.1	ND
8	22	M	Hepatitis B	14.6	1,580	237	4.5	ND[a]	—	0.5	ND	ND
9	39	F	Alcoholic liver cirrhosis	17.7	31	589	3.9	1.0	Vitamins B Folic acid Haloperidol Diazepam	0.7	ND	0.2
10	31	M	Alcoholic liver cirrhosis	6.2	30	268	4.4	0.8	Diazepam	0.5	0.3	ND
With spironolactone treatment												
11	62	M	Alcoholic liver cirrhosis with liver tumor	12.3	49	586	3.0	1.0	Spironolactone Furosemide Lactulose	1.5	ND	0.1

Patients with serum creatinine > 1.4 mg/dl											
Without spironolactone treatment											
12	74	F	Liver cirrhosis with liver malignoma	13.9	38	523	3.0	1.9	Vitamins B Lactulose Bisacodyl Triamteren Hydrochlorothiazide	1.5	0.6	ND
13	31	F	Sheehan syndrome, concomitant liver and renal failure with diffuse fatty liver and shock kidneys	15.4	214	336	3.5	3.0	Doxycylin Cimetidine Hydrocortisone Vitamin K Heparin Dopamine Thyroxine Furosemide Flunitrazepam Pancuronium Ticarcillin Metronidazol	3.6	1.9	ND
14	58	F	Alcoholic liver cirrhosis	43.6	36	293	3.2	1.6	Amikacin Paromomycin Ranitidine Furosemide Vitamins B Lactulose	1.0	0.7	0.1
15	87	F	Gastrointestinal tumor with liver metastases Renal failure Diabetes mellitus II	7.6	122	498	ND	3.7	—	0.8	0.5	ND
With concomitant spironolactone treatment											
16	53	F	Liver cirrhosis with coma	30.8	29	158	3.4	5.0	Spironolactone Furosemide Cefotaxime Ranitidine Vitamins D, K Paromomycin Nystatin	3.2	1.7	ND
17	56	M	Liver metastases	8.9	ND	863	2.8	1.5	Spironolactone Pentazocin Furosemide Paracetamol Imipramine	1.4	ND	ND

SGPT, serum-glutamate-pyruvate-transaminase; AP, alkaline phosphatase; ND, not determined.
[a]No creatinine concentration available; no evidence of renal failure.

(19) or some serum proteins (3,20) interfere with the immunological digoxin determinations.

In conclusion, our results demonstrate that in patients with hepatic disease, digoxin measurements can be erroneous. As determination by several different assays in our study gave divergent results for these samples, it is suggested that in cases when such artifactually elevated digoxin levels are suspected, determinations by two different methods should be performed.

Note added in proof: After submission of this article the presence of DLIS in patients with liver disease has also been reported by another group (21).

Acknowledgment: This work was supported by the Robert-Bosch-Foundation, Stuttgart. We want to thank Prof. Dr. U. Klotz for helpful discussions and the routine determination of digoxin levels. The excellent technical help of Ms. E. Deutschmann is highly appreciated. We would like to thank the physicians and nurses of the Robert-Bosch-Hospital and Prof. Dr. Dr. H. Wisser (Central Laboratory of the Robert-Bosch-Hospital) for their valuable help in collecting the plasma samples and Mrs. B. Grözinger for secretarial assistance.

REFERENCES

1. Aronson JK. Indications for the measurement of plasma digoxin concentrations. *Drugs* 1983;26:230–42.
2. Graves SW, Brown B, Valdes R. An endogenous digoxin-like substance in patients with renal impairment. *Ann Intern Med* 1983;99:604–8.
3. Heazlewood VJ, Heazlewood RL, Jellett LB. An endogenous digoxin-like substance and renal failure. *Ann Intern Med* 1984;100:618.
4. Gault MH, Vasdev SC, Longerich LL. Endogenous digoxin-like substance(s) and combined hepatic and renal failure. *Ann Intern Med* 1984;101:567–8.
5. Reisert PM, Kistner M. Klinisch wichtige Kreuzreaktionen bel der radioimmunologischen Bestimmung von Digoxin. *Fortschr Med* 1977;95:167–71.
6. Graves SW, Valdes R, Brown BA, Knight AB, Craig HR. Endogenous digoxin-immunoreactive substance in human pregnancies. *J Clin Endocrinol Metab* 1984;58:748–51.
7. Pudek MR, Seccombe DW, Whitfield MF. Digoxin-like immunoreactivity in premature and full-term infants not receiving digoxin therapy. *N Engl J Med* 1983;308:904–5.
8. Pudek MR, Seccombe DW, Jacobsen BE, Whitfield MF. Seven different digoxin immunoassay kits compared with respect to interference by a digoxin-like immunoreactive substance in serum from premature and full-term infants. *Clin Chem* 1983;29:1972–4.
9. Yatskoff RW, Desjardins PRE, Dalton JG. Digoxin-like immunoreactivity in the serum of neonates and uremic patients, as measured in the Abbott TDx. *Clin Chem* 1984;30:588.
10. Hicks JM, Brett EM. Falsely positive digoxin results in serum specimens from acute care infants. *Clin Chem* 1983;29:1249.
11. Rogers MC, Willerson JT, Goldblatt A, Smith TW. Serum digoxin concentrations in the human fetus, neonate and infant. *N Engl J Med* 1972;287:1010–3.
12. Sandor GGS, Reid G, Patterson MWH. Serum digoxin levels in neonates under 1500 grams [letter]. *Pediatr Pharmacol* 1983;3:57.
13. Lichey J, Schröder R, Rietbrock N. The effect of oral spironolactone and intravenous canrenoate-K on the digoxin radioimmunoassay. *Int J Clin Pharmacol* 1977;15:557–9.
14. Ochs HR, Greenblatt DJ, Bodem G, Harmatz JS. Dose-independent pharmacokinetics of digoxin in humans. *Am Heart J* 1978;96:507–11.
15. Balzan S, Clerico A, del Chicca MG, Montali U, Ghione S. Digoxin-like immunoreactivity in normal human plasma and urine, as detected by a solid-phase radioimmunoassay. *Clin Chem* 1984;30:450–1.
16. Gault MH, Vasdev SC, Longerich LL, et al. Plasma digitalis-like factor(s) increase with salt loading. *N Engl J Med* 1983;309:1459.
17. Hamlyn JM, Ringel R, Schaeffer J, et al. A circulating inhibitor of (Na^+ + K^+) ATPase associated with essential hypertension. *Nature* 1982;300:650–2.
18. Anonymous. Endogenous foxglove. *Lancet* 1983;2:1463–4.
19. Soldin SJ, Papanastasiou-Diamandi A, Heyes J, Lingwood C, Olley P. Are immunoassays for digoxin reliable? *Clin Biochem* 1984;17:317–20.
20. Vinge E, Molin L, Ekman R. Spurious results of digoxin radioimmunoassay. *N Engl J Med* 1984;310:725.
21. Nanji AA, Greenway DC. Falsely raised plasma digoxin concentrations in liver disease. *Br Med J* 1985;290:432–3.

Therapeutic Drug Monitoring
7:207–210 © 1985 Raven Press, New York

Determination of Chloroquine and its Desethyl Metabolite in Whole Blood: An Application for Samples Collected in Capillary Tubes and Dried on Filter Paper

Björn Lindström, *Örjan Ericsson, *Gunnar Alván, †Lars Rombo, Lena Ekman, *Margareta Rais, and *Folke Sjöqvist

*National Board of Health and Welfare, Department of Drugs, Uppsala, *Department of Clinical Pharmacology, Karolinska Institute, Huddinge University Hospital, Huddinge, and †Department of Infectious Diseases, Karolinska Institute, Roslagstull Hospital, Stockholm, Sweden*

Summary: A high performance liquid chromatography method for analysis of chloroquine and desethylchloroquine was adapted for 75 μl aliquots of whole blood obtained by finger-prick and dried on filter paper. The precision of the method was satisfactory at whole blood concentrations of 40 nmol/L (coefficient of variation, 5%). The dried samples were stable for at least 7 weeks at 20°C. The concentrations in venous whole blood and in dried samples correlated well. The correlation coefficient was 0.99 for chloroquine and 0.97 for desethylchloroquine. Chloroquine concentrations were marginally but significantly higher in venous whole blood. When fitted to a linear equation ($y = bx + a$) the relationship was $y = 0.96x + 0.03$. Desethylchloroquine concentrations did not differ significantly in venous whole blood and in finger-prick blood dried on filter paper. The method is specific and sensitive enough for pharmacokinetic studies and can be used in areas with limited technical facilities. **Key Words:** Chloroquine—Desethylchloroquine—High performance liquid chromatography—Microassay.

Chloroquine has been used for many years as an antimalarial medication and also for the treatment of rheumatoid arthritis. Chloroquine concentrations in blood and urine have been measured to establish the pharmacokinetic characteristics of the drug and to explore reasons for therapeutic failures in malaria. Many studies involving chloroquine concentrations have been made using spectrophotofluorometric methods which are not specific with respect to metabolites. Specific methods, such as gas or liquid chromatography, should always be preferred. It has been shown that the concentrations of chloroquine and its main metabolite, desethylchloroquine, are higher in serum than in plasma, and also that the measured concentration is dependent on the centrifugation force used when separating blood cells from plasma (1,2). A possible explanation for these observations is that both compounds have a strong tendency to bind to blood cells, especially to platelets (1).

The difficulties in standardizing the procedures for analysis of plasma or serum prompted us to modify the previously published high performance liquid chromatographic (HPLC) method (3) for whole blood analysis. As it is important to be able to analyze samples from children, the method was also evaluated for capillary size samples. The method is intended for use in areas with limited technical facilities. A procedure for analyzing dried samples, which are convenient to store and transport, was therefore developed.

Address correspondence and reprint requests to Dr. Ö. Ericsson at Department of Clinical Pharmacology, Huddinge University Hospital, S-141 86 Huddinge, Sweden.

MATERIALS AND METHODS

Instruments, Solvents, and Standards

The HPLC system was the same as described previously (3) with the exception that a model RF 530 fluorescence detector (Shimadzu, Kyoto, Japan) was used. The excitation and emission wavelengths of the detector were set to 335 and 380 nm, respectively.

The column (0.15 m × 4.6 mm internal diameter, packed with LiChrosorb Si 60 5 μm; Merck, Darmstadt, F.R.G.) was the same as described earlier (3) as was the eluent system (acetonitrile-methanol-diethylamine, 80:19.5:0.5, vol/vol). The mixture of acetonitrile and methanol was filtered through a column of silica (Kieselgel 60, 70–230 mesh ASTM; Merck) before the addition of diethylamine. About 60–70 ml of silica was used to filter 500 ml of the solvent mixture.

The internal standard used was 4-(4-dimethylamino-1-methylbutylamino)-7-chloroquinoline (3). Desethylchloroquine was a gift form Sterling-Winthrop, and chloroquine phosphate was supplied by Kabi-Vitrum, Stockholm, Sweden.

The diethylether used for extraction and the methanol for the eluent were of analytical grade. Acetonitrile was of HPLC grade.

Handling and Assay of Dried Samples

Sampling of blood was done with a capillary tube (75 μl heparinized tubes for microhematocrits; Drummond Scientific Company, PA, U.S.A.) directly from a fingertip. The contents of the tubes were emptied, absorbed on to a filter paper or a chromatography paper, and dried.

The dried blood spot on the paper was cut in pieces and put into a screw-capped tube together with 1 ml of a 0.1% aqueous solution of diethylamine and 100 μl of the internal standard solution (concentration of the internal standard was 850 nmol/L for samples with an expected chloroquine concentration of 150–1,500 nmol/L and 170 nmol/L when chloroquine concentration was expected to be 30–300 nmol/L). The mixture was exposed to ultrasonic treatment (10 min) and allowed to stand for 0.5 h. With the filter paper still in the tube, 0.5 ml of 1 *M* NaOH solution and 6 ml of diethylether were added, followed by extraction for 15 min. After centrifugation (5 min at 500 *g*) the ether phase was removed and evaporated under a stream of nitrogen. The residue was dissolved in 200 μl of the eluent mixture and filtered through a Pasteur pipette stoppered with fine glass wool, after which 50–100 μl was injected into the chromatograph.

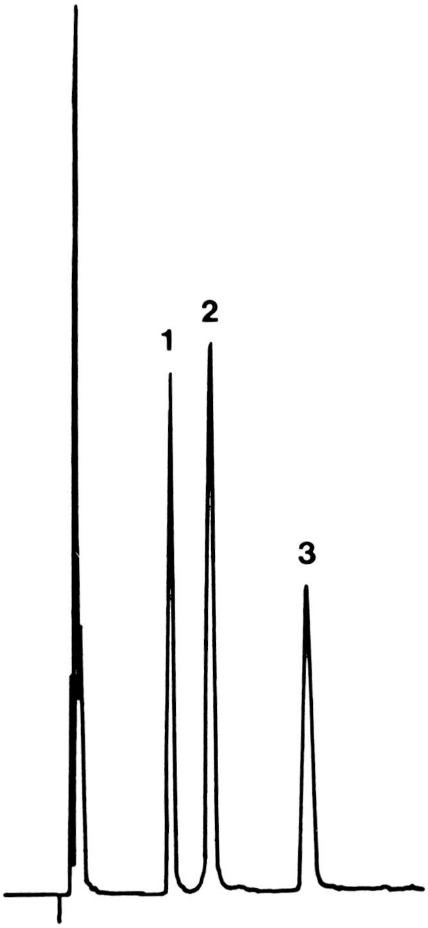

FIG. 1. Chromatogram of an extract of a blood sample dried on filter paper. Peak 1 is the internal standard (retention time 4.8 min), peak 2 is chloroquine (6.4 min), and peak 3 is desethylchloroquine (10.2 min). The chloroquine peak represents 3.3 μmol/L in whole blood.

Handling and Assay of Venous Whole Blood Samples

Venous blood was sampled in EDTA tubes (Vacutainer; Becton Dickinson, NY, U.S.A.). The blood

TABLE 1. *Precision[a] in the determination of chloroquine and desethylchloroquine*

	40 nmol/L	1,000 nmol/L
Venous blood		
Chloroquine	8	2
Desethylchloroquine	4	3
Dried samples		
Chloroquine	5	3
Desethylchloroquine	15	14

[a]Expressed as coefficient of variation (%); n = 10.

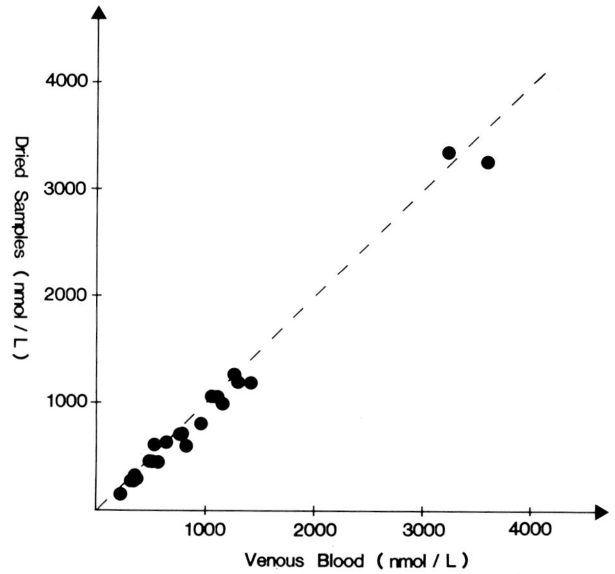

FIG. 2. Plot of whole blood chloroquine concentrations obtained in venous blood and in dried finger-prick capillary samples. The dashed line represents $y = x$.

was hemolyzed by dilution with 0.1% diethylamine (500 μl of blood in 3 ml of 0.1% diethylamine) and stored at −20°C until analyzed.

The hemolyzed blood samples were analyzed by adding 1.0 ml of 1 m NaOH and 100 μl of the internal standard solution to 1.0 ml of the hemolyzed blood and then processing the samples as described above.

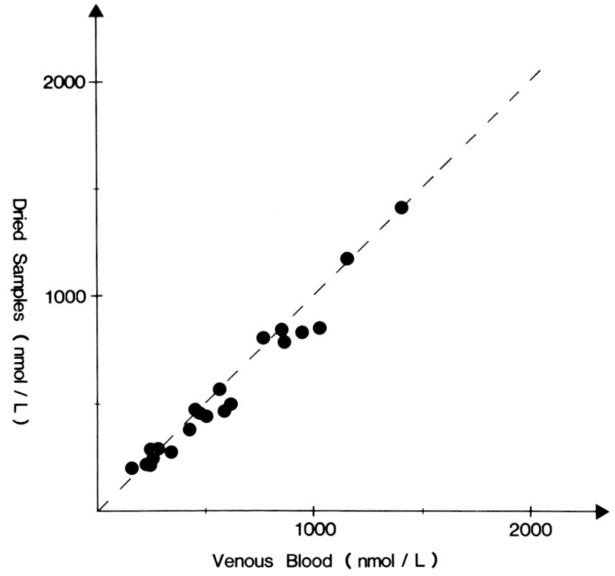

FIG. 3. Plot of whole blood desethylchloroquine concentrations obtained in venous blood and in dried finger-prick capillary samples. The dashed line represents $y = x$.

The precision and accuracy of the method were assessed by analyzing heparinized blood containing known concentrations of chloroquine and desethylchloroquine.

Comparisons of Concentrations Determined in Venous Whole Blood and in Capillaries Dried on Filter Paper

Venous whole blood and finger-prick capillary samples were obtained from 21 patients during or after antimalarial medication with chloroquine. The capillary tubes were immediately emptied onto filter papers, which were left to dry. All samples were stored at −20°C until analysis.

RESULTS AND DISCUSSION

Sample Handling and Extraction

The venous blood samples were hemolyzed by diluting the blood with an aqueous solution of diethylamine, followed by freezing. Chloroquine binds to glass and other materials (4,5), and if pure water is used for the hemolysis, serious adsorption losses will occur. Diethylamine at a concentration of 0.1% or more inhibits this adsorption. The extraction recovery of chloroquine and desethylchloroquine was 95 and 86%, respectively.

The capillary blood samples were taken in heparinized precision capillaries, immediately put on a filter paper, and allowed to dry. When analyzing the dried samples it was necessary to use sonication in order to remove chloroquine and desethylchloroquine quantitatively from the paper. As with the venous blood samples, diethylamine was used to prevent adsorption. A chromatogram is shown in Fig. 1.

The capillaries had a nominal volume of 75 μl. When the samples were applied to the paper, 2.4 ± 0.6% (SD) (n = 10, determined by weighing) remained in the tube.

Three different types of porous paper were tested, filter paper (Munktell) and two chromatographic papers (Whatman) of different thickness. No differences in results were observed.

During the investigations on the present method a similar procedure was published by Patchen et al. (6). Their method also utilizes samples dried on filter papers and a straight phase chromatographic system with an eluent containing diethylamine to enhance the fluorescence of the substances analyzed. The eluent was modified to enable the analysis of other antimalarials as well as chloroquine.

The extraction procedures of the dried samples are different in the two methods. In the method by Patchen et al., the filter paper is macerated in an acidic medium with a glass rod, after which the paper is removed and the medium made alkaline prior to extraction. Pilot investigations performed by us did not reveal any important differences between the two methods.

Storage of Samples

Samples were stored and analyzed after 1, 2, and 7 weeks to determine whether any change in the analytical results had occurred during this time period. The venous blood samples, which were stored in 10 ml tubes at 4 and − 30°C, showed no detectable decrease in the levels of chloroquine and desethylchloroquine. Similarly, the concentrations in the dried samples stored at 20°C were stable during the entire period.

Sensitivity and Precision

Data on the precision of the method are given in Table 1. The internal standard used is better suited for determination of chloroquine than for desethylchloroquine, and hence the precision in the determination of the parent drug is better than that for the metabolite. On the other hand, the internal standard used by Patchen et al. seems to be better suited for the determination of desethylchloroquine. The uncertainty in the determination of the metabolite will in most cases not be a limitation in the usefulness of the method.

Analysis of Venous Blood and Finger-Prick Blood Dried on Filter Paper

The mean chloroquine concentrations in blood dried on filter paper were significantly lower ($p < 0.01$, paired t test) than in venous blood. When fitted to a linear model, the relation was expressed as $y = 0.968x + 0.034$ (Fig. 2). The correlation coefficient was 0.99, and the standard deviation about the regression line ($S\ y/x$) was 0.108. Part of the difference is explained by the fact that some blood remains in the capillary tube when the sample is applied to the filter paper. The difference is marginal and is of no practical importance.

The corresponding desethylchloroquine concentrations were not significantly different from each other. The relation was expressed as $y = 0.944x + 0.013$, $S\ y/x = 0.0696$ and $r = 0.97$ (Fig. 3).

Applications

The use of dried finger-prick blood samples permits serial analyses of chloroquine concentrations, even in small children, under field conditions. During investigations of chloroquine resistance, determinations of chloroquine by this method are far more specific and also more sensitive than the qualitative urine tests previously used. Thus, this method is to be preferred both to detect recent medication with chloroquine before in vitro tests and to check ingestion of the drug during in vivo tests. The sensitivity of the method is sufficient for monitoring levels of chloroquine and desethylchloroquine during treatment of malaria and also for pharmacokinetic studies.

It should be remembered that hepatitis B virus may survive for several weeks in dried blood, and the samples must thus be handled as contagious material.

Acknowledgment: This work was supported by a grant from the Swedish Agency for Research Cooperation with Developing Countries.

REFERENCES

1. Bergqvist Y, Domeij-Nyberg B. Distribution of chloroquine and its metabolite desethyl-chloroquine in human blood cells and its implication for the quantitative determination of these compounds in serum and plasma. *J Chromatogr* 1983;272:137–48.
2. Rombo L, Ericsson Ö, Alván G, Lindström, B, Gustafsson LL, Sjöqvist F. Chloroquine and desethylchloroquine in plasma, serum, and whole blood. Problems in assay and handling of samples. *Ther Drug Monit* 1985;7:211–215.
3. Alván G, Ekman L, Lindström B. Determination of chloroquine and its desethyl metabolite in plasma, red blood cells and urine by liquid chromatography. *J Chromatogr* 1982;229: 241–7.
4. Staiger MA, Nguyen-Dinh P, Churchill FC. Sensitive high-performance liquid chromatographic analysis for chloroquine in body fluids. Application to studies of drug resistance in *Plasmodium falciparum*. *J Chromatogr* 1981;225:139–49.
5. Geary TG, Akood MA, Jensen JB. Characteristics of chloroquine binding to glass and plastic. *Am J Trop Med Hyg* 1983;32:19–23.
6. Patchen LC, Mount DL, Schwartz IK, Churchill FC. Analysis of filter-paper-absorbed, finger-stick blood samples for chloroquine and its major metabolite using high-performance liquid chromatography with fluorescence detection. *J Chromatogr* 1983;278:81–9.

Therapeutic Drug Monitoring
7:211–215 © 1985 Raven Press, New York

Chloroquine and Desethylchloroquine in Plasma, Serum, and Whole Blood: Problems in Assay and Handling of Samples

Lars Rombo, *Örjan Ericsson, *Gunnar Alván, †Björn Lindström, *Lars L. Gustafsson, and *Folke Sjöqvist

*Department of Infectious Diseases, Karolinska Institute, Roslagstull Hospital, Stockholm, *Department of Clinical Pharmacology, Karolinska Institute, Huddinge University Hospital, Huddinge, and †National Board of Health and Welfare, Department of Drugs, Uppsala, Sweden*

Summary: A spectrophotofluorometric method for determination of chloroquine in body fluids was compared with a recently developed high performance liquid chromatographic (HPLC) method. The spectrophotofluorometric method was found to codetermine the main metabolite desethylchloroquine and thus to give higher "chloroquine" concentrations than the HPLC method. The concentrations determined with spectrophotofluorometry roughly corresponded to the calculated sum of chloroquine and desethylchloroquine as determined with the HPLC method. The concentrations of chloroquine and desethylchloroquine were higher in serum, and considerably higher in whole blood, than in plasma. The duration and force of centrifugation greatly influenced the concentrations of chloroquine and desethylchloroquine found in plasma. The concentrations decreased as centrifugal force increased reaching relatively stable levels at 500 *g*. Increasing the centrifugation time partly compensated for lower *g* forces. These methodological problems can be avoided by using whole blood for determinations of chloroquine. Since the biological activities of desethylchloroquine and chloroquine are not the same, drug monitoring should be performed with a method distinguishing between the parent drug and the metabolite. **Key Words:** Chloroquine—Desethylchloroquine–High performance liquid chromatography—Spectrophotofluorometry—Centrifugation.

Chloroquine was introduced as an antimalarial drug in the late 1940s. Its basic pharmacokinetic properties were characterized at an early stage with a spectrophotofluorometric (SF) method (1–3). Much of this knowledge is still valid, but more specific and sensitive liquid chromatographic (LC) methods have been introduced (4–6). These methodological developments have permitted a reevaluation of the pharmacokinetics of chloroquine and its main metabolite, desethylchloroquine (7). It has been suggested that concentrations of chloroquine ought to be monitored to distinguish between resistance of *Plasmodium falciparum* to chloroquine and low drug concentrations during treatment (8–10). Since spectrophotofluorometry is still in use for this purpose, we have compared this method with LC. During the progress of this work, Bergqvist and Domeij-Nyberg (11) showed that the high content of chloroquine in blood platelets is another source of erroneous measurements of plasma levels of the drug unless the centrifugation force is standardized. Since

Address correspondence and reprint requests to Dr. L. Rombo at Department of Infectious Diseases, Roslagstull Hospital, Box 5651, S-114 89 Stockholm, Sweden.

this may be a significant technical problem under tropical field conditions, we have included a confirmatory study of this aspect of chloroquine determination.

MATERIALS AND METHODS

Materials and Instrumentation

Chloroquine phosphate (Klorokinfosfat) was obtained from Kabi-Vitrum, Stockholm, Sweden, and desethylchloroquine was provided by Sterling-Winthrop, Skärholmen, Sweden. Solvents and other chemicals were of analytical grade and used as obtained from the manufacturers. Spectrophotofluorometric determinations were made using an Aminco Bowman spectrophotofluorometer. The centrifuges were an IEC Centra 7 and a Beckman L5-65B ultracentrifuge.

Codetermination of Chloroquine and Desethylchloroquine by Spectrophotofluorometry

Desethylchloroquine was added to drug-free standardized serum to obtain five different concentrations (0, 0.3, 0.9, 1.8, and 3.0 μmol/L). The fluorescence after extraction according to the SF method was compared with the fluorescence after extraction of serum containing the same concentrations of chloroquine.

Comparison Between Spectrophotofluorometry and Liquid Chromatography

Blood for comparison of the two methods was drawn from 10 healthy Swedish volunteers, 3, 24, 96, 168, and 336 h after a single oral dose of 5 or 10 mg of chloroquine per kg body weight. All samples to be compared were taken during the same venepuncture in Vacutainer tubes. The tubes were inverted 10 times, kept at room temperature for 30 min, and then centrifuged at 2,000 *g* for 10 min. The lower 5 mm of plasma was left in the original tubes, while the rest was transferred into plastic tubes and stored at − 20°C until analysis.

Centrifugation

Whole blood was obtained in heparin and EDTA tubes. Blood was transferred to a glass flask, and known amounts of chloroquine and desethylchloroquine were added. The blood was gently agitated for 1 h at 37°C, transferred to glass tubes, and left standing at room temperature for 1–2 h before centrifugation. The samples were then centrifuged at 250, 500, or 1,000 *g* (IEC centra 7) for 5, 10, 20, or 40 min, or at 2,000, 4,000, and 8,000 *g* (Beckman L5-65B) for 10 min. The *g* force was calculated using the distance between the center of the centrifuge and the expected border between plasma and erythrocytes as radius.

Analysis

All analyses were made in duplicates. Standard curves were obtained by adding five different concentrations of chloroquine to drug-free serum. The LC method for analysis of chloroquine and desethylchloroquine has been described elsewhere (5). The SF method of McChesney (2) was modified as follows: 1 ml of 1 *M* NaOH, containing 17.5% NaCl, was added to 1 ml of serum. Chloroquine and desethylchloroquine were extracted into 12 ml of ethylene dichloride. The tubes were shaken for 30 min and centrifuged for 5 min at 800 *g*. The organic phase was then washed with 5 ml of 0.1 *M* NaOH. After reshaking for 10 min followed by 5 min of centrifugation, 10 ml of the organic phase was transferred into tubes containing 4 ml of 0.1 *M* HC1. After another 10 min of shaking and 5 min of centrifugation, 3 ml of the acidic phase was mixed with 0.3 ml of 1 *M* NaOH and 0.5 ml of borate buffer (1.55 g boric acid, 1.87 g KCl, and 15 ml of 1 *M* NaOH in distilled water to 100 ml, pH 9.3 ± 0.1). Fluorescence was read using an excitation wavelength of 340 nm and an emission wavelength of 384 nm. The lower sensitivity limit of the method is 0.03 μmol/L (coefficient of variation 9.4%; n = 10).

Statistical Evaluation

Statistical analysis was applied according to the principles stated by Westgard et al. (12).

RESULTS

Chloroquine and desethylchloroquine gave the same fluorescence when sera containing equal concentrations (0–3 μmol/L) were analyzed by the SF method. This method thus determines the sum of the drug and its main metabolite.

The comparison between the LC method and the SF method in vivo is presented in Table 1 and Fig. 1.The concentrations determined with the SF method correspond roughly to the sum of chloroquine and desethylchloroquine as determined by the LC method (Table 1). Concentrations of chloroquine and desethylchloroquine were generally higher in serum and considerably higher in whole blood than in plasma (Table 2).

TABLE 1. *Relationships between chloroquine determinations obtained with a liquid chromatographic* (x) *and a spectrophotofluorometric* (y) *method in serum, plasma, and whole blood samples (μmol/L)*

Biological medium	Number of paired samples	Mean		Standard deviation		Regression line	Standard deviation			Correlation coefficient
		x	y	S_x	S_y		Regression line	Slope	Intercept	
Chloroquine										
Serum	27	0.191	0.229	0.219	0.213	$y = 0.961x + 0.045$	0.034	0.030	0.001	0.988
Plasma	29	0.181	0.226	0.235	0.287	$y = 1.217x + 0.006$	0.032	0.026	0.007	0.994
Whole blood	35	0.604	0.830	0.668	0.954	$y = 1.373x + 0.001$	0.267	0.068	0.061	0.961
Chloroquine + desethylchloroquine										
Serum	27	0.257	0.229	0.272	0.213	$y = 0.780x + 0.028$	0.026	0.018	0.007	0.993
Plasma	29	0.262	0.226	0.335	0.287	$y = 0.849x + 0.009$	0.041	0.023	0.010	0.991
Whole blood	35	0.833	0.830	0.887	0.954	$y = 1.059x - 0.052$	0.168	0.032	0.039	0.985

The force and duration of centrifugation had major effects on the results (Fig. 2, top and bottom). The concentrations of chloroquine and desethylchloroquine were highest in plasma obtained after sedimentation of the blood cells for 3 h without centrifugation. The concentrations declined with increasing centrifugal force to reach relatively stable values at 500 *g*.

DISCUSSION

It is not possible to determine chloroquine and desethylchloroquine selectively with the SF method, since they have fluorescence at the same wavelength and cannot be separately extracted. The method described by McChesney et al. (2) involves an extraction procedure that gives some degree of selectivity for chloroquine, but about 20% of the desethylchloroquine is stated to be codetermined. The method used in this study was slightly different and determined the sum of chloroquine and desethylchloroquine. In many studies where spectrophotofluorometric methods have been used, the results have erroneously been given as chloroquine concentrations. As the metabolite possesses different biological activity from the parent compound against chloroquine resistant *P. falciparum* strains (13,14) and appears in appreciable concentrations in blood, a specific method, LC or gas chromatography, should always be preferred. In this study, the in vivo results obtained with the SF method were accepted as corresponding to the sum of chloroquine and desethylchloroquine obtained with the LC method.

Differences between two analytical methods for assay of endogenous compounds are often statistically evaluated by a paired *t* test. The result of the *t* test,

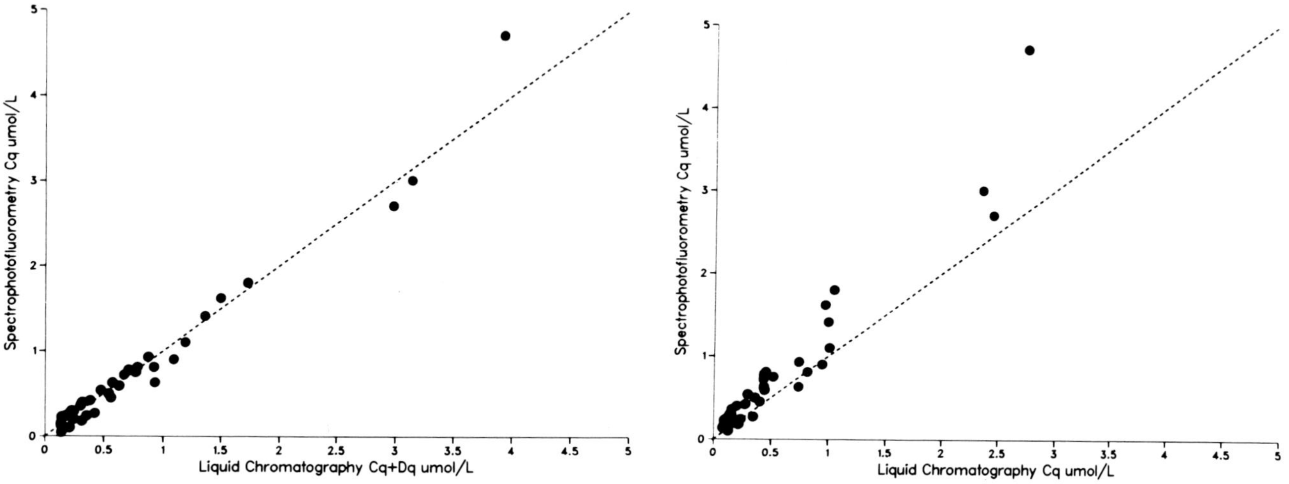

FIG. 1. Left: Plot of apparent "chloroquine" whole blood concentrations determined with the spectrophotofluorometric (SF) method versus the sum of chloroquine and desethylchloroquine concentrations determined with the liquid chromatographic (LC) method. The dashed line represents $y = x$. **Right:** Plot of apparent "chloroquine" whole blood concentrations determined with the SF method versus chloroquine determined with the LC method. The dashed line represents $y = x$.

TABLE 2. *Relationships between chloroquine and desethylchloroquine concentrations obtained in serum, plasma, and whole blood with liquid chromatography*

Body fluids compared (x/y)	Number of paired samples	Mean x	Mean y	Standard deviation S_x	Standard deviation S_y	Regression line	Standard deviation: Regression line	Standard deviation: Slope	Standard deviation: Intercept	Correlation coefficient
Chloroquine										
Plasma/serum	20	0.131	0.174	0.146	0.223	$y = 1.505x - 0.023$	0.041	0.065	0.013	0.984
Whole blood/serum	20	0.509	0.174	0.534	0.223	$y = 0.405x - 0.032$	0.059	0.025	0.018	0.966
Whole blood/plasma	24	0.615	0.175	0.676	0.239	$y = 0.343x - 0.035$	0.061	0.019	0.017	0.969
Desethylchloroquine										
Plasma/serum	20	0.054	0.064	0.051	0.063	$y = 1.123x + 0.003$	0.027	0.123	0.009	0.907
Whole blood/serum	20	0.178	0.064	0.181	0.063	$y = 0.339x + 0.003$	0.015	0.019	0.005	0.973
Whole blood/plasma	24	0.250	0.081	0.277	0.111	$y = 0.386x - 0.015$	0.032	0.024	0.009	0.960

however, is valid only for the means. When concentrations within a wide range are obtained, correspondence between two methods could also be evaluated from the regression equation (12). In our case, any concentration determined by LC is related to an SF concentration and an appropriate confidence interval. Unfortunately, the confidence interval is not constant, as it increases with the distance from the mean of the *x* parameter.

Many of the in vivo concentrations were low. Consequently, the slope was to a large extent determined by the values of a minor number of higher concentrations, and the slope obtained in the regression equations was less certain. The isolated high concentrations observed also resulted in misleadingly high correlations between the methods.

In the in vivo study, blood samples containing low concentrations of chloroquine had been drawn at later times after dosing. The half-life for desethylchloroquine in vivo is longer than for chloroquine, and consequently there are higher proportions of desethylchloroquine in such samples. For low concentrations, the codetermination of desethylchloroquine with the SF method thus results in less agreement with LC method and in nonlinear relationships between the SF and the LC methods.

The concentrations were found to be higher in serum and much higher in whole blood than in plasma. These observations, which are in gross accordance with those obtained by Bergqvist (15), may be explained by the extensive binding of chloroquine and desethylchloroquine to blood cells. The difference between serum and plasma is probably due to a release of the drug from platelets during the clotting process of serum (11,15).

It has been known for several years that basic drugs accumulate in platelets (16). Recently, Bergqvist and Domeij-Nyberg (11) showed that chloroquine binds to platelets, reaching a concentration of approximately 400 times that in erythrocytes. This phenomenon may cause the variations between results obtained in different laboratories. Most of the platelets will remain in plasma if the centrifugal force does not exceed 190 *g* for 15 min. However, 20,000 *g* for 30 min is needed to obtain platelet-free plasma (17). Thus, unknown

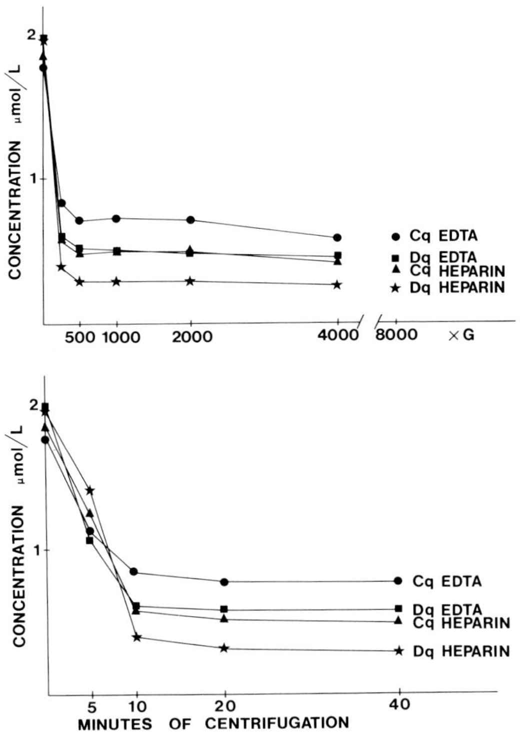

FIG. 2. Top: Effect of centrifugal force on chloroquine and desethylchloroquine concentrations in plasma. The samples were centrifuged for 10 min. **Bottom:** Effect of centrifugation time on chloroquine and desethylchloroquine concentrations in plasma. The centrifugal force was 250 *g*.

amounts of platelets will remain in plasma or serum with the centrifugation forces commonly used (250–2,000 *g*).

Our in vitro study confirms that the centrifugation force applied to separate plasma should be standardized whenever chloroquine is determined in plasma (and probably in serum). Increase of centrifugation time may partly compensate for a low centrifugal force.

Centrifugation errors and differences between plasma and serum could be avoided by using whole blood for analyses. Whole blood is also to be preferred because it contains higher concentrations of chloroquine and desethylchloroquine than serum or plasma. On the other hand, varying platelet and granulocyte counts might influence whole blood concentrations, as these cells contain more than half of the total chloroquine blood content (15). It is generally assumed that the pharmacological action of a drug is related to its unbound concentration in the blood. Thus, unbound concentrations would ideally be preferred for further studies of the relationship between pharmacokinetics and drug effects. However, a specific assay is a prerequisite for therapeutic drug monitoring, regardless of which blood compartment is used.

Acknowledgment: This work was supported by a grant from SAREC (Swedish Agency for Research Cooperation with Developing Countries). We thank Mrs. Emilia Sego and Mrs. Lena Ekman for skillful technical assistance.

REFERENCES

1. Brodie BB, Udenfriend S, Dill W, Chenkin T. The estimation of basic organic compounds in biological material. III. Estimation by conversion to fluorescent compounds. *J Biol Chem* 1947;168:319–25.
2. McChesney EW, Banks WF Jr, McAuliff JP. Laboratory studies of the 4-aminoquinoline antimalarials. II. Plasma levels of chloroquine and hydroxychloroquine in man after various oral dosage regimens. *Antibiot Chemother* 1962;12:583–94.
3. McChesney EW, Fasco MJ, Banks WF Jr. The metabolism of chloroquine in man during and after repeated oral dosage. *J Pharmacol Exp Ther* 1967;158:323–31.
4. Bergqvist Y, Frisk-Holmberg M. Sensitive method for the determination of chloroquine and its metabolite desethylchloroquine in human plasma and urine by high performance liquid chromatography. *J Chromatogr* 1980;211:119–27.
5. Alván G, Ekman L, Lindström B. Determination of chloroquine and its desethyl metabolite in plasma, red blood cells and urine by liquid chromatography. *J Chromatogr* 1982;229:241–7.
6. Staiger M, Nguyen-Dinh P, Churchill F. Sensitive high-performance liquid chromatographic analysis for chloroquine in body fluids. Application to studies of drug resistance in *Plasmodium falciparum*. *J Chromatogr* 1981;225:139–49.
7. Gustafsson LL, Walker O, Alván G, et al. Disposition of chloroquine in man after single intravenous and oral doses. *Br J Clin Pharmacol* 1983;15:471–9.
8. Faehlmann M, Rombo L, Hedman P. Serum concentrations of chloroquine in a patient with a late recrudescence of Kenyan *Plasmodium falciparum* malaria. *Trans R Soc Trop Med Hyg* 1981;75:362–4.
9. Jepsen S, Fogh S, Peterslund N, Black F. RII-RIII chloroquine resistant *Plasmodium falciparum* malaria from East Africa: studies of the in vivo and in vitro response to chloroquine. *Ann Trop Med Parasitol* 1983;77:349–54.
10. Herzog CH, Ellis CJ, Innes JA, Fletcher KA. Possible role of drug malabsorption in recrudescence of falciparum malaria. *Lancet* 1982;2:1157–8.
11. Bergqvist Y, Domeij-Nyberg B. Distribution of chloroquine and its metabolite desethyl-chloroquine in human blood cells and its implication for the quantitative determination of these compounds in serum and plasma. *J Chromatogr* 1983;272:137–48.
12. Westgard JO, de Vos DJ, Hunt MR, Quam EF, Garber CC, Carey RN. Concepts and practices in the evaluation of clinical chemistry methods III: statistics. *Am J Med Techn* 1978;44:552–71.
13. Aderounmu AF, Fleckenstein L. Pharmacokinetics of chloroquine diphosphate in the dog. *J Pharmacol Exp Ther* 1983;226:633–9.
14. Verdier F, Le Bras J, Clavier F, Hatin I. Blood levels and in vitro activity of desethyl chloroquine against *Plasmodium falciparum*. *Lancet* 1984;1:1186.
15. Bergqvist Y. Determination of chloroquine and its metabolites in various biological tissues and an evaluation of its disposition in man [Thesis]. Uppsala, Sweden. University of Uppsala, 1983.
16. Solomon HM, Zieve PD. The accumulation of organic bases by the human platelet. *J Pharmacol Exp Ther* 1967;155:112–6.
17. Malmgren R, Olsson P, Unge G. The effect of various inhibitors on the 5-HT binding and uptake by human platelets. *Thromb Res* 1981;22:469–80.

Therapeutic Drug Monitoring
7:216–221 © 1985 Raven Press, New York

A Sensitive Liquid Chromatographic Assay for Plasma Aspirin and Salicylate Concentrations After Low Doses of Aspirin

Roslyn A. Brandon, Mervyn J. Eadie, and Maree T. Smith

Department of Medicine, University of Queensland, Royal Brisbane Hospital, Brisbane, Australia

Summary: An original, highly sensitive and specific high performance liquid chromatographic method has been developed for the measurement of aspirin and salicylate in plasma. Minimum concentrations of 10 μg/L (aspirin) and 0.5 mg/L (salicylate) can be measured using 1 ml of plasma. After collection, plasma is first treated with physostigmine sulfate to inhibit enzymatic hydrolysis of aspirin to salicylate. Maximal recovery is achieved using an acid extraction into anhydrous diethyl ether with a subsequent drying-down step in an iced water bath. Aspirin and salicylate are separated by elution with a mixture of methanol, 1-butanol, orthophosphoric acid, and water on a reversed-phase octadecyl silane column at 47°C and detected at 234 nm by ultraviolet absorption. Quantitation is achieved using the peak height ratio of aspirin and salicylate to internal standard (*m*-anisic acid). The assay has been used for the study of simultaneous aspirin and salicylate pharmacokinetics after a single oral dose of 100 mg soluble glycinated aspirin for platelet antiaggregatory therapy in six subjects, one of whom was also studied after receiving a 600 mg dose. **Key Words:** Aspirin—Salicylate—Pharmacokinetics—Liquid chromatography—Thromboembolism.

Aspirin (ASA) has been widely used for decades for its analgesic, antiinflammatory, and antipyretic properties. Relatively recently, a new therapeutic use has been recognized based on the ability of ASA to prolong the bleeding time (1) by permanently acetylating the enzyme cyclooxygenase in blood platelets (2). Results from clinical trials suggest that ASA may be useful for the prevention of certain forms of thromboembolic arterial disease (3). Further evidence has been presented indicating that substantially lower doses of ASA may be as effective for this purpose (4,5) as the higher doses used for analgesic, antiinflammatory, antipyretic therapy and in the initial antithrombotic investigative trials.

An extensive but so far inconclusive search for a minimal effective dosage regimen in thromboembolic arterial disease has been made. However, few investigations have included the measurement of plasma concentrations of ASA, and little consideration has been given to possible differences in the bioavailability of ASA from different preparations. While the presently available methods for measuring plasma ASA and salicylate (SA) concentrations are adequate for measuring these substances following the ASA doses given for analgesic, antiinflammatory, antipyretic purposes (6–9), they are not sensitive enough to measure concentrations achieved following the lower doses currently being investigated for the platelet antiaggregatory action. The present study reports a simple, specific, and highly sensitive assay for ASA and SA using high performance liquid chromatography (HPLC). Low concentrations of ASA and its metabolite SA can be

Address correspondence and reprint requests to Dr. R. A. Brandon at Department of Medicine, University of Queensland, Royal Brisbane Hospital, Brisbane 4029, Australia.

measured in the plasma following the administration of small doses of ASA. The method permits study of the pharmacokinetics of the drug after oral doses of as little as 100 mg ASA.

MATERIALS AND METHODS

Reagents

ASA and SA were purchased from BDH Chemicals, Ltd. (Poole, England), *m*-anisic acid from Pfaltz and Bauer Inc. (Stamford, CT, U.S.A.) and physostigmine sulfate from Sigma (St. Louis, MO, U.S.A.). Anhydrous diethyl ether was supplied by Mallinckrodt Pty. Ltd. (South Oakleigh, Victoria, Australia) and peroxide-free diethyl ether by May and Baker Ltd. (Dagenham, England). Methanol was HPLC grade supplied by Waters Assoc. (Milford, MA, U.S.A.). All other chemicals were purchased commercially and were of analytical grade. Ether was discarded after 72 h of initial opening of the container.

Stock solutions of ASA, SA, and *m*-anisic acid were prepared in absolute methanol. Because of the instability of ASA in solution, new solutions were prepared before each analysis. SA was also freshly prepared. *m*-Anisic acid was stored at 4°C for no longer than 1 month. A stock solution of 20.26×10^{-3} *M* physostigmine sulfate (in saline) was stable for at least 2 months when stored at 4°C and protected from light.

Instrumentation

A model M6000A Solvent Delivery System, model U6K Universal Injector, and model 480 Absorbance Detector (all from Waters Assoc.) and a Tracor Instruments (Austin, TX, U.S.A.) column heating jacket were used.

The separations were achieved by use of a Waters 30 cm × 3.9 mm μBondapak 10 μ C_{18} (octadecyl silane) and a guard column (23 × 3.9 mm interior diameter) packed with μBondapak C18/Porasil B (Waters Assoc.). Peak heights at 234 nm were recorded with a dual-channel chart recorder using one channel at a setting of 10 mV and the other at either 100, 200, or 500 mV depending upon the concentration of the drug being measured. Chart speed was 0.5 cm/min, and all separations were carried out at 47°C.

Mobile Phase

The isocratic delivery system consisted of a single eluent that contained 0.13 ml orthophosphoric acid, 10 ml 1-butanol, 270 ml methanol, and 720 ml distilled water. This mixture was filtered through a glass filter (pore size, 0.5 μm; Millipore Corp., Bedford, MA, U.S.A.) and then degassed under reduced pressure. The flow rate was 1.8 ml/min.

Preparation of Standard Curves

Two standard curves each were prepared for ASA and SA because of the range of concentrations over which the method was operative. For the lower concentration range standards, aliquots of the methanolic stock solutions were added to glass centrifuge tubes (15 cm × 15 mm, with Teflon-lined screw caps) to give concentrations of 0.025–0.5 and 0.5–5.0 mg/L for ASA and SA, respectively. Similarly, for the high concentration range standards, aliquots were added to give concentrations of 0.5–10 and 5.0–70.0 mg/L for ASA and SA, respectively. Twenty-five microliters of a 50 mg/L solution of *m*-anisic acid was added to each tube as the internal standard. The methanol was evaporated to dryness under a stream of nitrogen at room temperature.

Plasma for standard curves contained a final concentration of 2×10^{-4} M physostigmine sulfate (6) and was known to be free of ASA and its metabolites. One milliliter plasma was then added to the tubes, followed by 0.2 ml 1.0 *M* HCl and 10 ml of anhydrous diethyl ether. Each tube was capped and the contents gently mixed for 5 min. After centrifugation at 1,500 *g* for 4 min, the organic phase was transferred to a ground glass stoppered tube. These tubes were then placed in an iced water bath, and a stream of nitrogen gas was blown over the solvent until the ether was evaporated to dryness; 0.2 ml of the mobile phase was added to each tube and the residue was dissolved by vortex-mixing for 90 s. Then, 5–100 μl of this extract was injected into the liquid chromatograph. Standard curves were constructed from peak height ratios of ASA or SA to internal standard.

Analytic Recovery Studies

Known amounts of ASA and SA in methanolic solution were added to ground glass stoppered tubes. The methanol was evaporated to dryness, and 0.2 ml of mobile phase was then added, vortex-mixed, and injected onto the chromatograph. These same concentrations of ASA and SA were extracted from plasma as described previously, and the peak height ratios to internal standard were compared with those from the nonextracted sample. Three replicates of six concentrations of ASA and SA were used.

Reproducibility Studies

Pooled samples of human plasma with known concentrations of ASA and SA were used for these studies. Six replicates were analyzed at each concentration. The peak height ratios of ASA and SA to internal standard were then converted to concentrations by use of the appropriate regression equations.

Specificity

Specificity of the method was studied by assaying plasma samples from patients receiving various commonly used drugs other than salicylates, plasma samples to which pure drug had been added, or directly injected alcoholic solutions of the substances under consideration.

Pharmacokinetic Study

Six informed, consenting volunteers (three men and three women) aged (mean ± SD) 26 ± 4.6 years and weight (mean ± SD) 67 ± 8.6 kg participated in the study after approval from the University of Queensland Ethics Committee. The subjects had not taken ASA or any other drug except oral contraceptives for at least 10 days prior to the study. All subjects fasted overnight and in the morning were given 100 mg of glycinated ASA (Solvin, Reckitt and Colman, Sydney, Australia). One male subject was also given a 600 mg dose of glycinated ASA on a separate occasion. The ASA was placed on the tongue to disperse within the mouth, and the subjects swallowed as desired.

Five to ten milliliters of venous blood was drawn through an indwelling Teflon catheter inserted into the cephalic vein and collected into lithium heparin tubes containing 100 μl of the stock solution of physostigmine sulfate (final concentration of approximately 2×10^{-4}) (6). Samples were centrifuged within 5 min of collection, and the plasma was separated and quick-frozen on dry ice before storage at −20°C. All samples were extracted and chromatographed (within 5 days of collection) in the same manner as spiked plasma for the standard curves. Internal standard was added in methanolic solution and evaporated to dryness in the bottom of the tube before the addition of the plasma.

Pharmacokinetic Analysis

Each set of unweighted paired plasma aspirin and salicylate concentration–time data was fitted simultaneously to linear equations for a one compartment pharmacokinetic model, using the iterative curve fitting program Multi (10) run on an Apple II plus microcomputer. The equations to which the data were fitted were:

$$C_{(ASA)} = \frac{\text{Dose}}{V} \frac{k_a}{(k_a - k)} (e^{-kt} - e^{-k_a t})$$

and

$$C_{(SA)} = \frac{k_a k_f D_{(SA)}}{V_{(SA)}} \left[\frac{e^{-kt}}{(k_a - k)(k_{(SA)} - k)} - \frac{e^{-k_a t}}{(k_a - k)(k_{(SA)} - k_a)} - \frac{e^{-k_{(SA)} t}}{(k_{(SA)} - k_a)(k_{(SA)} - k)} \right]$$

where V is the apparent volume of distribution of ASA, k_a is the absorption rate constant of ASA, k is the elimination rate constant of ASA, k_f is the formation rate constant for SA, $D_{(SA)}$ is the amount of SA formed, $V_{(SA)}$ is the apparent volume of distribution of SA, and $k_{(SA)}$ is the elimination rate constant for SA.

ASA area under the curve ($AUC_{0 \to \infty}$) was derived by calculating $AUC_{0 \to \infty}$ (where t was the latest time at which plasma ASA concentration was measurable) by trapezoidal rule integration, and adding to this result the value of $AUC_{t \to \infty}$, calculated as Ct/k. Because ASA hydrolysis occurs so rapidly one cannot be sure that the dose swallowed was the dose of ASA that was absorbed. Therefore, clearance and apparent volume of distribution values were not calculated. T_{max} and C_{max} values were read from the plasma concentration–time curves.

RESULTS

Figure 1 shows a typical chromatogram of a plasma sample spiked with 0.025 and 0.5 mg/L of ASA and SA, respectively. These concentrations represent the lowest calibration on the standard curve. However, for ASA, concentrations as low as 0.010–0.015 mg/L were measured accurately in plasma of subjects given 100 mg glycinated ASA orally. The retention time for each component was found to be constant at all con-

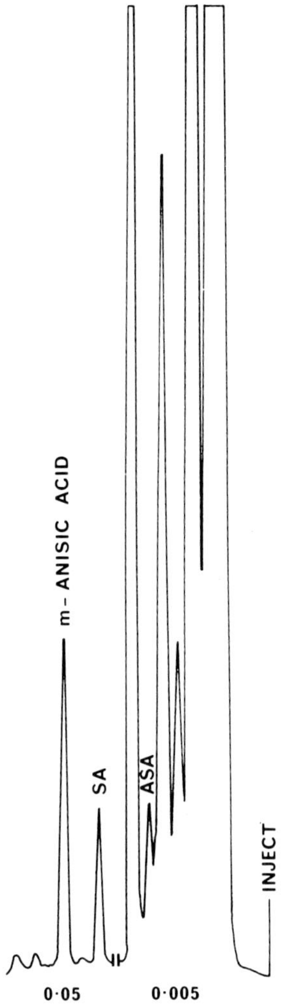

FIG. 1. Chromatogram of plasma extract; the compounds labeled in the figure are aspirin (ASA), salicylate (SA), and *m*-anisic acid (internal standard). Concentrations represented are 0.025, 0.5, and 1.25 mg/L for ASA, SA, and *m*-anisic acid, respectively. Chart speed was 0.5 cm/min. The numbers at the base of the chromatogram represent UV detector sensitivity setting.

centrations, and these values for ASA, SA, and *m*-anisic acid were 5.6, 8.0, and 9.6 min, respectively. Correlation coefficients for standard curves were in the range of 0.9980 to 0.9999 for six concentrations of ASA and SA.

Peaks that interfered with ASA were seen when anhydrous diethyl ether was used more than 72 h after container opening. Peroxide-free diethyl ether produced interfering peaks even when freshly opened.

When the ether extract was evaporated at ambient or higher temperature, erratic results, usually underestimations, were often obtained for SA. However, the results for SA became reproducible when the evaporation was carried out at lower temperatures by cooling the tubes in an iced water bath, thus minimizing SA losses by sublimation.

TABLE 1. *Results of reproducibility studies for aspirin and salicylate*

Aspirin concentration (mg/L)		Salicylate concentration (mg/L)	
Added	Recovered[a]	Added	Recovered[a]
0.025	0.025 ± 0.002	0.50	0.53 ± 0.03
0.050	0.049 ± 0.005	0.75	0.72 ± 0.04
0.100	0.101 ± 0.004	1.50	1.49 ± 0.06
0.200	0.201 ± 0.004	2.00	2.00 ± 0.06
0.350	0.349 ± 0.004	3.50	3.50 ± 0.05
0.500	0.497 ± 0.023	5.00	5.09 ± 0.22
1.000	1.020 ± 0.020	7.50	7.35 ± 0.21
2.500	2.480 ± 0.030	10.00	10.04 ± 0.24
5.000	4.937 ± 0.079	25.00	24.70 ± 0.47
7.500	7.611 ± 0.085	50.00	50.23 ± 0.33
10.000	9.964 ± 0.031	70.00	70.13 ± 1.80

[a]Means ± SD, n = 6.

Absolute recoveries of ASA ranged from 96.4 to 100.3%; similar studies on SA yielded recoveries from 76.7 to 91.2%. Table 1 shows the results of reproducibility studies. Interference by other drugs was studied with use of both solutions of the drug/metabolite and of samples from patients taking the medications listed in Table 2. Methyclothiazide was incompletely resolved from ASA.

Pharmacokinetic parameters were calculated from plasma concentration–time data for six subjects given a single dose of 100 mg glycinated ASA orally. The results for each subject, with the mean ± SD for the group, are shown in Table 3. It is noteworthy that ASA remained detectable at 3 h in all subjects following the 100 mg dose.

Figure 2 shows the time course of the concentrations of ASA and SA in plasma after the administration of 100 and 600 mg glycinated ASA to a male volunteer on separate occasions.

DISCUSSION

HPLC of plasma ASA and SA is more rapid and specific than fluorometric or colorimetric techniques, and unlike gas chromatography does not require derivatization of the drug for sensitivity and resolution to be adequate.

ASA is rapidly hydrolyzed in blood and plasma (11). To overcome the in vitro enzymatic hydrolysis of ASA, physostigmine sulfate was added to samples at collection. This procedure has been shown to be superior to the addition of fluoride for this purpose (6). However, to avoid acid-base hydrolysis of ASA,

TABLE 2. *Drugs tested for interference in plasma*

Tablet preparations and pure drugs/metabolites tested:	
Aminophylline	Methyclothiazide[a]
Amitriptyline	Methylphenobarbitone
Atenolol	Methylprednisolone
Carbamazepine	Metoprolol
Chlordiazepoxide	Mexiletine
Cimetidine	Midazolam
Clonazepam	Naphthoxyacetic acid
Desipramine	Nortriptyline
Dexamethasone	Oxazepam
Dicyclomine	Oxpranolol
Digoxin	Pentobarbitone
Disopyramide	Phenytoin
Ethosuximide	Prednisolone
Frusemide	Prednisone
Gentisic acid	Primidone
Glyceryl trinitrate	Procainamide
Haloperidol	Propranolol
Hydrocortisone	Quinidine
Imipramine	Salicyluric acid
Indomethacin	Spironolactone
Levodopa	Theophylline
Lignocaine	Valproic acid
Methdilazine	Warfarin
Plasma tested from patients receiving the following:	
Beclomethasone	Methysergide
Bromazepam	Metoclopramide
Caffeine	Nitrazepam
Chloral hydrate	Paracetamol
Codeine	Pethidine
Dextropropoxyphene	Prochlorperazine
Diazepam	Salbutamol
Doxycycline	Sulphamethoxazole
Ergotamine	Trimethoprim
Lithium carbonate	Verapamil

[a]Interferes with aspirin.

rapidity in the preparation of samples is important. Our sample preparation, although requiring more time than protein precipitation methods (6–8), involves only one short extraction step. The total sample preparation from collection to injection can be completed in less than 45 min and achieves maximal recovery of ASA.

The ASA sensitivity of our assay is five times greater than that reported by Buskin et al. (12), who use a back-extraction procedure, and is 50 times more sensitive than other previously reported assays which employ drying-down steps in their extraction procedure (9,13). Moreover, our assay retains the sensitivity for SA of the most sensitive of the previously reported assays (8,9,12,13).

It is often difficult to accurately measure small concentrations of ASA in the presence of large concentrations of SA in the same plasma sample using a single chromatograph injection. Our assay procedure has made this possible, using one internal standard at one concentration only, by the use of variations in a millivoltage setting on a dual pen chart recorder. In addition, this same procedure, using a lower UV detector sensitivity, allows concentrations that are achieved after higher, more conventional doses of ASA to be measured accurately.

Mean values for ASA (Table 3) of T_{max}, $t_{1/2\ elim}$, and $t_{1/2\ abs}$ were all in agreement with those previously reported (6,14,15) when oral doses of soluble ASA were administered. In the present study, the $t_{1/2\ elim}$ for SA (1.61 ± 0.79 h) was less than the 2.68 ± 0.63 h reported by Siebert et al. (15) after they had given a 600 mg dose of oral soluble ASA. The lower elimination half-life for SA following the 100 mg dose is presumably because of its dose-dependent elimination kinetics (16).

The present study reports a simple, specific, and highly sensitive method for the measurement of ASA and SA in plasma. This procedure is presently being

TABLE 3. *Pharmacokinetic parameters obtained from six normal subjects after a single oral dose of 100 mg glycinated aspirin*

		Aspirin					Salicylate			
Subject	r^2	C_{max} (mg/L)	T_{max} (min)	$T_{1/2\ elim}$ (min)	$T_{1/2\ abs}$ (min)	AUC (mg h/L)	C_{max} (mg/L)	T_{max} (h)	$T_{1/2\ elim}$ (h)	AUC (mg h/L)
1	0.971	0.96	45.0	45.6	46.4	1.8	7.09	3.25	1.16	31.0
2	0.985	1.63	30.0	7.5	7.6	1.1	4.77	0.75	3.18	27.2
3	0.985	2.20	20.0	10.7	31.1	2.3	8.71	1.50	1.62	33.9
4	0.994	1.46	30.0	15.6	18.9	1.6	5.29	1.25	1.17	15.6
5	0.984	1.84	20.0	5.3	35.3	2.1	6.76	2.00	1.46	25.5
6	0.976	2.20	15.0	3.5	25.0	2.1	7.18	1.25	1.09	19.9
Mean		1.7	26.7	14.7	27.4	1.8	6.63	1.67	1.61	25.5
±SD		0.47	10.8	15.7	13.5	0.4	1.42	0.88	0.79	6.8

C_{max}, maximum concentration; T_{max}, time of maximum concentration; $T_{1/2\ elim}$, elimination half-life; $T_{1/2\ abs}$, absorption half-life; AUC, area under concentration–time curve.

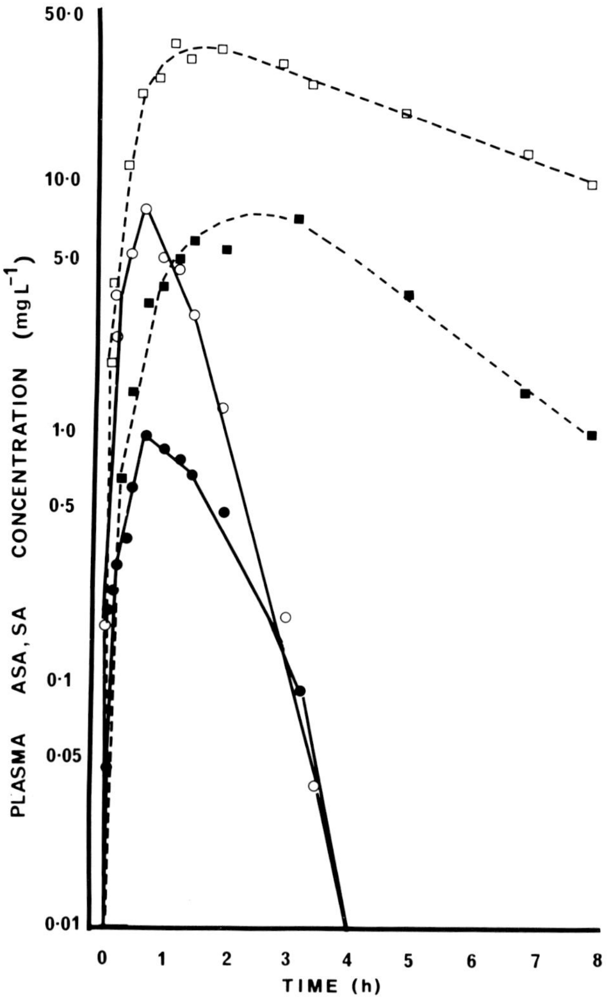

FIG. 2. Semilogarithmic plot of plasma aspirin (ASA) and salicylate (SA) concentrations (mg/L) against time (h) following oral administration of 100 and 600 mg glycinated aspirin to one male volunteer. 100 mg ASA (black circles) and SA (black squares); 600 mg of ASA (white circles) and SA (white squares).

used in our laboratory to determine the minimum plasma concentrations of ASA required to inhibit platelet aggregation for the purpose of ultimately defining a chronic therapeutic dosage regimen for the prevention of thromboembolic arterial disease. Previous to the development of this assay, to our knowledge there was no method available of sufficient sensitivity for this purpose.

Acknowledgment: Financial support was provided by the National Health and Medical Research Council (NHMRC) and the Pharmaceutical Division of Reckitt and Colman Ltd. We would like to thank Dr. R. Dickinson and Dr. W. Hooper for their invaluable technical assistance and guidance. Our thanks is also extended to the staff of Waters Assoc., Brisbane, for their advice.

REFERENCES

1. Quick AJ. Salicylates and bleeding: the aspirin-tolerance test. *Am J Med Sci* 1966;252:265–9.
2. Roth GJ, Majerus PW. The mechanism of the effect of aspirin on human platelets. I. Acetylation of a particulate fraction protein. *J Clin Invest* 1975;56:624–32.
3. Fields WS. Aspirin for prevention of stroke: a review. *Am J Med* 1983;74:61–5.
4. Hanley SP, Bevan J, Cockbill SR, Heptinstall S. Differential inhibition by low-dose aspirin of human venous prostacyclin synthesis and platelet thromboxane synthesis. *Lancet* 1981;1:969–71.
5. Masotti G, Galanti G, Poggesi L, Abbate R, Neri Serneri GG. Differential inhibition of prostacyclin production and platelet aggregation by aspirin. *Lancet* 1979;2:1213–7.
6. Cham BE, Ross-Lee L, Bochner F, Imhoff D. Measurement and pharmacokinetics of acetylsalicylic acid by a novel high performance liquid chromatographic assay. *Ther Drug Monit* 1980;2:365–72.
7. Rumble RH, Roberts MS. Determination of aspirin and its major metabolites in plasma by high-performance liquid chromatography without solvent extraction. *J Chromatogr* 1981;225:252–60.
8. Bakar SK, Niazi S. High-performance liquid chromatographic determination of aspirin and its metabolites in plasma and urine. *J Pharm Sci* 1983;72:1020–3.
9. Peng GW, Gadalla MAF, Smith V, Peng A, Chiou WL. Simple and rapid high-pressure liquid chromatographic simultaneous determination of aspirin, salicylic acid, and salicyluric acid in plasma. *J Pharm Sci* 1978;67:710–2.
10. Yamaoka K, Tanigawara Y, Nakagawa T, Uno T. A pharmacokinetic analysis program (Multi) for microcomputer. *J Pharm Dyn* 1981;4:879–85.
11. Morgan AM, Truitt EB. Evaluation of acetylsalicylic acid esterase in aspirin metabolism. Interspecies comparison. *J Pharm Sci* 1965;54:1640.
12. Buskin JN, Upton RA, Williams RL. Improved liquid-chromatography of aspirin, salicylate, and salicyluric acid in plasma with a modification for determining aspirin metabolites in urine. *Clin Chem* 1982;28:1200–3.
13. Low LY, Bye A. Specific and sensitive method for the determination of aspirin and salicylic acid in plasma using reversed phase high-performance liquid chromatography. *J Chromatogr* 1980;181:473–7.
14. Rowland M, Riegelman S, Harris PA, Sholkoff SD. Absorption kinetics of aspirin in man following oral administration of an aqueous solution. *J Pharm Sci* 1972;61:379–85.
15. Siebert DJ, Bochner F, Imhoff DM, et al. Aspirin kinetics and platelet aggregation in man. *Clin Pharmacol Ther* 1983;33:367–74.
16. Levy G, Tsuchiya T, Amsel LP. Limited capacity for salicyl phenolic glucuronide formation and its effect on the kinetics of salicylate elimination in man. *Clin Pharmacol Ther* 1972;13:258–68.

Therapeutic Drug Monitoring
7:222–228 © 1985 Raven Press, New York

Therapeutic Monitoring of Chlorpromazine I: Pitfalls in Plasma Analysis

J. W. Hubbard, J. K. Cooper, E. M. Hawes, *D. J. Jenden, *P. R. A. May, M. Martin, G. McKay, *T. Van Putten, and K. K. Midha

*College of Pharmacy, University of Saskatchewan, Saskatoon, Saskatchewan, Canada; and *Departments of Psychiatry and Pharmacology, University of California at Los Angeles, School of Medicine, Los Angeles, California, U.S.A.*

Summary: Pooled plasma from healthy volunteers was spiked with pure, synthetic chlorpromazine (CPZ), chlorpromazine sulfoxide (CPZSO), or chlorpromazine *N*-oxide (CPZNO), and then made alkaline with either sodium hydroxide or sodium carbonate. The samples were allowed to stand at room temperature for various timed intervals before extraction with organic solvent. It was found that CPZNO was reduced to CPZ in plasma made alkaline with sodium hydroxide, but not in protein-free buffer solution at high pH nor in plasma made alkaline with sodium carbonate. The reaction appears to take place through reducing equivalents generated by the action of sodium hydroxide on plasma proteins. Thus, apparent concentrations of CPZ in plasma from patients were elevated by as much as 343% when sodium hydroxide was used compared with concentrations in aliquots of the same plasma samples alkalinized with sodium carbonate. The amount of CPZ produced from CPZNO depends on the type of extraction procedure employed as well as on the quantity of sodium hydroxide added to the plasma. By contrast, no interconversion between CPZ and CPZSO or CPZNO and CPZSO was observed in plasma alkalinized and extracted under any of the conditions tested. **Key Words:** Chlorpromazine—Chlorpromazine sulfoxide—Chlorpromazine *N*-oxide—Plasma analysis, errors.

Most analytical methods for chlorpromazine (CPZ) require that plasma, serum (1), or whole blood be made alkaline before extraction of the drug with organic solvents. The most commonly used method for alkalinization is the addition of sodium hydroxide (1–14), although the number of milliequivalents of alkali added per milliliter of plasma, serum, or whole blood varies considerably. The use of sodium hydroxide appears to be rational, since it has been reported (7) that the efficiency of CPZ extraction was enhanced when whole blood samples were adjusted to a pH of 12 to 14 rather than to a pH of 9 to 11.

Address correspondence and reprint requests to Dr. K. K. Midha at College of Pharmacy, University of Saskatchewan, Saskatoon, Saskatchewan. S7N 0W0, Canada.

Dr. P. R. A. May is Professor, Della Martin Chair in Psychiatry, Neuropsychiatric Institute, Center for the Health Sciences, University of California, Los Angeles, California 90024, U.S.A.

Recently, we described a high–performance liquid chromatography (HPLC) method for the analysis of CPZ (15) in which the drug was extracted from plasma alkalinized by the addition of a saturated solution of sodium carbonate. In the course of developing this method, we found that the recovery of CPZ in pentane/3% isopropanol was similar (86%) between spiked plasma samples alkalinized with sodium carbonate and samples after alkalinization with sodium hydroxide. When we extracted specimen plasma samples from patients dosed with CPZ, however, the apparent concentrations of CPZ were much higher in the extracts of plasma aliquots alkalinized with sodium hydroxide than in those alkalinized with sodium carbonate. Thus, it appeared possible that metabolite(s) were being converted back into CPZ during the extraction at very high pH. This brought to mind that Krieglstein et al (16) had suspected that chlorpromazine *N*-oxide (CPZNO) was converted into CPZ and chlorpromazine sulfoxide (CPZSO) during their analytical procedure, which included an extraction step at pH 14. CPZNO and CPZSO are important metabolites that are present in the plasma of patients medicated with CPZ (17). We therefore carried out a series of experiments to investigate the effects of high pH on CPZNO, CPZSO, and CPZ in plasma.

METHODS

Materials

CPZ and CPZSO were kindly supplied by Poulenc Ltd. (Montreal, Quebec, Canada). CPZNO was synthesized in our laboratories by oxidation of CPZ with *m*-chloroperoxybenzoic acid (details to be reported elsewhere). The synthetic sample was identical [based on results of thin-layer chromatography (TLC) and ammonia chemical ionization–mass spectrometry (CI-MS)] with a reference sample kindly supplied by Dr. A. A. Manian. The purity and structural integrity of all three compounds was confirmed by TLC, CI-MS, proton magnetic resonance, infrared, and elemental analysis. All other chemicals were commercial analytical grade.

HPLC

HPLC equipment, mobile phase, and running conditions were as reported previously (15) except that the column was packed with 5-μm Spherisorb CN, not 10-μm Spherisorb CN. HPLC and all other operations were carried out in subdued light and at ambient temperature.

Collection of Plasma

Samples from three healthy volunteers were collected by venipuncture into evacuated heparinized tubes (Vacutainers; Becton-Dickinson, Mississauga, Ontario, Canada). Care was taken not to allow the blood to contact the rubber stopper (18). Blood from the three volunteers was decanted into a beaker and mixed. This was centrifuged immediately to separate the plasma. Freshly harvested plasma was used in all experiments and was collected as required from the same three volunteers.

Preparation of Samples

To 2.0 ml plasma was added 1.0 ml double-distilled water, followed by 40 μl acetonitrile containing 200 ng CPZ, CPZSO, or CPZNO. The sample was mixed, and the pH was adjusted by the addition of either 0.5 ml saturated sodium carbonate (condition 1) or 0.5 ml 10 *M* sodium hydroxide (condition 2). The final pH values were checked with a pH meter equipped with a combination glass–calomel electrode. Values obtained by such means are only approximations at very high pH. The pH meter readings were pH 11.7 under condition 1 and pH 13.6 under condition 2. The alkalinized samples were then allowed to stand at ambient temperature for the appropriate time (0, 15, 30, 45, 60, 90, and 120 min) before extraction. Three samples were prepared for each time point.

Extraction of Samples

The plasma samples were extracted with 5.0 ml *n*-pentane containing 3% isopropanol (PIP) by shaking (IKA Vibrax Shaker; Terochem Laboratories Limited, Edmonton, Alberta, Canada) for 15 min. The mixture was then centrifuged (1,500 *g*). The aqueous layer was separated and extracted with a second aliquot of PIP (5 ml) as described above. (In specified experiments, extraction with the second aliquot of PIP was omitted.) The aqueous layer was set aside for subsequent extraction with methylenedichloride (MDC).

To the combined PIP extracts was added an anti-bumping granule and 1.0 ml PIP containing 50 ng prochlorperazine as external standard. The mixture was then evaporated at 65°C (Thermolyne Dri-Bath; Fisher Scientific Company, Edmonton, Alberta, Canada). The residue was dissolved in 200 μl acetonitrile by mixing (Vortex-Genie; Fisher Scientific Company, Edmonton, Alberta, Canada). The acetonitrile solution (100 μl) was injected into the HPLC column.

The aqueous layer from above was transferred to a clean tube, to which 5.0 ml MDC was then added. The aqueous and MDC layers were mixed on a Multipurpose Rotator (Canlab, Edmonton, Alberta, Canada) for 30 min and then centrifuged (1,500 *g*). The MDC layer was removed and mixed with 1.0 ml PIP containing 50 ng prochlorperazine as an external standard. The solution was then concentrated to a small volume (~10 μl) at 40°C (Thermolyne Dri-Bath) in a stream of dry nitrogen. The concentrate was mixed (Vortex-Genie) with 200 μl acetonitrile, and an aliquot (100 μl) was injected into the HPLC column.

Calculations

All calculations for these absolute-recovery-type experiments were based on the absolute injection technique. The peak height of CPZ (or metabolite) was compared with the peak height of the corresponding

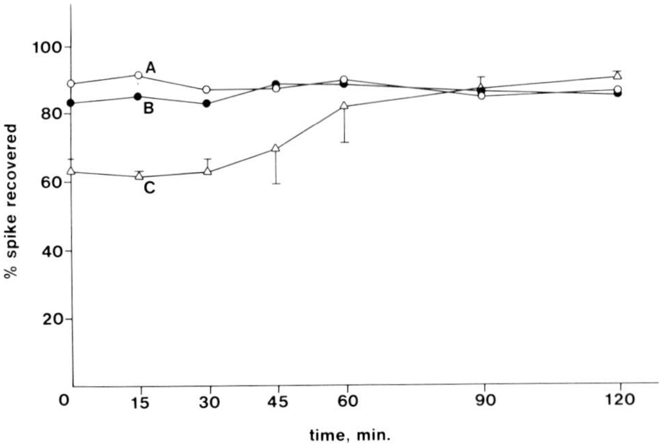

FIG. 1. Absolute recovery values for chlorpromazine from alkalinized plasma after the samples were allowed to stand at room temperature for various time intervals before extraction: **A**, alkalinization condition 1, extraction with two successive 5.0-ml aliquots of *n*-pentane containing 3% isopropanol (PIP), composite mean recovery 87.2 ± 2.2%; **B**, alkalinization condition 2, extraction with two successive 5.0-ml aliquots of PIP, composite mean recovery 85.2 ± 1.9%; **C**, alkalinization condition 1, extraction with a single 5.0-ml aliquot of PIP [mean absolute recovery values (n = 3) ± SD].

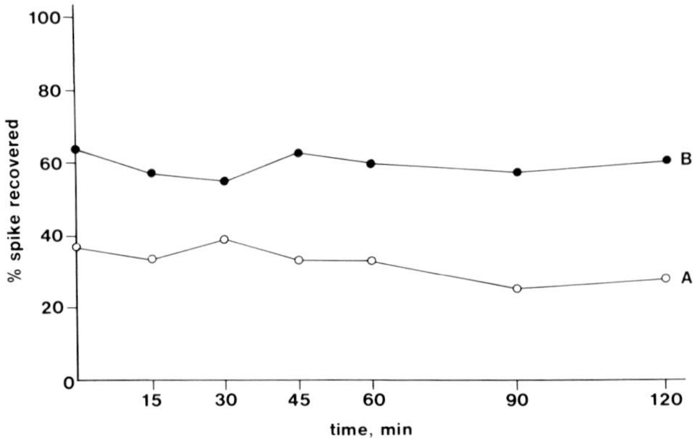

FIG. 2. Absolute recovery values for chlorpromazine sulfoxide from alkalinized plasma after the samples were allowed to stand at room temperature for various time intervals before extraction with two successive 5.0-ml aliquots of *n*-pentane containing 3% isopropanol: **A**, alkalinization condition 1, composite mean recovery 32.3 ± 4.4%; **B**, alkalinization condition 2, composite mean recovery 58.9 ± 2.6%.

standard in acetonitrile (100 μl). The external standard (prochlorperazine) was used to assure consistency in the relative retention times of CPZ and its metabolites.

RESULTS

Figure 1 shows the results of three experiments in which CPZ was added to human pooled plasma samples that were subsequently alkalinized under condition 1 or condition 2 before extraction with PIP. In two of these experiments (Fig. 1, curves A and B), where the samples were subsequently extracted with two successive aliquots of PIP, as described in Methods, the length of time for which the alkalinized spiked plasma samples were allowed to stand before extraction had no effect on recovery of CPZ. Results from these experiments can therefore be quoted as composite mean percentage recoveries (± SD). It is noteworthy that there was no significant difference between the composite mean recovery of CPZ samples alkalinized under condition 1 (87.2 ± 2.2%) and that of samples alkalinized under condition 2 (85.2 ± 1.9%).

In the third experiment, shown in curve C of Fig. 1, plasma samples alkalinized under condition 2 were extracted by shaking with a single aliquot of PIP for 15 min. Here the recovery of CPZ was markedly affected by the time for which the samples were allowed to stand before extraction. The recovery rose from ~65%, for samples extracted immediately after alkalinization, to 90%, for samples allowed to stand for 120 min. Thus, unless otherwise stated, all experiments were carried out by the use of two successive aliquots of PIP, as described in Methods.

In experiments in which plasma was spiked with CPZSO, the metabolite was recovered more efficiently in PIP after alkalinization under condition 2 (58.9 ± 2.6%; Fig. 2, curve B) than it was under condition 1 (32.3 ± 4.4%, Fig. 2, curve A). Note that only unchanged CPZSO was recovered. No CPZ or CPZNO was detected in any experiment in which CPZSO was added to plasma and subsequently alkalinized.

CPZNO was also recovered unchanged (53.8 ± 4.3%) in MDC extracts of plasma spiked with the *N*-oxide and alkalinized under condition 1 (Fig. 3). No CPZ or CPZSO was detected in either PIP or MDC extracts. By contrast, no unchanged CPZNO could be detected after alkalinization of plasma under condition 2. Instead, the PIP extracts, when injected into the HPLC column, gave a peak that corresponded in retention volume to CPZ. The HPLC eluate corresponding to this peak was collected and evaporated, and the residue was subjected to ammonia CI-MS by direct insertion probe. The mass spectrum was identical to that of an authentic reference sample of CPZ. It was concluded that CPZNO had undergone reduction to CPZ in plasma adjusted to very high pH under condition 2.

Figure 4 shows percentages of the CPZNO spike recovered as CPZ in two experiments. In the first experiment (Fig. 4, curve A), the spiked alkalinized

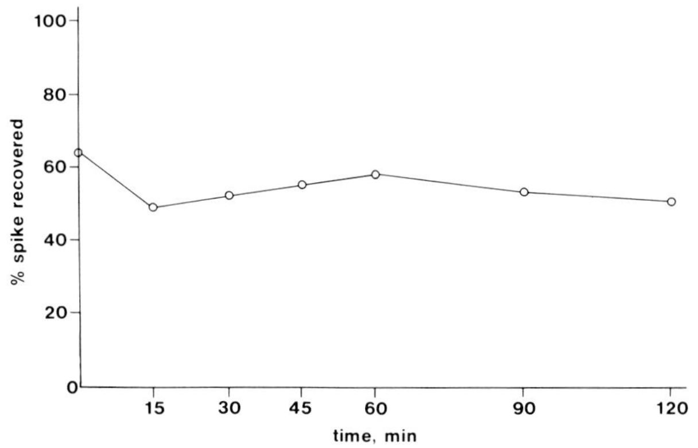

FIG. 3. Absolute recovery values (in methylenedichloride) for chlorpromazine *N*-oxide from alkalinized plasma (condition 1) after the samples were allowed to stand at room temperature for various time intervals before extraction (composite mean recovery 53.8 ± 4.3%).

(condition 2) plasma was extracted with a single aliquot of PIP. Note that very little CPZ was detected in extracts of plasma extracted immediately after alkalinization (time 0), although the amounts rose to 65% in alkalinized plasma samples allowed to stand for 30 min before extraction. By contrast, in the second experiment (Fig. 4, curve B), in which the plasma was extracted with two aliquots of PIP, the recovery of spike as CPZ was about 60% at time 0 and the composite mean recovery of spike as CPZ for this second experiment was 68 ± 6.2%.

In other experiments, the reduction of CPZNO to CPZ took place in 4% solutions of human serum albumin spiked with CPZNO and subsequently alkalinized under condition 2. A portion of the spike (32.1 ± 8.3%) was recovered as CPZ from the PIP extracts, and a further portion (13.3 ± 2.3%) was recovered as unchanged CPZNO in the MDC extracts. There was, however, no reduction of CPZNO in albumin solutions alkalinized under condition 1, or in protein-free solutions of CPZNO alkalinized under either condition.

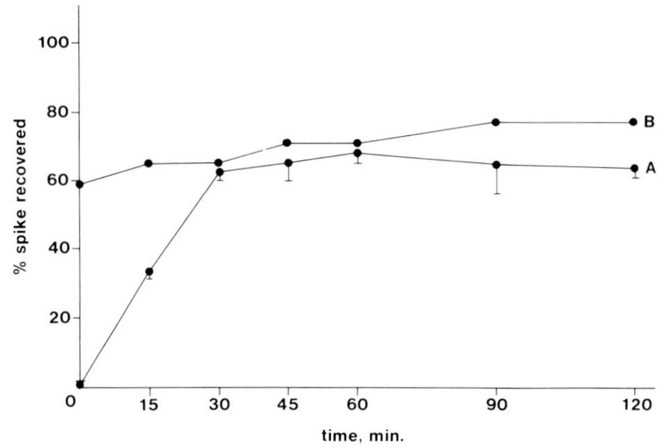

FIG. 4. Recovery of chlorpromazine from plasma spiked with chlorpromazine *N*-oxide, alkalinized (condition 2), and allowed to stand at room temperature for various time intervals before extraction with a single 5.0-ml aliquot of *n*-pentane containing 3% isopropanol (PIP) [mean values (n = 3) ± SD] (A), or two successive 5.0-ml aliquots of PIP (composite mean recovery 68 ± 6.2%) (B).

DISCUSSION

Figure 1 (curves A and B) shows that the extraction of CPZ with two successive aliquots of PIP gave good absolute recovery values whether the plasma was alkalinized under condition 1 or condition 2. Furthermore, the time between alkalinization and commencement of extraction had no effect on recovery under either condition. Extraction with a single aliquot of PIP, however, gave lower recovery values when the plasma samples were extracted within 30 min of alkalinization. The improvement in recovery of CPZ observed as the time between alkalinization and extraction was prolonged beyond 30 min may be related to a gradual breakdown of plasma proteins in the strongly alkaline medium. Presumably, after a long incubation period, there would be no remaining contribution from protein binding to the partitioning of the drug between aqueous and organic layers. Thus, after 120 min of incubation it was found that a single-aliquot extraction gave an absolute recovery value comparable to that obtained with the double-aliquot extraction method.

Extraction with two successive aliquots of PIP was not only more efficient than single-aliquot extraction, it also took at least 3 times as long to carry out, because of the extra centrifugation and transfer steps involved. Thus, even when the extraction procedure was begun immediately after alkalinization, unextracted plasma contents remained in contact with the alkali for at least 60–70 min before the extraction procedure was complete. These factors had the effect of making the recovery appear to be independent of any delay between alkalinization and extraction. The combination of the double-aliquot extraction method and strongly alkaline condition 2 not only masked the effects of the digestion of plasma proteins with alkali, but also provided a very harsh test system for the production of artifacts.

The conversion of CPZNO into CPZ requires a reduction reaction (19) that cannot be brought about merely by the treatment of CPZNO with strong alkali. Occurrence of an enzyme-catalyzed reduction under condition 2 is ruled out because of the very high pH of the medium. It is much more likely that the reduction of the tertiary amino *N*-oxide occurred as a result of chemical reaction between CPZNO and plasma constituents that had been modified under the strongly alkaline conditions. For example, it is known that disulfide bonds such as those in albumin (20) can be cleaved under alkaline conditions (21). Reactive groups generated by the cleavage of disulfide bonds can reduce susceptible functional groups such as *N*-oxides and sulfoxides (19). In the present experiments, however, we did not detect any reduction of CPZSO in strongly alkalinized plasma. Possibly this is because CPZSO is a cyclic diarylsulfoxide, whereas CPZNO is the *N*-oxide of an acyclic tertiary amine.

The hypothesis that the reduction of CPZNO is brought about by reducing equivalents generated in plasma by the action of strong alkali was supported by the observation that reduction occurred in albumin solutions alkalinized under condition 2. By contrast, there was no reduction of CPZNO to CPZ under either condition in buffer solutions that contained no albumin. This simple experiment confirms that plasma proteins such as albumin can participate in the reduction of CPZNO when subjected to strongly alkaline extraction conditions.

These data are consistent with the findings of Krieglstein et al. (16), who used a perfusion medium that contained 2% albumin in their experiments with isolated perfused rat brain preparations. They observed a rapid conversion of CPZNO into CPZ, but suspected that the reaction took place during their analytical procedure rather than as a metabolic reaction in the brain tissue. Their albumin solutions were reported to be adjusted to "pH 14" before extraction, which gives support to our observation that the combination of albumin and strong alkali is required to bring about the reduction of CPZNO. We are, however, unable to support the findings of Lewis and coworkers (22), who reported the conversion of CPZNO into CPZ in rat plasma or serum under physiological conditions. We duplicated as closely as possible the experimental and analytical methods described by Lewis et al. (22), but did not observe any conversion of CPZNO into CPZ in rat or human plasma incubated at physiological pH.

The implication of our results for the therapeutic monitoring of CPZ in plasma is that any analytical procedure that calls for adjustment of the plasma to a very high pH before extraction is likely to give spuriously high levels of CPZ. For example, in a previous study (9), CPZ was measured in the plasma of schizophrenics by a gas–liquid chromatography–mass spectrometry method. Before extraction with 3% isopropyl alcohol in heptane, the plasma samples (2.0 ml) were made alkaline by the addition of 0.5 ml 5 *M* sodium hydroxide (condition 3). Some plasma samples, from patients who withdrew from the study, had been retained in frozen storage (−20°C). Each of the samples was divided into two aliquots, which were alkalinized under condition 1 or condition 2 before extraction with PIP as described in Methods. Table 1 shows the results of this study, as well as CPZ concentrations determined (condition 3) at the time of the original study (9). The apparent CPZ concentrations were up to 270% higher in the plasma samples extracted under condition 3 than in the corresponding aliquots extracted under condition 1. After extraction under condition 2, the apparent concentrations of CPZ were even higher than those obtained in the condition 3 extracts, for which fewer equivalents of alkali were employed. Therefore, plasma samples from patients dosed with CPZ should be alkalinized by the addition of sodium carbonate (condition 1) rather than by the addition of sodium hydroxide (conditions 2 and 3).

In view of the widespread use of sodium hydroxide in published analytical methods for CPZ (1–14), we decided to reproduce a number of the reported conditions of alkalinization and to check their propensity to catalyze the conversion of CPZNO into CPZ. Thus, pooled plasma samples were spiked with CPZNO (200 ng/ml). The requisite volume of spiked sample was then alkalinized by the addition of the appropriate sodium hydroxide solution. After mixing, the samples were analyzed for CPZ and CPZNO as described in Methods. The results (Table 2) show that marked re-

TABLE 1. *Apparent chlorpromazine (CPZ) concentrations in plasma samples from patients medicated with CPZ*[a]

Sample no.	CPZ concentration (ng/ml) Condition 1	Condition 2	Condition 3
1	7.26	10.74	10.17
2	60.26	NS	162.2
3	2.44	3.3	2.86
4	11.72	26.58	20.03
5	12.82	29.30	25.12
6	181.26	333.9	216.9
7	199.76	423.2	284.9
8	8.8	39.02	10.49
9	17.52	42.76	31.16
10	17.00	32.66	23.21

NS, insufficient plasma.

[a]Each sample was divided into three aliquots, which were alkalinized under condition 1, 2, or 3.

TABLE 2. *Recovery of chlorpromazine (CPZ) from pooled plasma samples spiked with chlorpromazine* N-*oxide, alkalinized under a variety of conditions, and extracted immediately with two successive 5.0-ml aliquots of* n-*pentane containing 3% isopropanol*

Condition	Plasma volume (ml)	NaOH Volume (ml)	NaOH Concentration (*M*)	Recovery of CPZ (%)	Reference
4	1.5	1.5	1.0	55.1	14
5	1.0	1.0	1.0	53.9	6
6	1.0	1.0	1.25	57.8	1
7	2.0	1.0	1.25	40.6	2
8	3.0	1.0	1.25	30.8	3
9	4.0	1.0	1.25	23.0	4
10	5.0	1.0	1.25	14.1	5
11	3.0	0.1	1.0	0.4	3

duction of CPZNO to CPZ occurred under all but one condition. The single exception was condition 11, which calls for the addition of far less sodium hydroxide (0.033 mEq/ml plasma) than the other conditions. These data confirm that the use of alkalinization conditions that lead to very high pH values can give spuriously high concentrations of CPZ and correspondingly low values for CPZNO in clinical plasma samples.

In addition to the wide variation in the amount of sodium hydroxide added to plasma, published reports (1–14) on the analysis of CPZ also describe the use of a variety of solvent systems and extraction techniques. Some techniques are based on extractions with a single aliquot of organic solvent, whereas other methods use sequential extractions with two or more aliquots of organic solvent(s). In the present study, we carried out an experiment to compare the effects of two different extraction techniques on the amount of CPZNO reduced to CPZ. Aliquots of pooled plasma were spiked with pure CPZNO (200 ng/ml) and alkalinized under condition 9 (Table 2). The samples were then analyzed immediately, either by the double-aliquot extraction method described in Methods (shaking for 15 min each with two 5-ml aliquots of PIP) or by shaking for a period of 30 min with a single 10-ml aliquot of PIP. With the single-aliquot method, only 1.4% of the spike was recovered as CPZ, whereas the double-aliquot method gave 23.9% recovery of the spike as CPZ. The difference is undoubtedly due to the fact that the double-aliquot extraction method takes considerably longer to perform, because of the extra centrifugation and transfer steps involved. Hence, the *N*-oxide is in contact with the alkalinized plasma for much longer than in the corresponding single-aliquot method. The importance of the contact time is also illustrated dramatically in Fig. 4, where the data are from plasma alkalinized under condition 2. Here the double-aliquot method gave 60% recovery of the spike as CPZ, even when the extraction procedure was commenced immediately after alkalinization. By contrast, only ~1% of the spike was detected as CPZ in corresponding aliquots shaken for 15 min with a single aliquot of PIP.

In a practical situation, contact time will depend not only on the type of extraction method employed, but also on the number of samples being handled and on the efficiency of the technical staff. The larger the number of sample tubes there are to be dealt with, the longer it takes to complete any manipulation step for the whole set. Note that in the present study a highly competent technician was able to achieve respectable coefficient of variation (CV) values for recovery of CPZ produced by reduction of CPZNO. Thus, there may be nothing to alert an unsuspecting analyst concerned with the analysis of CPZ in patient samples when data are erroneous. Furthermore, in recent work, we have found that other tertiary amine *N*-oxides, such as those of trifluoperazine and doxepin, are also subject to reduction under similar conditions.

CONCLUSION

CPZNO is reduced to CPZ in plasma adjusted to high pH with sodium hydroxide. This can result in spuriously high concentrations of CPZ being obtained in clinical plasma samples, especially if the samples are subjected to a lengthy extraction procedure with a low-polarity solvent or are allowed to stand after the alkali has been added. It is preferable to alkalinize the plasma with sodium carbonate, since the use of this reagent does not lead to the reduction of CPZNO.

Acknowledgment: The authors gratefully acknowledge the Medical Research Council of Canada for Grant No. DG 248 to J. W. H. and Grant No. 7838 to K. K. M. Messrs. T. J. Jaworski and P. K. F. Yeung are thanked for their technical assistance.

REFERENCES

1. Curry SH. Determination of nanogram quantities of chlorpromazine and some of its metabolites in plasma using gas–liquid chromatography with electron capture detection. *Anal Chem* 1968;40:1251–5.
2. Tompsett SL. The spectrophotometric determination of phenothiazine drugs in blood serum. *Acta Pharmacol Toxicol (Copenh)* 1968;26:298–302.
3. Effron DH, Harris SR, Manian AA, Gaudette LE. Radioassay of chlorpromazine and its metabolites in plasma. *Psychopharmacologia* 1971;19:207–23.
4. MacKay AVP, Healy AF, Baker J. The relationship of plasma chlorpromazine to its 7-hydroxy and sulfoxide metabolites in a large population of chronic schizophrenics. *Br J Clin Pharmacol* 1974;1:425–30.
5. Alfredsson G, Wode-Helgodt B, Sedwall G. A mass fragmentographic method for the determination of chlorpromazine and two of its active metabolites in human plasma and CSF. *Psychopharmacology (Berlin)* 1976;48:123–31.
6. Davis CM, Meyer CJ, Fenimore DC. Improved gas chromatographic analysis of chlorpromazine in blood serum. *Clin Chim Acta* 1977;78:71–7.
7. Kaul PN, Whitfield LR, Clark ML. Chlorpromazine metabolism VIII: blood levels of chlorpromazine and its sulfoxide in schizophrenic patients. *J Pharm Sci* 1976;65:694–7.
8. Whitfield LR, Kaul PN, Clark ML. Chlorpromazine metabolism IX. Pharmacokinetics of chlorpromazine following oral administration in man. *J Pharmacokinetic Biopharm* 1978;6:187–96.
9. May PRA, Van Putten T, Jenden DJ, Cho AK. Test dose response in schizophrenia. *Arch Gen Psychiatry* 1978;35:1091–7.
10. Fekete J, Del Castilno P, Kraak JC. Reversed-phase liquid chromatography for the separation of chlorpromazine, imipramine and some of their metabolites. *J Chromatogr* 1981;204:319–27.
11. Sakurai Y, Takahashi R, Nakahara T, Ikenaga H. Prediction of response to and actual outcome of chlorpromazine treatment in schizophrenic patients. *Arch Gen Psychiatry* 1980;37:1057–62.
12. Gupta RN, Bartolucci G, Molnar G. Analysis of chlorpromazine in plasma: effects of specimin storage. *Clin Chim Acta* 1981;109:351–4.
13. Murakami K, Murakami K, Ueno T, Hijikata J, Shirasawa K, Muto T. Simultaneous determination of chlorpromazine and levopromazine in human plasma and urine by high performance liquid chromatography using electrochemical detection. *J Chromatogr* 1982;227:103–12.
14. Stevenson D, Reid E. Determination of chlorpromazine and its sulfoxide and 7-hydroxy metabolites by ion pair high pressure liquid chromatography. *Anal Lett (Biol)* 1981;14:741–61.
15. Cooper JK, McKay G, Midha KK. Subnanogram quantitation of chlorpromazine in plasma by high performance liquid chromatography with electrochemical detection. *J Pharm Sci* 1983;72:1259–62.
16. Krieglstein J, Rieger H, Schutz H. Effects of chlorpromazine and some of its metabolites on the EEG and on dopamine metabolism of the isolated perfused rat brain. *Eur J Pharmacol* 1979;56:363–70.
17. Craig JC, Gruenke LD, Hitzeman BA, Holaday J, Loh HH. Simultaneous determination of chlorpromazine and its major metabolites in plasma and red blood cells by a GC/MS method: clinical implications. In: Usdin E, Eckert H, Forrest IS, eds. *Phenothiazines and structurally related drugs*. New York: Raven Press, 1980:129–32.
18. Midha KK, Loo JCK, Rowe ML. The influence of blood sampling technique on the distribution of chlorpromazine and tricyclic antidepressants between plasma and whole blood. *Res Comm Psychol Psychiatry Behav* 1979;4:193–203.
19. Ohno A, Oae S. Thiols. In: Oae S, ed. *The organic chemistry of sulfur*. New York: Plenum Press, 1977:119–87.
20. Kragh-Hansen U. Molecular aspects of ligand binding to serum albumin. *Pharmacol Rev* 1981;33:17–53.
21. Field L. Disulfides and polysulfide. In: Oae S, ed. *The organic chemistry of sulfur*. New York: Plenum Press, 1977:303–82.
22. Lewis MH, Widerlov E, Knight PL, Kilts CD, Mailman RB. *N*-Oxides of phenothiazine antipsychotics: effects on in vivo and in vitro estimates of dopaminergic function. *J Pharmacol Exp Ther* 1983;225:539–45.

Therapeutic Drug Monitoring
7:229–235 © 1985 Raven Press, New York

Comparative Determination of Flupentixol in Plasma by Gas Chromatography and Radioimmunoassay in Schizophrenic Patients

A. E. Balant-Gorgia, L. P. Balant, Ch. Genet, and R. Eisele

Unité de Monitoring Thérapeutique, Department of Psychiatry, University of Geneva, Geneva, Switzerland

Summary: A new method of measuring flupentixol in plasma was developed using gas chromatography (GC) with a nitrogen-phosphorus detector. The minimal quantifiable concentration was 0.5 ng/ml and the day-to-day coefficient of variation was 9.4% at 2 ng/ml. A comparison of flupentixol concentrations measured with radioimmunoassay (RIA) and GC was undertaken on 100 plasma samples obtained from 50 schizophrenic patients. The RIA method tended to overestimate flupentixol concentrations compared with GC. The reasons for this discrepancy might be the presence in plasma of the inactive *trans*(E)-flupentixol isomer and metabolites of flupentixol, which would cross-react with the antibody. The results of this study show that GC can be used for therapeutic monitoring of flupentixol. **Key Words:** Flupentixol—Gas chromatography—Radioimmunoassay—Isomers—Plasma concentration—Schizophrenic patients.

cis(Z)-Flupentixol, the active principle of Fluanxol, is a thioxanthene used in the treatment of schizophrenia (1,2). The esterification of the hydroxy group in the piperazine side chain is the basis for a long-acting form of flupentixol, which is its decanoic ester dissolved in Viscoleo. This depot preparation is administered intramuscularly every 2–4 weeks. An average dose of the depot preparation is 20–40 mg every 2 weeks as based on the free drug. The long-term action of this ester is attributed to its slow release into the bloodstream, where it is rapidly hydrolyzed by esterases to the active free base.

The oral form of flupentixol, Fluanxol tablets or drops, is a 1:1 mixture of the active cis(Z)- and inactive trans(E)-isomer. It has been reported that the fate in the organism of the two isomers is the same, and the cis(Z)/trans(E) ratio remains constant at ~1 (3–5). The intramuscular preparation, Fluanxol Depot, contains only the decanoic ester of the pure cis(Z) isomer. The drug undergoes first-pass elimination (4), and the absolute bioavailability of the oral form compared with an intravenous infusion is ~50% (4,5), with a range of ~20–70% (5). Interindividual variability in the handling of flupentixol is marked, giving rise to fivefold differences between patients' plasma concentrations (6).

In recent years, there has been increased interest in relating blood levels of psychoactive drugs to clinical response and side effects. Therefore, a radioimmunoassay (RIA) for *cis*(Z)-flupentixol has been developed for this purpose (7). This method uses specialized equipment (i.e., scintillation counter), and the inactive isomer and the metabolites cross-react with the antibody. We have therefore adapted the gas chromatographic (GC) procedure for fluphenazine (8) to flupentixol. The procedure is specific and sufficiently sensitive for the determination of this drug in plasma during routine drug level monitoring.

This article describes the respective advantages and disadvantages of the two methods and may serve as a

Address correspondence and reprint requests to Dr. A. E. Balant-Gorgia, Unité de Monitoring Thérapeutique, Department of Psychiatry, University of Geneva C.M.U., CH–1211 Geneva 4, Switzerland.

preliminary evaluation of the possible value of monitoring flupentixol in plasma.

EXPERIMENTAL METHODS

Patients and Drugs

Both spiked plasma samples and plasma samples obtained from treated patients were used in the present study. The spiked samples were prepared with pure *cis*(Z)-flupentixol, *trans*(E)-flupentixol, or a 1:1 mixture of both diastereoisomers (gift from Lundbeck AG, Zurich). The investigation includes 50 patients suffering from schizophrenia, all of whose diagnoses were in conformity with the diagnostic criteria of the World Health Organization[1]. The 26 male and 24 female patients ranged in age from 15 to 63 years. Twenty-seven patients were hospitalized for an acute psychotic relapse and were treated with oral Fluanxol (4–12 mg daily) according to standard clinical criteria. Thirty chronically ill, schizophrenic outpatients were treated with Fluanxol Depot intramuscularly (20–40 mg every 2 weeks) as a maintenance medication to prevent relapse. Among these 30 outpatients, 23 had received the depot preparation for at least 1 year while the remaining 7 were on their first dose of Fluanxol Depot, having first been treated orally for at least 1 month as inpatients. The only concomitant medication for 23 of these 50 patients was levomepromazine (Nozinan), which does not interfere in the gas chromatographic assay.

Criteria of Good and Poor Clinical Response

The criteria of clinical improvement were based on an initial evaluation at the beginning of treatment using the Brief Psychiatric Rating Scale (BPRS) (9). We considered as responders those patients whose BPRS score was decreased by 40% during therapy (10). All patients who did not fulfill this criterion were considered poor responders or nonresponders. The BPRS for those patients considered stabilized and accordingly treated with the depot preparation remained unchanged during the duration of this medication, since these patients had already improved before the beginning of the maintenance treatment.

Materials and Reagents

The standard curve was prepared with flupentixol dihydrochloride. Usually the cis(Z) isomer was used. The internal standard was perphenazine dihydrochloride (gift from Schering Corp., USA). The solvents and reagents were of analytical grade (Merck-Darmstadt). The extraction solvent was prepared by mixing 9 volumes of heptane with 1 volume of 2-propanol. The acetylation mixture was prepared daily by mixing ethylacetate and acetic anhydride 9/1 V/V with 1% methanol. Round-bottom, conical-stoppered glass tubes were rinsed several times, first with bidistilled water and then with pure methanol to minimize drug adsorption.

A Hewlett-Packard 5880 or 5790 gas chromatograph equipped with a specific nitrogen-phosphorus detector was used for the analysis. Separation was obtained with a 0.9 m column (2 mm i.d.) packed with 2% OV 101 on Supelcoport 80–100 mesh. The injector port and detector were maintained at 300°C and the column at 250°C. Flow rates were 40 ml/min for the helium carrier gas, 100 ml/min for air, and 3.5 ml/min for hydrogen. Electrometer and attenuation were set at 1 and 4, respectively; and collector voltage was adjusted between 16 and 18 V to obtain adequate sensitivity for the 5790 chromatograph. For the 5880 chromatograph, the power applied to the collector element was set to a value of ~180 to obtain a baseline of 40 pA, which corresponds at attenuation 4 to a 10-cm shift on the chart of the integrator.

Standards

The 1 μg/ml standard solutions were prepared daily by diluting 1:100 with methanol stock solution of 100 μg/ml of flupentixol and perphenazine in methanol. The stock solution, stored at −20°C, was stable for 3 weeks. The same procedure was applied to the cis and trans isomers, and to the mixture of isomers.

Analytical Procedure

Two milliliters of plasma (unknown samples and plasma standards containing known amounts of the drug) was transferred to 20-ml glass tubes. The internal standard (perphenazine: 25 ng/ml) was added to the unknown samples and plasma standards. Each sample was analyzed in duplicate, and the mean of the two values was used for further calculations. To each tube 200 μl of 4 N NaOH and 5 ml of the extraction solvent were added. After mechanically shaking the tubes for 20 min, the two phases were separated by centrifugation at 3,500 r/min for 10 min. The upper organic layer was transferred to a 10-ml glass tube and 1 ml of 0.1 N HCl was added. The tubes were then shaken for 10 min and centrifuged

[1]Glossary of mental disorders and guide to their classification, 9th rev. 1975, Geneva, WHO (ICD–9).

for 5 min. The organic layer was discarded. The acid layer was transferred to a 10-ml glass tube, 0.1 ml of 6 N NaOH was added (pH 13), and the drugs were extracted into 0.5 ml of the extraction solvent. Following centrifugation, the organic layer was transferred to 10-ml conical glass tubes and evaporated to dryness at 40°C, with a gentle stream of nitrogen. Fifty microliters of acetylation mixture was added. The samples were heated for 40 min at 40°C, and 5 μl of this solution was injected directly into the gas chromatograph.

To enhance the chromatographic response, new columns are primed by repeated injections of 500 ng/ml of flupentixol and 500 ng/ml of internal standard followed by five injections of plasma extracts containing 50 ng/ml of flupentixol and 100 ng/ml of internal standard, acetylated as described above.

Plasma Samples

Blood was drawn from patients into tubes containing EDTA as an anticoagulant (Venoject, Terumo). The samples obtained from patients on the oral formulation were drawn in the morning, 10 h after the administration of the last dose of Fluanxol, before the next administration of the drug, and after a treatment of at least 5–7 days, which is sufficient to reach steady state since the half-life of the active principle is 19–39 h (4). For the intramuscular formulation, the blood samples were drawn 7 and 14 days following the injection of Fluanxol Depot. Plasma was separated and stored frozen until analysis. Assay standards of 0, 1, 2.5, and 10 ng/ml were routinely processed with patient samples according to the procedure described. Linear regression analysis of peak height ratio versus concentration of standards was performed, and flupentixol concentrations of patient samples were determined from peak height ratios and the equation for the standard curve.

Radioimmunoassay

The RIA kits were provided by IRE Belgium. The basic steps in the assay procedure are as follows: purification of plasma/serum by shaking with petroleum benzine at low pH, incubation of the reaction mixture for 16 h at room temperature, separation of free and antibody-bound *cis*(Z)-flupentixol by adsorption to dextran-coated charcoal by centrifugation, and counting the antibody-bound ^{3}H *cis*(Z)-flupentixol (supernatant). The antiserum against *cis*(Z)-flupentixol linked to bovine serum albumin through a carboxy group (7) has been raised in sheep.

For the comparison of the RIA and GC methods, several RIA kits were employed. The quality of the 15 kits used was found to be constant over the whole time range (12 months) of the present study.

Statistical Methods

A normal distribution of the measured parameters was assumed. For the comparison of the results obtained with the GC and the RIA methods, two regression lines were calculated by linear regression of the unweighted values, i.e., RIA versus GC and GC versus RIA. Confidence intervals were also calculated but were found to be of limited interest for the present discussion. An "averaged" slope was then estimated from the two slopes of the regression lines. This "average" regression line was used only for graphical purposes. This approach was used because, in the present case, it was not possible to decide which of the RIA or GC values should be considered the independent variable and the dependent variable, respectively. In addition, the "individual" slopes of each datum point were calculated assuming that the line passes through the origin. The slope (expressed as a fraction of 1) was obtained by the ratio of the RIA value to the GC value. This method of calculation is equivalent to the expression of the RIA values as percentages of the GC concentrations. It must be noted that the present work was not designed to calculate a transformation coefficient which would allow one to convert an RIA into a GC value and that, accordingly, these slopes have only a quantitative relevance.

RESULTS

Linearity and Sensitivity

The linearity of the method was demonstrated by correlation coefficients of peak height (or area) ratio versus flupentixol concentration of 0.99. The limit of detection (peak height being four times the background noise) was 0.5 ng flupentixol/ml plasma when a 2-ml plasma sample was used.

Recovery

The recovery of the compounds was calculated by comparison of peak height following direct injection of the acetylated substance with peak height following injection of substance extracted from plasma and acetylated, to which the same amount of substance had been added. The recoveries of flupentixol and perphenazine from plasma were constant over a range of 5–10 ng/ml and averaged 63.2 and 52.2% for the two substances, respectively. Perphenazine was added at a constant concentration and standard curves with five different concentrations of flupentixol were prepared for each assay (1, 2.5, 5, 7.5, and 10 ng/ml). These calibration curves were linear over the whole range studied and passed through the origin. This indicates that there is no mutual influence of the two substances during the extraction process.

Precision and Accuracy

Precision and accuracy of the method were determined by preparing flupentixol plasma standards of several concentrations for six samples. The results (Table 1) show that the overall accuracy of the procedure was satisfactory.

Selectivity of the GC Method

Evidence for the selectivity of the method was furnished by characteristic GC retention times of the reference compounds and the lack of interfering peaks in plasma extracts from subjects not treated with flupentixol (Fig. 1). Approximate retention times for flupentixol and perphenazine under the described conditions were 1.54 and 3.03 min, respectively. The method is, however, not selective for the cis and trans isomers. Spiked samples of the separate isomers, or of a 1:1 mixture of the two, showed that the GC procedure does not discriminate between the two isomers.

Eleven commonly used, psychoactive drugs were screened for interference in the assay of flupentixol and perphenazine by directly acetylating the methanolic solutions of the drugs and analyzing them under the conditions described. The retention times of the drugs relative to that of flupentixol are given in Table 2.

Comparison of the RIA and GC Methods

The two methods, RIA and GC, were first compared by measuring samples in which *cis*(Z)-flupentixol, alone, was added to normal plasma. There was excellent agreement between the two methods, the coefficient of correlation was 0.986 ($p < 0.001$) (Fig. 2).

A comparison of the RIA determination of flupentixol levels and flupentixol concentrations measured by GC was undertaken with samples obtained during drug monitoring in outpatients and inpatients. Sixty-one plasma samples from patients who received injections of Fluanxol Depot ranging from 20 to 40 mg were analyzed. The correlation between the two methods was fair ($r = 0.82$) (Fig. 3), but the slope of the "averaged" regression line was 1.2, indicating that the RIA results were 20% higher than those of the GC. This finding suggests that RIA overestimates flupentixol concentrations due to the relative nonspecificity of the antibody that binds the parent compound and probably some of its metabolites. The mean of the "individual" slopes (i.e., single RIA values versus GC values) was 2.46 ± 3.11. The higher value found by this calculation as compared to the "averaged" slope is due to some points with a very high RIA/GC ratio. In any case, the conclusion is the same for the two methods: The RIA seems to overestimate flupentixol concentrations. As discussed below, these estimations are based on the fact that it has been reported that in vivo the cis(Z)-/trans(E) isomer ratio does not seem to differ appreciably from 1 (3–5).

Another group of 39 plasma samples from patients treated orally with Fluanxol (4–12 mg daily), in which the two isomers are present in equal amounts, were analyzed by the RIA and the GC method. The correlation in this study was also fair ($r = 0.78$) (Fig. 4). The slope of the "averaged" regression line was 0.7. Since the GC method measures the two isomers

TABLE 1. *Precision and accuracy of the GC method*

Actual value (ng/ml)	Observed value[a] (ng/ml)						Mean	CV (%)
1	1.08	0.90	1.00	0.84	0.86	1.05	0.95	9.30
5	5.10	4.80	4.90	4.60	4.20	4.60	4.70	6.60
10	10.00	10.50	10.50	10.10	11.90	11.00	10.70	6.50

CV, coefficient of variation.

[a]Contrary to the measurements of plasma samples from patients, these observed values are obtained from a single determination of 6 spiked samples originating from the same pool. In addition, 12 samples of plasma containing 2 ng/ml were analyzed over a 2-week period. The day-to-day coefficient of variation was calculated to be 9.4%.

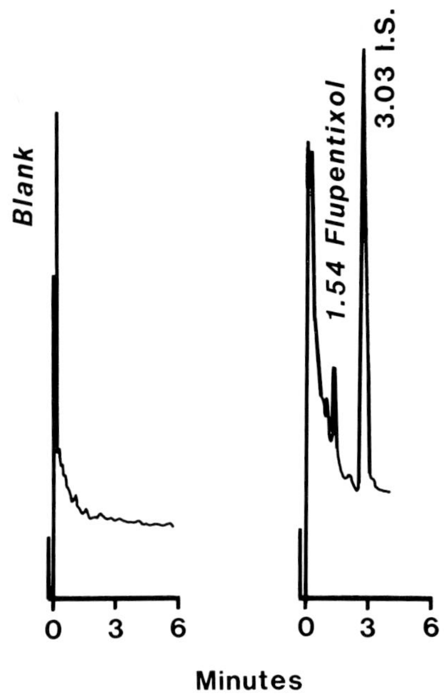

FIG. 1. Chromatograms obtained with a blank plasma sample **(left)** or a plasma sample from a patient treated with 40 mg Fluanxol Depot every 2 weeks (3.4 ng/ml) **(right).** Perphenazine (25 ng/ml) was added as internal standard. Retention times of *cis*(Z)-flupentixol and of the internal standard are shown.

and the RIA is specific for the active isomer, the slope of the theoretical regression line is 0.5. Accordingly, the RIA values were 40% higher than those measured by GC. This overestimation is probably due to cross-reactivity of the trans isomer and metabolites with the cis isomer. The same tentative conclusions are reached if the individual slopes (mean ± SD = 1.01 ± 0.51) are considered. As seen in Table 3, there was a weak relationship between the dosage of Fluanxol or Fluanxol Depot and plasma levels. The interindividual variability, however, was marked, confirming previous results (6).

TABLE 2. *Relative retention times of drugs*

Drug	Relative retention time
Flupentixol	1.00
Trifluoperazine	0.30
Desipramine	0.31
Desmethylclomipramine	0.50
Levomepromazine	0.55
Haloperidol	0.56
Thioridazine	0.84
Mesoridazine	1.70
Clopentixol	2.00
Perphenazine	2.07
Thiothixene	2.69

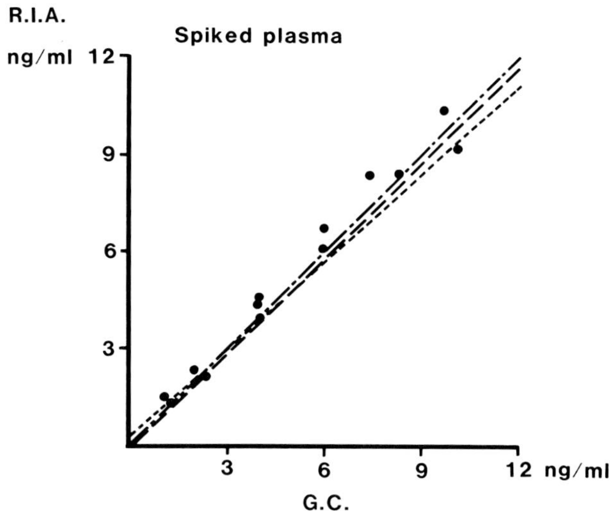

FIG. 2. Relationship between the results obtained with plasma samples spiked at different concentrations with *cis*(Z)-flupentixol: theoretical regression line with a slope of 1 (–·–·); two regression lines calculated from RIA vs. GC(----)and GC vs. RIA(–––).

DISCUSSION

Shader and Greenblatt (11) have presented guidelines for the appropriate use of plasma level monitoring of psychotropic drugs, which should aid in cost containment and reduce misuse of therapeutic drug monitoring in psychiatry. Among the basic requirements for such an approach to be clinically useful, these authors stressed the need for a "valid, reproducible method of analysis" and "prompt turn-around times" so that results can be used in clinical decision making.

Flupentixol has a narrow therapeutic range. It has a large interindividual variation in the steady-state plasma concentrations among patients receiving the same dose of the drug. Extrapyramidal side effects have been associated with high doses of the drug (6). The higher incidence of side effects was usually not associated with a significant improvement of the clinical status. Accordingly, flupentixol may be considered a good candidate for therapeutic drug monitoring (11–13).

A sensitive RIA has been developed for flupentixol. It is relatively specific for *cis*(Z)-flupentixol, since the trans isomer cross-reacts about 5–7%, according to IRE data and our results. It has been shown that neuroleptics, which have the same ring structure (thioxanthenes) or the same side chain as *cis*(Z)-flupentixol, cross-react to such a degree that flupentixol levels cannot be accurately measured if these drugs are given simultaneously. By contrast, the cross-reactivity caused by two flupentixol metabolites, *N*-dealkyl-flupentixol and flupentixol sulphoxide, is low and of little practical importance, according to IRE data. These two metabolites lack neuroleptic activity (4).

The within-assay precision of the RIA procedure is good, but when samples of pooled patients' sera were analyzed on different days, it appeared that between-assay standard deviation approached 20%, according to IRE data. Thus the manufacturer advises that samples must be run from the same series within the same assay. In addition, it must be stressed that if single samples are measured, the RIA procedure will be expensive.

It was of interest to see if an alternative analytical method would be suitable. When spiked plasma was measured (Fig. 2), the RIA and the GC methods gave essentially the same results, showing that they measure *cis*(Z)-flupentixol with good accuracy. This was, however, not the case with patients' plasma (Figs. 3 and 4). The presence in plasma of the trans(E) isomer after administration can be clearly seen from the fact that the "averaged" slope is 0.7, whereas it is 1.2 after the intramuscular administration of pure *cis*(Z)-flupentixol. The deviation from the theoretical slopes, 0.5 and 1, respectively, shows that the RIA method tends to overestimate the drug concentration, as compared with the GC method. The reasons for this discrepancy are unclear; but they could be caused by the presence in plasma of metabolites of flupentixol, which would cross-react with the antibody. On the other hand, it is also possible that *cis*(Z)- and *trans*(E)-flupentixol are not metabolized at the same rate, although it has been shown that the cis(Z)-/trans(E) isomer ratio does not differ appreciably from 1 (3–5). From these considerations, it appears that if the determination of flupentixol plasma concentrations were found to be a useful tool for better management of patients treated with Fluanxol, then the GC method presented herein would be a valid alternative, as compared with the RIA method, with regard to both turn-around time and financial considerations. The validity of this GC method has, however, not been tested in the context of pharmacokinetic studies, where these considerations play a minor role.

To optimize both the turn-around time and the cost of the assay, we have decided to introduce our GC method for the routine therapeutic monitoring of flupentixol in our inpatient and outpatient clinics. The GC method also offers the possibility of monitoring flupentixol in the exceptional cases in which patients must be treated with another neuroleptic that would interfere with the RIA.

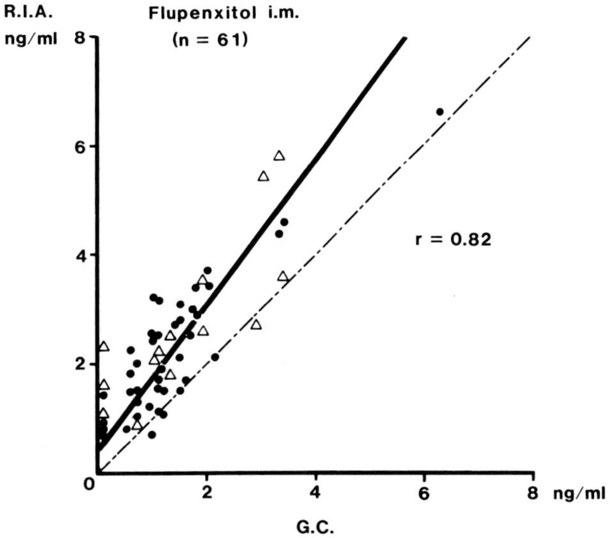

FIG. 3. Relationship between the results obtained with plasma from patients having received Fluanxol Depot: theoretical regression line with a slope of 1 (–·–·); "averaged" regression line (—). Patients who received only Fluanxol Depot (●) cannot be distinguished from patients who received another sedative neuroleptic (thioridazine or levomepromazine) (△).

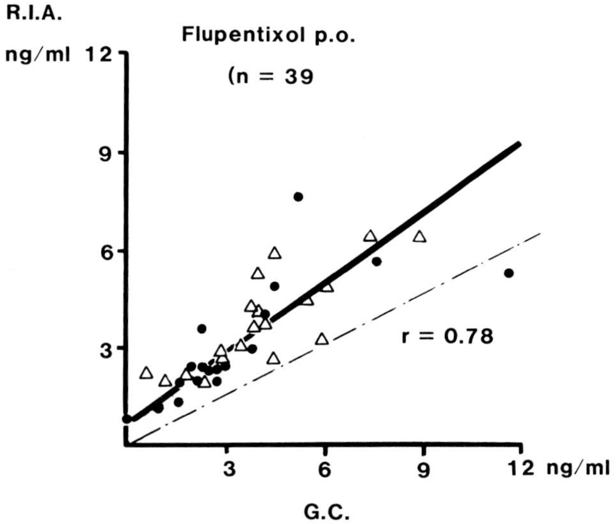

FIG. 4. Relationship between the results obtained with plasma from patients having received Fluanxol orally: theoretical regression line with a slope of 0.5 (–·–·); "averaged" regression line (—). Patients who received only Fluanxol orally (●) cannot be distinguished from patients who received another sedative neuroleptic (thioridazine or levomepromazine) (△).

TABLE 3. *Mean* cis*(Z)-flupentixol concentrations*

	No. of patients	Range (ng/ml)	Mean flupentixol level (ng/ml)	CV (%)
Oral dosage				
4	3	0.75–1.95	1.28	0.61
6	9	trace–2.75	1.57	0.88
8	11	0.80–3.70	1.96	0.75
10	11	0.30–5.85	2.19	1.72
12	5	1.00–3.80	1.90	1.12
Depot dosage				
0.71	10	trace–1.50	0.80	0.47
0.95	4	trace–1.90	1.02	0.73
1.33	3		trace	—
1.33	35	0.30–3.40	1.33	0.71
1.90	1		3.10	—
2.00	2	1.60–3.30	2.45	1.20
2.66	6	0.70–6.30	2.66	2.11

Trace indicates samples in which flupentixol could be detected but not quantified. For the calculation of the mean, an arbitrary value of 0.1 ng/ml was selected.

When flupentixol is given as Fluanxol Depot, the plasma concentrations are interpreted as such; whereas after oral administration, the measured values are divided by 2 to take into account the presence of inactive *trans*(E)-flupentixol. Although, from a clinical point of view, the presence of the trans(E) isomer does not seem to be important, it would certainly simplify flupentixol concentration measurements if the oral formulation contained only the active form of the drug.

Table 3 gives the mean *cis*(Z)-flupentixol concentrations measured over a period of 12 months. A preliminary analysis of these data, in view of the clinical files of the patients, indicates that drug concentrations below 1.5–2.0 ng/ml tend to be associated with a poor clinical response; whereas above a concentration of 4.5–5.0 ng/ml, the occurrence of adverse side effects tends to increase. However, it is premature to draw definitive conclusions from these data, as far as the final optimal concentration range of flupentixol is concerned. Indeed, among the many problems that must still be solved from a clinical point of view is whether it is imperative to determine if higher plasma concentrations of flupentixol are needed during the acute episodes of the disease than during the phases in which the patients are relatively stabilized.

In conclusion, the GC determination of flupentixol presented here offers clear advantages over the available RIA method and should thus be an acceptable alternative for routine plasma level monitoring of this neuroleptic when clinically desired.

Acknowledgment: The present study was performed through benefit of the budget of the Department of Psychiatry of the University of Geneva.

REFERENCES

1. Gottfries CG. Flupentixol and trifluoperazine: a double-blind investigation in the treatment of schizophrenia. *Br J Psychiatry* 1971;119:547–8.
2. Hall P, Coleman J. Flupentixol in the treatment of schizophrenia. *Br J Psychiatry* 1972;120:241–4.
3. Muusze RG, Visser-Van der Weel AJ, Verzijden R, Oei TT. Fluorimetrische bepaling os de dunne laag van de blodkoncentratie van thioxanthenen (Sordinol® en Fluanxol®) na orale en intramusculaire (depot) toediening. *Bulletin van de coördinatiecommissie biochemisch onderzoek van de sectie psychiatrische instituten van de nationale ziekenhuisraad* 1977;10:1–8.
4. Jorgensen A. Pharmacokinetic studies in volunteers of intravenous and oral cis(Z)-flupentixol and intramuscular cis(Z)-flupentixol decanoate in Viscoleo®. *Eur J Clin Pharmacol* 1980;18:355–60.
5. Jorgensen A, Andersen J, Bjorndal N, Dencker SJ, Lundin L, Malm U. Serum concentrations of cis(Z)-flupentixol and prolactin in chronic schizophrenic patients treated with flupentixol and cis(Z)-flupentixol decanoate. *Psychopharmacology* 1982;77:58–65.
6. McCreadie RG, Flanagan WL, McKnight J, Jorgensen A. High dose flupentixol decanoate in chronic schizophrenia. *Br J Psychiatry* 1979;135:175–9.
7. Jorgensen A. A sensitive and specific radioimmunoassay for cis(Z)-flupentixol in human serum. *Life Sci* 1978;23:1533–42.
8. Javaid JI, Dekirmejian H, Liskevych U, Lin RL, Davis JM. Fluphenazine determination in human plasma by a sensitive gas chromatographic method using nitrogen detector. *J Chromatogr Science* 1981;19:439–43.
9. Overall JE, Gorhaus DR. The brief psychiatric rating scale. *Psychol Rep* 1962;10:799–812.
10. Balant-Gorgia AE, Eisele R, Balant L, Garrone G. Plasma haloperidol levels and therapeutic response in acute mania and schizophrenia. *Eur Arch Psychiat Neurol Sci* 1984;234:1–4.
11. Shader RI, Greenblatt DJ. Clinical indication for plasma level monitoring of psychotropic drugs. *Am J Psychiatry* 1979;136:1590–1.
12. Sjöqvist F. Therapeutic drug monitoring—twenty years experience. In: Lemberger L, Reidenberg MM, eds. *Proceedings of the Second World Conference on Clinical Pharmacology and Therapeutics 1983, July 31–August 5, Washington DC.* Bethesda, Maryland: American Society for Pharmacology and Experimental Therapeutics, 1984:38–63.
13. Morselli PL. Clinical significance of neuroleptic plasma level monitoring. In: Usdin E, Dahl SG, Gram LF, Lingjaerde O, eds. *Clinical pharmacology in psychiatry.* London: Macmillan, 1981:199–209.

Therapeutic Drug Monitoring
7:236–238 © 1985 Raven Press, New York

Evaluation of Valproic Acid Fluoroimmunoassay and Comparison with a Gas Liquid Chromatographic Method

Sandra Tosoni, Costantino Signorini, and Alberto Albertini

Institute of Chemistry, Medical School, University of Brescia, Brescia, Italy

Summary: A method for monitoring valproic acid in serum with a fluoroimmunoassay is described. The evaluation was performed with run-to-run and within-run reproducibility, dilution, and recovery tests. The interferences of hemoglobin, bilirubin, and triglycerides were checked, and a comparison with a gas liquid chromatographic method was also performed. The between-run and within-run coefficients of variation were <5.2 and 2.6%, respectively. The method gave satisfactory results in dilution tests and a high correlation with a gas liquid chromatographic method (r = 0.98). The percentage of recovery was >97%. No interference from hemolysis, bilirubin, or triglycerides was observed. The accuracy and simplicity of this method make it suitable for routine laboratory use. **Key Words:** Fluoroimmunoassay—Valproic acid—Gas liquid chromatography.

Many methods have been developed for measuring valproic acid (VPA) in biological fluids of patients. The major assay procedures are high pressure liquid chromatography (HPLC) (1), gas liquid chromatography (GLC) (2–4), enzymoimmunoassay (EIA) (5), and the recent fluoroimmunoassay (FIA) (6). We have evaluated a commercial FIA kit (6) for determination of serum VPA concentrations. We studied within-run and between-run reproducibility and linearity of results for several dilutions of serum samples. We also performed a recovery test and checked interferences of normal serum constituents such as hemoglobin, bilirubin, and triglycerides. To validate the FIA procedure, we compared the values so obtained with those obtained with the GLC method.

MATERIALS AND METHODS

FIA Procedure

For the analysis we used a diluter and a dedicated filter fluorimeter (Fluorostat) equipped with a microprocessor (all from Ames Division, Miles Inc., Elkhart, IN, U.S.A.). Reagents were obtained from Ames Division (Miles Inc.) and used according to the manufacturer's instructions.

Address correspondence and reprint requests to Dr. S. Tosoni at Institute of Chemistry, Medical School, University of Brescia, 25100 Brescia, Italy.

GLC Method

The GLC was performed with a model F30 gas chromatograph equipped with flame ionization detector and a model 56 chart record (all from Perkin-Elmer Corp., Norwalk, CT, U.S.A.). The GLC determination did not require the derivatization of serum extract described previously (4).

Precision

Within-run precision was assessed by 10 replicates of each of three patient samples at low, medium, and high drug concentrations compared with the therapeutic level. The precision was expressed as coefficient of variation (%). Between run precision was determined by 12 replicates of each of the same patient samples, and it was also expressed as CV.

Accuracy

The accuracy of the method was checked by dilution and recovery experiments and by comparison with GLC assay. The dilution test was performed in

TABLE 1. *Fluoroimmunoassay summary of precision studies*

	Within-run				Between-run			
	Mean (mg/L)	SD (mg/L)	CV (%)	n	Mean (mg/L)	SD (mg/L)	CV (%)	n
Sample 1	27.9	0.74	2.6	10	28.7	1.50	5.2	12
Sample 2	55.1	1.09	1.9	10	57.7	2.30	3.9	12
Sample 3	132.6	1.08	1.5	10	130.4	4.17	3.2	12

TABLE 2. *Fluoroimmunosassay recovery of valproic acid added to buffer solution and to drug-free serum*

	Expected mean (mg/L)	Actual mean (mg/L)	n	Recovery (%)
Buffer	125	123.5	3	98
	100	96.0	3	96
	75	76.0	3	101
	50	49.2	3	98
	25	24.0	3	96
Serum	125	118.3	3	95
	100	97.2	3	97
	75	75.4	3	100
	50	48.4	3	97
	25	24.0	3	96

Mean recovery of valproic acid in buffer was 97.8%, and in serum 97.0%.

the following way: a high drug concentration serum was diluted several times with working buffer solution. The samples obtained were then analyzed three times in different runs, and the measured values were compared with the dilution factors. After adding 25–125 mg/L of authentic VPA (Sigma-Tau, Rome, Italy) to working buffer solution, we determine the amount of the drug three times and we calculated the percentage of recovery. Similarly, we added 25–125 mg/L of VPA to drug-free serum, we analyzed the obtained samples three times and computed the recovery rate. We also compared the mean recoveries of VPA in buffer solution with those in drug-free serum. The comparison between FIA and GLC procedures was performed by determining the VPA amounts in 105 patients' sera. Linear regression and Student's t test were used to examine the results.

Interferences

We added 100 mg/L of VPA to hemolytic samples containing as much as 5 g hemoglobin/L, to lipemic samples with high concentrations of triglycerides (as much as 3,000 g/L) and to patients' sera with hemolytic icterus (total bilirubin as much as 300 mg/L). We calculated the mean recovery rates for each interfering substance.

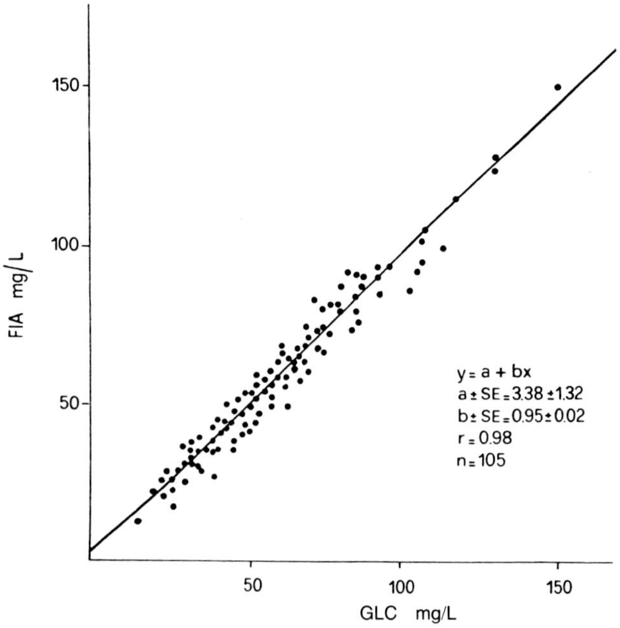

FIG. 1. Correlation between fluoroimmunoassay (FIA) *(y)* and gas liquid chromatography (GLC) *(x)* determinations in clinical serum samples. SE, standard error.

RESULTS AND DISCUSSION

The reproducibility of the FIA procedure is undoubtedly acceptable for clinical purposes. Within-run and run-to-run CVs were less than 3 and 6%, respectively (Table 1). The highest CV value (5.2%) was obtained in run-to-run experiments analyzing the low concentration in serum (mean 28.69 mg/L).

In the dilution test, the straight line obtained plotting measured concentrations *(y)* versus dilution factors *(x)* gave a slope of 156.44 mg/L, an intercept of 1.52 mg/L, and a correlation coefficient of 0.99. The dilution test indicates a good linearity over a wide range of concentrations that is from 156.44 to <40 mg/L, considerably below the therapeutic concentration interval (50–100 mg/L). Therefore, sera containing VPA amounts >150 mg/L can be diluted before the analysis.

The recovery test results gave a mean of 97.8% in the experiments performed in buffer solution and a mean of 97.0% in the presence of drug-free serum (Table 2). No significant difference was observed between results by the recovery test performed in buffer solution and those performed in serum, according to the Student's paired *t* test. Altogether the recovery studies gave satisfactory results within the range of the analytical variability.

The comparison with GLC results for 105 patients' sera shows a satisfactory correlation ($r = 0.98$, $p < 0.001$) (Fig. 1). The mean for the FIA procedure was 59.47 mg/L, and for GLC, 59.21 mg/L; the standard error of regression was 5.52. The statistical analysis by use of Student's *t* test on the slope of regression line gives a significant difference from unity. This could mean that with FIA lower values are measured than with GLC. On the other hand, this fact is also underscored by the recovery experiments in which we had a recovery rate of 97%. This could be due to a difference between the standards used for FIA and GLC procedures (we used the same authentic VPA to calibrate the GLC and to perform the recovery test). However, this disagreement is not important for clinical purposes.

No remarkable loss of VPA was observed in the interference studies, and the recovery rates were always >97% (i.e., 101% for hemolytic samples, 99.3% for lipemic samples, and 98.1% for bilirubinemic samples). Thus, with this procedure it is possible to analyze hemolytic, icteric, and lipemic samples.

There are several characteristics that make FIA attractive compared with GLC. There is no preliminary dilution or reconstitution of reagents, except for the buffer. The sample volume of 50 μl is small (this is important for pediatric patients) and does not require any pretreatment, such as extraction, or posttreatment, such as derivatization. Moreover, the time required to analyze five calibrators and 34 samples is about 1 h, from dispensing the reagents to recording the data. With GLC more time is employed for serum preparation and for analysis because the retention time of VPA is about 6 min (4). Also, the instrument requires a technician's attention and a long conditioning time.

REFERENCES

1. Farinotti R, Mahuzier G. Simultaneous determination of six anticonvulsants in serum by high-performance liquid chromatography. *J Liq Chromatogr* 1979;2:345–64.
2. Morita Y, Tsuen IR, Min LL, Atkinson AJ Jr. On a column propylation method for measuring plasma valproate concentrations by gas-chromatography. *Ther Drug Monit* 1981;3:193–9.
3. Gupta RN, Eng F, Gupta ML. Gas-chromatographic analysis for valproic acid as phenacyl esters. *Clin Chem* 1979;25:1303–5.
4. Tosoni S, Signorini C, Albtertini A. Gas-chromatographic determination of valproic acid in serum without derivatization. *Clin Chem* 1983;29:990.
5. Braun SL, Tausch A, Vogt W, Jacob K, Knedel M. Evaluation of a new valproic acid enzyme immunoassay and comparison with a capillary gas-chromatographic method. *Clin Chem* 1981;27:169–72.
6. Feinstein H, Hovav H, Fridlender B, Inbar D, Buckler RT. Substrate-labeled fluorescent immunoassay (SLFIA) for valproic acid. *Clin Chem* 1982;28:1665.

Therapeutic Drug Monitoring
7:239–241 © 1985 Raven Press, New York

Case Report

Desmethylimipramine Overdose: Nonlinear Kinetics in a Slow Hydroxylator

Edoardo Spina, Thomas K. Henthorn, *Lennart Eleborg, †Conny Nordin, and Juliette Säwe

*Departments of Clinical Pharmacology, *Anesthesiology, and †Psychiatry, Huddinge University Hospital, Huddinge, Sweden*

Summary: A case of desmethylimipramine (DMI) overdose is described. The analysis of DMI and its main metabolite, 2-hydroxydesmethylimipramine (2-OH-DMI), in plasma was performed by high performance liquid chromatography with fluorescence detection. Characterization of the elimination kinetics of DMI by using the SAAM 25 computer program indicated Michaelis-Menten kinetics. The patient was phenotyped with respect to debrisoquine hydroxylation and classified as a slow hydroxylator. Both nonlinear kinetics and slow hydroxylation might have contributed to the marked difference between the concentration of DMI and 2-OH-DMI in plasma in this patient. **Key Words:** Desmethylimipramine—Michaelis-Menten kinetics—Debrisoquine—Slow hydroxylation.

Tricyclic antidepressant (TCA) overdose is common and can be associated with severe, life-threatening symptoms. The major adverse reactions, including intraventricular conduction delays, respiratory depression, and seizures, are seen when TCA plasma levels exceed 1 μg/ml (~3,500 nmol/L) (1). Prolongation of the elimination half-life of the drug has been observed in cases of TCA overdose (2,3), but insufficiency of plasma data has prevented elucidation of the specific pharmacokinetic perturbations accounting for this observation. The following case report describes a patient who ingested a toxic quantity of desmethylimipramine (DMI). In this case, evaluation of plasma levels of the parent drug and its metabolite allowed a more complete kinetic analysis. Interestingly, the patient turned out to belong to the rare phenotype that hydroxylates certain drugs slowly.

CASE REPORT, PLASMA DETERMINATION, AND PHARMACOKINETIC ANALYSIS

A 44-year-old depressed woman was found unconscious in her home with several bottles of different psychoactive drugs nearby. Clinical examination, ~8 h after ingestion, revealed deep coma, no pain reactions, miosis, and weak pulse. The electrocardiogram showed aberrant and widened QRS complexes. Tracheal intubation, mechanical ventilation, and gastric lavage were immediately instituted. Activated charcoal was given. Sodium bicarbonate and dobutamine were administered, and diazepam was given to treat grand mal seizures. Over the subsequent 4 h after admission, the patient's hemodynamic status did not markedly improve, and hyperosmolar sodium bicarbonate treatment was then begun. Over the ensuing hour, the blood pressure, heart rate, and QRS configuration normalized. Seven hours after admission, 3 h of hemoperfusion over a carbon cartridge was performed. Approximately 18 h after drug intake, the patient was responsive but remained heavily sedated. Over the next 48 h, blood pressure and pulse rate were stable, but the patient was still sedated, and occasional seizures occurred. On the third day after admission, ventilatory support was discontinued, and the patient was extubated. On the fourth day, she was awake and alert, and no cardiac arrhythmias were noted. Treatment with oral thioridazine (50 mg/day) was started on the fifth day, at which time the patient

Address correspondence and reprint requests to Dr. J. Säwe at Department of Clinical Pharmacology, Huddinge University Hospital, S-141 86 Huddinge, Sweden.

was transferred to the psychiatric ward, where she was ambulatory but complained of tiredness.

Toxicologic screening for TCAs in the blood revealed high concentrations of DMI. A modification of the high performance liquid chromatography method of Sutfin and Jusko (4) was used to measure DMI and its main metabolite, 2-hydroxydesmethylimipramine (2-OH-DMI). The coefficient of variation was 1.8% for DMI and 5.3% for 2-OH-DMI. The lower limit of detection was about 40 nmol/L for DMI and about 60 nmol/L for 2-OH-DMI. The plasma concentrations of DMI and 2-OH-DMI during the 15 days following admission are shown in Fig. 1.

The postabsorption (from the fifth day onward) DMI plasma concentrations were fit to a one-compartment open model assuming a volume of distribution of 34 L/Kg (5) and parallel first-order and capacity-limited (Michaelis-Menten) elimination processes, as described by the following equation:

$$-dC_p/dt = K_e \cdot C_p + (V_m \cdot C_p/K_m + C_p)$$

where dC_p/dt is the rate of decline of the plasma concentration (C_p) at time t, K_e is the first-order elimination rate constant, V_m (nmol/h) is the theoretical maximum rate of drug elimination, and K_m (nmol/L) is the Michaelis constant (the plasma concentration at which the rate of elimination is half the theoretical maximum). Initial estimates of the parameters of this model were determined by graphic analysis (6). Least-squares best-fit estimates were calculated by the SAAM 25 computer program (7).

The nonlinear pharmacokinetic behavior of DMI is illustrated in Fig. 1. A significantly ($p < 0.01$) better fit was obtained with the Michaelis-Menten model as compared with a first-order model using the general linear test (8). The estimates for the elimination kinetic parameters were 32,655 nmol/h for V_m, 350 nmol/L for K_m, and a K_e of 0.00171 h-1.

Three months after the overdose intake, the patient was phenotyped with respect to debrisoquine hydroxylation according to Mahgoub et al. (9). She was given a single 10 mg oral dose of debrisoquine (D) and the ratio of D to its main metabolite, 4-hydroxydebrisoquine (4-OH-D), was determined by measuring D and 4-OH-D in urine collected during the 6 h after dose intake. A ratio below 12.6 is indicative of rapid hydroxylation, while a ratio above 12.6 is indicative of slow hydroxylation (10). Our patient was classified as a slow hydroxylator (D/4-OH-D ratio = 15).

DISCUSSION

The salient findings of the present report were the nonlinear decline in plasma concentration and the wide differences between DMI and 2-OH-DMI plasma concentrations.

The nonlinear pharmacokinetic solution indicates that, in overdose, plasma concentrations will initially decrease at a much slower rate (about 100 h for plasma concentrations to decrease by 50%) than is usually encountered following therapeutic doses, where a $t_{1/2}$ of 18 h has been reported (5). Gram and Kragh-Sørensen (11) found evidence for a dose-dependent effect on the disposition of DMI in elderly patients receiving increasing doses of its parent drug, imipramine, but another study shows conflict on this issue (12). A prolonged half-life following overdose has been previously reported (3), but plasma concentra-

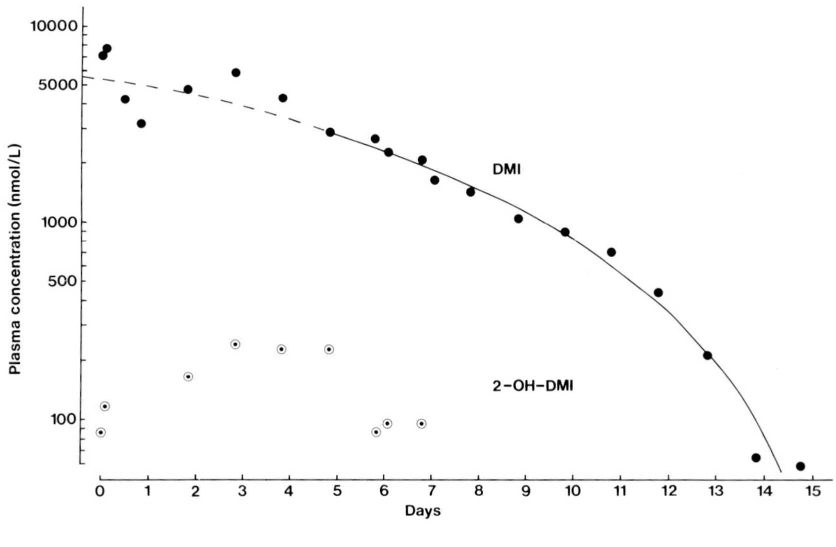

FIG. 1 Plasma concentrations of desmethylimipramine (DMI) (●) and 2-hydroxydesmethylimipramine (2-OH-DMI) (⊙) in the patient. The first sample was obtained approximately 8 h after intake of the overdose and is referred to as 0 on the x-axis. The analytical method did not permit measurement of 2-OH-DMI after 7 days. The solid line represents the computer-fitted least-squares solution, and the dashed line is extrapolated from the equation of that solution, as the data points prior to day 5 were not used in the fit.

tion data were insufficient to demonstrate nonlinear kinetics. Our analysis indicates that with DMI overdose, one should anticipate a markedly prolonged elimination half-life as the drug metabolizing processes are saturated. This nonlinearity could also result from prolonged gastrointestinal absorption, possibly enhanced by anticholinergic effects of TCAs themselves, or metabolic inhibition by other drugs.

In 47 patients receiving chronic treatment with DMI, Bock et al. (13) found that the average plasma concentration ratio of unconjugated 2-OH-DMI to DMI was about 0.5. In our patient, this ratio never exceeded 0.08. The wide differences we observed between the parent drug and the metabolite concentrations could be explained if the metabolism of DMI were saturated and/or if our patient had a decreased ability to hydroxylate DMI. Environmental and nutritional factors, concomitant diseases, and coadministration of other drugs are important determinants of drug-metabolizing ability. Concurrent treatment with neuroleptics (13), for instance, inhibits the metabolism of DMI. However, recent findings indicate that deficient hydroxylation of certain drugs, of which debrisoquine (9) and sparteine (14) are the prototypes, is mainly genetically determined. Recent studies in vivo and in vitro have indicated that the rates of hydroxylation of the monomethylated TCA nortriptyline and DMI are dependent on the individual's hydroxylation phenotype, as determined with these prototype drugs (15,16). Our patient was phenotyped with debrisoquine and found to be a slow hydroxylator. Both nonlinear kinetics and slow hydroxylation may have contributed to the marked difference between the concentration of drug and its metabolite in plasma. Enzymatic saturation may occur already at low DMI concentrations in slow hydroxylators. Our estimate of Km being 350 nmol/L indicates that elimination kinetics in a slow hydroxylator may appear to be nonlinear within the plasma concentration range (200–500 nmol/L) usually encountered in the treatment of depressed patients. As a pharmacokinetic analysis has not been performed in an overdose of a rapid hydroxylator, it remains uncertain whether K_m, V_m, or both are changed in slow hydroxylators.

Our case appears to be the first documentation of drug intoxication in a slow hydroxylator, the phenotype at risk to develop adverse reactions already at therapeutic doses. It is tempting to suggest that such individuals are more likely to succumb from TCA overdoses than rapid hydroxylators.

Acknowledgment: This study was supported by grants from the Swedish Medical Research Council (04X-03902). Dr. E. Spina was recipient of a fellowship awarded by Fidia Research Laboratories, Abano Terme, Italy.

REFERENCES

1. Spiker DG, Weiss AN, Chang SS, Ruwitch JF, Biggs JT. Tricyclic antidepressant overdose: clinical presentation and plasma levels. *Clin Pharmacol Ther* 1976;19:725–31.
2. Pedersen OL, Gram LF, Kristensen CB, et al. Overdosage of antidepressants: clinical and pharmacokinetic aspects. *Eur J Clin Pharmacol* 1982;23:513–21.
3. Sawyer WT, Caudill JL, Ellison MJ. A case of severe acute desipramine overdose. *Am J Psychiatry* 1984;141:122–3.
4. Sutfin TA, Jusko WJ. High performance liquid chromatographic assay for imipramine, desipramine and their 2-hydroxylated metabolites. *J Pharm Sci* 1979;68:703–5.
5. Alexanderson B. Pharmacokinetics of desmethylimipramine and nortriptyline in man after single and multiple oral doses. *Eur J Clin Pharmacol* 1972;5:1–10.
6. van Ginneken CAM, Rossum JM, Fleuren HLM. Linear and nonlinear kinetics of drug elimination. I. Kinetics on the basis of a single capacity-limited pathway of elimination with or without simultaneous supply-limited elimination. *J Pharmacokin Biopharm* 1974;2:395–415.
7. Berman M, Weiss MF. *SAAM 25 manual.* Washington, DC: United States Government Printing Office, 1974, publication no. (PHS) 1703.
8. Boxenbaum HG, Riegelman S, Elashoff RM. Statistical estimations in pharmacokinetics. *J Pharmacokin Biopharm* 1974;2:133–48.
9. Mahgoub A, Idle JR, Dring LG, Lancaster R, Smith RL. Polymorphic hydroxylation of debrisoquine in man. *Lancet* 1977;2:584–6.
10. Price Evans DA, Mahgoub A, Sloan TP, Idle JR, Smith RL. A family and population study of the genetic polimorphism of debrisoquine oxidation in a white British population. *J Med Genet* 1983;17:102–5.
11. Gram LF, Kragh-Sørensen P. Pharmacokinetics and plasma level/effect relationships of tricyclic antidepressants—an update. In: Usdin E, Dahl E, Gram LF, Lingjaerde O, eds. *Clinical pharmacology in psychiatry: neuroleptic and antidepressant research.* London: MacMillan, 1981:241–52.
12. Potter WZ, Zavadil AP, Kopin IJ, Goodwin FK. Single-dose kinetics predict steady-state concentrations of imipramine and desipramine. *Arch Gen Psychiatry* 1980;37:314–20.
13. Bock JL, Craig Nelson J, Gray S, Jatlow PI. Desipramine hydroxylation: variability and effect of antipsychotic drugs. *Clin Pharmacol Ther* 1983;33:322–8.
14. Eichelbaum M, Spannbrucker N, Steinke B, Dengler HS. Defective N-oxidation of sparteine in man: a new pharmacogenetic defect. *Eur J Clin Pharmacol* 1979;16:183–7.
15. Mellström B, Bertilsson L, Säwe J, Schulz H-U, Sjöqvist F. E- and Z-hydroxylation of nortriptyline: relationship to polymorphic debrisoquine hydroxylation. *Clin Pharmacol Ther* 1981;30:189–93.
16. Spina E, Birgersson C, von Bahr C, et al. Phenotypic consistency in the hydroxylation of desmethylimipramine and debrisoquine in healthy volunteers and in human liver microsomes. *Clin Pharmacol Ther* 1984;36:677–682.

Therapeutic Drug Monitoring
7:242–243

Short Communication

Analysis of Tricyclic Antidepressants in Serum and Plasma Yields Similar Results

E. Spina, Ö. Ericsson, and *C. Nordin

*Departments of Clinical Pharmacology and *Psychiatry, Huddinge University Hospital, Huddinge, Sweden*

Determination of some drugs in serum and plasma gives different results. As an example, chloroquine concentrations in serum are about twice as high as those in plasma (1). Disopyramide and quinidine are also present in higher concentrations in serum than in plasma (2). On the other hand, serum and plasma yield identical results for phenytoin, carbamazepine, and valproic acid (3). It is not always possible for a drug monitoring laboratory to have full control over the sampling procedure. Even though plasma is recommended for the analysis of a particular drug, serum may sometimes be obtained. It is therefore essential to know the influence of the sampling procedure on the result of analysis.

Most data concerning kinetics and concentration-effect relationships for tricyclic antidepressants are based on measurements of drug concentrations in plasma (4). Plasma has been commonly used for therapeutic monitoring of these drugs; nevertheless, laboratories frequently receive serum samples from psychiatric clinics. To our knowledge it has not been demonstrated that plasma and serum concentrations of the antidepressant drugs differ. We have therefore analyzed both serum and plasma samples from patients treated with amitriptyline or chlorimipramine, two widely prescribed tricyclic antidepressants.

The samples were obtained from patients treated with amitriptyline (Tryptizol) or chlorimipramine (Anafranil) at the psychiatric clinic at Huddinge Hospital. Serum and plasma samples were drawn simultaneously from the same patient. Serum samples were drawn in plain Vacutainer tubes and plasma samples in heparinized Venoject tubes. The samples were kept at room temperature for 30 min and then centrifuged for 10 min at 700 *g*. Ten serum and plasma samples were collected for each drug. The concentrations of the parent drugs and their demethylated metabolites nortriptyline and desmethylchlorimipramine were determined using the high performance liquid chromatography method by Mellström and Braithwaite (5). This method is routinely used for the analysis of patient samples at Huddinge Hospital.

TABLE 1. *Plasma and serum concentrations of tricyclic antidepressants*

	Plasma (nmol/L)	Serum (nmol/L)
Amitriptyline	211 ± 114	201 ± 124
Nortriptyline	183 ± 57	169 ± 54
Chlorimipramine	197 ± 78	190 ± 65
Desmethylchlorimipramine	357 ± 230	324 ± 204

Mean ± SD; n = 10. No significant difference was found between plasma and serum concentrations (paired *t* test).

The results of the analysis of antidepressants in serum and plasma were compared using a *t* test for paired values (Table 1).

There is a tendency toward higher concentrations in plasma than in serum, but the difference is not statistically significant. It should be recalled that for chloroquine, quinidine, and disopyramide, the concentrations are higher in serum than in plasma. This is believed to be due to release of the drug from platelets during the clotting process (1). The slightly higher concentration of the tricyclic antidepressants in plasma may depend on the higher protein content in plasma compared with serum.

This study was performed using amitriptyline and chlorimipramine and their demethylated metabolites. However, all the tricyclic antidepressants have similar physicochemical properties and can be expected to

Address correspondence and reprint requests to Dr. Ö. Ericsson at Department of Clinical Pharmacology, Huddinge University Hospital, S-141 86 Huddinge, Sweden.

behave in a similar way. We conclude that both serum and plasma can be used for therapeutic drug monitoring of tricyclic antidepressant drugs.

Acknowledgment: This study was supported by a grant from the Swedish Medical Research Council (04X-03902).

REFERENCES

1. Bergqvist Y, Domeij-Nyberg B. Distribution of chloroquine and its metabolite desethylchloroquine in human blood cells and its implication for the quantitative determination of these compounds in serum and plasma. *J Chromatogr* 1983;271:137–48.
2. Bergqvist Y, Eckerbom S, Funding L. Ger analys i serum och plasma samma läkemedelskoncentrationer? *Farmaceutisk Årskongress.* Stockholm Apotekarsocieteten, 1982.
3. Godolphin W, Trepanier J, Farrel K. Serum and plasma for total and free anticonvulsant drug analyses: effects on EMIT assays and ultrafiltration devices. *Ther Drug Monit* 1983;3:319–23.
4. Sjöqvist F, Bertilsson L, Åsberg M. Monitoring tricyclic antidepressants. *Ther Drug Monit* 1980;2:85–93.
5. Mellström B, Braithwaite R. Ion-pair liquid chromatography of amitryptyline and metabolites in plasma. *J Chromatogr* 1978;157:379–85.

Therapeutic Drug Monitoring
7:244–246 © 1985 Raven Press, New York

Book Reviews

Free Radicals in Molecular Biology, Aging, and Disease. (Vol. 27) *Armstrong, D., Sohal, R. S., Cuter, R. G., Slater, T. F. (eds.).* Raven Press, New York, 1984. 432 pp., $69.50.

This book is Volume 27 in a series on aging and is designed to summarize current information in regard to the molecular biology of free radicals and their possible relationship to aging and disease. The volume, which is a collection of symposium papers, is not immediately relevant to those engaged in therapeutic drug monitoring and clinical pharmacology. However, the volume may be of indirect interest because some drugs, especially at toxic levels, might cause tissue damage through free radical formation. If the theoretical relationship between aging and free radical formation and lipofuscin pigment is correct, then excessive or toxic amounts of clinical drugs could enhance the aging process. Correlations between the metabolic rate, rate of lipofuscin accumulation, cell loss, and life span have previously suggested that lipofuscin pigment of postmitotic cells may represent an important cellular marker for normal aging, as well as a variety of age-related diseases. In addition, considerable evidence has also recently been found that suggests a close, or at least a casual, link between age pigments and the free radicals that are generated as a result of sequential oxygen reduction during aerobic respiration. To date, evidence for oxygen free radical damage of cells in vivo is substantial but only offers indirect proof of a link between oxygen free radical damage of cells and aging. Recent evidence suggests that abnormal free radical activity with increasing age and in certain diseases may represent an important cause of cellular damage leading to the breakdown of cells. Age-related changes in molecular oxygen, trace metals, and antioxidant activity have also been studied in relation to the generation of free radicals, lipopigment accumulation, and cell death. Free radicals are thought to cause peroxidation of polyunsaturated lipids of membranes resulting in lipopigment accumulation, cell loss, and tissue breakdown. If this idea is correct, than age- and disease-related tissue and cell breakdown may represent a result of increasingly abnormal free radical activity. There is also the possibility that this cellular breakdown may trigger even greater free radical activity as well as tissue damage. Because of this possible age-related breakdown of cell structure and function, the topic of free radicals has become increasingly important in molecular biology and certainly relates to nutrition, pharmacology, and pathology, as well as clinical practice.

The main goal of this volume is to bring together both the background basic information as well as the most recent information on free radicals in aging and disease. The book contains 24 chapters including an introductory chapter by Dr. Dennis Harman, one of the important pioneers in this area of research. Dr. Harman describes free radicals and the origination, evolution, and present status of the free radical theory of aging. The next 23 chapters of the book are divided into four sections which include: free radicals; basic reactions; free radicals in aging; free radicals, effects of antioxidants; and free radicals in disease. Closing remarks are then made by Dr. Trevor F. Slater. The chapters specifically deal with the free radical theories of aging, basic chemistry of free radical reactions, effects on lipopigments, free radicals in age-related diseases and antioxidant defense mechanisms. The chapters in this book should help those who wish to plan and conduct research on the causes or mechanisms of aging, ranging from the molecular to levels of the entire organism. Due to the marked increase in the proportion of the elderly in our population, the search for causes of aging in the area of molecular biology should attract a greater number of investigations from many areas of research.

The volume does attain its stated goals and should be of special interest to students, physicians, biochemists, nutritionists, pharmacologists, and other scientists who are interested in relating the aging process to the molecular biology of free radicals. These studies might have useful applications in the area of nutritional and chemical intervention.

Raymond J. Shamberger

Benzodiazepine Recognition Site Ligands: Biochemistry and Pharmacology. *Biggio, G., and Costa, E. (eds.).* Raven Press, New York, 1983. 272 pp., $31.00.

In June, 1983, the Third Capo Boi Conference on Neuroscience was held in Villasimius, Italy. This volume of *Advances in Biochemical Psychopharmacology* represents the proceedings of that symposium, prepared and published within 6 months of the symposium's completion. As those who have attempted to elicit, edit, and publish symposia manuscripts will attest, such prompt publication can only be attained by the herculean efforts of contributors, editors, and publishers.

A total of 58 participants have contributed 22 manuscripts to this book, which is presented in photo-offset form. Nearly every major group involved in benzodiazepine receptor research is represented and most of the principal subject areas are covered and reviewed in some detail. These areas include: primary description and characterization of the receptors, evaluation of receptor subpopulations, coupling to chloride channels, relation to γ-aminobutyric acid neurotransmission, agonists and antagonists, the search for endogenous ligands, peripheral binding sites, and the relation of receptor binding to in vivo behavioral and pharmacologic effects. The most important, and as yet unanswered, question is posed by Dr. Costa in the final chapter, where he asks whether benzodiazepine receptors actually mediate anxiolytic or anxiogenic behavior via an endogenous ligand, or whether they are just drug receptor sites.

This book is primarily for basic and clinical scientists actively engaged in receptor research. It is not of direct value to persons involved in therapeutic drug monitoring. Because benzodiazepine receptor science is developing at a very rapid pace, this book will be rendered of mostly historical interest within a few years.

David J. Greenblatt

Compendium of Pharmaceuticals and Specialties, 19th Ed. Canadian Pharmaceutical Association, Ottawa, Ontario, Canada. U.S. distribution by Marcel Dekker, New York, 1984. 908 pp., $65.00.

The *Compendium of Pharmaceuticals and Specialties* (CPS) is a reference source containing up-to-date information on more than 3,000 drugs available in Canada. The information is presented in monograph format and is based primarily on information contained in the manufacturer's Official Product Monograph; many monographs contain additional clinical, pharmacological, and/or pharmacokinetic information from the published literature. The approach used to cumulate information for CPS monographs differs from that used in the publishing of the popular *Physicians Desk Reference* (PDR), in which only the drug monographs approved by the Food and Drug Administration (FDA) are used.

The well-organized layout of the book facilitates the task of information retrieval. The drug monographs are arranged in alphabetical order by both the trade and generic names of the drugs. The typical entry includes the trade name, manufacturer, generic name, and therapeutic category (i.e., sympathomimetic, antihistamine, corticosteroid) followed by a drug monograph format containing the following categories of information: pharmacology, indications, contraindications, warnings, precautions, adverse effects, overdose symptoms and treatment, drug dosage, and how the drug is supplied. The depth of information presented in each monograph is sufficient for the reader to learn the drug's medical indications, under what conditions the drug is contraindicated, and which adverse reactions to expect with the use of the drug. Additional basic and clinical pharmacology should be obtained from other reference sources, such as Goodman's and Gilman's *The Pharmacological Basis of Therapeutics* or Melmon's and Morelli's *Clinical Pharmacology*. The quality and quantity of pharmacokinetic and biopharmaceutic information contained in the drug monographs is very good, considering that the CPS is a general drug reference book. The information presented is clear, concise, and easy to locate because of the standardized format of each monograph.

The CPS also contains several helpful indexes. The blue section contains clinically relevant information such as alcohol content of pharmaceuticals, sodium content of drugs, and nomograms for body surface area. There is also a comprehensive set of charts comparing the contents of over 250 multiple vitamin preparations available in Canada. A therapeutic index contains drugs listed in a particular therapeutic class (i.e., β blockers, allergy therapy, analgesics). Manufacturers pay a fee to have their drugs listed in this section. A product recognition section contains full-color photographs of tablets and capsules of the more popular drug products in Canada and is intended to serve as a quick guide to drug identification. A manufacturers index contains a listing of the addresses and telephone numbers of manufacturers and distributors of Canadian pharmaceuticals along with a list of their products. Other indexes include a cross-reference index of brand and generic names for single entity drugs, and a directory of regional poison control centers in

Canada. The CPS is available in either French or English editions.

The CPS must be on the bookshelf of those engaged in therapeutic drug monitoring, clinical pharmacology, pharmacy, medicine, and nursing in Canada. For practitioners in the United States, the CPS would be a useful supplement to the PDR, since its monographs appear to contain more clinical pharmacology and pharmacokinetic information than is normally found in the official FDA-approved monograph.

Alan W. Bakst

Neurotransmitters, Seizures and Epilepsy II. *Fariello, R.M., Morselli, P.L., Lloyd, K.G., Quesney, L.F., Engel, J. Jr. (eds.).* Raven Press, New York, 1984. 371 pp., $57.50.

This book is a collection of manuscripts written by the participants in The Second Workshop on Neurotransmitters and Epilepsy, held in April, 1983. Following each article is a transcript of the comments made by the participants at the time the material was presented at the workshop. The book is a photo-offset of the typescript.

A major focus of this conference was the effect of manipulations of γ-aminobutyric acid mechanisms in various experimental models of epilepsy. Additional areas of interest pertain to catecholaminergic systems, excitatory amino acids, and opioids and other neuropeptides. The strength of the volume is its relative timeliness, quality and variety of presentations, juxtaposition of contradictory data from different researchers, and discussion by the conference participants regarding these discrepancies. The last of these, in particular, is helpful in defining the current state of knowledge, and of agreement, in the field. The verbatim proceedings of the discussion contain typographical errors, colloquialisms, and syntax errors. Certainly these could have been re-edited, but the reader has no trouble understanding what the participants were trying to say and such review would have only delayed final publication. However, I would have preferred that the references had included article titles.

For the readers of this journal, the conference could be characterized as one dealing with the monitoring of therapeutics and therapeutic efficacy as opposed to the study of therapeutic drug monitoring per se. However, the study of basic mechanisms today is directly relevant to the development of therapeutic drugs tomorrow. As such, this book will be of interest to everyone interested in the development of improved treatments for intractable epilepsy.

Ronald P. Lesser

Guide to Clinical Studies and Developing Protocols. *Spilker, B.* Raven Press, New York, 1984. 319 pp., $45.00.

The successful design and implementation of a clinical study require attention to a host of decisions ranging from ethical considerations to protocol adjustments when subjects are kept home by bad weather. It is remarkable to see the scope of the clinical study design produced in detail by Bert Spilker in *Guide to Clinical Studies and Developing Protocols.* Because the compact volume is intended for both new and experienced investigators as well as others involved in cinical investigations, a wide variety of issues are raised, defined, and explained in detail. In his preface, Spilker states that the book can be viewed as a "peripheral memory," thus saving investigators the need to newly develop or recall procedures for documentation, subject recruitment, drug monitoring, packaging and dispensing, and data collection.

Because of its nuts-and-bolts approach, which amplifies the understanding of the tasks of each participant, this book will be very helpful for all persons involved in a clinical study, regardless of their level of current expertise. Special attention is given to the challenges of multicenter trials, and the author suggests a number of ways to plan for uniformity of data collection, analysis, and information-sharing. The same detailed approach is used throughout whether psychometric testing, pharmacokinetics, laboratory examinations, or interacting with FDA and pharmaceutical auditors is being discussed.

The volume could be enhanced by consideration of the subject's and family's experiences from participating in a study and the support of a subject through a successful or unsuccessful trial. As a clinical trial nurse, I find that the information in this book closely parallels my own experiences. This book will serve as an excellent reference to all persons involved in clinical trials.

Diane Friedman

Therapeutic Drug Monitoring
7:247–254 © 1985 Raven Press, New York

Blood–Brain Barrier Transport of CI-912: Single-Passage Equilibration of Erythrocyte-Borne Drug

Eain M. Cornford and Kristin P. Landon

Southwest Regional Veterans Administration Epilepsy Center, Research and Neurology Services, Veterans Administration Wadsworth Medical Center, and Department of Neurology, Reed Neurological Research Center, University of California at Los Angeles, School of Medicine, Los Angeles, California, U.S.A.

Summary: Brain capillary transit of CI-912 was studied in vivo after a single capillary transit by the intracarotid injection technique. Brain permeability of ^{14}C-drug was measured relative to that of tritiated water, a highly diffusible reference substance. The brain uptake index of CI-912 was measured at concentrations ranging from 5 to 400 μg/ml in different regions of the rat brain. Brain uptake was not via a saturable, carrier-mediated mechanism, but was attributable to lipid-mediated transport. The octanol/saline partition coefficient determined in vitro was 3.9, and the blood–brain barrier permeability times surface area product was 0.26 ml min^{-1} g^{-1} (in vivo). In the rat brain, efflux of CI-912 after intracarotid injection was found to be minimal, suggesting that this drug is retained in brain tissues. This drug is weakly bound to plasma proteins (75–79% of the drug is freely dialyzable in 4% human serum albumin at 5 μg/ml), and protein binding does not affect brain uptake. In contrast, the drug is highly bound to erythrocytes. At concentrations that approximate the predicted optimum therapeutic range (6–40 μg/ml), it has been demonstrated that in addition to exchange of plasma-borne drug, erythrocyte-borne CI-912 is able to equilibrate across the blood–brain barrier in the course of a single transcapillary transit. Approximately one half of the drug gaining access to brain in a single transcapillary passage is erythrocyte-borne. **Key Words:** Brain capillary permeability—Zonisamide—AD-810—Erythrocyte-carried drug—Anticonvulsant.

The experimental anticonvulsant sulfonamide drug CI-912 (3-sulfamoylmethyl-1,2-benzisole; also known as AD-810, or the generic name zonisamide) is currently being clinically evaluated in phase I trials. Like other sulfonamides, CI-912 is preferentially taken up by erythrocytes. Erythrocyte/plasma partition ratios ranging from 6 to 18 have been reported, and the uptake process includes a saturable transport system in the erythrocyte (1).

Several saturable, carrier-mediated transport mechanisms have been identified in vivo in the blood–brain barrier, and these carriers facilitate brain uptake of nutrients (2). The blood–brain barrier and erythrocyte exhibit remarkable similarities when facilitated diffusion systems are compared (3). Thus, the present studies were initiated to determine whether or not a facilitated diffusion system could be kinetically defined in the brain capillary (i.e., a saturable, carrier-mediated transport mechanism) or whether drug entry into brain could be attributed to lipid-mediated transport.

It has been recently established that albumin-bound ligands (4), including anticonvulsant drugs (5), are able to dissociate and equilibrate into the brain during a single transcapillary transit. A second objective was to ascertain whether or not plasma-borne and eryth-

Address correspondence and reprint requests to Dr. E. M. Cornford at 691-W127B Epilepsy Center, VA Wadsworth Medical Center, Los Angeles, CA 90073, U.S.A.

rocyte-borne fractions of CI-912 shared this characteristic; thus, we focused upon the transcapillary exchange of drug, and on the effects of red blood cell binding upon drug uptake at the target site. Specifically, blood–brain barrier permeability of zonisamide has been measured in vivo using the single-pass, intracarotid injection technique. Data demonstrate, for the first time, the rapid exchange of erythrocyte-borne drug into brain tissue during a single transcapillary transit.

MATERIALS AND METHODS

Animal Methods

Brain uptake indices were measured in ketamine-anesthetized adult rats as described previously (6). A mixture of 95% ketamine HCl (Ketalar; Parke-Davis, Morris Plains, NJ, U.S.A.) and 5% xylazine (Rompun; Bayvet Division, Cutter Laboratories, Shawnee, KS, U.S.A.) was injected intraperitoneally to administer 175 mg/kg ketamine in conjunction with 1.75 mg/kg xylazine. All animal studies were performed in the morning and completed by early afternoon. The common carotid artery was surgically exposed under anesthesia and cannulated with a 27 gauge needle. An intraarterial bolus injection (0.20 ml), containing tritiated water as a diffusible reference, a ^{14}C-drug, and a plasma volume reference consisting of [^{113m}In]EDTA was performed. The mixture of isotopes injected was routinely buffered with 10 m*M* Hepes (Sigma Chemical Company, St. Louis, MO, U.S.A.). The rat was decapitated 5 s after injection (or later, when the washout of drug or ^{3}H-water from brain was under study). It has been demonstrated that the injected bolus is almost completely washed from the brain vasculature by this time, and that no dilution artifacts are caused by mixing of the injection bolus with the circulating rat plasma (7). After decapitation, the brain was removed, and the hemisphere ipsilateral to the carotid injection was sampled and prepared for simultaneous ^{3}H, ^{14}C, and ^{113m}In counting.

The rate-constant of efflux of water and drug from specific brain regions was determined using methods that have been previously described for both brain (8) and liver (9). Cerebral blood flow rates (CBF) were determined in brains and brain regions of the ketamine-anesthetized rat from the relationship CBF $= kV'/E$, where k is the rate constant for efflux of water (min^{-1}), V' is the distribution volume of water in brain relative to blood (0.83 ml g^{-1}), and E is the maximal fraction of water extracted by the brain.

Blood

Human blood was freshly drawn from normal adult volunteers. Red blood cells were separated after centrifugation at 2,000 *g* for 15 min at 5°C. The cells were resuspended in Ringers saline and washed three times. For injections into the carotid arteries of rats, the cell suspensions were adjusted to give a hematocrit reading of 40% unless otherwise stated. Rat blood was drawn from ether-anesthetized animals and similarly prepared. Lots of human serum albumin (HSA, essentially fatty acid free) were purchased (as <0.005% fatty acids) from Sigma Chemical Company to compare single-pass brain uptake of erythrocyte-borne and albumin-borne drug. The partitioning of CI-912 between (a) human erythrocytes and saline and (b) rat erythrocytes and rat plasma was determined from isotopic analyses of the two phases after separation in a standard hematocrit tube.

Octanol/Saline Partition Coefficient

The partition coefficient of CI-912 was determined as described previously (10). Approximately 0.1–0.2 μCi of the ^{14}C-drug was added to 2.0 ml of saline. The 2.0 ml of labeled saline was placed in a glass culture tube with a Teflon-lined cap. An equal volume of *n*-octanol (octyl alcohol; J. T. Baker Chemical Company, Phillipsburg, NJ, U.S.A) was added, and the tube was vortex-mixed for 1 min at high speed and then centrifuged for 10 min at ~2,000 *g* to separate the oil and saline phases. The phases were carefully separated, and three 200-μl aliquots were taken from each phase and placed in preweighed 20-ml scintillation vials. The vials were then weighed and prepared for scintillation counting as described below. The first octanol/saline partition was discarded routinely as a wash because large variations tended to occur in the initial washings. One milliliter of the phase containing the greatest quantity (cpm) of the compound being partitioned was then removed, made up to 2.0 ml, added to a fresh aliquot of the opposite phase, vortex-mixed, centrifuged, and sampled as above. This procedure was performed on duplicate tubes and repeated until the partition coefficient had stabilized (typically, two or three washes). The partition coefficient was then determined (from the final rinse of each phase) as the ratio of [(^{14}C dpm g^{-1} octanol)/(^{14}C dpm g^{-1} saline)].

Free and Bound Drug

Equilibrium dialysis in vitro was performed for 3 h at 37.5°C in a system with 1 vol serum (spiked with

0.1–0.2 μCi of ^{14}C-CI-912) dialyzed against 10 vol Ringer's saline (with 10 m*M* Hepes buffer, pH 7.55, and 0.05% sodium azide). Aliquots of the serum and saline were prepared for scintillation counting after 3 h, and the system was reestablished with fresh saline for overnight equilibrium dialysis. Sixteen hours later, samples of the serum and saline solutions were again taken for analysis, and the percentages of free and bound drug were calculated. The dialysis was repeated in any instance where the 3-h and overnight values differed by more than 5%. In some instances, duplicate dialysis systems were established (either with or without sodium azide) so that the same serum and drug sample used for in vitro dialysis could be utilized for in vivo measurements of brain uptake. These duplicates never differed by >2%.

Chemicals and Radioisotopes

All chemicals used were reagent grade. Hepes buffer was obtained from Sigma Chemical Company. The tritiated water was obtained from New England Nuclear Corporation (Boston, MA, U.S.A.). The ^{14}C-labeled CI-912 was a gift from the Pharmaceutical Research Division, Warner-Lambert Company (Ann Arbor, MI, U.S.A.); specific activity 31 μCi mg^{-1}). The ^{113m}indium generator was purchased from New England Nuclear Corporation Radiopharmaceuticals Division (North Billerica, MA, U.S.A.). Each 1.0 ml of indium eluted from the generator was chelated by the addition of 10 μl of sterile disodium edetate (150 mg ml^{-1}) solution (Endrate; Abbott Laboratories, North Chicago, IL, U.S.A.). This indium-EDTA chelate solution was then titrated with 1.0 *N* NaOH to neutrality (about 40 μl) and adjusted to pH 7.55 by addition of 200 m*M* Hepes buffer. The final concentration of drug injected into the artery was adjusted through the addition of unlabeled CI-912 (lot U) supplied by the Warner Lambert Company.

Liquid Scintillation Counting

The digested brain tissue, or the sample dissolved for partition coefficient determination, was mixed with 10 ml of scintillation fluid (Econofluor Packard Instruments, Downers Grove, IL, U.S.A.). Glacial acetic acid had been freshly added (7 ml/L of scintillation fluid) to neutralize the strongly basic tissue solubilizer, and minimize chemiluminescence. The indium was then counted (0.5–1.0 min counts) in a Beckman LS5800 liquid scintillation counter with one channel adjusted for peak indium efficiency as described by Oldendorf and Szabo (11). Days later, after most of the ^{113m}In ($t_{1/2}$ = 100 min) had decayed, the vials were recounted for determination of ^{3}H and ^{14}C content. The net indium counts were obtained by subtraction and appropriate decay correction (each successive vial is decay-corrected for the elapsed counting time). The ^{14}C and tritium counts are expressed as dpm by comparison with stored standard curves in the microprocessor unit.

Brain Uptake Indices

Brain capillary transfer, that is, the brain uptake index (BUI), was determined as previously described in Animal Methods (6) from the following relationship:

$$\mathrm{BUI} = \left[\frac{(^{14}\text{C-drug}/^{3}\text{H-water})\ \text{brain}}{(^{14}\text{C-drug}/^{3}\text{H-water})\ \text{mix}} - \frac{([^{113m}\text{In}]\text{EDTA}/^{3}\text{H-water})\ \text{brain}}{([^{113m}\text{In}]\text{EDTA}/^{3}\text{H-water})\ \text{mix}}\right] \times 100\%$$

where mix is the isotope mixture injected into the carotid artery. In this equation the minuend, or the uncorrected BUI, represents the total radioactivity present both within the brain and in the vasculature. The subtrahend, or IUI (indium-EDTA uptake index), is an estimate of the test substance that remains exclusively in the vasculature.

The BUI, more simply, is a function of the single-pass extraction (E%) of these compounds, i.e., $(E_{drug} - E_{In\text{-}EDTA})/E_{water}$. Thus, the single-pass extraction of CI-912 can be derived from (BUI)(E_{water}). The permeability times surface area (PS) product (measured in ml min^{-1} g^{-1}) can therefore be derived from Crone's equation $PS = -\mathrm{CBF} \cdot \ln[1 - E]$, where CBF is cerebral blood flow rate, as described previously in Animal Methods (6).

All data were reduced to the mean ($\bar{x}$), standard deviation (SD), and sample number (n). Linear regression analyses were performed using a Hewlett-Packard 97 desk-top calculator.

RESULTS

Brain Uptake Indices

The BUI of saline borne CI-912 was determined to be about 30% (Table 1) in initial studies of the rat

TABLE 1. *Brain uptake index of saline-borne and albumin-borne CI-912 in cerebral hemisphere*

Concentration	Brain uptake index (%)	
	Buffered saline (n)	4% HSA (n)
5.6	27.7 ± 2.1 (3)	20.3 ± 1.1 (3)
15.0	29.3 ± 5.2 (3)	23.2 ± 7.0 (8)
50.0	30.1 ± 4.9 (3)	34.4 ± 3.9 (3)
400.0	31.6 ± 4.5 (3)	29.6 ± 4.3 (4)

HSA, human serum albumin.

cerebral hemisphere. The PS product was determined to be 0.26 ml min^{-1} g^{-1}, similar to values previously determined for the anticonvulsant drugs phenytoin (PS 0.16) and valproic acid (PS 0.34) (12).

The possibility that uptake in the rat brain might be due to the presence of a saturable, facilitated diffusional mechanism was examined. No reduction in BUI was observed when the injected concentration of zonisamide was adjusted from 5.6 to 400 μg/ml (Table 1). Thus, although this drug may enter erythrocytes via a facilitated diffusion mechanism (1), no saturable, carrier-mediated transport system is apparent in the rat blood-brain barrier. This observation has been tested in both the forebrain (Table 1) and the cortical gray matter. In the frontoparietal cortex, the BUI of HSA-borne CI-912 was 41.6 ± 6.0 (n = 3) at a concentration of 5.6 μg/ml, and 45.7 ± 4.1 (n = 4) at 400 μg/ml. Further confirmation is suggested by the observation that the BUI in rats previously dosed with drug to a plasma concentration of 6 μg/ml (26.8 ± 1.9%; n = 4) was not different from that in naive control animals (BUI of 27.6 ± 2.1; n = 4).

In Vitro Partition Coefficient in Octanol:Saline

The partition coefficient (in triplicate trials) ranged from 3.50 to 4.11, with a mean of 3.86 ± 0.59 (log PC = 0.59). Thus, CI-912 acid is a reasonably hydrophobic compound, and its ability to gain access to brain by virtue of its lipophilic properties is consistent with the absence of a carrier-mediated uptake mechanism.

Uptake and Washout From the Adult Rat Brain

Once it gains access to the brain, CI-912 is not washed out. In contrast to ^{3}H-water, efflux of this drug was so low that a rate constant could not be defined (Fig. 1). These data suggest that CI-912 is either bound, or retained by brain tissue. Furthermore, the drug is retained in the colliculi, cortical gray matter, midbrain, and hippocampus, suggesting no regional specificity of drug retention (Table 2). In contrast, water washout rate constants were determined. Measurements made from the cortical gray matter (0.51 min^{-1}), hippocampus (0.37 min^{-1}), colliculi (0.58 min^{-1}) and forebrain (0.50 min^{-1}) indicate the degree of CBF variation in these regions.

It is also apparent that while water is rapidly washed out from the brain ($t_{1/2}$ = 1–2 min), 90–98% of the CI-912 is sequestered by the brain during this period (Table 2). This suggests that the drug may be bound or retained in the central nervous system.

Effects of Serum Binding on Transcapillary Exchange of CI-912

It has been previously demonstrated (7,13,14) that virtually no mixing of the injected solution with ani-

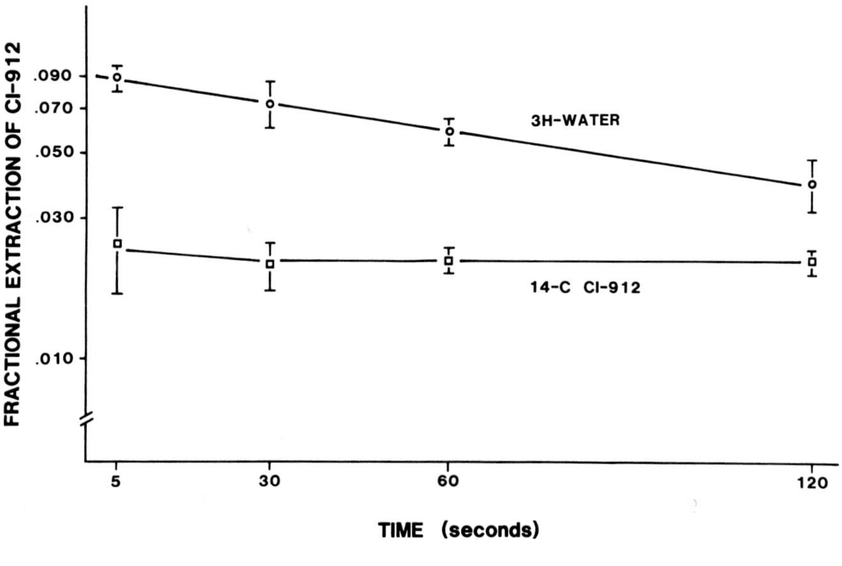

FIG. 1. Fractional extraction of ^{14}C-CI-912 and ^{3}H-water in the rat forebrain. Determination of the rate constant for efflux of ^{3}H-water (0.50 min^{-1}) suggests a cerebral blood flow rate of 0.64 ml min^{-1} g^{-1}, given $E^{3}H$ water = 0.65 (17) in ketamine-anesthetized animals. In contrast, there are no significant differences in the quantity of ^{14}C-CI-912 remaining in brain during the period from 5–120 s after intracarotid injection, suggesting that this drug is bound or retained in brain tissue.

TABLE 2. *Retention of CI-912 in brain after intracarotid injection: extraction of CI-912 by region (15 μg/ml in 4% HSA)*

Brain region	Time after injection (s) 5	30	60	120
Cortex	0.065 ± 0.048	0.045 ± 0.017	0.044 ± 0.009	0.057 ± 0.020
Colliculi	0.038 ± 0.019	0.041 ± 0.012	0.031 ± 0.007	0.029 ± 0.005
Midbrain	0.025 ± 0.011	0.019 ± 0.007	0.018 ± 0.006	0.020 ± 0.004
Hippocampus	0.042 ± 0.008	0.036 ± 0.014	0.034 ± 0.007	0.037 ± 0.010
Forebrain	0.036 ± 0.018	0.024 ± 0.008	0.025 ± 0.006	0.028 ± 0.013
Hemisphere	0.036 ± 0.017	0.025 ± 0.007	0.026 ± 0.006	0.028 ± 0.012

n = 4–6 for all points. HSA, human serum albumin.

mal plasma occurs prior to the time that the isotopes first traverse the capillary bed. For this reason, comparative measurements of zonisamide uptake in the presence of buffered saline, and drug uptake in the presence of serum (where uptake may be inhibited by binding to the plasma proteins), permit the in vivo study of the effects of plasma protein binding. For example, the BUI of a trace concentration (5.6 μg/ml) of CI-912 in the presence of 4% HSA is only slightly less than the BUI of saline-borne drug (Table 1). At higher drug concentrations (15, 50, and 400 μg/ml), differences in BUI of saline- and albumin-borne drug are not statistically significant (Table 1). These data are consistent with in vitro observations (1) (Table 3) that CI-912 was only 25% weakly bound to serum proteins in our equilibrium dialysis measurements (Table 4).

In the presence of 4% HSA and 100 μg/ml valproic acid, the BUI of CI-912 (15 μg/ml) was 21 ± 1%, compared with an observed BUI of 19 ± 1% without valproate. The retention of CI-912 in brain after intracarotid injection was not altered by coadministration of valproic acid (Table 4).

Erythrocyte-Borne Equilibration of CI-912 into the Brain

At a concentration of 15 μg/ml, CI-912 is highly bound to human erythrocytes. Our in vitro measurements indicate that when the saline solution contains 40% erythrocytes, 73% of the drug partitions into red blood cells and the remaining 27% is saline-borne (Table 3). If only the unbound fraction of drug was available to equilibrate across the blood–brain barrier in vivo, then the BUI in the presence of erythrocytes would be expected to be 73% less than the BUI of saline-borne CI-912. Since the BUI in saline is 27%, a 73% reduction would predict the BUI of erythrocyte-borne drug to be about 8%. The observed BUI of erythrocyte-borne drug was 16% (Table 5). Thus, half of the drug gaining access to brain is saline-borne, and the other half is attributable to brain uptake of erythrocyte-borne CI-912.

At a subtherapeutic drug concentration (6 μg/ml), there is also evidence for brain uptake of erythrocyte-borne drug. The predicted BUI (5%) is considerably lower than the observed BUI (9%), suggesting that almost one half of the drug equilibrating into the central nervous system at this concentration is erythrocyte-borne (Table 5). At 50 μg/ml, in addition to brain uptake of saline-borne drug, some erythrocyte-borne CI-912 apparently gains access to the brain (Table 5).

To ensure that transport of erythrocyte-borne drug was not a cross-species artifact attributable to some interaction of human erythrocytes with the rat brain capillaries, the study was repeated with rat red blood cells and rat plasma instead of human erythrocytes in buffered saline. At a drug concentration of 15 μg/ml, 77% of the zonisamide partitions into (or is bound to) erythrocytes in vitro and the remaining 23% in the plasma (Table 3). If only the plasma-borne drug fraction equilibrated across brain capillaries in vivo, then

TABLE 3. *Regional extraction of CI-912 in the presence of 100 μg/ml valproic acid (CI-912 concentration: 15 μg/ml in 4% HSA)*

Tissue	Time after injection (s) 5	30	60
Cortex	0.057 ± 0.013	0.048 ± 0.007	0.070 ± 0.011
Colliculi	0.032 ± 0.004	0.035 ± 0.005	0.035 ± 0.011
Midbrain	0.034 ± 0.005	0.026 ± 0.008	0.028 ± 0.004
Hippocampus	0.047 ± 0.002	0.039 ± 0.017	0.054 ± 0.014
Forebrain	0.025 ± 0.002	0.023 ± 0.005	0.023 ± 0.003

HSA, human serum albumin.

TABLE 4. *In vitro partitioning of CI-912 (percentage of CI-912 bound to ligand)*

Ligand	Dialysate	CI 912 concentration (μg/ml) 5.6	15	50	100
4% HSA	Saline	21.3%	23.9%	20.1%	21.3%[a]
20% human erythrocytes[b]	Saline	ND	37.2	30.0	ND
40% human erythrocytes[b]	Saline	81.4[c]	72.8	51.5	53.4[d]
Rat blood	Rat plasma	ND	76.5	ND	51.0

HSA, human serum albumin; ND, not determined.
[a]CI-912 concentration = 400 μg/ml.
[b]Partitioning % = [dpm g^{-1} of erythrocytes or HSA)/total dpm g^{-1} in both phases] × 100%.
[c]Determined at 6 μg/ml.
[d]Determined at 115 μg/ml. Partitioning at 22 μg/ml was also measured and found to be 64.4%, further demonstrating the trend of decreasing binding to the erythrocyte with increasing drug concentration.

the BUI of CI-912 in erythrocytes would be anticipated to be 77% less than the BUI of plasma-borne drug (18%, Table 6). Instead of the predicted BUI of 4% for erythrocyte-borne CI-912, the observed BUI was 12% (Fig. 2). Further evidence that erythrocyte-borne CI-912 traverses the blood–brain barrier comes from the observation that (when the drug concentration is 100 μg/ml) the BUI of plasma-borne CI-912 (21 ± 5%) is not significantly different from that of erythrocyte-borne CI-912 (BUI of 20 ± 4%), even though 51% of the drug is bound to erythrocytes in vitro at this concentration (Fig. 2). Equilibration of erythrocyte-borne CI-912 into the brain during a single transcapillary transit has also been demonstrated in regional studies of cortical gray matter, colliculi, midbrain, and hippocampus (Table 6). Collectively, these data indicate that at drug concentrations ranging from 15 to 100 μg/ml, more than one half of the drug gaining access to the brain is erythrocyte-borne CI-912 (Table 6, Fig. 2).

DISCUSSION

The present work demonstrates (a) that blood–brain barrier transport of CI-912 is not a carrier-mediated process, but is rather attributable to lipid mediation; (b) that this drug is sequestered by brain, analagous to propanolol and lidocaine (15) and steroid hormones (4) but in contrast to valproic acid (16); and (c) that zonisamide is bound primarily to erythrocytes rather than plasma proteins, however, erythrocyte-borne drug in vivo is available for distribution to tissues. Combinations of the ability of this drug to sequester in the central nervous system, and the availability of erythrocyte-borne drug to equilibrate across brain capillaries, are characteristics that lead to a favorable distribution of CI-912 to the target site.

Equilibrium dialysis measurements obtained in the present study compare favorably with those in previous reports. CI-912 is generally considered to be <35% bound to human serum at low to moderate concentrations (1). The present measurements of human serum (75–79% free) and 4% HSA (76–79% free) may be a reflection of the different techniques employed. In addition, the rate constants of water efflux estimated in the present study are comparable to those of Pardridge and Fierer (17), who reported 0.69 min^{-1} in ketamine-anesthetized rats. Minor differences can be tentatively attributed to differences in dosage and route of administration of the anesthetic.

Binding of this drug to erythrocytes is believed to occur via a two-component system. One component is a saturable mechanism with a half-saturation constant of 1.58 μg/ml; the other is a nonsaturable component (H. Bockbrader, personal communication). The

TABLE 5. *Brain uptake indices (BUI) of CI-912 determined in the presence of human erythrocytes*

Concentration	In saline	In 20% erythrocytes	In 40% erythrocytes Predicted[a]	In 40% erythrocytes Observed
5.6, forebrain	28	ND	5	9.07 ± 1.25
15.0, forebrain	29	16.28 ± 1.82	8	15.79 ± 3.59
50.0, forebrain	30	19.34 ± 1.56	15	15.94 ± 0.72

Erythrocytes were washed free of plasma proteins, and injected in buffered saline solution. ND, not determined.
[a]BUI predicted if erythrocyte-borne drug does not equilibrate into brain during a single transcapillary passage; based on in vitro measurements of drug partitioning (Table 4).

TABLE 6. *Brain uptake indices (BUI) of CI-912 in rat plasma and rat whole blood*

Brain region	Concentration (μg CI-912/ml)	BUI in the presence of rat plasma (n)	BUI in heparinized rat blood: Predicted[a]	Observed	(n)
Forebrain	15.0	18.19 ± 1.03 (3)	4.3	11.64 ± 2.21	(3)
Forebrain	100.0	21.48 ± 5.05 (4)	10.5	20.39 ± 4.10	(5)
Cortex	100.0	25.47 ± 7.28 (4)	12.5	29.97 ± 8.44	(5)
Colliculi	100.0	25.01 ± 4.80 (3)	12.3	25.49 ± 2.84	(3)
Midbrain	100.0	28.20 ± 9.78 (3)	13.8	21.68 ± 0.30	(3)
Hippocampus	100.0	26.74 (2)	13.1	25.09	(2)

[a]BUI that would be predicted assuming that erythrocyte-bound drug is not available to the brain. Based on partitioning determined in vitro (Table 4).

observation that erythrocyte-borne CI-912 equilibrates across the blood–brain barrier at the lowest drug concentrations we could test (6 μg/ml) suggests that the drug available for brain capillary transport is associated with the nonsaturable erythrocyte pool, rather than with the saturable binding component of erythrocytes. We have no evidence suggesting CI-912 bound to the saturable binding site can dissociate from the red blood cell and equilibrate into the brain in a single capillary transit. In contrast, when the saturable binding site becomes fully impregnated with drug, CI-912 which is taken up by the erythrocytes via the nonsaturable component is apparently readily available to the brain during a transcapillary passage. Presumably, the rate of drug-erythrocyte association via the nonsaturable component is slow relative to blood–brain barrier transport; thus, brain uptake of erythrocyte-borne drug occurs primarily at higher CI-912 concentrations (>5 μg/ml). If this hypothesis is true, then delivery of CI-912 to the central nervous system, and the therapeutic effect of this drug, may be significantly enhanced at plasma drug levels that imbrue the saturable binding site in red blood cells; i.e., more than threefold the half-saturation constant. In clinical studies (1,18), workers have measured both plasma and whole blood drug levels; our data underscore the use of whole blood drug levels, especially in estimating CI-912 delivery to the brain.

Many workers have suggested that red blood cells, or even red cell ghosts, may serve as carriers of drugs and facilitate delivery of agents to a desired site (19). In addition to protection from in vivo degradation, this erythrocyte encapsulation can effect delayed or controlled kinetics of release as well as increased specificity of delivery to target sites (19). At plasma drug levels near the half-saturation constant for CI-912 binding to erythrocytes (1–2 μg/ml), delayed drug release of this drug would be predicted. There is very

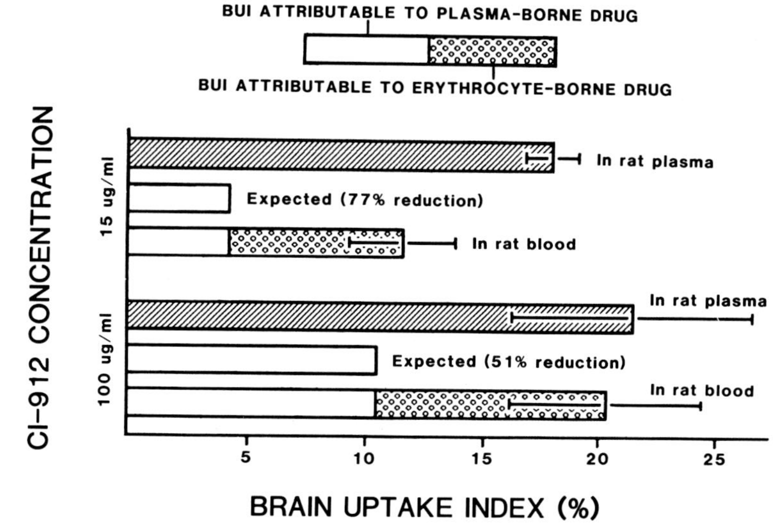

FIG. 2. At a concentration of 15 μg/ml, 77% of the CI-912 is bound to rat erythrocytes in vitro; the remaining 23% is in the plasma (Table 4). The brain uptake index (BUI) of CI-912 in rat plasma was determined to be 18 ± 1% (Table 6). In the presence of erythrocytes, if only the plasma-borne fraction was available to the brain in vivo, a 77% reduction in the BUI would be expected, resulting in a predicted BUI of 4%. The observed BUI was 12 ± 2%. Thus, more than one half of the total CI-912 equilibrating into the brain during a single transcapillary passage was erythrocyte-borne drug. Similarly, at a CI-912 concentration of 100 μg/ml, 51% of the drug is erythrocyte-bound in vitro; yet, the observed BUI in the presence of erythrocytes (20 ± 4%) is not significantly different from the BUI of plasma-borne drug (21 ± 5%).

little information describing erythrocyte-carried drugs, metabolites, or enzymes to the central nervous system. Jacquez (20) has indicated that the erythrocyte has a tremendous capacity to carry glucose. It is noted that the glucose transport capacity is 12,000 times greater than the glucose utilization rate in red blood cells. He concludes it is theoretically possible that red blood cells may facilitate glucose transport across the blood–brain barrier in adult primates, although experimental demonstrations have not yet been made. Studies of isolated dog brains, however, suggest that certain erythrocyte-borne amino acids can equilibrate with the central nervous system (21). The present study indicates that erythrocyte-borne drugs can equilibrate across the blood–brain barrier in vivo.

It is assumed that the drug binding reaction with the red blood cell measured in vitro is near steady-state. These in vitro binding measurements will predict in vivo distribution (a) if brain capillary membrane transport is not high enough to act as a sink, or (b) if the erythrocyte binding is not altered in vivo during the transcapillary passage. The observed 30% BUI of saline-borne CI-912 is not consistent with sink-effect distribution of this drug. Data presented in Fig. 2 suggest that further studies are needed to address the possibility that drug binding may be rapidly altered as the erythrocyte squeezes through the capillary. Presumably, a factor may be transiently generated (either by the endothelial or red blood cell) that inhibits erythrocyte binding during capillary transit. This catalytic factor generated in vivo may be either a chemical or a physical mechanism generated through the intimate cell-to-cell contacts formed in a transcapillary passage.

In summary, our data indicate that (a) at therapeutic concentrations of CI-912, approximately one half of the drug reaching the target site is erythrocyte-borne; and (b) to our knowledge, this represents the first in vivo demonstration that erythrocyte-borne ligand can equilibrate into brain during a single transcapillary passage.

Acknowledgment: This study was funded by the Department of Health, Education and Welfare under contract number N01-NS-0-2332, and supported by the Veterans Administration. We thank Dr. William M. Pardridge for discussions of this study and for providing unpublished manuscripts, and Dr. John McLean and Dr. Howard Bockbrader of the Warner-Lambert Parke Davis Company for supplying the CI-912.

REFERENCES

1. Wilensky AJ, Friel PN, Ojemann LM, Almes MJ, Levy RH, Buchanan RA. Pharmacokinetics of CI-912 in epileptic patients. In: Levy RH, Pitlick WH, Eichelbaum M, Meijer J, eds. *Metabolism of antiepileptic drugs*. New York: Raven Press, 1984:206–16.
2. Pardridge WM. Transport of nutrients and hormones through the blood–brain barrier. *Fed Proc* 1984;43:201–4.
3. Cornford EM, Oldendorf WH. Blood–brain barrier permeability to amines and amine precursors. In: Mosnaim AD, Wolf ME, eds. *Noncatecholic phenylethylamines. Part 2: phenylethanolamine, tyramines, and octopamine*. New York/Basel: Marcel Dekker, 1980:21–51.
4. Pardridge WM. Transport of protein-bound hormones into tissues in vivo. *Endocr Rev* 1981;2:103–23.
5. Cornford EM. Blood-brain barrier permeability to anticonvulsant drugs. In: Levy RH, Pitlick WH, Eichelbaum M, Meijer J, eds. *Metabolism of antiepileptic drugs*. New York: Raven Press, 1984:129–42.
6. Cornford EM, Pardridge WM, Braun LD, Oldendorf WH. Increased blood–brain barrier transport of protein-bound anticonvulsant drugs in the newborn. *J Cereb Blood Flow Metab* 1983;3:280–6.
7. Pardridge WM, Landaw EM. Tracer kinetic model of blood–brain barrier transport of plasma protein-bound ligands. Empiric testing of the free hormone hypothesis. *J Clin Invest* 1984;74:745–52.
8. Bradbury MWB, Patlak CS, Oldendorf WH. Analysis of brain uptake and loss of radiotracers after intracarotid injection. *Am J Physiol* 1975;229:1110–25.
9. Cornford EM, Pardridge WM, Braun LD, Oldendorf WH. Blood flow rate and cellular influx of glucose and arginine in mouse liver in vivo. *Am J Physiol* 1980;238:H533–60.
10. Cornford EM, Braun LD, Oldendorf WH, Hill MA. Comparison of lipid-mediated blood–brain barrier penetrability in neonates and adults. *Am J Physiol* 1982;243:C161–8.
11. Oldendorf WH, Szabo J. Amino acid assignment to one of three blood–brain barrier neutral amino acid carriers. *Am J Physiol* 1976;230:94–8.
12. Cornford EM. The blood–brain barrier. A dynamic regulatory interface. *Molec Physiol* 1985 (in press).
13. Oldendorf WH. Brain uptake of radiolabeled amino acids, amines, and hexoses after arterial injection. *Am J Physiol* 1971;221:1621–39.
14. Pardridge WM, Mietus LJ. Transport of steroid hormones through the rat blood–brain barrier. Primary role of albumin bound hormone. *Clin Invest* 1979;64:145–54.
15. Pardridge WM, Sakiyama R, Fierer G. Transport of propanolol and lidocaine through the rat blood-brain barrier. Primary role of globulin-bound drug. *J Clin Invest* 1983;71:900–8.
16. Cornford EM, Diep CP, Pardridge WM. Blood–brain barrier transport of valproic acid. *J Neurochem* 1985 44:1,541–50.
17. Pardridge WM, Fierer G. Blood–brain barrier transport of butanol and water relative to *n*-isopropyl-*p*-iodoamphetamine (IMP) as the internal reference. *J Cereb Blood Flow Metabol* 1985;5:275–81.
18. Wagner JG, Sackellares JC, Donofrio PD, Berent S, Sakmar E. Nonlinear pharmacokinetics of CI-912 in adult epileptic patients. *Ther Drug Monit* 1984;6:277–83.
19. Ihler GM. Erythrocyte carriers. *Pharmacol Ther* 1983;20:151–69.
20. Jacquez JA. Red blood cell as glucose carrier: significance for placental and cerebral glucose transfer. *Am J Physiol* 1984;246:R289–98.
21. Drewes LR, Conway WP, Gilboe DR. Net amino acid transfer between plasma and erythrocytes and perfused dog brain. *Am J Physiol* 1977;233:E320–25.

Therapeutic Drug Monitoring
7:255–257 © 1985 Raven Press, New York

Evaluation of Amitriptyline Pharmacokinetics During Peritoneal Dialysis

*Jerry J. Tasset, †Satwant Singh, and *†‡Amadeo J. Pesce

**Department of Pathology and Laboratory Medicine, ‡Division of Nephrology, Department of Medicine, University of Cincinnati Medical Center, and †Division of Nephrology, Veterans Administration Medical Center, Cincinnati, Ohio, U.S.A.*

Summary: The pharmacokinetics of a single oral dose of amitriptyline were examined in five functionally anephric patients undergoing continuous ambulatory peritoneal dialysis (CAPD). The concentration of the parent drug and its major metabolite nortriptyline in plasma were measured by high performance liquid chromatography. Patients on CAPD did not have a significantly extended elimination half-life ($t_{1/2}$) as compared to literature controls. However, the variation in $t_{1/2}$ was extremely large in both the CAPD and normal renal function groups (range 15–34 h and 24–70 h, respectively). No statistically significant change was observed ($p < 0.05$). Although a major route of elimination was removed and there was no change in $t_{1/2}$, the drug levels in these patients should be closely monitored because of the large variability in patient metabolism. **Key Words:** Amitriptyline—Peritoneal dialysis—Pharmacokinetics.

The prevalence of chronic renal failure is ~19 per 100,000 patients, of which four per 100,000 require dialysis for survival (1). Despite the common occurrence of depressive symptoms in chronic renal failure (2), there is considerable disagreement over the actual incidence of primary depressive illness. It has also been demonstrated that dialysis patients who are psychiatrically ill have a decreased life span (3). These facts would suggest that some effective psychiatric treatment is necessary.

When a psychotropic medication is indicated, tricyclic antidepressant drugs may be useful (4). The patient's response to these medications has not been studied systematically (5), but it has been reported that chronic renal failure patients who also suffer concurrent endogenous depression respond less to antidepressant drug therapy than do control patients (6). More investigation into this area is warranted.

Amitriptyline (AMI) is a tricyclic antidepressant commonly employed in the treatment of depression. The toxicity associated with high plasma levels of this drug include an elevation of heart rate, electrocardiogram (ECG) changes (7–9), hypotension, seizure, and coma (7), necessitating the monitoring of plasma concentration during treatment. Significant increases in patient plasma concentration may be associated with cardiotoxicity (7–10).

Amitriptyline and its metabolites are excreted in the urine via glomerular filtration (11). The presence of renal insufficiency may create difficulty in establishing a proper dosage regimen that maximizes the benefit to toxicity ratio. Investigation into possible changes in nortriptyline pharmacokinetics while patients were undergoing hemodialysis showed no statistically significant ($p < 0.05$) difference between the dialyzed and normal renal function groups (12). The purpose of this investigation was to evaluate any change in AMI $t_{1/2}$ in patients with end-stage chronic renal failure undergoing continuous ambulatory peritoneal dialysis (CAPD) compared with patients with normal renal function.

METHODS

A single 100 mg oral dose of AMI hydrochloride (Merck, Sharp and Dohme, West Point, PA, U.S.A.)

Address correspondence and reprint requests to Dr. J. Tasset at Department of Pathology and Laboratory Medicine, University of Cincinnati Medical Center, 234 Goodman Street, Cincinnati, OH 45267-0714, U.S.A.

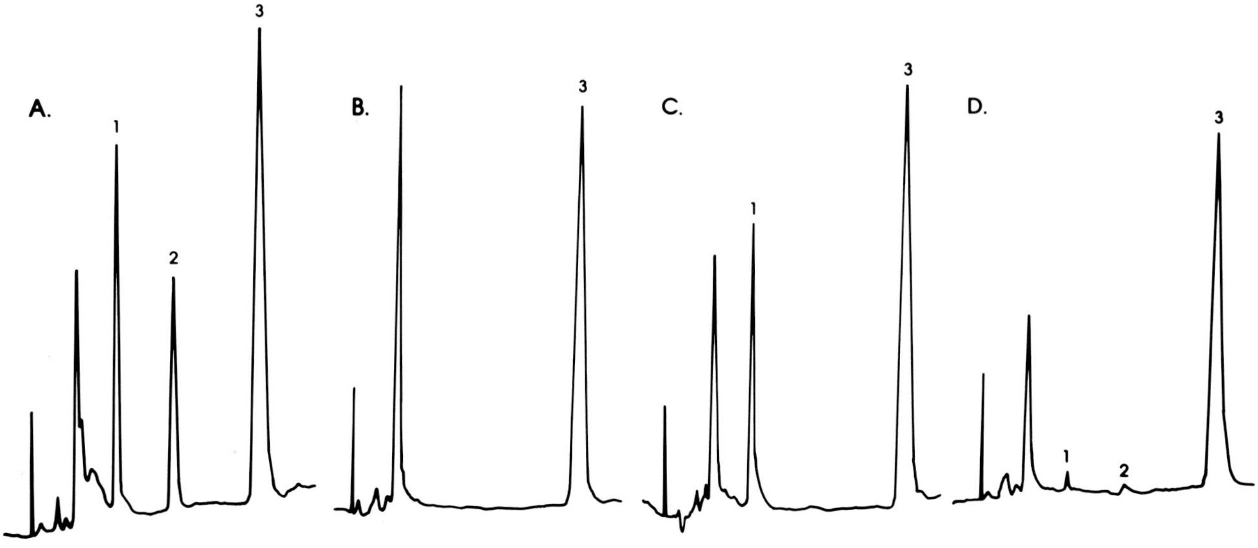

FIG. 1. High performance liquid chromatographic tracings from patient 3 undergoing continuous ambulatory dialysis following an oral 100 mg dose of amitriptyline. **A**, 200 ng/ml standard; **B**, patient blank; **C**, patient peak concentration after dosage; **D**, patient concentration 24 h after dosing; 1, amitriptyline; 2, nortriptyline; 3, protriptyline (internal standard).

was given following the introduction of a 2 L exchange of dialysate "for a 24 hour period" (Dianeal 137 with 1.5% dextrose, Travenol Laboratories). A 10 ml blood sample was then drawn at 0, 0.5, 1, 2, 4, 8, 12, and 24 h postingestion for AMI quantitation. All blood samples were immediately centrifuged, and the plasma was frozen at −20°C until the time of assay.

AMI plasma concentrations were determined by high performance liquid chromatography (HPLC) (13). The samples were thawed, extracted, and analyzed at 254 nm. The system utilized a Waters M-6000 pump, 710B Waters Intelligent Sample Processor (WISP), Waters μPorasil Normal Phase Column, Model 441 Absorbance Detector and OmniScribe, Houston Instrument, strip chart recorder.

By use of these measurements, a log-plasma AMI concentration versus time was constructed for each patient. A linear least squares regression analysis was used to fit individual plasma data onto the elimination phase line. From this line, the plasma AMI $t_{1/2}$ was calculated.

RESULTS

Figure 1 shows the HPLC elution profiles at the peak (C) and 24 h (D) after administration of AMI as compared with a 200 ng/ml standard (A) and a patient not receiving AMI (B). No nortriptyline was observed except in patient 3. This is in agreement with other studies of single dose AMI with subjects possessing normal function. Therefore, the metabolism, as far as this type of observation could establish, was not significantly altered. The five patients depicted in Fig. 2 and Table 1 show considerable vari-

TABLE 1. *Details of five patients receiving an oral 100 mg dose of AMI while undergoing continuous peritoneal dialysis*

Patient number	Age (yr)	Sex	Weight (kg)	Cause of renal failure	Coadministered drugs	AMI half-life (h)
1	65	M	96.7	Glomerulonephritis	None	24
2	44	M	56.0	Diabetic glomerulonephritis	None	22
3	58	M	65.0	Atheromatous embolization of kidney	None	15[a]
4	56	M	81.0	Interstitial nephritis	None	34
5	65	M	80.5	Hypertensive nephrosclerosis	None	18

AMI, amitriptyline.
[a]Trace amounts of nortriptyline present.

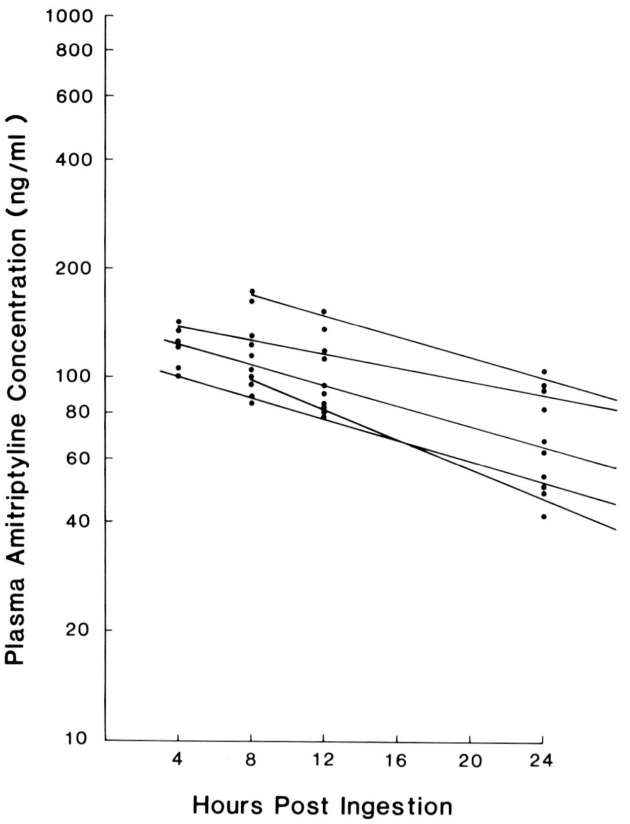

FIG. 2. Elimination profiles of amitriptyline in end-stage renal patients undergoing continuous ambulatory peritoneal dialysis. Amitriptyline plasma concentrations done in duplicate, each represented by a black dot.

ability in their AMI $t_{1/2}$ lives. The range of AMI $t_{1/2}$ is 15–34 h, whereas that of non–renal disease patients is 24–70 h. From these data, changes in AMI $t_{1/2}$ in patients undergoing CAPD were not marked and were well within the reported range of normal values.

DISCUSSION

The pharmacokinetics of AMI were evaluated during CAPD. No decrease in AMI elimination was noted, even though ~20–40% of the active portions of AMI and its metabolites are excreted through the kidney (14). Desmethyl metabolites were found in only one of five patients in this single dose study. It is assumed that these metabolites would accumulate following multiple doses. Thus, an alteration in kinetics would be expected. Any lack of action of tricyclic antidepressant drugs that might be observed in this group of endogenously depressed CAPD patients is not due to a change in AMI elimination.

REFERENCES

1. McCornich M, Navarro J. Prevalence of chronic renal failure and access to dialysis. *Int J Epidemiol* 1973;2:247–55.
2. Tyler HR. Neurological disorders in renal failure. *Am J Med* 1968;4:734–48.
3. Farmer CJ, Snowden SA, Parsons J. The prevalence of psychiatric illness among patients on home haemodialysis. *Psychol Med* 1979;4:509–14.
4. Cramand WA, Knight PR, Lawrence JR, et al. Psychological aspects of the management of chronic renal failure. *Br Med J* 1968;1:539–43.
5. Czaczkes JW, De Nour AK.. *Chronic haemodialysis as a way of life*. New York: Brunner/Mazel, 1978.
6. Buchanan DC, Abram HS, Wells C, Teschore P. Psychosis and pseudodementia associated with haemodialysis. *Int J Psychiatr Med* 1977;8:85–97.
7. Scoggins BA, Maquire KP, Norman TR, Burrows GD. Measurement of tricyclic antidepressants. Part II: applications of methodology. *Clin Chem* 1980;26:805–15.
8. Smith RC, Chojnacki M, Hu R, Mann E. Cardiovascular effects of therapeutic doses of tricyclic antidepressants: importance of blood level monitoring. *J Clin Psychiatry* 1980;41:57–63.
9. Petit JM, Spilur DG, Biggs JT. Psychiatric diagnosis and tricyclic plasma levels in 36 hospitalized overdosed patients. *J Nerv Ment Dis* 1976;163:289–93.
10. Gutler NR, Heiser JF. The tricyclic antidepressants. *JAMA* 1978;240:2264–6.
11. Jaivik M. Drugs used in the treatment of psychiatric disorder. In: Goodman LS, Gilman A, eds. *The pharmacological basis of therapeutics*. New York: MacMillan, 1980:186–92.
12. Dawling S, Lynn K, Rosser R, Braithwaite R. The pharmacokinetics of nortriptyline in patients with chronic renal failure. *Br J Pharmacol* 1981;12:39–45.
13. Hassan M, Ditzel CA, Manon D, Judd RL, Pesce AJ. Use of high-performance liquid chromatography for therapeutic drug monitoring. In: Kaplan LA, Pesce AJ, eds. *Nonisotopic alternatives to radioimmunoassay: principles and applications*. New York: Marcel Dekker, 1981:23–34.
14. Orsulak P. Tricyclic and tetracyclic antidepressants. In: Gerson B, ed. *Essentials of therapeutic drug monitoring*. New York: Izaku-Shinon, 1983:149–73.

Therapeutic Drug Monitoring
7:258–264 © 1985 Raven Press, New York

Experience with a Computer-Based Technique for Estimating Pharmacokinetic Constants from Limited Data

K. Bachmann, V. Pongsin, *R. Forney Jr., and †G. Gronau

*Department of Pharmacology, University of Toledo College of Pharmacy and Departments of *Pathology and †Data Services, Medical College of Ohio, Toledo, Ohio, U.S.A.*

Summary: A computer-based approach for estimating pharmacokinetic data and predicting plasma drug concentrations based on two measurements of plasma drug concentrations was compared with a standard two-point method for estimating aminoglycoside (AG) pharmacokinetic parameters. The computer-based technique was also used to predict a theophylline steady-state nadir from two preceding ones. The computer-based and standard two-point methods provided similar estimates for mean (±SD) values of elimination rate constant (λ) (0.172 ± 0.103 h^{-1} and 0.179 ± 0.010 h^{-1}, respectively) and apparent volume of distribution (*V*) (22.7 ± 9.9 L and 23.3 ± 11.5 L, respectively). The mean (±SD) of predicted AG troughs was 1.3 ± 0.5 mg/L for the standard method and 1.3 ± 0.6 mg/L for the computer-based method. Neither was significantly different from the actual AG trough mean of 1.3 ± 0.7 mg/L. Both methods exhibited a slightly negative bias in their predictions of actual AG troughs. When applied to theophylline data from patients or subjects receiving multiple-dose theophylline, the computer-based method effectively predicted trough theophylline concentrations for three formulations of theophylline. Mean prediction errors ranged from 0.1 to 0.5 mg/L, and root mean squared error ranged from 1.1 to 1.2 mg/L. This computer-based technique may be useful in dose individualization since relatively few constraints are placed on the type of data required for its application. **Key Words:** Pharmacokinetic parameters—Computers—Two-point methods—Individualized dosing.

Interindividual and intraindividual variations in drug disposition and the factors that condition them are becoming increasingly well recognized as causes for apparently anomalous drug responses (1,2). One tool for coping with variability in drug disposition in the clinical environment is therapeutic drug monitoring (TDM); measuring a plasma or salivary drug concentration to ascertain whether it lies within acceptable limits for a given patient. If the measured value deviates from an acceptable range and response to the drug is also unacceptable, then a dosage modification aimed at returning monitored drug levels to within acceptable limits is invoked. To minimize the frequency of dosage manipulations and subsequent TDM, individualized estimates of appropriate pharmacokinetic parameters ought to be secured. Since, as a practical matter, routine multisample data collection under rigidly controlled conditions is not possible, individualized estimates of pharmacokinetic parameters must be undertaken with the collection of very few samples and for the most part under conditions dictated by prevailing clinical exigencies. Exciting new approaches including some programmable calculator and computer-based ones have recently evolved to accommodate such limited data. Examples include the two-point method for adjusting intravenous theophylline doses described by Chiou et al. (3), the single point methods described by Love et al. (4) and Slat-

Address correspondence and reprint requests to Dr. Kenneth Bachmann at Professor of Pharmacology, The University of Toledo College of Pharmacy, 2801 W. Bancroft, Toledo, Ohio 43606, U.S.A.

tery et al. (5); the three-point protocol outlined by Slattery for establishing targeted steady-state trough concentrations (6); a two-point method using peak and trough concentrations for adjusting aminoglycoside (AG) doses (7); an unstructured two-point method for one-compartment drugs obeying first-order kinetics (8); and an adaptive feedback strategy requiring one or two sample points and estimates of population mean values and measures of dispersion for relevant kinetic parameters (9).

The purpose of the work described herein was to (a) compare a new two-point, computer-based method for individual pharmacokinetic parameter estimation, Pharmatrol, with a standard two-point method used for estimating AG parameters (7); (b) assess the effect of small (10%) errors in the measurement of AGs on Pharmatrol's estimates of the parameters; and (c) compare Pharmatrol-predicted theophylline trough values with actual trough values measured in subjects who had participated in multiple dose theophylline bioavailability studies.

MATERIALS AND METHODS

Pharmatrol

Pharmatrol is a series of computer programs currently written in BASIC and operating on a Hewlett-Packard 3354 computer. Utilizing two appropriate drug concentration values, Pharmatrol provides estimates for kinetic parameters after iteratively searching for them beginning at population mean values for healthy, young adults (10). It is not necessary to specify whether a patient belongs to a distinct subpopulation, e.g., renal failure, smoker, etc.; however, neonates are not accommodated unless suitable mean neonatal values are first specified. Iterations cease when the differences between observed and calculated plasma concentrations are minimized. It is similar in broad strategy to other computer-based, two-point methods (11,12). Assumptions on which Pharmatrol operates are as follows: (a) The disposition of theophylline and AG antibiotics can be adequately described by a one-compartment open model. (b) The plasma disappearance of theophylline and AG antibiotics can adequately be described by first-order kinetics. (c) The infusion of AG is zero-order. (d) The absorption of theophylline is first-order. [For further information about Pharmatrol write to Dr. Robert Forney Jr., Associate Professor of Pathology, at Department of Pathology, Medical College of Ohio, C.S. 10008, Toledo, Ohio 43699. U.S.A.]

Estimates of AG Parameters

Patients treated with AGs from January 1983 until March 1983 at a teaching hospital in northern Ohio were used as the source of AG blood level data provided that the patient's total body weight was known; at least two AG levels had been measured during AG treatment, one peak followed by one trough measurement (not necessarily during the same dosing interval); and times of drug administration and blood sampling were indicated. Serum concentration pairs were obtained at steady-state. For the purposes of the following comparisons it was assumed that drug administration times and blood sampling times were charted accurately. Patients' weights ranged from 45.5 to 185 kg (mean 78.6 kg). A total of 25 data pairs (peak/trough) were available from 16 patients (9 men, 7 women). Peak samples were drawn 0.8 ± 0.7 h (±SD) after infusions ended, and trough samples were drawn 0.6 ± 0.5 h before the next dose. Three patients received gentamicin; all others received tobramycin.

Assays were performed in accordance with customary TDM procedures at the institution. AGs were measured with a fluorescence polarization immunoassay technique (TDx, Abbott) that exhibited between-run coefficients of variation of 2.8 and 3.4% for gentamicin and tobramycin, respectively.

Estimates of apparent volume of distribution *(V)* and elimination rate constant (λ) were made by using a standard two-point method (7) and Pharmatrol. Parameters estimated by both methods were compared by a paired *t* test, and were used to predict steady-state trough values for each of 16 patients for whom such additional data had been harvested. Predicted steady-state trough values, $\hat{C}_{\min\,\mathrm{ss}}$, by both methods were compared with actual steady-state trough values, $\hat{C}_{\min\,\mathrm{ss}}$. Bias and precision of those predictions were evaluated by calculating mean prediction errors and RMSEs, respectively (13).

Estimates of AG Parameters with Errant Data

To determine the impact of 10% errant assay data on the estimates of pharmacokinetic parameters, 13 peak/trough pairs were randomly selected from the values reported for eight patients and were either increased or decreased by 10% from the measured values. Application of the two-point method and Pharmatrol was otherwise as described. Estimates of *V* and λ using errant data were compared with estimates of *V* and λ for the same patients using actual AG values, and the latter were considered the standards against which estimates of precision and bias could be made. Parameters calculated using errant data were also compared against those using measured AG values by a paired *t* test.

Predictions of Trough Theophylline Concentrations

The data used in this study were provided, in part, by the authors of a bioavailability study of theophylline products (14). Additional data from Dasta et al. (15) were also used. Subjects in the Meyer study (14) (study A) had a mean age of 24.4 yr (21–32 yr) and mean weight of 77.4 kg (68–93 kg). All were healthy, nonsmoking men. Theophylline concentrations were measured by an enzyme immunoassay technique (EMIT, Syva) with a reported coefficient of variation <10%. Ten patients (4 men, 6 women) were used in the Dasta study (study B); they had a mean age of 39.8 yr (25–53 yr) and a mean weight of 66.8 kg (46.3–89.4 kg). Eight patients had asthma, and two had bronchitis.

Each subject's weight, dosage regimen, and two steady-state trough theophylline concentrations were used in arriving at Pharmatrol estimates of V, λ, and a third steady-state theophylline concentration, $\hat{C}_{min\ SS3}$. Precision and bias estimates of Pharmatrol-predicted $\hat{C}_{min\ SS3}$ values were calculated. Predictions using three different oral theophylline formulations were made. In study A, Aminodur and Elixophyllin Elixir were the formulations for which predictions were made. Aminophyllin was used in study B.

TABLE 1. *Pharmacokinetic parameters and predicted troughs determined by two-point method and Pharmatrol*

Patient	Sample[a] peak/trough (mg/L)	Method used in calculation: Two-point λ(h^{-1})	Two-point V(L)	Pharmatrol λ(h^{-1})	Pharmatrol V(L)	$C_{ss\ min}$ actual trough (mg/L)	Predicted trough: Two-point (mg/L)	Predicted trough: Pharmatrol (mg/L)
1	3.0/0.8	0.214	43.1	0.219	41.1	1.4	0.8	0.7
2	4.7/2.5	0.100	35.0	0.096	36.2	2.5	2.2	2.5
						2.6	2.3	2.4
	3.4/0.4	0.476	16.6	0.467	16.9	0.7	0.8	0.8
3	3.1/0.7	0.458	20.8	0.453	21.2	1.0	0.8	0.8
						0.7	0.6	0.7
	7.4/3.9	0.157	27.9	0.128	28.7	0.5	1.2	1.3
4	2.8/1.3	0.171	16.4	0.192	15.2	1.0	1.0	0.9
	7.2/1.0	0.190	13.4	0.190	13.3	0.9	1.1	1.1
5	4.6/2.2	0.071	18.0	0.077	17.4	—	—	—
6[b]	8.6/3.8	0.127	16.4	0.138	16.1	2.2	1.5	1.4
	6.6/2.2	0.100	16.9	0.103	14.6	2.2	1.7	2.0
7	4.4/1.3	0.188	22.3	0.194	19.0	—	—	—
8	3.7/1.2	1.190	16.4	0.185	17.2	0.9	1.5	1.4
9	6.3/1.0	0.245	17.4	0.245	14.0	—	—	—
	7.2/3.2	0.133	15.0	0.087	18.5	—	—	—
	4.8/1.2	0.205	10.5	0.133	11.8	—	—	—
10	1.5/0.7	0.131	24.0	0.129	24.1	0.6	0.5	0.5
	0.8/0.6	0.064	52.0	0.072	43.3	0.9	1.2	1.2
11	4.2/0.8	0.255	21.7	0.250	19.5	—	—	—
12	4.3/2.1	0.108	23.3	0.109	21.0	2.0	1.8	1.9
	4.9/2.0	0.111	19.8	0.120	17.0	—	—	—
13	4.3/1.5	0.156	23.2	0.150	23.7	—	—	—
	2.2/1.0	0.116	55.3	0.133	49.7	—	—	—
14[b]	2.6/0.7	0.219	25.4	0.214	26.0	1.0	1.0	1.0
15[b]	6.7/2.1	0.183	17.4	0.184	16.9	—	—	—
16	3.3/1.9	0.099	14.1	0.040	24.1	—	—	—
Mean ± SD		0.140 ± 0.051	25.7 ± 13.6	0.144 ± 0.049	23.9 ± 11.7	1.3 ± 0.7	1.3 ± 0.5	1.3 ± 0.6

λ, elimination rate constant; V, volume of distribution.
[a]Peak and trough used for calculation in both methods.
[b]Patients taking gentamicin.

TABLE 2. *Performance of two-point method and Pharmatrol in predicting steady-state troughs from peak/trough aminoglycoside data*

Parameter	Two-point method	Pharmatrol
mpe (mg/L)	−0.07 (−0.28, 0.14)	−0.03 (−0.24, 0.18)
RMSE (mg/L)	0.39	0.38

mpe, mean prediction error; RMSE, root mean squared error. Values in parentheses denote 95% confidence interval.

RESULTS

AG Pharmacokinetic Parameters and Trough Values

The peak and trough AG levels used in the estimate of pharmacokinetic parameters and prediction of $\hat{C}_{\mathrm{min\ ss}}$ values are shown in Table 1. Peak and trough concentrations were obtained at steady-state. Mean ± SD estimates for λ and *V* were 0.179 ± 0.101 h^{-1} and 23.3 ± 11.5 L, respectively, by the standard two-point method, and 0.172 ± 0.103 h^{-1} and 22.7 ± 9.9 L, respectively, for the Pharmatrol method. These were not significantly different. The mean of measured trough AG levels was 1.3 ± 0.7 mg/L; not different from the mean of trough values predicted by the standard two-point method, 1.3 ± 0.5 mg/L, or the mean of the trough values predicted by the Pharmatrol method, 1.3 ± 0.6 mg/L. Precision and bias of the Pharmatrol-predicted troughs evaluated against the actual AG troughs and the standard two-point method-predicted troughs against the actual AG troughs are presented in Table 2. Both methods exhibited a slightly negative bias in their estimates of $\hat{C}_{\mathrm{min\ ss}}$.

Estimates of AG Parameters Using 10% Errant Data

Thirteen peak/trough AG pairs adjusted at random either up or down by 10% are given in Table 3 along with values of *V* and λ computed by the standard two-point method and Pharmatrol using the errant data. The mean ± SD values for λ were 0.145 ± 0.061 h^{-1} and 0.154 ± 0.072 h^{-1} estimated by the standard two-point and Pharmatrol methods, respectively. These compare with means of 0.140 ± 0.051 h^{-1} and 0.144 ± 0.049 h^{-1} estimated by the standard and Pharmatrol methods, respectively, for matching nonerrant peak/trough pairs (Table 1). Mean ± SD values for *V* based on errant data were 24.4 ± 11.1 L and 23.5 ± 12.6 L, respectively, estimated by the standard two-point and Pharmatrol methods. These compared with values of 25.7 ± 13.6 L and 23.9 ± 11.7 L for matching nonerrant peak/trough pairs. For neither method were differences between estimates based on errant vs. nonerrant data significantly different. Both methods exhibited a slightly positive bias in their estimates of λ and a slightly negative bias in their estimates of *V* when 10% errant data were used (Table 4).

Pharmacokinetic Parameters and Steady-State Trough Predictions for Three Formulations of Theophylline

Individualized estimates of theophylline kinetic parameters and actual and predicted trough values are shown in Tables 5, 6, and 7 for Aminodur, Elixophyllin Elixir, and Aminophyllin, respectively. Preci-

TABLE 3. *Pharmacokinetic parameters determined by two-point method and Pharmatrol using 10% errant data*

Patient	10% errant samples	Two-point method λ (h^{-1})	Two-point method V(L)	Pharmatrol λ(h^{-})	Pharmatrol V(L)
2	5.2/2.3	0.129	26.3	0.125	26.9
4	2.5/1.2	0.163	19.0	0.268	13.5
	7.9/0.9	0.209	11.8	0.215	11.5
6	7.7/4.2	0.094	22.6	0.094	22.8
	7.3/2.0	0.118	14.1	0.124	12.1
8	3.3/1.1	0.186	18.7	0.200	17.9
10	1.7/0.8	0.129	21.4	0.127	21.6
	0.9/0.7	0.056	52.6	0.039	57.6
11	4.6/0.7	0.290	16.7	0.291	16.4
12	3.9/1.9	0.108	25.6	0.107	23.7
	4.4/2.2	0.086	26.1	0.098	21.5
13	4.7/1.7	0.151	21.7	0.153	21.2
	2.4/0.9	0.163	40.4	0.167	39.3
Mean ± SD		0.145 ± 0.061	24.4 ± 11.1	0.154 ± 0.072	23.5 ± 12.6

λ, elimination rate constant; *V*, volume of distribution.

TABLE 4. *Performance of two-point method and Pharmatrol in estimating aminoglycoside kinetic parameters from errant peak/trough data when compared to estimates from actual peak/trough data*

Parameter	λ Two-point method	λ Pharmatrol	V Two-point method	V Pharmatrol
mpe	0.005	0.011	−1.3	−0.4
95% CI	(−0.009, 0.019)	(−0.009, 0.031)	(−4.9, 2.3)	(−4.3, 3.5)
RMSE	0.023	0.033	5.8	6.3

λ, elimination rate constant; *V*, volume of distribution; mpe, mean prediction error; RMSE, root mean squared error; CI, confidence interval. Units are h^{-1} for λ and L for *V*.

sion and bias estimates of the forecasted troughs, $\hat{C}_{min\ SS3}$, are given in Table 8. Mean prediction errors show a slightly positive bias ranging from 0.1 mg/L for Aminodur to 0.4 mg/L for Elixophyllin Elixir and 0.5 mg/L for Aminophyllin. RMSE for the predicted theophylline troughs for each formulation were 1.1, 1.1, and 1.2 mg/L, respectively. Similar results occurred when data from the three formulations were analyzed collectively. When formulation was ignored and all 34 data pairs were used, the mean prediction error was 0.3 mg/L with a 95% confidence interval of −0.1 to 0.7 mg/L. RMSE was 1.2 mg/L.

DISCUSSION

The computer-based estimates of pharmacokinetic parameters of the AGs tobramycin and gentamicin were comparable to estimates produced by a standard two-point method (7) when the same peak/trough data pairs were used. Both methods were comparable in predicting future trough AG concentrations, and neither method was especially sensitive to small (10%) errors in AG measurements providing that both peaks and troughs of the errant data were too high or too low. Similarly, the Pharmatrol-predicted theophylline troughs were very close to the actual trough values measured for each of three oral formulations of theophylline given in multiple doses. In fact, RMSEs ranged from 1.1 to 1.2 mg/L, and deviations of this magnitude might almost be anticipated by virtue of sampling and assay error.

That the Pharmatrol method provided estimates of AG pharmacokinetic parameters and equally accurate prediction of steady-state nadirs as a standard two-

TABLE 5. *Individual pharmacokinetic parameters and predicted next trough for Aminodur[a]*

Patient[b]	Weight (kg)	Sample[c] (mg/L) Tr/Tr	λ (h^{-1})	V (L)	Actual[d] trough (mg/L)	Predicted trough (mg/L)
SA	80	5.1/4.3	0.116	40.0	5.9	5.2
EB	84	8.5/11.6	0.054	42.4	9.4	11.1
JD	73	7.1/9.5	0.076	36.7	10.6	9.0
JC	75	6.4/5.6	0.100	37.5	7.1	6.5
MS	68	6.9/5.6	0.105	33.9	8.1	6.8
TM	93	9.2/9.3	0.080	31.2	10.0	10.0
BR	86	8.2/8.0	0.080	35.6	8.2	8.7
MA	82	11.3/11.4	0.080	25.4	11.1	12.2
AW	68	8.8/5.7	0.092	33.8	9.3	7.9
MH	73	9.0/8.2	0.080	33.5	8.7	9.3
SB	70	11.9/11.5	0.080	24.6	11.8	12.6
JJ	77	11.9/15.9	0.040	39.2	14.7	16.5
Mean ± SD			0.082 ± 0.021	34.5 ± 5.4	9.6 ± 2.3	9.7 ± 3.1

λ, elimination rate constant; *V*, volume of distribution.
[a]The data of Meyer et al. (14).
[b]Dosage regimens for all patients were entered into Pharmatrol as 236 mg every 8 hours for 9 doses.
[c]Two troughs drawn just before and 8 h after the seventh dose were used in calculating λ and *V*.
[d]Drawn 8 h after the ninth dose.

TABLE 6. *Individual pharmacokinetic parameters and predicted next trough for Elixophyllin Elixir*[a]

Patient[b]	Sample[c] (mg/L) Tr/Tr	λ (hr⁻¹)	V (L)	Actual[d] trough (mg/L)	Predicted trough (mg/L)
SA	4.5/5.3	0.079	60.3	5.1	5.0
EB	8.9./9.8	0.062	42.0	10.0	9.8
JD	6.8/8.1	0.080	39.4	8.2	7.6
JC	5.0/5.0	0.113	37.5	4.9	5.0
MS	6.7/8.2	0.080	39.4	7.7	7.6
TM	8.8/8.6	0.080	33.9	10.1	8.8
BR	7.1/6.5	0.080	43.0	5.8	6.9
MA	8.6/10.4	0.061	41.9	9.8	9.9
AW	9.3/9.4	0.075	34.0	6.8	9.5
MH	8.0/9.9	0.073	36.5	7.2	9.2
SB	7.5/14.0	0.064	35.5	10.3	11.2
JJ	13.8/13.9	0.080	21.2	14.5	14.1
Mean ± SD		0.077 ± 0.014	38.7 ± 8.4	8.4 ± 2.7	8.7 ± 2.6

λ, elimination rate constant; *V*, volume of distribution; Tr, trough.
[a]The data of Meyer et al. (14).
[b]Dosage regimens for all patients were entered into Pharmatrol as 250 mg every 8 h for 9 doses.
[c]Two troughs drawn just before and 8 h after the seventh dose were used in calculating λ and *V*.
[d]Drawn 8 h after the ninth dose.

point method is important. In the foregoing comparisons Pharmatrol was constrained to use peak/trough pairs since (a) such data are customarily acquired for pharmacokinetic dose adjustment of AGs and (b) that is the data required for implementation of the standard two-point method. However, by virtue of its application of superpositioning, Pharmatrol has some flexibility as has already been demonstrated for an unstructured two-point program (8) and can therefore operate on the somewhat less structured data that are often on hand when AG and other drugs are monitored. For example, it can operate on two trough values, two peak values, two mid-dose values, or trough/peak values. Successive values can be employed even if harvested several dosing cycles apart providing that one might reasonably expect a particular patient's drug dispositional processes to remain relatively constant over that time. Moreover, samples drawn during different dosing regimens can be accommodated. One must, however, be equipped with an accurate account of the dosing regimens and the blood sampling times.

Pharmatrol accurately predicted steady-state theophylline concentrations from two preceding trough values. It did so for three different oral formulations

TABLE 7. *Individual pharmacokinetic parameters and predicted next trough for Aminophyllin*[a]

Patient	Weight (kg)	Dose[b] (mg/6 h)	Sample[c] (mg/L) Tr/Tr	λ (h⁻¹)	V (L)	Actual[d] (mg/L) trough	Predicted trough (mg/L)
EJ	89.4	500	21.0/20.5	0.080	30.4	19.3	22.5
RB	61.6	400	17.5/16.6	0.080	30.5	17.6	17.9
RM	58.0	300	4.5/6.4	0.079	74.2	4.5	5.6
DH	70.2	200	7.9/9.5	0.068	35.1	8.9	9.3
BH	68.2	400	10.4/12.9	0.080	47.4	5.5	5.8
DS	69.6	400	10.4/12.9	0.070	51.1	12.6	12.4
LH	74.2	200	3.7/4.5	0.079	81.1	4.5	3.4
PS	77.3	200	3.8/4.0	0.079	67.5	3.7	4.1
DE	73.4	200	9.3/5.8	0.080	36.1	6.2	7.5
JW	46.3	200	4.3/3.5	0.189	23.2	4.5	3.9
Mean ± SD				0.088 ± 0.036	47.7 ± 20.3	8.7 ± 5.8	9.2 ± 6.5

λ, elimination rate constant; *V*, volume of distribution; TR, trough.
[a]The data of Dasta et al. (15).
[b]Aminophyllin dose is equivalent to 80% theophylline.
[c]Two troughs drawn just before and 6 h after the first dose given upon admission to the hospital.
[d]Drawn 6 h after the second dose.

TABLE 8. *Performance of Pharmatrol in predicting theophylline trough concentrations from two preceding trough values*

	Aminodur (n = 12)	Elixophyllin Elixir (n = 12)	Aminophyllin (n = 10)	Collective data (n = 34)
mpe (mg/L)	0.1	0.4	0.5	0.3
95% CI	(−0.7, 0.8)	(−0.4, 1.1)	(−0.3, 1.4)	(−0.1, 0.7)
RMSE (mg/L)	1.1	1.1	1.2	1.2

mpe, mean prediction error; RMSE, root mean squared error; n, number; CI, confidence interval.

of theophylline including a sustained-release formulation. Its effectiveness in estimating pharmacokinetic parameters (upon which blood concentration predictions for drugs are based) for other formulations of theophylline is untested at this time. In addition to its ability to cope with nonrigidly collected data (i.e., data likely to be available in the TDM laboratory) Pharmatrol and related computer-based methods for estimating pharmacokinetic parameters with two data points (11,12,16) can utilize presteady-state values.

In conclusion, Pharmatrol accurately estimated pharmacokinetic parameters of AGs when parameter estimates were compared with those estimated by a standard two-point method, effectively predicted future trough AG concentrations, and accurately predicted steady-state trough concentrations of theophylline from two preceding trough measurements. Like other computer-based techniques for individualizing drug dosages, Pharmatrol holds some promise for its application to TDM and dose individualization since there are relatively few constraints on the type of data required for its application. Its effectiveness in dose individualization is being tested prospectively.

REFERENCES

1. Morselli P, Franco-Morselli R. Clinical pharmacokinetics of antiepileptic drugs in adults. *Pharmacol Ther* 1980;10:65–101.
2. Breimer D. Interindividual variations in drug disposition: clinical implications and methods of investigation. *Clin Pharmacokin* 1983;8:371–7.
3. Chiou W, Radalla M, Peng G. Method for the rapid estimation of the total body drug clearance and adjustment of dosage regimens in patients during a constant-rate intravenous infusion. *J Pharmacokinet Biopharm* 1978;6:135–51.
4. Love B, Tsuei S, Thomas J, Nation R. The single-point method of dosage prediction: pharmacokinetic basis and method optimization. *Biopharm Drug Dispo* 1982;3:191–201.
5. Slattery J, Gibaldi M, Koup J. Prediction of maintenance dose required to attain a desired drug concentration at steady-state from a single determination of concentration after an initial dose. *Clin Pharmacokin* 1980;5:377–85.
6. Slattery J. A pharmacokinetic model-independent approach for estimating dose required to give desired steady-state trough concentrations of drug in plasma. *J Pharmacokinet Biopharm* 1980;8:105–10.
7. Zaske D, Irvine P, Strand L, Strate R, Cipolle R, Rotschafer J. Wide interpatient variations in gentamicin dose requirements for geriatric patients. *JAMA* 1982;248:3122–6.
8. Ball W. Unstructured two-point estimation of one- compartment linear pharmacokinetic parameters. *J Clin Pharmacol* 1982;22:326–34.
9. Sheiner L, Beal S, Rosenberg B, Marathe V. Forecasting individual pharmacokinetics. *Clin Pharmacol Ther* 1979;26:294–305.
10. Benet L, Massoud N, Gambertoglio J: *Pharmacokinetic Basis for Drug Treatment*. New York: Raven Press, 1984:419–40.
11. Koup J, Killen T, Bauer L. Multiple dose non-linear regression analysis program: aminoglycoside dose prediction. *Clin Pharmacokin* 1983;8:456–62.
12. Kelman A, Whiting B, Bryson S. OPT: a package of computer programs for parameter optimisation in clinical pharmacokinetics. *Br J Clin Pharmacol* 1982;14:247–8.
13. Sheiner L, Beal S. Some suggestions for measuring predictive performance. *J Pharmacokinet Biopharm* 1981;503–12.
14. Meyer M, Straughn A, Lieberman P. Multiple-dose study of sustained-release theophylline and aminophylline. *Chest* 1980;78:300–3.
15. Dasta J, Mirtallo J. Comparison of standard and sustained release theophylline tablets in patients with chronic obstructive pulmonary disease. *Am J Hosp Pharm* 1979;36:613–7.
16. Sheiner L. ADVISE Users Guide. Version 1.1. San Francisco: Regents of University of California, 1981.

Therapeutic Drug Monitoring
7:265–268 © 1985 Raven Press, New York

Nomogram for Bretylium Dosing in Renal Impairment

Joseph Adir, *Prem K. Narang, and †John Josselson

*College of Pharmacy and Pharmacol Sciences, Howard University, Washington, D.C.; and *Clinical Pharmacokinetics Research Laboratory, Pharmacy Department, Clinical Center, National Institutes of Health, Bethesda, and †Department of Nephrology, School of Medicine, University of Maryland at Baltimore, Baltimore, Maryland, U.S.A.*

Summary: Bretylium (Bretylol), an antiarrhythmic agent, is currently being used in the prophylaxis and treatment of patients with life-threatening ventricular fibrillation and tachycardia not responsive to conventional therapy. Because bretylium has a delayed onset of action that commonly causes hypotension and may increase ventricular irritability, its use in patients (especially patients with renal impairment) must be exercised with caution. Our results show that the maximum plasma concentration (C_{max}) observed at the end of bretylium infusion, when normalized to the dose, increases significantly as renal function diminishes. Significant reductions in renal and total body clearance of bretylium have been observed in patients with renal insufficiency. In order to minimize the risk of potential toxicity following multiple dosing in such patients, dosage adjustments are necessary. Based on correlations developed between the total body clearance of bretylium and renal function, we present a nomogram herein that can be effectively used for adjusting the dosage of bretylium in patients with renal impairment. **Key Words:** Bretylium—Dosing scheme—Renal impairment—Drug monitoring.

Bretylium tosylate (Bretylol; American Critical Care, IL, U.S.A.), a bromobenzyl quaternary ammonium compound, is approved for treatment of refractory ventricular tachycardia and other recurrent life-threatening ventricular arrhythmias. Substantial evidence in the literature suggests that bretylium exhibits poor absorption following oral administration (1), stability to metabolism (2), and predominant elimination via the renal route involving both the glomerular filtration and active secretion processes (1,3). Oral use of bretylium is still under investigation. Clinical experience has suggested its widespread use in both short- and long-term settings (4). Its major electrophysiologic effect is reflected by the prolongation of both the action potential and the effective refractory period of the tissues of the heart.

Address correspondence and reprint requests to Dr. P. K. Narang at Clinical Pharmacokinetics Research Laboratory, Room 1D-37, Pharmacy Department, Clinical Center, National Institutes of Health, Bethesda, MD 20205, U.S.A.

We have recently reported the pharmacokinetics of bretylium in normal volunteers (5) and in patients with renal insufficiency (6) following a constant infusion of bretylium tosylate. A significant reduction in total body clearance (TBC), amount of unchanged drug recovered in the urine, and renal clearance (RC) of bretylium was observed in patients with renal dysfunction (6); however, nonrenal clearance (NRC) did not differ. A reduction in the elimination capacity of the kidneys in patients with renal disease can lead to drug accumulation following prolonged administration, thereby significantly enhancing the risk of associated toxicity. Dosage adjustments are therefore necessary in patients with compromised renal function in order to maintain drug levels between the therapeutic indices. A review of the available literature indicates that the optimal therapeutic range of bretylium concentration has not yet been clearly established and that it might vary based on the type of arrhythmia.

The purpose of this report is to present a nomogram for adjusting the dosage of bretylium in patients with impaired renal function based on their creatinine clearances (CL_{cr}).

MATERIALS AND METHODS

Male subjects ($n = 9$) who participated in the study were nonobese by the criterion of desirable weights of adults (7) and ranged in age from 20 to 63 years. They included four normal volunteers and five renally impaired patients (two with end-stage renal disease who underwent hemodialysis for a period of 6 h). One patient was reevaluated within a 1-year period following further deterioration of his renal function. Thus, a total of 10 studies were performed. Baseline value of renal function in each participant was obtained by monitoring CL_{cr} in three sequential 12-h urine specimens immediately preceding drug administration. Informed consent was obtained from all those who participated in the study.

A single dose (4 mg/kg) of bretylium tosylate was administered as a constant i.v. infusion (5 mg/min). Subjects with $CL_{cr} < 30$ ml/min × 1.73 M^2 received only 2 mg/kg drug. Blood samples were collected for up to 8 days. Both plasma and urine samples were stored at −20°C until analysis. Subjects were kept supine for a period of at least 12 h after drug administration, and vital signs were monitored throughout the study. Plasma and urine samples were analyzed for unchanged bretylium content by a specific and sensitive electron capture gas chromatographic procedure (8). The injection port and column temperatures employed for routine laboratory analysis were 250° and 236°C, respectively. The assay procedure has a sensitivity limit of 5 ng/ml and an overall coefficient of variation of <7%.

Plasma bretylium concentration and urinary excretion data for each participant were simultaneously fitted by a two-compartment open model using a digital computer program, SAAM-27 (9). Model selection was achieved by using an F-test that evaluates the weighted sum of squared differences between the two model outputs (10) and by evaluating the randomness of residuals around the model output (11). Clearance parameters obtained from the analysis of areas and model-dependent approaches were compared for significant differences at the $p < 0.05$ level for model validation. Details and the results of these analyses have been reported previously (5,6).

Attempts were made to correlate renal function with clearances and other pharmacokinetic parameters of bretylium in order to gain insight into appropriate dosing strategies. Univariate linear regression of RC, TBC, elimination constant (k_{el}), hybrid disposition rate constant (β), and apparent distribution volume (V_c) was performed as a function of CL_{cr} to examine the influence of renal disease on these parameters. Employing regression estimates of correlation between TBC and CL_{cr}, a nomogram was developed to optimally compute rate of bretylium tosylate administration (R_o) for patients with varying degrees of renal insufficiency.

TABLE 1. *Comparative pharmacokinetics of bretylium in subjects with normal and impaired renal function*

Parameter	Group: Normal (range)		Group: Renally impaired (range)	
CL_{Cr} (ml/min)	108.4	(99.6–129.0)	32.7	(<1.0–83.0)
C_{max} (ng/ml/dose)	9.4	(6.8–15.0)	14.3	(9.2–18.7)
k_{el} (h^{-1})	0.56	(0.44–0.75)	0.18	(0.06–0.37)
β (h^{-1})	0.09	(0.085–0.10)	0.036	(0.008–0.067)
RC (L/h)	38.9	(35.5–44.0)	7.8	(0.01–20.8)
NRC (L/h)	7.5	(1.5–13.2)	4.6	(2.0–11.8)
TBC (L/h)	46.5	(44.2–51.9)	12.4	(2.7–23.1)
$V_{d\,ss}$ (L/kg)	5.9	(4.9–6.8)	4.3	(3.3–5.1)
Dose in urine (%)	77.0	(65.3–84.2)	36.8	(0.22–88.2)
		(n = 4)		(n = 5)

CL_{cr}, creatinine clearance; C_{max}, maximum plasma concentration; k_{el}, elimination constant; β, hybrid disposition rate constant; RC, renal clearance; NRC, nonrenal clearance; TBC, total body clearance; $V_{d\,ss}$, volume of distribution at steady-state; n, number.

RESULTS

Plasma bretylium concentrations, following a zero-order input as an infusion, increased rapidly in each subject and reached a maximum (C_{max}) at the end of infusion. Semilogarithmic plots of postinfusion bretylium data showed a biphasic exponential decay in both the plasma and urinary excretion rate profiles (6). Kinetic analysis using empiric models and based on area analysis gave consistent clearance parameters. Table 1 concisely shows the mean and the range of some important pharmacokinetic parameters in the normal and the renally-insufficient group. Figure 1 shows a plot of C_{max} (normalized to the dose) as a function of CL_{cr}. The negative slope ($r = 0.81$, $p < 0.01$) indicates the existence of an inverse relationship between C_{max} and CL_{cr}. This observation is corroborated by the reduced amount of unchanged drug recovered in the urine of subjects with renal insufficiency (Table 1).

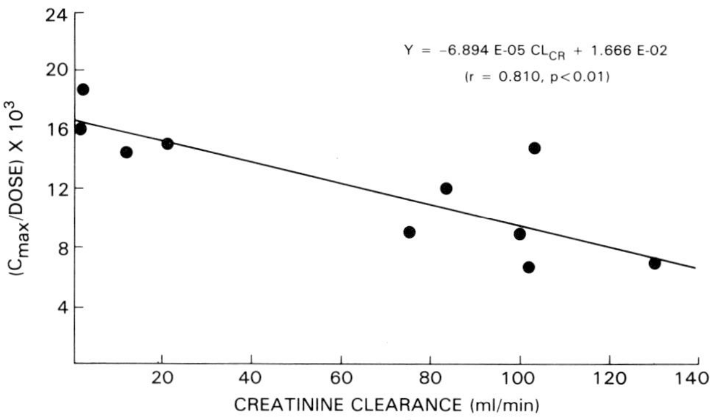

FIG. 1. A dose normalized plot of maximum plasma concentration (C_{max}) of bretylium in plasma at the end of infusion as a function of subject's creatinine clearance (CL_{cr}).

The decrease ($p < 0.025$) in steady-state volume distribution ($V_{d\ ss}$) associated with the disease suggests a possible decrease in intracellular volume and/or tissue binding. Significant reduction in both RC and TBC is also evident in patients with renal impairment (Table 1). The large values of distribution volumes suggest that the drug is highly bound to tissues and negligibly bound to plasma proteins.

Figure 2 shows that TBC of bretylium is highly dependent ($r = 0.93$, $p < 0.001$) on renal function. The linear relationship also reveals that the extrarenal (nonrenal) clearance accounts for ~10–15% of the TBC of bretylium. In addition to TBC other statistically significant correlations were observed between k_{el}, RC, β, and CL_{cr}. Although not significant, V_c appeared to be reduced in subjects with renal impairment.

The nomogram shown in Fig. 3 is based on the correlation observed between the CL_{cr} of the patients studied with the TBC of bretylium. Given a patient with compromised renal function, whose CL_{cr} is known, R_o of bretylium tosylate can be obtained from the intersection on Scale C of the line joining the CL_{cr}

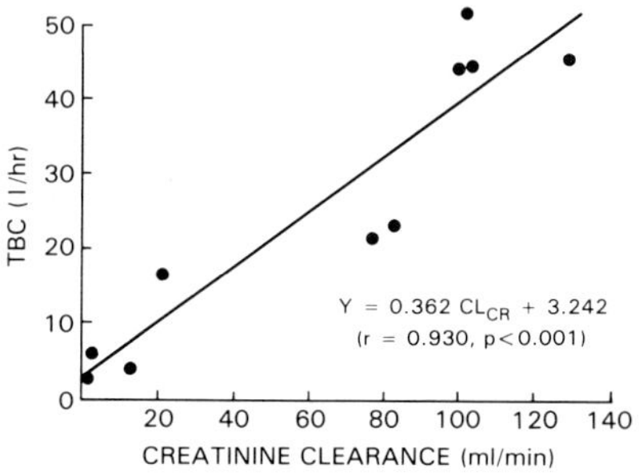

FIG. 2. Relationship between total body clearance (TBC) of bretylium and creatinine clearance (CL_{cr}) of subjects with varying degrees of renal function.

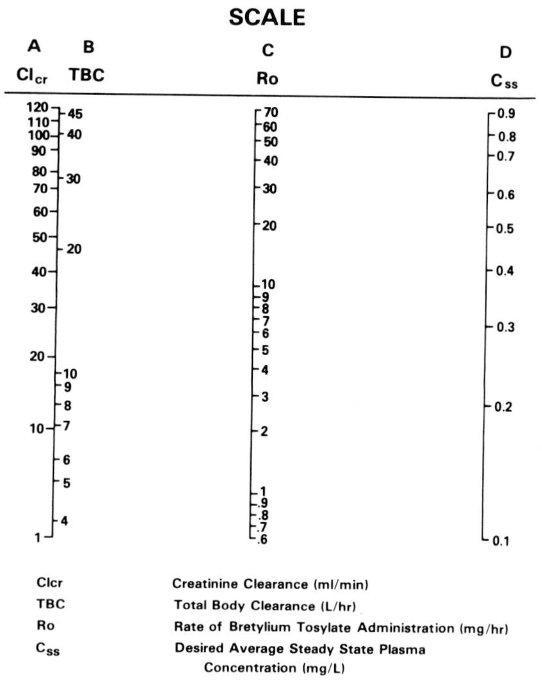

FIG. 3. A nomogram for computing appropriate rate of bretylium tosylate administration (R_o) to obtain desired average steady-state plasma concentration (C_{ss}).

(Scale A, Fig. 3) with the desired average steady-state plasma concentration (Scale D, Fig. 3). A CL_{cr} value of 120 ml/min is considered to represent normal renal function.

DISCUSSION

We have previously described the pharmacokinetics of bretylium in normal volunteers (5) and in patients with renal insufficiency (6) following i.v. infusion. A two compartment empiric model, with elimination from the central compartment and renal and nonrenal components for drug elimination, was found to adequately describe the pharmacokinetics of bretylium, based on model discriminating statistical evaluations. The mean half-life of drug in normal volunteers was 7.8 h compared to 33.4 h in patients with impaired renal function. TBC of bretylium in normal subjects averaged 46.5 L/h with RC accounting for almost 85% of this value. Estimated RC of bretylium (~800 ml/min) approaches renal blood flow and suggests that the drug is completely cleared from blood during a single pass through the kidney. Significant reductions in RC and TBC observed in patients with renal disease (Table 1) suggest a need for dosage adjustment. Since bretylium is eliminated predominantly via the renal route, reductions in its clearance in renal disease can lead to significant drug accumulation in renally impaired patients. Prolongation of the half-life of bretylium due to diminished TBC in renal disease suggests that dosage should be adjusted in these patients to avoid toxicity during prolonged or repeated drug administration. Anderson et al. (12) also made similar recommendations in an earlier report.

Before developing a rational therapeutic dosage regimen for bretylium, it is important to consider the relationship between its pharmacodynamics and its time course in the body by means of pharmacokinetics. From a pharmacodynamic view point, the therapeutic range for bretylium required for the treatment of ventricular arrhythmia has not been clearly established. There are suggestions in the literature that the therapeutic range may even differ for various tachyrhythmias. However, an insight into this range may be gained from an earlier report (13) in which Romhilt et al. evaluated the antiarrhythmic effect of bretylium as a function of its plasma concentration following the i.m. administration of a 4 mg/kg dose of the drug. These investigators observed that the onset of the pharmacologic effect coincided with a plasma concentration corresponding to one-half the peak level of 1.2 mg/L. Since the antiarrhythmic effect lasted ~12 h and the observed mean half-life in eight patients was 10 h, it can be deduced that the therapeutic range for bretylium lies between 0.2 and 0.6 mg/L. It should be noted, however, that no toxicity has been observed or reported with plasma bretylium levels as high as 1.0 mg/L (5,12,14).

It is evident from the data in Fig. 1 that administration of the same dose of bretylium leads to significantly higher drug concentration, reflective of the diminished clearance of the drug, in renally impaired patients (Fig. 2). The data also support the existence of a linear relationship between TBC and CL_{cr} of these subjects. It is apparent from Fig. 2 that renal function alone accounts for 86% of the total variability in the TBC data. The remaining unexplained 14% may be due to the error associated with the quantitation of creatinine. Analytical error in assay of bretylium is relatively small and may have contributed <7% (8).

In cases in which it is desired to achieve a desired average steady-state plasma concentration (C_{ss}) quickly, a bolus of bretylium containing twice the maintenance dose can be administered. Two simultaneous infusions, an approach similar to that suggested for theophylline (15), can also be employed. Since oral absorption and/or bioavailability of bretylium is poor (15–20%), its administration by this route is not recommended (1,12). We are cognizant of the fact that pharmacodynamics of different arrhythmias may differ and that dosage requirements may vary; however, there is potential need for such information when it is necessary to administer bretylium to patients with renal insufficiency. This report presents a nomogram for adjusting therapeutic dosage regimens of bretylium in patients with impaired renal function based on their CL_{cr} in a clinical setting.

REFERENCES

1. Dollery CT, Emslie-Smith D, and McMichael J. Bretylium tosylate in the treatment of hypertension. *Lancet* 1960;1:296–9.
2. Duncombe WG, McCoubrey A. The excretion and stability to metabolism of bretylium. *Br J Pharmacol* 1960;15:260–4.
3. Kuntzman R, Tsai I, Chang R, Conney AH. Disposition of bretylium in man and rat. *Clin Pharmacol Therap* 1970;11:829–37.
4. Koch-Weser J. Drug therapy. Bretylium. *N Engl J Med* 1979;300:473–7.
5. Narang PK, Adir J, Josselson J, Yacobi A, Sadler J. Pharmacokinetics of bretylium in man after intravenous administration. *J Pharm Biopharm* 1980;8:363–72.
6. Josselson J, Narang PK, Adir J, Yacobi A, Sadler J. Bretylium pharmacokinetics in renal insufficiency. *Clin Pharmacol Ther* 1983;33:144–50.
7. Scientific Tables, *Documenta* 7th ed. Geigy, Ardsley, New York: Geigy Pharmaceuticals 1972:712.
8. Lai CM, Kamath BL, Carter JE, Erhardt P, Look ZM, Yacobi A. A GLC determination of bretylium in biological fluids. *J Pharm Sci* 1980;69:681–3.
9. Berman M, Weiss MF. Statistical Analysis and Modeling Manual. Washington D.C.: 1978; DHEW publication no. (NIH)–78–180.
10. Daniel C, Wood FS. *Fitting Equations to Data*, New York: Wiley-Interscience, 1971.
11. Mandel J. *The Statistical Analysis of Experimental Data*, New York: Interscience 1964.
12. Anderson JL, Patterson E, Wagner JG, Stewart JR, Behm HL, Lucehesi BR. Oral and intravenous bretylium disposition. *Clin Pharmacol Therap* 1980;28:468–78.
13. Romhilt DW, Bloomfield SS, Lipicky RJ, Welch RM, Fowler NO. Evaluation of bretylium tosylate for the treatment of premature ventricular contractions. *Circulation* 1972;45:800–7.
14. Bacaner MB. Treatment of ventricular fibrillation and other acute arrhythmias with bretylium tosylate. *Am J Cardiol* 1968;21:530–43.
15. Mitenko PA, Ogilvie RI. Pharmacokinetics of intravenous theophylline. *Clin Pharmacol Therap* 1973;14:509–13.

Therapeutic Drug Monitoring
7:269–273 © 1985 Raven Press, New York

Carbamazepine Protein Binding and Disposition in Pregnancy

M. S. Yerby, P. N. Friel, and D. Q. Miller

Epilepsy Center, Department of Neurological Surgery, School of Medicine, University of Washington, Seattle, Washington, U.S.A.

Summary: The pregnancies of five women with epilepsy treated with carbamazepine monotherapy were studied prospectively. Free and total serum concentrations of carbamazepine and its epoxide and dihydrodiol metabolites were analyzed at monthly intervals from the first trimester through 8 weeks postpartum. Assays were by high performance liquid chromatography, and free compounds were separated by ultrafiltration. The mean intrinsic clearance of carbamazepine (clearance of free drug corrected for changes in maternal body weight) did not change appreciably during pregnancy and the postpartum period. The mean free fractions of carbamazepine and the epoxide were elevated during pregnancy (0.25 and 0.50) compared with postpartum (0.22 and 0.43). Mean total maternal carbamazepine and epoxide concentrations were 40 and 48% higher than neonatal levels at birth, but maternal and neonatal free concentrations agreed closely. The ratio of epoxide to parent drug increased during pregnancy, as reported by other authors. Evidence is presented that this may be a result of inhibition of further biotransformation of the epoxide rather than of increased production. Two patients missed at least one dose of carbamazepine during labor, resulting in markedly reduced serum concentrations at delivery. **Key Words:** Pregnancy—Carbamazepine—Protein binding—Free drug levels.

Antiepileptic drug disposition in pregnancy is of major concern for the epileptic mother and her physician. There is a tendency for serum antiepileptic drug levels to decline during pregnancy, and seizure frequency is exacerbated in approximately one of three pregnancies (1). The mechanism for declining serum levels is poorly understood, but it may involve factors such as noncompliance and changes in drug absorption, metabolism, or distribution (2,3). Maternal weight gain, without a change in the amount of medication prescribed, must also be taken into account. This report describes a pilot study of pregnancy in five epileptic women treated with carbamazepine monotherapy. Carbamazepine is a favorable drug for this type of study because it is relatively widely used in pregnancy and because serum concentrations and protein binding of two important metabolites, as well as of the parent drug, can be monitored (Fig. 1). Monotherapy is also advantageous because it minimizes interindividual variation in disposition due to drug interactions (4,5). The aims of this study were to determine the effects of pregnancy on the serum protein binding and metabolism of carbamazepine, and to compare neonatal and maternal drug and metabolite concentrations at birth.

METHODS

Five epileptic women treated with carbamazepine monotherapy were followed prospectively throughout their pregnancies. The mean age at entry into the study was 29 years (range 24–32 years). The carba-

Address correspondence and reprint requests to Dr. M. S. Yerby at Epilepsy Center ZA-50, Harborview Medical Center, 325 9th Ave., Seattle, WA 98104, U.S.A.

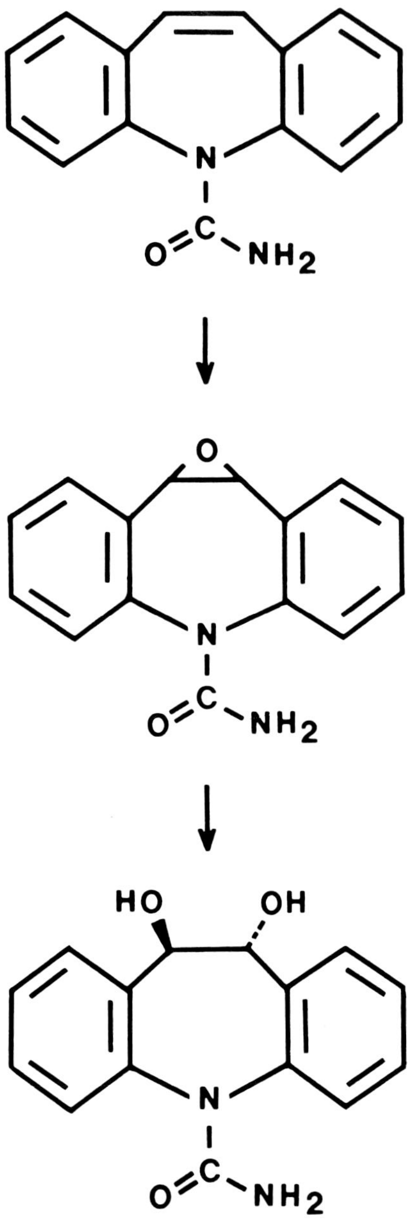

FIG. 1. Sequential biotransformation of carbamazepine to the epoxide and dihydrodiol metabolites.

mazepine dose was constant in four patients (400, 800, 800, 1000 mg/dl). In the fifth patient it was increased from 1,200 mg/dl to 1,400 mg/dl from the 28th week of pregnancy until delivery. Three patients entered the study during their first trimesters, and the remaining two entered early in the second trimester. All pregnancies were carried to term. Blood samples were collected monthly at the same time in the dosing interval (± 1 h) for each patient for analysis of carbamazepine, carbamazepine-10,11-epoxide, and carbamazepine-10,11-*trans* diol. Assays were performed by high performance liquid chromatography (6,7). Free drugs were separated by ultrafiltration (8). Day-to-day coefficients of variation were <9% for all compounds. Maternal and neonatal cord blood was collected at birth in three cases. Postpartum blood samples were collected at 1 and 2 months after delivery. Medication compliance was good throughout the study, based on specific interviews by the study physician at each visit.

Free fractions were calculated as the ratio of free concentration to total concentration. Clearances were calculated by these formulas (9):

$$\text{Plasma clearance} = \frac{\text{Daily dose}}{\text{Total serum concentration} \times 24\ \text{h} \times \text{body weight}}$$

$$\text{Intrinsic clearance} = \frac{\text{Daily dose}}{\text{Free serum concentration} \times 24\ \text{h} \times \text{body weight}}$$

This study did not permit the determination of bioavailability, so for the purpose of the clearance calculations it was assumed to be 100%. Statistical comparisons were made with the one-sided sign test.

RESULTS

As shown in Table 1, mean total serum carbamazepine concentrations declined during the second and third trimesters, were markedly lower at delivery, and increased during the postpartum period ($p < 0.05$). Delivery values must be interpreted cautiously for two reasons: Samples were obtained for only three patients, and two of those patients reported that at least one carbamazepine dose was missed during labor. In contrast to the parent drug, mean total epoxide levels showed no consistent change during pregnancy or the postpartum period. The epoxide/carbamazepine ratio increased in the third trimester, consistent with reports of other investigators (10). Total levels of the dihydrodiol metabolite paralleled those of the parent drug.

When free concentrations were evaluated (Table 1; Fig. 2) a somewhat different pattern was observed. Free carbamazepine concentrations declined, but to a lesser extent than total levels. The mean free epoxide concentration actually was increased by about 15% compared with postpartum values. Mean free dihy-

TABLE 1. *Carbamazepine disposition during pregnancy (mean (SD))*

	First trimester	Second trimester	Third trimester	Delivery	Postpartum
Number of patients	3	5	5	3	5
Number of samples	6	13	15	3	10
Serum carbamazepine					
Free (μg/ml)	2.0 (0.6)	1.8 (0.5)	1.8 (0.5)	1.4 (0.4)	2.0 (0.5)
Total (μg/ml)	8.7 (2.9)	7.0 (2.1)[a]	7.0 (1.7)[a]	5.5 (1.6)	8.9 (1.8)
Free fraction	0.24 (0.03)	0.25 (0.01)[a]	0.25 (0.01)[a]	0.26 (0.01)	0.22 (0.02)
Serum epoxide					
Free (μg/ml)	0.80 (0.42)	0.74 (0.39)	0.84 (0.33)	0.85 (0.47)	0.69 (0.33)
Total (μg/ml)	1.8 (1.0)	1.5 (0.9)	1.7 (0.7)	1.7 (0.7)	1.6 (0.7)
Free fraction	0.49 (0.11)	0.52 (0.04)[a]	0.50 (0.03)[a]	0.50 (0.05)	0.43 (0.03)
Serum dihydrodiol					
Free (μg/ml)	1.8 (0.2)	1.4 (0.6)	1.4 (0.5)	1.5 (0.7)	1.9 (0.5)
Total (μg/ml)	2.8 (0.5)	2.3 (0.9)	2.2 (0.6)	2.4 (1.1)	3.0 (0.9)
Free fraction	0.62 (0.03)	0.61 (0.04)	0.62 (0.06)	0.62 (0.05)	0.63 (0.03)
Expoxide/carbamazepine					
Free	0.37 (0.11)	0.42 (0.14)	0.47 (0.12)[a]	0.61 (0.28)	0.34 (0.08)
Total	0.19 (0.07)	0.20 (0.08)	0.24 (0.07)[a]	0.32 (0.13)	0.17 (0.04)
Clearance (L/h/kg)					
Plasma	0.07 (0.01)	0.09 (0.03)	0.07 (0.02)[a]	—	0.06 (0.02)
Intrinsic	0.29 (0.08)	0.30 (0.03)	0.29 (0.08)	—	0.28 (0.09)
Body weight (kg)	59 (5)	64 (6)	72 (6)[a]	—	64 (5)
Serum albumin (g/dl)	4.4 (0.1)	3.7 (0.3)[a]	3.6 (0.3)[a]	—	4.4 (0.3)

[a]Significantly different from postpartum value, $p < 0.05$, sign test.

drodiol concentrations paralleled concentrations of the parent drug, except at delivery, where data were not at steady state because of missed doses.

Free fractions of carbamazepine and the epoxide metabolite were consistently higher during pregnancy (means 0.25 and 0.50) than during the postpartum period (means 0.22 and 0.43). Second and third trimester values were significantly higher than postpartum values. The mean free fraction of the dihydrodiol was stable at ~0.62.

In order to estimate any changes in carbamazepine metabolism that might have occurred during pregnancy, we calculated plasma clearance and intrinsic clearance. Since carbamazepine is removed from the circulation almost entirely by metabolism, clearance values are proportional to the rate of metabolism.

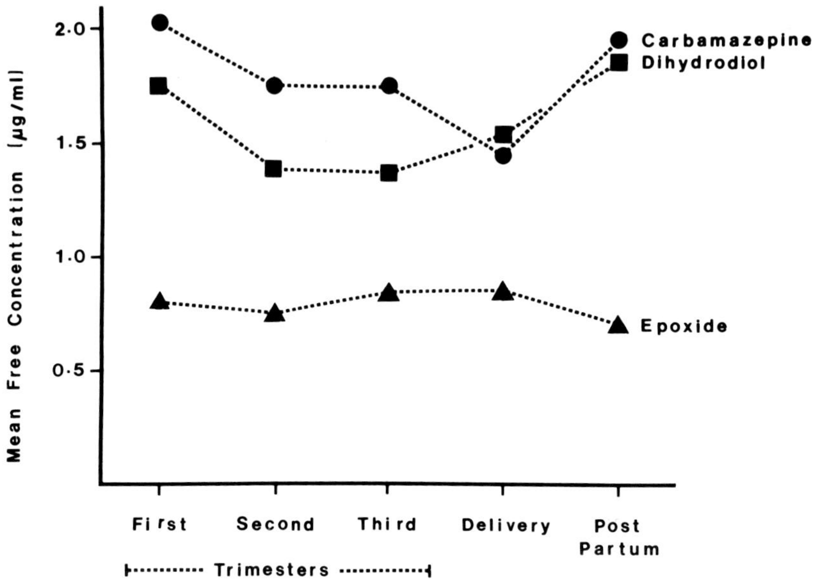

FIG. 2. Mean free concentrations of carbamazepine and its epoxide and dihydrodiol metabolites during pregnancy and delivery and to 2 months postpartum. Drug and metabolite concentrations at delivery were determined for three of five patients and were not at steady state.

TABLE 2. *Transplacental passage of carbamazepine and metabolites*

	Maternal	Neonatal cord
Total concentration (μg/ml)		
Carbamazepine	5.5 (1.6)	3.9 (0.8)
Epoxide	1.7 (0.7)	1.1 (0.3)
Dihydrodiol	2.4 (1.1)	2.4 (0.8)
Free concentration (μg/ml)		
Carbamazepine	1.4 (0.4)	1.4 (0.3)
Epoxide	0.9 (0.5)	0.7 (0.2)
Dihydrodiol	1.5 (0.7)	1.5 (0.6)
Free fraction		
Carbamazepine	0.26 (.01)	0.35 (.03)
Epoxide	0.50 (.05)	0.61 (.09)
Dihydrodiol	0.62 (.05)	0.63 (.04)

Blood samples collected at birth. Mean (SD), n = 3.

Mean plasma clearance (clearance of total drug/kg body weight) was higher during pregnancy than during the postpartum period ($p < 0.05$, third trimester versus postpartum). However, when changes in protein binding were taken into account by calculating the intrinsic clearance (clearance of free drug/kg body weight), the mean did not change appreciably during pregnancy or the postpartum period (Table 1). The intrinsic clearance values of individual patients were stable throughout pregnancy and the postpartum period in one patient, slightly higher during pregnancy in two, and slightly higher in the postpartum period in two.

The delivery values of carbamazepine and metabolites in maternal and neonatal cord serum are shown in Table 2. Maternal total levels of the parent drug and epoxide metabolite were consistently higher than neonatal levels. Free levels tended to agree more closely. The parent drug and the epoxide were less extensively bound in neonatal serum than maternal serum, but dihydrodiol binding appeared to be similar in mother and newborn.

DISCUSSION

Our pilot study confirms previous observations that the ratio of epoxide metabolite to carbamazepine concentration rises during pregnancy and falls postpartum, and that parent drug and metabolites are detectable in neonatal serum at birth (10,11). In addition, we found a small but consistent increase in the free fractions of carbamazepine and the epoxide metabolite during pregnancy. This finding is consistent with previous observations on phenobarbital and phenytoin binding during pregnancy, which appear to decrease in parallel with reductions in maternal serum albumin (12). Our results are especially useful because in contrast to most previous studies, where drugs were added in vitro to serum collected from pregnant nonepileptic women, we have measured binding in patients actually treated with the drug of interest.

Measurement of free drug concentrations allowed us to calculate the intrinsic clearance of carbamazepine, which is the best measure of clearance for highly bound drugs with low extraction ratios. Our finding of a stable mean intrinsic clearance suggests that in an "average" patient the metabolism of carbamazepine itself changes little, if any, during pregnancy.

If the intrinsic clearance of carbamazepine undergoes little or no change in pregnancy, how can the increase in the epoxide/parent drug ratio be explained? An increase in the concentration of a metabolite may be explained by an increase in production, a decrease in further metabolism, or a combined effect on production and further metabolism. In the present case, the stable intrinsic clearance of carbamazepine suggests no change in epoxide production, with a decrease in biotransformation to the dihydrodiol metabolite by epoxide hydrolase. If this is the case, one would expect epoxide and dihydrodiol levels to vary inversely; i.e., dihydrodiol levels should drop while epoxide levels rise. If, on the other hand, epoxide production is increased without a change in further biotransformation, epoxide and dihydrodiol levels should rise in parallel. As can be seen in Fig. 2, our data tend to support the concept of inhibition of epoxide hydrolase, since mean epoxide and dihydrodiol levels vary inversely. Inhibition of oxidative metabolism during pregnancy has been shown previously in the cases of antipyrine and caffeine (13,14). Inhibition of epoxide hydrolase during pregnancy, if confirmed by further studies, might have major implications for the study of antiepileptic drug-induced dysmorphogenesis, since epoxide intermediates may be embryotoxic (4).

Our findings suggest that in the "average" monotherapy patient, if carbamazepine doses are adjusted to remain constant on a mg/kg/day basis throughout pregnancy, free (and pharmacologically active) levels of the parent drug will be stable, while free levels of the epoxide metabolite will rise by ~35% by the third trimester. Since it is thought that the epoxide metabolite has pharmacological activity comparable with that of the parent compound (15), this dosing approach would result in an increase in total drug load to the patient. An alternative approach would be to maintain a constant carbamazepine dose in mg/day and monitor levels and clinical status closely throughout pregnancy. This strategy would result in a modest decrease in free carbamazepine (~15%) and a modest increase in free epoxide (~25%). One unexpected finding in this study was that at least two of our patients missed at least one carbamazepine dose during labor. Patients should be reminded that carbamazepine has a relatively short half-life, and that missed doses could result in increased risk of seizures during labor and delivery.

It should be emphasized that our findings are preliminary and based on a small sample size. The epoxide-diol metabolic pathway accounts for only 30–60% of a dose of carbamazepine during chronic therapy, so changes in other metabolic pathways cannot be ruled out. We were fortunate in being able to study a group of patients treated homogeneously with monotherapy. It is likely that the situation in pregnant patients treated with polytherapy is much more complex. We did not address bioavailability in this study. Nevertheless, we were able to describe the pattern of free carbamazepine and metabolite concentrations as they occur in typical monotherapy patients in the clinic. We are now conducting a much larger study in an attempt to replicate and expand upon the present findings.

Acknowledgment: The advice of Drs. R. H. Levy and R. E. Ramsey is gratefully acknowledged. Ms. Jane Shofer provided expert biostatistical assistance. This study was supported by NINCDS Grant No. 17111.

REFERENCES

1. Schmidt D, Canger R, Avanzini G, et al. Change of seizure frequency in pregnant epileptic women. *J Neurol Neurosurg Psychiatry* 1983;46:751–5.
2. Nau H, Kuhnz W, Egger HJ, Rating D, Helge H. Anticonvulsants during pregnancy and lactation. Transplacental, maternal and neonatal pharmacokinetics. *Clin Pharmacokinet* 1982;7:508–43.
3. Philbert A, Dam M. The epileptic mother and her child. *Epilepsia* 1982;23:85–9.
4. Lindhout D, Hoppener RJEA, Meinardi H. Teratogenicity of antiepileptic drug combinations with special emphasis on epoxidation (of carbamazepine). *Epilepsia* 1984;25:77–83.
5. Bourgeois BFD, Wad N. Carbamazepine-10,11-diol steady-state serum levels and renal excretion during carbamazepine therapy in adults and children. *Ther Drug Monit* 1984;6:259–65.
6. Sawchuk RJ, Cartier LL. Simultaneous liquid chromatographic determination of carbamazepine and its epoxide metabolite in plasma. *Clin Chem* 1982;28:2127–30.
7. Wad N. Simultaneous determination of eleven antiepileptic compounds in serum by high performance liquid chromatography. *J Chromatogr* 1984;305:127–33.
8. Levy RH, Friel PN, Johno I, et al. Filtration for free drug level monitoring: carbamazepine and valproic acid. *Ther Drug Monit* 1984;6:67–76.
9. Levy RH. General principles. Drug absorption, distribution, and elimination. In: Woodbury DM, Penry JK, Pippenger CE, eds. *Antiepileptic Drugs*. 2nd ed. New York: Raven Press, 1982:11–29.
10. Dam M, Christiansen J, Munck O, Mygind KI. Antiepileptic drugs: metabolism in pregnancy. *Clin Pharmacokinet* 1979;4:53–62.
11. Kuhnz W, Jager-Roman E, Rating D, Deichl A, Kunze J, Helge H. Carbamazepine and carbamazepine-10,11-epoxide during pregnancy and postnatal period in epileptic mothers and nursed infants: pharmacokinetics and clinical effects. *Pediatr Pharmacol* 1983;3:199–208.
12. Perucca E, Crema A. Plasma protein binding of drugs in pregnancy. *Clin Pharmacokinet* 1982;7:336–52.
13. Chiba K, Ishizaki T, Tabuchi T, Wagatsuma T, Nakazawa Y. Antipyrine disposition in relation to lowered anticonvulsant plasma level during pregnancy. *Obstet Gynecol* 1982;60:620–6.
14. Cummings AJ. A survey of pharmacokinetic data from pregnant women. *Clin Pharmacokinet* 1983;344–54.
15. Tomson T, Bertilsson L. Potent therapeutic effect of carbamazepine-10,11-epoxide in trigeminal neuralgia. *Arch Neurol* 1984;41:598–601.

Therapeutic Drug Monitoring
7:274–276 © 1985 Raven Press, New York

Carbamazepine and Carbamazepine-Epoxide Serum Protein Binding in Newborn Infants

James B. Groce III, *Daniel T. Casto, and Peter Gal

*Moses H. Cone Memorial Hospital, Greensboro Area Health Education Center, Greensboro, North Carolina; *College of Pharmacy and Department of Pediatrics, University of Texas at Austin, Austin, and University of Texas Health Science Center at San Antonio, San Antonio, Texas, U.S.A.*

Summary: To evaluate the serum protein binding of carbamazepine (CBZ) and its active metabolite carbamazepine-10,11-epoxide (CBZ-E) in newborns, cord serum was obtained from 20 infants at the time of birth. Each of the samples was spiked to concentrations of CBZ 12 + CBZ-E 3 μg/ml, and CBZ 4 + CBZ-E 1 μg/ml and then subjected to analysis for total and free drug concentrations. Total drug concentrations were determined by high pressure liquid chromatography (HPLC), and free drug concentrations were determined by ultrafiltration and subsequent HPLC. The mean percentage of CBZ unbound, calculated as (free drug concentration ÷ total drug concentration) × 100, was 30.6 and 29.8% at the high and low concentrations, respectively. Results for CBZ-E were 52.0 and 47.5% at the high and low concentrations, respectively. Compared with previously published values for protein binding in older children and adults, neonates appear to bind CBZ to a lesser degree and CBZ-E to the same degree. The lower binding of CBZ suggests that the therapeutic range of total CBZ in neonates may differ from that in older patients; however, this will have to be determined through clinical study. As previously demonstrated in older patients, CBZ and CBZ-E binding was variable. Monitoring of free CBZ serum concentrations in neonates appears advisable because of this variability. **Key Words:** Carbamazepine—Carbamazepine-10,11-epoxide—Protein binding.

Carbamazepine (CBZ) is effective in the treatment of generalized tonic-clonic and complex partial seizures in adults (1,2) and children (3,4). Optimal serum concentrations in these patient populations are purported to be 4 to 12 μg/ml (5), and it is generally recommended that doses be adjusted to achieve concentrations within this range. Although CBZ use in newborns has been limited, this agent may prove to be valuable in neonates with refractory seizures (6). In this study the serum protein binding of CBZ in neonates was examined in order to determine whether changes in the optimal therapeutic range due to altered protein binding should be considered. Additionally, we examined the protein binding of the active metabolite of CBZ, carbamazepine-10,11-epoxide (CBZ-E), which may reach concentrations of up to half those of the parent compound (7).

METHODS

From each of 20 newborn infants a 15–25 ml cord blood sample was collected at the time of birth. In all cases the delivery was vaginal and uncomplicated. Blood samples were collected with a syringe and then placed in nonheparinized blood collection tubes. Each sample was allowed to clot, centrifuged, the serum recovered and then stored in nonheparinized, stoppered glass tubes at − 20°C until the time of laboratory investigation.

Address correspondence and reprint requests to Dr. D. T. Casto at Clinical Pharmacy Programs, Department of Pharmacology, University of Texas Health Science Center, 7703 Floyd Curl Drive, San Antonio, TX 78284, U.S.A.

CBZ and CBZ-E were dissolved in HPLC grade methanol (Fisher Scientific, Inc.) to provide a stock solution containing 400 and 100 μg/ml, respectively. This solution was used to prepare a high and a low spiked sample for each serum specimen collected. High concentrations were 12 μg/ml for CBZ and 3 μg/ml for CBZ-E; low concentrations were 4 μg/ml for CBZ and 1 μg/ml for CBZ-E. An appropriate amount of stock solution was pipetted into a clean screw-cap glass culture tube, the methanol was evaporated under a stream of nitrogen, and 2.5 ml of serum was added. The tubes were capped, mixed on a rotary mixer (Scientific Industries, Inc.) for 30 min and then allowed to stand at room temperature for a minimum of an additional 60 min prior to duplicate HPLC analysis for CBZ and CBZ-E in serum and serum ultrafiltrate.

Chromatographic equipment used included a 4.6 mm × 25 cm octadecylsilane 10 μ column (Alltech Associates, Inc.), a U6K injector, M6000 solvent delivery unit, a model 440 UV detector equipped with an extended wavelength module, and a 730 Data Module (all from Waters Associates, Inc.). The mobile phase consisted of methanol and distilled, deionized water (55:45), and was pumped at a rate of 1.7 ml/min. Detection was at 214 nm and 0.02 − 0.05 AUFS.

Total CBZ and CBZ-E concentrations were determined using a modified HPLC method of Dalton et al. (8), which employs cyheptamide as an internal standard. To a glass culture tube 200 μl of serum, 300 μl of acetonitrile, and 75 μl of methanol containing cyheptamide (50 μg/ml) were added. The mixture was vortexed for 30 s, then centrifuged at 2,000 rpm for 5 min. The resulting supernatant was transferred to another tube, diluted with 3 ml of 0.01 *M* phosphate buffer (pH 4.0), and aspirated through an octadecylsilane extraction column (J. T. Baker Chemical Co.). The column was prepared by twice washing with 1 ml of methanol and twice rinsing with 1 ml of distilled, deionized water. The diluted sample was then added, the column washed with three 1 ml additions of distilled, deionized water, and after a 1–2 min drying period, the sample was finally eluted with two 75 μl additions of methanol. A 15–25 μl portion of the eluate was then injected into the chromatograph. Drug concentrations were determined by relating peak height ratios of CBZ and CBZ-E to internal standard, to those of known reference standards ranging from 0.6 to 14.4 μg/ml for CBZ and from 0.15 to 3.6 μg/ml for CBZ-E. Day-to-day coefficient of variation of the assay was ≤4.4% for CBZ at a concentration of 1.2 μg/ml and ≤6.0% for CBZ-E at a concentration of 0.3 μg/ml.

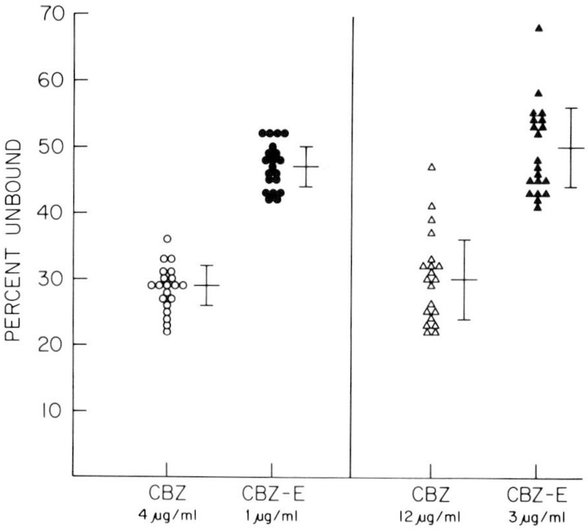

FIG. 1. Protein binding of carbamazepine (CBZ), open figures, and carbamazepine-10,11-epoxide (CBZ-E), shaded figures, in spiked cord serum. Low concentration samples are represented by circles, high concentration samples are represented by triangles.

Free drug concentrations were determined by pipetting ~1 ml of spiked serum into a Filter I ultrafiltration device (Syva Co.) and centrifuging at maximum speed (3,300 rpm) for 20 min at room temperature, in an angle-head centrifuge (Adams Dynac). The ultrafiltrate was then subjected to the same extraction procedure and HPLC analysis employed for total drug concentration, using cyheptamide 10 μg/ml as the internal standard. The free percentages of CBZ and CBZ-E were calculated as (free drug concentration ÷ total drug concentration) × 100.

RESULTS

The free percentages in cord serum at concentrations of 4 and 12 μg/ml for CBZ, and 1 and 3 μg/ml for CBZ-E are depicted in Figure 1. The mean percentage of CBZ unbound was 29.8 (range 22.0–36.2) at 4 μg/ml and 30.6 (range 22.1–47.6) at 12 μg/ml. For CBZ-E the mean free percentage was 47.5 (range 42.0–52.8) at 1 μg/ml and 52.0 (range 42.0–67.7) at 3 μg/ml. Protein binding was not statistically different at the low and high concentrations of either CBZ or CBZ-E (paired *t* test, $p > 0.05$).

DISCUSSION

The protein binding of drugs in newborns is often less than that in adults and older children (9). This difference in binding may require a modification of the optimal therapeutic range of total drug concentrations to reflect comparable concentrations of unbound drug. Results of the current investigation indicate that the protein binding of CBZ, but not of CBZ-E, is slightly different in newborns from that in older patients (10–12). The mean percentage of unbound CBZ in cord serum in our study (~30%) is somewhat greater than the mean values of 24.9% found by Lawless et al. (10) in adults and 24.3% reported by MacKichan et al. (12) in children. Our results are, however, in agreement with those of Kuhnz et al. (13) who reported a mean CBZ unbound of 31.5% in the serum of neonates, compared with 28.4% in the serum of their mothers, and 26.5% in the serum of adult volunteers. Whether the difference in protein binding of CBZ in neonates is sufficient to warrant an alteration of the usual therapeutic range for total CBZ in this age group is still unknown; this will have to be determined through clinical trials.

The percentage of CBZ-E unbound in cord serum in our study (~50%) was lower than the 61.5 ± 3.1% observed in the study of Kuhnz et al. (13). Our free percentages were similar to the value of 55.1 ± 5.0% in mothers and 49.1 ± 5.7% in the control subjects of this earlier report. Reasons for the discrepancy between the results are not readily apparent. We conducted our study at room temperature, whereas Kuhnz et al. (13) conducted their investigations at 37°C. Temperature can have a pronounced effect on drug protein binding (14), and the different conditions employed in the two studies may account for the disparate results. It is puzzling, however, that the different conditions did not provide a similar difference in the results obtained for CBZ.

Our results indicated a twofold difference in the percentage of CBZ unbound in cord blood. Some, but not all, studies conducted in older patients have previously demonstrated extensive variability in binding (10,14). For example, unbound CBZ in patients studied by Lawless et al. (10) ranged from 10 to 50% of the total serum concentration. Part of the variability noted in our study could possibly be attributable to a saturation of protein binding at higher concentrations of CBZ. Although there was no significant difference in the mean percentage unbound at the high and low concentrations, variability was greater at the high concentration, and several patients' samples showed a distinctly greater percentage unbound at the higher concentration. Based on our results, it appears that monitoring of total CBZ concentrations may not be adequate in neonates and that measurement of free-drug concentrations may be important for optimal management.

CONCLUSION

Neonates appear to bind CBZ to a slightly lesser degree than children and adults. Whether this difference in binding is of clinical significance remains to be determined. Serum protein binding of CBZ-E was not altered in the neonates we studied.

Acknowledgment: We wish to thank the labor and delivery nurses at Moses H. Cone Memorial Hospital for their assistance with collection of cord blood.

REFERENCES

1. Ramsay RE, Wilder BJ, Berger JR, Bruni J. A double-blind study comparing carbamazepine with phenytoin as initial seizure therapy in adults. *Neurology* 1983;33:904–10.
2. Pynnonen S, Sillanpaa M, Frey H, Iisalo E. Carbamazepine and its 10,11-epoxide in children and adults with epilepsy. *Eur J Clin Pharmacol* 1977;11:129–33.
3. Troupin A, Ojemann LM, Halpern L, et al. Carbamazepine—a double-blind comparison with phenytoin. *Neurology* 1977;27:511–9.
4. Sillanpaa M, Pynnonen S, Laippala P, Sako E. Carbamazepine in the treatment of partial epileptic seizures in infants and young children: a preliminary study. *Epilepsia* 1979;20:563–9.
5. Troupin A. Carbamazepine epilepsy. In: Klawans HL, ed. *Clinical Neuropharmacology*, Vol. 3. New York: Raven Press, 1978;15–40.
6. Rey E, Athis P, Lauture D, Dulac O, Aicardi J, Olive G. Pharmacokinetique de la carbamazepine chez le nouvae-ne et l'enfant. In: Olive G, Matthieu H, Pontohnier G, eds. *Pharmacologic du Development*, Vol. 89. France: Institut national de la sante et de la recherche medicale, 1979;421–34.
7. Pynnonen S, Kanto J, Sillanpaa M, Erkkola R. Carbamazepine: Placental transport, tissue concentrations in foetus of newborns, and levels in milk. *Acta Pharmacol Toxicol* 1977;41:244–53.
8. Dalton M, Powell JR, Donn K, Messinheimer J. The influence of cimetidine on single dose carbamazepine pharmacokinetics. *Epilepsia* 1985;26:127–30.
9. Morselli PL, Morselli RF, Bossi L. Clinical pharmacokinetics in newborns and infants—age related differences and therapeutic implications. *Clin Pharmacokin* 1980;5:485–627.
10. Lawless LM, DeMonaco HJ, Muido LR. Protein binding of carbamazepine in epileptic patients. *Neurology* 1982;32:415–8.
11. DiSalle E, Pacifici GM, Morselli PL. Studies on plasma protein binding of carbamazepine. *Pharmacol Res Commun* 1974;6:193–202.
12. MacKichan JJ, Duffner PK, Cohen ME. Salivary concentrations and plasma protein binding of carbamazepine and carbamazepine 10,11-epoxide in epileptic patients. *Br J Clin Pharmacol* 1981;12:31–7.
13. Kuhnz W, Steldinger R, Nau H. Protein binding of carbamazepine and its epoxide in maternal and fetal plasma at delivery: comparison to other anti-convulsants. *Dev Pharmacol Ther* 1984;7:61–72.
14. Hooper WD, Dubetz DK, Bochner F, Cotter LM, Smith GA, Eady MJ, Tyrer JH. Plasma protein binding of carbamazepine. *Clin Pharmacol Ther* 1975;17:433–40.

Therapeutic Drug Monitoring
7:277–282 © 1985 Raven Press, New York

Lateral Gaze Nystagmus in Carbamazepine-Treated Epileptic Patients: Correlation with Total and Free Plasma Concentrations of Parent Drug and Its 10,11-Epoxide Metabolite

R. Riva, M. Contin, F. Albani, *E. Perucca, G. Ambrosetto, G. Procaccianti, M. Santucci, and A. Baruzzi

*Laboratory of Neuropharmacology, Institute of Neurology, University of Bologna, Bologna, and *Institute of Medical Pharmacology, University of Pavia, Pavia, Italy*

Summary: The incidence of lateral gaze nystagmus and its correlation with free and total plasma concentrations of carbamazepine (CBZ) and carbamazepine-10,11-epoxide (CBZ-E) were examined in 97 epileptic patients receiving chronic treatment with CBZ alone (n = 54) or in combination with phenobarbital (PB) (n = 43). All patients had plasma CBZ concentrations within the clinically optimal range (<50 μmol/L). Nystagmus was seen in 26% of patients receiving monotherapy and in 33% receiving combination therapy. Within each group, however, nystagmus was much more frequent among patients with higher CBZ concentrations. For patients receiving PB in combination the CBZ levels above which nystagmus was particularly frequent appeared to be lower than in the monotherapy patients—a finding that could not be attributed to differences in plasma PB concentrations. The correlation of CBZ-E levels (or the sum of CBZ + CBZ-E) with the occurrence of nystagmus was no better than that observed with CBZ levels alone. Free drug levels did not appear to be superior to total levels in discriminating between patients with or without nystagmus. These results indicate that the occurrence of nystagmus is concentration-dependent within the therapeutic plasma CBZ concentration range and suggest that the threshold at which this neurological sign appears is reduced in the presence of PB, possibly as a result of a pharmacodynamic interaction. **Key Words:** Carbamazepine—Carbamazepine-10,11-epoxide—Nystagmus—Drug interaction.

Nystagmus is the neurological sign most frequently observed in patients taking carbamazepine (CBZ). Unless it is associated with toxic symptoms such as dizziness or diplopia, it is not generally regarded as an index of overdosage (1–3) and does not cause any subjective disturbance. In previous reports, a wide interindividual variability in the plasma CBZ concentrations at which nystagmus appears (2,4) has been indicated. This may be due to the influence of compounding factors such as the effect of comedication, concentration of the active 10,11-epoxide metabolite, patient's age, rate at which dosage is increased and duration of therapy, fluctuations in plasma drug level between time of sampling and time of assessment, wide variability in the fraction of free, pharmacologically active drug in plasma, associated disease, and pharmacodynamic variation. Despite this, in a recent study on the relationship between diurnal plasma CBZ fluctuations and transient side effects in a small group of patients, it was suggested that there may be a threshold concentration of free and total drug above which nystagmus is more likely to occur (5). Since information on this topic is largely restricted to occasional case reports or uncontrolled clinical observations, we set up a prospective investigation aimed at documenting the

Address correspondence and reprint requests to Dr. R. Riva at Laboratory of Neuropharmacology, Institute of Neurology, University of Bologna, via Foscolo 7, 40123 Bologna, Italy.

correlation between free and total CBZ and carbamazepine-10,11-epoxide (CBZ-E) concentration and appearance of nystagmus in a large population of patients.

As nystagmus is an objective measure of drug effect, we also considered that such a study would provide useful information on the theoretical but as yet unproven superiority of measuring free instead of total plasma CBZ concentrations as an indicator of a central effect.

PATIENTS AND METHODS

All patients who attended the Epilepsy Clinic of the Institute over a 6-month period were considered for the study. Inclusion criteria were: (a) chronic (>6 months) treatment with CBZ alone or in combination with phenobarbital (PB); (b) no changes in drug dosage during the preceding 4 weeks; (c) absence of associated neurological disease or other conditions interfering with the clinical examination; and (d) aged >3 years.

Details of the 97 patients (54 receiving monotherapy) who fulfilled the inclusion criteria are given in Table 1. All patients were on t.i.d. dosing schedule (8 a.m., 1 p.m., and 8 p.m.).

Blood samples were collected in heparinized tubes (8—10 I.U. heparin/ml blood) at 11 a.m., 3 h after the first daily dose, and the plasma was separated by centrifuging at 4°C within 30 min. Immediately before sampling, all patients underwent a brief neurological examination aimed at documenting possible side effects on an especially designed check-list. The evaluation criteria for nystagmus were aimed at discriminating drug-induced nystagmus from the normal physiological gaze-evoked condition. Nystagmus was considered drug-induced when observed at intermediate gaze angle or if well evident and inexhaustible at the extreme lateralities in both right and left gaze. No attempt was made to quantify the severity of nystagmus. All examinations were carried out by the same neurologist, who was unaware of drug dosage and plasma drug levels. The plasma was stored immediately at −20°C and analyzed within 2 weeks. This collection and storage procedure does not alter plasma CBZ and CBZ-E binding (unpublished observations).

Plasma filtrates (300 μl) were obtained at 25°C in duplicate from 1 ml plasma aliquots by using the Free Level System (Syva, Palo Alto, CA, U.S.A.) according to the procedure recommended by the manufacturer.

The concentrations of CBZ and CBZ-E in whole plasma (for total levels) and plasma filtrates (for free levels) were determined in each sample by high performance liquid chromatography (HPLC) (6). Statistical analysis was carried out by using the Student's *t* test or the χ^2 test whenever appropriate.

RESULTS

Among the patients included in the study, 54 were receiving CBZ alone (monotherapy group) and 43 CBZ + PB (polytherapy). Twenty-eight patients showed a lateral gaze nystagmus (monotherapy group, 26%; polytherapy group, 33%; $p < 0.05$). In two patients (one receiving CBZ alone) nystagmus was associated with diplopia. The remaining 69 patients were apparently free of side effects.

Within both groups the CBZ dosage in the patients with nystagmus was similar to that in the patients

TABLE 1. *Details of the patients included in the study*

	Patients without nystagmus		Patients with nystagmus	
	CBZ alone	CBZ + PB	CBZ alone	CBZ + PB
Sex	19 men, 21 women	14 men, 15 women	9 men, 5 women	11 men, 3 women
Age (yr)	24.4 ± 17.9	23.4 ± 15.7	23.3 ± 15.1	27.8 ± 15.3
CBZ dose (mg/kg/day)	14.2 ± 5.5	14.3 ± 4.3	13.6 ± 2.6	17.0 ± 4.0
Total CBZ concentration (μmol/L)	29.4 ± 6.9[a]	26.7 ± 6.9[b]	35.0 ± 6.3	33.7 ± 9.2
Free CBZ concentration (μmol/L)	5.1 ± 1.3[a]	4.5 ± 1.1[b]	6.3 ± 1.5	5.9 ± 1.5
Total CBZ-E concentration (μmol/L)	4.8 ± 1.3	5.1 ± 1.6[b]	5.5 ± 1.8	6.6 ± 1.8
Free CBZ-E concentration (μmol/L)	1.8 ± 0.6	1.9 ± 0.5[b]	2.1 ± 0.7	2.5 ± 0.7

Values are means ± SD.
[a] $p < 0.05$ vs. patients with nystagmus.
[b] $p < 0.01$ vs. patients with nystagmus.

without nystagmus whereas total and free plasma CBZ concentrations were slightly but significantly higher in the former (Table 1). The free and total CBZ-E concentrations were higher in the patients with nystagmus only in the polytherapy group (Table 1). To determine whether the frequency of nystagmus was related to drug or metabolite concentrations, patients were divided into three groups according to the plasma level of the compound in question. The ranges used were determined empirically, i.e., for each group of patients (mono- or polytherapy) mean concentrations were calculated for subjects with or without nystagmus (as shown in Table 1, mean values were invariably higher for the subjects with nystagmus).

For each group the two mean values were used to identify three subgroups: A, subjects with levels below the lower mean value; B, subjects with levels between the two mean values; C, subjects with levels above the upper mean value.

When total CBZ concentrations were considered (Fig. 1), the frequency of nystagmus was found to be significantly ($p < 0.05$) higher in group C (50%) as compared to groups A and B (16% in both) for monotherapy patients and in groups B and C (50% in both) as compared to group A (10%) for polytherapy patients. The frequency of nystagmus was significantly ($p < 0.05$) higher in group B patients receiving polytherapy than in group B patients receiving monotherapy (50 vs. 16%, respectively) despite CBZ concentrations being lower in patients receiving polytherapy.

When free levels were considered (Fig. 1), nystagmus was also found to be more frequent in the patients receiving monotherapy with the highest concentrations (group C) than in the other two monotherapy groups (54 vs. 18 and 19%, respectively, $p < 0.05$). Among patients receiving polytherapy, nystagmus increased gradually with increasing free CBZ concentrations (group A, 11%; group B, 37%; group C, 67%; $p < 0.05$ for group C vs. A).

Among monotherapy patients, neither total nor free CBZ-E levels appeared to correlate with the frequency of nystagmus (Fig. 2). Among polytherapy patients the frequency of nystagmus tended to increase with increasing CBZ-E concentrations (16% at low, 33% at intermediate, and 65% at high concentrations, $p < 0.01$ for high vs. low). It should be noted, however, that in both the mono- and the polytherapy groups, CBZ-E concentrations correlated positively with CBZ concentrations ($r = 0.80$ and 0.70, respectively). When the sums of CBZ and CBZ-E were considered, the relationship to the frequency of nystagmus was similar but slightly less clear cut than that observed for CBZ alone (data not shown). A meaningful comparison of the relative frequency of nystagmus at different CBZ concentrations in polytherapy patients requires evaluation of the plasma PB levels in the various subgroups.

Phenobarbital levels (see figure legends) were similar in all subgroups considered. Invariably, no relationship was found between plasma PB and nystagmus. In fact, within all subgroups, PB levels in patients with nystagmus were similar to those in patients without nystagmus.

Overall, mean PB levels ($\pm$ SD) in patients with and without nystagmus were 102 ± 30 and 96 ± 33 μmol/L, respectively.

DISCUSSION

Although clinically important adverse effects (ataxia, diplopia, dizziness, etc.) are usually associated with high plasma CBZ levels (over 50 μmol/L), nystagmus has been reported to occur at levels as low as 6 μmol/L (2,7). In our study we found a positive relationship between plasma CBZ concentrations within the clinically occurring range and the presence of nystagmus. Although one group of patients was receiving PB, it is unlikely that PB itself was directly responsible for the nystagmus since there was clearly no relationship between this sign and blood levels of PB. On the other hand, nystagmus was relatively infrequent at lower CBZ levels (~15% irrespective of presence or absence of PB), but it was seen in as many as 50% of the patients in the subgroups with the highest CBZ levels. Since nystagmus was not instrumentally recorded, the possible correlation between the severity of this sign and drug plasma concentrations could not be established. Overall, the incidence of nystagmus was quite considerable (30%) and in good agreement with previously reported estimates (1). These data are particularly interesting when it is considered that our population was representative of chronically treated, brain-undamaged patients whose plasma CBZ level distribution was not dictated by chance but rather by the clinician's skill aided by regular drug monitoring. Previous optimization of therapy explains why all patients had therapeutic plasma levels (<50 μmol/L) and only two showed clinically relevant signs of toxicity. An additional explanation for the lack of toxicity lies in the fact that the assessment was made in the morning whereas, due to diurnal fluctuations in plasma CBZ concentrations, transient side effects tend to occur later in the day (5,8).

Although the overall frequency of nystagmus was only slightly increased in the comedication group,

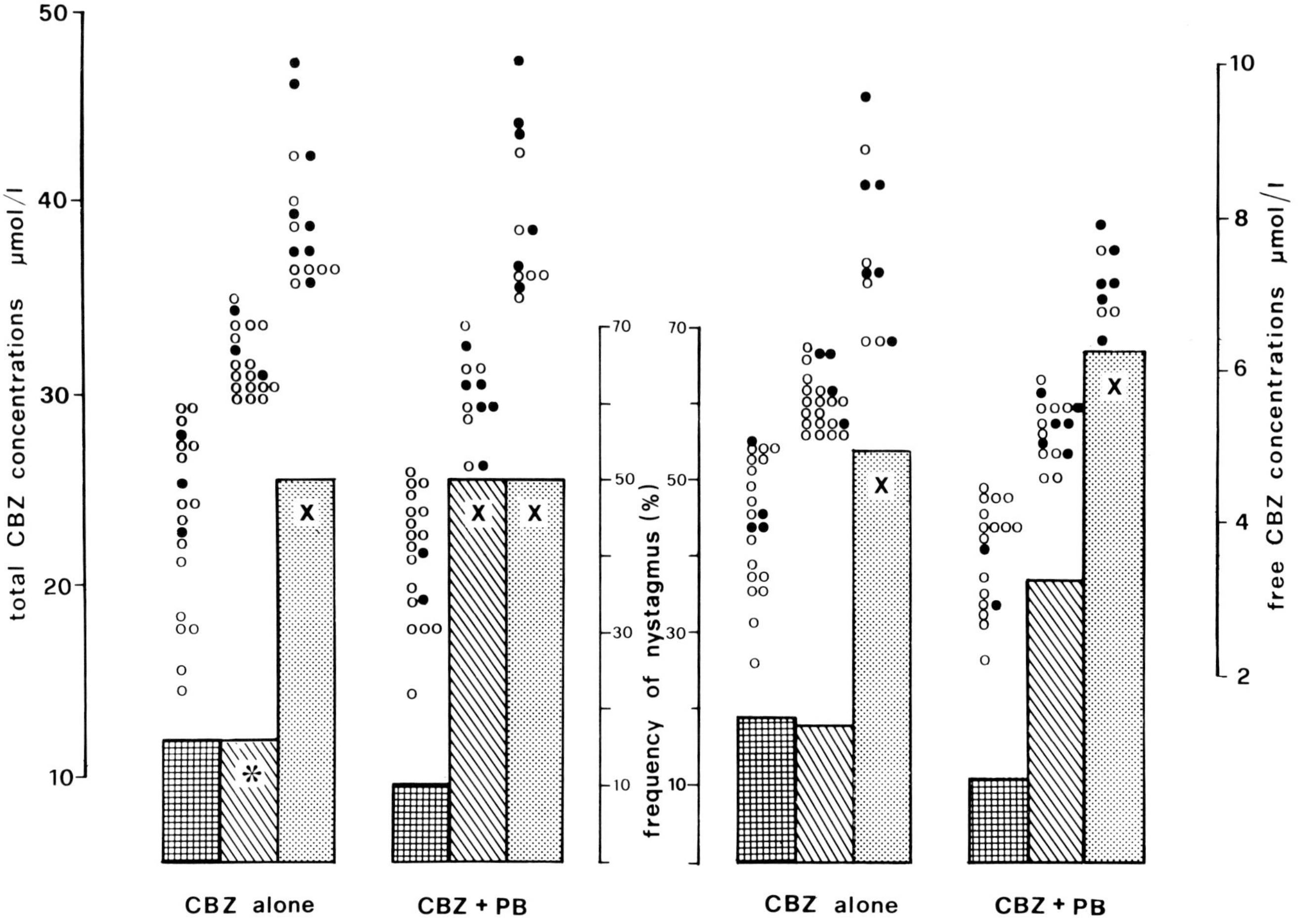

FIG. 1. Relationship between total (left) and free (right) plasma CBZ concentrations and lateral gaze nystagmus. Bars indicate the percentage of subjects showing nystagmus in subgroups with lower (squared bars), intermediate (lined bars), and higher (shaded bars) concentrations [see text for explanation of the concentration ranges]. Symbols indicate individual concentration values (filled and open circles identify patients with or without nystagmus, respectively). X, $p < 0.05$ vs. frequency of nystagmus at lower levels (except for free concentrations in CBZ + PB subgroup in which the frequency of nystagmus is significantly higher only vs. subgroup A); *, $p < 0.05$ vs. frequency of nystagmus in the same subgroup of the CBZ + PB group. The mean PB concentrations (± SD) in the polytherapy subgroups with lower, intermediate and higher CBZ levels were 110 ± 38, 89 ± 29, and 89 ± 18 µmol/L, respectively (groups divided according to total CBZ levels) or 105 ± 38, 97 ± 36, and 92 ± 18 µmol/L, respectively (groups divided according to free CBZ levels).

some evidence for an interactive effect of PB was found. As shown in Fig. 1, the threshold CBZ level above which the incidence of nystagmus appeared to be particularly frequent was lower in patients receiving PB in combination than in those receiving monotherapy. Although the criteria used to divide patients into subgroups were somewhat arbitrary, it should be noted that the cut-off limits of CBZ levels for each subgroup were lower in patients receiving CBZ and PB than in those treated with CBZ alone. This strengthens the evidence for a lower threshold for nystagmus in the polytherapy group.

A reduced tolerability to CBZ in patients receiving other antiepileptic drugs was reported previously by Masland (3), whereas Kutt et al. (1) noted that the toxic effects of CBZ were enhanced at phenytoin concentrations above 80 µmol/L. Our finding of a lower nystagmus threshold in the comedication group confirms these observations, although it should be stressed that by itself nystagmus cannot be regarded as a toxic effect. The apparently increased sensitivity to nystagmus in patients taking PB and CBZ could be explained by a pharmacokinetic and/or pharmacodynamic interaction between these two drugs. A pharmacodynamic interaction is plausible since PB itself can induce nystagmus, especially at toxic concentrations (9). Although our patients had PB concentrations in the range of 40–130 µmol/L and, as discussed herein, PB was

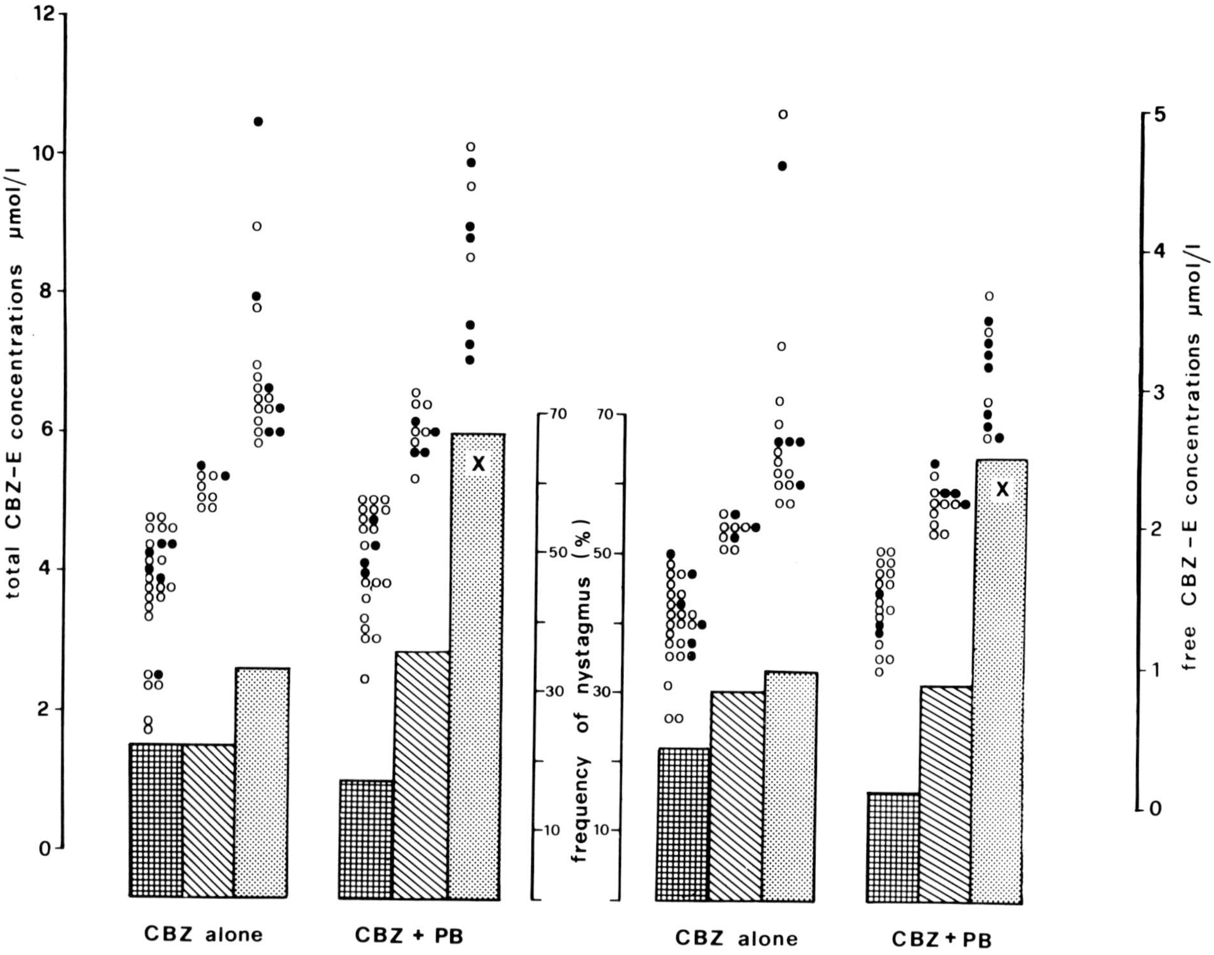

FIG. 2. Relationship between total and free plasma CBZ-E concentrations and lateral gaze nystagmus. Bars indicate the percentage of subjects showing nystagmus in each concentration subgroup. For explanation of bars and symbols see the legend for Fig. 1. X, $p < 0.01$ vs. frequency of nystagmus in subgroup A. The mean PB concentrations (± SD) in the polytherapy subgroups with lower, intermediate, and higher CBZ-E levels were 103 ± 32, 94 ± 31, and 92 ± 20 µmol/L, respectively (groups divided according to total CBZ-E levels) or 108 ± 35, 94 ± 36, and 93 ± 22 µmol/L, respectively (groups divided according to free CBZ-E levels).

unlikely to cause the nystagmus directly, it is possible that PB contributed to the sign by adding to or facilitating CBZ action. At the pharmacokinetic level, PB is known to induce CBZ metabolism and to decrease the ratio between parent drug and its possibly active 10,11-epoxide metabolite in plasma. For this reason, some investigators postulated that CBZ-E might play a significant role in determining the difference in CBZ plasma level-effect relationship between patients receiving monotherapy and patients receiving polytherapy (10). The contribution of CBZ-E to the overall CBZ effect in epileptic patients, however, is still unproved (8) even though the compound is active in trigeminal neuralgia (11) and increased toxicity has recently been reported in patients with abnormally high plasma CBZ-E levels, e.g., during comedication with valpromide (12).

A role of CBZ-E in precipitating signs of CBZ toxicity in comedicated patients was postulated recently by Schoeman et al. (13). The side effects observed by these investigators, however, could have been ascribed easily to associated drugs, including valproic acid (14), and no proof for a direct role of the CBZ metabolite was provided. In our own study, we found no evidence that CBZ-E contributed to the lower nystagmus threshold in PB-treated patients. In fact, CBZ-E concentrations for groups B in Fig. 1 were similar in patients receiving CBZ alone and in those receiving CBZ + PB (total values 5.2 ± 0.8 vs. 5.6 ± 1.3 µmol/L, respectively; mean ± SD) although the frequency of nystagmus was significantly different. Moreover in the monotherapy group CBZ-E concentrations seemed to be unrelated to the frequency of nystagmus. Although these data argue against a role of CBZ-E in the pathogenesis of nystagmus, a definitive conclusion cannot be drawn because the concentrations of the metabolite correlated with those of CBZ. A precise estimate of the activity of the epoxide will be obtained only by direct administration of the compound itself. In this respect, it is of interest that Tomson and Bertilsson (11) found no evidence of side effects in patients with trigeminal neuralgia given CBZ-E at dosages yielding plasma levels up to 12 μmol/L.

As far as free level monitoring is concerned, inspection of Figs. 1 and 2 shows that for both CBZ and CBZ-E results were virtually superimposable to those obtained with total levels. Although there was a trend for free CBZ levels to show less overlap between patients with nystagmus and those without nystagmus in the polytherapy group, the difference was slight and overall free concentrations did not appear to be superior to total concentrations in discriminating between the presence or absence of the sign. It should be noted, however, that the correlation of free and total CBZ and CBZ-E levels with other central effects (e.g., toxic or therapeutic) and the influence of comedication may be different from that observed with nystagmus.

In conclusion, the results of this study indicate that (a) the occurrence of lateral gaze nystagmus is concentration-dependent within the clinically optimal range of CBZ levels. No evidence for a role of CBZ-E in the pathogenesis of nystagmus could be found; (b) free CBZ levels do not appear to be superior to total CBZ concentrations in discriminating between affected and nonaffected patients; (c) nystagmus tends to develop at lower CBZ levels in patients taking both PB and CBZ than in those taking CBZ alone. Further studies, preferably supplemented by quantitative electronystagmographic recording, will be required to confirm and clarify the nature of the potentiating action of associated drugs.

Acknowledgment: This work was part of the "Progetto Finalizzato Medicina Preventiva e Riabilitativa" of the National Research Council of Italy, Grant N.83.02528.56. We appreciate the excellent technical assistance provided by Miss C. Tonello and Mrs. E. Zoni.

REFERENCES

1. Kutt H, Solomon G, Wasterlain C, Peterson H, Louis S, Carruthers R. Carbamazepine in difficult to control epileptic out-patients. *Acta Neurol Scand* 1975;60(suppl):27–32.
2. Meinardi DL. Other antiepileptic drugs: carbamazepine. In: Woodbury DM, Penry JK, Schmidt RP, eds. *Antiepileptic Drugs, 1st ed.* New York: Raven Press, 1973:487–96.
3. Masland RL. Carbamazepine: neurotoxicity. In: Woodbury DM, Penry JK, Pippenger CE, eds. *Antiepileptic Drugs, 2nd ed.* New York: Raven Press, 1982;521–31.
4. Kutt H. Use of blood levels of anticonvulsant drugs in clinical practice. *Pediatrics* 1974;53:557–60.
5. Riva R, Albani F, Ambrosetto G, Contin M, Cortelli P, Perucca E, Baruzzi A. Diurnal fluctuations in free and total steady state plasma levels of carbamazepine and correlation with intermittent side effects. *Epilepsia* 1984;25:476–81.
6. Contin M, Riva R, Albani F, Perucca E, Baruzzi A. Determination of total and free plasma carbamazepine concentrations by enzyme multiplied immunoassay: interference with the 10,11-epoxide metabolite. *Ther Drug Monit* 1985;7:46–50.
7. Schneider H. Carbamazepine: an attempt to correlate serum levels with antiepileptic and side effects. In: Schneider H, Janz D, Gardner-Thorpe, Meinardi H, Sherwin AL, eds. *Clinical Pharmacology of Antiepileptic Drugs.* New York: Springer-Verlag, 1975;151–8.
8. Riva R, Contin M, Albani F, et al. Free and total plasma concentrations of carbamazepine and carbamazepine 10-11-epoxide in epileptic patients: diurnal fluctuations and relationship with side effects. *Ther Drug Monit* 1984,6:408–13.
9. Mattson RH, Cramer JA. Phenobarbital toxicity. In: Woodbury DM, Penry JK, Pippenger CE, eds. *Antiepileptic drugs, 2nd ed.* New York: Raven Press, 1982;351–63.
10. Hvidberg EF, Dam M. Clinical pharmacokinetics of anticonvulsants. *Clin Pharmacokinet* 1976;1:161–88.
11. Tomson T, Bertilsson L. Potent therapeutic effect of carbamazepine-10,11-epoxide in trigeminal neuralgia. *Arch Neurol* 1984;41:598–601.
12. Meijer JWA, Binnie CD, Debets RM Chr, Van Parys JAP, deBeer-Pawlikowski NKB. Possible hazard of valpromide-carbamazepine combination therapy in epilepsy. *Lancet* 1984;1:802.
13. Schoeman JF, Elyas AA, Brett EM, Lascelles PT. Correlation between plasma carbamazepine-10,11-epoxide concentration and drug side-effects in children with epilepsy. *Dev Med Child Neurol* 1984;26:756–64.
14. Zaccara G, Paganini M, Campostrini R, et al. Effect of associated antiepileptic treatment on valproate-induced hyperammonemia. *Ther Drug Monit* 1985;7: in press.

Therapeutic Drug Monitoring
7:283–289 © 1985 Raven Press, New York

Extent of Urinary Excretion of *p*-Hydroxyphenytoin in Healthy Subjects Given Phenytoin

R. G. Dickinson, W. D. Hooper, M. Patterson, M. J. Eadie, and *B. Maguire

*Department of Medicine, University of Queensland, Brisbane, and *Parke-Davis Pty. Ltd., Sydney, Australia*

Summary: Urinary excretion of *p*-hydroxyphenytoin and its glucuronide conjugate was measured in eight healthy young adults in a comparative bioavailability study of oral sodium phenytoin (~5 mg/kg/dose). Among these subjects the percentage of the phenytoin dose converted to *p*-hydroxyphenytoin and appearing in urine was relatively similar (mean 79%, range 67–88%). The great majority of the *p*-hydroxyphenytoin appeared in urine as conjugates; only 1.4–3.4% of the excreted *p*-hydroxyphenytoin was in the form of unconjugated metabolite. The proportion of a single phenytoin dose excreted in urine as *p*-hydroxyphenytoin or its conjugate increased from the first dose (mean ± SD) 74.9 ± 4.6% to the second dose, given 2 weeks later 79.3 ± 4.6% ($p < 0.05$). This finding suggests that autoinduction of phenytoin metabolism may occur after relatively brief exposure to the drug. **Key Words:** Autoinduction—Bioavailability—Metabolism—Phenytoin.

It is generally accepted that *p*-hydroxyphenytoin (*p*-HPPH), 5-(*p*-hydroxyphenyl)-5-phenylhydantoin, is the major metabolic product of the anticonvulsant phenytoin in several animal species, including humans (1). There have been a number of published measurements of the extent of conversion of phenytoin to *p*-HPPH in humans (Table 1). Many of these measurements were made under presumedly steady-state conditions in patients taking the drug for epilepsy. Some of the published figures show considerable intersubject variation in the extent of *p*-HPPH formation, which may in part reflect the variety of circumstances under which the measurements were made, e.g., different subject ages and different concurrent medications. Sometimes clear distinctions were not drawn between the phase I metabolite, *p*-HPPH, and its phase II glucuronide conjugate, which is the main metabolite excreted in urine.

Address correspondence and reprint requests to Prof. M. J. Eadie at University of Queensland Department of Medicine, Clinical Sciences Building, Royal Brisbane Hospital, Herston, Brisbane, Australia 4029.

During an oral bioavailability study of conventional design comparing batches of phenytoin sodium prepared to conform to British Pharmacopoeal specifications, on the one hand, and to United States Pharmacopoeal specifications, on the other, we have taken the opportunity to study quantitative aspects of the formation of *p*-HPPH from phenytoin in a relatively homogeneous population of noncomedicated healthy young adult volunteers. It was hoped that such a study would yield useful reference values for the extent of formation of *p*-HPPH in the young healthy adult, as well as providing support for any conclusions drawn about oral phenytoin bioavailability from analysis of the plasma concentration–time data.

MATERIALS AND METHODS

Subjects

Studies were carried out in eight healthy young adult volunteers (six men, two women) who gave informed consent to participation in the investigation, which had been approved by the University of

TABLE 1. *Published data on percentage of phenytoin dose excreted in urine as* p*-hydroxyphenytoin (unconjugated and conjugated)*

Authors	Number of subjects	Phenytoin dose	Circumstances of study	Percentage excreted as *p*-HPPH
Eadie et al. (2)	4 adults (3 possible slow metabolizers)	100–500 mg/day p.o.	Steady-state measurements after different doses in the same subject	30–80% (tended to fall with increasing dose)
Kutt et al. (3)	3 slow metabolizers and 4 controls	1.4–7.3 mg/kg p.o.	Steady state	48%, 49.3%, 54%—slow metabolizers; 60.5–73.26%—controls
Glazko et al. (4)	5 adults	250 mg i.v.	Single dose	Mean 76% (65–81%)
Mascher and Bernhardt (5)	—	—	—	Mean 60%
Borofsky et al. (6)	8 children (5–17 yr)	3.5–7.5 mg/kg/day p.o.	Steady-state normals	Mean 72% (59–88%)
	7 subjects (2–20 yr) with unusual plasma phenytoin levels relative to dose	3.1–14.7 mg/kg/day p.o.	Steady state	28, 44%; 86%; 91%; 40%; 27%; 64%; 65%
Karlen et al. (7)	2	4 mg/kg/day p.o.	Steady state	Mean 81%
Bochner et al. (8)	3 subjects (2 controls and 1 slow metabolizer)	p.o.	Single dose	95%, 70%, 45%[a]
Borga et al. (9)	4 adults	100 mg/day p.o.	Steady state	Mean 77% (52–94%)
Witkin et al. (10)	3 adults	300–400 mg/day p.o.	Steady state	62%, 72%, 17%
Landon and Kirkley (11)	5 pregnant women	100–400 mg/day p.o.	Steady state	Mean 38%
Kochenour et al. (12)	5 postpartum women	p.o.	Steady state	60 ± 20%
Glazko et al. (13)	4 long half-life and 5 short half-life volunteers	300 mg/day p.o.	Steady state (after 14 days)	Mean 64.9%—long half-life; mean 75.5%—short half-life
Present study	8 adults	5 mg/kg p.o.	Single dose	Mean 79% (67–88%)

[a]Value for slow metabolizer.

Queensland's Human and Animal Experimentation Ethics Committee. Details concerning individual subjects are provided in Table 2. No subject took any concurrent medication and all subjects abstained from consumption of alcoholic beverages during the studies.

Investigational Protocol

Each subject was studied twice, at 2 week intervals. On one occasion the subject received sodium phenytoin manufactured to British Pharmacopoeal (B.P.) specifications and contained in 100-mg capsules. On the other occasion the subject received sodium phenytoin manufactured to United States Pharmacopoeal (U.S.P.) specifications, again supplied in 100-mg capsules. Each subject received the number of 100-mg capsules that most nearly provided him or her with a sodium phenytoin intake of 5 mg/kg body weight. The order of administration of the two preparations was arranged so that

TABLE 2. *Personal data of individual subjects studied*

				Sodium phenytoin dose		Order of administration	
Subject	Age (yr)	Sex	Weight (kg)	(mg)	(mg/kg)	B.P.	U.S.P.
A	23	M	90	500	5.55	1	2
B	25	M	84	400	4.76	1	2
C	23	M	79	400	5.06	1	2
D	24	F	61	300	4.92	1	2
E	23	F	46	200	4.08	2	1
F	23	M	84	400	4.76	2	1
G	23	M	74	400	5.41	2	1
H	23	M	75	400	5.33	2	1

B.P., British Pharmacopoeal preparation; U.S.P., United States Pharmacopoeal preparation.

TABLE 3. *Individual $AUC_{0\rightarrow 80}$ and $AUC_{0\rightarrow\infty}$ values (mg L^{-1} h) for the plasma concentration–time data for each subject in each study*

	Subject								
	A	B	C	D	E	F	G	H	Mean curve
B.P.									
$AUC_{0\rightarrow 80}$	212.315	157.425	180.536	217.700	126.800	216.275	130.164	183.050	177.956
$AUC_{0\rightarrow\infty}$	221.918	164.832	190.319	231.009	129.859	249.832	131.175	194.178	186.576
U.S.P.									
$AUC_{0\rightarrow 80}$	193.029	153.150	154.875	172.450	129.875	219.875	121.555	163.875	166.840
$AUC_{0\rightarrow\infty}$	205.390	158.752	160.374	189.342	131.847	231.134	122.526	175.003	175.496

$AUC_{0\rightarrow 80}$, Area under concentration–time curve for period from 0 to 80 h; $AUC_{0\rightarrow\infty}$, AUC for period from 0 h to infinity; other abbreviations as in Table 2.

half the subjects took the B.P. preparation first, and the other half took the U.S.P. preparation first. Details of the actual dosages and orders of administration are provided in Table 2. The mean dose (± SD) was 4.98 ± 0.47 mg/kg.

After an overnight fast, each subject took the oral phenytoin dose at 8 a.m. A light breakfast was eaten 2 h later. Thereafter subjects followed their normal patterns of activity and food intake over the 80-h study period. Venous blood was collected from the forearm for phenytoin assay at the following times: 0, 0.5, 1.0, 1.5, 2, 3, 4, 6, 8, 12, 24, 32, 48, 56, 72, and 80 h. All urine passed was collected separately over the following intervals: 0–8, 8–16, 16–24, 24–48, and 48–80 h.

Assay of Phenytoin in Plasma

To 1 ml plasma in Teflon-lined, screw-capped glass test tubes was added 100 μl hydrochloric acid (0.2 *M*) and 5 ml chloroform containing 10 μg of the internal standard 5-phenyl-5(*p*-tolyl) hydantoin (TPH). The tubes were shaken for 30 s and centrifuged at 1,000 *g* for 2 min; the upper aqueous layer was then aspirated to waste. The chloroform was transferred to a clean tapered test tube, and evaporated to dryness under a stream of nitrogen. The residue was reconstituted in 50–100 μl methanol, and 20 μl was injected onto a high performance liquid chromatography (HPLC) system comprising a Tracor model 950 pump, a Rheodyne 7120 injector, a Waters μBondapak C-18 column (10 μm), a Tracor model 970 A variable wavelength UV detector, and a Shimadzu R-201 strip chart recorder. The mobile phase was acetonitrile–water (40:60) at a flow rate of 1 ml/min, and the relevant peaks, which were detected at 215 nm, eluted at 6.5 (phenytoin) and 8.5 min (TPH).

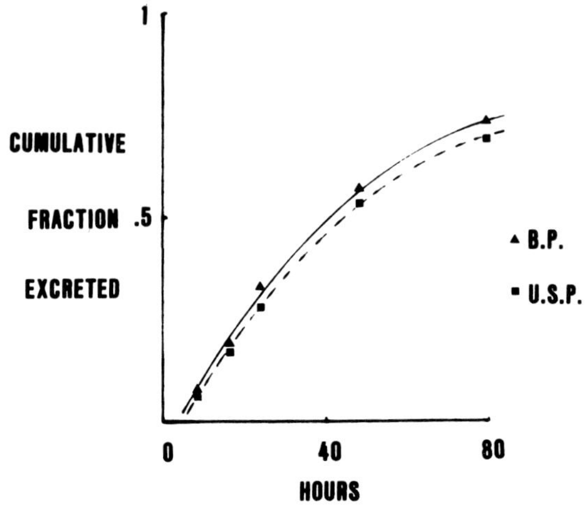

FIG. 1. Plot of mean cumulative excretion of *p*-hydroxyphenytoin (unconjugated plus conjugated), expressed as a molar fraction of the original phenytoin dose, versus time. B.P., British Pharmacopoeal preparation; U.S.P., United States Pharmacopoeal preparation.

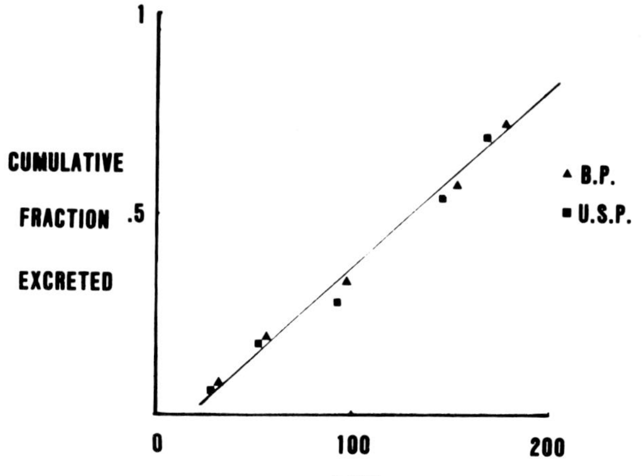

FIG. 2. Plot of mean cumulative excretion of *p*-hydroxyphenytoin (conjugated plus unconjugated), expressed as a molar fraction of the original phenytoin dose, versus area under the plasma phenytoin concentration–time curve (AUC) from time zero to *t*. Abbreviations as in Fig. 1.

TABLE 4. *Individual subject data for fraction of phenytoin dose excreted in urine as unconjugated* p-*hydroxyphenytoin* (p-*HPPH*) *(a), conjugated* p-*HPPH (b), and total* p-*HPPH (c) as a function of time*

	Subject[a]														
	A			B			C			D			E		
Time (h)	a	b	c	a	b	c	a	b	c	a	b	c	a	b	c
B.P. sodium phenytoin															
0–8	0.001	0.086	0.087	0.002	0.080	0.082	0.001	0.046	0.047	0.001	0.027	0.028	0.001	0.125	0.126
8–16	0.001	0.103	0.104	0.003	0.113	0.116	0.001	0.111	0.112	0.001	0.052	0.053	—	—	—
16–24	0.002	0.135	0.137	—	—	—	0.002	0.139	0.141	0.002	0.139	0.141	0.001	0.168	0.169
24–48	0.003	0.236	0.239	0.005	0.278	0.283	0.003	0.270	0.273	0.007	0.232	0.239	0.002	0.262	0.264
48–80	0.002	0.128	0.130	0.002	0.124	0.126	0.003	0.168	0.171	0.003	0.159	0.162	0.000	0.152	0.152
80–∞	0.003	0.031	0.034	0.001	0.028	0.029	0.000	0.040	0.040	0.001	0.049	0.050	0.000	0.017	0.017
Total	0.012	0.719	0.731	>0.013	>0.623	>0.636	0.010	0.774	0.784	0.015	0.658	0.673	>0.004	>0.724	>0.728
U.S.P. sodium phenytoin															
0–8	0.001	0.050	0.051	0.003	0.049	0.052	0.002	0.079	0.081	0.002	0.058	0.060	0.001	0.059	0.060
8–16	{0.005	0.229	0.234}	0.003	0.084	0.087	0.001	0.110	0.111	0.002	0.113	0.115	0.001	0.112	0.113
16–24				0.004	0.092	0.096	0.001	0.140	0.141	0.001	0.069	0.070	0.002	0.121	0.123
24–48	0.005	0.272	0.277	—	—	—	0.004	0.258	0.262	0.006	0.271	0.277	0.003	0.296	0.299
48–80	0.003	0.122	0.125	0.007	0.126	0.133	0.006	0.173	0.179	0.007	0.203	0.210	0.000	0.089	0.089
80–∞	0.001	0.043	0.044	0.000	0.013	0.013	0.000	0.027	0.027	0.002	0.070	0.072	0.000	0.010	0.010
Total	0.015	0.716	0.731	>0.010	>0.371	>0.381	0.014	0.787	0.801	0.020	0.784	0.804	0.007	0.687	0.694

B.P., British Pharmacopoeal preparation; U.S.P., United States Pharmacopoeal preparation.
[a]For order of administration see Table 2.
[b]Means were calculated only for subjects for whom data collection was complete.

Assay of Phenytoin and *p*-HPPH in Urine

Urinary phenytoin and unconjugated *p*-HPPH concentrations were assayed concurrently, using a minor modification of the above procedure. This involved the substitution of ethyl acetate for chloroform and of 0.2 ml acetate buffer (0.1 *M*, pH 5) for hydrochloric acid, to make the procedure equivalent to that used for total *p*-HPPH assay. The *p*-HPPH eluted at 5 min.

Total urinary *p*-HPPH was assayed by a similar procedure after hydrolysis of the conjugated *p*-HPPH using β-glucuronidase. In this instance 100 μl methanol solution containing 10 μg TPH was added to the assay tube and the methanol was removed under nitrogen. An aliquot (generally 200 μl) of urine was added, then 200 μl acetate buffer (0.1 *M*, pH 5) and ~1,000 units β-glucuronidase. The solution was incubated at 37°C for a minimum of 4 h, but usually overnight. Ethyl acetate (5 ml) was added, and the sample was thereafter handled exactly as for the plasma phenytoin assay described above.

Data Analysis

Plasma concentration–time data were fitted to one- and two-compartment linear pharmacokinetic models with first-order absorption and a lag time. For all subjects a two-compartment model yielded better fits than a one-compartment model. Hence the equation finally fitted to the plasma concentration–time data was of the form

$$C = ae^{-\alpha t} + be^{-\beta t} - ce^{-\gamma t}.$$

The plasma concentration–time data were analyzed on a microcomputer by the least-squares iterative curve-fitting program MULTI (14). The area under the plasma concentration–time curve over the period of measurement ($AUC_{0\rightarrow 80}$) was calculated by trapezoidal-rule integration (taking cognizance of the absorption lag time), and $AUC_{0\rightarrow\infty}$ by adding to $AUC_{0\rightarrow 80}$ the value of $AUC_{80\rightarrow\infty}$ ($= C_{80/\beta}$). It was recognized that the elimination kinetics of phenytoin are better described by Michaelis–Menten than by linear kinetics. However, there are major difficulties in calculating accurate Michaelis–Menten parameter values from concentration–time data obtained after a single dose of phenytoin (15). Therefore it was decided to work with a phenytoin dose low enough to provide peak plasma phenytoin levels below the likely K_m values for the drug. In these circumstances linear kinetics have a better chance of approximating the true situation than if higher plasma phenytoin levels are used.

Rates of urinary excretion of *p*-HPPH and *p*-HPPH glucuronide were calculated as molar fractions of the administered phenytoin dose, with corrections for bioavailability differences and for incomplete late-stage collections of metabolites (as explained below in Results).

TABLE 4. *(contd.)*

Subject[a]											
F			G			H			Mean ± SD[b]		
a	b	c	a	b	c	a	b	c	a	b	c
B.P. sodium phenytoin *(contd.)*											
0.001	0.068	0.069	0.003	0.092	0.095	0.002	0.064	0.066	0.002 ± 0.001	0.074 ± 0.030	0.075 ± 0.030
0.002	0.082	0.084	0.009	0.236	0.245	0.002	0.100	0.102	0.003 ± 0.003	0.114 ± 0.058	0.117 ± 0.061
0.003	0.104	0.107	0.002	0.095	0.097	0.002	0.147	0.149	0.002 ± 0.001	0.132 ± 0.025	0.134 ± 0.025
0.007	0.237	0.244	0.009	0.318	0.327	0.003	0.191	0.194	0.005 ± 0.003	0.253 ± 0.038	0.258 ± 0.039
0.011	0.188	0.199	0.006	0.105	0.111	0.005	0.216	0.221	0.004 ± 0.003	0.155 ± 0.036	0.159 ± 0.038
0.004	0.105	0.109	0.000	0.007	0.007	0.000	0.044	0.044	0.001 ± 0.002	0.040 ± 0.030	0.040 ± 0.031
0.028	0.784	0.812	0.029	0.853	0.882	0.014	0.762	0.776	0.018 ± 0.008	0.758 ± 0.067	0.775 ± 0.072
U.S.P. sodium phenytoin *(contd.)*											
0.001	0.036	0.037	0.000	0.088	0.088	—	—	—	0.001 ± 0.001	0.060 ± 0.018	0.061 ± 0.018
0.002	0.084	0.086	0.008	0.162	0.170	0.002	0.117	0.119	0.003 ± 0.002	0.112 ± 0.026	0.114 ± 0.028
0.001	0.089	0.090	0.006	0.152	0.158	0.001	0.082	0.083	0.002 ± 0.002	0.106 ± 0.031	0.109 ± 0.033
0.004	0.250	0.254	0.010	0.126	0.136	0.003	0.263	0.266	0.005 ± 0.002	0.248 ± 0.056	0.253 ± 0.054
0.007	0.186	0.193	0.001	0.210	0.211	0.003	0.204	0.207	0.004 ± 0.003	0.164 ± 0.046	0.168 ± 0.047
0.000	0.036	0.036	0.000	0.006	0.006	0.001	0.045	0.046	0.001 ± 0.001	0.031 ± 0.022	0.032 ± 0.022
0.015	0.681	0.696	0.025	0.744	0.769	>0.010	>0.711	>0.721	0.016 ± 0.006	0.733 ± 0.046	0.749 ± 0.050

Student's *t* tests were used to evaluate the statistical significances of differences in means.

RESULTS

Comparative Bioavailability

Bioavailability data are given only insofar as they bear on the urinary metabolite data.

Comparison of $AUC_{0\rightarrow\infty}$ values for the plasma phenytoin concentration–time curves showed a statistically significant ($t = 3.5557$, $df = 7$, $p < 0.05$) difference in mean $AUC_{0\rightarrow\infty}$ value between the B.P. and U.S.P. sodium phenytoin given in the same oral dose to the same subjects (Table 3). Assay of the 100-mg capsules used showed mean sodium phenytoin contents of 100.8 (B.P.) and 101.9 (U.S.P.) mg. The B.P. sodium phenytoin was ~8% more bioavailable than the U.S.P. sodium phenytoin. This knowledge was used in assessing the urinary metabolite data. Individual $AUC_{0\rightarrow 80}$ and $AUC_{0\rightarrow\infty}$ values for each preparation are shown in Table 3. The individual values are used in correcting the urinary metabolite data to obtain *p*-HPPH excretion values to time infinity.

Urinary Metabolite Data

Individual subject data for urinary *p*-HPPH, *p*-HPPH glucuronide, and total *p*-HPPH excretion over the various urine collection times, expressed as molar fractions of the administered phenytoin dose, are given in Table 4. Mean total cumulative *p*-HPPH excretion (as a fraction of ingested phenytoin dose) is plotted against time in Fig. 1, and against the plasma $AUC_{0\rightarrow t}$ value in Fig. 2. It can be seen that cumulative excretion of *p*-HPPH tends to rise asymptotically with time, and is directly proportional to plasma $AUC_{0\rightarrow t}$ value to at least 80 h. In view of this latter relation, it has been assumed that cumulative *p*-HPPH excretion to time infinity would also be directly proportional to AUC calculated to time infinity. The urinary *p*-HPPH excretion data up to 80 h for each study in each subject were therefore corrected for the consequences of an insufficiently long urine collection period by multiplying the excretion figure for 0–80 h by the corresponding $AUC_{0\rightarrow\infty}/AUC_{0\rightarrow 80}$ ratio. The total cumulative excretion figures may be found in Table 4. Regression analysis showed no statistically significant relation between total *p*-HPPH excretion and total sodium phenytoin dose.

Unconjugated *p*-HPPH constituted only 1.4–3.4% of the total *p*-HPPH excretion, and cumulative excretion of *p*-HPPH and its conjugate increased with time, suggesting that glucuronidation of the phase I metabolite was rapid. The cumulative excretion of total *p*-HPPH showed relatively little variation among the subjects. The mean value (± SD) in subjects in whom urine collection was complete (calculated with the U.S.P. preparation data from Table 4 corrected for the mean 8% bioavailability difference) was 0.792 ± 0.063 (range 0.673–0.882).

The bioavailability difference between the two sodium phenytoin products was paralleled by a difference in the mean fraction of the nominal molar phenytoin dose excreted as unconjugated plus conjugated p-HPPH. For B.P. phenytoin the fraction was 0.776 ± 0.072, and for U.S.P. phenytoin, 0.749 ± 0.050. However, this 3.5% difference was not statistically significant (t = 0.7411; df = 10; $p > 0.05$), unlike the bioavailability difference calculated from the plasma phenytoin AUC data, which was statistically significant, though so small as to be unlikely to be important clinically.

When patterns of cumulative p-HPPH excretion in subjects taking sodium phenytoin for the first time were compared with the patterns obtained when these same subjects took the drug for the second time a difference emerged. A slightly, but statistically significantly, greater proportion (mean ± SD) of the dose was excreted as p-HPPH plus p-HPPH glucuronide following the second exposure to the drug (first-exposure 0.724 ± 0.046, second-exposure 0.793 ± 0.058, paired t = 2.8894, df = 5, $p < 0.05$). In this comparison, subject B with two incomplete collections and subject H with an incomplete collection favoring higher excretion on the second occasion were excluded, but subject E with a higher excretion on the second occasion despite known incomplete collection was included.

DISCUSSION

There are a number of known metabolites of phenytoin in humans (16). It appears likely that the drug is metabolized by several parallel pathways, of which the dominant one is oxidation, catalyzed by the liver monooxygenase system, to form the phenolic derivative p-HPPH. Much of the p-HPPH formed then appears to be conjugated with glucuronic acid in the liver. This glucuronide and some unconjugated p-HPPH are excreted in urine. In addition, both may be excreted into bile. The conjugate in bile is probably cleaved in the intestine by β-glucuronidase activity. Much of the p-HPPH so formed may be reabsorbed, but some, and perhaps some intact p-HPPH glucuronide, may be lost in feces. Therefore measurement of the total amount of p-HPPH (unconjugated and conjugated) that appears in urine may underestimate to some extent the body's total conversion of phenytoin to p-HPPH. It is also conceivable that renal excretion is a rate-limiting step in the appearance of p-HPPH or its glucuronide in urine. However, this possibility would be unlikely to invalidate the findings of the present study, since cumulative p-HPPH excretion approached a plateau before the measurements ended, by which time phenytoin levels in plasma had become almost immeasurably small.

Phenytoin is eliminated by a process that appears to follow Michaelis–Menten kinetics under clinically relevant circumstances in humans. Because of this, steady-state plasma phenytoin concentrations rise disproportionately with increasing drug dose. When the drug is metabolized by a number of parallel pathways, the relative amounts of the phenytoin dose that follow the various pathways may vary with the plasma and tissue drug concentrations. Some evidence consistent with this possibility has been described (2). In the present study all subjects received reasonably similar phenytoin dosages relative to body weight (and similar to the usual therapeutic dose), and all achieved relatively similar plasma phenytoin concentrations. Therefore the quantitative conclusions reached in the study may not necessarily apply at all phenytoin dosages and plasma phenytoin concentration ranges.

The group of healthy young adults studied showed relatively little intersubject variation in apparent capacity to oxidize phenytoin to p-HPPH. The extent of conversion ranged from at least 67 to at least 88% of the ingested dose (mean 79%). The actual figure for the conversion may be somewhat higher, in that some p-HPPH may have been lost in feces and some of the urine collections on which the figures are based may have been incomplete, despite attempts to obtain all urine passed. These figures are compared in Table 1 with other published data on the proportion of a phenytoin dose excreted in urine as conjugated plus unconjugated p-HPPH. Nearly all the latter data were obtained under presumedly steady-state conditions, and involved metabolite measurements in each subject after one or several 24-h urine collections. Some of the data conform well with the findings of the present study, but others show significantly lower portions of the dose to be excreted as unconjugated plus conjugated p-HPPH. To some extent this greater variation in estimated p-HPPH formation may reflect the study of patients suspected of abnormal phenytoin metabolism on the basis of unusual relationships between their plasma phenytoin levels and phenytoin doses. Other factors, such as possible bioavailability differences between the preparations used by various investigators and undetected incomplete urine collections, may have been involved. If allowance is made for these possibilities, the findings of the present study may be regarded as providing a representative value (at least for the first phenytoin dose taken) for the conversion of phenytoin to p-HPPH, as estimated from urinary excretion data, in healthy young adults.

It is necessary to add the reservation about the first dose because of the increased excretion of p-HPPH after the second phenytoin dose. This apparent increase in phenytoin metabolism to *p*-HPPH on reexposure to the drug after a single phenytoin dose raises the question (among others) of autoinduction of phenytoin metabolism. We have not found any previous clear evidence of this phenomenon in humans in relation to phenytoin. Pharmacokinetic studies have provided data consistent with autoinduction of metabolism of other anticonvulsants, e.g., carbamazepine (17,18). However, such a pharmacokinetic approach to demonstrating autoinduction would not be suitable for phenytoin, because of the difficulty in obtaining reliable estimates of Michaelis–Menten parameters after a single dose of a drug that follows saturable elimination kinetics (15). Given these circumstances, measurement of metabolite formation after a spaced series of single phenytoin doses would be a more suitable means of demonstrating autoinduction of metabolism. The present study has accidentally approached such an experimental design and has provided findings consistent with autoinduction. Extended studies should be carried out to see whether additional evidence of this phenomenon can be obtained.

REFERENCES

1. Chang T, Glazko AJ. Quantitative assay of 5,5-diphenylhydantoin (Dilantin) and 5-(*p*-hydroxyphenyl)-5-phenylhydantoin by gas–liquid chromatography. *J Lab Clin Med* 1970;75:145–55.
2. Eadie MJ, Tyrer JH, Bochner F, Hooper WD. The elimination of phenytoin in man. *Clin Exp Pharmacol Physiol* 1976;3:217–24.
3. Kutt H, Wolk M, Scherman R, McDowell F. Insufficient parahydroxylation as a cause of diphenylhydantoin toxicity. *Neurology* 1964;14:542–8.
4. Glazko AJ, Chang T, Baukema J, Bill WA, Goulet JR, Buchanan RA. Metabolic disposition of diphenylhydantoin in normal human subjects following intravenous administration. *Clin Pharmacol Ther* 1969;10:498–504.
5. Mascher J, Bernhardt W. Uberwachung der Langzeitmedikation mid Diphenylhydantoin. Gaschromatische Bestimmung von Diphenylhydantoin und Hydroxy-Diphenylhydantoin. *Zeitschrift fur Neurologie* 1973;204:1790–2.
6. Borofsky L, Louis S, Kutt H. Diphenylhydantoin in children. Pharmacology and efficacy. *Neurology* 1973;23:967–72.
7. Karlen B, Garle M, Rane A, Gutover M, Lindborg B. Assay of the major (4-hydroxylated) metabolites of diphenylhydantoin in human urine. *Eur J Clin Pharmacol* 1975;8:359–63.
8. Bochner F, Hooper WD, Eadie MJ, Tyrer JH. Decreased capacity to metabolise diphenylhydantoin in a patient with hypersensitivity to warfarin. *Aust NZ J Med* 1975;5:462–6.
9. Borga O, Hoppel C, Odar-Cederlof I, Garle M. Plasma levels and renal excretion of phenytoin and its metabolites in patients with renal failure. *Clin Pharmacol Ther* 1979;265–306–14.
10. Witkin KM, Bius DL, Teague BI, Wiese LD, Boyles LW, Dudley KH. Determination of 5-(*p*-hydroxyphenyl)-5-phenylhydantoin and studies relating to the disposition of phenytoin in man. *Ther Drug Monit* 1979;1:11–34.
11. Landon MJ, Kirkley M. Metabolism of diphenylhydantoin (phenytoin) during pregnancy. *Br J Obstet Gynaecol* 1979;86:125–32.
12. Kochenour NK, Emery MG, Sawchuk RJ. Phenytoin metabolism in pregnancy. *Obstet Gynecol* 1980;56:577–82.
13. Glazko AJ, Peterson FE, Chang T, Dill WA, Smith TC, Buchanan RA. Phenytoin metabolism in subjects with long and short plasma half-lives. *Ther Drug Monit* 1982;4:281–92.
14. Yamaoka K, Tanigawa Y, Nakagawa T, Uno T. A pharmacokinetic analysis program (MULTI) for microcomputer. *J Pharmacobiodyn* 1981;4:879–85.
15. Metzler CM, Tong DDM. Computational problems of compartment models with Michaelis–Menten-type elimination. *J Pharm Sci* 1981;70:733–7.
16. Eadie MJ. Metabolism of anticonvulsant drugs. *Rev Drug Metab Drug Interact* 1981;3:317–47.
17. Eichelbaum M, Ekbom K, Bertilsson L, Ringberger VA, Rane A. Plasma kinetics of carbamazepine and its epoxide metabolite in man after single and multiple doses. *Eur J Clin Pharmacol* 1975;8:337–41.
18. Pitlick WH, Levy RH, Troupin AS, Green JR. Pharmacokinetic model to describe self-induced decreases in steady-state concentrations of carbamazepine. *J Pharm Sci* 1976;65:462–3.

Therapeutic Drug Monitoring
7:290–294 © 1985 Raven Press, New York

Chronic Valproic Acid Therapy and Incidence of Increases in Venous Plasma Ammonia

Dan Haidukewych, Geetha John, Janusz J. Zielinski, and Ernst A. Rodin

Epilepsy Center of Michigan, Detroit, Michigan, U.S.A.

Summary: Results are described on the association of elevated ammonia (NH_3) with valproic acid (VPA) therapy in a large group (n = 157) of randomly selected, chronically medicated (>2 years) outpatients. The highest incidence (45.5%) of elevations occurred in patients comedicated with VPA-phenobarbital (PB)–phenytoin (PHT) combinations, followed by VPA-PB (33.3%) and VPA-PHT (15.4%). No NH_3 elevations were detected in all patients (n = 38) on chronic VPA monotherapy. Considering the total sample (n = 157), NH_3 concentrations were found to be linearly and directly correlated with VPA plasma concentration (n = 125, r = 0.249, $p < 0.001$), PB concentration (n = 86, r = 0.411, $p < 0.001$), sum of VPA-PB concentration (n = 60, r = 0.721, $p < 0.001$), and sum of VPA-PB-PHT concentration (n = 33, r = 0.802, $p < 0.001$). When patients in the subgroups (n = 73) that included all the patients with elevated NH_3 were separated into one group (n = 47) with normal NH_3 ($\leq$0.70 μg/ml) and one group (n = 26) with elevated NH_3 ($\geq$0.71 μg/ml), Student's t tests for equality of means showed that the group with elevated NH_3 had a significantly higher mean plasma concentration for VPA, PB, sum of VPA-PB, and sum of VPA-PB-PHT (all at $p < 0.001$) when compared with the normal group. Furthermore, there was a linear and direct correlation with elevated NH_3 and VPA concentrations (n = 26, r = 0.606, $p < 0.001$), sum of VPA-PB (n = 24, r = 0.486, $p < 0.001$), and sum of VPA-PB-PHT (n = 15, r = 0.525, $p < 0.001$). None of the patients had NH_3 elevations higher than thrice the upper limit of normal. Medication with VPA is a necessary but not sufficient condition for increased incidence of venous plasma NH_3 elevations in chronically medicated patients. Patients on VPA and coanticonvulsant therapy (especially PB) are the most likely group to show NH_3 elevations. At highest risk are those patients with relatively high VPA and PB plasma concentrations who are also medicated with PHT. **Key Words:** Valproic acid—Coanticonvulsants—Venous plasma ammonia elevation—Statistical correlations.

Recently, extensive interest has been shown in blood ammonia (NH_3) concentration of epileptic patients medicated with valproic acid (VPA) alone or with coanticonvulsants (1–13). In general, it appears that some patients treated with VPA therapy may show elevated NH_3 concentration in the absence of abnormal liver enzyme activities, and if this asymptomatic and reversible hyperammonemia is recognized early, altered mental status or gastrointestinal symptoms may be avoided by reducing the dosage of VPA (12). Patients receiving multiple anticonvulsants, especially phenobarbital (PB) may be at highest risk (6). The increased incidence of elevated NH_3 for VPA-treated patients has been identified even after 3 years of chronic therapy (3). Nevertheless, the chronic affect of VPA is difficult to evaluate, since (as a rule) the

Address correspondence and reprint requests to Dr. D. Haidukewych at Epilepsy Center of Michigan, 3800 Woodward Avenue, Detroit, MI 48201, U.S.A.

patients were medicated with coanticonvulsants, small number of patients were studied, and no correlation has been found between VPA plasma concentration and the extent of NH_3 elevation (13). Furthermore, several pitfalls have been recognized in assaying NH_3 (13,14), and high carbohydrates (11), protein load (2), or exercise (15) may contribute to elevated NH_3.

To shed more light on the association of elevated NH_3 with VPA therapy, we describe here results from venous plasma NH_3 concentration determinations in a large group (n = 157) of randomly selected, chronically medicated, (>2 years) epileptic patients.

MATERIALS AND METHODS

One hundred fifty-seven patients with epilepsy (73 women, 84 men) with a mean age of 15 years (range, 3–69 years) were screened for venous plasma NH_3 concentration. All patients had epilepsy for which they were treated as outpatients of the Epilepsy Center of Michigan. One hundred twenty-one (77%) came to the Center's Pediatric Seizure Clinic for routine anticonvulsant level determination for maintenance therapy or for adjustment of dosages because of seizures or clinical toxicity. To establish a normal range of NH_3 concentration, plasma from apparently healthy employee volunteers (n = 15) was obtained and assayed concurrently with plasma from the patients, including those not on VPA therapy (n = 32) and in whom no NH_3 elevation was expected. Plasma levels of VPA, PB, phenytoin (PHT), and carbamazepine (CBZ) were determined using Abbott Diagnostics reagents with the TDx automated fluorescence polarization analyzer.

Determination of Ammonia

An ammonia reagent kit (Sigma Diagnostics, St. Louis, MO, U.S.A.) was used as specified in Procedure No. 170-UV enclosed with the kit and as modified for use with the Abbott VP Analyzer. NH_3 concentrations were determined on specimens from patients arriving after breakfast (e.g., after morning doses of medication) and before lunch. None of the patients experienced seizures within 2 days of blood collection or were involved in any unusual physical activity. Blood (5 ml, Venojet #T-2065SLH) was collected from the forearm in a normal fashion, immediately centrifuged (3 min, 10,000 *g*) and refrigerated at 4–8°C for as long as 2.5 h before batch NH_3 determination. Visibly hemolyzed specimens were rejected. These conditions applied to all patients, including those not on VPA medication and normal employee volunteers. With each daily batch of specimens, a specimen of solution obtained by mixing 5 ml of distilled water with an "empty" Venojet tube was included for NH_3 assay. All NH_3 determinations were made in triplicate, and only acceptable averages (<5% CV) were used for statistical analysis. Background NH_3 for blanks was never >0.02 μg/ml.

RESULTS AND DISCUSSION

Statistical data by drug combination subgroups for 157 patients chronically medicated with anticonvulsants and screened for venous plasma NH_3 are shown in Table 1. As is evident, the highest incidence (45.5%) of elevations occurred in patients medicated with VPA-PB-PHT combination (Table 1A), followed by VPA-PB combination (33.3%; Table 1B), and VPA-PHT combination (15.4%; Table 1C). Patients with VPA-CBZ combination (Table 1D) showed no NH_3 elevation. It is interesting to note that all patients on chronic VPA monotherapy (n = 38, Table 1E) showed no elevation of NH_3. Therefore, it appears that medication with VPA is a necessary but not sufficient condition for increased incidence of venous NH_3 elevations in chronically medicated patients. Patients medicated with PB-PHT (n = 32, Table 1F) as expected, showed no NH_3 elevations, but their samples were assayed concurrently with all other specimens as an internal quality control for methodology used and any effect of plasma storage (as long as 2.5 h at 4–8°C). Recognizing the pitfalls associated with assaying NH_3 (13,14), we found it essential to include the plasma from patients not treated with VPA (Table 1F) as indicators of possible artifactual NH_3 elevation.

Correlation between the indicated variables and venous plasma NH_3 concentration for all patients (n = 157) is shown in Table 2. NH_3 concentrations were found to be linearly and directly correlated with VPA plasma concentration (n = 125, r = 0.249, $p < 0.001$), PB concentration (n = 86, r = 0.721, $p < 0.001$), sum of VPA-PB (n = 60, r = 0.721, $p < 0.001$), and sum of VPA-PB-PHT concentrations (n = 33, r = 0.802, $p < 0.001$). No correlation was found between NH_3 and PHT or CBZ plasma concentration.

The data for the patients in the combined three subgroups (n = 73, Table 1A–C) that included all the patients with elevated NH_3 were then separated into two groups. Group I consisted of patients (n = 47) with normal NH_3 (≤0.70 μg/ml) and group II of patients (n = 26) with elevated NH_3 (≥0.71 μg/ml). Two-sample Student's t tests for equality of means

TABLE 1. *Statistical data by drug combination subgroups for 157 patients chronically dosed with anticonvulsants and screened for ammonia*[a]

Medication	n[b]	No. of patients with elevated ammonia	Ammonia (μg/ml)[c]	Plasma (μg/ml)			
				VPA	PB	PHT	CBZ
A. VPA + PB + PHT	33	15	0.80 ± 0.47 (33)	64.81 ± 33.41 (33)	25.91 ± 8.34 (33)	12.30 ± 5.23 (33)	—
B. VPA + PB	27	9	0.58 ± 0.31 (27)	63.20 ± 29.45 (27)	24.08 ± 5.24 (27)	—	—
C. VPA + PHT	13	2	0.64 ± 0.22 (13)	72.98 ± 36.21 (13)	—	14.28 ± 6.79 (13)	—
D. VPA + CBZ	14	0	0.33 ± 0.17 (14)	75.86 ± 23.97 (14)	—	—	8.39 ± 2.76 (14)
E. VPA[d]	38	0	0.34 ± 0.19 (38)	86.46 ± 48.42 (38)	—	—	—
F. PB + PHT	32	0	0.46 ± 0.14 (32)	—	18.63 ± 6.08 (26)	10.28 ± 4.32 (16)	—

VPA, valproic acid; PB, phenobarbital; PHT, phenytoin; CBZ, carbamazepine.
[a]All values are means ± SD; number of interpatient data points in parentheses.
[b]Number of comedicated patients.
[c]Established normal ammonia range in our laboratory, 0.14 to 0.70 μg/ml; literature reported normal range, 0.18 to 0.80.
[d]Includes 11 patients comedicated with ethosuximide.

TABLE 2. *Correlation between indicated variable and venous plasma ammonia concentration for 157 patients chronically medicated with anticonvulsants*

Variable	Ammonia (μg/ml plasma) Mean	SD	n	Correlation (r)	F statistic	Significance (p)
VPA (μg/ml plasma)	73.28	37.98	125	0.249	8.2	<0.001
PB (μg/ml plasma)	23.13	7.41	86	0.411	17.1	<0.001
Sum of VPA and PB (μg/ml plasma)	89.01	33.29	60	0.721	62.8	<0.001
Sum of VPA, PB, and PHT (μg/ml plasma)	102.99	35.18	33	0.802	56.2	<0.001
PHT (μg/ml plasma)	12.18	5.47	62	−0.077	0.4	NS
CBZ (μg/ml plasma)	8.39	2.76	14	−0.032	0.0	NS

VPA, valproic acid; PB, phenobarbital; PHT, phenytoin; CBZ, carbamazepine; NS, not significant.

were compared for the indicated variables, as shown in Table 3. The statistical trend, probably implicating elevated venous NH_3 concentration with increased concentration of anticonvulsants in plasma, is evident again. Group II (abnormal NH_3) patients showed statistically significant higher mean plasma concentration for VPA, PB, sum of VPA-PB, and sum of VPA-PB-PHT, when compared with the normal group I. Furthermore, there was a linear and direct correlation with elevated NH_3 and VPA, sum of VPA-PB, and sum of VPA-PB-PHT concentration (data summarized in the footnote of Table 3). It should be noted that the magnitude of NH_3 elevations was rather low. No subjects had elevations greater than thrice the upper limit of normal NH_3.

It is of particular interest to comment on the clinical status of the 26 patients with elevated venous plasma NH_3. For the majority of the patients (n = 21), elevated NH_3 was not suspected and the patients showed no signs of obtundation. Fifteen patients had had seizures (mostly myoclonic, astatic-atonic, and complex partial) in the 6-month period prior to assay for NH_3. Ten patients had normal liver enzyme activities [serum glutamic-oxaloacetic transaminase (SGOT) and serum glutamic-pyruvic transaminase (SGPT)]; four had mildly elevated SGOT and SGPT, and three had mild SGPT elevation. No enzyme data was available for nine patients.

We concluded that (a) patients on chronic VPA monotherapy are unlikely to show elevated NH_3, and (b) patients on VPA and coanticonvulsant therapy (especially PB) are the most likely group to show elevated NH_3. At highest risk are those patients with relatively high VPA and PB plasma concentration who are also comedicated with PHT.

The synergistic effect of VPA on increased PB accumulation in plasma is well known and is attributed to decreased metabolism of PB in the liver. For VPA-PB patients, PB dosages are usually reduced soon after initiation with VPA treatment. Nevertheless, for patients with difficult-to-control seizures requiring three drugs (e.g., VPA-PB-PHT), the tendency is not only to drive VPA plasma concentration to the upper therapeutic limit, but also to keep PB concentration as high as possible without overt intoxication. One result of this may be a decreased urea synthesis and consequent increase of NH_3 in plasma.

As a matter of practical approach, determination of venous plasma NH_3 concentration may be justified in only those patients with clinical signs of obtundation

TABLE 3. *Variables with significant differences by Student's* t *tests for normal (group I) and abnormal (group II) ammonia in 73 patients*[a]

Variable	Normal ammonia (n = 47) (0.41 ± 0.18 μg/ml)	Abnormal ammonia (n = 26) (1.16 ± 0.31 μg/ml)[b]	p value = 0.0000
VPA (μg/ml plasma)	52.64 ± 25.21 (47)	88.85 ± 30.88 (26)	<0.001 (t = 5.109)
PB (μg/ml plasma)	22.64 ± 5.21 (36)	29.35 ± 7.55 (24)	<0.001 (t = 4.016)
Sum of VPA and PB (μg/ml plasma)	71.56 ± 23.01 (36)	115.58 ± 28.14 (24)	<0.001 (t = 6.3736)
Sum of VPA, PB, and PHT (μg/ml plasma)	80.22 ± 22.12 (18)	130.37 ± 27.60 (15)	<0.001 (t = 5.6785)

VPA, valproic acid; PB, phenobarbital; PHT, phenytoin; CBZ, carbamazepine.

[a]All values are means ± SD; number of interpatient data points in parentheses.

[b]Linear regression analyses for group II (abnormal ammonia) in relation to anticonvulsants produced direct significant correlation. For VPA, r = 0.606, n = 26 (p < 0.001); for sum of VPA and PB, r = 0.486, n = 24 (p < 0.001); and for sum of VPA, PB, and PHT, r = 0.525; n = 15 (p < 0.001).

who have relatively high VPA and PB plasma concentration. Preliminary results of a study in progress may indicate that epileptic patients with mental retardation seem to show more pronounced intoxication in spite of nearly the same magnitude of NH_3 elevations as normal epileptics.

REFERENCES

1. Coulter DL, Allen RJ. Secondary hyperammonaemia: a possible mechanism for valproate encephalopathy. *Lancet* 1980;1:1310–1.
2. Rawat S, Borkowski WJ, Swick HM. Valproic acid and secondary hyperammonemia. *Neurology* 1981;31:1172–4.
3. Coulter DL, Allen RJ. Hyperammonemia associated with valproic acid. *Ann Neurol* 1981;10:307.
4. Murphy JV, Marquardt K, Swick HM. Hyperammonemia in children receiving valproic acid. *Neurology* 1981;31:142.
5. Batshaw ML, Brusilow SW. Valproate-induced hyperammonemia. *Ann Neurol* 1982;11:319–21.
6. Zaret BS, Beckner RR, Marini AM, Wagle W, Passarelli C. Sodium valproate–induced hyperammonemia without clinical hepatic dysfunction. *Neurology* 1982;32:206–8.
7. Sugimoto T, Yasuhara A, Matsumura T, Hara K, Sakane Y, Tamiuchi K. Hyperglycinemia and hyperammonemia following administration of valproate sodium. In: Akimoto H, Kazamaturi H, Seino M, Ward A, eds. *Advances in epileptology: XIII epilepsy international symposium.* New York: Raven Press, 1982:297–300.
8. Warter JM, Marescaux Ch, Brandt Ch, et al. Sodium valproate associated with phenobarbital: effects on ammonia metabolism in humans. *Epilepsia* 1983;24:628–633.
9. Warter JM, Brandt Ch, Marescaux Ch, et al. The renal origin of sodium valproate–induced hyperammonemia in fasting humans. *Neurology* 1983;33:1136–40.
10. Williams CA, Tiefenbach S, McReynolds JW. Valproic acid–induced hyperammonemia in mentally retarded adults. *Neurology* 1984;34:550–3.
11. Warter JM, Marescaux Ch, Chabrier G, et al. Increase of valproate-induced hyperammonemia in normal subjects by carbohydrate intake. *Neurology* 1984;34:1487–9.
12. Zaccara G, Campostrim R, Paganini M, et al. Acute changes in blood ammonia may predict short-term adverse effects of valproic acid. *Neurology* 1984;34:1518–21.
13. Zaret BS, Marini AM. Standardization in VPA-induced hyperammonemia. *Neurology* 1985;35:136–7.
14. Howanitz JH, Howanitz PJ, Skrodzki CA, Iwanski JA. Influence of specimen processing and storage conditions on results for plasma ammonia. *Clin Chem* 1984;30:906–8.
15. Allen SI, Conn HO. Observations on the effect of exercise on blood ammonia concentration in man. *Yale J Biol Med* 1960;33:133.

Therapeutic Drug Monitoring
7:295–298 © 1985 Raven Press, New York

Organization and Efficacy of a Therapeutic Drug Monitoring Consultation Service in a Pediatric Hospital

*Gideon Koren, †Steven J. Soldin, and *Stuart M. MacLeod

**Division of Clinical Pharmacology, The Research Institute, and †Therapeutic Drug Monitoring Laboratory, The Hospital for Sick Children, and Departments of Pediatrics and Pharmacology, University of Toronto, Ontario, Canada*

Summary: On July 1, 1982, a therapeutic drug monitoring (TDM) consultation service was instituted in the hope of improving the decision-making of clinicians with respect to drug therapy. Thirteen different drugs are monitored daily, with an average load of 1,600 inpatient samples per month. The team consists of clinical pharmacology fellows and staff who are available 7 days a week to monitor all drug levels that are outside the putative therapeutic range. In order to evaluate the efficacy of this service in preventing development of potentially toxic drug concentrations, the TDM data from July 1982 to December 1983 have been reviewed. The percentage of toxic levels from the total sample load was significantly lower in the period of July–December 1983 compared with July–December 1982 at the beginning of the service (2.25% vs. 4.25%, $p < 0.01$). Since January 1983, the percentage has been maintained at <3%. A TDM consultation service can help to optimize the use of drug monitoring data by physicians and may lead to improved prescribing in a hospital setting. **Key Words:** Therapeutic drug monitoring—Pediatrics.

Unlike clinical chemistry and hematology, which have been practiced and taught in medical schools for centuries, therapeutic drug monitoring (TDM) is a relatively new field often unknown to pediatricians. In 1981, the Hospital for Sick Children in Toronto instituted a TDM consultation service (TDM-CS) in order to better control the safety of drug therapy in children. It was hoped that such a service would facilitate the introduction of pharmacokinetic principles and therapeutic rationale to the house staff.

In the present communication we discuss our TDM-CS and assess its efficacy during the first year and a half (July 1982 through December 1983).

THERAPEUTIC DRUG MONITORING CONSULTATION SERVICE (TDM-CS)

Our TDM-CS is composed of teams of clinical pharmacologists (physicians) and clinical pharmacists (BsC Pharm, MsC Pharm, or Pharm D). Each team includes a fellow and a staff person from the Division of Clinical Pharmacology. Seven days a week, 24 h a day, the fellow on call is paged by the TDM laboratory for any drug level that is above the therapeutic range. Table 1 summarizes all drugs measured daily in the TDM laboratory and the upper therapeutic level for each drug. The fellow is expected to identify the problem by reading the chart and discussing the case with the physician in charge, and to detect the reason for the high level, such as inappropriate sampling time, drug overdose, or disease state. Table 2 summarizes various reasons that must be considered in any such case. The fellow discusses the possible mechanisms with the house staff, suggesting the necessary changes in drug regulation, and is responsible for following up the case in the days ahead. In addition, a record is kept at the Division of Clinical Pharmacology indicating the team's activity in each case.

Serum drug concentrations lower than the therapeutic range are dealt with only in special cases at the request of the responsible clinician. In such cases, a pharmacokinetic investigation is often deemed nec-

Address correspondence and reprint requests to Dr. G. Koren at Division of Clinical Pharmacology, The Hospital for Sick Children, 555 University Avenue, Toronto, Ontario, Canada M5G 1X8.

TABLE 1. *Drugs measured daily at the therapeutic drug monitoring laboratory in Toronto and their therapeutic concentrations*

	Drug	Therapeutic serum concentration (1)
Antibiotics	Gentamicin	trough <2–3 mg/L, peak <10 mg/L
	Tobramycin	trough <2–3 mg/L, peak <10 mg/L
	Amikacin	trough 5–10 mg/L, peak 15–30 mg/L
Cardiovascular	Digoxin	0.9–2 mg/ml
	Quinidine	2.3–5 mg/ml
Anticonvulsants	Phenobarbital	15–40 mg/L
	Phenytoin	6–20 mg/L
	Ethosuximide	40–100 mg/L
	Primidone	5–12 mg/L
	Valproic acid	50–100 mg/L
	Carbamazepine	4–8 mg/L
Other drugs	Theophylline	10–20 mg/L
	Methotrexate	minimal >0.01 μM potentially toxic 5 μM

essary in order to detect the reason for the difficulty in achieving therapeutic levels. For example, difficulties were experienced in achieving therapeutic serum concentrations of salicylates in Kawasaki disease, and a study was performed indicating impaired bioavailability of acetylsalicylic acid as the reason for this condition (11).

METHODS

Assessment of Efficacy of TDM-CS

In order to evaluate the efficiency of our TDM-CS over a period of one and a half years, we calculated the percentage of supratherapeutic concentrations (levels above the accepted therapeutic range) of the total number of drug tests performed on inpatients every month between July 1982 and December 1983. Thirteen different drugs are monitored daily, with an average load of 1,600 inpatient samples per month. Phenobarbital was not included in the analysis because phenobarbital coma is a common therapeutic practice in our pediatric intensive care unit. In many other cases, neonates and children in seizure are loaded with high doses of phenobarbital. Therefore, a supratherapeutic serum concentration of phenobarbitone could not necessarily be considered as an erroneous event to be corrected. Of the total number of assessments, the percentage of supratherapeutic levels was compared between months by the χ^2 test.

RESULTS

Figure 1 summarizes the percentage of supratherapeutic levels for each month between July 1982 and December 1983. There was the highest percentage of supratherapeutic levels in the first month of the TDM-CS (6.4%). Thereafter, the percentage gradually decreased to 2.65% in December 1982. The percentage of supratherapeutic levels of all samples analyzed was significantly higher in July–December 1982 compared with July–December 1983 (4.25% vs. 2.25%, $p < 0.01$). The percentage for each month during the summer of 1983 was significantly lower than for the summer of 1982 [July 1983 (3.7%) < July 1982 (6.4%), $p = 0.02$; August 1983 (2.9%) < August 1982 (4.6%), $p = 0.02$; September 1983 (2.9%) < September 1982 (4.6%), $p = 0.04$]. Beginning in January 1983, the percentage of supratherapeutic levels fell below 3% until a new peak in July 1983 (3.7%), which was significantly higher than the previous month (June 1983; month 2.6%) < ($p = 0.05$). Thereafter, the percentage again decreased.

TABLE 2. *Common reasons for supratherapeutic serum concentrations of drugs*

Reason	Examples and references
Wrong sampling time	Sampling after a bolus and not before a predose as requested (1) Peak level drawn before distribution is complete
Overdose	Errors 10fold error in calculation of drug dose (2); accidental administration Too high dose stemming from ignorance or lack of information on the particular drug in the particular age group (3,4), e.g., gentamicin or digoxin in preterm infants
Drug-disease interaction	Impairment of theophylline metabolism caused by influenza virus, causing toxicity (5) Renal failure causing accumulation of digoxin or aminoglycosides (6)
Drug-drug interaction	Interaction between digoxin and quinidine, verapamil, or amiodarone causing digoxin toxicity (7) Erythromycin inhibition of theophylline metabolism (8)
Increased bioavailability	Improvement in preparation of phenytoin (9)
Increased compliance	Improvement in compliance due to disturbing symptoms of the disease (10)

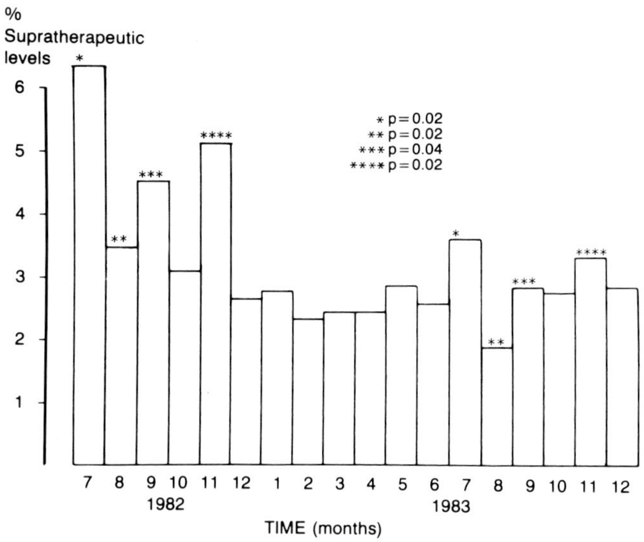

FIG. 1. Percentage of supratherapeutic levels of all samples analyzed monthly; a significant decrease in July–December 1983 compared with July–December 1982.

Gentamicin by far exceeded all other drugs in the number of supratherapeutic drug levels (38%) during July 1982 through December 1983. In conjunction with amikacin and tobramycin, aminoglycosides caused 59% of the supratherapeutic levels. Theophylline contributed 25% of the potentially toxic levels, followed by phenytoin (8%) and digoxin (8%).

DISCUSSION

In trying to assess the efficacy of our TDM-CS, we searched for an objective end point that would allow us to compare longitudinal performance in different months. We assumed that the percentage of supratherapeutic levels from the total number of assessments for each month may reflect the TDM performance of the house staff, and therefore putative improvement initiated by our teams. However, several confounding factors must be considered in this context: Each July, one third of the residents in our hospital leave the hospital, and new residents take their place. Therefore, the performance during this month is anticipated to be the poorest with respect to TDM, as it is with other diagnostic and therapeutic functions. Therefore, we had to assume that improvement in percentage of supratherapeutic levels in August, September, and October 1982 would occur regardless of the function of the TDM-CS. The new "peak" in percentage of supratherapeutic levels in July 1983 supports our assumption that new residents perform less efficiently with respect to TDM. However, we believe that the fact that the performance in each month during summer 1983 was significantly better than in summer 1982 can at least in part be attributed to the activity of the TDM-CS. More importantly, there was a twofold decrease in supraoptimal levels in July–December 1983 as compared with July–December 1982.

On a subjective basis, there were many instances where a thorough discussion with a resident on pharmacokinetic principles governing drug dosing was followed by better understanding and fewer future errors. Furthermore, it is suggested that the concept of an interactive system, which is activated in each case of a potentially toxic level, certainly has a psychological impact on the house staff; supratherapeutic levels have the connotation of errors, and everyone would try to prevent these iatrogenic events. In addition to improving the percentage of supratherapeutic levels by explaining and discussing each case with the house staff, a TDM-CS is efficient in detecting problems on larger scales and in trying to solve them prospectively. Two examples are given here: (a) Gentamicin was involved in significantly more supratherapeutic levels than any other measured drug. Moreover, many of these events occurred in the neonatal intensive care unit, where many of the infants are treated with gentamicin for suspected or proven gram-negative sepsis. This prompted a prospective study, which has shown that in very low birth weight infants, gentamicin clearance is significantly lower, and therefore they need smaller doses of gentamicin (12). (b) In reviewing cases of high digoxin and gentamicin serum concentrations in preterm infants, we have demonstrated that indomethacin, by impairing renal function, causes accumulation of these drugs if appropriate reduction of digoxin dose does not take place (3,4).

CONCLUSION

We have described the function of our TDM-CS. During the first year and a half of this service, the rate of potentially toxic levels has dropped in our hospital to one half. We believe that the fact that our teams initiate the consultations, and do not wait to be invited by the clinicians, helps to uncover most cases of potential toxicity and to deal with them appropriately.

REFERENCES

1. Taylor WJ, Finn A, eds. *Individualizing drug therapy.* New York: Gross, Townsend, Frank, Inc., 1981.
2. Koren G, Barzilay Z, Modan M. Errors in computing drug doses. *Can Med Assoc J* 1983;129:721–3.
3. Koren G, Zarfin Y, Perlman M, MacLeod SM. Effects of indomethacin pharmacokinetics in preterm infants. *Pediatr Pharmacol* 1984;4:25–30.

4. Zarfin Y, Koren G, Maresky D, Perlman M, MacLeod SM. Possible indomethacin-aminoglycoside interaction in preterm infants. *J Pediatr* 1985;106:511–3.
5. Kraemer MJ, Furukawa CT, Koup JR, Shapiro GG, Pierson WE, Bierman CW. Altered theophylline clearance during an influenza B outbreak. *Pediatrics* 1982;69:476–9.
6. Balant L, Fabre J. Renal failure, drug pharmacokinetics, and drug action. In: Gibaldi M, Prescott L, eds. *Handbook of clinical pharmacokinetics*. New York: ADIS Health Science Press, 1983:Section III,212–34.
7. Koren G. Interaction between digoxin and commonly coadministered drugs in children. *Pediatrics* 1985;75:1,032–7.
8. Renton KW, Gray JD, Hung OR. Depression of theophylline elimination by erythromycin. *Clin Pharmacol Ther* 1981;30:422–6.
9. Tozer TN, Winter ME. Phenytoin. In: Evans WE, Schentag JJ, Jusko WJ eds. *Applied pharmacokinetics*. 1980:217–78.
10. Haynes RB, Taylor DW, Sackett DL. *Compliance in health care*. Baltimore: Johns Hopkins University Press, 1979:49–78.
11. Koren G, MacLeod SM. Difficulty in achieving therapeutic serum concentrations of salicylate in Kawasaki disease. *J Pediatr* 1984;105:991–5.
12. Koren G, Leeder S, Harding E, Jacques D, MacLeod SM. Optimization of gentamicin therapy in very low birth weight infants. *Pediatr Pharmacol* 1985;5:79–87.

Therapeutic Drug Monitoring
7:299–302 © 1985 Raven Press, New York

Experience with a Specific Request Form for Antidepressant Drug Monitoring

Albert D. Fraser

Division of Clinical Chemistry, Victoria General Hospital; and Dalhousie University Halifax, Nova Scotia, Canada

Summary: With the introduction of an antidepressant drug monitoring service in this hospital, it became necessary to have a completed request form prior to analysis. The importance of ordering these tests selectively and of basic pharmacokinetics for antidepressants was stressed through special lectures and a newsletter. This study was undertaken to assess whether the use of this form assisted in optimizing drug monitoring of antidepressants. Information provided on the form was used to assist in interpretative reporting and to improve clinical use of the results. Requested information included the name, age, sex, height, and weight of the patient; time of last dose; date therapy started at present dose; reason for the request; and a list of concurrent medications. Results obtained for 600 specimens in 18 months showed that the form was completed fully, sampling time was appropriate, and drug concentration was at steady state 82, 73, and 95% of the time, respectively. Major reasons for requesting analysis were suspicion of subtherapeutic (52%), uncertain (20%), above therapeutic (15%), and toxic (10%) ranges. The most popular monitoring requests were for imipramine (40%), doxepin (28%), amitriptyline (14%), and desipramine (11%). Clinical impression of efficacy in the treatment of endogenous depression agreed with plasma levels 60% of the time in the subtherapeutic range, but agreement was only 32% above the therapeutic range. It was concluded that a special request form helps to assure appropriate sampling, explain observed drug interactions, and facilitate interpretative reporting for the medical and nursing staff. **Key Words:** Request form—Antidepressants—Drug monitoring.

Therapeutic drug monitoring has been shown to provide valuable information for individualizing drug therapy over the past 15 years.

With the expansion of drug monitoring services, several reports have documented inappropriate use of therapeutic drug monitoring (1,2). Inability to alter dosing regimens, based on inappropriate monitoring, has been reported up to 60% of the time (3,4). Major sources of error include the collection of specimens before achieving the steady-state concentration and at the wrong time in the dosing interval.

Address correspondence and reprint requests to Dr. A. D. Fraser at Division of Clinical Chemistry (Toxicology), Victoria General Hospital, 1278 Tower Road, Halifax, Nova Scotia, Canada B3H 2Y9.

One approach aimed at improving the clinical usefulness of drug monitoring is the issuance of a specific request/report form (5–7).

Initiation of antidepressant monitoring program in our laboratory 18 months ago required that a specific request form accompany all the specimens. The usefulness of routine monitoring of antidepressant medications used in the treatment of endogenous depression is still controversial since there is no consensus concerning the relationship between the concentration of the antidepressant in plasma and clinical response (8). Individualizing therapy by monitoring plasma concentrations is considered important in patients with renal or hepatic disorders, in patients who fail to respond to moderate doses, in the elderly, and in assessing noncompliance.

Name:

Age:

Sex:

Height (cm):

Weight (Kg):

M.S.I. No.:

TRICYCLIC ANTIDEPRESSANT
DRUG MONITORING FORM

Analysis will only be performed when this completed form (and a yellow Toxicology requisition) are received along with a blood specimen collected in a B.D. royal blue stoppered tube (#6526) or a red stoppered Venoject tube.

Analysis Requested__________

Time of Last Dose__________h (prior to collection) Time of collection__________h

Last Dose__________mg Date of collection__________ Y M D

Total Daily Dose __________mg

Therapy with drug at present dose commenced on __________ Y M D

Reason for request: ? Toxicity__________ ? Subtherapeutic__________

? Compliance__________ Other__________

? Above Therapeutic__________

Concurrent Medications Received: Please specify which drug(s)

Barbiturates__________ Corticosteroids__________

Benzodiazepines__________ Antiepileptics__________

Phenothiazines__________ Anticholinergic__________

Thyroid Drugs__________ Methylphenidate__________

Other__________ __________ __________

Does the patient smoke?__________ No. of packs/day__________

Physician's Signature__________

For clarification on any concerns about antidepressant analysis contact:__________

FIG. 1. Request form for antidepressant drug monitoring used at the Victoria General Hospital Toxicology Laboratory.

A special form was considered important since basic pharmacokinetic principles are often ignored, thus making analysis of little value. In addition, few of the antidepressant medications have an accepted therapeutic window for endogenous depression. A list of concurrent medications was requested since many drugs

TABLE 1. *Antidepressant drug analyses available and therapeutic range*

Drug	Therapeutic range μmol/L	ng/ml
Amitriptyline/nortriptyline	250–720	70–200
Nortriptyline	190–570	50–150
Imipramine/desipramine	450–900	125–250
Desipramine	450–900	125–250
Doxepin/desmethyldoxepin	540–1000	150–280
Clomipramine/desmethylclomipramine	800–1600	250–500
Maprotiline/desmethylmaprotiline	650–1450	180–400

can interfere with the analysis, and certain drug interactions have been observed involving antidepressant medications.

METHODS

The request form (Fig. 1) included space for patient demographics, basic pharmacokinetic data, reason for requesting the analysis, list of concurrent medications, and smoking history. A list of the assays available and "working" therapeutic ranges are found in Table 1.

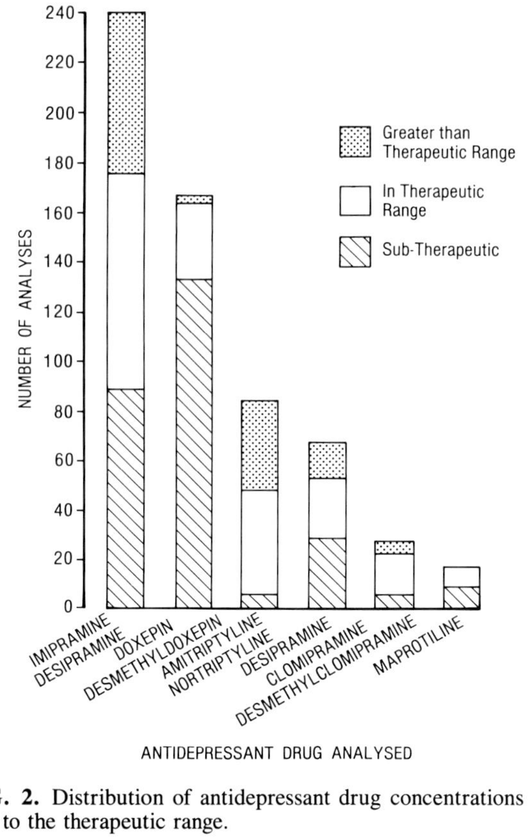

FIG. 2. Distribution of antidepressant drug concentrations relative to the therapeutic range.

RESULTS

This retrospective study was based on forms submitted with 600 specimens for analysis. The request form was completed fully, the sampling time after dose was appropriate, and the plasma drug level was at steady state concentration 82, 73, and 95% of the time, respectively. The information provided on the forms was considered correct.

Major reasons for requesting analysis were suspicion of subtherapeutic (52%), uncertain (20%), greater than therapeutic (15%), and toxic (10%) ranges.

Benzodiazepines were prescribed for 20% of the patients and a phenothiazine (mainly chlorpromazine) for 14%. One third of the patients smoked cigarettes.

The most common drugs for monitoring were imipramine (40%), doxepin (28%), amitriptyline (14%), and desipramine (11%). A summary of plasma concentrations measured relative to their tentative therapeutic ranges is given in Fig. 2.

A comparison of clinical impression of efficacy relative to drug plasma level showed a 60% agreement when the level was in the subtherapeutic range, but clinical impressions were correct only 32% of the time at higher than therapeutic concentrations.

DISCUSSION

Overall, the request forms were completed satisfactorily. They were mainly completed by psychiatry residents, and interaction with the laboratory was positive.

Administering a constant daily dose for a minimum of 7 days was the guideline for assuming that steady state concentrations had been reached. Except for cases of suspected overdose, most specimens were submitted for analysis >10 days after the last dose change.

It was of interest that 33% of the patients smoked cigarettes regularly. No correlation between low values and smoking was observed even though smoking is known to decrease the steady-state concentration of antidepressant drugs, presumably by induction of the hepatic mixed function oxidase system (9).

No obvious relationship between plasma levels and concurrent medications was found except for the well-documented increase in secondary amine metabolites in the presence of phenothiazines due to impaired hepatic hydroxylation (10).

The large number of doxepin values in the subtherapeutic category may be due to the fact that our working therapeutic range is too high (11,12), or may reflect inadequate dosing.

Better correlation between the clinical impression of efficacy and plasma drug concentration was found within the subtherapeutic range rather than above the therapeutic range. This may indicate that inadequate therapy is easier to assess clinically than the nonspecific clinical indices of increasing toxicity.

Optimal therapeutic drug monitoring requires analytical reliability, appropriate specimen collection, and interpretative reporting. Implementation of this request form helped to assure appropriate sample collection, improved laboratory-clinician interaction when discussing individual cases, and thereby made drug analyses more useful clinically.

REFERENCES

1. Woodcock AA, Johnson MA, Geddes DM. Theophylline prescribing, serum concentrations, and toxicity. *Lancet* 1983;2:610–2.
2. Floyd RA, Taketomo R. Serum drug level usage review—a clinical pharmacy service. *Drug Intell Clin Pharm* 1979;13:44–45.
3. Guest K, McLean AJ, Wellington CV. Drug assay services and therapeutic drug use in a general hospital. *Med J Aust* 1980;1:167–70.
4. Elenbaas RM, Rayne VW, Bauman JL. Influence of clinical pharmacist consultations on the use of drug blood level tests. *Am J Hosp Pharm* 1980;37:61–4.
5. Svirbely JR, Speicher CE. The importance of request and report forms in the interpretation of therapeutic drug monitoring data. *Ther Drug Mont* 1980;2:211–16.
6. Sohn D. The clinician-laboratory connection, the vital link: comments regarding the NCCLS proposed standards for clinical laboratory requisition forms. *Ther Drug Monit* 1979;1:453–7.
7. Pippenger CE. Editorial. *Ther Drug Monit* 1979;1:451–2.
8. Asberg M, Sjoqvist F. Therapeutic monitoring of tricyclic antidepressants: clinical aspects. In: Richens A, Marks V, eds. *Therapeutic drug monitoring*. Edinburgh: Churchill Livingstone, 1981:224–38.
9. Perel JM, Stiller RI, Glassman AH. Studies on plasma level/effect relationships in imipramine therapy. *Commun Psychopharmacol* 1978;2:429–39.
10. Gram LF, Overo KF, Kirk L. Influence of neuroleptics and benzodiazepines on metabolism of tricyclic antidepressants in man. *Am J Psychiat* 1974;131:8–12.
11. Green DO. Clinical importance of doxepin antidepressant plasma levels. *J Clin Psychiat* 1978;5:481–2.
12. Biggs JT. Clinical pharmacology and toxicology of antidepressants. *Hosp Pract* 1978;13:79–84.

Therapeutic Drug Monitoring
7:303–307 © 1985 Raven Press, New York

Aminoglycoside Monitoring: Timing of Peak Levels Is Critical

Jürg Blaser, *Hans Peter Simmen, *Hans Ruedi Gonzenbach, †Wolfgang Sonnabend, and Ruedi Lüthy

*Department of Medicine, University Hospital of Zürich, Zürich, *Department of Surgery, Cantonal Hospital of St. Gallen, and †Institute of Medical Microbiology St. Gallen, St. Gallen, Switzerland*

Summary: Recommendations for optimal therapeutic peak concentrations of aminoglycosides are often not differentiated with respect to duration of infusion and timing of peak sample thereafter. To document the relevance of the timing, 139 dose intervals were analyzed in 58 patients during administration of gentamicin, amikacin, and netilmicin. Serum concentrations measured immediately after 30-min infusions were compared with concentrations obtained 90 min later (2 h values). The ratio of 30 min/2 h concentrations showed considerable variability. This ratio was <1.5 in 15% of the dose intervals analyzed and >3 in 8% of the intervals. The poor correlation between concentrations measured at 30 min and at 2 h was documented by the coefficients of variation of 0.82, 0.30, and 0.67 for gentamicin, amikacin, and netilmicin, respectively. This variability was not explained by interindividual differences, renal function, or drug half-life. However, the initial decrease in concentrations was significantly lower in patients with impaired renal function ($p < 0.001$). These data suggest that timing is critical for the sampling of serum to determine peak levels in patients and the definition of optimal therapeutic concentrations. **Key Words:** Aminoglycoside antibiotics—Pharmacokinetics—Drug monitoring—Peak concentrations.

The inter- and intraindividual variability of the serum-kinetics of aminoglycoside antibiotics has already been described by a number of investigators (1-6). Most research concludes that aminoglycosides should be monitored during therapy because of their narrow therapeutic range and the lack of consistent predictability of their pharmacokinetics. However, no uniform timing has been established thus far for the sampling of serum for the determination of the so-called peak serum concentration of the aminoglycosides.

Serum concentrations of antibiotics decline sharply immediately after the end of intravenous infusions due to distribution processes (7,8). This phenomenon may appear less substantial when plotting the time course of serum concentrations on semilogarithmic rather than linear scales. Nevertheless, this observation must be considered when defining optimal therapeutic peak concentrations. Sampling times for the determination of these peak levels should therefore be specified properly with respect to the mode of administration (p.o., i.m., i.v.), the duration of intravenous infusion, and the exact timing of the sample obtained for determination of the peak concentration thereafter.

A variety of different sampling times for the determination of peak levels are recommended, ranging from 0 up to 90 min after the end of an intravenous infusion (9,10). Because of the rapid decline in serum concentrations immediately after the end of infusion, different sampling times for the peak concentrations would also require different recommendations for op-

Address correspondence and reprint requests to Dr. J. Blaser at Department of Medicine, University Hospital of Zürich, CH–8091 Zürich, Switzerland.

timal levels as a function of time. However, this appears useful only when excellent correlations exist between peak concentrations determined at various sampling times. Thus, serum concentrations 2 h after the beginning of a 30 min i.v. infusion should be predictable on the basis of the maximal concentration achieved immediately after stopping the infusion and vice versa. However, if substantial variations occur in the ratios of 30 min to 2 h serum concentrations, then recommendations for peak serum concentrations should be limited to one specific sampling time in order to achieve reproducible serum concentration time profiles.

We assessed the influence of the sampling time on serum peak levels of three aminoglycosides by determining inter- and intraindividual variations of the decrease in serum concentrations immediately after intravenous infusions. [These results were presented in part at the 23rd Interscience Conference on Antimicrobial Agents and Chemotherapy held in Las Vegas October 24–26, 1983.]

MATERIALS AND METHODS

Serum kinetics of 33 men and 25 women with severe systemic infections were investigated. In patients treated with a combination of an aminoglycoside and a beta-lactam antibiotic, the two drugs were not administered simultaneously to avoid chemical interactions between these antibiotics at high drug concentrations (11). A total of 139 dose intervals were analyzed in the course of therapies with gentamicin (49 intervals analyzed in 17 patients), amikacin (46 intervals, 27 patients), and netilmicin (44 intervals, 14 patients). During the course of therapy, doses of aminoglycosides were adjusted to achieve the desired serum concentrations (9). Every 2 to 3 days, three serum samples were analyzed per dose interval. They were sampled immediately after the end of a 30-min intravenous infusion, 90 min later (2 h values) and 8 h after beginning the infusion. Exact timing of the samples was strictly enforced. Each serum sample obtained with a delay of 5 min or more was excluded from data analysis. Gentamicin and netilmicin were administered by drip infusion and amikacin by a volumetric infusion pump.

Blood samples were drawn either through an indwelling winged needle placed in the forearm contralateral to the infusion site or directly through the infusion catheter, after flushing it thoroughly with physiologic saline solution. Once clotting had occurred at room temperature, the specimens were centrifuged at 4°C to obtain the serum.

Concentrations of gentamicin and netilmicin were analyzed by single determinations by fluorescence polarization immunoassay (TDx, Abbott Laboratories, Chicago, IL, U.S.A.). The precision of this assay was determined by fivefold measurements of 12 spiked samples with concentrations selected in the range of 2 to 21 mg/L. The coefficient of variation averaged 3.4 and 1.6% for gentamicin and netilmicin, respectively. The accuracy was established by determining the concentrations of 12 spiked specimens in two different laboratories. The relative difference of the results of these duplicate assays averaged 4.7 and 9.2% for gentamicin and netilmicin, respectively.

Amikacin was measured in quintuplicate by a large plate agar diffusion method (12). Standards in the range of 2–64 mg/L were prepared from pooled antibiotic-free human serum. Samples and standards were frozen in liquid nitrogen and measured within one week. The assay organism was *Bacillus subtilis* when amikacin was used alone and a multiresistant strain of *Klebsiella pneumoniae* when amikacin was combined with another antibiotic. The precision of the assay was determined by fivefold measurements of nine spiked samples in the range of 2 to 64 mg/L. The coefficient of variation was lower than 5.1% for all concentrations and both assay organisms. After the study was completed, the accuracy of this microbiological assay was determined by reassaying 18 serum specimens from 12 patients in another laboratory (Laboratory of Pharmaceutical Microbiology, Ghent, Belgium) using a different microbiological technique (13). The relative difference of the results of these duplicate assays averaged 8.5%.

Half-life was calculated based on the concentrations determined 2 h and 8 h after the infusion was started, assuming an exponential decline of the serum concentration within this time period.

RESULTS

The ratio of 30 min/2 h serum concentrations (mean ± SD) averaged 2.21 ± 0.70, 2.12 ± 0.56, and 2.18 ± 0.62 for gentamicin, amikacin, and netilmicin, respectively. The large individual variations are illustrated by the respective ranges of this ratio: 1.06–4.8, 1.11–3.6, and 1.14–3.6 (Fig. 1). The ratio of 30 min/2 h concentrations was <1.5 in 15% of the dose intervals analyzed and >3 in 8% of the intervals. The poor correlation between concentrations after 30 min and 2 h was documented by the coefficients of correlation of 0.82, 0.30, and 0.67 for gentamicin, amikacin, and netilmicin.

Serum concentrations decreased between 30 min and 2 h significantly less in patients with a serum

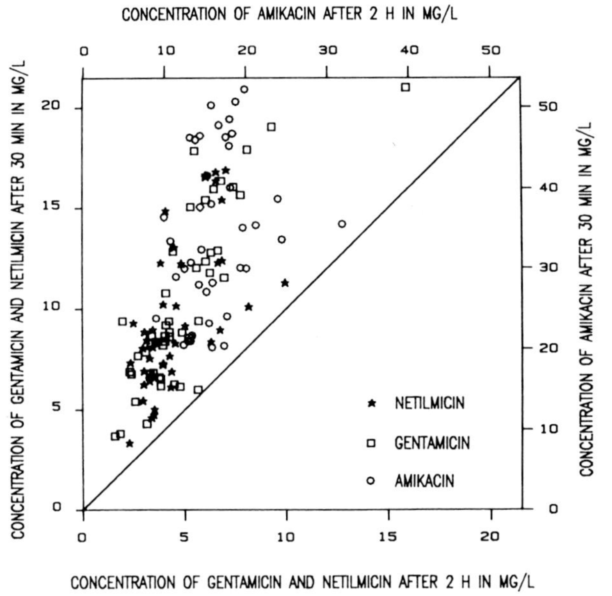

FIG. 1. Correlation between the aminoglycoside concentration of serum samples drawn 30 min and 2 h after the start of 30-min infusions.

creatinine of >1.4 mg/100 ml ($p < 0.001$) than in patients with lower serum creatinine levels. However, differences in the elimination rate may only partially explain individual variations in the initial decrease. Figure 2 demonstrates that the initial decrease in concentration varied considerably even in patients with similar elimination half-lives. For example, in patients with serum half-lives of ~4 h, the ratio of 30 min/2 h concentrations varied between 1.4 and 2.8. Moreover, these variations are not limited to interindividual observations. Figure 3 shows the intraindividual fluctuations of the ratios of 30 min/2 h concentrations that were observed on different days during the course of netilmicin therapies. In two of these 14 patients, the ratio of 30 min/2 h serum concentrations was >4 on one day and <1.5 on the other day.

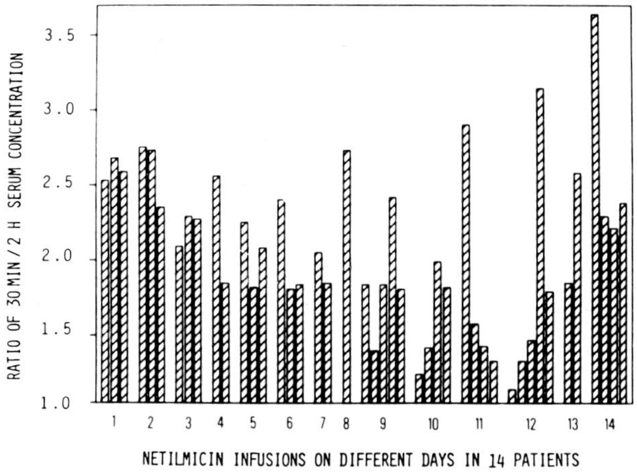

FIG. 3. Intraindividual variations of the ratio of 30 min/2 h serum concentrations of netilmicin observed following infusions on different days during therapy in 14 patients.

These intraindividual variations may not be explained by changes in renal function during therapy as shown for gentamicin in Fig. 4. Both the ratios of 30 min/2 h concentrations and the serum creatinine levels are plotted for different days during therapy in 14 patients. Despite the stability of serum creatinine for patient 14, there were remarkable variations in the 30 min/2 h concentration ratio. On the other hand, substantial changes in serum creatinine did not seriously influence this ratio in patients 6 and 10. With none of the three aminoglycosides studied did the ratio

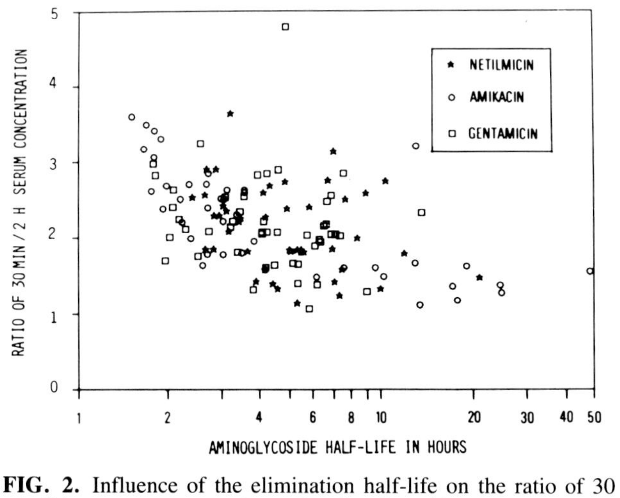

FIG. 2. Influence of the elimination half-life on the ratio of 30 min/2 h serum concentrations of aminoglycosides.

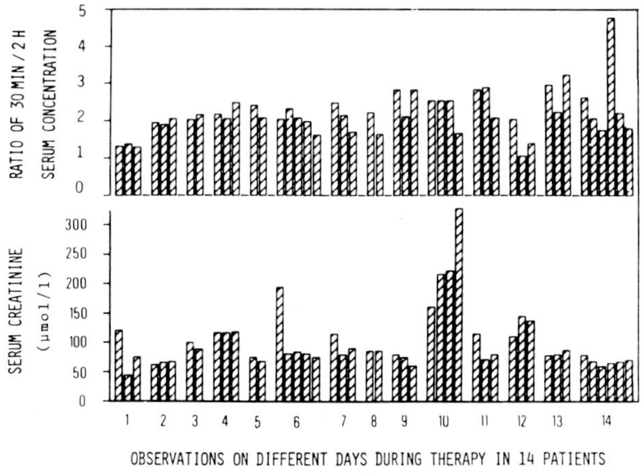

FIG. 4. Ratio of 30 min/2 h serum concentrations of gentamicin (upper panel) and serum creatinine level (lower panel) measured on different days during therapy in 14 patients.

of 30 min/2 h concentration show a tendency to decrease or increase during the course of therapy.

DISCUSSION

Despite exact timing of the aminoglycoside serum concentrations and the acceptable reproducibility of drug analysis, poor correlation was found between the concentrations measured at the end of infusion and 2 h after the start of the infusion. Similar variability of the ratios of 30 min/2 h concentrations was observed for all three aminoglycosides, even though serum concentrations of gentamicin and netilmicin were studied at a different center (Cantonal Hospital St. Gallen) and measured by a different assay technique (fluorescence polarization immunoassay) than amikacin (University Hospital Zurich, biological assay). Therefore the lack of good correlation reflects biological rather than analytical variability.

The rapid decrease in serum concentration that is observed immediately after an infusion is a result of both distribution of the drug into different body compartments and elimination of the drug from the body. Since the elimination rate of aminoglycosides is fairly stable within one dose interval (5,7), the variations of the ratio of 30 min/2 h concentrations must be mainly attributed to variations in the process of drug distribution.

Since there is considerable variability in serum kinetics of aminoglycosides during the first 2 h after the administration of the dose, a uniform time for drawing samples for the determination of peak levels should be established to determine optimal therapeutic serum levels. It has not been established whether efficacy and toxicity correlate better with the peak concentration measured immediately after the end of infusion or 90 min later. Therefore, the dilemma exists as to which peak level offers more information for aminoglycoside monitoring.

Several pharmacokinetic arguments favor the concept of measuring serum levels 60 min after either intramuscular injections or the start of short intravenous infusions of 15 to 30 min. Such 60 min levels are (a) representative of maximal concentrations achieved in interstitial fluid (14), (b) less sensitive to errors in exact timing than samples drawn earlier, (c) less affected by individual differences in drug elimination than samples drawn later, and (d) also used for monitoring drug levels after intramuscular administrations. This concept of measuring peak serum concentrations is supported by a number of other investigators (1,2,4,11).

Another possibility of measuring the peak concentrations was suggested by Zaske et al. (10), who proposed to sample serum specimens immediately at the end of 60-min infusions. The relatively long infusion time of 60 min allows for a more complete equilibration of the distribution process. Because of the simultaneous termination of the infusion and the drawing of the sample, this might be a feasible and practical procedure.

CONCLUSION

There is considerable variability in serum concentrations of aminoglycosides during the first 2 h after the start of 30-min infusions. This variability is not explained by intra- and interindividual differences, renal function, or drug half-life. Therefore the timing of drug administration and the collection of samples for determining peak levels is critically important. A uniform time should be established to determine optimal therapeutic serum concentrations for aminoglycosides.

Acknowledgment: We thank B. Joos, J. Pijck, and H. Soep for analyzing serum specimens to determine the accuracy of the assays used. We also thank S. H. Zinner for critically reading the manuscript and J. McClain for secretarial assistance.

REFERENCES

1. Riff LJ, Jackson GG. Pharmacology of gentamicin in man. *J Infect Dis* 1971;124:S98–105.
2. Kaye D, Levison ME, Labovitz ED. The unpredictability of serum concentrations of gentamicin: pharmacokinetics of gentamicin in patients with normal and abnormal renal function. *J Infect Dis* 1974;130:150–4.
3. Barza M, Brown RB, Shen M, Gibaldi M, Weinstein L. Predictability of blood levels of gentamicin in man. *J Infect Dis* 1975;132:165–74.
4. Siber GR, Echeverria P, Smith AL, Paisley JW, Smith DH. Pharmacokinetics of gentamicin in children and adults. *J Infect Dis* 1975;132:637–51.
5. Blaser J, Rieder H, Niederer P, Lüthy R. Biological variability of multiple dose pharmacokinetics of netilmicin in man. *Eur J Pharmacol* 1983;24:399–406.
6. Schentag JJ, Jusko WJ, Vance JW, Cumbo TJ, Abrutyn M, Delattre M, Gerbracht LM. Gentamicin disposition and tissue accumulation on multiple dosing. *J Pharmacokin Biopharm* 1977;5:559–77.
7. Blaser J, Rüttimann R, Bhend HJ, Lüthy R. Increase of amikacin half-life during therapy in patients with renal insufficiency. *Antimicrob Agents Chemother* 1983;23:888–91.
8. Lüthy R, Münch R, Blaser J, Bhend HJ, Siegenthaler W. Human pharmacology of cefotaxime (HR 756), a new cephalosporin. *Antimicrob Agents Chemother* 1979;16:127–33.
9. Lüthy R. Basis for an adequate dosage of aminoglycoside antibiotics. *Infection* 1980;8(suppl 1):S558–61.
10. Zaske E, Cipolle JC, Rotschafer LD, Solem NR, Mosier NR, Strate RG. Gentamicin pharmacokinetics in 1640 patients: Method for control of serum concentrations. *Antimicrob Agents Chemother* 1982;21:407–11.

11. Ristuccia A, Cunha BA. The aminoglycosides. *Med Clin North Am* 1982;66:303–12.
12. Bennett JV, Brodie JL, Benner EJ, Kirby WMM. Simplified, accurate method for antibiotic assay of clinical specimens. *Appl Microbiol* 1966;14:170–7.
13. Pijck J, Hallynck T, Soep H, Baert L, Daneels R, Boelaert J. Pharmacokinetics of amikacin in patients with renal insufficiency: Relation of half-life and creatinine clearance. *J Infect Dis* 1976;134(suppl):S331–41.
14. Schreiner A, Hellum KB, Digranes A, Bergman I. Transfer of penicillin G and ampicillin into human skin blisters induced by suction. *Scand J Infect Dis* 1978;14(suppl):233–7.

Therapeutic Drug Monitoring
7:308–312 © 1985 Raven Press, New York

Case Report

Evidence Supporting 3(S)-3-Hydroxyquinidine-Associated Cardiotoxicity

Larry D. Bowers, Kay M. Nelson, Robert Connor, Cynthia J. Lais, and Elliot Krauss

Department of Laboratory Medicine and Pathology, University of Minnesota, Minneapolis, Minnesota, U.S.A.

Quinidine has been used since 1749 as a medication for atrial fibrillation and ventricular premature complexes and tachycardia. Despite this long therapeutic history, the mechanism of action of quinidine has not been fully elucidated, nor has its role in "quinidine syncopy" (1) and the associated "sudden death" been described. The pharmacologic activity of the quinidine metabolites and their role in toxicity have been debated (2–6). No reports of toxicity in humans attributable to metabolites have been forthcoming. We present here evidence to support the action of (3S)-3-hydroxyquinidine (3-OHQ) in life-threatening cardiotoxicity, including a case report of the episode that prompted this investigation.

CASE REPORT

A 47-year-old white woman was admitted in July, 1981, for treatment of idiopathic congestive cardiomyopathy. A left anterior hemiblock and first degree A-V block were diagnosed by electrocardiogram. An echocardiogram showed a dilated left ventricle with diffuse hypokinesis and low ejection fraction. The patient was being treated at admission with aminophylline and oral potassium iodide for asthma. Treatment following admission included digoxin (0.125 mg), furosemide (120 mg b.i.d.), isosorbide dinitrate (40 mg q.i.d.), hydralazine (100 mg q.i.d.), and potassium supplements.

Two weeks after initiation of this therapy, the patient experienced several short runs of ectopic ventricular activity. Lidocaine (1 mg/min) and quinidine (300 mg each 6 h) were given. Lidocaine was discontinued the following day to resolve symptoms of toxicity. Steady-state trough quinidine concentrations were <0.5 mg/L. The quinidine dose was increased stepwise to offset suspected poor absorption (Table 1), in an attempt to achieve a therapeutic serum concentration (1.5–5.0 mg/L for quinidine in our laboratory). On day 29, the patient developed ventricular tachycardia resulting in cardiac arrest. The patient was cardioverted, but experienced a second arrest <12 h later. The patient was again successfully resuscitated. In each case, the ventricular tachycardia occurred between 2 and 3 h after the quinidine dose. The quinidine was discontinued after consultation with the laboratory and with clinical pharmacology, and the patient was started on procainamide. The patient improved, with no subsequent arrhythmias. During the period of cardiotoxicity, serum digoxin concentrations were in the 1.0–1.2 ng/ml range, and serum potassium concentrations ranged from 4.0 to 5.1 m*M*.

After the patient had cleared all of the quinidine, a 1,000 mg oral dose was administered; serum concentrations of quinidine and 3-OHQ were measured.

METHODS

Analysis of Samples

The concentrations of quinidine and 3-OHQ are measured using a reversed-phase high performance liquid chromatographic (HPLC) method with fluorescence detection similar to that of Drayer et al. (7). One milliliter of quinine sulfate internal standard (0.6 mg/L) in 0.2 *M* NaOH is added to 100 μl of serum or standard, and the resulting solution is placed on a Dupont type W (polystyrene divinylbenzene) cartridge. The quinidine and 3-OHQ are extracted on the Dupont Prep I, using program 3 with acetone as the eluting solvent. The samples are reconstituted with 20 μl of methanol, and 10 μl is injected into the HPLC

Address correspondence and reprint requests to Dr. L. D. Bowers at Department of Laboratory Medicine and Pathology, University of Minnesota, Minneapolis, MN 55455, U.S.A.

TABLE 1. *Quinidine concentrations and electrocardiographic observations*

Day	Dose	Quinidine (mg/L)	3-hydroxyquinidine (mg/L)	QRS complex (s, $\times 10^3$)	PR interval (s, $\times 10^3$)	QT_c (s, $\times 10^3$)
1	—	—	—	153	200	553
18	300 mg q. 6 h	<0.5	1.15	—	—	—
21	400 mg q. 6 h	<0.5	0.92	153	210	483
25	600 mg q. 6 h	<0.5	1.37	—	—	—
28	800 mg q. 6 h	0.9	2.48			
29[a]	1,000 mg q. 6 h	1.4	4.05	177	232	481
30[b]	1,000 mg q. 6 h	1.5	4.5	200	260	—
32	—	<0.5	0.6	—	—	—
36	—	<0.5	0.5	150	200	—

q., each.
[a]800 mg dose administered 1200 h; arrest occurred 0240 h; blood drawn 0315 h; 1,000 mg dose administered 1800 h.
[b]1,000 mg dose administered 0015 h; arrest occurred about 0300 h; blood drawn 0729 h.

system. The recovery for both quinidine and 3-OHQ was >94%.

The chromatographic system consists of a Waters model 6000 A solvent delivery system, Rheodyne 7120 injection valve, and μ-Bondapak C-18 column. A Perkin Elmer MPF-44A spectrofluorometer is used to monitor the fluorescence of the eluting peaks (λ_{ex} = 350 nm; λ_{em} = 447 nm). The mobile phase is 13/87 acetonitrile/0.01 *M* KH_2PO_4 and 2 g/L tetramethylammonium chloride, adjusted to pH 2.20 with H_3PO_4. The flow rate is 2.5 ml/min ($\Delta P \approx$ 4,000 psi).

The mass spectrometry data were obtained using a Hewlett Packard 5985B mass spectrometer. The 3-OHQ used for standardization was a gift from Beckman Instruments. Samples of 2′-quinididone, quinidine-*N*-oxide, and quinidine-10,11-diol were graciously provided by Dr. Sidney Riegelman's group at the University of San Francisco and used without further purification to identify the retention times of the metabolites. The diol compound was resolved into two distinct peaks, both of which were present in human serum samples (Fig. 1).

Retrospective Chart Review

A retrospective review of the medical records of any of 150 patients who had quinidine measurements ordered during a 6-month study period was undertaken if any of the following occurred: (a) the concentration of 3-OHQ was ⩾2.0 mg/L, (b) the ratio of 3-OHQ to quinidine concentration was >1.0, or (c) the sum of the quinidine and 3-OHQ concentration was >5.0 mg/L. These levels were chosen after a retrospective review of laboratory data taken from archives indicated that ~95% of the concentrations in our files were less than the selection limits. Additional rationale for selection criteria (b) and (c) were obtained from the literature (4,8). The charts selected (14 of 150) were perused for health professionals' notes of minor or serious toxicity, sodium and potassium concentrations, and drug concentrations (particularly other cardioactive drugs) at the time of the

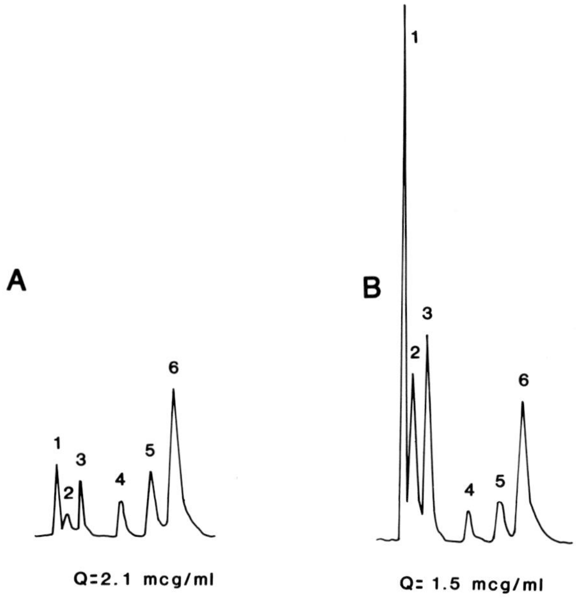

FIG. 1. Chromatogram obtained with the reported high performance liquid chromatographic assay for a typical patient (**A,** quinidine = 2.1 mg/L) and for the case report patient (**B,** quinidine = 1.5 mg/L). The peaks correspond to (1) and (2) quinidine-10,11-diol (1.45 and 1.60 min, respectively), (3) 3-hydroxyquinidine (2.05 min), (4) quinidine-*N*-oxide (3.50 min), (5) quinidine (4.55 min), and (6) quinine (5.40 min) (internal standard). 2′-quininidone (14.5 min) is not shown on this plot and was not detected in this or the other patients reported here. *o*-Desmethylquinidine (2.7 min) was likewise not detected.

unusual quinidine result. During the study, any result meeting criteria (b) was immediately brought to the attention of the clinician.

RESULTS AND DISCUSSION

Quinidine is frequently used as an antiarrhythmic agent. It is extensively metabolized after oral administration, the major metabolites being 3OHQ and 2′-quininidone (2′OXO). Three minor metabolites, *o*-desmethylquinidine, quinidine-*N*-oxide (9), and a 10, 11-diol (8) product are present in small amounts in human serum. There has been some debate regarding the pharmacologic and toxic activity of the metabolites.

Both 3-OHQ and 2′-OXO have activity equivalent to quinidine against chloroform- and hypoxia-induced ventricular fibrillation in mice (3). In $BaCl_2$-induced ventricular arrhythmias in rabbits, 2′-OXO and quinidine exhibited equivalent activity, whereas 3-OHQ was only a third as active and exhibited toxicity in a third of the animals (3). Neither activity nor toxicity could be demonstrated in administration of 3-OHQ to human volunteers (6). More recently, however, it was found that the first pass metabolism of quinidine caused a broadening of the QT interval in humans relative to an equivalent intravenous dose (5).

In the HPLC method used, six peaks are routinely observed in patients administered quinidine, as shown in Fig. 1. Our experience with quinidine analysis indicated that the patient in question had an unusually high concentration of the constituent present in the third peak. Although the diol metabolites are also elevated, this type of pattern, without the elevation in the third peak, has been observed in a number of patients with no serious toxic manifestations. We therefore concentrated on identifying and quantifying the metabolite that was notably increased in the first case of toxicity. Material isolated from this peak gave a mass spectrum consistent with 3-OHQ (10). Subsequent procurement of pure metabolites allowed assignment of the peak identities and the quantitation of the 3-OHQ reported in Table 1. It should be noted that under the conditions used, *o*-desmethylquinidine does not fluoresce efficiently and is thus not detected.

The most striking feature of Table 1 is the high concentration of 3-OHQ relative to quinidine. In earlier work, the ratio of 3-OHQ to quinidine was never observed to exceed 1.0 (4). Nevertheless, it was reported that 3-OHQ made a significant contribution to the effect of quinidine, since 3-OHQ is 74% protein bound compared with 89% protein binding for quinidine (3). Thus, the free concentrations observed could be quite high compared with the free concentration of quinidine. A second finding of note was the coincident timing of the tachycardia and cardiac arrests after the quinidine dose and the peak of the 3-OHQ concentration after a 1 g oral dose was given to the patient reported above (Fig. 2). In light of these results, the peak concentration of 3-OHQ on day 30 could have approached 10 mg/L.

To ascertain the frequency of elevated 3-OHQ concentrations, a study of all quinidine analyses requested during a 6-month period was undertaken. During that period, 295 determinations were made on samples from 150 patients. A histogram of the ratio of the concentrations of 3-OHQ to quinidine is shown in Fig. 3. In contrast to an earlier report (4), seven patients (5%) had a total of 16 measurements in which the ratio was greater than one (Table 2). In five of seven cases, the patients had, or developed, broadened QRS or QT_c intervals or other symptoms of quinidine toxicity (nausea, emesis). In three of these patients, quinidine was discontinued on the basis of clinical signs prior to prospective laboratory contact; of the remaining four patients who were carefully monitored after laboratory consultation, two failed to develop any clinical signs of toxicity. In five of the seven patients, "normal" ratios were observed at least once before the elevations occurred. The reason for this apparent change in metabolism or clearance of quinidine and its metabolites is under further study. Two of the seven had significant changes in their 3-OHQ/quinidine ratio after changing medication form (e.g., quinidine sulfate to gluconate). Whether this has a cause-and-effect relationship will require further study. The differences in peak concentrations and times observed by Greenblatt et al. (11) for quinidine sulfate and gluconate may be attributable to a difference in

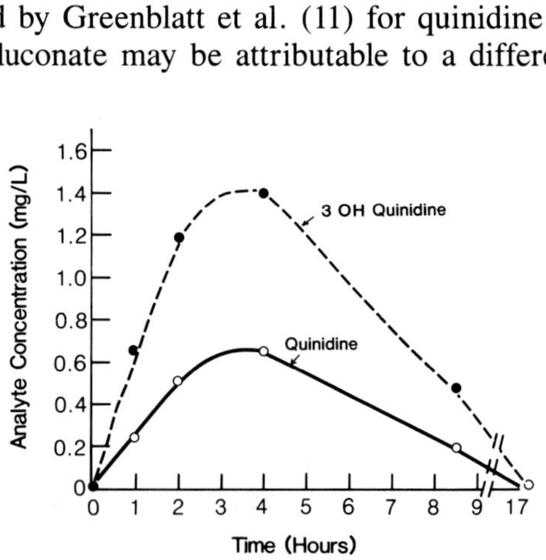

FIG. 2. Time course of quinidine and 3-hydroxyquinidine concentrations in the reported patient after a 1,000 mg oral dose.

TABLE 2. *Summary of clinical and laboratory data on seven patients exhibiting fast metabolism*

Patient	Quinidine (mg/L)	3-OHQ/Q	Comments
1	2.0	3.3	Severe toxicity[a] with an increased QRS interval
2	1.9	1.4	No toxicity documented; QS → QG[b]
3	1.5	1.6	Mild toxicity[c]
4	1.9	1.7	QS → QG[b]
5	1.6	1.5	No toxicity documented
6	0.4	3.1	Mild toxicity[c]
7	1.7	2.0	Severe toxicity[a] with an increased QRS interval

3-OHQ/Q, 3(S)-3-hydroxyquinidine/quinidine ratio.
[a]Cardiovascular arrhythmias.
[b]Change of medication from quinidine sulfate (QS) to quinidine gluconate (QG) within 2 days of elevated ratio. Ratios prior to the change were <1.0.
[c]Includes rash, nausea, emesis.

metabolism of the two drugs due to the nonspecific method used and may support this observation.

It should be emphasized that the laboratory method used to quantify the quinidine has an important role in the clinical interpretation of the concentrations. The fluorescence method of Cramer and Isaksson (12), which has a quoted "therapeutic range" of 2.0–5.0 mg/L, has been shown to measure quinidine and a fraction of the 3-OHQ (13). HPLC methods, such as that used in the present studies, are specific for quinidine but can detect unusual metabolic patterns. Immunochemical methods can be specific for quinidine or can measure a sum of quinidine and metabolites. In either case, the results obtained may vary from lot to lot of antibody.

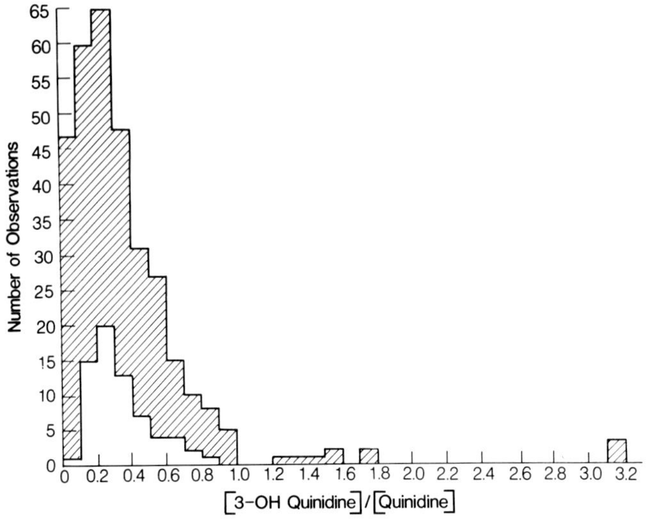

FIG. 3. Histogram of the 3-hydroxyquinidine/quinidine concentration ratio. The clear area represents data previously reported by Drayer et al. (3,4). Lined area represents the results of the present 6-month study.

We attempted to assess whether a particular concentration of 3-OHQ or a sum of quinidine and 3-OHQ concentrations, analogous to the situation for procainamide and *N*-acetylprocainamide, could be shown to be consistently coincident with clinical toxicity. A retrospective chart review of the 150 patients noted above failed to produce any consistent correlations. This may have been due to the relatively small population of patients, to the fact that we only considered 3-OHQ and quinidine, or to the well-known variability in patient response with electrolyte or myocardium status. It is impossible to attribute the toxic manifestations observed solely to 3-OHQ for similar reasons. It is apparent, however, that some patients may produce concentrations of 3-OHQ significantly greater than the quinidine concentration. Although we could document increases in diol concentration, we were unable to detect significant increases in the concentration of the other metabolites. This could have been related to either methodological or pharmacological factors. In any case, it appears that monitoring of the quinidine metabolites, in particular 3-hydroxyquinidine, may be important in the therapeutic monitoring of quinidine.

REFERENCES

1. Selzer A, Wray HW. Quinidine syncopy. Paroxysmal ventricular fibrillation during treatment of chronic atrial arrhythmias. *Circulation* 1964;30:17–26.
2. Drayer DE, Cook CE, Reidenberg MM. Active quinidine metabolites. *Clin Res* 1976;24:623A.
3. Drayer DE, Lowenthal DT, Restivo KM, Schwartz A, Cook CE, Reidenberg MM. Steady-state serum levels of quinidine and active metabolites in cardiac patients with varying degrees of renal function. *Clin Pharmacol Ther* 1978;24:31–9.
4. Drayer DE, Hughes M, Lorenzo B, Reidenberg MM. Prevalence of high (3S)-3-hydroxyquinidine/quinidine ratios in serum, and clearance of quinidine in cardiac patients with age. *Clin Pharmacol Ther* 1980;27:72–5.

5. Holford NHG, Coates PE, Guentert TW, Riegelman S, Sheiner LB. The effect of quinidine and its metabolites on the electrocardiogram and systolic time intervals: concentration-effect relationships. *Br J Clin Pharmacol* 1981;11:187–95.
6. Huffman DG, Hignite GE, Ischanz C. The relationship betwen quinidine, 3-OH quinidine, and the QT_c interval in man. *Clin Res* 1977;25:553A.
7. Drayer DE, Restivo K, Reidenberg MM. Specific determination of quinidine and (3S)-3-hydroxyquinidine in human serum by high-pressure liquid chromatography. *J Lab Clin Med* 1977;90:816–22.
8. Rakhit A, Holford NHG, Guentert TW, Riegelman S. Pharmacokinetics of quinidine and its metabolites in man after i.v. administration and multiple oral doses. *APhA Academy of Pharmaceutical Sciences Meeting*, [Abstracts]. San Antonio, TX. 1980;10:75.
9. Guentert TW, Coates PE, Riegelman S. Isolation and identification of a new quinidine metabolite. *APhA Academy of Pharmaceutical Sciences Meeting*, [Abstracts]. 1978;8:137.
10. Palmer KH, Martin B, Baggett B, Wall ME. The metabolic fate of orally administered quinidine gluconate in humans. *Biochem Pharmacol* 1969;18:1845–60.
11. Greenblatt DJ, Pfeiffer HJ, Ochs HR, MacLaughlin DS, Smith TW, Koch-Weser J. Pharmacokinetics of quinidine in humans after intravenous, intramuscular, and oral administration. *J Pharmacol Exp Ther* 1977;202:365–78.
12. Cramer G, Isaksson B. Quantitative determination of quinidine in plasma. *Scand J Clin Lab Invest* 1963;15:553–6.
13. Guentert TW, Upton RW, Holford NHG, Riegelman S. Divergence in pharmacokinetic parameters of quinidine obtained by specific and nonspecific assay methods. *J Pharmacokinet Biopharm* 1979;7:303–10.

Therapeutic Drug Monitoring
7:313–314 © 1985 Raven Press, New York

Rapid Protein Determinations on Ultrafiltrates Prepared for Free Phenytoin Quantification

Charles P. Turley and Tammy Milligan

Pediatric Pathology Laboratory, Arkansas Children's Hospital, Little Rock, Arkansas, U.S.A.

Summary: Ultrafiltration techniques for the separation of bound and free ligand are dependent on minimal amounts of protein-bound drug leakage through the membrane devices. A dye-impregnated test strip protein assay (Chemstrip-9) provides a rapid, visual assessment of membrane protein leakage. The test strips are sensitive to 200 mg/L of albumin in ultrafiltrates and do not react with as much as 4 mg/L of phenytoin. **Key Words:** Ultrafiltration—Free phenytoin.

The measurement of physiologically active drug concentrations is becoming an increasingly popular tool for assessing therapeutic status, especially in cases of suspected alterations in drug-protein binding. The ultrafiltration techniques provide a rapid, convenient means of separating bound from free ligand that is suitable for clinical and service pharmacology laboratories.

Leakage of protein-bound drug through defective membranes and into the ultrafiltrate can lead to spuriously elevated free phenytoin concentrations. One ultrafiltration device manufacturer recommends that replicate filtrations be performed to check for leakage (1). Alternatively, microprotein quantification can be used to determine whether leakage has occurred. We evaluated the performance of a test-strip method for protein, originally designed for urinary protein measurements, on ultrafiltrates prepared for free phenytoin assays.

MATERIALS AND METHODS

Serum from children receiving therapeutically administered phenytoin was collected in barrier-free tubes (2) and pooled. Ultrafiltrates were prepared by centrifuging 0.5 ml samples in Centrifree filters (Amicon, Danvers, MA, U.S.A.) in a fixed angle centrifuge at 2,000 *g*, 25 ± 3°C for 20 min. Some devices were intentionally damaged by punching one, three, or six holes in the membranes with a 25 gauge needle. Free phenytoin determinations were conducted by TDx fluorescence polarization immunoassay (Abbott Laboratories, North Chicago, IL, U.S.A.). Protein was measured on the Ektachem 400 (Kodak, Rochester, NY, U.S.A.), Chemstrip-9 (Bio-Dynamics, Indianapolis, IN, U.S.A.), and by a modified Lowry method (3).

RESULTS AND DISCUSSION

We assessed the sensitivity limits of the Chemstrip-9 protein strip on ultrafiltrates by spiking an ultrafiltrate (containing 50 mg/L protein by the modified Lowry procedure) with 100, 200, and 300 mg/L bovine albumin. A faint but discernible color change on the Chemstrip-9 protein test strip was observed in 67% of the filtrates containing 100 mg/L protein. It was difficult to assess whether the change was "negative" rather than "trace." The 200 mg/L filtrate had a noticeable color change and was clearly "trace." The filtrates spiked with 300 mg/L protein gave a 1+ reading, equivalent to the color change the test strips give with urine proteins. We concluded that the test strips could easily detect 200 mg/L of protein in the

Address correspondence and reprint requests to Dr. C. P. Turley at Pediatric Pathology Laboratory, Arkansas Children's Hospital, 804 Wolfe Street, Little Rock, AR 72202, U.S.A.

TABLE 1. *Protein and free phenytoin levels in ultrafiltrates prepared from devices having damaged membranes*

Number of holes in membrane	Free phenytoin[a] (mg/L)	Total protein[b] (g/L)	Test strip protein[c]
0	0.60	0.05	Negative
1	2.7	21.0	>3+
3	7.6	63.0	>3+
6	7.9	65.0	>3+

[a]Free phenytoin was measured on the Abbott TDx analyzer. Samples having >4 mg/L phenytoin were diluted before analysis.
[b]Total protein was measured on the Kodak Ektachem 400 analyzer or by the Lowry technique.
[c]Test strip protein was measured on Chemstrip-9. A 3+ reading is equivalent to 5 g/L protein.

ultrafiltrate. Given the test strip sensitivity, we calculate that 0.3% protein leakage can be detected, assuming a serum total protein concentration of 70 g/L.

We then measured free phenytoin and protein concentrations in ultrafiltrates prepared from patent and damaged membranes. Free phenytoin concentrations of as much as 4 mg/L did not cause a color change in the dye-impregnated test strips. The free phenytoin concentrations in the ultrafiltrates prepared from devices having damaged membranes increased linearally with the extent of damage and correlated with the filtrate protein concentrations (r = 0.99) as shown in Table 1. All filtrates prepared from the damaged membranes had >3+ protein by test strip. It was readily apparent that the filtrates prepared from the extensively damaged membranes (three and six holes) were dubious because they had the gross appearance of serum. The moderately damaged membrane (one hole) had a slight yellow hue and best demonstrates the utility of the test strip protein assay. The free phenytoin level of 2.7 mg/L in this specimen could be considered elevated, but was not unexpected in some cases of altered drug-protein binding. The positive test strip protein would, however, alert the analyst to the erroneous result. The 21 g/L total protein content of this filtrate represents leakage of 32% of the total serum protein (65 g/L). We estimate from regression analysis of these data that a twofold elevation in free phenytoin could occur with a protein leakage of 8.3 mg/L (13% leakage). This would be detected as a >3+ protein reading on the test strip.

The test strip methodology is based on the "protein error of indicator dyes" and is most sensitive to albumin, the protein to which phenytoin is primarily bound. We conclude that strips should prove to be a useful, rapid, and inexpensive tool in screening ultrafiltrates for protein contamination, especially in drug monitoring laboratories not equipped with microprotein testing capabilities.

REFERENCES

1. Centrifree micropartition system. Package insert. Danvers, Massachusetts: Amicon Corp. 1984.
2. Quattrocchi F, Karnes HT, Robinson JD, Hendeles L. Effect of serum separator blood collection tubes on drug concentrations. *Ther Drug Monit* 1983;5:359–62.
3. Lowry OH, Rosenbrough NJ, Farr AL, Randall RJ. Protein measurement with the Folin phenol reagent. *J Biol Chem* 1951;193:265.

Therapeutic Drug Monitoring
7:315–320 © 1985 Raven Press, New York

Analysis of 6-Mercaptopurine in Serum or Plasma Using High Performance Liquid Chromatography

*†C. E. Whalen, †‡H. Tamary, †‡M. Greenberg, †‡A. Zipursky, and *†§S. J. Soldin

*Departments of *Clinical Biochemistry, §Pharmacology, and ‡Pediatrics, University of Toronto, and †Research Institute, The Hospital for Sick Children, Toronto, Ontario, Canada*

Summary: The analysis of 6-mercaptopurine (6-MP) by a rapid, sensitive, and specific high performance liquid chromatographic assay is described. This method does not require any derivatization and allows for direct quantitation of the drug. Only 200 μl of serum or plasma is needed, and concentrations as low as 10 ng/ml can be reliably quantitated. Analytical recoveries of 83% for 6-MP and 71% for the internal standard, 6-thioguanine, are obtained. Between-day precision studies at three plasma concentrations of 6-MP produce a mean coefficient of variation of 7.2%. This assay will be clinically useful for pharmacokinetic studies of 6-MP in patients in remission of acute lymphoblastic leukemia. **Key Words:** 6-Mercaptopurine—High performance liquid chromatography—Acute lymphoblastic leukemia.

6-Mercaptopurine (6-MP) (Fig. 1) has been used as an antineoplastic agent since it was first synthesized and developed by Elion and Hitchings in 1951 (1). Today, the daily oral administration of 6-MP forms the backbone of maintenance chemotherapy for acute lymphoblastic leukemia (ALL).

Induction therapy using prednisone and vincristine is successful in producing a complete remission in 90% of patients with ALL (2); however, response to maintenance therapy with 6-MP is variable, with 35% of these patients relapsing (3). Studies recently completed have shown that there are great individual differences in the pharmacokinetics of 6-MP in patients with ALL (4). These differences may explain some of the unpredictable responses to maintenance therapy.

The 6-MP plasma concentrations are found to be unexpectedly low and highly variable, with marked individual differences found in the peak plasma concentration and the time to peak concentration. Perhaps of greatest importance is the existence of a greater than fivefold variation in the area under the plasma concentration-time curve (4). These variations result in unpredictable exposure to the drug after a uniform oral dose. Therefore, by monitoring the 6-MP concentration over time, we can individualize dosage regimens, thereby ensuring the adequate drug exposure required to prolong remission.

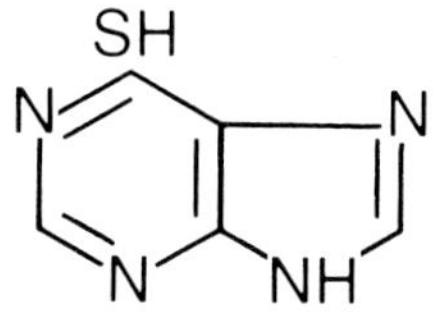

FIG. 1. Structure of 6-mercaptopurine.

6-MP is a purine analogue whose metabolites are responsible for the biological effects of the drug. 6-MP must be converted intracellularly to thioinosinic acid before it can exert any antileukemic or toxic effect (5) (Fig. 2). The relationship between plasma levels of the parent compound and intracellular levels of the metabolite has not yet been determined; however, it can be expected that useful information may be obtained by studying the relationship between the

Address correspondence and reprint requests to Dr. S. J. Soldin at Department of Biochemistry, The Hospital for Sick Children, 555 University Avenue, Toronto, Ontario M5G 1X8, Canada.

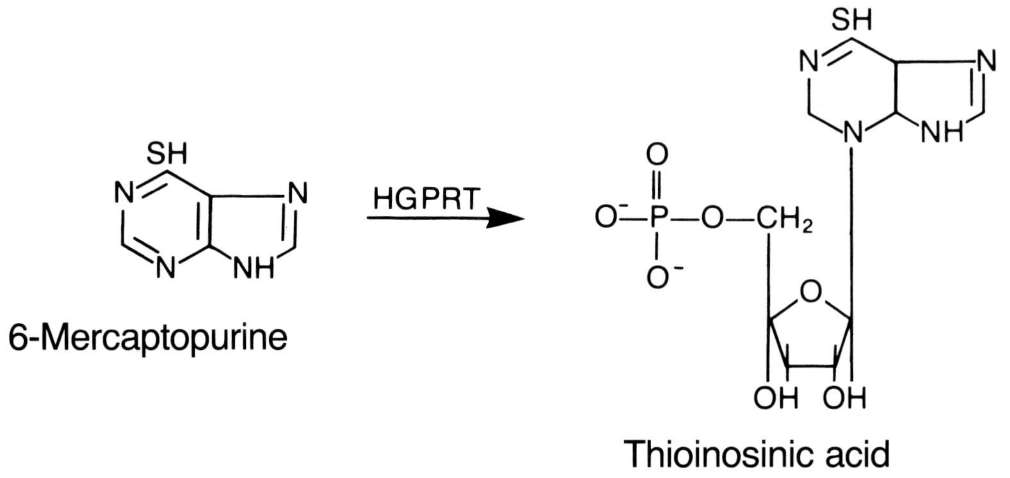

FIG. 2. The anabolic conversion of 6-mercaptopurine to thioinosinic acid (6-MP riboside-5′-phosphate) by hypoxanthine guanine phosphoribosyl transferase (HGPRT).

AUC (concentration × time) of 6-MP versus the biological effects.

There are a variety of published methods for the analysis of 6-MP. Fluorometric detection has been used in several instances; however, the methods by Maddocks (6), Finkel (7), and Tawa et al. (8) require many time-consuming analytical steps and do not allow for the direct quantitation of 6-MP, but rather measure the concentration of the 6-MP derivatives, purine-6-sulfonates. Colorimetric (9) and gas chromatographic (10) methods have also been devised; however, their lower limit of sensitivity of 200 and 500 ng/ml, respectively, makes these procedures impractical for clinical use. A gas-chromatographic–mass-spectrometric method by Rosenfeld et al. (11) has a maximal 6-MP recovery of only 40%.

Several high performance liquid chromatographic (HPLC) methods have also been published. The procedures developed by Lin et al. (12) and Day et al. (13) have a lower limit of sensitivity of 258 and 200 ng/ml, respectively, which severely restricts their use in most clinical trials. The methods by Narang et al. (14), Abreu et al. (15), and Ding and Benet (16) all require larger sample volumes, a greater number of analytical steps, and a longer time for sample analysis than the procedure reported in this paper. Furthermore, the method published by Ding and Benet has a recovery for 6-MP of only 12%.

The HPLC method presented in this paper is simple, allows for the direct quantitation of 6-MP in 200 μl of either serum or plasma, and is both sensitive and specific enough to monitor 6-MP pharmacokinetics in a clinical situation.

METHODS

Apparatus

This study used a model 6000 A solvent delivery system (Waters Associates Inc., Milford, MA, U.S.A.) with a Model U6K injector (Waters Associates, Inc.). The columns used were connected in series and were the 7.5 cm × 4.6 mm ID Altex Ultrasphere with 3μ-octadecylsilane particles (Beckman Instruments, Berkeley, CA, U.S.A.) and a 30 cm × 4 mm reverse phase μ-Bondapak C-18 column with 10 μm particles (Waters Associates, Inc.) The model 441 absorbance detector (Waters Associates, Inc.) was set to a full scale absorbance of 0.005, and a fixed wavelength of 313 nm was used. The spectrophotometer was attached to a Houston Instrument, Omniscribe model B5217-Al strip chart recorder (Houston Instruments, Austin, TX, U.S.A.). The absorption spectra of 6-MP were obtained with a Zeiss spectrophotometer PMQII (Carl Zeiss, Oberkochen, G.F.R.).

Reagents

Toluene (T324B), hydrochloric acid, sodium hydroxide (NaOH), and potassium phosphate (KH_2PO_4) were purchased from the Fisher Scientific Co. (Chemical Manufacturing Division, Fair Lawn, NJ, U.S.A.). Ethyl acetate (Omniscribe, glass distilled) was purchased from BDH Chemicals (Toronto, Ontario, Canada), and methanol (UV cutoff 204 nm) from Caledon Laboratories Ltd. (Georgetown, Ontario, Canada). 6-MP, 2-amino-6-mercaptopurine (6-thioguanine), phenylmercuric acetate, and dithiothreitol were obtained from the Sigma Chemical Co. (St. Louis, MO, U.S.A.).

The mobile phase was a 98/2 volume mixture of a 10 m*M* KH_2PO_4 buffer, pH 2.5, and methanol, respectively. The mobile phase also contained a 1 m*M* concentration of dithiothreitol.

Stock solutions of 1 mg/L 6-MP and 20 mg/L 6-thioguanine (internal standard) were made in methanol. These stock solutions were then used to make aqueous standard solutions of 1 mg/L 6-MP and 10 mg/L 6-thioguanine. A 0.4 N NaOH solution was made in distilled water. These solutions remained stable for several weeks when stored at 4°C. A solution of 0.03% phenylmercuric acetate was made in ethyl acetate. This solution remained stable for 1 week when stored at 4°C.

Extraction Procedure

The extraction procedure developed centers on the sulfhydryl group of the 6-MP molecule and is a modification of the method described by Maddocks (6). The thiol group of 6-MP, in alkalinized plasma, reacts with the mercury atom of phenylmercuric acetate, creating the complex, 6-phenylmercury mercaptopurine. This complex is less polar than the parent 6-MP and therefore is more soluble in an organic solvent. When the organic layer is shaken with dilute hydrochloric acid, the complex dissociates and 6-MP is regenerated.

This assay requires only 200 μl of plasma or serum. The internal standard, 6-thioguanine (10 μl), is added to the sample before the extraction to give a concentration of 0.48 mg/L. The procedure is as follows: to the plasma is added 400 μl ethyl acetate containing a concentration of 0.03% phenylmercuric acetate, 400 μl toluene, and 20 μl 0.4 N NaOH. This is vortex-mixed for 15 sec and centrifuged at 12,000 *g* for 2 min, and 600 μl of the clear organic layer is then transferred to a second tube, where 100 μl 0.1 N hydrochloric acid is added. This tube is then vortex-mixed for 15 sec and centrifuged at 12,000 *g* for 1 min, and 80 μl of the acid phase is then injected into the system (Fig. 3). The conditions of chromatography are shown in Table 1.

All volumes stated allow for the highest possible recovery for both 6-MP and 6-thioguanine.

A typical chromatogram for a serum sample containing 0.1 μg/ml 6-MP is illustrated in Fig. 4.

To 200 μL of plasma or serum add:

↓

10 μL 6-thioguanine (internal std)
400 μL toluene
400 μL ethyl acetate containing 0.03% PMA
20 μL 0.4N sodium hydroxide

↓

Vortex
Centrifuge

↓

Transfer 600 μL of the overlying clear organic layer

↓

Add 100 μL 0.1N hydrochloric acid

↓

Vortex
Centrifuge

↓

Inject 80 μL of acid phase

FIG. 3. Schematic representation of the extraction procedure. PMA, phenylmercuric acetate.

Method of Calculation

Three standard serum pools were prepared with the addition of 0.025, 0.05, and 0.1 mg/L 6-MP. These pools were analyzed each day, and the peak height ratio of 6-MP to 6-thioguanine was determined. These ratios were then divided by the concentration of drug known to be in the sample. A mean of the three resulting factors was calculated and then used to cal-

TABLE 1. *Conditions of analysis*

Parameter	Assay conditions
Mobile phase	98/2, 10 m*M* potassium phosphate pH 2.5/methanol; 1 m*M* dithiothreitol
Columns	Altex Ultrasphere 7.5 cm × 4.6 mm ID connected to μBondapak C-18 4 mm × 30 cm
Temperature	Ambient
Pressure	2000 psi
Absorbance full scale	0.005
Flow rate	1.0 ml/min
Wavelength	313 nm
Internal standard	6-thioguanine
Retention time (6-mercaptopurine)	13 min
Retention time (thioguanine)	11 min

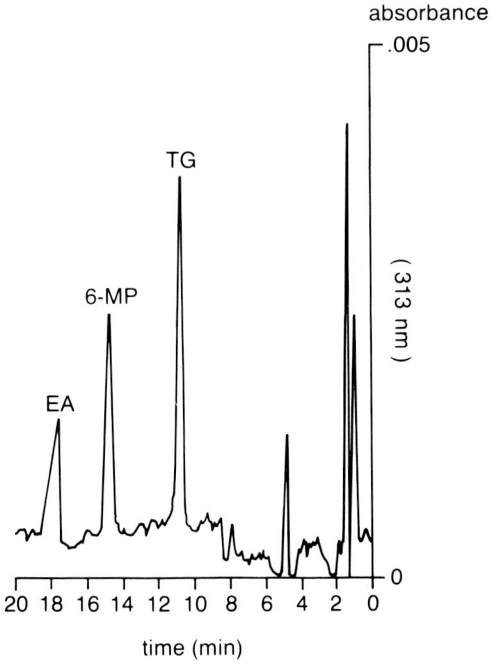

FIG. 4. Chromatogram of a serum sample containing 0.1 μg/ml 6-mercaptopurine and 0.48 mg/L 6-thioguanine. The peak due to ethyl acetate is also shown.

culate the unknown concentration of drug in the patient samples, as shown below:

$$\frac{\text{peak height of 6-MP in unknown}}{\text{peak height of internal standard in unknown}} \times \frac{1}{\text{mean factor}} = \text{concentration of 6-MP in mg/L}$$

Recovery Studies

The recovery of both 6-MP and thioguanine was determined by the following procedure. Known concentrations of aqueous standards were injected to obtain standard peak heights for both thioguanine and 6-MP. Plasma aliquots containing 6-MP at concentrations of 0.025, 0.05, and 0.1 mg/L were each analyzed 12 times, as described previously. The concentrations chosen cover the clinically relevant range for 6-MP. The percentage analytical recovery was then calculated from the peak height obtained as compared with those obtained by the direct injection of standard. Results are shown in Table 2.

RESULTS AND DISCUSSION

Detector Wavelength

This system uses a mercury vapor lamp at a fixed wavelength of 313 nm. Although the absorbance of 6-MP at 313 nm is only 80% of the maximum absorbance, the greater stability and more constant intensity of the signal using the mercury line enable us to work at a greater sensitivity than would be possible employing a variable wavelength detector with a deuterium lamp.

TABLE 2. *Recovery studies*

Concentration	Number analyzed	Analytical recovery (%)[a]
6-Mercaptopurine		
0.025 mg/L	12	87
0.05 mg/L	12	80
0.1 mg/L	12	81
Thioguanine		
1.0 mg/L	20	71

[a]Average, 83%.

Mobile Phase

It was noted that the separation of 6-MP and 6-thioguanine is highly dependent upon the pH and the solvent used. Resolution between the two compounds increased as the pH was decreased. The lower limit for the columns, pH 2.5, allows for optimal separation of the two compounds. Methanol was preferred to acetonitrile as the solvent, as it provides better resolution of the drug and internal standard, with an optimal separation being achieved at a methanol concentration of 2%.

Dithiothreitol (DTT) is a reducing agent that acts to stabilize the thiol group of 6-MP. Without the addition of DTT, the 6-MP was unstable in the mobile phase.

Optimal Phenylmercuric Acetate Conditions

A concentration of 0.03% phenylmercuric acetate (PMA) was made in ethyl acetate. This particular concentration was chosen because any increased amounts of PMA interacted with the binding sites on the columns, and the 6-MP peak heights then decreased over a period of several injections. The 0.03% PMA concentration minimized the binding interactions and allowed for optimal 6-MP recovery. This concentration differs significantly from the 0.3% reported by Maddocks (6).

Ethyl acetate was preferred to toluene, water, or diethyl ether and was chosen as the solvent for PMA because it easily dissolved the PMA and allowed for the highest possible recovery of the drug.

Columns

This procedure requires two columns run in series. The Altex Ultrasphere is responsible for the separation of 6-MP from the ethyl acetate peak which appears in the extraction chromatogram. The Altex column follows the Waters 30 cm column, which is required for the separation of 6-MP from thioguanine. No single column could be found to separate the three peaks after all parameters had been varied.

Precision

The between-day precision of this assay was determined over a period of 20 consecutive days using three 6-MP plasma concentrations covering the clinically relevant range. At concentrations of 0.025, 0.05, and 0.1 mg/L, the method yielded coefficients of variation of 7.9%, 7.3%, and 6.6% respectively.

Stability

Oxidation of the thiol group of 6-MP appears to cause an instability of the aqueous standard when maintained at room temperature over a period of several hours. By maintaining the standard in an ice bath, this instability has been eliminated. This instability was also noted in extracted samples not immediately analyzed. Therefore, all samples are extracted just prior to their injection into the system. When frozen, 6-MP is not stable in plasma. This is demonstrated in Fig. 5. This problem has been eliminated by partial extraction of each sample before freezing with the addition of ethyl acetate containing the PMA. The ethyl acetate solution containing the 6-MP complex formed with the PMA is stable for at least 1 week.

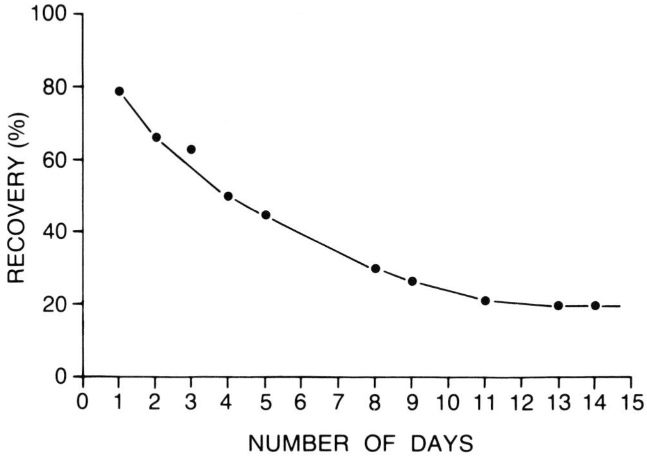

FIG. 5. 6-Mercaptopurine (6-MP) stability curve showing the decrease in 6-MP recovery over a period of 2 wk when the serum is not partially extracted before being frozen.

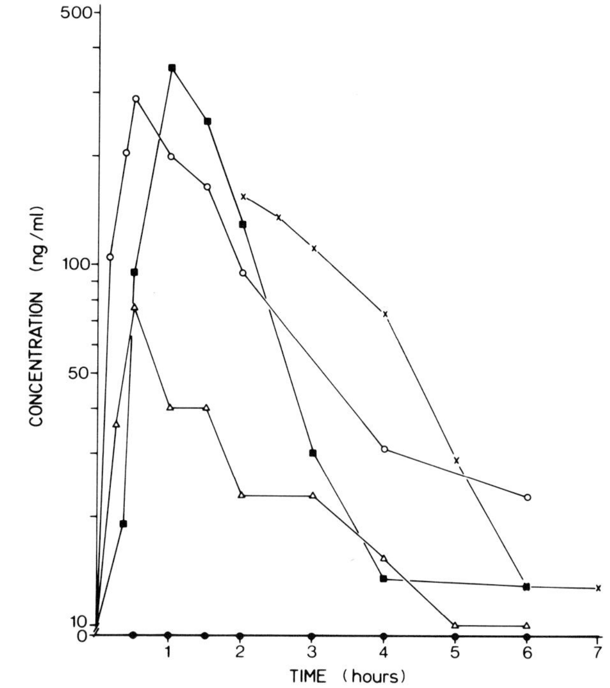

FIG. 6. Pharmacokinetic profile of the plasma concentration of 6-mercaptopurine (6-MP) versus time in five subjects after oral administration. Patients B.P. (black circles), K.B. (white triangles), N.B. (black squares), B.K. (white circles), and S.S. (x-x) all received 75 mg/m² 6-MP.

Interference Studies

A series of 20 patient samples, none of which contained 6-MP, was extracted and analyzed. No peaks were found to interfere with 6-MP or thioguanine. Direct injection of methotrexate, sulfamethazine, sulfadiazene, sulfamerazine, digoxin, acetylsalicylic acid, cyclophosphamide, bleomycin, vinblastine, nitrogen mustard, and Septra (trimethoprim and sulfamethoxazole), all dissolved in distilled water, showed no peaks that would interfere with either 6-MP or thioguanine. Patient samples containing digoxin, phenobarbital, phenytoin, carbamazepine, methotrexate, cyclophosphamide, cis-platinum, adriamycin, gentamicin, theophylline, valproic acid, primidone, trimethoprim, sulfamethoxazole, ethosuximide, caffeine, and their metabolites were run through the extraction procedure. No peaks with the retention times of 6-MP or thioguanine were observed.

Preliminary Clinical Studies

Serum concentrations of 6-MP were measured in five patients over a 6-h period post oral dose. The results of the study are shown in Fig. 6 and summarized in Table 3. The patients were each in remission

TABLE 3. *Pharmacokinetic values of oral 6-mercaptopurine in patients*

Patient	Age/sex (yr)	Weight (kg)	Peak plasma concentration (ng/ml)	Time to plasma peak (min)	$t_{1/2}$ (min)	AUC (μM min)
B.P.[a]	9/M	26.6	—	—	—	0
K.B.	2.75/M	12.5	75	30	100	57.6
N.B.	7/M	24.2	350	60	36	196
B.K.	3.5/M	14.9	290	30	65	211
S.S.[b]	4/M	20	—	—	67	185

[a]The pharmacokinetic study was completed twice; the area under the plasma concentration curve (AUC) was zero in both cases.
[b]The first 2 h of sample collection were unavailable; therefore, the AUC is approximate only.

from ALL and were receiving 75 mg/m^2 of 6-MP daily. Marked individual differences are demonstrated.

After oral administration, the mean elimination half-life was 67 ± 23 min (range 36–100 min). The mean peak plasma concentration of 6-MP was found to be 238 ± 118 ng/ml, and the mean area under the plasma concentration curve (AUC) was 130 ± 85 μM min (range 0–211 μM min).

The AUC, a measure of exposure of tissues to drug as delivered by the systemic circulation, was noted to have a greater than 10-fold variation because one patient had an AUC of zero. A greater than fourfold variation in the peak plasma concentration and a two-fold variation in time to peak plasma concentration also existed between individuals. This variability resulted in unpredictable plasma concentrations after a uniform oral dose and may explain the unpredictable response to maintenance therapy.

We are in the process of correlating serum concentrations of 6-MP and methotrexate with both toxicity and relapse-free interval. Should good correlations exist, we will then individualize dosage regimens, thereby ensuring an adequate drug exposure required to prolong remission.

REFERENCES

1. Elion GB, Hitchings, GE, Vanderwerff H. Antagonists of nucleic acid derivatives. VI. Purines. *J Biol Chem* 1951;192:505–18.
2. Ortega JA, Nesbit ME, Donaldson MH. L-asparaginase, vincristine and prednisone for induction of first remission in acute lymphoblastic leukemia. *Cancer Res* 1977;37:535.
3. Simone JV. The treatment of acute lymphoblastic leukemia. *Br J Haematol* 1980;45:1.
4. Zimm S, Collins J, Riccardi R, et al. Variable bioavailability of oral mercaptopurine. Is maintenance chemotherapy in acute lymphoblastic leukemia being optimally delivered? *N Engl J Med* 1983;308:1005–9.
5. Elion GB, Hitchings GH. Metabolic basis for the action of analogues of purines and pyrimidines. *Adv Chemotherapy* 1965;2:91–177.
6. Maddocks J. Assay of azathioprine, 6-mercaptopurine and a novel thiopurine metabolite in human plasma. *Br J Clin Pharmacol* 1979;8:273–8.
7. Finkel J. A fluorometric method for the estimation of 6-mercaptopurine in serum. *Anal Biochem* 1967;21:363–71.
8. Tawa R, Takeshima S, Hirose S. The use of xanthine oxidase for a specific and sensitive fluorometric determination of 6-mercaptopurine in serum. *Biochem Med* 1984;32:303–10.
9. Loo TI, Phil D, Luce SK, Sullivan MP, Frei III E. Clinical pharmacologic observations on 6-mecaptopurine and 6-methylthiopurine ribonucleoside. *Clin Pharm Ther* 1968;9:180–94.
10. Bailey D, Wilson T, Johnson G. A gas chromatographic method for measuring 6-mercaptopurine in serum. *J Chromatogr* 1975;111:305.
11. Rosenfeld J, Jaguchi V, Hillcoat B, Kawai M. Determination of 6-mercaptopurine in plasma by mass spectrometry. *Anal Chem* 1977;49:725–7.
12. Lin S-N, Jessup K, Floyd M, et al. Quantitation of plasma azathioprine and 6-mercaptopurine levels in renal transplant patients. *Transplantation* 1980;29:290–4.
13. Day JL, Tterliktis L, Niemann R, Mobley A, Spikes C. Assay of mercaptopurine in plasma using paired-ion high performance liquid chromatography. *J Pharm Sci* 1978;67:1027–8.
14. Narang P, Yeager R, Chatterji D. Quantitation of 6-mercaptopurine in biologic fluids using high performance liquid chromatography: a selective and novel procedure. *J Chromatogr* 1982;230:373–80.
15. Abreu R, Van Baal J, Schouten T, Schretlen E. High performance liquid chromatographic determination of plasma 6-mercaptopurine in clinically relevant concentrations. *J Chromatogr* 1982;227:526–33.
16. Ding TL, Benet L. Determination of 6-mercaptopurine and azathioprine in plasma by high performance liquid chromatography. *J Chromatogr* 1979;163:281–8.

Therapeutic Drug Monitoring
7:321–323 © 1985 Raven Press, New York

Reversed-Phase High Performance Liquid Chromatographic Determination of Nifedipine in Human Plasma

B. J. Gurley, Robert G. Buice, and Paramjeet Sidhu

Department of Pharmaceutics, University of Tennessee Center for the Health Sciences, Memphis, Tennessee, U.S.A.

Summary: A reversed-phase high performance liquid chromatographic method is presented by which the calcium channel blocker, nifedipine (NFP), may be measured in human serum using 17-α-ethinylestradiol as an internal standard. A mobile phase of phosphate buffer (0.01 *M*, pH 6.1)/methanol/acetonitrile (20:35:45) passed through a μBondapak C-18 column at 1.0 ml/min produced symmetrical bands for nifedipine and internal standard. A rapid and simple chloroform extraction of NFP from 1 ml serum samples proved to be efficient and reproducible. Recovery over a concentration range of 5–100 ng/ml was 92.3 ± 5.1% (mean ± SD, n = 6). Ultraviolet absorbance detection at 235 nm was sensitive to serum NFP concentrations of 5 ng/ml. Between-day coefficients of variation at 100 and 5 ng/ml were 4.0 and 11.4%, respectively (n = 10). Serum concentration data from NFP-treated subjects are presented. **Key Words:** Nifedipine—Liquid chromatography.

Nifedipine (NFP) is a calcium channel blocker that has recently become available for clinical use. NFP increases cardiac output, reduces peripheral resistance, and is an effective coronary vasodilator (1). NFP may be administered intravenously although the oral route is more common. It is extensively metabolized to inactive products with only a small fraction of the administered dose being excreted unchanged (1,2). In solution NFP is both thermally unstable and light-sensitive, undergoing photo-oxidation by daylight to form the nitrosopyridine homologue and by UV light to form the nitropyridine homologue (3).

In the past NFP concentrations in biological fluids have been successfully measured by gas liquid chromatography, but a recent trend toward high performance liquid chromatography (HPLC) has produced several methods. For our purposes these methods were found to be less than adequate because they produce poor quality chromatograms (4,5), require excessive sample volumes (4), elevate column temperatures (6), involve complicated extraction procedures with long turnaround times (3,4,5,6), or result in less than adequate sensitivity (7). In the present report we describe a rapid and relatively simple HPLC method for the quantitation of NFP in human plasma. Plasma concentration data from NFP-treated subjects are presented.

METHODS

The instrumentation consisted of a U6K injector, a model 6000A solvent delivery system, a μBondapak C-18 column, and a model 481 variable wavelength detector (235 nm) (Waters Associates, Milford, MA, U.S.A.). The mobile phase [0.01 *M* phosphate buffer, pH 6.1/methanol/acetonitrile (20:35:45)] was passed through the column at a flow rate of 1.0 ml/min. Analytical samples of NFP were supplied by Pfizer, Inc. (New York, NY, U.S.A.) and the internal standard (17-α-ethinylestradiol) was purchased from Sigma Chemical Co. (St. Louis, MO, U.S.A.). All solvents

Address correspondence and reprint requests to Dr. Robert G. Buice at Department of Pharmaceutics, University of Tennessee Center for the Health Sciences, Memphis, TN 38163, U.S.A.

were HPLC grade and all reagents were analytical grade. All work was performed in subdued light, and any glassware used throughout the procedure was wrapped in foil.

Prior to HPLC analysis, NFP was separated from plasma by solvent extraction. Calibration standards of NFP in methanol were prepared in concentrations of 5 to 100 ng/ml, and 1 ml of each standard was added to a separate 20 ml silanized screw-cap tube. Following the addition of 50 μl of internal standard [17-α-ethinylestradiol (7.5 gm/ml in methanol)], the contents of each tube were evaporated to dryness under nitrogen, 1 ml normal human plasma was added, and each tube was vortexed 45 s yielding calibration samples containing NFP in serum over a concentration range of 5–100 ng/ml.

For patient samples containing NFP, 50 μl of internal standard was added to each of a series of 20 ml silanized screw-cap tubes, methanol was evaporated to dryness under nitrogen, 1 ml patient plasma was added, and each tube was vortexed 45 s. To each 1 ml calibration sample and each 1 ml patient sample was added 2 ml sodium carbonate (0.5 *M*) and 10 ml water-saturated chloroform. Tubes were shaken 20 min and centrifuged 10 min at 3,000 rpm. The aqueous phase was removed by aspiration, and 8 ml of the chloroform phase was transferred to a 15 ml silanized conical tube. Chloroform was evaporated to dryness under nitrogen, the contents of each tube were reconstituted in 100 μl mobile phase, and a 10 μl aliquot was injected. Peak height ratios of drug/internal standard were used for NFP quantitation. Efficiency and between-day precision of the extraction procedure, over a concentration range of 5–100 ng/ml, were assessed daily for 6 days by comparing calibration curve slopes (extracted spiked serum vs. NFP standards simulating 100% recovery). Between-day precision of the method was further assessed by replicate assays (n = 10) of human serum containing NFP (100 and 5 ng/ml).

Plasma NFP concentrations in subjects participating in a clinical study were measured by this method. NFP was administered orally to each subject in the form of a 10 mg capsule. Blood samples (6 ml) were obtained by venipuncture and collected in heparinized glass vials wrapped in foil. Plasma was separated by centrifugation (3,000 rpm for 10 min) and stored in the dark at −20°C until assay. Each sample was assayed in duplicate.

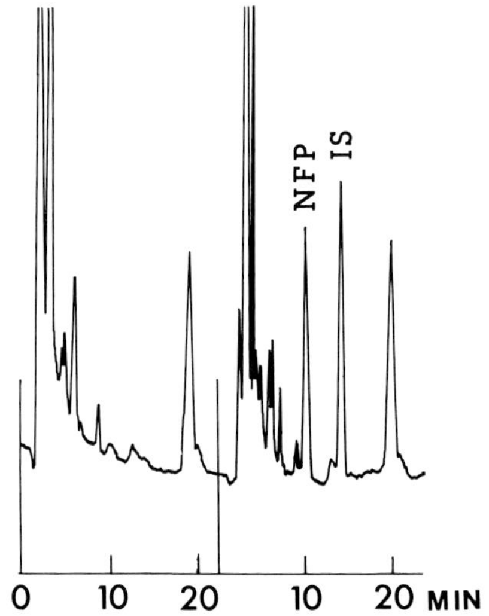

FIG. 1. High performance liquid chromatograms from the analysis of plasma containing nifedipine (NFP) (25 ng/ml, 0.002 aufs) compared with that of blank plasma. IS, internal standard.

RESULTS AND DISCUSSION

Chromatograms presented in Fig. 1 compare the analysis of plasma containing NFP with that of blank plasma. UV detection at 235 nm was sensitive to NFP concentrations as low as 5 ng/ml. Cross-interference studies with other drugs were not performed, but analysis of numerous normal human and patient plasma blanks revealed no chromatographic bands that interfere with the measurement of NFP in the proposed concentration range. Moreover, analysis of photodegradation products (nitrosopyridine and nitropyridine) suggested no potential interference with drug or internal standard. In vitro degradation studies in this laboratory have shown that NFP in methanol exposed to normal room lighting (~50 fc, daylight fluorescent) decomposes at a rate of ~4%/h. Therefore samples containing NFP should be carefully protected from light during each phase of sample preparation and chromatographic analysis. Calibration plots over a 6-day period were linear from 5 to 100 ng/ml (correlation coefficient 0.9969 ± 0.0019, mean ± SD, n = 6). Analytical recovery from 5 to 100 ng/ml over the same time period was found to be 92.3 ± 5.1% (mean ± SD, n = 6), representing a between-day coefficient of variation of 5.5%. Replicate assays of plasma containing 100 and 5 ng/ml revealed between-day coefficients of variation of 4.0 and 11.4%, respectively (n = 10). Representative data from NFP-treated subjects are given in Table 1.

TABLE 1. *NFP concentrations in plasma taken 1 h after administration of a 10 mg oral capsule (each sample assayed in duplicate)*

Subject	Plasma concentrations (ng/ml)
1	35.3, 39.2
2	84.7, 95.2
3	47.6, 47.6
4	43.1, 43.1
5	43.1, 51.0
6	58.2, 52.9
7	58.2, 58.2
8	37.0, 37.0

This method affords several advantages over previously reported HPLC methods for NFP. Adequate resolution of symmetrical bands is evidenced in Fig. 1. Detection is sensitive to 5 ng/ml using only 1 ml plasma. The simplicity of the extraction permits a turn around time of <2 h. Thus the method is adequate for therapeutic monitoring of NFP-treated patients as well as pharmacokinetic/bioavailability studies.

REFERENCES

1. Henry PD. Comparative pharmacology of calcium antagonists: nifedipine, verapamil, and diltiazem. *Am J Cardiol* 1980;46:1047–58.
2. Stone PH, Antman EM, Muller JE, Braunwald E. Calcium channel blocking agents in the treatment of cardiovascular disorders. Part II. Hemodynamic effects and clinical applications. *Ann Intern Med* 1980;93:886–904.
3. Pietta P, Rava A, Biondi P. High performance liquid chromatography of nifedipine, its metabolites and photochemical degradation products. *J Chromatogr* 1981;210:516–21.
4. Sadanaga T, Hikida K, Tameto K, Matsushima Y, Ohkura Y. Determination of nifedipine in plasma by high performance liquid chromatography. *Chem Pharm Bull* 1982;30:3807–9.
5. Dokladolova J, Tykal JA, Coco SJ, Durkee PE, Quercia GT, Korst JJ. Occurrence and measurement of nifedipine and its nitropyridine derivative in human blood plasma. *J Chromatogr* 1982;231:451–8.
6. Bach PR. Determination of nifedipine in serum or plasma by reversed-phase liquid chromatography. *Clin Chem* 1983; 29:1344–8.
7. Miyazaki M, Kohri N, Arita T, Shimono H, Katoh K, Nomura A, Yasuda H. High performance liquid chromatographic determination of nifedipine in plasma. *J Chromatogr* 1984;310:219–22.

Therapeutic Drug Monitoring
7:324–328 © 1985 Raven Press, New York

Quantitative Liquid Chromatography of Allopurinol and Oxypurinol in Human Plasma and Urine

*J. M. Failler, *†R. Farinotti, and *A. Dauphin

**Service Pharmaceutique, C.H.U. Bichat, Paris, and †Laboratoire de Chimie Analytique II, Faculté de Pharmacie, Chatenay Malabry, France*

Summary: A high performance liquid chromatographic (HPLC) assay is described for allopurinol and oxypurinol determination in human plasma and urine, in the range expected during therapy. The procedure involves addition of trichloroacetic acid to samples, followed by centrifugation. The supernatant is then neutralized and analyzed by reversed-phase HPLC. Characteristics of the method are reported, and data are presented on its application to the pharmacokinetics studies. Separation is optimal with an octadecylsilane (ODS) stationary phase and a sodium acetate mobile phase adjusted to pH 7.2 for plasma and pH 5 for urine. **Key Words:** Allopurinol—Oxypurinol—Plasma—Urine—High performance liquid chromatography.

Allopurinol (A) is a purine analog drug that inhibits the formation of uric acid from xanthine and hypoxanthine by an action on xanthine oxidase. Furthermore, the major oxidative metabolite, oxypurinol (O), is also an inhibitor of the enzyme and thus leads to a reduction in plasma and urinary uric acid levels. It appears that much of the effectiveness of treatment of gout with A may be due to the activity of O (1). Assay procedures suitable for biochemical and pharmacological studies are based on high performance liquid chromatography (HPLC) (2–5). The sample preparation steps necessitate ligand exchange chromatography (2) or chemical deproteinization with perchloric or trichloracetic acids (3–5). Separations are realized with an ion exchange (2) or a reversed-phase mode (3,5–8). These methods require ultraviolet (2,4–6,9) or electrochemical (7) detection. In order to study the pharmacokinetics of A and O, we report a rapid and sensitive HPLC technique. The procedure involves deproteinization of samples with trichloroacetic acid, centrifugation, and neutralization of the supernatant prior to injection. The method discriminates between the naturally occurring purines and is suitable for simultaneous determination of A and O in serum and urine.

Address correspondence and reprint requests to Dr. J. M. Failler at Service Pharmaceutique, C.H.U. Bichat, 46, rue H. Huchard, 75018 Paris, France.

MATERIALS AND METHODS

Chemicals and Reagents

The following materials were used: 1.22 *M* sodium hydroxide; sodium acetate 3 H_2O (Prolabo); trichloroacetic acid 20%; 1 *M* pH 4.5 acetate buffer; and A, O, xanthine, and hypoxanthine (Sigma). Stock standard solutions of A (100 mg/L) and O (1 g/L) were prepared in distilled water. Dissolution required addition of a drop of 1 *M* sodium hydroxide.

Material and Chromatographic Conditions

The liquid chromatographic system used consisted of a Chromatem model 380 pump (Touzart et Matignon), a Wisp (Waters intelligent sample processor), a detector Schoeffel model 757 (used at a wavelength of 254 nm), and a data module recording integrator

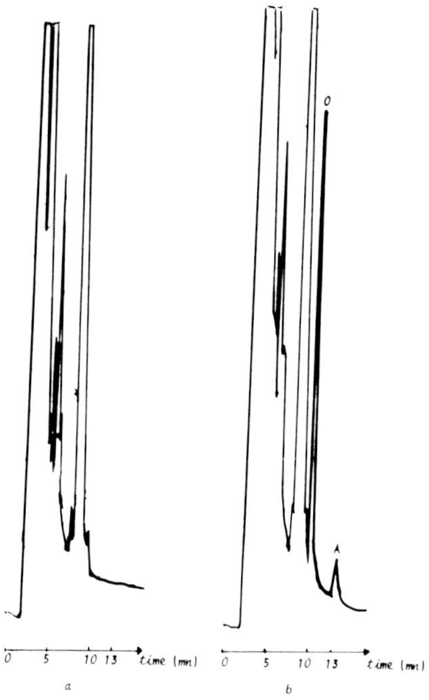

FIG. 1. Chromatogram of a blank plasma **(a)** and of a plasma spiked with allopurinol (0.5 mg/L) and oxypurinol (5 mg/L) **(b)**.

HP 3390 A (Hewlett Packard). The guard column and column (Brownlee) were filled with the same sorbent. The cartridge was a RP 18-5 μm, 4.6 × 220 mm type. For plasma analysis, the separation was performed isocratically, employing a 0.02 *M*, pH 7.2 sodium acetate mobile phase. For urine samples, the pH of the solution was adjusted to 5 with acetic acid. In all cases, the flow rate was 1.3 ml min^{-1}. The mobile phase was filtered through a HA 0.45 μm filter (Millipore). Pure water and acetonitrile were used at the end of each day to purge the column.

Biological Sample Collection and Storage

Blood and urine samples were obtained from healthy volunteers treated with different doses of A. Plasma was collected into tubes containing disodium EDTA and immediately centrifuged. All plasma and urine samples were stored at − 20°C until analysis.

Preparation of Working Standards

For plasma standards, 10, 25, 50, 75, and 150 μl of stock solution of A and 10, 25, 50, 75, and 100 μl of stock solution of O, respectively, were added to normal human plasma from volunteers not receiving this drug. The final volume was adjusted to 5 ml with plasma. These plasma standards were produced containing the range 0.20–3.00 mg/L of A and 2–20 mg/L of O.

Urine standards were prepared similarly with 25, 50, 150, and 300 μl of stock solution of A, and with 10, 25, 50, 100, and 150 μl of stock solution of O, to obtain the range 0.5–6 mg/L of A and 2–30 mg/L of O. We adjusted final volume to 5 ml with a pool of blank urine diluted 10-fold with distilled water.

Sample Preparation

Samples were prepared by adding 100 μl of 20% trichloroacetic acid to 0.5 ml of plasma or 0.5 ml of a 10-times-diluted urine. After mixing 30 sec on a Vortex mixer and centrifugation at 3,000 *g* for 10 min at 4°C, 0.2 ml of the supernatant was neutralized with 50 μl of 1.22 *M* sodium hydroxide and 50 μl of 1 *M* pH 4.5 acetate buffer. Twenty-five microliters of this solution was injected in the chromatograph. However, 50 μl of the solution was injected to analyze quantitatively the 24 and 48 h O amounts of the pharmacokinetics studies. The final concentration in urine was obtained including the 10 dilution factor.

RESULTS

Plasma Analysis

Figure 1 illustrates chromatograms obtained from a blank plasma and a spiked plasma sample. As can

TABLE 1. *Reproducibility of allopurinol and oxypurinol: determination in spiked plasma (n = 5)*

Concentration of allopurinol (mg/L)	CV (%)		Concentration of oxypurinol (mg/L)	CV (%)	
	Within-day	Day-to-day		Within-day	Day-to-day
0.20	4.2	8.5	2	5.3	8.4
0.50	3.5	6.6	5	3.7	7.5
1.00	3.2	5.9	10	3.8	7.6
1.50	3.6	5.8	15	3.3	5.5
3.00	2.6	5.6	20	1.9	4.0

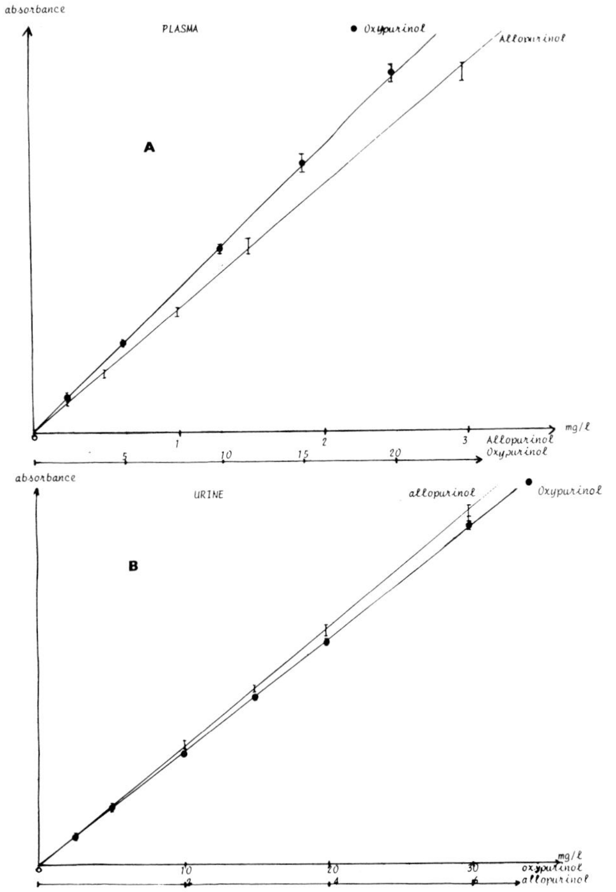

FIG. 2. Calibration curves. **A:** Plasma calibration curve. **B:** Urine calibration curve.

be seen, there are no interfering peaks at retention times corresponding to those of A and O. Reproducibility was determined on spiked plasma over a concentration range of 0.2–3 mg/L for A and 2–20 mg/L for O, by assaying five plasma samples at each concentration. Within-day and between-day precision of the assay was assessed by determining the coefficient of variation (CV) at each of several A and O concentrations. The data in Table 1 clearly demonstrate that the CV of the method is <6% for both drugs at each concentration in the intraassay and <10% in the day-to-day assay. Calibration curves were linear from 0 to 20 mg/L for O and from 0 to 10 mg/L for A (Fig. 2). Under these conditions, the lower limit of quantitative sensitivity is 0.02 mg/L for A and 0.15 mg/L for O. In order to evaluate the recovery of any compound after deproteinization, we analyzed five samples of plasma at different concentrations based on comparison with aqueous mixed standards (Table 2). It can be seen that A is more adsorbed on protein precipitate (83%) than O (95%). We studied the elution of A, O, and other xanthines, as uric acid, xanthine, and hypoxanthine, on the C_{18} column as a function of pH of the eluent (Table 3). There is a change in the capacity factors (k′ values) of all peaks, but the change was most significant for uric acid. Concentration of sodium acetate in the mobile phase did not modify the capacity factors of O and A (Table 4).

As an example, we report the concentration profiles for A and O in the plasma following the administration of 300 mg A orally to a volunteer (Fig. 3). The drug was rapidly absorbed, reaching a peak of 1.70 mg/L at 1 h, and eliminated with a half-time of ~0.92h; and O reached a maximal concentration of 5.80 mg/L at 3 h followed by a slow elimination with a half-time of ~20 h. These results were in good agreement with findings by previous workers (3).

Urine Analysis

Figure 4, a chromatogram of a urine fraction (0–3 h) from a volunteer who had received 100 mg of A, shows an absence of interfering peak relatively to blank urine.

As for plasma, a good linearity of response (Fig. 2) and a good reproducibility (Table 5) were obtained.

TABLE 2. *Analytical recoveries of standards from five treated plasma specimens*

Concentration of allopurinol (mg/L)	Recovery (%)	Concentration of oxypurinol (mg/L)	Recovery (%)
0.2	83	2	98
0.5	81	5	93
1.0	81	10	93
1.5	83	15	94
3.0	89	20	98
mean ± SD	83.4 ± 3.3	mean + SD	95.2 ± 2.6

TABLE 3. *Variation of capacity factors (k′) of allopurinol, oxypurinol, uric acid, xanthine, and hypoxanthine at different pH values*

	pH			
	4	5	6	7.2
k′ Oxypurinol	7.1	8.4	10.4	9.1
k′ Allopurinol	8.2	10.2	12.9	12.3
k′ Uric acid	3.8	3.8	2.1	1.2
k′ Xanthine	6.0	7.2	7.0	5.6
k′ Hypoxanthine	5.0	5.8	6.2	6.2

TABLE 4. *Variation of capacity factors (k′) of allopurinol, oxypurinol, and uric acid vs sodium acetate concentration in mobile phase* (*C**) (pH = 7.2)

	*C** (mol/L)		
	$5 \cdot 10^{-3}$	10^{-2}	$2 \cdot 10^{-2}$
k′ Oxypurinol	8.8	9.5	9.1
k′ Allopurinol	12.2	12.1	12.3
k′ Uric acid	0.8	1.1	1.2

DISCUSSION

Reproducibility of the method is very dependent on the deproteinization step. This phase does not occur as an important loss of A and O during precipitation; the supernatant solution injected does not reduce the column life, and its selectivity must be sufficient to eliminate interfering compounds contained in the biological fluid. The procedure is completed by neutralization of the supernatant before injection. This treatment does not change the chromatographic conditions and reduces the loss in efficiency of the column. At the end of each analytical day, we washed the column with water and then with acetonitrile. Because of the nature of the sample preparation procedure and the excellent reproducibility of injection, the use of an internal standard proposed by some authors was deemed unnecessary.

Chromatographic conditions were established in a reversed-phase system, varying the nature, the ionic strength, and the pH of the mobile phase. Many investigators (5,6,9) used phosphate buffer at various pH values to elute uric acid and other interfering substances near the void volume. In our procedure, use of organic buffer as sodium acetate was easier, limiting the risks of microcrystallization.

Varying the concentration from 5 to 20 m*M* of the sodium acetate mobile phase (keeping the pH at 7.2) revealed an increase in k′ values (Table 4); however, this fact is not very important. In each case, uric acid eluted very rapidly. A better elution was obtained with the concentration of 20 m*M*. Under these conditions, the retention times also increased by changing the pH from 4 to 7.2.

For A and O, k′ values are greater at pH 7.2 than at pH 4. Uric acid is eluted rapidly at pH 7.2, and other endogenous or exogenous derivatives—xanthines (xanthine, hypoxanthine, theophylline, theobromine) or drugs such as phenylbutazone, indomethacin, ketoprofen, antineoplastic (5-fluorouracil, methotrexate, doxorubicine)—do not interfere with the measurement. For plasma analysis, the best result was obtained at pH 7.2. The urine analysis was performed with a mobile phase at pH 5, which offered a better resolution (Fig. 4B).

CONCLUSION

This method offers the advantages of speed and sensitivity. Quantitative recoveries are obtained without internal standard by a sample extraction procedure. Sodium hydroxide and acetate buffer yield a fairly neutral pH of the supernatant without undue dilution of sample. This advantage was associated with the use of an organic buffer, as the mobile phase reduces column deterioration.

Furthermore, the aqueous nature of the eluent limits the baseline fluctuations usually due to its absorb-

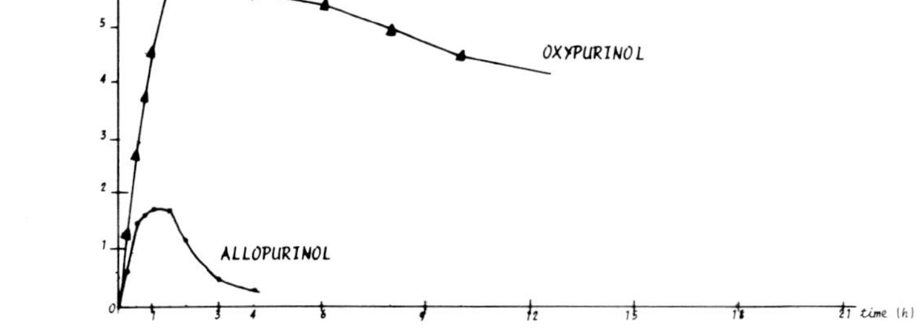

FIG. 3. Plasma concentration time profile of allopurinol (small dots) and oxypurinol (triangles) after oral administration of 300 mg of allopurinol.

TABLE 5. *Reproducibility for allopurinol and oxypurinol determination in spiked urine (n = 5)*

	Concentration of allopurinol (mg/L)						Concentration of oxypurinol (mg/L)					
	0.5	1	2	3	4	6	2.5	5	10	15	20	30
CV%	9.0	5.4	4.7	2.1	2.5	3.0	3.0	3.0	1.5	1.0	1.7	3.1

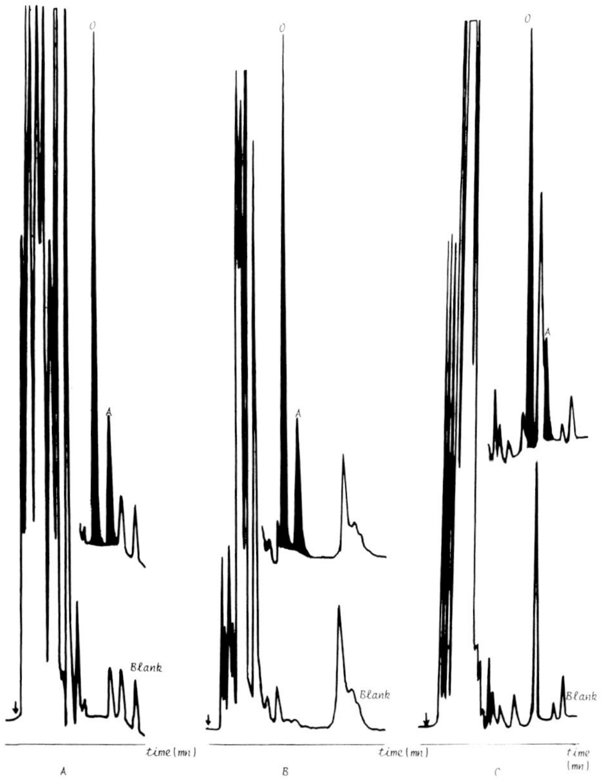

FIG. 4. Retention time variations of oxypurinol (O), allopurinol (A), and endogenous interfering compounds in urine. **A:** pH = 6. **B:** pH = 5. **C:** pH = 4.

ance or the pump pulsations. Also, the method is suitable for clinical analysis of large number of biological specimens, and it is used in our laboratory to study the influence of associated drugs on oxypurinol pharmacokinetics in gouty patients.

REFERENCES

1. Massey V, Komai H, Palmer G. On the mechanism of inactivation of xanthine oxidase by allopurinol and other pyrazolo-(3,4-d)-pyrimidines. *J Biol Chem* 1970;245:2837–44.
2. Brown M, Bye A. The determination of allopurinol and oxopurinol in human plasma and urine. *J Chromatogr* 1977;143:195–202.
3. Sved S, Wilson DL. Analysis of allopurinol and oxypurinol in plasma and its application to metabolic studies. *Biopharm Drug Dispos* 1980;1:111–7.
4. Wung WE, Howell SB. Simultaneous liquid chromatography of 5-fluorouracil, uridine, hypoxanthine, xanthine, uric acid, allopurinol, and oxipurinol in plasma. *Clin Chem* 1980;26:1704–8.
5. Kramer WG, Feldman S. Apparent metabolism of allopurinol by blood—a preliminary report. *Res Commun Chem Pathol Pharmacol* 1977;18:781–4.
6. Boulieu R, Bory C, Baltassat P. Simultaneous determination of allopurinol, oxipurinol, hypoxanthine and xanthine in biological fluids by high-performance liquid chromatography. *J Chromatogr* 1984;307:469–74.
7. Palmisano F, Desimoni E, Zambonin PG. High-performance liquid chromatography with polarographic and voltammetric anodic detection: simultaneous determination of allopurinol, oxipurinol and uric acid in body fluids. *J Chromatogr* 1984;306:205–14.
8. Taylor A, Dady PJ, Harrap KR. Quantitative high-performance liquid chromatography of nucleosides and bases in human plasma. *J Chromatogr* 1980;183:421–31.
9. Chang SL, Kramer WG. Improvements to a high-performance liquid chromatographic assay for allopurinol and oxipurinol in plasma. *J Chromatogr* 1980;181:286.

Therapeutic Drug Monitoring
7:329–335 © 1985 Raven Press, New York

Determination of Warfarin in Human Plasma by High Performance Liquid Chromatography and Photodiode Array Detector

Per Magne Ueland, Gry Kvalheim, *Per Eystein Lønning, and *Stener Kvinnsland

*Clinical Pharmacology Unit, Department of Pharmacology and *Department of Oncology, University of Bergen, Norway*

Summary: A simple liquid chromatographic method for the determination of warfarin in human plasma is described. The method involves precipitation of plasma proteins with acetonitril. No further processing of samples is required. The supernatant was analyzed on a short (10 cm) 3-μm reversed-phase column eluted with 23% acetonitril in 100 m*M* ammonium formate, pH 3.5. The method takes advantage of the fact that warfarin dissolved in this mobile phase has a characteristic absorbance spectrum with distinct peaks at 271, 281, and 305 nm. Using an online photodiode array detector, the UV spectrum could be recorded during analysis without interrupting the flow of the mobile phase. This spectral information improves identification possibilities and evaluation of the purity of the chromatographic peaks. Warfarin was separated from other UV-absorbing compounds in plasma in <3 min, and there was no interference from numerous drugs given to patients. The standard curve (305 nm) was linear in the concentration range observed after oral intake of the single dose of warfarin and for a time corresponding to several half-lives. The detection limit of the method was about 0.1 μg/ml when the absorbance was recorded at 305 nm. At this wavelength, the solvent front was small relative to that observed at lower wavelengths. The precision of the method, given as coefficient of variation, was 6.4%. The method was used for the determination of plasma half-lives of R- and S-warfarin in humans. **Key Words:** Warfarin—High performance liquid chromatography—Photodiode array detector.

Warfarin (3-(α-acetonylbenzyl)-4-hydroxycoumarin) is an extensively used peroral anticoagulant. This drug has an asymmetric carbon atom and exists in two enantiomeric forms, R- and S-warfarin. The clinical form of the drug is a racemate, but the S-form is more effective as an anticoagulant than the R-form (1). Warfarin undergoes stereoselective hydroxylation catalyzed by hepatic mixed function oxidase (1–3).

The therapeutic effect of warfarin and other coumarin anticoagulants has usually been monitored from prothrombin times (4). Recently, it has been demonstrated that a significant correlation exists between suppression of prothrombin complex activity and total warfarin in plasma, suggesting that plasma warfarin monitoring may represent a guideline for the design of warfarin dosage regimens (5). In addition, plasma warfarin assays are occasionally required to check patient compliance to therapy, to quantify covert anticoagulant ingestion, to monitor warfarin resistance, and to study warfarin drug interactions (4).

Widely used methods for the determination of warfarin in plasma involve spectrophotometry, thin-layer chromatography, or gas chromatography. These methods suffer from complex sample processing or low sensitivity and specificity (6–11). Recently, several

Address correspondence and reprint requests to Dr. P. M. Ueland at Clinical Pharmacology Unit, Laboratory of Clinical Biochemistry, 5016 Haukeland sykehus, Bergen, Norway.

convenient high performance liquid chromatography (HPLC) assays for warfarin in plasma have been developed. These methods include extraction of warfarin in plasma into an organic phase, followed by analysis of the extract by reversed-phase liquid chromatography. The absorbance of the effluent is recorded by either a fixed or a variable wavelength detector (12–18).

UV-visible photodiode array detectors for HPLC have recently been introduced. This detector allows continuous recording of absorbance spectra of the compounds eluting from the column within 40 ms without interrupting the flow of the mobile phase. The advantages of this detector in screening for drugs and drug metabolites in biological material have recently been pointed out by Overzet et al. (19).

Warfarin has a rather characteristic absorption spectrum with three absorbance maxima in the range 200–400 nm. The spectral properties of this drug allow the evaluation of the purity and indicate the identity of the warfarin peak in plasma. This makes warfarin an ideal drug for HPLC analysis involving a photodiode array detector.

MATERIALS AND METHODS

Chemicals and Drugs

HPLC-grade acetonitril was purchased from Ratburn Chemicals, Ltd. (Peeblesshire, Scotland). R-warfarin, S-warfarin, and warfarin racemate (sodium salts) were gifts from Chemoswed AB (Malmø, Sweden). O.D.S. Hypersil 3 μm microparticle medium for reversed-phase chromatography was obtained from Shandon Southern Products Ltd. (Cheshire, England) and Pelliquard LC-18 (40 μm) from Supelco, Inc. (Bellefonte, PA, U.S.A.). The analytical column was slurry-packed with O.D.S. Hypersil at 9,000 psi, using a Shandon column packer. The guard column was dry-packed and subjected to mechanical compression, as described previously (20).

Standards

R-warfarin or S-warfarin was dissolved in 100% acetonitril at a concentration of 0.2–10 mg/ml. The compounds were diluted in acetonitril to known concentrations.

Spectrophotometry

Warfarin (5 mg/ml racemate) was dissolved in 23% acetonitril in 100 m*M* ammonium formate, pH 3.5, or in acetonitril. The absorbance spectrum was recorded between 190 nm and 600 nm using a recording spectrophotometer from Kontron, model 810.

Sample Processing

Plasma was mixed with equal volumes of 100% acetonitril. The precipitated protein was removed by centrifugation, and the supernatant was transferred to sample vials for HPLC analysis.

Instruments

A Spectra-Physics SP 8700 solvent delivery system was connected to a Perkin-Elmer ISS 100 autosampler for HPLC, equipped with a coolable sample tray. The column outlet was connected to a photodiode array detector, model HP 1040 A, from Hewlett Packard. In some experiments a variable wavelength detector, model Spectroflow 773 from Kratos, was used. The chromatographic profiles were routinely recorded and integrated by a reporting integrator (Spectra Physics model SP 4270 or Hewlett Packard model HP 3390A). The absorbance spectra of the upslope, top, and downslope of the warfarin peaks were monitored and stored on floppy discs (model HP 82901 M from Hewlett Packard). The spectra (and the chromatograms) were recorded by a X-Y plotter (model HP 7470 A from Hewlett Packard).

HPLC

Samples of 25 μl were injected into a 3 μm O.D.S. Hypersil column (10 cm) equipped with a guard column (2.5 cm). The sample tray was cooled (0–2°C) by circulating 20% ethanol. The column was eluted isocratically at ambient temperature with a mobile phase composed of 23% acetonitril in 100 m*M* ammonium formate, pH 3.5. The flow rate was 2 ml/min, corresponding to a back pressure of 3,500 psi. The retention time was 2.6 min for both R- and S-warfarin.

RESULTS

Extraction of Warfarin from Plasma

Human plasma was supplemented with warfarin (racemate) at concentrations in the range found in plasma from patients receiving a single dose (about 0.3 mg/kg) of the drug. Warfarin was extracted from plasma by mixing plasma with equal volumes of acetonitril. The recovery of warfarin, determined by

TABLE 1. *Recovery of exogenously added warfarin from plasma*

Concentration of warfarin (μg/ml)	Recovery (%)
10	101.2 ± 1.1
2	100.4 ± 1.9
0.2	95.0 ± 2.1

A concentrated solution (1 mg/ml) of warfarin in acetonitril was diluted in plasma to 10 μg/ml and was further diluted with plasma to the concentrations given in the table. In a parallel experiment, the same concentrated standard was diluted according to the same procedure, except that plasma was replaced with distilled water. The recovery of warfarin from plasma was determined by comparison of the peak area of standards in water vs. standard extracted from plasma. The values are given as mean ± SEM of four determinations.

comparison of the peak area of standard in water versus standard extracted from plasma, was 95% (Table 1).

Absorbance Spectrum

The absorbance spectrum of racemate warfarin was identical with that of the separate enantiomers and was dependent on the medium in which the drug was dissolved (data not shown). Warfarin in a solution with the same composition as the mobile phase (23% acetonitril in 100 m*M* ammonium formate, pH 3.5) showed a characteristic spectrum with three distinct maxima (at 271, 281, and 305 nm) and a shoulder at 317 nm. This spectrum (Fig. 1), obtained by conventional scanning photometer equipped with a deuterium and tungsten lamp, was equal to that obtained by HPLC and a photodiode array detector (Fig. 3).

Reversed-Phase Liquid Chromatography

The reversed-phase column was routinely subjected to refilling and mechanical compression (20) each 100 injections to prevent peak splitting during unattended analysis.

Figure 2 shows chromatograms of plasma from a patient treated with warfarin (panels to the left) or plasma from the same patient before treatment (panels to the right). The absorbance was recorded simultaneously at eight different wavelengths, and the profiles obtained at 254, 271, 281, and 305 nm are shown in the figure. Warfarin eluted as a single sharp peak at a retention time of 2.6 min. Warfarin was separated from interfering material at 271, 281, and 305 nm, but a peak eluted close to warfarin at 254 nm. The solvent front was less pronounced at higher wavelengths (Fig. 2).

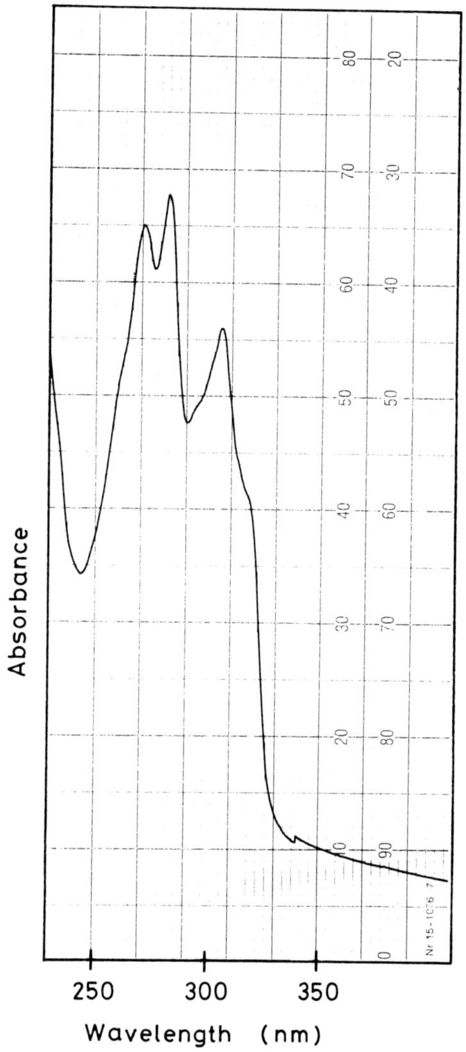

FIG. 1. The absorbance spectrum of warfarin. Warfarin (racemate) was dissolved in 100 m*M* ammonium formate, pH 3.5, containing 23% acetonitril. The absorbance was recorded between 230 and 400 nm using a conventional recording spectrophotometer equipped with a deuterium and tungsten lamp.

Identification and Purity of the Chromatographic Peak

The warfarin peak in plasma obtained from persons receiving single doses of warfarin p.o. cochromatographed with authentic warfarin (racemate) in several systems (15–30% acetonitril in 100 m*M* ammonium formate, pH 3.5).

The absorbance spectrum of warfarin in plasma from patients receiving this drug was routinely recorded. Figure 3 shows the spectrum at the upslope, maximum, and downslope of the warfarin peak in plasma. The chromatogram of the same plasma is shown in Fig. 2. The spectra were identical with each

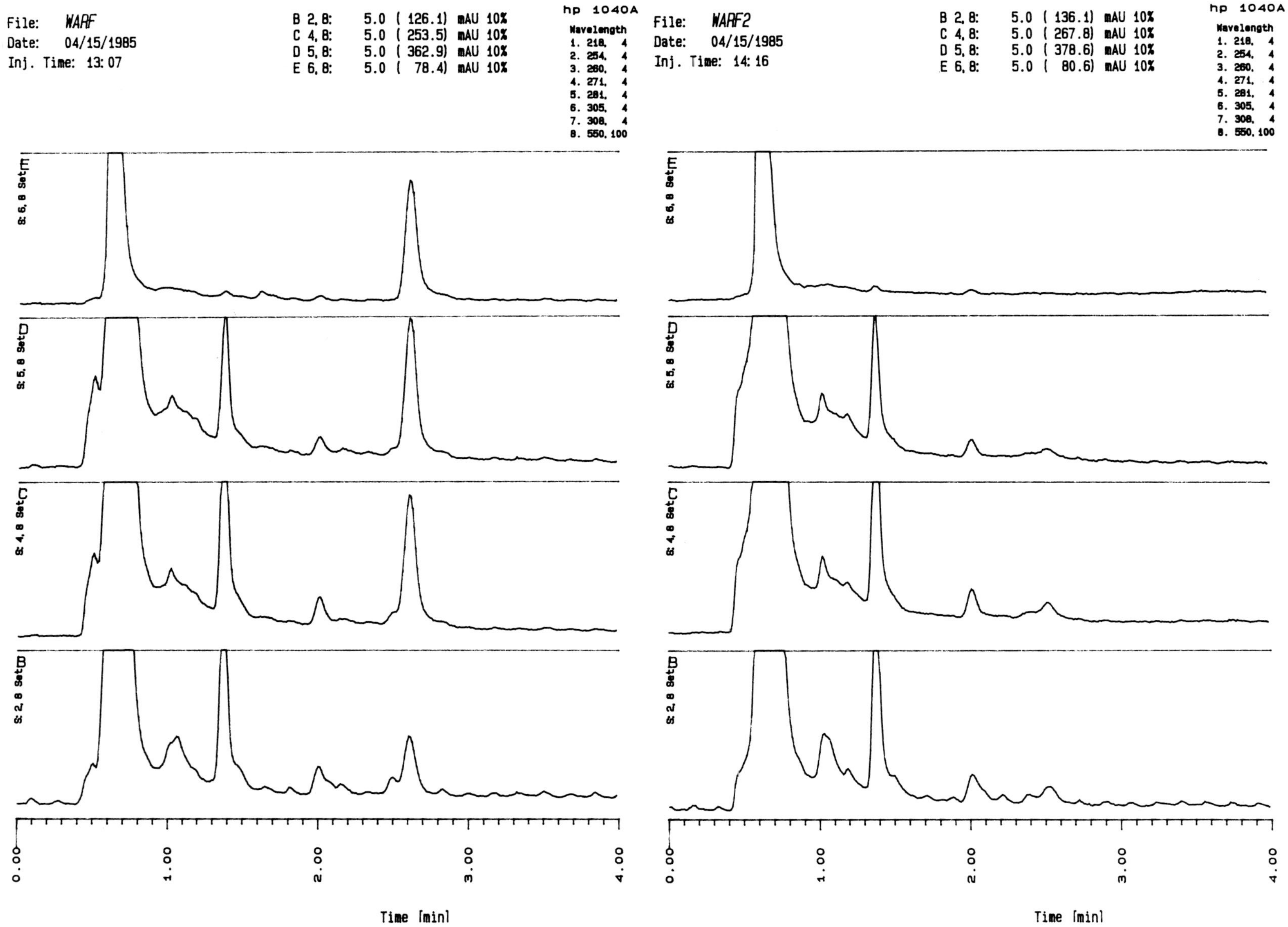

FIG. 2. Multiple signal plot of plasma containing warfarin (panels to the left) or containing no drug (panels to the right). Plasma from a patient was subjected to analysis by reversed-phase liquid chromatography, before and after initiation of warfarin treatment. The absorbance of the effluent was recorded by a photodiode array detector simultaneously at the eight wavelengths given in the upper right corner of each set. The chromatographic profiles obtained at 254 nm (lower panels, **B**), 271 nm (panels **C**), 281 nm (panels **D**) and 305 nm (upper panels, **E**) are shown.

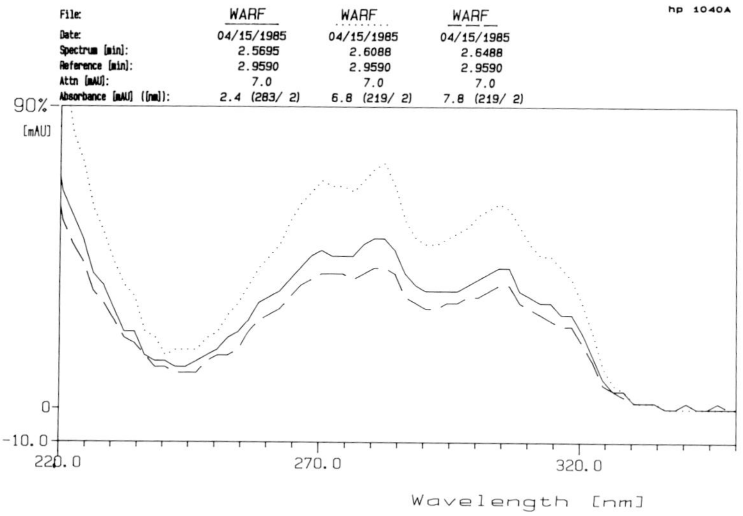

FIG. 3. Absorbance spectra of the warfarin peak in plasma. The absorbance spectrum of the chromatographic peak tentatively identified as warfarin in Fig. 2 was recorded at the upslope (solid line), apex (dotted line) and downslope (interrupted line) of the peak.

other (Fig. 3) and with the spectrum obtained by injection of warfarin standard (data not shown). The comparison of the spectra of the various parts of the chromatographic peak was facilitated by computerized overlay of the separate spectra. In Fig. 3, the attenuations were selected to slightly separate the spectra.

The data in Fig. 3 show that the sensitivity of the photodiode array detector allows the recording of an absorbance spectrum of high quality of warfarin in plasma from a patient treated with this drug. The main details of the spectrum were also apparent in chromatograms of plasma 2–3 half-lives after the patient received a single dose (about 20 mg) of warfarin (data not shown).

Standard Curves, Detection Limit, and Precision of the Method

The standard curves of warfarin in plasma were constructed at three wavelengths, corresponding to the absorbance maxima of warfarin, i.e., at 271, 281, and 305 nm (Fig. 4). Linear standard curves were obtained at these wavelengths, and the detection limit was about 0.07 μg warfarin per ml plasma.

Experiments were carried out to compare the photodiode array detector with a conventional variable wavelength detector, characterized by low noise. The detection limit of the latter detector was about the same at all wavelengths corresponding to the absorbance maxima of warfarin (271, 281, and 305 nm), and the detection limit was about 20% of that observed with the photodiode array detector (data not shown). Because of the small solvent front at 305 nm and no interference at this wavelength (Fig. 2), the pilot signal was routinely recorded at 305 nm.

The within-run precision of the method was determined by analyzing 10 samples of the same plasma containing warfarin (2μg/ml). The coefficient of variation was 6.4%.

Interference with Various Drugs

Interference with various drugs was tested for by analysis of plasma from patients taking therapeutic doses of these drugs, but not warfarin. None of the drugs listed in Table 2 caused interference with the warfarin assay (305 nm).

Plasma Concentration Curves

Patients were given a single dose of either R-warfarin (0.33 mg/kg) or S-warfarin (0.20 mg/kg), and

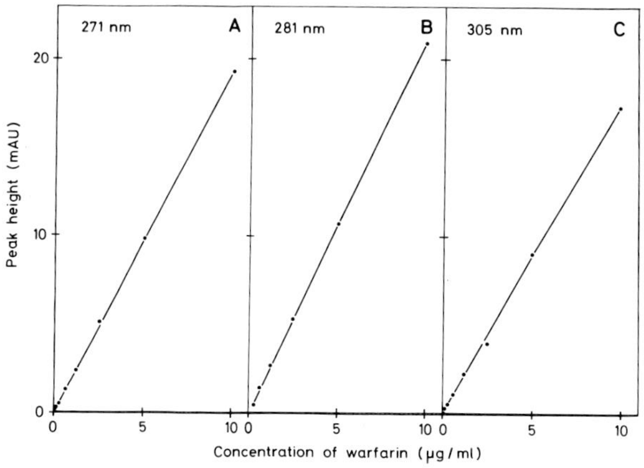

FIG. 4. Standard curves for warfarin at various wavelengths. The standard curve for warfarin was constructed from the absorbance (peak height) obtained at 271 nm (**A**), 281 nm (**B**), and 305 nm (**C**) using a photodiode array detector. The band width was 4 nm.

TABLE 2. *Drugs tested for interference with the warfarin assay*

Phenoxymethylpenicillin
Nitrazepam
Glibenclamid
Dexamethasone
Digitoxin
Furosemide
Hydrochlorothiazide
Piroxicam
Propranolol
Indomethacin
Chlorpromazine
Methadone chloride
Morphine chloride
Naproxen
Tamoxifen
Paracetamol
Codeine phosphate
Prednisone
Flunitrazepam
Buprenorphine chloride
Diazepam

the amount of drug in plasma was determined at various time points. The terminal plasma half-lives were ~40 h for R-warfarin and 20 hours for S-warfarin (Fig. 5). These data are in accordance with the half-lives for warfarin published by others (1).

DISCUSSION

The present report describes a simple liquid chromatographic method for the determination of warfarin in human plasma. No extraction of plasma with organic phase was required, and the plasma samples were only deproteinized with acetonitril prior to HPLC analysis. This simple sample processing ensures quantitative transfer of the drug to the solution subjected to HPLC, and no internal standard was required.

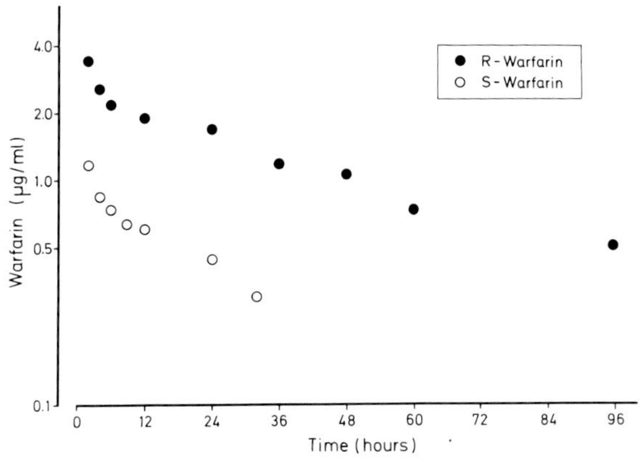

FIG. 5. Plasma concentration curves for R-warfarin and S-warfarin after oral administration (0.33 mg/kg R-warfarin; 0.20 mg/kg S-warfarin, single dose).

Published HPLC methods for warfarin include more or less laborious extraction procedures to remove interfering material (14,16–18). We observed no interference from compounds present in normal plasma when the absorbance of the effluent was recorded at 305 nm (Fig. 2). This may be related to both the mobile phase (low pH and high ionic strength) and the column (short microparticulate O.D.S. column) used. However, routine analysis of crude plasma extract should include continuous evaluation of the purity of the chromatographic peak. This possibility is offered by the photodiode array detector recording the spectral properties of the warfarin peak in plasma. Because of the rather complex and characteristic absorbance spectrum of warfarin (Figs. 1 and 3), this spectral information confirms the identity and purity of the warfarin peak. Thus, determination of warfarin in plasma is an example of the versatility of the photodiode array detector in the analysis of drugs in biological material.

The sensitivity of the present method equalled that obtained with other HPLC assays and ordinary UV detectors (14,17,18) and allows the determination of warfarin in plasma and the elimination curves of the drug (Fig. 5). A new generation of variable wavelength detectors for HPLC, characterized by low noise (about 2×10^{-5} absorbance units full scale at 0.1 s response time), has recently been introduced. The detection limit with this type of detector is 1/5 to 1/3 of that obtained with the photodiode array detector, but multiple injections or stopped flow are required to obtain the absorbance spectrum of a particular peak.

We have used the present warfarin assay for the assessment of the induction of drug metabolism, as judged by half-lives of R- and S-warfarin (Fig. 5), in patients receiving various dosage regimens with aminoglutethimide against advanced breast cancer. Such investigations require a large number of analyses over a wide concentration range for the construction of numerous plasma elimination curves. On a few occasions, the method has been used for the diagnosis of covert warfarin ingestion.

In conclusion, UV detection using a photodiode array detector for HPLC is the basis of a rapid HPLC assay for warfarin in plasma, which includes simple sample processing and fast analysis (retention time of <3 min). Several hundred samples could be subjected to unattended analysis per day, and the number of samples was in fact only limited by the capacity of the sample tray (100) or the mechanical stability of the reversed-phase column.

Acknowledgment: The technical assistance of Halvard Bergesen is highly appreciated. This work was supported by grants from the Norwegian Cancer Society and the Norwegian Society for Fighting Cancer.

REFERENCES

1. Kelley JG, O'Malley K. Clinical pharmacokinetics of oral anticoagulants. *Clin Pharmacokinet* 1979;4:1–15.
2. Kaminsky LS, Fasco MJ, Guengerich FP. Comparison of different forms of purified cytochrome P-540 from rat liver by immunological inhibition of regio- and stereoselective metabolism of warfarin. *J Biol Chem* 1980;255:85–91.
3. Kaminsky LS, Guengerich FP, Dannan GA, Aust SD. Comparison of warfarin metabolism by liver microsomes of rats treated with a series of polybrominated biphenyl congeners and a component-purified cytochrome P-450 isozymes. *Arch Biochem Biophys* 1983;225:398–404.
4. Orme MLE, Breckenridge AM. Coumarin anticoagulants. In: deWolff FA, Mattie H, Breimer DD, eds. *Therapeutic relevance of drug assays*. Leiden University Press, 1980:95–103.
5. Mungall D, Ludden TM, Marshall J, Crawford M, Hawkins D. Relationship between steady-state warfarin concentrations and anticoagulant effect. *Clin Pharmacokinet* 1984;9(suppl 1):99–100.
6. Welling PG, Lee KP, Khanna U, Wager JG. Comparison of plasma concentrations of warfarin measured by both simple extraction and TLC methods. *J Pharm Sci* 1970;59:1621–5.
7. Cole ER, Bachmann F. Spectrophotometric assays for warfarin sodium and dicumarol. *Arch Intern Med* 1976;136:474–9.
8. Corn M, Berberich R. Rapid fluorometric assay for plasma warfarin. *Clin Chem* 1967;13:126–31.
9. Kaiser DG, Martin RS. GLC determination of warfarin in human plasma. *J Pharm Sci* 1974;10:1579–81.
10. Hanna S, Rosen M, Eisenberger P, Rasero L, Lachmann L. GLC determination of warfarin in human plasma. *J Pharm Sci* 1978;67:84–6.
11. Midha KK, McGilveray, Cooper JK. GLC determination of plasma levels of warfarin. *J Pharm Sci* 1974;63:1725–9.
12. Vesell ES, Shively CA. Liquid chromatographic assay of warfarin: similarity of warfarin half-lives in human subjects. *Science* 1974;184:466–8.
13. Mundy DE, Quick MP, Machin AF. Determination of warfarin in animal relicta and feeding-stuffs by high-pressure liquid chromatography with confirmation of identity by mass spectrometry. *J Chromatogr* 1976;121:335–42.
14. Bjornsson TD, Blaschke TF, Meffin PJ. High-pressure liquid chromatographic analysis of drugs in biological fluids I. Warfarin. *J Pharm Sci* 1977;66:142–4.
15. Fasco MJ, Piper LJ, Kaminsky LS. Biochemical application of a quantitative high-pressure liquid chromatographic assay of warfarin and its metabolites. *J Chromatogr* 1977;131:365–73.
16. Small U, Nipper HC. A high performance liquid chromatographic method for the rapid determination of warfarin and its metabolites in serum. *Clin Chem* 1977;23:1138.
17. Wong LT, Solomonraj G, Thomas BH. Analysis of warfarin in plasma by high-pressure liquid chromatography. *J Chromatogr* 1977;135:149–54.
18. Welle-Watne A, Jahren G. Analysis of warfarin in plasma by high performance liquid chromatography. *Med Norsk Farm Selsk* 1980;42:45–52.
19. Overzet F, Rurak A, Van der Voet H, Drenth BFH, Ghijsen RT, De Zeeuw RA. On-line diode array UV-visible spectrometry in screening for drugs and drug metabolites by high-performance liquid chromatography. *J Chromatogr* 1983;267:329–45.
20. Ueland PM, Solheim E. Simple method for increasing the life-time of 3 μm particulate columns for reversed-phase liquid chromatography. *J Chromatogr* 1983;276:157–62.

Therapeutic Drug Monitoring
7:336–343 © 1985 Raven Press, New York

Determination of Valproic Acid in Plasma or Serum by Solid-Phase Column Extraction and Gas-Liquid Chromatography

Wen-nuei Lin and Annetta R. Kelly

Division of Pharmacology/Toxicology, Department of Pathology, Henry Ford Hospital, Detroit, Michigan, U.S.A.

Summary: A simple, fast, sensitive, and inexpensive method is described for routine therapeutic monitoring of both total and free valproic acid (VPA) at therapeutic concentrations in seizure patients. The method uses solid-phase (Bond Elut) columns for the preliminary extraction of 100 μl plasma or serum and gas-liquid chromatography (GLC) analysis, using 10% Carbowax 6000 on a Chromosorb WAW 80/100 column and α-methyl-α-ethylcaproic acid as an internal standard. The extraction efficiency for VPA at a concentration of 70 μg/ml is 98 ± 4%. The calibration curve is linear in the range of 1.0–280 μg/ml. The detection limit of VPA is 1.0 μg/ml. Syva enzyme multiplied immunoassay technique (EMIT) Free-Level filters were used in the analysis of free VPA from plasma. The described Bond Elut · GLC (BE · GLC) method was used to determine total drug concentrations in 56 VPA-treated patients, and the results were compared with those obtained by conventional liquid-liquid extraction · GLC analysis. The 44 sera involved were also analyzed by EMIT. In addition, BE · GLC was compared with the Abbott TDx system on an additional 21 specimens. Statistical agreement was excellent between BE · GLC and TDx, but poor between BE · GLC and liquid-liquid extraction · GLC. Agreement with the EMIT method was intermediate. **Key Words:** Valproic acid—Free and total drug concentrations—Therapeutic drug monitoring—Bond Elut column—Gas-liquid chromatography.

Valproic acid (VPA) has become one of the first-choice antiepileptic drugs (1). Since it is used in children with petit mal seizures, a sensitive microtechnique for its quantitation is necessary. VPA is also used in conjunction with other antiepileptic drugs and may cause drug interaction problems (2–7). Due to the lack of correlation between plasma concentrations and observed clinical effects (1–8), routine monitoring of total VPA plasma concentrations in epileptic patients seems to be of limited value. Determination of free VPA in plasma is necessary for optimum therapeutic assessment of this highly (90–95%) protein-bound drug (3,5).

Evaluation of free drug concentrations has been routinely performed in some laboratories. Ultra-Free filters (Worthington Diagnostics Systems Inc., Freehold, NJ, U.S.A.) and Centriflo CF 50 cones (Amicon Corp., Danvers, MA, U.S.A.) have been used for the assay of free VPA (3,6). Ultra-Free filters and enzyme multiplied immunoassay technique (EMIT) Free-Level filters (Syva Corp., Palo Alto, CA, U.S.A.) have been used to assay free phenytoin (9,10) and free carbamazepine (9). Numerous gas-liquid chromatography (GLC) methods (10–29) and high performance liquid chromatography (HPLC) procedures (30,31) have been described for the estimation of VPA in plasma. Most of these procedures require large specimen volumes

Address correspondence and reprint requests to Dr. W. Lin at Division of Pharmacology/Toxicology, Department of Pathology, Henry Ford Hospital, 2799 W. Grand Blvd., Detroit, MI 48202, U.S.A.

and are time consuming (11,13,21). Some methods are complicated by the necessity of forming a derivative (11,12,15,23). Derivatization of VPA is required for HPLC procedures (30,31) to overcome the problem of poor analytic absorbance in the ultraviolet region. Several GLC procedures (14,16–20) employ small volumes of extracting solvent to avoid an evaporation step. A GLC analysis of VPA has been reported (23) that uses Clin-Elut columns (Analytichem International, Inc., Harbor City, CA, U.S.A.) for extraction and on-column methylation and requires 0.5 ml serum.

The study reported in this article deals with the development of a rapid, simple, and accurate procedure that involves one-tube extraction and eliminates the problems of emulsion formation, phase transfer, and organic phase evaporation. This procedure is reproducible and sensitive, requiring only a small volume (100 μl) of plasma or serum. It can therefore be applied to free VPA quantitation.

MATERIALS

Specimens

Fifty-six samples of serum or heparinized plasma were obtained from inpatients and outpatients receiving VPA therapy in a 900-bed hospital. Total VPA concentrations were determined by the Bond Elut extraction · GLC method (as described in Equipment and Methods) and compared with those obtained by conventional liquid-liquid extraction (19) · GLC analysis. Forty-four of these samples (sera) were also analyzed by an immunoassay technique (EMIT; Syva Corp.). VPA levels of 21 additional specimens obtained by Bond Elut · GLC and fluorescence polarization immunoassay (TDx; Abbott Laboratories, Diagnostics Division, North Chicago, IL, U.S.A.) were compared. All samples were analyzed within 2 to 4 h of collection and measured with SMI Micro/pettors (Scientific Manufacturing Industries, Emeryville, CA, U.S.A.).

Reagents

Methanol distilled in glass was from Burdick & Jackson Laboratories, Inc. (Muskegon, MI 49442, U.S.A.). Acetone, chloroform, isoamyl alcohol, and sulfuric acid were Baker analyzed reagents (J. T. Baker Chemical Co., Phillipsburg, NJ 08865, U.S.A.). Phosphoric acid was 85% analytical reagent (Mallinckrodt Chemical Works, St. Louis, MO, U.S.A.). A 12 N solution of sulfuric acid was prepared by adding 10 ml 24 N sulfuric acid to 10 ml double-distilled water. A 0.7 *M* solution of phosphoric acid was prepared by diluting 4.76 ml 85% (14.7 *M*) H_3PO_4 to 100 ml with double-distilled water.

Standards

VPA (1.0 mg/ml in methanol) was purchased from Supelco, Inc. (Bellefonte, PA, U.S.A.). A standard solution of VPA (0.1 mg/ml in methanol) was prepared by diluting 1.0 ml stock solution to 10 ml with methanol. The internal standard, α-methyl-α-ethylcaproic acid, was purchased from the K & K Life Science Division of ICN Pharmaceuticals, Inc. (Plainview, NJ, U.S.A.). A stock solution (1.0 mg/ml) of the internal standard was prepared by dissolving 10 mg α-methyl-α-ethylcaproic acid in 10 ml methanol. Internal standard solution A (10 μg/ml in chloroform) was prepared by diluting 1.0 ml stock solution to 100 ml with chloroform, and was stored in a brown bottle at 4°C. Internal standard solution B (100 μg/ml in 0.7 *M* H_3PO_4) was prepared by diluting 1.0 ml stock solution to 10 ml with 0.7 *M* H_3PO_4. Internal standard solution C (10 μg/ml in 0.7 *M* H_3PO_4) was prepared by diluting 1.0 ml internal standard solution B to 10 ml with 0.7 *M* H_3PO_4. Toxicology controls (midrange anticonvulsants containing 70 μg/ml VPA, and high-range anticonvulsants containing 140 μg/ml VPA) were purchased from Utak Lab (Saugus, CA, U.S.A.). Drug free serum (Normal Human Clinical Chemistry Control Serum) was purchased from Fisher Scientific Company (Diagnostic Division, Orangeburg, NJ, U.S.A.).

Immunoassay Kits

EMIT

The G6019 VPA assay kit, calibrators, and controls were purchased from Syva Corp. The six calibrators contain 0, 10, 25, 50, 100, and 150 μg/ml VPA. The control contains 75 μg/ml VPA.

TDx

The no. 9514–20 VPA reagent pack; no. 9514–01 calibrators containing 0, 12.5, 25, 50, 100, and 150 μg/ml VPA; and no. 9514–10 VPA controls were purchased from Abbott Laboratories.

EQUIPMENT AND METHODS

Extraction Methods

Bond Elut Extraction of Total VPA

Bond Elut C-18 columns (BE 6001) and a Vac Elut vacuum manifold were purchased from Analytichem International (Harbor City, CA, U.S.A.). The Bond Elut columns were placed in the manifold and suction was applied from a standard laboratory vacuum line. A 1-L vacuum flask was inserted between the vacuum pump and the Vac Elut manifold as a trap to collect the waste materials. The columns were washed twice with methanol and twice with distilled water. The vacuum line was disconnected, allowing the aqueous layer to remain 0.2 mm above the surface of the resin bed. One hundred microliters of plasma and 40 μl internal standard solution B (100 μg/ml) were added to the Bond Elut columns. Suction was reestablished and both sample and internal standard were drawn through the columns. After each column was washed with a single column volume of distilled water, the vacuum line was disconnected. To avoid cross contamination from the water phase, the stainless steel tips of the Vac Elut apparatus were dried before labeled collection tubes were placed beneath each of the Bond Elut columns. One hundred microliters of acetone was added to each column, followed by a 1-min equilibration period. Suction was resumed and the solvent was allowed to pass completely through the columns into the collection tubes. Suction was discontinued and a second 100 μl acetone was added to each column, followed again by a 1-min equilibration period. Suction was reapplied a final time and the eluates were collected in their respective collection tubes. Five microliters of each of the eluates was injected into the GLC system. Up to 10 Bond Elut columns could be processed simultaneously.

Extraction of Free VPA

EMIT Free-Level filters were purchased from Syva Corp. For the determination of free VPA, these filters were assembled according to the supplied instructions for obtaining plasma ultrafiltrates. One hundred microliters of the ultrafiltrate obtained from 1.0 ml of each plasma sample was transferred to a Bond Elut column. Forty microliters of internal standard solution C (10 μg/ml in 0.7 *M* H_3PO_4) was added and eluted twice with 70 μl acetone. Five microliters of the eluate was injected into the GLC system.

Liquid-Liquid Extraction of Total VPA

The liquid-liquid extraction method employed was a modification of Löscher's method (19). One milliliter of plasma or serum and 200 μl 12 N sulfuric acid were added to a 60-ml extraction bottle containing 10 ml internal standard solution A (10 μg/ml in chloroform). The bottle was shaken for 10 min on a mechanical platform shaker. The organic layer was transferred to a 15-ml conical centrifuge tube and 100 μl isoamyl alcohol was added. The chloroform was evaporated under an air stream. The isoamyl alcohol (2 μl) was used for the analysis.

Analytical Methods

GLC

Quantitative determination of VPA was performed on a Varian model 2100 series gas chromatograph (Varian Instrument Co., Walnut Creek, CA, U.S.A.) equipped with dual columns, dual flame ionization detectors, and a linear temperature programmer. A glass column (6 ft × 2 mm inner diameter) packed with 10% Carbowax 6000 on Chromosorb WAW 80/100 (Applied Science Lab, Inc., State College, PA, U.S.A.) was conditioned at 200°C for 18 h (19). Temperatures of the column, injector block, and flame ionization detector were 170, 200, and 200°C, respectively. Nitrogen, hydrogen, and air flow rates were 30, 30, and 300 ml/min, respectively. Attenuations for quantitation of total and free VPA were 1×10^{-10} and 1×10^{-11} A/mV, respectively. An Omni Scribe model B 5217–1 recorder (Houston Instrument, Austin, TX, U.S.A.) was used to record the chromatograms. Quantitation of VPA was achieved by relating the VPA/internal standard peak height ratio in the unknown sample to that of a standard of known concentration.

Homogeneous Enzyme Immunoassay

Employing the well-established standard Syva EMIT technique (32) and reagents specifically designed for use with the EMIT, VPA was quantitated using a digital reading microsample spectrophotometer with a 3017T Thermal Control Unit (Gilford Instruments, Oberlin, OH, U.S.A.), a data microprocessor (Syva model 1000), and a Syva model 1500 pipetter–diluter. Optimum sensitivity range of the assay is 10–150 μg/ml VPA.

Fluorescence Polarization Immunoassay (FPIA)

All reagents were specifically designed for use with the Abbott TDx fluorescence polarization analyzer and were used according to the manufacturer's instructions. The underlying principles of fluorescence polarization and the operational features of the Abbott TDx analyzer have been reported previously (33,34). The lowest measurable VPA concentration distinguishable from 0 with 95% confidence is 0.7 μg/ml.

Statistical Methods

Analysis, Comparisons, and Tolerance Limits

Analysis was performed using the statistical packages MIDAS (35) and SAS (36). Comparisons included paired *t* tests and least-squares linear regression. Tolerance limits were also computed (37) for each value obtained with Bond Elut · GLC.

Standard Deviation Index (SDI)

The Proficiency Service of the College of American Pathologists computed these indices, a measure of accuracy of results, for three test specimens [Therapeutic Drug Monitoring (TDM) Survey Set Z-B] analyzed by the Bond Elut · GLC method in comparison with results obtained by other, accepted GLC specimen preparation methods. The index is calculated as follows:

$$\text{SDI} = \frac{\text{Test method result} - \text{mean of accepted method}}{\text{SD of accepted method}}$$

Values of $< \pm 1$ SD are considered good, values of $\pm$ 1–1.5 acceptable, and values of $> \pm 1.5$ unacceptable.

RESULTS

Linearity and Recovery

Figure 1 shows chromatograms of the blank serum, serum with 48.0 μg/ml VPA, and serum with 4.6 μg/ml free VPA. Figure 2 demonstrates linearity of the peak height ratios of VPA to internal standard solution B (100 μg/ml α-methyl-α-ethylcaproic acid in 0.7 *M* H_3PO_4) in plasma at VPA concentrations in the range 14–280 μg/ml. A standard curve was also established for the quantitative analysis of free VPA in plasma by extracting 100 μl plasma containing 1.0, 2.0, 3.5, 7.0, and 14.0 μg/ml VPA and 40 μl internal standard solution C (10 μg/ml α-methyl-α-ethylcaproic acid in 0.7 *M* H_3PO_4). Peak height ratios of VPA to this internal standard were linear. VPA concentrations (μg/ml) and resultant ratios were as follows: 1, 0.15; 2, 0.32; 3.5, 0.53; 7, 1.07; and 14, 2.17. The calibration curve was linear from 1.0 to 280 μg/ml, or from low therapeutic through toxic concentrations, for both total and free VPA.

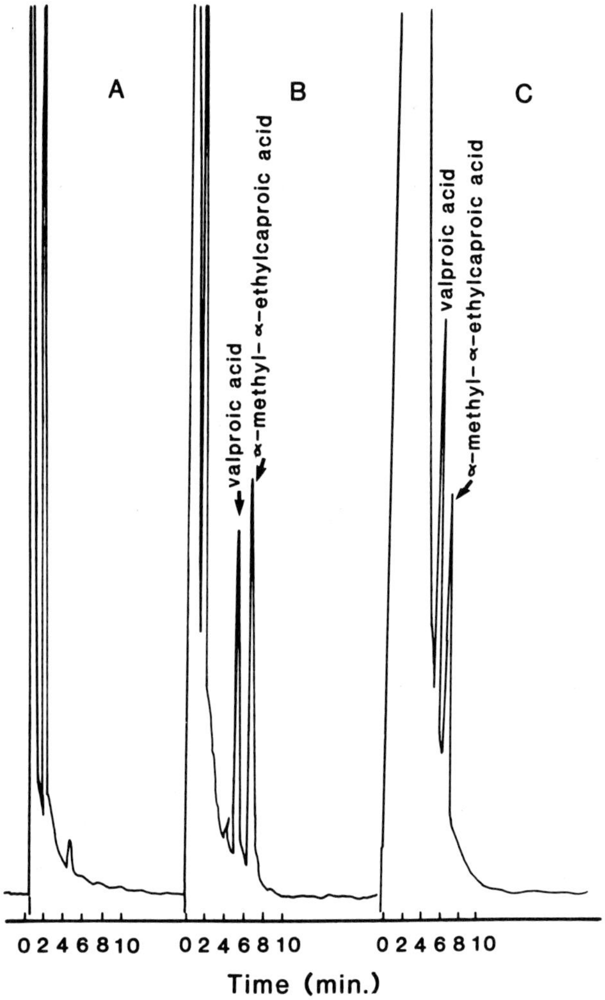

FIG. 1. Gas chromatograms of blank serum (**A**), serum with 48.0 μg/ml valproic acid and 40.0 μg/ml α-methyl-α-ethylcaproic acid (**B**), and serum with 4.6 μg/ml free valproic acid and 4.0 μg/ml α-methyl-α-ethylcaproic acid (**C**). Attenuation: A and B, 1×10^{-10} A/mV; C, 1×10^{-11} A/mV.

Recoveries were 92 ± 5% (2 μg/ml), 93 ± 5% (7 μg/ml), 98 ± 4% (70 μg/ml), and 97 ± 2% (140 μg/ml). The detection limit for the determination of VPA was 1.0 μg/ml [n = 10, CV = 8.67%, mean ± 2 SD = 1.01 ± 0.1775].

Precision

Within-run reproducibility of the procedure was determined by analyzing the toxicology control (high-range anticonvulsants) with concentrations of 2, 7, 14, 70, and 140 μg/ml VPA. A summary of these data is given in Table 1. CVs ranged from 1.68 to 3.19%.

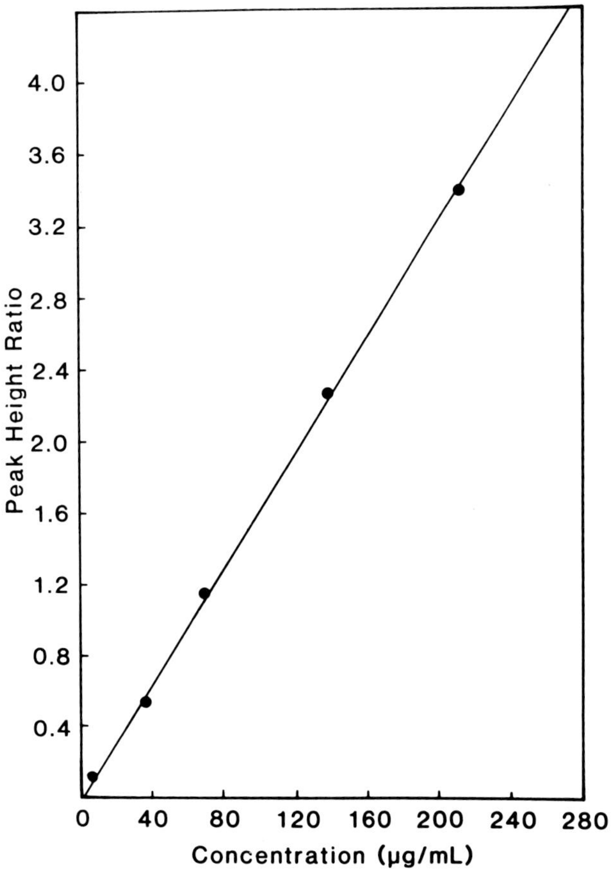

FIG. 2. Calibration curve for measuring valproic acid (VPA) in serum. Peak height ratio (VPA/internal standard solution B) is plotted against VPA concentration.

SD of 0.22 μg/ml (CV = 2.24%) at a concentration of 9.63 μg/ml was observed for free VPA extracted from six aliquots of a single patient's specimen after filtration with EMIT Free-Level filters and analysis by the Bond Elut · GLC method. For the day-to-day precision, 100 μl toxicology control (midrange anticonvulsants), 70 μg/ml, analyzed in 12 consecutive runs, gave an average CV of 2.33%.

TABLE 1. *Precision of Bond Elut · GLC method*

VPA conc. (μg/ml)	n	Mean	SD (μg/ml)	CV (%)
Within assay				
2	10	1.99	0.05	2.59
7	10	6.62	0.11	1.68
14	9	14.50	0.43	3.00
70	12	68.54	2.19	3.19
140	14	141.58	4.44	3.13
Day-to-day				
70	12	69.42	1.62	2.33

VPA, valproic acid.

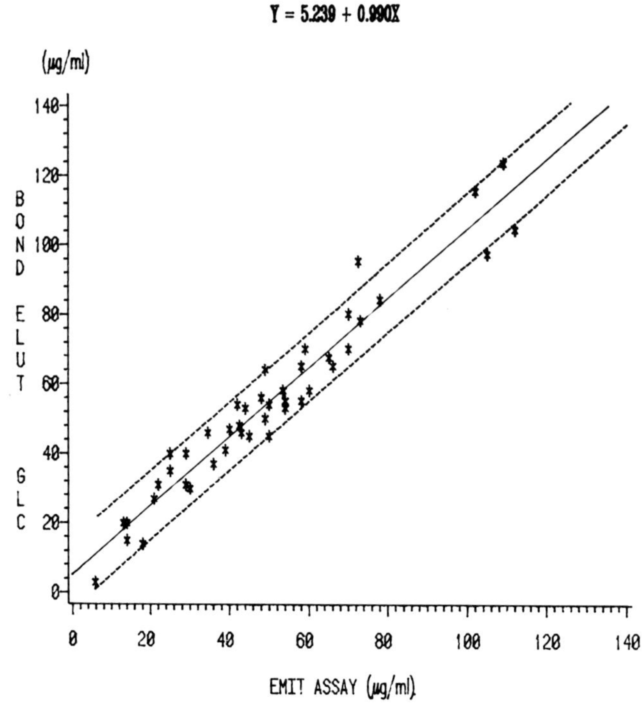

FIG. 3. Comparison of serum valproic acid levels measured by Bond Elut extraction · gas-liquid chromatography (GLC) analysis and enzyme multiplied immunoassay technique (EMIT) assay. The least-squares regression line is shown with the tolerance limits (dashed lines) computed for each value from Bond Elut · GLC.

SDI values were 0.4, 0.0, and 0.6 at concentrations of 80, 128, and 120 μg/ml, respectively, for the analysis of the CAP TDM Survey Set Z-B, supplied in July 1982.

Statistical Results

To assess the performance of the Bond Elut · GLC method, plasma from VPA-treated patients with VPA levels in the range of 3–130 μg/ml were analyzed and the results compared with those obtained by liquid-liquid extraction · GLC, EMIT, and FPIA (TDx). Statistical results for VPA comparison studies are summarized in Table 2 and Figs. 3–5.

The Bond Elut · GLC method was considered as the dependent variable in fitting three regression equations using each of the other three methods as the independent variable. Perfect agreement would result in a line with a slope of 1 and an intercept of 0. The test of this joint hypothesis showed that this result can be considered valid only for the FPIA (TDx) procedure. Further analysis indicated that the intercept was not 0 for comparison with EMIT, and the slope was significantly different from 1 for comparison with the liquid-liquid extraction · GLC method. It appears that the Bond Elut · GLC method gives concentrations

TABLE 2. *Statistical comparison of valproic acid (VPA) determination methods*

Methods	VPA conc. (μg/ml) (mean ± SD)	Paired *t* test	Linear regression
Bond Elut · GLC *(y)* Liquid-liquid extraction · GLC *(x)*	55.5 ± 28.5 51.4 ± 25.1	$t = 3.77$, n = 56, $p < 0.001$	Slope = 1.097[a], intercept = −0.984, $r = 0.964$, $p < 0.001$
Bond Elut · GLC *(y)* EMIT *(x)*	54.2 ± 26.3 49.5 ± 25.7	$t = 4.77$, n = 44, $p < 0.001$	Slope = 0.990, intercept = 5.239[b], $r = 0.968$, $p < 0.001$
Bond Elut · GLC *(y)* TDX *(x)*	56.9 ± 24.1 56.3 ± 24.2	$t = 1.92$, n = 21, $p < 0.07$	Slope = 0.992, intercept = 1.052, $r = 0.998$, $p < 0.001$

EMIT, Enzyme multiplied immunoassay technique; GLC, gas-liquid chromatography.
[a]Significantly different from unity ($p < 0.05$).
[b]Significantly different from 0 ($p < 0.05$).

somewhat higher than does either the EMIT or the liquid-liquid extraction · GLC method. This is further confirmed by a paired *t* test, which indicates significant ($p < 0.05$) differences between the methods.

Tolerance limits were constructed and are included in Figs. 3–5. For a particular value of *x*, the tolerance limit has a 90% chance of covering 90% of the distribution of the corresponding fitted value of *y*. The liquid-liquid extraction · GLC method shows values outside the tolerance limit of Bond Elut · GLC at a wide range of concentrations, which indicates poor agreement between the two. The FPIA (TDx) method is in excellent agreement with the Bond Elut · GLC method, while agreement of the EMIT method is intermediate.

Interferences

Normal constituents of plasma and serum, as well as other commonly used antiepileptic drugs, did not produce interfering peaks in the region of VPA or its internal standard. Table 3 lists drugs checked for in-

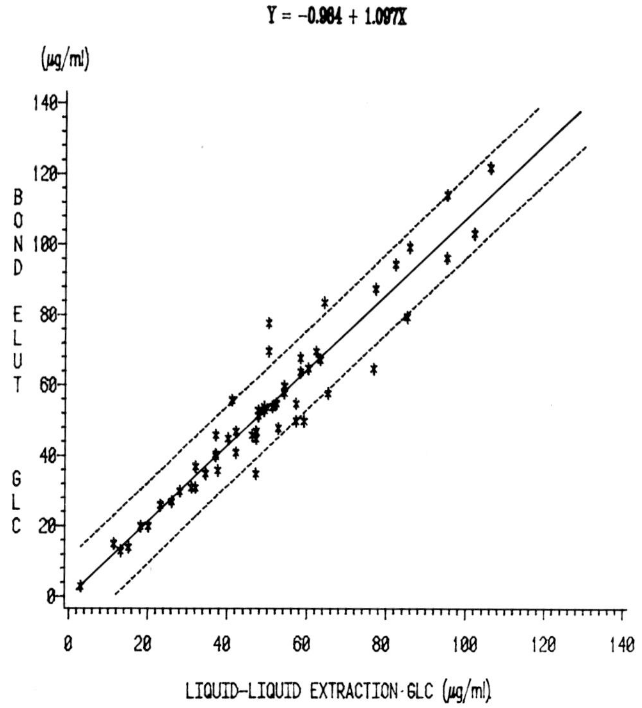

FIG. 4. Comparison of serum valproic acid levels measured by Bond Elut extraction · gas-liquid chromatography (GLC) analysis and liquid-liquid extraction · GLC analysis. The least-squares regression line is shown with the tolerance limits (dashed lines) computed for each value of Bond Elut · GLC.

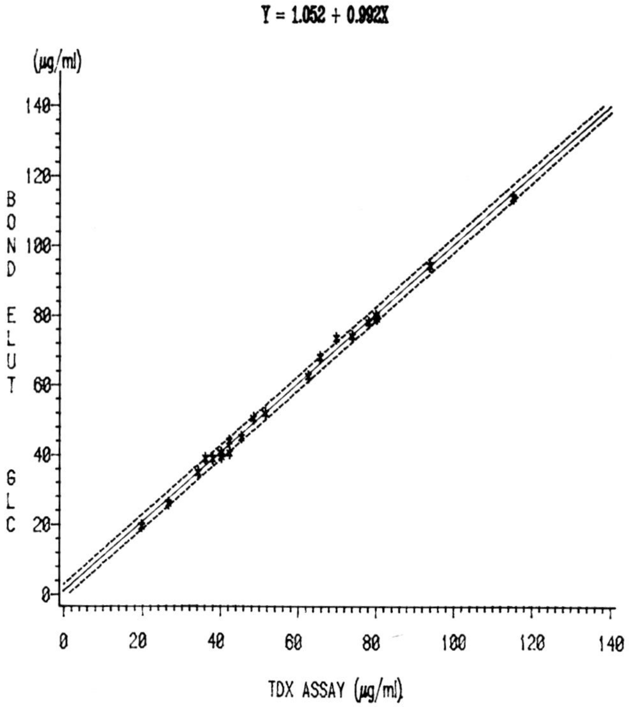

FIG. 5. Comparison of serum valproic acid levels measured by Bond Elut extraction · gas-liquid chromatography (GLC) analysis and TDx assay. The least-squares regression line is shown with the tolerance limits (dashed lines) computed for each value of Bond Elut · GLC.

TABLE 3. *Interference studies*

Compound	Amount injected (μg)	Retention time (min)
Acetaminophen	2.0	—
Caffeine	0.5	—
Carbamazepine	0.6	—
Dimethadione	1.0	—
Ethchlorvynol	0.5	2.0
Ethosuximide (Zarontin)	0.6	20.0
Ethylphenylhydantoin	1.0	—
Glutethimide	1.0	—
Ibuprofen (Motrin)	0.6	—
Mephenytoin	0.6	—
Mephobarbital	0.6	—
Meprobamate	2.0	—
Methaqualone	0.5	—
Metharbital (Gemonil)	0.5	—
Methsuximide (Celontin)	0.5	25.0
α-Methyl-α-ethylcaproic acid (valproic acid internal standard)	0.4	6.0
α-Methyl-α-phenylsuccinimide	0.5	—
Methyprylon	0.5	—
Pentobarbital	0.6	—
Phenobarbital	0.6	—
Phenytoin	0.8	—
Primidone	0.6	—
Salicylamide	1.0	—
Salicylic acid	1.0	—
Theophylline	0.6	—
Thiopental	0.6	—
Trimethadione	0.5	1.5
Valproic acid	0.4	5.0

Dash signifies no peak between 1.0 and 30 min.

terference in this GLC procedure. Ethosuximide eluted at 20.0 min and methsuximide at 25.0 min.

Reusability of the Bond Elut Columns

The reusability of Bond Elut columns was studied by repeated extraction on the same column. One hundred microliters of toxicology control (high-range anticonvulsants) was diluted to 1,000 μl with drug free control serum. One hundred microliters of this solution (containing 14 μg/ml VPA) was extracted and eluted from the same column five times. Recoveries were reproducible with a SD value of 2.30%. Resulting chromatograms showed no additional peaks.

DISCUSSION

Extraction of VPA from plasma or serum by the method described has definite advantages over other methods. Disadvantages of previous methods are the relatively large volumes of serum or plasma needed, which is especially a problem with newborns and infants, and the necessity for time-consuming solvent extraction and evaporation. In spite of careful mixing during solvent extraction, an emulsion forms which is not easy to break. Although several microtechniques have been developed, it is difficult to obtain extracts that are completely free of the aqueous phase and syringe needles often become plugged when passing through the aqueous phase into the lower organic layers. By use of Bond Elut columns, extraction time is shortened due to elimination of tube transfers. Preparation of 10 specimens using Bond Elut columns can be accomplished within 20 min. The volume of acetone with which VPA is eluted from the column is as small as 100–200 μl. Because evaporation is not required, loss of VPA, a volatile compound, is minimized. The capacity of the Bond Elut columns is remarkably high and recoveries are linear even above 300 μg/ml. The significant problem caused by emulsion formation in liquid-liquid extraction is avoided. Small volumes (50–100 μl) of plasma or serum are used. Such quantities are suitable not only for routine monitoring of free VPA but also for quantitating the drug in pediatric patients.

It is possible to reuse Bond Elut columns up to five times without impairing VPA recoveries. However, if the biological fluid contains particles that occlude the filter even partially, the column is no longer suitable for use.

The polar liquid phase of the GLC column (10% Carbowax 6000) permits the same column to be used for analysis of other volatile antiepileptic drugs, such as ethosuximide, allowing more efficient use of the instrument.

The EMIT VPA method is simple and rapid but can be used only on serum or heparinized plasma. Anticoagulation with EDTA significantly increases values, and citrate and oxalate reduce VPA concentrations by 15–30% (38,39). Analysis by FPIA (TDx) is fast and accurate, but more expensive than analysis by GLC.

CONCLUSIONS

Our method for determination of serum VPA uses Bond Elut extraction columns and gas chromatography on a 10% Carbowax 6000 column using α-ethyl-α-methylcaproic acid as the internal standard. This sensitive microtechnique offers excellent reproducibility, detection limits, linearity, and specificity. The procedure is suitable for routine monitoring of total and free VPA in microsamples and should be useful in clinical laboratories. Free drug concentrations in plasma correlate well with observed clinical effects.

Acknowledgment: The authors wish to thank Dr. Peter D. Frade for critiquing the manuscript.

REFERENCES

1. Schobben F, van der Kleijn E, Vree TB. Therapeutic monitoring of valproic acid. *Ther Drug Monit* 1980;2:61–71.
2. Friel PN, Leal KW, Wilensky AJ. Valproic acid–phenytoin interaction. *Ther Drug Monit* 1979;1:243–8.
3. Cramer JA, Mattson RH. Valproic acid: in vitro plasma protein binding and interaction with phenytoin. *Ther Drug Monit* 1979;1:105–16.
4. Perucca E, Hebdige S, Frigo GM, Gatti G, Lecchini S, Crema A. Interaction between phenytoin and valproic acid: plasma protein binding and metabolic effects. *Clin Pharmacol Ther* 1980;28:779–89.
5. Levy RH. Monitoring of free valproic acid levels? *Ther Drug Monit* 1980;2:199–201.
6. Haidukewych D, Rodin EA. Variable in vivo binding of valproic acid in epilepsy patients being medicated with other anticonvulsants. *Clin Chem* 1980;26:1634–5.
7. Rodin EA, DeSousa G, Haidukewych D, Lodhi R, Berchou RC. Dissociation between free and bound phenytoin levels in presence of valproate sodium. *Arch Neurol* 1981;38:240–2.
8. Zimmerman CL, Patel IH, Levy RH, Edwards D, Nelson SD, Hutchinson M. Protein binding of valproic acid in the presence of elevated free fatty acids in patient and normal human serum. *Epilepsia* 1981;22:11–7.
9. Cronin M, Chegwidden K, Kabakoff D. Performance and validation of the EMIT free level system for phenytoin and carbamazepine. *Clin Chem* 1981;27:1093.
10. Joern WA. Gas-chromatographic assay of free phenytoin in ultrafiltrates of plasma: test of a new filtration apparatus and specimen stability. *Clin Chem* 1981;27:417–21.
11. Willox S, Foote SE. Simple method for measuring valproate (Epilim) in biological fluids. *J Chromatogr* 1978;151:67–70.
12. Chan SC. Monitoring serum valproic acid by gas chromatography with electron-capture detector. *Clin Chem* 1980;26:1528–30.
13. Kwong T, Bacharach A, Kankoski T, Mirabella F, Martinez R, Keller J. A rapid gas–liquid chromatographic assay for valproic acid in serum. *Clin Chem* 1980;26:1053.
14. Goudie JH, Reed K, Ayers GJ, Burnett D. Improved extraction of valproic acid from serum before chromatography. *Clin Chem* 1980;26:1929.
15. Gupta RN, Eng F, Gupta ML. Gas-chromatographic analysis for valproic acid as phenacyl esters. *Clin Chem* 1979;25:1303–5.
16. Freeman DJ, Rawal N. Extraction of underivatized valproic acid from serum before gas-chromatography. *Clin Chem* 1980;26:674–5.
17. Berry DJ, Clarke LA. Determination of valproic acid (dipropylacetic acid) in plasma by gas-liquid chromatography. *J Chromatogr* 1978;156:301–7.
18. Kumps A, Mardens Y. Simplified simultaneous determination of valproic acid and ethosuximide in serum by gas–liquid chromatography. *Clin Chem* 1980;26:1759.
19. Löscher W. Rapid determination of valproate sodium in serum by gas-liquid chromatography. *Epilepsia* 1977;18:225–7.
20. Jakobs C, Bojasch M, Hanefeld F. New direct micro-method for determination of valproic acid in serum by gas chromatography. *J Chromatogr* 1978;146:494–7.
21. Sioufi A, Colussi D, Marfil F. Gas chromatographic determination of valproic acid in human plasma. *J Chromatogr* 1980;182:241–5.
22. Hershey AE, Patton JR, Dudley KH. Gas chromatographic method for the determination of valproic acid in human plasma. *Ther Drug Monit* 1979;1:217–41.
23. Gast B, Thoma J. GLC analysis of valproic acid using an extube extraction and on-column methylation. *Clin Chem* 1979;25:1118.
24. Odusote KA, Sherwin AL. A simple, direct extraction method for gas-liquid chromatographic determination of valproic acid in plasma. *Ther Drug Monit* 1981;3:103–6.
25. Kupferberg HJ. Gas–liquid chromatographic quantitation of valproic acid. In: Pippenger CE, Penry JK, Kutt H, eds. *Antiepileptic drugs: quantitative analysis and interpretation*. New York: Raven Press, 1978:147–51.
26. Schmidt D, Ferrandes B, Grandjean D, et al. Interlaboratory variability of valproic acid determinations. *Arzneimittelforsch* 1977;27:1078–81.
27. Frederick DL, Kelly BR, Fowler MW, Altmiller DH. A rapid gas-liquid chromatographic analysis for valproic acid in serum. *Clin Chem* 1979;25:1118.
28. Fullinfaw RO, Marty JJ. Gas chromatography of valproic acid, with benzyl alcohol as internal standard. *Clin Chem* 1981;27:1776.
29. Kumps AH, Kumps-Grandjean B, Mardens Y. Enzyme immunoassay and gas-liquid chromatography compared for determination of valproic acid in serum. *Clin Chem* 1981;27:1788–9.
30. Van der Wal S, Bannister SJ, Dolan JW, Snyder LR. Codetermination of ethosuximide and valproate by high performance liquid chromatography on the Technicon fast-LC™ system. *Clin Chem* 1980;26:1006.
31. Gupta RN, Keane PM, Gupta ML. Valproic acid in plasma, as determined by liquid chromatography. *Clin Chem* 1979;25:1984–5.
32. Bastiani RJ, Phillips RC, Schneider RS, et al. Homogeneous immunochemical drug assays. *Am J Med Technol* 1973;39:211–6.
33. Jolley ME. Fluorescence polarization immunoassay for the determination of therapeutic drug levels in human plasma. *J Anal Toxicol* 1981;5:236–40.
34. Jolley ME, Stroupe SD, Schwenzer KS, et al. Fluorescence polarization immunoassay. III. An automated system for therapeutic drug determination. *Clin Chem* 1981;27:1575–9.
35. Fox DJ, Guire KE. Documentation for MIDAS. In: *Statistical research laboratory, 3rd ed*. Ann Arbor: University of Michigan, 1976:1–203.
36. Ray AA, ed. *SAS user's guide: statistics, 1982 ed*. Cary, NC: SAS Institute, Inc., 1982:1–584.
37. Leurgans S. Evaluating laboratory measurement techniques. In: Miller RG, Efron B, Brown BW, Moses LE. *Biostatistics casebook*. New York: John Wiley & Sons, 1980:190–219.
38. Godolphin W, Trepanier J, Farrell K. Serum and plasma for total and free anticonvulsant drug analysis: effects on EMIT assays and ultrafiltration devices. *Ther Drug Monit* 1983;5:319–23.
39. Cloyd JC, Leppik IE. Valproic acid: therapeutic use and serum concentration monitoring. In: Taylor WJ, Finn AL, eds. *Individualizing drug therapy*, vol 2. New York: Gross Townsend, Frank, 1982:88–108.

Therapeutic Drug Monitoring
7:344–350 © 1985 Raven Press, New York

Radioimmunoassay for Clonidine in Human Plasma and Urine Using a Solid Phase Second Antibody Separation

Peter R. Farina, Carol A. Homon, Chien T. Chow, James J. Keirns, *Paul A. Zavorskas, and *Henry J. Esber

*Department of Biochemistry, Research and Development, Boehringer Ingelheim, Ltd., Ridgefield, Connecticut; and *EG&G Mason Research Institute, Worcester, Massachusetts, U.S.A.*

Summary: A reliable, sensitive, and specific radioimmunoassay (RIA) procedure for the quantitation of clonidine in plasma and other biological fluids was developed. The detection limit of the assay is 2 pg based on a 200 μl sample. Nine commonly used drugs were found not to interfere with the RIA. The utility of the assay was demonstrated in a bioavailability study of clonidine conducted with 24 healthy subjects. Clonidine was readily quantitated in plasma over 4 half-lives. This assay is suitable for pharmacokinetic and bioavailability studies as well as therapeutic drug monitoring of patients. **Key Words:** Clonidine—Radioimmunoassay—Therapeutic drug monitoring—Pharmacokinetic and bioavailability studies.

Clonidine hydrochloride [2-(2,6-dichlorophenylamine)-2-imidazoline hydrochloride] is a widely used anti-hypertensive drug whose effects are mediated through central α-adrenergic mechanisms (1,2,3). The blood pressure regulatory centers of the brain appear to be the site of action leading to a decrease in sympathetic tone to the periphery and a concomitant increase in vagal tone. Clonidine has also been investigated in many indications other than hypertension. Its most notable uses are in the treatment of acute opiate withdrawal symptoms (4), post-menopausal flushing (5), migraine prophylaxis (6,7), and Gilles de Tourette syndrome (8).

The pharmacokinetics of clonidine has been extensively studied (9–12). The drug is rapidly absorbed with little first pass metabolism. Bioavailability of the drug is high when administered in tablet form and is equivalent to oral reference solution (13). In humans substantial amounts of the drug are excreted in urine (13–16) accompanied by small amounts of metabolites including *p*-hydroxyclonidine (14). The wide applicability of this drug and its low oral dosage (0.1–0.3 mg) have stimulated interest in developing analytical procedures for monitoring the drug in biofluids. Keranen et al. (10) have observed that side effects of clonidine, such as dry mouth and drowsiness, follow the time course of plasma levels. Several reports on gas chromatographic or mass spectrometric methods have been published, but these reports share common problems associated with extraction, handling of large sample sizes and often, inadequate sensitivity (17–21). Arndts et al. (15,16) have developed a radioimmunoassay (RIA) method that employs an ^{125}I-labeled derivative of clonidine and a specific antibody which permits quantitation to 50 pg/ml and eliminates the need for extraction due to reported low levels of cross-reacting metabolites (15,16).

The need at our research center to increase sensitivity and routinely assay large numbers of clinical samples for clonidine has prompted us to modify the published RIA by further purification of the radiolabeled clonidine and incorporation of a solid phase second antibody separation in place of the charcoal method originally described (16). These modifications

Address correspondence and reprint requests to Dr. P. R. Farina at Department of Biochemistry, Research and Development, Boehringer Ingelheim Pharmaceuticals, Inc., 90 East Ridge, Ridgefield, CT 06877, U.S.A.

allow for direct counting of the antibody bound phase, which reduces nonspecific binding; eliminates the need for additional pipetting, otherwise required; and enhances the detectability and sensitivity of the assay procedure.

This method has been successfully employed to monitor clonidine levels in plasma and urine in a study of 24 healthy humans receiving a single Combipres tablet (Boehringer Ingelheim, Ltd., Ridgefield, CT, U.S.A.) containing clonidine in combination with the diuretic, chlorthalidone. Also reported here is our clinical experience with the solid phase RIA for clonidine in association with blood collection methods, assay validation, and precision and stability studies.

MATERIALS AND METHODS

The conjugate was prepared by reacting the *N*-hydroxysuccinimide ester of *p*-carboxyclonidine (ST 1984) with bovine serum albumin (BSA) in a 35:1 molar ratio according to the method of Anderson et al. (22). Spectrophotometric determination of the hapten to BSA ratio after extensive diafiltration was performed as described by Erlanger (23,24) and indicated 8 clonidine molecules per mole of protein.

American Dutch rabbits were each immunized subcutaneously at multiple sites with 1 mg of the conjugate in Complete Freunds Adjuvant followed by monthly boosters in incomplete adjuvant. Antibody titers after 6 months ranged from 1 in 10,000 to 1 in 80,000. All antisera were stored at − 80°C.

4-Carboxyclonidine-tyrosyl-methyl-ester (ST 1984-TME), a gift of Dr. Arndts (Boehringer Ingelheim KG) was iodinated by a modification of the chloramine T method (16). The mono-iodinated product was isolated by Sephadex G-25 column chromatography. Since de-esterification of this methyl ester occurred during isolation and storage at 4°C in the elution buffer (sodium citrate, 0.1 *M*, pH 6.0), additional purification to the more stable mono-iodo 4-carboxyclonidine-tyrosine was performed by preparative thin layer chromatography (silica gel 60, F–254 EM Reagents, Cincinnati, OH, U.S.A.) using methanol/ethyl acetate (1:1, v/v). The mono-iodo acid product was recovered by scraping and extracting twice with ethanol (5 ml, each) after identification of the most polar band by autoradiography and by comparison with an authentic nonradioactive standard. After centrifugation, the ethanolic solution was concentrated to 3–4 ml with a nitrogen stream and stored at − 20°C. The mono-iodinated product was used for assays for 1 month without appreciable change noted in the standard curve.

The following reagents were used: sodium phosphate buffer, 0.1 *M*, pH 7.4; immunobead second antibody, goat anti-rabbit immunoglobulin (Bio-Rad Laboratories, Richmond, CA, U.S.A.), reconstituted as directed by manufacturer; standards, urine samples, and antiserum were diluted in plasma prepared by mixing 20 parts heparinized with 80 parts citrated plasma (20/80 NHP); plasma samples containing heparin were diluted with citrated plasma (1:5); clonidine (Boehringer Ingelheim Ltd.) stock solution (200 μg/ml) was prepared by dissolving 23.255 mg of clonidine hydrochloride in 100 ml of water. Serial dilutions of the stock were made to prepare standards of 1.0, 0.5, 0.1, 0.05, and 0.01 ng/ml in 20/80 NHP.

Unknown plasma samples, controls, and clonidine standards (0.2 ml) were allowed to equilibrate for 18 h at 4°C in 12 × 75 mm polypropylene tubes with 0.1 ml of [^{125}I]clonidine label (10,000 cpm), 0.4 ml of phosphate buffer, and 0.1 ml of the diluted antibody (50% binding). Following a second incubation with immunobeads (0.5 ml) for 2 h at room temperature, the tubes were centrifuged at 3000 *g* for 10 min, supernatants were discarded and the remaining pellets counted in a Packard Gamma Spectrometer, Model 5520. Calculations were performed using a Wang Computer 2200T and a Wang spline-fit or logit program.

The crossreactivity of clonidine antiserum was evaluated for four known metabolites (obtained from Boehringer Ingelheim KG) present in urine: 2,6-dichlorophenyl-guanidine (ST 2075), *p*-hydroxyclonidine (ST 666), 1-(2,6-dichloro-4-hydroxyphenyl)-guanidine (ST 2236), and 2-(2,6-dichlorophenyl)-imino-imidazolidine-4-one (ST 2245). Chlorthalidone was spiked into both human plasma (2,000 ng/ml) and urine (4,000 ng/ml) samples containing known amounts of clonidine to determine whether the diuretic would interfere in the assay. In addition, plasma (4 h post-dose) from a subject who received a 25 mg commercial tablet of chlorthalidone was spiked with clonidine at the same concentrations used in the precision study and assayed. This study was performed to determine whether chlorthalidone metabolites might crossreact with the antiserum.

Interference by several commonly used drugs was tested at the therapeutic concentration of the drug and at a toxic or extremely high concentration. The drugs were added as solutions to heparinized plasma samples of clonidine at both 0.5 and 1.0 ng/ml. These solutions were then further diluted resulting in a final concentration of heparinized plus citrated plasma (1:4).

Clonidine was spiked into human plasma at 0.5, 0.2, and 0.05 ng/ml and into human urine at 40, 8, 4, and 0.4 ng/ml. After analysis of the fresh samples, aliquots were stored at −20°C and assayed thereafter at 1, 2, 4, 6, 9, and 12 months.

Human blood was collected from 10 subjects by either glass or plastic syringe or by commercial evacuated tubes containing various anticoagulants. After separation of the formed elements, clonidine was spiked into each individual's plasma to a final theoretical concentration of 0, 0.05, 0.15, 0.3, 0.5, and 1.0 ng/ml.

Either one Combipres (0.3 mg clonidine hydrochloride/15 mg chlorthalidone) or one 0.1/15 mg tablet were administered to 24 healthy males in a single dose crossover design. These subjects ranged in age from 18 to 43 years (mean 28.8 years), in height from 164 to 185 cm (mean 174.5 cm) and in weight from 62.6 to 85.0 kg (mean 72.3 kg). Each subject was healthy as confirmed by a complete medical history, physical examination, and blood test. All subjects were within their normal weight range. At 6:00 a.m., following a fast of ≥10 h, the subjects received 400 ml of water and then at 7:00 a.m. one Combipres tablet plus 222 ml of water. Forty minutes later and every hour thereafter for 8 h, a minimum of 100 ml of water was given. Four hours and 30 min after initial drug administration, all subjects received a standard light meal. The next meal was at 8 h following drug administration, after which there were no further restrictions on meals. Subjects remained recumbent until 2 hours after drug administration. For each test period, blood samples were collected in an evacuated tube containing heparin immediately prior to and at 0.5, 1, 1.25, 1.5, 1.75, 2, 2.5, 3, 4, 6, 8, 12, 24, 48, 72, and 96 h after the open label administration of treatment. In addition, urine samples were collected at baseline and 0–2, 2–4, 4–6, 6–8, 8–12, 12–24, 24–48, 48–72, 72–96, and 96–120 h after administration of treatment. No drugs were allowed to be taken within 14 days of the first test day nor during the entire testing period including the 2-week washout period between treatments. On each test day coffee, tea, and cola beverages were withheld from subjects for 12 h prior to treatment administration and until the blood sampling was completed.

RESULTS

Clinical plasma samples containing heparin as an anticoagulant were routinely diluted in citrated blood bank plasma (1:5) to eliminate background interference. Urine samples were generally diluted 1:50 (ratio never <1:10) in 20/80 NHP to reduce urine matrix effects which could result in erroneously elevated clonidine values.

TABLE 1. *Between-assay and within-assay precision data for clonidine radioimmunoassay*

Concentration (ng/ml)	n	Mean assayed value (ng/ml)	SD	CV (%)	Recovery (%)
		Between-assay			
0.640	17	0.638	0.065	10	100
0.160	17	0.153	0.020	13	96
0.040	17	0.040	0.004	10	100
0.010	17	0.0090	0.0010	11	90
		Within-assay			
0.640	10	0.649	0.018	2.8	101
0.160	10	0.161	0.010	6.2	101
0.040	10	0.036	0.003	8.3	90
0.010	10	0.011	0.001	9.1	110

CV, coefficient of variation; SD, standard of deviation.

Sensitivity

The detection limit of this assay is 2 pg based on a 200 μl sample volume and a final clonidine dilution in 20/80 NHP to 0.010 ng/ml. Clinical samples in heparinized plasma can therefore be assayed to 0.050 ng/ml, because of the initial dilution (1:5) with citrated plasma.

Precision

Control 20/80 NHP samples (0.64, 0.16, 0.04, and 0.01 ng/ml) were prepared in sufficient quantities to allow one set of controls to be analyzed with each assay. Coefficients of variation ranged from 10 to 13% over the 6 month period of analysis of the Combipres study (Table 1). Intra-assay precision was determined by replicate analysis of four concentrations of clonidine. The results of this study are presented in Table 1.

Stability

The analytical results of the spiked clonidine samples stored in aliquots at −20°C showed no statistically significant trend ($p < 0.05$) over the course of the 1 year study.

Specificity

The crossreactivity profiles of the available synthetic metabolites evaluated in comparison to a clonidine standard curve are shown in Fig. 1. Three metabolites (ST 2075, ST 2236, and ST 2245) did

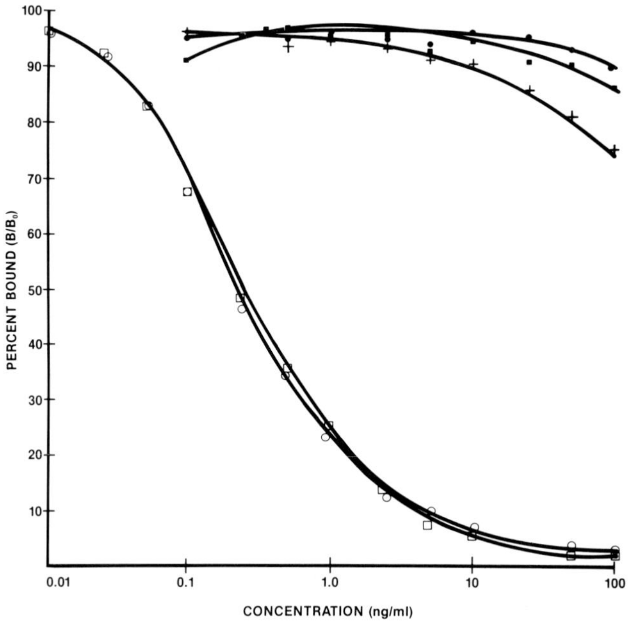

FIG. 1. Crossreaction profile of clonidine antiserum comparing clonidine with the major metabolites. Clonidine (ST 155), open circles; *p*-hydroxyclonidine (ST 666), open squares; 2,6-dichlorophenyl-guanidine (ST 2075), filled circles; 1-(2,6-dichloro-4-hydroxyphenyl)-guanidine (ST 2236), filled squares; 2-(2,6-dichlorophenyl)-imino-imidazolidine-4-one (ST 2245), crosses.

not show any appreciable displacement of radiolabeled clonidine up to 100 ng/ml. However, *p*-hydroxyclonidine (ST 666) was 100% crossreactive and equivalent to clonidine in immunoreactivity. Chlorthalidone did not interfere in the determination of either plasma or urine clonidine levels (Table 2) at levels of the diuretic which exceeded the highest concentration expected for the Combipres formulation. No interference was noted in the analysis of clonidine spiked into plasma from a subject who received a 25 mg tablet of chlorthalidone. This indicates that chlorthalidone metabolites in plasma pose no problem in the RIA for clonidine. Nine commonly used drugs tested for interference at two clonidine concentrations did not alter the amount of clonidine assayed; however, salicylic acid at higher concentrations may lead to erroneously low values for clonidine (Table 3).

Blood Collection Methods and Anticoagulants

No discernible effect on the clonidine RIA was noted from the study conducted with 10 subjects comparing various blood collection methods and anticoagulants. Intersubject variation increased substantially at spiked concentrations of clonidine of 0.150 ng/ml and below (Table 4). A positive bias was observed in measured clonidine at only the lower concentrations.

Validation Studies

Clonidine hydrochloride was spiked into human heparinized plasma and urine over the expected clinical range to prepare unknowns for blinded analysis at the Central Clinical Laboratory (EG&G Mason Research Institute, Worcester, MA, U.S.A.). Table 2 contains the validation results for clonidine RIA determination in plasma and urine with and without chlorthalidone. As can be seen from these results, excellent correlations were obtained for both the spiked plasma and the spiked urine samples, values ranging from 0.991 to 0.999.

Clinical Experience

The solid phase RIA has been used to quantitate clonidine levels in several thousand plasma and urine samples from various pharmacokinetic, bioavailability, and medical studies. The results of plasma and urine determinations of clonidine in a single dose crossover study of Combipres 0.1 mg clonidine/15 mg chlorthalidone and 0.3/15 tablets administered to 24

TABLE 2. *Validation results for clonidine radioimmunoassay determinations for plasma and urine*

Biofluid	Analyte	Range studied (ng/ml)	Least squares equation	Correlation
Plasma[a]	Clonidine	0–1.30	$y = 1.194(x) - 0.028$	0.998 (n = 6)
Plasma[a]	Clonidine + 2000 ng/ml chlorthalidone	0–1.30	$y = 1.274(x) + 0.048$	0.998 (n = 6)
Urine	Clonidine	0–100	$y = 1.198(x) - 1.864$	0.991 (n = 7)
Urine	Clonidine + 4000 ng/ml chlorthalidone	0–100	$y = 1.158(x) + 0.132$	0.999 (n = 7)

[a]Heparin used as anticoagulant.

TABLE 3. *Evaluation of potential interference of several drugs at therapeutic and toxic levels with the clonidine radioimmunoassay*

Drug tested	Concentration (μg/ml)	Assay results spiked clonidine samples (ng/ml) 1.0	0.5
Acetaminophen	300	0.890	0.460
	15	0.860	0.485
Cimetidine	10	0.975	0.530
	1	0.990	0.490
Diazepam	10	0.830	0.485
	0.6	0.930	0.445
Digitoxin	0.04	0.985	0.500
	0.01	1.010	0.540
Digoxin	0.003	0.935	0.520
	0.001	0.985	0.565
Indomethacin	10	1.015	0.530
	2	0.960	0.550
Dilantin	25	1.065	0.510
	10	1.010	0.530
Propranolol	0.2	1.070	0.580
	0.02	1.020	0.540
Theophylline	25	0.915	0.460
	5	0.960	0.495
Clonidine controls (n = 5)		0.984 ± 0.059	0.522 ± 0.010
Salicylic acid[a]	200	0.720	0.410
	150	0.795	0.415
	100	0.865	0.420
	50	0.805	0.475
	10	0.885	0.480
	0	1.03	0.500

[a]Expanded study performed at a later date.

healthy males are shown in Fig. 2 and 3. Clonidine was readily quantitated over 4 half-lives ($t_{1/2}$ = 12–14 h) for both the low and high dose formulations. Dosage proportionality and parallelism were observed over the time course studied. Cumulative urinary excretion for unchanged clonidine was found to be 36–

TABLE 4. *Effect of blood collection methods and anticoagulants on clonidine values*

Blood collection method	Anticoagulant	Clonidine ng/ml (CV %)[a] 1.00	0.500	0.300	0.150	0.050
Vacutainer	heparin	1.20 (16)	0.580 (15)	0.361 (16)	0.192 (23)	0.081 (33)
Venoject	heparin	1.07 (7)	0.516 (17)	0.312 (17)	0.181 (32)	0.079 (33)
Plastic syringe	heparin	1.07 (9)	0.528 (15)	0.362 (16)	0.169 (18)	0.074 (32)
Glass syringe	heparin	1.12 (9)	0.557 (11)	0.355 (11)	0.188 (20)	0.087 (31)
Venoject	EDTA	1.02 (12)	0.520 (14)	0.348 (14)	0.197 (25)	0.084 (28)
Venoject	citrate	0.912 (19)	0.439 (10)	0.320 (8)	0.189 (22)	0.061 (24)
Vacutainer	none (serum)	1.07 (13)	0.541 (13)	0.356 (13)	0.219 (20)	0.091 (34)
Vacutainer	heparin	1.07 (15)	0.503 (10)	0.356 (14)	0.204 (15)	0.078 (17)

[a]Two separate studies performed on different days.

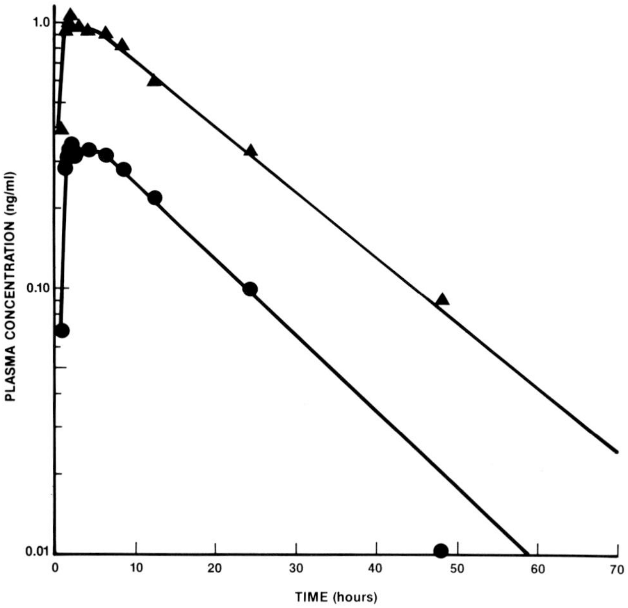

FIG. 2. Mean plasma levels of clonidine from 24 subjects following a single oral dose of either 0.1 (circles) or 0.3 (triangles) mg Combipres tablets.

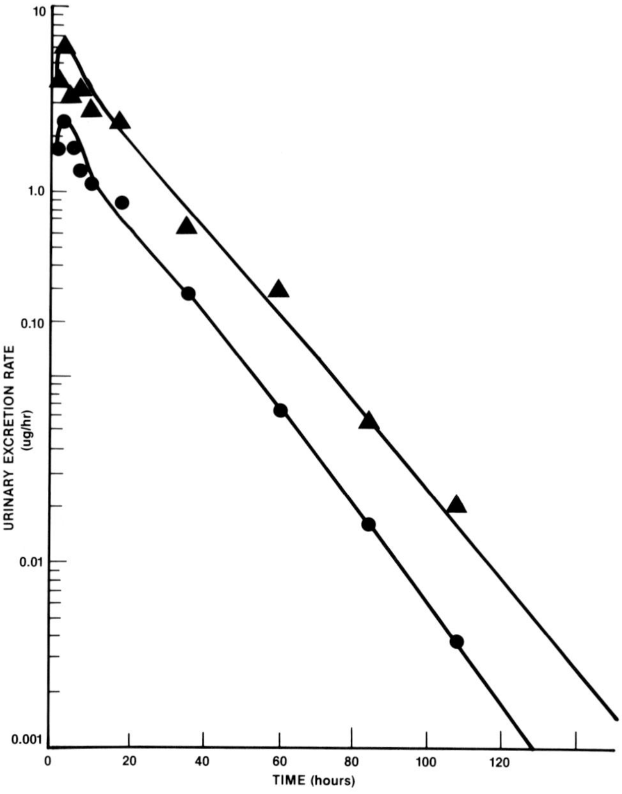

FIG. 3. Mean urinary excretion rates for clonidine following a single oral dose of either 0.1 (circles) or 0.3 (triangles) mg Combipres tablets.

39% of the dose. These pharmacokinetic parameters were in good agreement with values reported by others using gas chromatographic methods (11,12,25).

DISCUSSION

Determination of clonidine concentrations obtained during pharmacokinetic and bioavailability studies requires an assay that is sensitive, specific, and reliable as well as cost efficient. These assay requirements led to development of an RIA that maintained both the sensitivity and specificity of previous assays while producing greater flexibility and reliability with a high degree of sample throughput. The mono-iodinated radiolabel was purified to a single product, which achieved consistency of the specific activity and therefore of the standard curve. Introduction of the second antibody technique for separation of the bound and free phases resulted in lower nonspecific binding, simplified the procedure, and increased sample throughput. This present method has been used to analyze several thousand clonidine samples including plasma from a 24-subject Combipres bioavailability study. Clonidine could be quantitated over 4 half-lives after subjects received a single 0.1 mg Combipres tablet. Combipres also contains the diuretic chlorthalidone, which did not affect the quantitation of clonidine. In addition, several other commonly used therapeutic agents were tested for interference in the RIA. At therapeutic concentrations none of the drugs affected the quantitation of clonidine; however, salicylic acid at higher concentrations did lead to lower assay levels of clonidine. Three of the four known metabolites of clonidine (ST 2075, ST 2236, and ST 2245) did not crossreact with the clonidine antiserum. *p*-Hydroxy-clonidine (ST 666), which significantly crossreacts, should not interfere with the analysis of clonidine in plasma samples by the RIA since no significant levels of the metabolite in plasma from both normal subjects and subjects experiencing chronic renal failure have been found (D. Arndts, personal communication). Darda (14) has observed low levels of ST 666 in urine that may cause some interference in the RIA. In conclusion, this assay has been proven adequate to reliably determine clonidine concentrations for either single dose pharmacokinetic studies or to monitor compliance during chronic dosing.

Acknowledgment: We would like to thank Mr. A. Thor for the preparation of the non-radioactive mono-iodo-4-carboxyclonidine tyrosine, Ms. A. Gladczuk Graham for preparation of the immunogens, Mr. P. Kinkade for determining the purity of the methyl-ester label, and J. Arnold,

M.D., of the Quincy Research Center, Kansas City, MO, for performing the clinical study. The assistance of Ms. K. Matzek and Mr. T. MacGregor in the pharmacokinetic analysis of the Combipres data is also greatly appreciated.

REFERENCES

1. Lawrence I. Clonidine in the central nervous system: site and mechanism of hypotensive action. *J Cardiovasc Pharmacol* 1980; 2(suppl 1):S5–S19.
2. Houston MC. Clonidine hydrochloride: review of pharmacologic and clinical aspects. *Prog Cardiovasc Dis* 1981;23:337–50.
3. Kobinger W. Central α-adrenergic systems as targets for hypotensive drugs. *Rev Physiol Biochem Pharmacol* 1978;81:39–100.
4. Gold MS, Redmond DE, Kleber HD. Clonidine blocks acute opiate withdrawal symptoms. *Lancet* 1978;2:599–602.
5. Buckingham L, Davidson G, Greenwood D, Mather B. Menopausal flushing an alternative to oestrogen therapy. *Med J Aust* 1976;2:546.
6. Wall MC, Wilkinson M. Clonidine against migraine. *Lancet* 1973;2:510.
7. Brogden RN, Pinder RM, Sawyer PR, Speight TM, Avery GS. Low-dose clonidine (Dixarit) an independent report of its use for migraine prophylaxis. *Curr Ther* 1976;17:25–31.
8. Cohen DJ, Nathanson JA, Young JG, Shaywitz BA. Clonidine in Tourette's syndrome. *Lancet* 1979;2:551–3.
9. Lowenthal DT. Pharmacokinetics of clonidine. *J Cardiovasc Pharmacol* 1980;2(suppl 1):S29–37.
10. Keranen A, Nykanen S, Taskinen J. Pharmacokinetics and side-effects of clonidine. *Eur J Clin Pharmacol* 1978;13:97–101.
11. Frisk Holmberg M, Edlund PO, Paalzow L. Pharmacokinetics of clonidine and its relation to the hypotensive effect in patients. *Br J Clin Pharmacol* 1978;6:227–32.
12. Davies DS, Wing LMH, Reid JL, Neill E, Tippett P, Dollery CT. Pharmacokinetics and concentration-effect relationships of intravenous and oral clonidine. *Clin Pharmacol Ther* 1977;21:593–601.
13. Arndts D, Doevendans J, Kirsten R, Heintz B. New aspects of the pharmacokinetics and pharmacodynamics of clonidine in man. *Eur J Clin Pharmacol* 1983;24:21–30.
14. Darda VS, Forster HJ, Stahle H. Metabolischer abbau von clonidin. *Arzneimittelforsch* 1978;28:255–9.
15. Arndts D, Stahle H, Struck CJ. A newly developed precise and sensitive radioimmunoassay for clonidine. *Arzneimittelforsch* 1979;29:532–8.
16. Arndts D, Stahle H, Forster HJ. Development of a RIA for clonidine and its comparison with the reference methods. *J Pharmacol Methods* 1981;6:295–307.
17. Davies DS, Neill E, Reid JL. Applications of deuterium labelling in pharmacokinetic and concentration-effect studies of clonidine. In: Baillie TA, ed. *Stable isotopes*. London: Macmillan. 1978;45–54.
18. Draffan GH, Clare RA, Murray S, Bellward GD, Davies, DS, Dollery CT. The determination of clonidine in human plasma. In: Frigerio A, ed. *Advances in mass spectrometry in biochemistry and medicine, vol. II*. New York: Spectrum Publications, 1976;389–94.
19. Murray S, Waddell KA, Davies DS. The measurement of clonidine in human plasma and urine by combined gas chromatography mass spectrometry with ammonia chemical ionization. *Biomed Mass Spectrom* 1981;8:500–2.
20. Chu LC, Bayne WF, Tao FT, Schmitt LG, Shaw JE. Determination of submicrogram quantities of clonidine in biological fluids. *J Pharm Sci* 1979;68:72–4.
21. Edlund PO. Determination of clonidine in human plasma by glass capillary gas chromatography with electron-capture detection. *J Chromatogr* 1980;187:161–9.
22. Anderson GW, Zimmerman JE, Callahan FM. The use of esters of N-hydroxysuccinimide in peptide synthesis. *J Am Chem Soc* 1964;86:1839–42.
23. Erlanger BF, Borek F, Beiser SM, Lieberman S. Steroid protein conjugates, I. preparation and characterization of conjugates of bovine serum albumin with testosterone and with cortisone. *J Biol Chem* 1957;228:713–27.
24. Erlanger BF, Borek F, Beiser SM, Lieberman S. Steroid protein conjugates, II. preparation and characterization of conjugates of bovine serum albumin with progesterone, deoxycorticosterone and estrone. *J Biol Chem* 1958;234:1090–4.
25. Frisk-Holmberg M, Paalzow L, Edlund PO. Clonidine kinetics in man—evidence for dose dependency and changed pharmacokinetics during chronic therapy. *Br J Clin Pharmacol* 1981;12:653–8.

Therapeutic Drug Monitoring
7:351–354 © 1985 Raven Press, New York

Evaluation of Fluorescence Polarization Immunoassay for Quantitation of Serum Salicylates

H. Thomas Karnes and Larry A. Beightol

Department of Pharmacy and Pharmaceutics, Virginia Commonwealth University/Medical College of Virginia, Richmond, Virginia, U.S.A.

Summary: A fluorescence polarization immunoassay (FPIA) for serum salicylates that has been developed for use with the Abbott TDx analyzer is evaluated with regard to precision, accuracy, and stability of the standard curve. The FPIA method is also compared with a well-established high performance liquid chromatography (HPLC) technique in a clinical laboratory environment. The FPIA demonstrates excellent precision, and the standard curve is sufficiently stable to perform reproducible measurements over a 29-day period without recalibration. Superior accuracy of the FPIA method is indicated for salicylate concentrations between 50 and 800 μg/ml by recovery studies and by favorable comparison with the reference method. The performance of the FPIA for salicylate concentrations between 0 and 50 μg/ml is somewhat less favorable and should be used with caution in this range. The present method is more appropriate than HPLC for the management of patients receiving chronic high doses of salicylates or in cases of acute salicylate overdose and is also more rapid. **Key Words:** Salicylates—Fluorescence polarization immunoassay—Acetylsalicylic acid.

The availability of rapid, accurate, and precise methods for the quantitation of salicylates in blood serum is necessary for the proper management of salicylate poisoning, which may arise from chronic high doses of salicylates or from acute overdose. Chronic high doses of salicylates are indicated for the therapy of rheumatoid arthritis, and salicylate overdoses are frequently observed because of the availability of the drugs in over-the-counter dosage forms (1). Salicylates (primarily sodium salicylate and acetylsalicylic acid) produce their analgesic, antipyretic, and antiinflammatory action through conversion to salicylic acid, which is metabolized primarily in the liver by conversion to its glucuronide and glycine conjugates. Therapeutic levels of salicylates in patients undergoing therapy for rheumatoid arthritis are maintained at 150–300 μg/ml, and levels >300 μg/ml are considered toxic (2). The toxic effect of salicylates can reduce salicylate elimination through acidification of the urine (3), and salicylates demonstrate dose-dependent pharmacokinetics (4). Both of these aspects of salicylate pharmacokinetics can cause unexpected rises in serum salicylate levels, an occurrence that makes monitoring very important to prevent toxicity.

Several methods are available for the measurement of salicylate concentrations. These methods include gas-liquid chromatography (5–7), high performance liquid chromatography (HPLC) (8–11), thin layer chromatography (12), fluorescence spectroscopy (13), and spectrophotometry (14). These methods have been primarily applied to the collection of pharmacokinetic data from blood components, or, in many cases, to the assay of urine containing salicylic acid and its metabolites. Virtually all of these methods require some pretreatment of the sample and are not optimal for drug monitoring situations because of the relatively

Address correspondence and reprint requests to Dr. Karnes at Department of Pharmacy and Pharmaceutics, Medical College of Virginia, Box 581, MCV Station, Richmond, VA 23298-0001, U.S.A.

long analysis time required. Fluorescence polarization immunoassay (FPIA) with the aid of the automated TDx analyzer provides a method that is more rapid than existing methods and less susceptible to variations in operator technique, which is ideal for routine clinical monitoring.

The FPIA developed by Abbott Laboratories uses the principle of competitive binding to a limited supply of salicylate selective antibody (15). The salicylate molecules in a sample compete with a known quantity of fluorescent-labeled salicylate molecules, producing an equilibration of the system in which the amount of labeled molecules bound to the antibody is inversely related to the amount of sample molecules. The antibody bound fraction of fluorescent-labeled salicylate molecules exhibits a greater degree of fluorescence polarizability relative to the free fraction of labeled molecules because of their restricted motion upon binding. Hence, the resulting fluorescence polarization measurement from the equilibrated reaction mixture is inversely related to serum salicylate concentration and serves as the basis for quantitation. The fluorescence polarization measurement is made with the TDx analyzer, which is fully automated and uses a unique system of liquid crystals to quantitate polarization of fluorescence (16,17).

MATERIALS AND METHODS

Forty serum samples from normal volunteers and 51 serum samples from clinical subjects were obtained from an in-house pharmacokinetic study and Abbott Laboratories, respectively. All samples were stored at −20°C for as long as 5 months and assayed by both HPLC and the TDx method over a 29-day testing period.

Abbott TDx salicylate kits (lot no. 15960-20), calibrators (lot no. 15696-49), and controls (lot no. 15696-49) were supplied by Abbott Laboratories (Abbott Park, IL, U.S.A.) as part of a field evaluation study, and all reagents, calibrators, and controls were stored at 4°C when not in use. The FPIA was performed using the TDx automated analyzer according to the protocol outlined in the procedures for operation section of the Abbott TDx system operation manual. A standard curve was constructed by running in duplicate each of the six TDx calibrators which contained 0.0, 50.0, 100.0, 200.0, 400.0, and 800.0 μg/ml of salicylate in normal human serum. The curve was stored in the microprocessor memory of the TDx analyzer and used throughout the testing period. TDx controls containing 75.0, 300.0, and 600.0 μg/ml of salicylate in normal human serum were assayed with each set of samples.

Analysis by HPLC was carried out with a procedure developed in-house, using a Spherisorb S-5-ODS (25 cm × 3.2 mm internal diameter) column and a mobile phase consisting of 45% methanol and 55% phosphate buffer (0.05 *M*, pH 2.5). A Varian model 5000 liquid chromatograph equipped with a Gilson model HM Holochrome variable wavelength detector set at 313 nm was used at a flow rate of 1.0 ml/min. Serum samples, standards, and controls (250 μl) were extracted by addition of 500 μl of acetonitrile containing 0.5 mg/ml of the *o*-anisic acid internal standard. These mixtures were vortex-mixed and centrifuged, and 250 μl of the supernate was evaporated to dryness at room temperature under dry nitrogen. The residue was reconstituted with 500 μl of the mobile phase, and 50 μl of this solution was injected onto the column. A standard curve was constructed by plotting the peak area ratios of the salicylate standard peaks (observed at a retention time of 7.3 min) to corresponding internal standard peaks (retention time 6.0 min) versus concentration of the standards. Standards for HPLC analysis contained 0, 2, 10, 50, 100, 200, and 800 μg/ml of salicylate in citrated normal plasma.

RESULTS

The stability of the standard curve was tested by assaying the five nonzero TDx calibrators in duplicate at 7 days and 14 days subsequent to the initial calibration. Deviations from the target values of 50, 100, 200, 400, and 800 μg/ml were −8.76, −5.38, −5.42, −4.59, and −4.38%, respectively, for calibrators run on the seventh day and −7.06, −3.26, −3.73, −4.24, and −4.24%, respectively, for calibrators run on the 14th day. The fact that all of these deviations were negative indicates a slight drift of the standard curve, although the magnitude of drift was consistently less than 10% and would not cause significant error in sample evaluation. In addition, there were no shifts or trends in quality control data collected over the 29-day study period, which further indicates the stability of the standard curve.

The within-run precision of the FPIA method was evaluated by running 20 replicates of each TDx control sequentially on the same day. Between-run precision was determined by 30 singlet runs of each TDx control in order of increasing concentration over a period of 27 days. The results of the precision studies (Table 1) indicate excellent reproducibility at all three concentrations studied.

TABLE 1. *Precision of the TDx salicylate assay*

	Mean (μg/ml)	SD (μg/ml)	CV (%)
Within run (n = 20)	77.04	1.57	2.04
	298.87	5.50	1.84
	611.11	21.88	3.58
Between run (n = 30)	75.89	2.71	3.57
	289.86	5.73	1.98
	579.12	15.73	2.72

See text for further description of within run and between run.

The accuracy of the TDx method was evaluated by assaying citrated normal plasma spiked at various concentrations with salicylate six times each over a period of 2 days. The results of this study are presented in Table 2 and indicate good recovery throughout the concentration range of 50–800 μg/ml. Recovery from samples spiked with salicylate at concentrations lower than 50 μg/ml was somewhat low, and the results were also relatively imprecise. To investigate the possibility of an interfering substance in the citrated plasma matrix that may have covered the observed low recovery, the 50 μg/ml TDx calibrator was serially diluted with the zero calibrator to yield concentrations of 25, 12.5, and 6.25 μg/ml and assayed in duplicate by the FPIA method. The percent recoveries for these three dilutions were 81.76, 66.00, and 66.8%, respectively. The TDx calibrators and controls were also assayed by the HPLC method using standards in citrated plasma to detect any differences in matrix from that of the normal serum matrix used for the TDx method. Salicylate recovery from the 50, 75, 100, 200, 300, 400, 600, and 800 μg/ml TDx calibrators and controls, as evaluated by HPLC, were 104.44, 104.27, 101.77, 103.50, 100.94, 101.63, 100.95, and 100.73, respectively. The results of both of these evaluations indicate that the low recovery observed was probably not a matrix effect and was due to inferior reliability of the standard curve in that region.

TABLE 2. *Recovery of salicylate by the TDx method from spiked citrated plasma (n = 16)*

Spiked concentration (μg/ml)	Recovery (μg/ml)	Mean percentage recovery
800	757.09 ± 55.95	94.63
400	387.76 ± 3.56	96.94
200	195.22 ± 4.06	97.61
50	48.07 ± 1.88	96.15
20	16.78 ± 2.60	83.90
10	6.66 ± 1.13	66.63
5	1.83 ± 1.21	36.60

Potential interference from salicylate metabolites, drugs that may be used in conjunction with salicylates, and other commonly used drugs was investigated by assaying aqueous solutions (1,000 μg/ml) of several of these compounds in duplicate by the TDx method. The compounds propranolol, salicyluric acid, cimetidine, acetaminophen, chlorpheniramine, pseudoephedrine, theophylline, caffeine, ibuprofen, salicylamide, benzoic acid, and diazepam all demonstrated less than 0.1% interference, whereas gentisic acid demonstrated an interference of 73%.

The ability of the automated TDx analyzer to internally dilute high samples was tested by selecting 15 samples that had concentrations above 400 μg/ml and assaying them according to the dilution protocol outlined in the Abbott TDx system operation manual. This study showed a mean percentage difference of +6.26 ± 1.64 for a 1:4 dilution protocol as compared with the 1:2 dilution protocol. The study samples ranged from 408.30 to 1556.47 μg/ml of salicylate, and none of the samples studied demonstrated differences >10%.

The TDx method *(y)* was compared with the HPLC method *(x)* by assaying the 91 test samples by both methods and analyzing the results by linear regression. Regression analysis provided the equation $y = 0.974x + 1.32$, with a correlation coefficient *(r)* of 0.998, indicating excellent agreement between the two methods. The concentrations of salicylate in these samples ranged from 3.91 to 1,556.47 μg/ml.

DISCUSSION

The performance characteristics of the TDx salicylate assay, as indicated by this study, ranged from acceptable to excellent. The calibration curve prepared from the TDx reagents is sufficiently stable for measurement of serum samples for at least a 29-day period. The shape of the calibration curve is such that a greater slope is observed at the low concentration end. This may explain the relatively poor recovery for very low concentrations, since very small errors in calibration could lead to large measurement errors. This problem could be overcome by calibration with several standards in the concentration range of 0–50 μg/ml. This is not necessary for patient management, however, since salicylate monitoring is done almost exclusively when ranges are >50 μg/ml, and the TDx method seems to perform optimally in this region. Measurements <50 μg/ml should simply be regarded as subtherapeutic, and caution should be exercised in interpreting these results in quantitative terms.

The precision of control measurements was excellent over the range of salicylate concentrations studied, and acceptable accuracy was indicated in both recovery and comparison studies. The TDx method can be used to reliably quantitate citrated plasma samples, and no interferences were noted in slightly hemolyzed, lipemic, or icteric sera. Interference from the salicylate metabolites and other drugs studied was not a significant problem, except for gentisic acid, which differs from the analyte by only one hydroxyl substituent. The dilution protocol appears to be effective in extending the upper range of sample measurement to 2,400 μg/ml, which is adequate for almost any incidence of overdose.

The TDx salicylate assay has a distinct advantage when compared with HPLC for patient management. The analysis time for nine single samples by TDx with a stored calibration curve is approximately 10 min; whereas an HPLC result would require at least 3 h for a similar analysis. This becomes very important when a fast analysis time is needed to monitor the effectiveness of treatment in overdose cases, and the TDx salicylate assay should prove to be a valuable tool for the clinical laboratory in this regard.

Acknowledgment: This study was supported by Abbott Diagnostics, which provided funds and TDx reagents necessary for this work. The authors would also like to thank Willie Kiang of Abbott for her expert assistance.

REFERENCES

1. Woodbury DM, Final E. Analgesic-antipyretics, anti-inflammatory agents, and drugs employed in the theory of gout. In: Goodman LS, Gilman A, eds. *The pharmacological bases of therapeutics*. 5th ed. New York: Macmillan, 1975:326–39.
2. Ireland G, ed. *Drug monitoring data pocket guide*. 1st ed. Washington: American Association for Clinical Chemistry, 1980:43–5.
3. Proudfoot AT. Toxicity of salicylates. *Am J Med* 1983;75:99–102.
4. Levy G. Pharmacokinetics of salicylates in man. *Drug Metab Rev* 1979;9:3–19.
5. Walter LJ, Biggs DF, Coutts RT. Simultaneous GLC estimation of salicylic acid and aspirin in plasma. *J Pharm Sci* 1974;63:1754–8.
6. Blakley ER. Gas chromatography of phenolic acids. *Anal Biochem* 1966;15:350–4.
7. Tischio JP. Determination of salicylates by GLC. *J Pharm Sci* 1976;65:1530–3.
8. Bekersky I, Boxenbaum HG, Whitson MH, et al. Simultaneous determination of salicylic acid and salicyluric acid in plasma and urine by high pressure liquid chromatography. *Anal Lett* 1977;10:539–50.
9. Peng GW, Gadalla MAF, Smith V, et al. Simple and rapid high-pressure liquid chromatographic simultaneous determination of aspirin, salicylic acid and salicyluric acid in plasma. *J Pharm Sci* 1978;67:710–2.
10. Cham BE, Johns D, Bochner F, Imhoff DM, Rowland M. Simultaneous liquid-chromatographic quantitation of salicylic acid, salicyluric acid and gentisic acid in plasma. *Clin Chem* 1979;25:1420–5.
11. Mason WD, Gillilan R. Revised method for determination of aspirin and salicylic acid in human plasma by high pressure liquid chromatography. *Anal Lett* 1983;16:903–12.
12. Morrison JC, Orr JM. Analysis of selected pharmaceuticals by quantitative thin layer chromatography. *J Pharm Sci* 1966;55:936–41.
13. Saltzman A. Fluorophotometric method for the estimation of salicylates in blood. *J Biol Chem* 1948;174:399–404.
14. Furman M, Finberg L. A rapid method for estimation of salicylate in serum. *J Pediatr* 1967;70:287–89.
15. Jolley ME, Stroupe SD, Wang CJ, et al. Fluorescence polarization immunoassay I. Monitoring aminoglycoside antibiotics in serum and plasma. *Clin Chem* 1981;27:1190–7.
16. Popelka SR, Miller DM, Holen JT, Kelso DM. Fluorescence polarization immunoassay II. Analyzer for rapid, precise measurement of fluorescence polarization with use of disposable cuvettes. *Clin Chem* 1981;27:1198–201.
17. Jolley ME, Stroupe ME, Schwenzer KS, et al. Fluorescence polarization immunoassay III. An automated system for therapeutic drug determination. *Clin Chem* 1981;27:1575–9.

Therapeutic Drug Monitoring
7:355–357 © 1985 Raven Press, New York

Evaluation of a Mouse Monoclonal Antibody for the Determination of Serum Theophylline by Fluorescence Polarization Immunoassay

*Catherine A. Ross, †Cheryl J. Kraft, §Min Hwa Lee, and *‡David B. Haughey

**Regional Kidney Disease Program, Hennepin County Medical Center, †Lufkin Medical Laboratories, and ‡College of Pharmacy, University of Minnesota, Minneapolis, Minnesota, U.S.A., and §Seoul National University, College of Pharmacy, Seoul, Korea*

Summary: Theophylline concentrations in spiked human serum and serum specimens obtained from patients with normal and impaired renal function were measured by fluorescence polarization immunoassay (FPIA) using a mouse monoclonal antitheophylline antibody. The interday coefficients of variation of the assay after 14 days were 4.2, 3.3, and 2.4% at serum theophylline concentrations in pooled human serum of 7.1, 12.2 and 26.9 mg/L. Theophylline concentrations determined by FPIA and high performance liquid chromatography (HPLC) were used to generate the following linear regression equations relating the corresponding theophylline concentrations measured by each method in serum specimens from 50 patients with normal renal function (FPIA = 1.00 HPLC + 1.01, r = 0.98) and 50 patients with end-stage renal disease (FPIA = 1.04 HPLC + 0.08, r = 0.99). In contrast to previous studies performed with a polyclonal antitheophylline antibody, the precision, accuracy, and specificity of the FPIA were adequate for analysis of theophylline in serum specimens obtained from patients with end-stage renal disease. **Key Words:** Theophylline—Fluorescence polarization immunoassay—End-stage renal disease.

Theophylline serum concentrations are frequently monitored to adjust theophylline dosage because (a) the therapeutic serum concentration range is narrow (1), (b) the intersubject variability in total body clearance and dosage requirements is pronounced (2,3), and (c) theophylline metabolism is complex and may be dose dependent in some patients (4). Several methods for determining theophylline concentrations in clinical serum specimens are currently used, including high performance liquid chromatography (HPLC) (5,6), radioimmunoassay (7), homogeneous enzyme immunoassay (8), laser nephelometry (9), and fluorescence polarization immunoassay (FPIA) (10). The last (FPIA) is a relatively new technique, which is purported to be fast and accurate. The accuracy of FPIA for theophylline (TDx, Abbott Diagnostics Division) was questioned (11) when discrepancies were noted between serum theophylline concentrations determined by HPLC and corresponding theophylline concentrations measured on the TDx Analyzer using a polyclonal antitheophylline antibody (TDx, Abbott Diagnostics Division). The disparate results were observed in serum specimens obtained from patients with elevated serum creatinine concentrations (11). The present study was performed to determine the precision, accuracy, and specificity of FPIA using a mouse monoclonal antitheophylline antibody to measure serum theophylline concentrations. The results obtained with a monoclonal antibody demonstrated that theophylline concentrations measured by FPIA were in good agreement with corresponding theophylline concentrations measured by HPLC in serum

Address correspondence and reprint requests to Dr. D. Haughey at Renal Laboratory, Regional Kidney Disease Program at Hennepin County Medical Center, 701 Park Avenue, Minneapolis, MN 55415, U.S.A.

Presented in part at the 36th National Meeting of the American Association for Clinical Chemistry, Washington, DC, August, 1984.

specimens obtained from patients with normal renal function and in serum specimens from patients with end-stage renal disease.

METHODS

Blood specimens from 50 dialysis patients and 50 patients with no clinical evidence of renal impairment were obtained by direct venipuncture and allowed to clot in red-top Corvac tubes (Sherwood Medical, St. Louis, MO, U.S.A.). The resulting serum was gathered and stored at − 20°C until analysis. Blood urea nitrogen concentrations were measured by a conductivity rate method, and serum creatinine determinations were performed by an alkaline picrate method on the Astra-8 (Beckman Instruments, Brea, CA, U.S.A.). HPLC was performed with a Waters 6000 A Solvent Delivery System, a Waters Model 480 Lambda Max UV detector set at 280 nm, and a Waters M730 Data Module integrating recorder set in the peak height mode (Waters Associates, Milford, MA, U.S.A.). Serum samples were prepared and extracted into chloroform:2-propanol according to the method of Jusko and Poliszczuk (5). Chromatography was performed on a Dupont Zipax 30 μm column, 2.1 mm × 100 cm (Dupont Company, Wilmington, DE, U.S.A.) as described previously (5). The FPIA was performed on the Abbott TDx Analyzer (Abbott Laboratories, Diagnostics Division, Irving, TX, U.S.A.). Theophylline calibrators in human serum containing 0–40 mg/L theophylline (lot 57-122SV), human serum control specimens containing 7.0, 12.0, and 26.0 mg/L theophylline (lot 57-125SV), and theophylline reagent packs containing pretreatment solution, theophylline mouse monoclonal antiserum, and theophylline-fluorescein tracer (lot 15193-157) were kindly provided by Abbott Laboratories.

Assay Validation and Precision

Standards for HPLC were prepared in human serum at theophylline concentrations of 0.0, 0.75, 1.5, 7.5, 15.0, and 30.0 mg/L. Cross-validation of the methods was performed by analyzing the TDx theophylline calibrators in quadruplicate by HPLC and the HPLC serum standards in quadruplicate on the TDx Analyzer. The within-day and between-day precision of the FPIA was determined by analyzing the theophylline TDx control serum specimens in quintuplicate on 14 different days. Blank human serum was spiked with 12.5–100 mg/L caffeine and analyzed in duplicate by FPIA to determine cross-reactivity of the monoclonal antitheophylline antibody with caffeine.

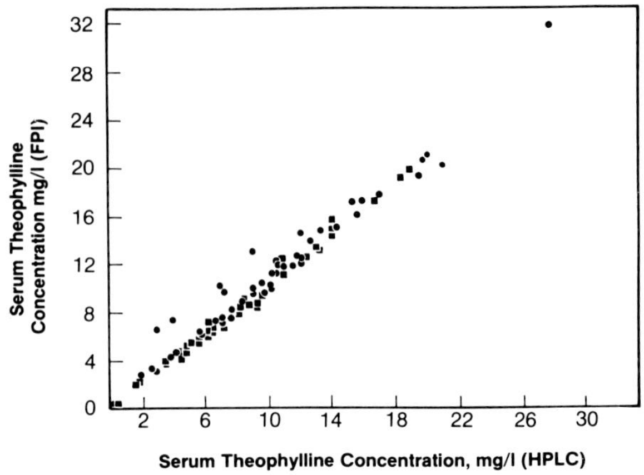

FIG. 1. Comparison of serum theophylline concentrations determined by high performance liquid chromatography (HPLC) and fluorescence polarization immunoassay (FPI) in specimens obtained from dialysis patients (black squares) and patients with normal renal function (black circles).

Analysis of Patient Specimens

Serum theophylline concentrations in specimens obtained from patients with normal and impaired renal function were determined in duplicate by FPIA and singly by HPLC. The duplicate serum theophylline concentrations measured by FPIA were averaged and compared with corresponding values measured by HPLC. Ordinary least-squares linear regression analysis and perpendicular weighted least-squares regression analysis were used to compare the two methods (12). The level of significance chosen for all statistical tests was $p < 0.05$ (two-tailed).

RESULTS

The theophylline concentrations measured by each method in serum standards were in good agreement with the corresponding nominal concentration for serum standards used to perform the HPLC assay ($FPIA_{measured} = 1.03\ HPLC_{nominal} - 0.07$, $r = 0.99$, $n = 28$) and the FPIA ($HPLC_{measured} = 1.01\ FPIA_{nominal} + 0.01$, $r = 0.99$, $n = 24$). Blank human serum spiked to achieve caffeine concentrations ranging from 12.5 to 100 mg/L showed no cross-reactivity with the monoclonal antitheophylline antibody. The within-day precision of the FPIA was determined on each of 14 days. The within-day coefficients of variation ranged from 0.9 to 3.1, 0.3 to 2.7, and 0.7 to 3.3% at corresponding serum theophylline concentrations of 7.1, 12.2, and 26.9 mg/L. The between-day coefficients of variation were 4.2, 3.3, and 2.4% at corresponding serum theophylline concentrations in pooled human serum of 7.1,

TABLE 1. *Comparison of theophylline concentrations determined by high performance liquid chromatography and fluorescence polarization immunoassay using linear regression (OLS) and perpendicular weighted least-squares regression (PWL) analysis*

	Slope (SE)		*y*-intercept (SE) (mg/L)		*r*
Normal (OLS)	1.00	(0.03)	1.01	(0.22)[a]	0.98
Uremic (OLS)	1.04	(0.02)	0.08	(0.14)	0.99
Combined (OLS)	1.02	(0.02)	0.44	(0.18)[a]	0.98
Normal (PWL)	1.03	ND	0.65	ND	0.98
Uremic (PWL)	1.05	ND	0.01	ND	0.99
Combined (PWL)	1.05	ND	0.20	ND	0.99

ND, not determined.
[a] $p < 0.05$ vs. a *y*-intercept value of zero.

12.2, and 26.9 mg/L. Linear regression analysis and perpendicular weighted least-squares regression analysis were used to compare the corresponding serum theophylline concentrations measured by FPIA and HPLC in specimens obtained from patients with normal and impaired renal function (Table 1, Fig. 1). The blood urea nitrogen and serum creatinine concentrations determined in specimens obtained from patients with end-stage renal disease averaged 55.8 ± 21.3 mg/dl (range 10–90 mg/dl) and 7.5 ± 4.0 mg/dl (range 0.7–15.3), respectively.

DISCUSSION

The specificity of an analytical method is difficult to ascertain with any degree of certainty because the extent to which drug metabolites, endogenous compounds, or other potentially interfering substances accumulate in biologic specimens cannot be anticipated. Theophylline concentrations in patient specimens measured by FPIA using the TDx monoclonal antibody were in good agreement with corresponding concentrations determined by HPLC. These findings suggest that the monoclonal antibody used in the present study to analyze uremic specimens was more specific than that reported for a polyclonal antitheophylline antibody in a previous study of serum theophylline concentrations in specimens from patients with elevated serum creatinine concentrations (11). An excellent correlation was noted (Table 1) between corresponding theophylline concentrations measured by the two analytical methods. The analytical error of the FPIA was acceptable, and no bias was noted in the determination of serum theophylline concentrations by FPIA in dialysis patient specimens when compared with HPLC. The mouse monoclonal antitheophylline antibody provided analytical results that were precise, accurate, and suitable for the analysis of specimens from selected patients with normal and impaired renal function.

Acknowledgment: The authors wish to thank Abbott Laboratories for providing the monoclonal antibody used in the present study.

REFERENCES

1. Jacobs M, Senior R, Kessler G. Clinical experience with theophylline. Relationships between dosage, serum concentration and toxicity. *JAMA* 1976;235:342–5.
2. Jusko WJ, Gardner MJ, Mangione A, et al. Factors affecting theophylline clearances: age, tobacco, marijuana, cirrhosis, congestive heart failure, obesity, oral contraceptives, benzodiazepines, barbiturates, and ethanol. *J Pharm Sci* 1979;68:1358–66.
3. Anonymous. IV Dosage guidelines for theophylline products. *FDA Drug Bull* 1980;10:4–6.
4. Dan-Shya Tang Lui D, Williams RL, Riegelman S. Nonlinear theophylline elimination. *Clin Pharmacol Ther* 1982;19:358–69.
5. Jusko W, Poliszczuk A. High pressure liquid chromatographic and spectrophotometric assays of theophylline in biologic fluids. *Am J Hosp Pharm* 1976;33:1193–6.
6. Butrimovitz GR, Raisys VA. An improved micromethod for theophylline determination by reversed phase liquid chromatography. *Clin Chem* 1979;25:1461–4.
7. Cook CE, Twine MD, Myers M, et al. Theophylline radioimmunoassay: synthesis of antigen and characterization of antiserum. *Res Commun Chem Pathol Pharmacol* 1976;13:497–505.
8. Chang J, Gotcher S, Gushaw J. Homogeneous enzyme immunoassay for theophylline in serum and plasma. *Clin Chem* 1982;28:361–7.
9. Nishikawa T, Kubo H, Saito M. Competitive nephelometric immunoassay of theophylline in plasma. *Clin Chem Acta* 1979;91:59–65.
10. Jolley ME, Stroupe SD, Schwenzer KS, et al. Fluorescence polarization immunoassay III. An automated system for therapeutic drug determination. *Clin Chem* 1981;27:1575–9.
11. Nelson KM, Mathews SM, Bowers LD. Theophylline concentrations may be falsely high in serum of uremic patients. *Clin Chem* 1983;29:2125–6.
12. Riggs DS, Guarnieri JA, Adelman S. Fitting straight lines when both variables are subject to error. *Life Sci* 1978;22:1305–60.

Therapeutic Drug Monitoring
7:358–363 © 1985 Raven Press, New York

Assessment of Blood Collection Systems for the High Performance Liquid Chromatography Measurement of Propranolol

Steven H. Y. Wong, *William B. White, Rosinda Fernandes, *†Robert Holden, ‡F. C. Lin, and ‡S. Narayanan

*Drug Analysis Division, Department of Laboratory Medicine, *Department of Medicine, University of Connecticut School of Medicine, Farmington, †Mount Sinai Hospital, Hartford, Connecticut; and ‡Becton-Dickinson Vacutainer Systems, Rutherford, New Jersey, U.S.A.*

Summary: The effect of blood collection devices on the high performance liquid chromatography (HPLC) measurement of propranolol was assessed. Blood was collected from hypertensive patients treated with propranolol for at least 7 days. Two venipunctures (opposite arm technique) were performed on each patient using the reference (syringe/silanized, ethylene diamintetraacetate tubes) procedure and the Vacutainer Brand Tubes (lavender-, royal blue-, green-, and red-stoppered) that were free of tris(2-butoxyethyl) phosphate. Propranolol concentrations were determined utilizing a published HPLC procedure. This study showed that in the four evacuated tubes, propranolol concentrations in serum or plasma were highly correlated to those of the reference procedure (correlation coefficients, 0.986 to 0.997; and slope, 0.912 to 1.013). Mean propranolol concentrations of the red-stoppered tube serum were lower (7.5%) than that of the reference syringe ($0.01 < p < 0.05$). Thus, lavender-, royal blue-, green-, and red-stoppered tubes would be acceptable for propranolol monitoring. **Key Words:** Blood collection—Propranolol—Antihypertensives—β-blocker—High performance liquid chromatography assay.

Propranolol, a β-adrenergic blocker, has been used in the treatment of hypertension, angina pectoris, cardiac arrhythmias, and thyrotoxicosis (1–3). Additionally, a recent multicenter study entitled the β-blocker Heart Attack Trial demonstrated the usefulness of propranolol in patients who had experienced recent myocardial infarction and who did not show contraindication to β-blockade (4,5). Oral administration of propranolol may be effective in preventing recurrent gastrointestinal bleeding in patients with cirrhosis (6).

It may be useful to correlate plasma levels of propranolol with clinical response (3,7). In studying propranolol disposition in man, Cotham and Shand (8) discovered spuriously low plasma concentrations of propranolol. Propranolol concentrations were determined by using a fluorometric procedure that might lack specificity as compared to a high performance liquid chromatography (HPLC) assay. A substance, possibly eluted from the rubber stopper of the evacuated blood collection tubes, caused a redistribution of the drug in whole blood. As a result, the drug migrated into the erythrocytes, resulting in a relatively higher drug concentration in erythrocytes and a relatively lower concentration in plasma. Borga et al. (9) later identified a plasticizer, tris(2-butoxyethyl) phosphate (TBEP), that selectively displaced some basic drug binding to α-1-acid glycoprotein. Additionally, several published assays of propranolol and metabolites by Walle et al. (10), Jatlow et al. (11), Wong et al. (12), and Lo and Riegelman (13) showed that 4-

Address correspondence and reprint requests to Dr. S. H. Y. Wong at Department of Laboratory Medicine, University of Connecticut School of Medicine, Farmington, CT 06032, U.S.A.

Presented in part at the 35th Annual Meeting of the American Association of Clinical Chemistry, July 24–29, 1983, New York, NY, U.S.A.

hydroxy-propranolol, a pharmacologically active metabolite of propranolol, was not stable in neutral or acidic pH and that an antioxidant such as sodium hydrogen sulphite was added to the plasma to ensure stability. At present, there is a lack of data on the suitability of commercially available, TBEP-free blood collection devices for propranolol monitoring.

The effect of TBEP on drug binding has also been observed for other groups of drugs such as the antidepressants, lidocaine, alprenolol, meperidine, and quinidine (14–19). In addition, heparin could also cause the same effect for tricyclic antidepressants (TCA) as described by Scoggins et al. (20). Since then, several studies (21–23) have examined the suitability of various alternative blood collection systems for TCA and thioridazine (24). The results demonstrated that an evacuated blood collection tube with powdered disodium salt of ethylene diamintetraacetic acid (EDTA) would yield plasma suitable for TCA assays by either gas-liquid chromatography (GLC) (21) or HPLC (23) procedures. Lai et al. (25) evaluated the effect of blood collection methods on in vitro dopamine-receptor-blocking activities as measured by a radioreceptor assay for six neuroleptic drugs—thioridazine, trifluoperazine, haloperidol, chlorpromazine, thiothixene, or fluphenazine. From this study, it was found that the royal blue-stoppered evacuated tube without additive was adequate for blood collection for all but one of these drugs, thioridazine, which would require the green-stoppered evacuated tube. Again, TBEP was implicated in that it affected drug binding and inhibited the nonspecific binding of the tracer tritiated spiperone to plasma proteins, and thus decreased blocking activities. Thus, blood collection tubes without additives were recommended for the assay. Shang-Qiang and Evenson (26) evaluated the effects of contaminants in several commercially available blood collection devices for 25 commonly used drugs. TBEP and other contaminants were identified by gas chromatography-mass spectrometry in some of these devices. The resulting increases in coefficients of variation ranged from 5 to over 20%. These investigators cautioned against the use of inappropriate blood collection devices.

Slockbower (27) and Narayanan and Lin (28) recently reviewed the various general problems in sample collection. Logistic problems, such as requisitions, identification, and technical problems, were considered. Winek and Paul (29) showed that alcohol samples of blood from living humans may be held up to 14 days. Frazer et al. (30) cautioned on the use of capillary technique for neonatal theophylline monitoring. Quattrocchi et al. (31) reported on the bias of the serum separator tube (SST) (Becton-Dickinson) for lidocaine, pentobarbital, and phenytoin, and recommended the processing of a minimum of 2 ml of sample within the hour.

The purpose of the present investigation was to assess the various TBEP-free blood collection devices for monitoring patients on steady state therapy of propranolol for the treatment of hypertension. Various evacuated blood collection tubes were compared to a reference syringe tube procedure using the opposite arm technique. Based upon the experience of a previous study on blood collection systems for TCA monitoring (23), the adopted reference procedure of using a syringe-EDTA-silanized tube—would yield noninterfering plasma (HPLC analysis of drug-free extract would not show any interference peak). An established propranolol HPLC assay (32) was used to quantitate the plasma concentrations in order to avoid interference from other drugs, metabolites, and endogenous chemicals. This study identified propranolol concentrations of lavender-stoppered tubes with EDTA to be comparable to those obtained with the reference procedure. Other suitable devices are the green-, royal blue-, and red-stoppered tubes. Preliminary results using these devices have been presented elsewhere (33).

MATERIALS AND METHODS

Patient Selection

Fifty hypertensive patients, treated with varying dosages of propranolol (40–480 mg/day) for at least 7 days, were included in this study. In order to measure steady-state trough levels, sampling time was ~6 h after the dose and ~0.5 h before ingestion of the next dose.

Blood Collection

An opposite arm venipuncture technique was used (the reference procedure and the procedure with two evacuated tubes were performed on separate arms). The pair usually consisted of either evacuated tubes *1* and *2*, or *3* and *4* as designated in the following paragraph. The reference procedure utilized a Monoject syringe (Sherwood Medical Company, St. Louis, MO, U.S.A.) to draw 10 ml of blood. After removing the needle from the syringe, the entire content was immediately transferred into an EDTA powder (15 mg), glass test tube (these tubes had been silanized to minimize drug adsorption to the tube) with a polypropylene cap. This sample was then inverted gently to avoid hemolysis. A venipuncture was performed on the other arm with an adaptor and two evacuated tubes.

The following four evacuated tubes were used: *1*–lavender-stoppered with powder EDTA (disodium EDTA, 10 ml; lot 1E611, catalog no. A3200Q); *2*–green-stoppered (sodium heparin, 7 ml; lot 1A102, catalog no. 6483); *3*–red-stoppered (nonadditive, 7 ml; lot 1F740, catalog no. 6431); and *4*–royal blue-stoppered (nonadditive, 10 ml; lot 1D102, catalog no. 6526) Vacutainer tubes. These Vacutainers were obtained from Becton, Dickinson and Co. (Rutherford, NJ, U.S.A.). According to the manufacturer, the stoppers did not contain the plasticizer, TBEP, in the rubber formulation.

Immediately after the venipuncture the lavender-stoppered tube was gently inverted several times to allow complete mixing with EDTA in order to avoid hemolysis. The other sample tubes were treated in the routine manner. No attempt was made to ensure or to avoid the contact of blood with the inside surface of the rubber stoppers. These specimens were allowed to stand at room temperature from 0.5 to 1 h and were then centrifuged. The serum or plasma was transferred by using silanized pipettes into a series of marked polypropylene test tubes. Then these samples were capped and frozen for later analysis. From another hospital laboratory the serum or plasma samples were transported in ice packs to our laboratory within 2 weeks of collection.

Chromatographic Analysis

The chromatographic assay was adapted from a published procedure of Hackett and Dusci using promazine as the internal standard (32). In order to minimize adsorption, test tubes and pipettes were silanized. Briefly, plasma was alkanized and extracted with *n*-heptane/isoamyl alcohol (98.5:1.5). The organic layer was transferred and evaporated. The residue was reconstituted in mobile phase for injection. Chromatographic parameters were: column = μBondapak C-18 with a guard column packed with Bondapak/Corasil C_{18} (Waters Associates, Milford, MA, U.S.A.), mobile phase = 65% KH_2PO_4, 0.045 *M*, pH = 3.0 and 35% acetonitrile, detection wavelength = 230 nm and flow rate = 1.5 ml/min. Using the peak height ratios of standard/internal standard, patient propranolol concentrations were estimated.

ANALYSIS OF RESULTS

Correlation of propranolol serum or plasma concentrations from various evacuated tubes with those of the reference procedure was evaluated by linear regression. Statistical significance was evaluated at $p < 0.05$ by the two-tailed paired *t* test.

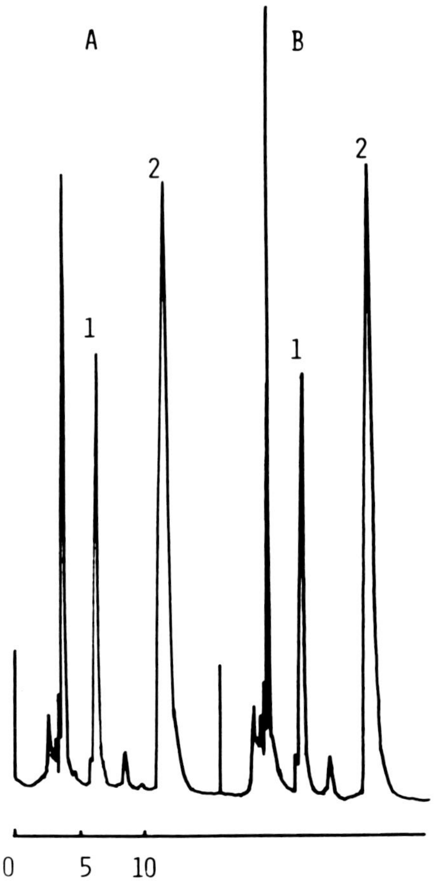

FIG. 1. Chromatograms of extracts of serum or plasma from a patient. **A**, plasma (from reference procedure tube) containing 90 μg/L of propranolol; **B**, serum (from royal blue-stoppered tube) containing 85 μg/L of propranolol. Peak identification: 1, propranolol; 2, internal standard.

RESULTS

In designing this study an established HPLC assay of propranolol was used in order to avoid interferences that might occur in a fluorometric method (8). A typical chromatogram of the extract of a patient's plasma is shown in Fig. 1. Retention volumes of propranolol and promazine were 9.8 and 17.6 ml, respectively. Figures 2–5 show the correlation plots for patient propranolol concentrations obtained from the reference and various blood collection tubes, and Table 1 shows the data of the correlation and paired *t* test analyses. Percentages of plasma concentration <25

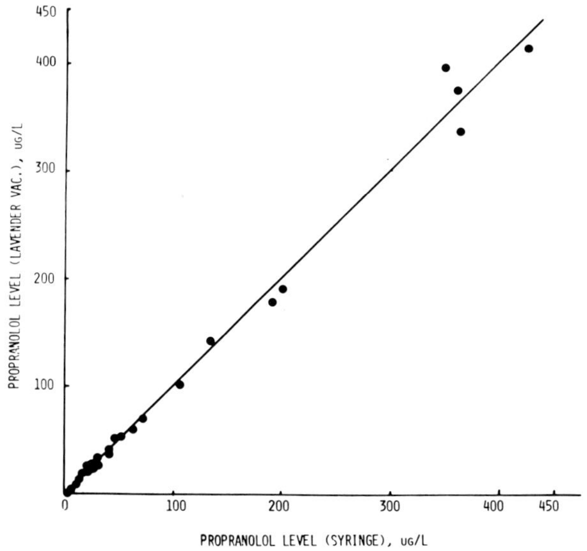

FIG. 2. Correlation of patient propranolol concentrations from two blood collection protocols, reference (syringe/tube) and lavender-stoppered tube.

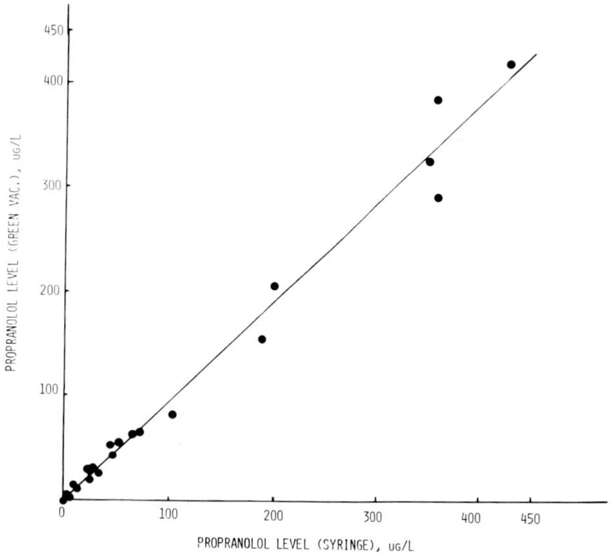

FIG. 4. Correlation of patient propranolol concentrations from two blood collection protocols, reference (syringe/tube) and green-stoppered tube.

μg/L were as high as 30% (e.g., 9/30 for lavender-stoppered group).

DISCUSSION

Correct sampling techniques are essential for the specialty of therapeutic drug monitoring and toxicology. As pointed out in the introduction, the measurement of various groups of drugs may be affected (8–20). The plasticizer, TBEP, causes spurious lowering of the plasma concentration of β-blocking agents and others. Thus, TBEP was eliminated in most of the recent rubber stopper manufacturing processes. This study focuses on the suitability of selected TBEP-free evacuated tubes for the monitoring of propranolol.

In carrying out this study the selection and sampling of patients from our clinic and another hospital and the sample processing and transportation were designed to be as close as possible to a "real-life" clinical setting so that the findings of this study would be useful for routine clinical propranolol monitoring. After 7 days of propranolol therapy, the selected hypertensive patients had supposedly achieved steady state propranolol levels. Thus, a correlation of the plasma concentrations with response could have been achieved with this study. In retrospect, the substantial number

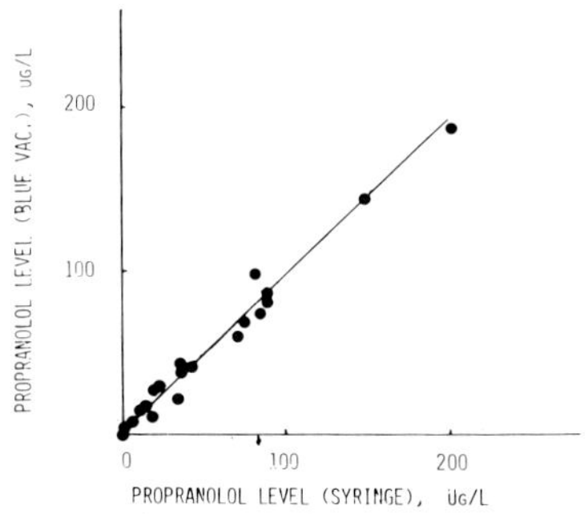

FIG. 3. Correlation of patient propranolol concentrations from two blood collection protocols, reference (syringe/tube) and royal blue-stoppered tube.

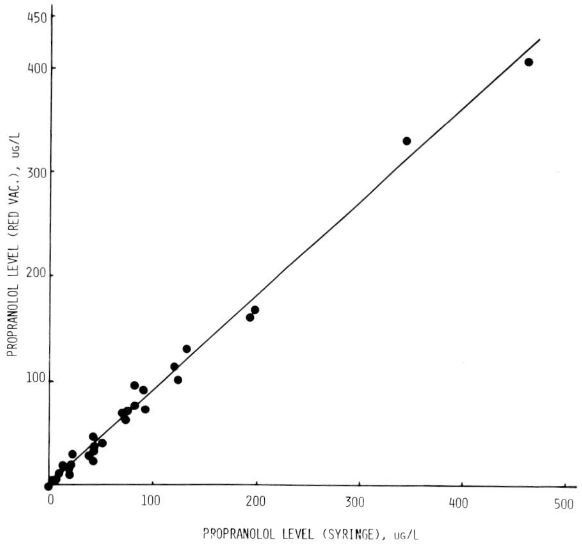

FIG. 5. Correlation of patient propranolol concentrations from two blood collection protocols, reference (syringe/tube) and red-stoppered tube.

TABLE 1. *Comparison of propranolol concentrations obtained from the reference (syringe/tube) and evacuated tubes procedures*

Procedures	Propranolol mean (μg/L)	Propranolol range (μg/L)	n	*r*	Slope	Intercept	Paired *t* test
Reference Lavender	88.1 90.6	<10 to 426	30	0.997	1.013	1.35	NS
Reference Royal Blue	52.7 51.8	<10 to 200	21	0.986	0.972	0.061	NS
Reference Green	97.3 93.4	<10 to 426	25	0.992	0.949	1.10	NS
Reference Red	81.5 75.4	<10 to 460	31	0.995	0.912	1.10	<0.05[a]

NS = Not significant at $p < 0.05$ by two-tailed paired *t* test; n, number.
[a]$p = 0.013$.

of patients with propranolol levels <25 μg/L could possibly be due to patient noncompliance, and propranolol measurement could serve as a useful check.

After performing the previously described "normal" blood drawing protocol, the serum or plasma was transferred to a polypropylene tube and kept frozen for later analysis or transport to our laboratory from the other hospital (a process similar to sending out samples to a reference laboratory). As pointed out by Walle et al. (10), and from our experience in developing an HPLC assay for 4-hydroxy-propranolol (34) in frozen plasma, both propranolol and 4-hydroxy-propranolol would be stable. Thus the described sampling procedure, using the lavender-stoppered EDTA tube, would yield plasma that could be useful for the clinical monitoring and pharmacokinetic studies involving propranolol and 4-hydroxy-propranolol.

In avoiding interindividual and technical variations, HPLC assay of propranolol was carried out by a single laboratory technologist, with the normal precautions such as periodic guard-column packing changes and column washing after each run. With the day-to-day coefficient of variation (CV) <10%, the chromatographic assay did not contribute substantially to the imprecision of the study.

The correlation data show that for propranolol monitoring the following blood collection devices would be preferable: lavender-, royal blue-, and green-stoppered tubes, based upon the slope of the correlation and the paired *t* test analyses. The red-stoppered tubes, when compared to the reference tubes, yield lower (7.5%) mean plasma concentrations ($0.01 < p < 0.05$) that would not be clinically significant when compared with day-to-day CV of the HPLC assay, as indicated previously. Thus, red-stoppered tubes might also be used for clinical monitoring of propranolol. Since serum is obtained from both red- or blue-stoppered tubes, the rubber formulation might account for the observed minor difference. The blue stopper is manufactured with nitrile butyl rubber with acid-washing to prevent trace metal contamination, whereas the red-stopper is manufactured with butyl rubber. As evidenced in Figs. 2–4 and Table 1, the number of patients in each group differs because of unavoidable clinical situations in which, occasionally, the amount of blood (<5 ml) collected in some of the evacuated stoppered tubes was insufficient. Consequently, such samples were not included for propranolol quantitation.

Lai et al. (25) demonstrated that the blue top was suitable for five of six neuroleptic drugs. Our study showed that blue top is also clinically efficacious for propranolol monitoring. However, it should be emphasized that these findings should not be extrapolated for other drugs. And before choosing a TBEP-free tube for monitoring new drugs, a systematic study should be carried out to evaluate various blood collection devices.

Acknowledgment: This study was funded by the Becton-Dickinson Vacutainer systems. We wish to thank Drs. J. Perel, R. Stiller and J. G. Fink for many helpful discussions.

REFERENCES

1. Nies A, Shand DG. Clinical pharmacology of propranolol. *Circulation* 1975;52:6–15.
2. Pine M, Farrot L, Smith S, McDonald K, Chidsey CA. Correlation of plasma propranolol concentration with therapeutic response in patients with angina pectoris. *Circulation* 1975;52:886–93.
3. Hollifield JW, Sherman K, Zwagg RV, Shand DG. Proposed mechanisms of propranolol's antihypertensive effect in essential hypertension. *N Engl J Med* 1976;295:68–73.
4. β-blocker Heart Attack Trial Research Group. A randomized

trial of propranolol inpatients with acute myocardial infarction. I. Mortality results. *JAMA* 1982;247:1707–14.
5. β-blocker Heart Attack Trial Research Group. A randomized trial of propranolol in patients with acute myocardial infarction II. Morbidity results. *JAMA* 1983;250:2814–9.
6. Lebrec D, Poynard T, Hillon P, Benhamou JP. Propranolol for prevention of recurrent gastrointestinal bleeding in patients with cirrhosis. *N Engl J Med* 1981;305:1371–4.
7. Chidsey C, Pine M, Farrot L, et al. The use of drug concentration measurements in studies of the therapeutic response to propranolol. *Postgrad Med J* 1976;52(suppl):26–32.
8. Cotham RH, Shand D. Spuriously low plasma propranolol concentrations resulting from blood collection methods. *Clin Pharmacol Ther* 1976;18:535–8.
9. Borga O, Piafsky KM, Nilsen OG. Plasma protein binding of basic drugs. I. Selective displacement from alpha-1-acid glycoprotein by tris(2-butoxyethyl) phosphate. *Clin Pharmacol Ther* 1977;22:539–44.
10. Walle T, Morrison J, Walle K, Conradi E. Simultaneous determination of propranolol and 4-hydroxypropranolol in plasma by mass fragmentography. *J Chromatogr* 1975;114:351–9.
11. Jatlow P, Bush W, Hochster H. Improved liquid-chromatographic determination of propranolol in plasma, with fluorescence detection. *Clin Chem* 1979;25:777–9.
12. Wong L, Nation R, Chiou WL, Mehta PK. Plasma concentrations of propranolol and 4-hydroxypropranolol during chronic oral propranolol therapy. *Br J Clin Pharmacol* 1979;8:163–7.
13. Lo M, Riegelman S. Determination of propranolol and its major metabolites in plasma and urine by high-performance liquid chromatography without solvent extraction. *J Chromatogr* 1980;183:213–20.
14. Fremstad D, Beregrud K. Plasma protein binding of drugs as influenced by blood collection methods. *Acta Pharmacol Toxicol* 39:570–2.
15. Piafsky KM, Borga O. Inhibition of drug-protein binding in vacutainers. *Lancet* 1976;2:963–4.
16. Brunswick DJ, Mendels J. Reduced levels of tricyclic antidepressants in plasma from vacutainers. *Commun Psychopharmacol* 1977;1:131–4.
17. Jennison TA, Chinn D, Crouch J, Tatcher GW, Hemphill G. The effects of blood collection tubes on the plasma, sera, and blood levels of amitriptyline and nortriptyline. *Clin Chem* 1978;24:1059.
18. Kessler KM, Leech RC, Spann JF. Blood collection techniques, heparin, and quinidine protein binding. *Clin Pharmacol Ther* 1979;25:204–10.
19. Midha KK, Loo JCK, Rowe ML. The influence of blood sampling technique on the distribution of chlorpromazine and tricyclic antidepressants between plasma and whole blood. *Res Commun Psychol Psychiatr Below* 1979;4:193.
20. Scoggins BA, Maguire KP, Norman TR, Burrows GD. Measurement of tricyclic antidepressants. Part I. A review of methodology [Abstract]. *Clin Chem* 1980;26:5–17.
21. Stiller RL, Perel JM, Lin FC, Narayanan S. A comparative study of serum versus plasma for tricyclic antidepressant drugs. *Clin Chem* 1980;26:1000.
22. Levy S, Kaufman G, Dioso C, Sternschein P, Lin FC, dePolo G, Narayanan S. Whole blood to plasma distribution ratio of tricyclic antidepressants [Abstract]. *Clin Chem* 1981;27:1102.
23. Wong SH, Jain N, Jain P, Santiago C, Lin FC, Narayanan S. Effect of anticoagulants in blood collection system on the analysis of tricyclic antidepressant (TCA) by high performance liquid chromatography (HPLC) [Abstract]. *Clin Chem* 1982;28:1644.
24. Stiller RL, Perel JM, Lin FC, Narayanan S. Effect of specimen collection and preparation on the radioimmunoassay (RIA) of thioridazine [Abstract]. *Clin Chem* 1983;29:1210.
25. Lai AA, Fleck RJ, Patzke JV, Glueck BG, Shaskan EG, Rosenberg BJ. Influence of blood sampling methods on dopamine-receptor-blocking activities as determined by a radioreceptor assay. *Ther Drug Monit* 1982;4:89–93.
26. Shang-Qiang J, Evenson MA. Effects of contaminants in blood collection devices on measurements of therapeutic drugs. *Clin Chem* 1983;29:456–61.
27. Slockbower JM. Blood collection problems: factors in specimen collection that contribute to laboratory error. *Am Assoc Clin Chem—TDM* October 1982:1–6.
28. Narayanan S, Lin FC. Sampling technique. In: Wong SHY, ed. *Therapeutic Drug Monitoring and Toxicology by Liquid Chromatography*. New York: Marcel Dekker, 1985:79–88.
29. Winek CL, Paul LJ. Effect of short-term storage conditions on alcohol concentrations in blood from living human subjects. *Clin Chem* 1983;29:1959–60.
30. Frazer JF III, Stasiowski P, Boyd GK. A clinically useful capillary blood-sampling technique for rapid determination of therapeutic levels of theophylline. *Ther Drug Monit* 1983;5:109–12.
31. Quattrocchi F, Karnes HT, Robinson JD, Hendeles L. Effect of serum separator blood collection tubes on drug concentration. *Ther Drug Monit* 1983;5:359–62.
32. Hackett LP, Dusci LJ. The analysis of propranolol in human serum using high-performance liquid chromatography. *Clin Toxicol* 1979;15:63–6.
33. Wong SH, White WB, Holden R, Narayanan S, Lin FC. Effect of blood collection systems on the analysis of propranolol [Abstract]. *Clin Chem* 1983;29:1236.
34. Wong SH, Chamberlin E. Simultaneous determination of propranolol and 4-hydroxy-propranolol by reversed-phase liquid chromatography [Abstract]. *Clin Chem* 1984;30:1014.

Therapeutic Drug Monitoring
7:364–368 © 1985 Raven Press, New York

Measurement of Vitamin E in Serum and Plasma by High Performance Liquid Chromatography with Electrochemical Detection

M. C. Castle and W. J. Cooke

Department of Pharmacology, Eastern Virginia Medical School, Norfolk, Virginia, U.S.A.

Summary: A deficiency of vitamin E has been associated with a wide variety of pathological conditions, many of them involving neonates. Previously published methods for the quantitation of vitamin E require large sample volumes as well as extensive extraction and concentration procedures. The present work describes a method for the quantitation of vitamin E in small volumes (≤50 μl) of serum or plasma without the need for extraction or concentration of the sample. With further optimization, even smaller volumes (≤10 μl) can be employed. Sample preparation consisted of precipitation of plasma proteins with absolute ethanol. After centrifugation, a small volume (10 to 50 μl) of the supernatant was injected directly onto the high performance liquid chromatography (HPLC) column. A dual channel electrochemical detector was used for quantitation of the vitamin E. Pooled serum or plasma was used to determine within-day (8.43 ± 0.19 mg/L) and between-day (8.49 ± 0.34 mg/L) precision. Analytical recovery of added vitamin E (4–16 mg/L) averaged 102 ± 7.0%. No interfering peaks were observed. Linearity was demonstrated over 0.5 to 800 ng. Vitamin E acetate is not detected by this method. HPLC with electrochemical detection is a highly sensitive and specific method for the quantitation of vitamin E in plasma or serum. This procedure is rapid and simple, and can be performed with very small sample volumes. **Key Words:** Vitamin E—α-Tocopherol—High performance liquid chromatography—Electrochemical detection—Plasma levels.

A deficiency of vitamin E (α-tocopherol) has been implicated in a wide variety of pathological conditions including hematological disorders, cardiovascular disease, and bronchopulmonary dysplasia (1). In addition, a purported association exists between vitamin E deficiency and numerous specific abnormalities in premature infants. These include hemolytic anemia, retrolental fibroplasia, hyperbilirubinemia, bronchopulmonary dysplasia, and intraventricular hemorrhage.

In most of these conditions, the evidence to support the role of vitamin E deficiency in the pathogenesis and control of these abnormalities is equivocal. This has been especially true in neonates, since the determination of blood levels of vitamin E is complicated by difficulties in obtaining sufficient volumes of blood for quantitative analysis of vitamin E.

Quantitation of vitamin E levels in plasma and serum have included colorimetric and fluorometric assays as well as gas chromatography. In addition, numerous methods have employed high performance liquid chromatography (HPLC) with ultraviolet (2–9) or fluorometric detection (10,11). These methods have one or more of the following drawbacks: (a) requirements of large sample volume, (b) extensive sample preparation and sample cleanup, (c) lack of specificity, and (d) lack of reproducibility.

Address correspondence and reprint requests to Dr. M. C. Castle at Department of Pharmacology, Eastern Virginia Medical School, P.O. Box 1980, Norfolk, VA 23501, U.S.A.

The purpose of the investigations reported here was to develop a method for the analysis of vitamin E that would satisfy the following requirements: (a) small sample volume (e.g., <50 μl of serum or plasma), (b) high degree of specificity and reproducibility, (c) rapid and simple sample preparation, and (d) rapid and simple method of quantitation. The results of this work have been presented previously in abstract form (12).

METHODS

Reagents

Vitamin E was a gift from the Henkel Corp. (Kankakee, IL, U.S.A.). Tetraethylammonium perchlorate was prepared by the combination of equimolar amounts of tetraethylammonium hydroxide (Eastman Kodak Company, Rochester, NY, U.S.A.) and perchloric acid. HPLC-quality acetonitrile and isopropyl alcohol were purchased from Burdick and Jackson Laboratories, Inc. (Muskegon, MI, U.S.A.).

Apparatus

The electrochemical detector (ECD) was a Model 5100A Coulochem dual electrode detector (ESA, Inc., Bedford, MA, U.S.A.) with T1 set at + 180 mV and T2 set at + 500 mV. A typical setting for the gain was 4,000 for both channels (maximum setting for this instrument is 10,000). The pump was a model M600 (Waters Associates, Milford, MA, U.S.A.) equipped with a model 7125 injector (Rheodyne Corp, Cotati, CA, U.S.A.). The column was a reversed-phase Ultrasphere ODS Minicolumn (Beckman Corp., Berkley, CA, U.S.A.) 45 mm in length and 4.6 mm inside diameter, and contained packing material with a 5 μm particle size. A Hewlett Packard model 3390 reporting integrator was used for calculations of the area under the curve of the chromatographic tracings.

HPLC Parameters

The mobile phase (2 ml/min) consisted of 50% isopropyl alcohol, 30% acetonitrile, and 20% water. Tetraethylammonium perchlorate (5 m*M*), was added and the final solution was adjusted to pH 4.0 with perchloric acid. Injection volumes were typically 5 or 10 μl.

Standards and Sample Preparation

Vitamin E standards were prepared daily by pipetting the stock solution into absolute alcohol. Pooled blood or blood from individual donors was collected into tubes containing heparin. The plasma was separated and frozen at − 20°C until assayed. At the time of analysis, plasma was allowed to thaw at room temperature. An aliquot was mixed with an equal amount of water, and 100 μl of the mixture was added to a 1.5 ml siliconized polypropylene centrifuge tube (W. Sarstedt, Princeton, NJ, U.S.A.) containing 400 μl of absolute ethanol. The tube was vortex-mixed for 30 s and then centrifuged at 5,000 *g* for 2 min in a model 59 centrifuge (Fisher Scientific, Pittsburg, PA, U.S.A.). The supernatant was injected onto the HPLC column.

Method of Calculation

Quantitation was routinely performed by manual measurement of peak heights and comparison to a standard curve. The accuracy of this method was checked by comparing the results with those obtained after integration of the area under the curve of the vitamin E peak. Recoveries were determined by adding vitamin E (4.0, 8.0, or 16.0 μg/ml) to pooled plasma. The addition of vitamin E to pooled plasma was performed by dissolving vitamin E in absolute ethanol and adding 50 μl to 0.95 ml of plasma.

Calculations were performed by subtracting the concentration of vitamin E in the unspiked plasma from the total concentration of the spiked samples.

RESULTS

Chromatography

Previously published methods for the separation of vitamin E by HPLC utilized very high percentages of methanol or acetonitrile. These methods are not suitable for use with ECD, because these detectors require the presence of ions in the mobile phase to permit a flow of electrons during the oxidation process. To overcome this problem, we have employed a short column (45 mm) to achieve a separation of vitamin E with a mobile phase containing 5 m*M* tetraethylammonium perchlorate as the ionic species. Figure 1 shows representative chromatograms of vitamin E standard (A) and extracted plasma (B).

Electrochemical Detection

In order to determine the appropriate parameters for the ECD, the flow of current generated by the injection of a given amount of vitamin E (5 ng) was measured at different voltages. As shown in Fig. 2, no oxidation of vitamin E occurs until the voltage

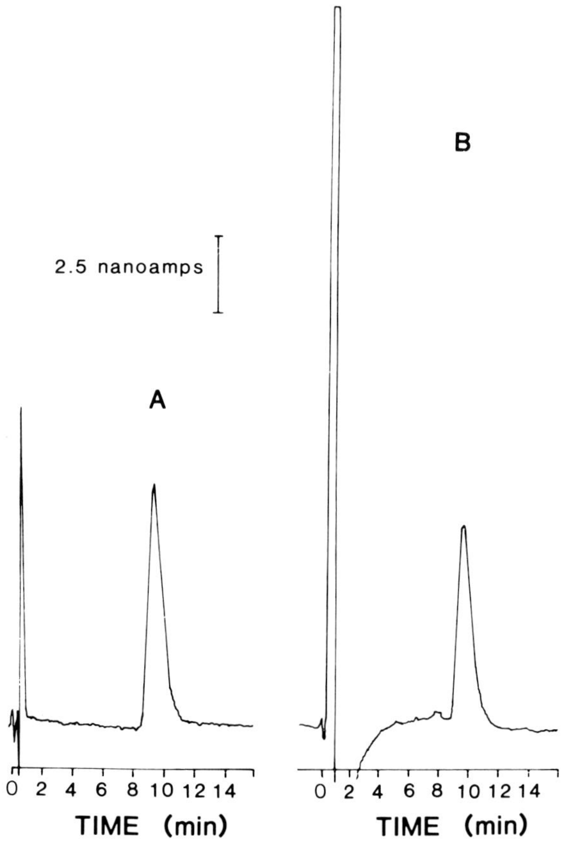

FIG. 1. High performance liquid chromatogram of vitamin E and plasma extract. **A**, injection of 10 ng of vitamin E standard. **B**, injection of 10 μl of an extract (450 μl absolute ethanol) of 50 μl of plasma. The calculated plasma concentration of vitamin E was 8.25 μg/ml.

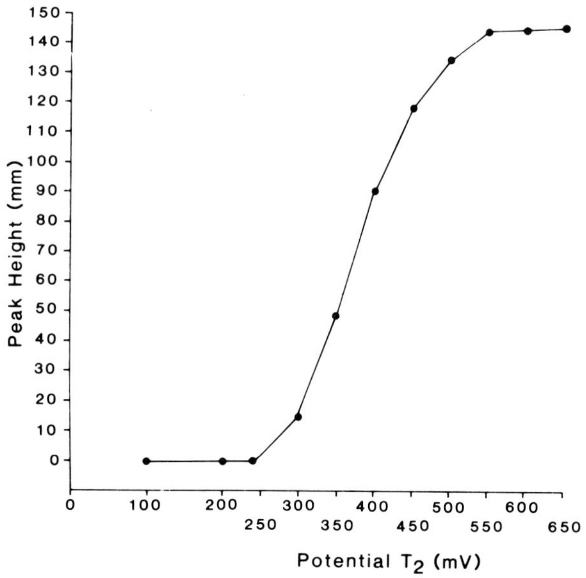

FIG. 2. Current-voltage curve for the oxidation of vitamin E. Peak heights (mm) are those measured after an injection of 5 ng of vitamin E at different electrical potentials on electrode two. Electrode one (T_1) was set at zero.

reaches 250 mV. Oxidation reaches a maximum at ~550 mV. We chose to set T1 at + 180 mV and T2 at + 500 mV.

Linearity

Figure 3 illustrates the linearity of the chromatographic analysis over a range of 0.5 to 30 ng. Optimization of chromatographic and electrochemical parameters would permit quantitation of considerably smaller or larger amounts of vitamin E.

Recovery

The recovery of vitamin E added to pooled plasma is shown in Table 1. There were no significant differences in recovery among the three groups of spiked samples. Recovery of vitamin E from samples containing <8 μg/ml cannot be predicted from the present studies.

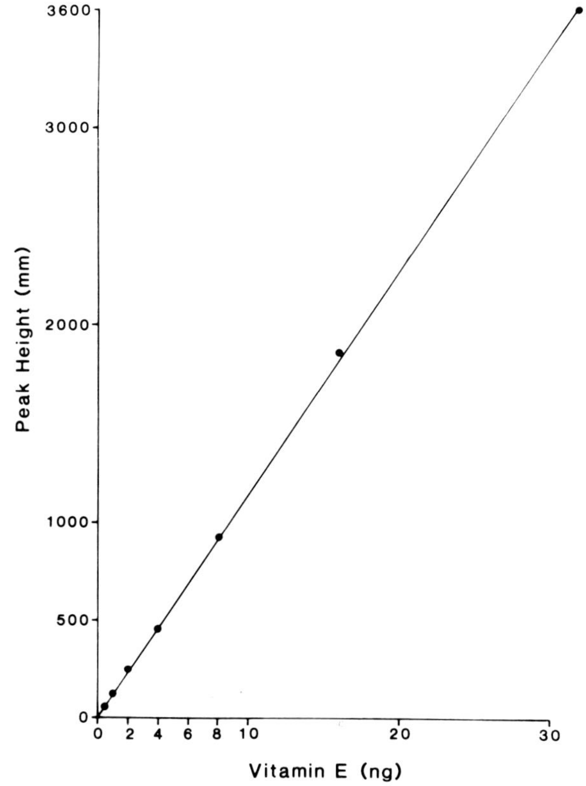

FIG. 3. Linearity of vitamin E measurement by high performance liquid chromatography with electrochemical detection. Peak heights (mm) shown are those calculated for different amounts of vitamin E at a constant gain of 800 nanoamps full scale.

TABLE 1. *Analytical recovery of vitamin E added to plasma*[a]

Added vitamin E (μg/ml)	Total vitamin E measured (μg/ml)	Recovery of added vitamin E (%)
0.0	8.16 ± 0.44	
4.0	12.34 ± 0.48	105 ± 2.45
8.0	16.14 ± 6.98	102 ± 11.43
16.0	24.09 ± 1.58	100 ± 6.98

[a]Values represent mean ± SD (n = 4).

Precision

The reproducibility of this method of analysis within the same day and from day to day is shown in Table 2. Even with the single determinations used in the present studies, the range of values is such that all samples fall within 10% of the mean. Since this method of analysis of vitamin E is simple and rapid, precision could be greatly enhanced by performing the assay in duplicate.

DISCUSSION

The ability of a drug to be oxidized, and thus produce a flow of electrons, has often been employed for quantitative analysis. However, previous methods were difficult to use and lacked specificity and sensitivity. These drawbacks have been overcome in recent years by combining ECD with HPLC for the analysis of a wide variety of drugs. The primary advantage of ECD over other detectors such as ultraviolet is greatly enhanced sensitivity (in many cases by a factor of 100-fold or more). In addition, the dual channels available in modern ECD permit the first channel to serve as a screen to eliminate potentially interfering compounds and greatly enhance the specificity provided by HPLC. In the present work, we have combined these two techniques to develop a method for the analysis of vitamin E that is much more sensitive than previously published methods.

TABLE 2. *Reproducibility of vitamin E measured by HPLC-ECD*

Within day (μg/ml)	Day to day (μg/ml)
8.7	8.72 ± 0.16
8.6	8.00 ± 0.30
8.6	8.55 ± 0.25
9.0	8.45 ± 0.05
7.7	
8.3	
8.49 ± 0.34[a]	8.43 ± 0.27[a]

HPLC-ECD, high performance liquid chromatography with electrochemical detector.
[a]Mean ± SD.

The specificity of this method is derived from both the HPLC and the ECD. The HPLC isolates vitamin E from potentially interfering compounds such as drugs and endogenous lipids. The ECD measures only those substances that can be oxidized at the selected voltage potential. The specificity of the ECD can be illustrated by the fact that vitamin E acetate is not detectable by this method, since the acetate moiety occupies the site of oxidation of vitamin E (the phenol group). In addition, the dual channel detector permits a "window" to be set so that only substances that are oxidized at a specific voltage will be measured. It is highly unlikely that a compound will have both the same elution time and the same electrochemical properties as vitamin E. Thus, there is very little chance that the presence of interfering compounds would lead to inaccurate determinations of vitamin E. An appropriate internal standard for the HPLC-ECD analysis of vitamin E is not readily apparent, since such a compound must have electrochemical properties similar to those of vitamin E and must behave similar to vitamin E in HPLC analysis. Although other tocopherols may useful as an internal standard in some situations, they would not be useful for individuals ingesting certain vitamin E preparations that contain these tocopherols.

The markedly increased sensitivity and specificity provide several advantages in the analysis of serum or plasma levels of vitamin E. The extensive extraction and concentration procedures employed with most other methods are not required with the present method. A simple precipitation of plasma proteins with ethanol provides a sample sufficiently clean to enable the supernatant to be directly injected onto the HPLC. This simple extraction technique, combined with the short elution time of vitamin E on the HPLC, means that between six and 10 specimens can be analyzed in 1 h. Optimization of the various steps in this procedure (i.e., extraction, separation by HPLC, and detection by ECD) would permit the use of extremely small sample volumes (e.g., <10 μl of serum or plasma). The ability to use very small sample volumes would be especially valuable in monitoring vitamin E levels in neonates. By this method, blood obtained from a heel prick and collected in a capillary tube would provide a sufficient volume of serum for analysis of vitamin E. Alternately, very low levels of vitamin E (<0.1 μg/ml) could be quantitated in the unlikely event that such low levels should occur.

In conclusion, HPLC with ECD is a highly sensitive, specific, and reproducible method for the determination of vitamin E in serum or plasma. The procedure requires very little sample preparation and can be adapted for very small sample volumes.

REFERENCES

1. Bieri JG, Corash LC, Hubbard VS. Medical uses of vitamin E. *N Engl J Med* 1983;308:1063–71.
2. Bieri JG, Tolliver TJ, Catignani GL. Simultaneous determination of α-tocopherol and retinol in plasma or cells by high-pressure liquid chromatography. *Am J Clin Nutr* 1979;32:2143–9.
3. de Leenheer AP, de Bevere VO, Cruyl AA, Claeys AE. Determination of serum α-tocopherol (vitamin E) by high-performance liquid chromatography. *Clin Chem* 1978;24:585–90.
4. Driskell WJ, Neese JW, Bryant CC, Bashor MM. Measurement of vitamin A and vitamin E in human serum by high-performance liquid chromatography. *J Chromatogr* 1982;231:439–44.
5. Howell SK, Wang Y-M. Quantitation of physiological a-tocopherol, metabolites, and related compounds by reversed-phase high-performance liquid chromatography. *J Chromatogr* 1982;227:174–80.
6. Koskas J-P, Cillard J, Cillard P. Separation of α-tocopherol, α-tocopherolquinone and α-tocopherol dimer by reversed-phase high-performance liquid chromatography. *J Chromatogr* 1984;287:442–6.
7. Stump DD, Roth EF, Gilbert HS. Simultaneous determination by high-performance liquid chromatography of tocopherol isomers, α-tocopherol quinone, and cholesterol in red blood cells and plasma. *J Chromatogr* 1984;306:371–6.
8. Rammell CG, Cunliffe B, Kieboom AJ. Determination of alpha-tocopherol in biological specimens by high-performance liquid chromatography. *J Liquid Chromatogr* 1983;6:1123–30.
9. Hatam LJ, Kayden HJ. A high-performance liquid chromatographic method for the determination of tocopherol in plasma and cellular elements of the blood. *J Lipid Res* 1979;20:639–45.
10. Catignani GL, Bieri JG. Simultaneous determination of retinol and α-tocopherol in serum or plasma by liquid chromatography. *Clin Chem* 1983;29:708–12.
11. Zapel BJ, Csallany AS. Determination of alpha-tocopherol in tissue and plasma by high-performance liquid chromatography. *Anal Biochem* 1983;130:146–50.
12. Castle MC, Cooke WJ. Measurement of vitamin E (VIT E) in serum by high-performance liquid chromatography (HPLC) with electrochemical detection (ECD) [Abstract]. *Clin Chem* 1984;30:1008.

Therapeutic Drug Monitoring
7:369–370 © 1985 Raven Press, New York

Short Communication

Daily Variations in Plasma Levels of Lidocaine During Local Anaesthesia in Dental Practice

Bernard Bruguerolle and Roger Isnardon

Laboratoire de Pharmacologie Clinique, Marseille, France

Several factors may influence lidocaine concentration, the time of administration appearing to be of particular interest since the efficacy of this drug has been reported to exhibit circadian changes (1).

The aim of our study was to investigate possible circadian variations in the plasma concentrations of lidocaine during its use in dental surgery. Our subjects were 24 men (mean body weight = 66.0 ± 2.0 kg, mean age = 35.0 ± 3.5 years). All had normal hepatic, cardiac, and renal functions and were not taking other drugs.

METHODS

Subjects were divided randomly into four groups (n = 6) corresponding to an hourly administration. During dental surgical interventions (tooth extractions), local anaesthesia was achieved by injection of a single dose (0.65 mg/kg of body weight) of lidocaine. The four groups of subjects were injected at different times of day, i.e., at 0930, 1230, 1530, or 1830 h. Blood samples (2ml) were collected in the antecubital vein at 5, 10, 15, 20, 25, and 30 min after drug injection. The plasma was separated and kept frozen until assayed. Total lidocaine plasma levels were determined by an immunoenzymatic method (EMIT-CAD). Single pharmacokinetic parameters such as maximal concentration (C_{max}) and time to reach maximal concentration (T_{max}) were estimated. The area under the plasma concentration curve (AUC) was calculated by using the trapezoidal rule. Means ± SEM of these data were compared by analysis of variance (ANOVA) statistical analysis.

Address correspondence and reprint requests to Dr. B. Bruguerolle at Laboratoire de Pharmacologie Clinique, CHU Timone, 27 Bd J. Moulin, F 13385 Marseille Cedex 5, France.

RESULTS AND DISCUSSION

As shown in Table 1, C_{max} and T_{max} values did not vary significantly with time of day although they were somewhat higher at 1530 h. However our data reveal a significant variation of the AUC during the day since this value is highest when the drug is injected at 1530 h.

Circadian rhythms in drug action have been reported for local anaesthetic agents. Reinberg and Reinberg (1) demonstrated that duration of anaesthesia after lidocaine or betoxycaine was two to three times longer in man when the drug was adminstered at 1500 compared to 0900 h. Other studies of local anaesthetic use in dental practice confirm these observations (2).

Our data indicate that C_{max} of lidocaine is obtained when the drug is given at 1530 h and disagree with those of Reinberg and Reinberg (1) or Pollman (2) since the highest local anaesthetic activity occurred at 1500 h. The lack of correspondence between the effect of lidocaine and circadian kinetics may indicate that circadian changes of local anaesthetic activity are only related to circadian changes of cell membrane properties and/or to circadian rhythm in catecholamine secretion (1).

Nevertheless our results suggest that under conditions of daily dental practice the hour of administration of lidocaine may affect its concentration in plasma.

TABLE 1. *Maximal plasma level (C_{max}, μg ml^{-1}), maximal time to reach C_{max} (T_{max}, h) and area under the plasma concentration curve (AUC_{exp}, μg ml^{-1} h) of total lidocaine after a single dose of 0.65 mg kg^{-1} injected at 0930, 1230, 1530, or 1830 h in men (n = 24) during dental surgical interventions*

	0930 h	1230 h	1530 h	1830 h	ANOVA
C_{max}	0.88 ± 0.11	0.78 ± 0.08	1.21 ± 0.21	0.85 ± 0.02	NS
T_{max}	0.16 ± 0.03	0.15 ± 0.01	0.16 ± 0.03	0.12 ± 0.01	NS
AUC_{exp}	0.665 ± 0.074	0.625 ± 0.059	0.900 ± 0.066	0.718 ± 0.034	$p < 0.025$

ANOVA, analysis of variance; NS, not significant.

REFERENCES

1. Reinberg A, Reinberg MA. Circadian changes of the duration of action of local anaesthetic agents. *Naunyn-Schmiedeberg's Arch Pharmacol* 1977;297:149–52.
2. Pollman L. Circadian changes in the duration of local anaesthesia. *J Interdiscipl Cycle Res* 1981;12:187–92.

Therapeutic Drug Monitoring
7:371 © 1985 Raven Press, New York

Editorial

Cyclosporine Quality Control Program

It is with great pleasure that we call to our readers' attention a second cyclosporine quality control program. Again, we urge every reader who is analyzing cyclosporine to participate in the available external quality control programs. The following announcement outlines the United Kingdom Quality Assessment Scheme:

The scheme is open to all laboratories in the United Kingdom measuring cyclosporine, irrespective of methodology; there is no charge for membership. Enquiries from other centres outside the United Kingdom are welcome.

Each laboratory is identified by a code number known only to themselves and the co-ordinating laboratory. Three samples are supplied each month either as whole blood or plasma.

A variety of samples are circulated ranging from those containing no cyclosporine to pools collected from patients receiving the drug and samples spiked with known cyclosporine concentrations.

A number of variables are tested periodically, including assay sensitivity, accuracy, recovery of added cyclosporine, and reproducibility both within and between assay.

Results are circulated monthly giving details of methodology used by each centre and individual results. Mean results are calculated on the basis of sample and method type.

Further information on this scheme can be obtained from the organiser, Dr. David W. Holt, Principal Biochemist, Poisons Unit, Guy's Hospital, London SE1 9RT, United Kingdom.

C. E. Pippenger
Cleveland, Ohio

Therapeutic Drug Monitoring
7:372–376 © 1985 Raven Press, New York

Interaction Between Digoxin and Nifedipine at Steady State in Patients with Atrial Fibrillation

*†C. H. Kleinbloesem, †P. van Brummelen, ‡J. Hillers, §A. J. Moolenaar, and *D. D. Breimer

**Center for Bio-Pharmaceutical Sciences, Division of Pharmacology, University of Leiden, and Departments of †Nephrology, ‡Cardiology, and §Chemical Pathology, University Hospital, Leiden, The Netherlands*

Summary: The possible kinetic and hemodynamic interactions between digoxin and nifedipine were evaluated in nine patients with atrial fibrillation who were receiving chronic digoxin. After 2 control weeks, nifedipine (20 mg b.i.d.), in a new formulation with sustained release characteristics, was added to the therapeutic regimen for 2 weeks. Trough serum digoxin concentrations and peak nifedipine concentrations were determined repeatedly. On the same days, resting blood pressure and heart rate were measured. During nifedipine administration, serum digoxin levels increased by 15% from 0.87 ± 0.38 to 1.04 ± 0.37 ng/ml (mean ± SD, $p < 0.05$). This was accompanied by a reduction in systolic and diastolic blood pressure of 16 ± 6 ($p < 0.01$) and 12 ± 5 mm Hg ($p < 0.001$), respectively. In two patients, noncardiac side effects were reported. In two other patients, nifedipine was discontinued because of skin rash and severe headache, respectively. In conclusion, plasma digoxin levels were elevated slightly in the presence of nifedipine, but this probably has little clinical relevance. **Key Words:** Nifedipine—Digoxin—Interaction.

The combined use of digoxin and the calcium channel blocker nifedipine in cardiac patients is not uncommon in clinical practice. Because of the relatively narrow therapeutic index of cardiac glycosides, it is relevant to know whether the kinetics of digoxin are influenced by nifedipine. The data in the literature are rather conflicting. In single-dose experiments in healthy subjects no influence of nifedipine on serum kinetics of digoxin could be demonstrated, whereas the effect on urinary excretion of digoxin was small (1). During chronic digoxin use in healthy subjects, increased as well as unaltered steady-state digoxin concentrations have been reported during combined treatment with nifedipine (2,3). Recently it was shown in two studies in patients receiving long-term digoxin therapy that the serum levels of digoxin were not influenced by the addition of nifedipine (4,5).

In the present study, we have investigated the influence of a new formulation of nifedipine, with a different kinetic and dynamic profile (6), on the steady-state serum levels of digoxin in patients with atrial fibrillation.

METHODS

Subjects

Nine patients with atrial fibrillation, treated chronically with digoxin for at least 6 months, participated in the study. Patient characteristics, concomitant medication that was continued throughout the study, and the daily dose of digoxin are given in Table 1. All patients had normal hepatic and renal function, but some took other cardiovascular drugs (Table 1). The

Address correspondence and reprint requests to Prof. D. D. Breimer at Center for Bio-Pharmaceutical Sciences, Sylvius Labs, P. O. Box 9503, 2300 RA Leiden, The Netherlands.

TABLE 1. *Patient characteristics, concomitant medication, and reported side effects during nifedipine*

Patient	Age (yr)	Sex	Daily digoxin dose (mg)	Concomitant diagnosis	Concomitant medication	Pre-nifedipine treatment blood pressure (mm Hg)	Side effects
N	42	M	0.25	—	Phenprocoumon	120/71	Nausea, blurred vision
F	55	M	0.25	Essential hypertension	Endralazine, atenolol, chlorthalidone	140/78	—
S	59	F	0.375	—	Quinidine	145/78	Nausea, dizziness[a]
A	66	M	0.25	Essential hypertension	Phenprocoumon, propranolol, chlorthalidone	143/80	—
D	61	M	0.25	Arthritis	Amiodarone, propranolol, ibuprofen	159/90	—
J	67	M	0.25	—	Phenprocoumon, nitrazepam	143/73	—
K	68	M	0.50	Essential hypertension	Pindolol, hydrochlorothiazide, phenprocoumon, triamterene	174/100	Nausea, blurred vision
T	39	F	0.25	Essential hypertension	Pindolol, furosemide, phenprocoumon	180/106	Skin rash[b]
E	70	M	0.25	Essential hypertension	Pindolol, phenprocoumon	112/84	—

[a]Patient dropped out after first dose of nifedipine (see Results).
[b]Patient dropped out after 1 week of nifedipine (see Results).

purpose and nature of the study were explained prior to the study and all subjects have their consent. The protocol was approved by the Ethical Committee of the Hospital.

Study Design

The study consisted of two 2-week periods in which the drugs were given in an open manner. During the first period, all subjects continued their daily digoxin use. They were seen at the same times on days 1, 8, and 15, and digoxin tablets were taken immediately after the hospital visit. During the second period, nifedipine tablets (Bayer AG, Leverkussen, F.R.G.) with slow-release characteristics (6) were added to the treatment regimen. These tablets were ingested every 12 h, and ~3 h before the hospital visit (total daily dose 40 mg). In this period, subjects were seen 3, 7, and 14 days after the start of nifedipine.

At each visit, supine systolic and diastolic blood pressure and heart rate were measured, and patients were asked about side effects. One blood sample was obtained by venipuncture for determination of trough digoxin and also during the second study period for expected peak serum nifedipine concentrations.

Analytical Methods

Blood samples were drawn in tubes without additives, and serum was separated after immediate centrifugation and stored at −20°C until analyzed within 1 month. In order to prevent photodegradation of nifedipine, blood samples were carefully protected from light by aluminum foil. Serum concentrations of digoxin were determined by [^{125}I] digoxin radioimmunoassay (Becton Dickinson Labware, Oxnard, CA, U.S.A.). The standard deviation of the assay was less than 5%, and the samples were measured blindly. The minimum level of quantification was 0.2 ng/ml. It was found that nifedipine, using real samples in concentrations up to 300 ng/ml, did not interfere. Nifedipine levels were determined in serum by a selective high performance liquid chromatography procedure (7).

Hemodynamic Measurements

All subjects remained recumbent for 10 min before and during measurement of blood pressure and heart rate. Blood pressure was measured with an automatic device (Bosch EBM 500; F.R.G.). Blood pressure figures used for analysis represented the mean of three consecutive measurements. Heart rate was measured by pulse frequency counting.

Statistical Analysis

Statistical methods used included two-way analysis of variance, followed by Newmans-Keuls test where appropriate (8).

RESULTS

In our study population there were two dropouts. Patient S discontinued nifedipine treatment after the first dose as a result of severe subjective side effects (i.e., headache, flush, dizziness). Data from this patient are not included in the statistical calculations. Patient K stopped nifedipine after 1 week because of a skin rash, which disappeared after nifedipine treatment was discontinued.

Individual digoxin concentrations before and during nifedipine are represented in Table 2 and mean values are shown in Fig. 1. Stable pre-nifedipine digoxin levels were found in all patients. After 3 days of nifedipine, digoxin levels had increased from 0.87 ± 0.38 to 1.05 ± 0.4 ng/ml ($p < 0.05$) and remained elevated during continued treatment. Nifedipine peak levels are shown in Fig. 1. No correlation was found between the plasma levels of nifedipine and the changes in digoxin levels. During nifedipine administration, systolic and diastolic blood pressure were significantly reduced. Heart rate was not significantly influenced by nifedipine (Fig. 1). Side effects were reported exclusively during nifedipine and included dizziness, blurred vision, skin rash, and nausea (Table 1).

DISCUSSION

The results of the present study suggest that serum digoxin levels increase slightly when nifedipine is used concomitantly. Because of the open study design, the possibility cannot be excluded that the increase in serum digoxin levels was due to improved patient compliance with the therapeutic regimen. However, this explanation seems unlikely, since the obtained steady-state digoxin trough levels were relatively stable both before and during nifedipine (Table 2). The increase in serum digoxin levels found in the present study, using nifedipine tablets, are just between the results of Belz et al. (2) on one hand and Schwartz et al. (3) and Kuhlmann (5), who found no change, on the other hand. Differences in study populations and study design probably account for these divergent results.

The kinetic mechanisms by which serum digoxin concentrations were increased in the present study are not completely understood. Interference of nifedipine and/or metabolites with the digoxin assay was excluded by appropriate in vitro experiments. Changes in volume of distribution of digoxin are not likely, since these would result only in transient changes in digoxin steady-state levels. Reduced renal or extrarenal digoxin clearance is probably responsible for increased digoxin levels (1,2), although changes in drug absorption cannot be excluded.

The pharmacodynamic consequences of elevated digoxin serum levels during treatment with calcium antagonists are considered to be clinically relevant (2). We used nifedipine tablets with slow-release characteristics. As a result of slowly increasing plasma nifedipine concentrations, blood pressure is lowered, but counter-regulation mechanisms, e.g., a baroreceptor-mediated increase in heart rate, are much less stimulated than after using nifedipine capsules (6). A sympathetic contribution to inotropism evoked by nifedipine is therefore less pronounced. Since digitalis glycosides enhance intracellular calcium, antagonism of nifedipine to digoxin inotropism is quite possible

TABLE 2. *Digoxin serum concentrations (ng/ml) before and during concomitant nifedipine use (trough values)*

Patient	Before nifedipine			During nifedipine		
	Day 1	Day 8	Day 15	Day 3	Day 7	Day 14
N	0.5	0.5	0.6	0.7	0.8	0.8
F	0.8	0.9	0.9	1.1	0.8	1.0
S[a]	—	—	—	—	—	—
A	1.5	1.5	1.3	1.8	1.8	1.6
D	0.7	0.5	0.7	0.8	0.8	0.8
J	1.1	1.4	1.1	1.2	1.2	1.1
K	0.5	0.3	0.4	0.5	0.6	—
T	1.0	1.2	1.1	1.3	1.2	1.3
E	0.8	0.8	0.9	1.0	1.1	1.2
Mean	0.86	0.88	0.87	1.05[b]	1.04[b]	1.03[b]
SD	0.33	0.45	0.30	0.40	0.37	0.34

[a]Patient withdrawn from study (see Results).
[b]$p < 0.05$.

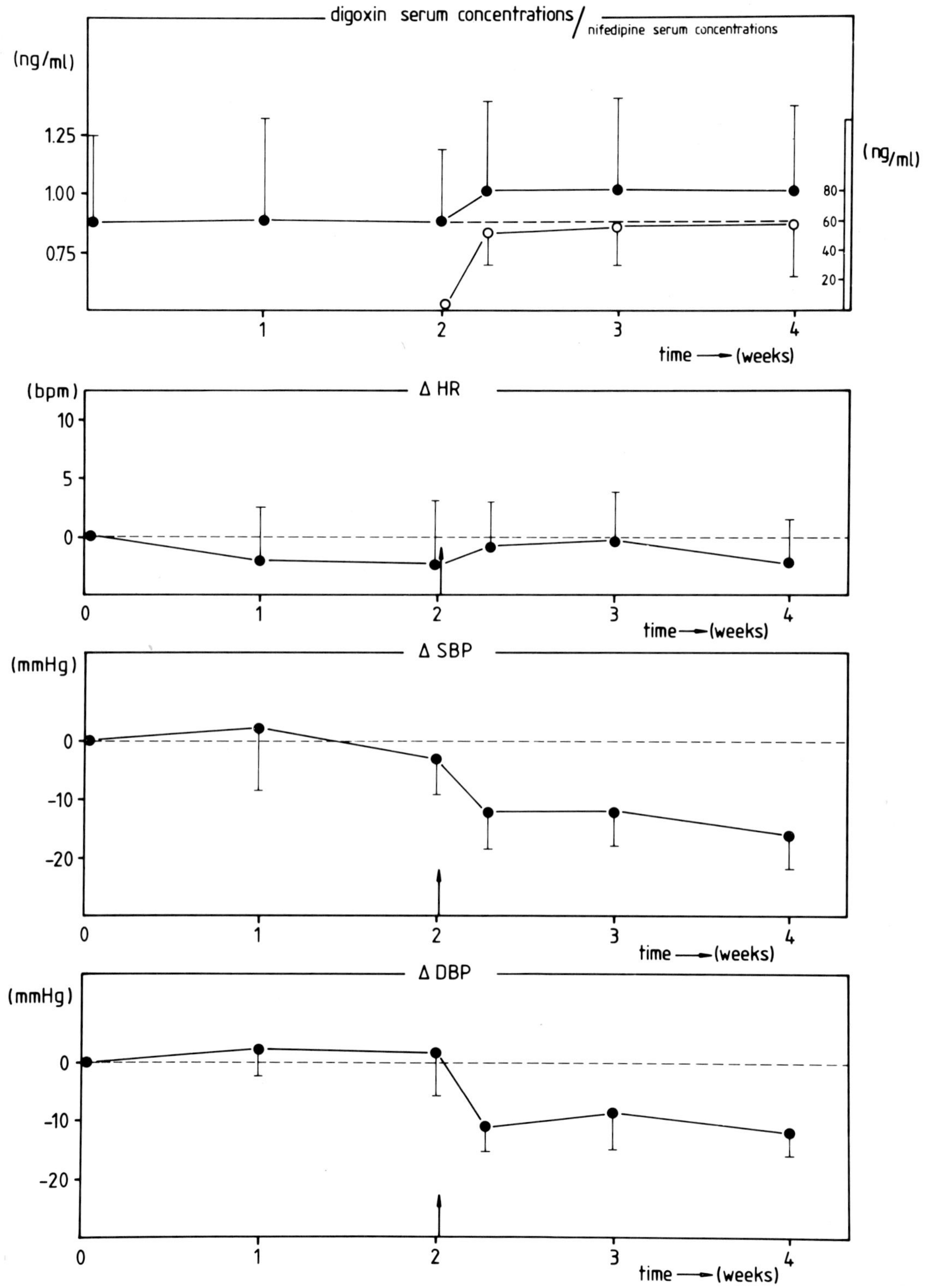

FIG. 1. Trough serum digoxin concentrations (filled circles) before and during concomitant nifedipine use, as well as mean nifedipine peak serum concentrations (open circles) (mean ± SD). Changes in heart rate (HR), systolic blood pressure (SBP), and diastolic blood pressure (DBP) versus time. Time of nifedipine administration is indicated by arrow.

(9). On the other hand, the beneficial effect of afterload reduction, and the increase in digoxin concentrations induced by nifedipine, should be considered. However, it is unlikely that noncardiac side effects of digoxin, like nausea and blurred vision, would be antagonized by nifedipine. In the two patients with those symptoms, serum digoxin concentrations were within the normal range.

In our patients, nifedipine serum concentrations were twice as high as might be expected from single-dose studies (6). As reported previously, nifedipine levels after oral administration vary considerably between patients, which is caused, at least partially, by the existence of slow and rapid metabolizers (10). However, some influence of digoxin, or of the other drugs taken by our patients, on the serum levels of nifedipine cannot be excluded.

It can be concluded from the present study that nifedipine in tablet formulation elevated digoxin levels by ~15%. However, for most patients this interaction probably has no clinical relevance.

Acknowledgment: The authors wish to thank Mrs. H. C. N. Kappelle-de Vries for typing the manuscript and H. Faber for technical assistance. The study was supported in part by a grant from Bayer AG, Wuppertal, F.R.G.

REFERENCES

1. Pedersen KE, Klitgaard NA, Nielsen-Kudsk F. Effect of nifedipine on digoxin kinetics in healthy subjects. *Clin Pharmacol Ther* 1982;32:562–5.
2. Belz GG, Doering W, Munkes R, Matthews J. Interaction between digoxin and calcium antagonists and antiarrythmic drugs. *Clin Pharmacol Ther* 1983;33:410–7.
3. Schwartz JB, Raizner AE, Aker S. The effect of nifedipine on serum digoxin concentrations in patients. *Am Heart J* 1984;107:669–73.
4. Schwartz JB, Migliore PJ. Effect of nifedipine on serum digoxin concentration and renal digoxin clearance. *Clin Pharmacol Ther* 1984;36:19–24.
5. Kuhlmann J. Effects of nifedipine and diltiazem on plasma levels and renal excretion of beta-acetyldigoxin. *Clin Pharmacol Ther* 1985;37:150–6.
6. Kleinbloesem CH, Van Brummelen P, Van de Linde JA, Voogd PJ, Breimer DD. Nifedipine: kinetics and dynamics in healthy subjects. *Clin Pharmacol Ther* 1984;35:742–9.
7. Kleinbloesem CH, Van Harten J, Van Brummelen P, Breimer DD. Liquid chromatographic determination of nifedipine in plasma and of its main metabolite in urine. *J Chromatogr Biomed Appl* 1984;308:209–16.
8. Barr AJ, Goodnight JH, Sall JP, Blair WH, Chilko DH. In: *Statistical analysis system*. Raleigh, North Carolina: SAS Institute, Inc., 1979.
9. Hansen PB, Buch J, Rasmussen OØ, Waldorff S, Steiness E. Influence of atenolol and nifedipine on digoxin-induced inotropism in humans. *Br J Clin Pharmacol* 1984;18:817–22.
10. Kleinbloesem CH, Van Brummelen P, Faber H, Danhof M, Breimer DD. Variability in nifedipine pharmacokinetics and dynamics: a new oxidation polymorphism in man. *Biochem Pharmacol* 1984;33:3721–4.

Therapeutic Drug Monitoring
7:377–386 © 1985 Raven Press, New York

New and Simple Method to Predict Dosage of Drugs Obeying Simple Michaelis-Menten Elimination Kinetics and to Distinguish Such Kinetics from Simple First Order and from Parallel Michaelis-Menten and First Order Kinetics

John G. Wagner

College of Pharmacy and Upjohn Center for Clinical Pharmacology, The University of Michigan Medical Center, Ann Arbor, Michigan, U.S.A.

Summary: It has been found empirically that either average or minimum steady-state plasma concentrations (C_{ss}) of drugs obeying Michaelis-Menten elimination kinetics give essentially linear plots on semilogarithmic graph paper when C_{ss} is plotted versus the maintenance dose *(D)* or dose rate *(R)*. The equations of such straight lines may be converted to the following nonlinear equation: $C_{ss} = ab^D$ which fits the C_{ss},D data essentially as well as $D = V_m C_{ss}/(K_m + C_{ss})$. The parameter *b* is analogous to unity plus the interest fraction in logarithmic growth or compound interest calculations, and each drug appears to have a characteristic value of this parameter, with extremely small intersubject variation. From the above equation the following equation, $D_{n+1} = D_n + \ln(C_{n+1}/C_n)\ln b$ can be derived, which forms the basis of predicting the needed dosage, D_{n+1}, to obtain a desired steady-state concentration, C_{n+1}, using one initial steady-state concentration, C_n, obtained with dose, D_n, and using a population value of *b* for the drug. It appears that it is the value of the "initial capital" (i.e., *a* in relation to the initial dose) rather than the "interest fraction" (i.e., $b - 1$) that causes most of the intersubject variation in C_{ss} of a given drug. Several drugs illustrate the usefulness of the method. A semilogarithmic plot also appears to be an excellent method to distinguish simple Michaelis-Menten kinetics from parallel Michaelis-Menten and first order elimination kinetics and from simple first order kinetics with steady-state data in the range 0.3–3 K_m. **Key Words:** Dose prediction—Michaelis-Menten kinetics—Pharmacokinetics—Plasma levels.

Some simplified methods have been published (1–3) to aid in predicting and adjusting the dosage of drugs that obey linear pharmacokinetics. In 1972, phenytoin was shown to obey Michaelis-Menten elimination kinetics (4). Since that time, various methods have been proposed to estimate the parameters V_m and K_m of the Michaelis-Menten equation—most of them based on linear transformations of the nonlinear Michaelis-Menten equation. Many investigators do not appear to realize that such linear transforms weight the data points in peculiar manners and, because of this, provide biased estimates of the parameters. The approach of several investigators (5–10 has been to publish nomograms to aid in initial dosage and dosage adjustment of phenytoin. However, as pointed out by Grasela et al. (11), the utility of these nomograms is highly dependent on the accuracy of the population pharmacokinetic parameters (i.e., V_m

Address correspondence and reprint requests to Dr. J. G. Wagner at The Upjohn Center for Clinical Pharmacology, The University of Michigan Medical Center, Ann Arbor, MI 48109-1065, U.S.A.

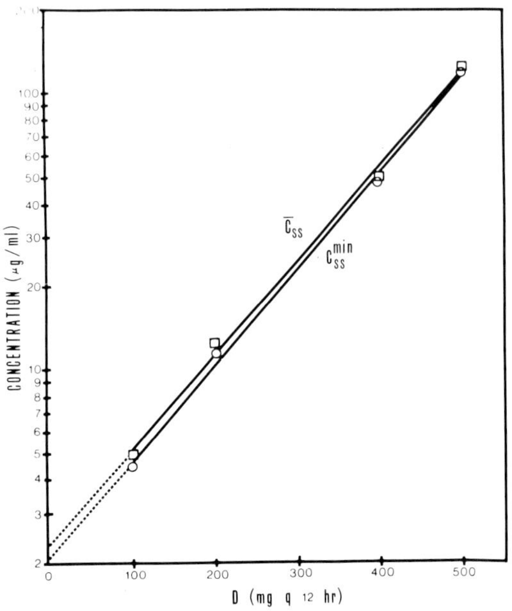

FIG. 1. Data simulated using approximately the average parameters of zonisamide (CI-912) in 10 epileptic patients (17). Lines through points are based on Eq. 2 with parameters given in the text.

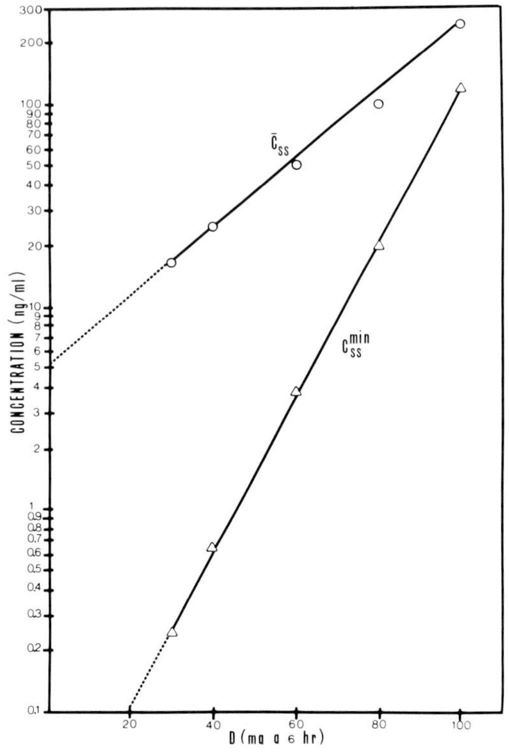

FIG. 2. Data simulated using approximately the average parameters of propranolol in four normal volunteers (18,19). Lines through points are based on Eq. 2 with parameters given in text.

and K_m) used to construct them and the similarity between the study population and the patients for whom the nomogram is to be used. Moreover, optimal adjustment of dosage regimens, based on measured steady-state phenytoin concentrations, requires information regarding the interindividual variability of the parameters (12). More recently, Sheiner and colleagues (11,13,14) have analyzed phenytoin data with the digital computer program NONMEM, which involves both pharmacokinetics and rather complicated statistics.

The author has found that steady-state concentration–maintenance dose data, which obeys the Michaelis-Menten equation, gives linear ascending plots when plotted on simple semilogarithmic graph paper (Fig. 1 and 2). Thus, the C_{ss},D data are described by the simple logarithmic growth or "compound interest" function. This has been pursued via both simulated data and application to four drugs that obey Michaelis-Menten kinetics at steady state, namely, phenytoin, propranolol, nicardipine, and adinazolam.

METHODS

Equations

In the context of this article, the Michaelis-Menten equation is written as

$$D = \frac{V_m C}{K_m + C} \tag{1A}$$

or

$$C = \frac{K_m D}{V_m - D} \tag{1B}$$

The author and colleagues have recently shown (15) that Eqs. 1A and 1B apply to a two-compartment open model as well as the one-compartment open model. In Eqs. 1A and 1B $D = n\tau R =$ the maintenance dose per day where n is the number of dosage intervals per day, τ is the dosage interval, and R is the dose rate per hour; or $D = R\tau$ (i.e., amount per dosage interval), V_m is the maximal velocity of metabolism with same dimensions as D, K_m is the Michaelis constant, and C is the steady-state concentration (either the average steady-state concentration, symbolized by $\bar{C}_{ss}$, or the minimum steady-state concentration, symbolized by C_{ss}^{min}).

If the C,D data are linear on semilogarithmic graph paper, then one can apply linear least squares regression with the equation:

$$\ln C = I + SD \tag{2}$$

where ln C is the ordinate or y value, D is the abscissa or x value, I is the intercept of the line corresponding to $D = 0$, and S is the slope of the line.

Based on Eq. 2 we may also write

$$C = ab^D \tag{3}$$

where $a = e^I$ and $b = e^S$ (with e being the base of natural logarithms). Hence this investigation has indicated that Eq. 3 fits the same data as well as, or nearly as well as, Eq. 1A or 1B, and, in certain instances, the fit is better.

If a ratio is made of two equations like Eq. 3, with C_n corresponding to dose D_n, and C_{n+1} corresponding to D_{n+1}, with the parameters a and b remaining constant, then a cancels out and the following equation is obtained:

$$\frac{C_{n+1}}{C_n} = \frac{b^{D_{n+1}}}{b^{D_n}} \tag{4}$$

$$C_{ss} = \frac{1}{2k_e}\left[\left(\frac{R}{V} - \frac{V_m}{V} - k_e K_m\right) + \sqrt{\left(\frac{R}{V} - \frac{V_m}{V} - k_e K_m\right)^2 + 4k_e \frac{R}{V} K_m}\right] \tag{10}$$

Taking natural logarithms of both sides of Eq. 4 and rearranging one term yields:

$$\ln C_{n+1} = \ln C_n + \ln b(D_{n+1} - D_n) \tag{5}$$

Solving for D_{n+1} in Eq. 5 gives

$$D_{n+1} = D_n + \frac{\ln(C_{n+1}/C_n)}{\ln b} \tag{6}$$

Hence, Eq. 6 provides a method of estimating the dose, D_{n+1}, necessary to give a desired steady-state concentration C_{n+1} if one knows a single steady-state concentration C_n corresponding to the maintenance dose D_n and if a population value of b is used. It turns out that the parameter b has very small intersubject variation, unlike the relatively large intersubject variation of both V_m and K_m of Eqs. 1A and 1B.

The coefficients of determination (r^2) reported in this article were estimated as follows

$$r^2 = 1 - \frac{\Sigma dev^2}{Sy^2} \tag{7}$$

where dev is the difference between the model-predicted and observed values of the y (i.e., ordinate values) and Sy^2 is the corrected sum of squares of the Y values (i.e., $Sy^2 = \Sigma y^2 - (\Sigma y)^2/N$). In comparing r^2 values it is important that like things be compared—i.e., when the ordinates are the same, but the functions fitting the data differ.

The minimum steady-state concentrations for the simulations were obtained as follows (16):

$$C_{ss}^{min} = \frac{D}{V_d}\left[\frac{1}{e^Q - 1}\right] \tag{8}$$

$$Q = \frac{V_m \tau - D}{V_d K_m} \tag{9}$$

The average steady-state concentrations for the simulations were obtained with Eq. 1B.

For the one-compartment open model with parallel Michaelis-Menten and first order elimination kinetics, steady-state concentrations were calculated by use of Eq. 10 (16),

where R is the zero order input rate and k_e is the first order rate constant for the parallel path.

Simulations

Two sets of C_{ss}^{min} and $\overline{C}_{ss}$ values were simulated using Eqs. 1B, 8, and 9. The first set were generated using parameter values very close to the mean parameter value of zonisamide or CI-912 (17), namely $V_m = 600$ mg/12 h, $K_m = 25$ μg/ml, $V_d = 100$ L, $\tau = 12$ h, and $D = 100$, 200, 400, and 500 mg/12 h. Equations 8 and 9 gave the circle points in Fig. 1, while Eq. 1B gave the squares in Fig. 1.

The second set of C_{ss}^{min} and $\overline{C}_{ss}$ values were simulated using parameter values very close to the mean parameter values of propranolol, reported by Wagner (18) and calculated from the data of Silber et al. (19), namely, $V_m = 120$ mg every 6 h, $K_m = 0.05$ mg/L, $V_d = 300$ L, $\tau = 6$ h, and $D = 30$, 40, 60, 80, and 100 mg every 6 h. Equation 1B gave the circle points in Fig. 2, while Eqs. 8 and 9 gave the diamonds in Fig. 2.

An example of data simulated with Eq. 10 employed the parameters $V_m = 600$ mg every 12 h, $V_m/V_d = 200$ mg/(L × h), $K_m = 25$ μg/ml, $V_d = 100$ L, $k_e = 0.004$ h^{-1} (which is 20% of $k_{el} = V_m/VK_m = 0.02$ h^{-1}), $\tau = 12$ h, and $R = 100$, 200, 400, and 500 mg every 12 h.

Wilkinson's method (20) was used to fit data to Eq. 1A. The author has shown that this method gives

TABLE 1. *Fitting of phenytoin data of Murphy et al. (20) to the logarithmic growth function and the Michaelis-Menten equation and comparison of coefficients of determination* (D *in mg phenytoin sodium per day*)

Subject No.		$\ln C_{ss} = I + SD$ (Eq. 2) Slope (S) (SE slope)	Intercept (I) (SE intercept)	r^2	$C_{ss} = ab^D$ (Eq. 3) $a = e^I$	$b = e^S$	r^2	$D = \frac{V_m C_{ss}}{K_m + C_{ss}}$ (Eq. 1A) V_m (mg/day)	K_m (μg/ml)	r^2	$C_{ss} = \frac{K_m D}{V_m - D}$ (Eq. 1B) r^2
1	5	0.005521	0.1008	0.975	1.106	1.00554	0.969	745	8.72	0.975	0.969
		(0.000510)	(0.151)					(98.5)	(2.04)		
2	3	0.009349	−2.2771	0.950	0.103	1.00939	0.957	688	4.21	0.975	0.983
		(0.00215)	(1.186)					(27.2)	(0.828)		
3	3	0.005306	−1.0944	0.901	0.305	1.00532	0.915	806	2.86	0.911	0.939
		(0.00175)	(0.968)					(112)	(1.25)		
4	3	0.008550	−1.0671	0.951	0.344	1.00859	0.913	496	2.82	0.929	0.751
		(0.00195)	(0.608)					(94.2)	(1.56)		
7	3	0.005570	0.4821	0.913	1.619	1.00558	0.921	691	11.0	0.945	0.891
		(0.00172)	(0.638)					(190)	(6.70)		
8	3	0.01068	0.1530	0.957	1.165	1.01074	0.969	397	9.67	0.939	0.940
		(0.00227)	(0.561)					(60.1)	(3.97)		
9	4	0.006550	−0.1133	0.943	0.893	1.00657	0.896	630	7.13	0.945	0.893
		(0.00113)	(0.364)					(131)	(3.14)		
11	3	0.01154	−1.6404	0.990	0.194	1.01161	0.990	473	3.66	0.9995	0.993
		(0.00117)	(0.412)					(3.52)	(0.107)		
12	3	0.007147	−0.4869	0.997	0.615	1.00717	0.994	628	5.80	1.000	1.000
		(0.000360)	(0.153)					(1.01)	(0.0303)		
13	3	0.007487	0.08340	0.990	1.087	1.007515	0.990	568	9.20	0.994	0.995
		(0.000756)	(0.266)					(26.4)	(1.14)		
Mean		0.00777	−0.5860	0.957	0.746	1.0078025	0.951	612	6.51	0.961	0.936
CV (%)		28.4	154.0	3.4	67.3	2.2	3.9	21.0	46.8	3.3	8.0
Pooled data of 10 subjects											
	33	0.002807	1.2013	0.244	3.324	1.00281	—	474[a]	2.28	—	—
		(0.000887)	(0.341)					(41.5)	(0.787)		

[a] Very poor estimate, since in 8 of 10 subjects the individual subject V_m values are larger than this value of 474, and 7 of 33 of the D values exceed this V_m value.

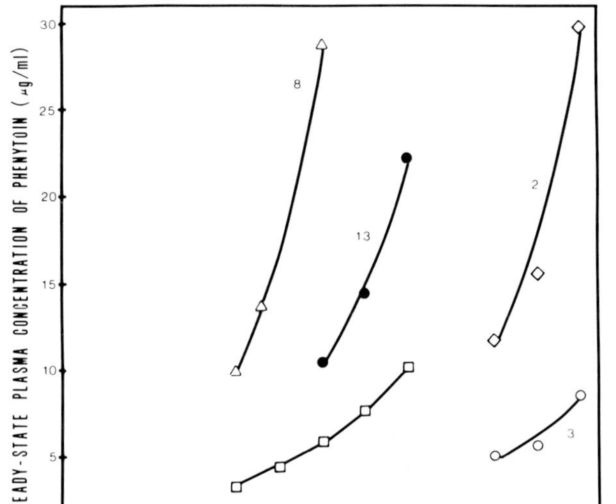

FIG. 3. Representative plots of the phenytoin data of Murphy et al. (21). Lines through points are based on Eq. 3 with parameters given in Table 1 for the subjects indicated by the numbers on the curves.

essentially identical estimates and errors of the parameters as nonlinear least squares. An r^2 value for each fit was obtained with $y = D$ (see Eq. 1B and text), then the same parameter values were used in Eq. 1B and a new r^2 value calculated with $y = C$.

Linear least squares regression was used to fit data to Eq. 2. An r^2 value was calculated with $y = \ln C$. Then the parameters I and S were converted to a and b, respectively, as indicated in the text following Eq. 3, and another r^2 value was calculated using $y = C$.

Fitting of Real Data

Estimates of the dose D_{n+1} needed to produce a steady-state concentration C_{n+1} using the initial concentration C_n obtained with dose D_n and a population value of b were made with Eq. 6.

Individual subject phenytoin data of Murphy et al. (21), where three to five steady-state concentrations were measured, were fitted to both 1A and 2. Similar fittings were performed with the propranolol C_{ss} values reported by Wagner (18) and calculated from the data of Silber et al. (19); for each of four subjects, average steady-state concentrations were measured for multiple doses of 40, 80, 160, 240, and 320 mg/day. Similar fittings were performed with three subjects' adinazolam C_{ss}^{min} values following multiple oral doses of 1, 2, and 3 mg of adinazolam mesylate administered hourly for 12 h after loading doses (unpublished observations). In this case D was the 12-h dose given at a constant rate. Calculations were also made on unpublished data on nicardipine in humans.

RESULTS

Simulations

The least squares line (Eq. 2) drawn through the $\bar{C}_{ss}$ squares in Fig. 1 has an I = 0.8717 (SE = 0.107), S = 0.007824 (SE = 0.000316), and r^2 = 0.997. Conversion to Eq. 3 gave a = 2.391 and b = 1.00785 with r^2 = 0.994. The least squares line (Eq. 2) drawn through the C_{ss}^{min} circles in Fig. 1 has an I = 0.7505 (SE = 0.107) and S = 0.008026 (SE = 0.00035) with r^2 = 0.997. Conversion to Eq. 3 gave a = 2.118 and b = 1.00806 with r^2 = 0.994. The two lines in Fig. 1 are close together since there is little difference between peaks and nadirs as a result of the long limiting elimination half-life, $t_{1/2} = 0.693V_dK_m/V_m$ = 34.15 h.

Fitting of the C_{ss}^{min} data of Fig. 1 to Eq. 1A gave V_m = 591 (SE = 3.12) and K_m = 22.58 (SE = 0.373) with r^2 = 0.99993. Conversion to Eq. 1B gave r^2 = 0.997.

The least squares line (Eq. 2) drawn through the $\bar{C}_{ss}$ circle points in Fig. 2 has an I = 1.6695 (SE = 0.0831), S = 0.03878 (SE = 0.00124) with r^2 = 0.997. Conversion to Eq. 3 gave a = 5.3095 and b = 1.03854 with r^2 = 0.989. The least squares line drawn through the C_{ss}^{min} diamonds in Fig. 2 has I = − 3.9737 (SE = 0.0543) and S = 0.08752 with r^2 = 0.9998. Conversion to Eq. 3 gave a = 0.0188 and b = 1.0915 with r^2 = 0.99994.

Fitting of the C_{ss}^{min} data of Fig. 2 to Eq. 1A gave V_m = 87.76 (SE = 8.23) and K_m = 0.770 (SE = 0.319) with r^2 = 0.872. In this case, the logarithmic growth equation gave a considerably better fit than the Michaelis-Menten equation. Application of Wilkinson's method (20) to the $\bar{C}_{ss}$ data of Fig. 2 gave the original parameter values exactly. The two lines in Fig. 2 are quite far apart, since the peak-nadir difference in this case is large as a result of the short limiting $t_{1/2}$ of 0.52 h in relation to the dosage interval of 6 h.

Fitting of Real Data

Table 1 gives the results of fitting the phenytoin data of Murphy et al. (21). It should be noted that the parameter b of Eq. 3 has a coefficient of variation of only 2.2%, which is quite remarkable for phar-

TABLE 2. *Estimation of maintenance dose per day of phenytoin sodium needed to produce a steady-state concentration of phenytoin of 10 μg/ml using a population value of the parameter* b *and one measured phenytoin concentration and comparison of the estimate with dose predicted using all the data for each subject (used* b = *1.0078025 and ln* b = *0.007772)*

Subject	D_n (mg/day)	C_n (μg/ml)	$D_{n+1} = D_n + \frac{\ln[10/C_n]}{0.00777}$	Predicted D_{n+1} values using all data: $\frac{10\,V_m}{K_m + 10}$	Predicted D_{n+1} values using all data: $\frac{\ln 10 - I}{S}$	% deviation: Col. 4 vs. Col. 5	% deviation: Col. 4 vs. Col. 6
1	200	3.2	347	398	399	− 12.8	− 13.0
2	500	11.7	500	484	490	3.3	2.04
3	500	5.0	589	627	640	− 6.06	− 7.97
4	200	1.7	428	387	394	10.6	8.63
7	300	7.8	332	329	327	0.91	1.53
8	200	9.0	214	202	201	5.94	6.47
9	200	3.0	355	368	369	− 3.53	− 3.79
11	300	6.4	357	346	342	3.18	4.39
12	300	5.3	382	397	390	− 3.78	− 2.05
13	300	10.5	294	296	296	− 0.68	− 0.68
Mean			380[a,b]	383[a]	385[b]	5.1[c]	5.1[c]
CV (%)			27.7	29.5	30.4	—	—

Col., columns of this table.
[a]Paired t test = 0.42 ($p > 0.25$).
[b]Paired t test = 0.57 ($p > 0.25$).
[c]Mean absolute (sign ignored) deviation.

macokinetic analysis. The coefficients of determination that should be compared are those in columns 8 and 12 of Table 1 since the y value, namely C_{ss}, was the same in calculation of these two values. The comparison shows nearly identical mean r^2 values of 0.951 and 0.961 for Eq. 3 and 1B, respectively; in five of the 10 subjects, the r^2 value for Eq. 3 is either equal to or greater than that for Eq. 1B. Note the footnote to Table 1, which indicates that pooling the data of the 10 subjects gives a poor result for a population V_m of Eq. 1A and that pooling gave an r^2 value of only 0.244 when Eq. 2 was employed. In this case, mean parameter values are much better population values obtained by pooling data of different subjects.

Figure 3 shows representative plots of five of the 10 subjects of Murphy et al. (19) showing the measured phenytoin steady-state concentrations fitted with Eq. 3 using the parameters a and b given in Table 1.

Table 2 shows applications of Eq. 6 to predict the maintenance dose of phenytoin sodium needed to produce a steady-state concentration of 10 μg/ml using the first measured steady-state concentration C_n corresponding to dose D_n and the population value of b taken as the mean of the b values in Table 1. The predicted values have a mean absolute deviation of 5.1% when compared with predicted doses based on all the data for each subject. Thus, the average error is of the same order of magnitude as the assay error.

Table 3 gives results of fitting the propranolol data (18,19). Again, it is the r^2 values in columns 8 and 12 of Table 3 that should be compared, since the y value, namely $\overline{C}_{ss}$, was the same in the calculation of these two values. Again, the mean of 0.984 in column 8 does not differ significantly from the mean of 0.993 in column 2. In this case, the pooled data (N = 20) for the four subjects gave S and I values essentially the same as the corresponding mean parameter values, and the b value from the pooled data is the same as the mean b value. Figure 4 shows the plots based on Eq. 2 for the four individual subjects. Table 4 shows applications of Eq. 6 to predict the maintenance dose of propranolol needed to produce a steady-state plasma concentration of 50 ng/ml using the C_n corresponding to D_n = 40 mg/day and using the population value of b = 1.0105, which is the mean of the four b values in Table 3. The predicted values have a mean absolute deviation of 12.3 and 13.4% when compared with estimates of the needed dose using Eq. 1A and 2 for all the data for each subject. These deviations are higher than those obtained for phenytoin (Table 2) but still are respectable for therapeutic drug monitoring.

TABLE 3. *Fitting of propranolol data of Silber et al. (18) to the logarithmic growth function and the Michaelis-Menten equation and comparison of coefficients of determination (D in mg propranolol per day); data are plotted in Fig. 4*

		$\ln \overline{C}_{ss} = I + SD$ (Eq. 2)			$\overline{C}_{ss} = ab^D$ (Eq. 3)			$D = \frac{V_m \overline{C}_{ss}}{K_m + \overline{C}_{ss}}$ (Eq. 1A)			$C_{ss} = \frac{K_m D}{V_m - D}$ (Eq. 1B)
Subject	No.	S (SE of S)	I (SE of I)	r^2	$a = e^I$	$b = e^S$	r^2	V_m (SE of V_m) (mg/day)	K_m (SE of K_m) (μg/ml)	r^2	r^2
A	5	0.01243	1.3123	0.997	3.718	1.0125	0.988	377	37.7	0.993	0.999
		(0.000517)	(0.102)					(17.4)	(4.69)		
B	5	0.01164	0.8520	0.950	2.344	1.0117	0.973	437	31.7	0.989	0.997
		(0.00154)	(0.303)					(33.4)	(5.31)		
C	5	0.009529	1.6916	0.969	5.428	1.00957	0.990	518	64.6	0.988	0.985
		(0.000980)	(0.193)					(54.4)	(12.6)		
D	5	0.008246	1.8545	0.974	6.389	1.00828	0.983	684	90.8	0.987	0.992
		(0.000782)	(0.154)					(104)	(20.1)		
Mean concentration	5	0.01051	1.4635	0.985	4.321	1.0106	0.998	446	46.5	0.968	0.994
		(0.000736)	(0.145)					(29.3)	(6.63)		
Mean of 4 subjects		0.01046	1.4276	0.972	4.470	1.0103	0.984[a]	504	56.2	0.989	0.993[a]
CV (%)		18.3	31.2	—	40.2	2.1	0.8	26.4	48.3	—	0.6
Pooled data of 4 subjects		0.01046	1.4275	0.954	4.168	1.0105	0.749	431	41.14	0.998	0.856
								(25.6)	(4.92)		

[a] Paired t test = 1.64 ($p < 0.10$).

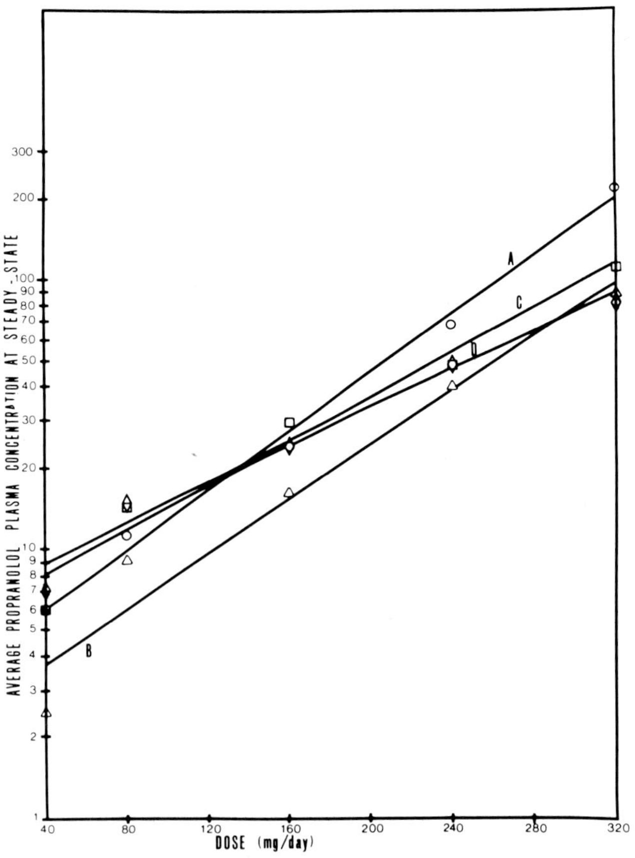

FIG. 4. Semilogarithmic plots of propranolol data of Silber et al. (19), calculated by Wagner (18), in conformity with Eq. 2. See Table 3 for parameters (slopes and intercepts) of the lines drawn through the points.

Table 5 gives results, in the same format as used in Tables 1 and 3 and plotted in Fig. 5, for adinazolam administered hourly at three dose rates (1, 2, and 3 mg/h) for 12 h after initial loading doses. The dose in this case was the amount ingested in 12 h at a constant rate, namely, 12, 24, and 36 mg of adinazolam mesylate.

Parallel Michaelis-Menten and First Order Kinetics

The salicylate data of Günsberg et al. (22) and the theophylline data of Massey et al. (23) gave plots on semilogarithmic graph paper that were initially markedly curved, but the terminal data became linear. In an attempt to explain these observations, steady-state data were simulated with the appropriate Eq. 12 (16). A rectilinear plot of these data is shown inset in Fig. 6. Wilkinson's method applied to these $C_{ss}, R_0/V$ data gave an excellent fit with V_m = 6.572 mg every 12 h (SE = 0.0488), K_m = 27.73 μg/ml (SE = 0.482) and r^2 = 0.99985. The line drawn through the inset points is based on Eq. 1B with these parameter values and r^2 = 0.9975. Hence, the parallel Michaelis-Menten and first order paths pool to give a pooled V_m and a pooled K_m, which were not the same as the original parameter values. Such pooling was discussed previously by Wagner (24). Hence, with the rectilinear plot simple Michaelis-Menten kinetics could not be distinguished from parallel Michaelis-Menten and first order elimination kinetics. However, plotting of the same $C_{ss}, R_0/V$ data on semilogarithmic paper gave an initially curved plot, which became linear for terminal data as shown in Fig. 6. Thus, the semilogarithmic plot apparently is more useful in discriminating between simple Michaelis-Menten kinetics and parallel Michaelis-Menten and first order kinetics than a rec-

TABLE 4. *Estimation of maintenance dose per day of propranolol needed to produce an average plasma concentration of 50 μg/ml using a population value of the* b *and one measured average plasma concentration of propranolol corresponding to a dose of 40 mg/day and comparison of the estimate with the dose predicted using all the data for each subject (used* b = *1.0105 and ln* b = *0.010455)*

Subject	D_n (mg/day)	C_n (ng/ml)	$D_{n+1} = D_n + \dfrac{\ln[50/C_n]}{0.010445}$	Predicted D_{n+1} values using all the data: $\dfrac{50\ V_m}{K_m + 50}$	Predicted D_{n+1} values using all the data: $\dfrac{\ln 50 - I}{S}$	% deviation: Col. 4 vs. Col. 5	% deviation: Col. 4 vs. Col. 6
A	40	6.05	242	215	209	12.6	15.8
B	40	2.47	328	267	263	22.8	24.7
C	40	6.16	240	226	233	6.19	3.0
D	40	7.21	225	243	250	−7.41	−10.0
Mean			259	238	239	12.3[a]	13.4[a]
CV (%)			18.1	9.5	9.8	—	—

Col., columns of this table.
[a]Mean absolute deviations.

TABLE 5. *Fitting of mean steady-state minimum plasma concentration of adinazolam for three normal volunteers to the logarithmic growth equation and the Michaelis-Menten equation and comparison of the coefficients of determination; data are plotted in Fig. 5*

	$\ln C_{ss}^{min} = I + SD$ (Eq. 2)			$C_{ss}^{min} = ab^D$ (Eq. 3)			$D = \frac{V_m C_{ss}^{min}}{K_m + C_{ss}^{min}}$ (Eq. 1A)			$C_{ss}^{min} = \frac{K_m D}{V_m - D}$ (Eq. 1B)
Subject	S (SE of S)	I (SE of I)	r^2	$a = e^I$	$b = e^S$	r^2	V_m (SE of V_m) (mg/12h)	K_m (SE of K_m) (μM)	r^2	r^2
3	0.06891 (0.000252)	2.5400 (0.0654)	0.999	12.680	1.07134	0.999	62.28 (8.77)	110 (28.8)	0.991	0.996
5	0.05088 (0.00133)	3.1829 (0.0346)	0.999	24.117	1.05220	0.999	139 (57.2)	419 (206)	0.991	0.992
6	0.05182 (0.00164)	3.2874 (0.0425)	0.999	26.773	1.05319	0.999	131 (47.7)	443 (199)	0.992	0.993
Mean	0.05720	3.0034	0.999	21.190	1.0589	0.999	111	324	0.991	0.994
CV (%)	17.7	13.5	—	35.3	1.0	—	38.0	57.3	—	—

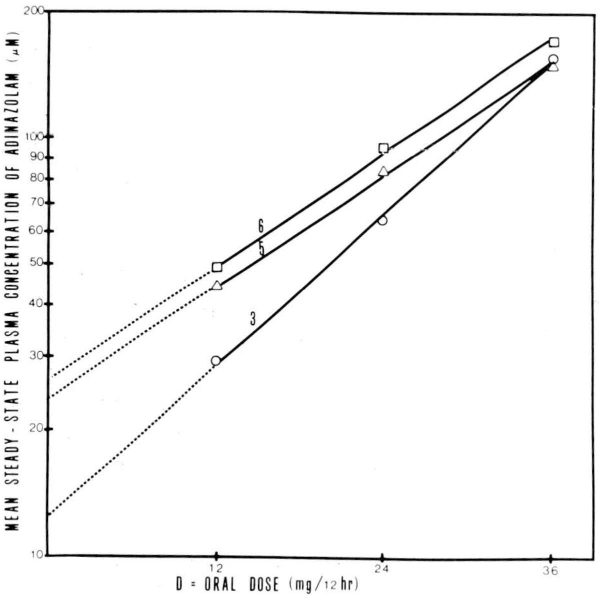

FIG. 5. Semilogarithmic plots of adinazolam data for three subjects (3, 5, and 6). Lines through points are based on Eq. 2. See Table 5 for parameters of the lines drawn through the points.

tilinear plot of the steady-state concentration versus the zero order input rate.

First Order Kinetics

The semilogarithmic plot distinguishes Michaelis-Menten kinetics not only from parallel Michaelis-Menten and first order kinetics, but also from simple first order kinetics. The triangles in Fig. 6 give an example of first order kinetics where the clearance is 0.1; hence, the equation for these points was $C_{ss} = 10\ R_0/V_d$. These points form a continuous curving line on the semilogarithmic graph paper. Hence, this distinguishes the first order kinetics from parallel first order and Michaelis-Menten kinetics (the circles in Fig. 6), where there is curvature, at first, which later becomes a straight line, and simple Michaelis-Menten kinetics where the plot is entirely linear (Fig. 1, 2, 4, and 5).

Accumulation Percentages

The value of 100(b − 1) is the accumulation percentage and is analogous to the compound interest percentage of logarithmic growth. It appears that each drug obeying Michaelis-Menten elimination kinetics has its own characteristic population values of the accumulation percentage, which has low intersubject variability. Accumulation percentages for four drugs in normal volunteers are given in Table 6.

DISCUSSION

The utilities of semilogarithmic plots of steady-state drug concentrations versus corresponding maintenance doses have been shown (a) to distinguish simple Michaelis-Menten kinetics from parallel Michaelis-Menten and first order kinetics and from simple first order kinetics, (b) to predict steady-state concentrations as a function of maintenance dose, and (c) to make predictions of the maintenance dose of a specific drug needed to produce a desired steady-state drug concentration. With respect to (a), simple Michaelis-Menten kinetics is characterized by the semilogarithmic C_{ss} versus D plot being essentially linear throughout the whole dose range, while parallel Michaelis-Menten and first order kinetics are characterized by

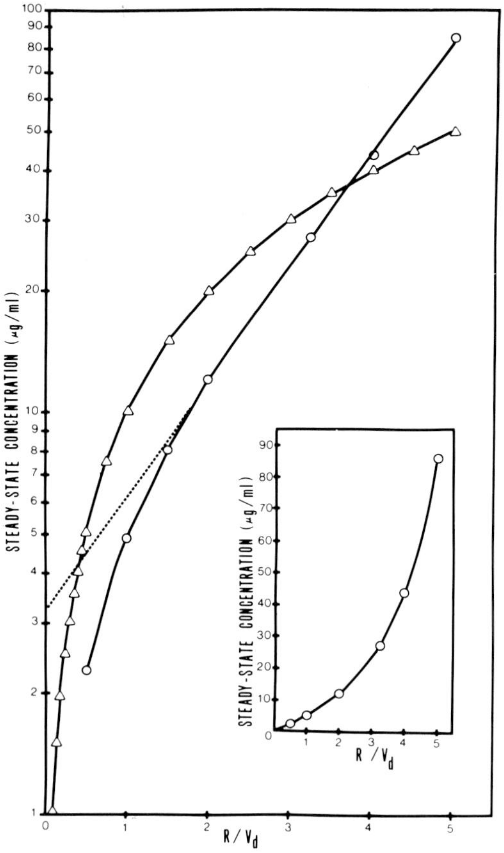

FIG. 6. The circles resulted from a simulation of parallel Michaelis-Menten and first order kinetics—which on the main semilogarithmic plot gave an initially curved line, that later became linear; inset are the same data plotted on rectilinear graph paper, and the fitted line is based on the equation: $C_{ss} = 27.73\ R/V_d\ (6.57 - R/V_d)$, which indicates, falsely, simple Michaelis-Menten kinetics. The diamonds resulted from a simulation of first order kinetics with equation: $C_{ss} = 10\ R/V_d$, and the trend line is continuously curving over the whole range of R/V_d values.

an initial curved C_{ss} versus D plot at low doses, which becomes linear for terminal C_{ss},D data. Simple first order kinetics give a continuously curving line on semilogarithmic graph paper. The above holds only in the range of concentration 0.3–3 K_m.

With respect to (b), it should be carefully noted that this author does not recommend estimating the S of the semilogarithmic C_{ss},D plot from the first two measured $\overline{C}_{ss}$ or C_{ss}^{min} values using a rearrangement of Eq. 5, namely $\ln b = \ln(C_{n+1}/C_n/(D_{n+1} - D_n)$. As can be seen from the $\overline{C}_{ss}$ data in Fig. 2 and all data in Fig. 4, such a method would lead to very large errors in the S values. Rather, the author recommends that the S and corresponding b parameter values be determined for each drug from a study population of patients for whom predictions are to be made, as recommended by Grasela et al. (11) and Vozeh et al. (12). Suppose that such a population value of b has been determined and the first steady-state drug concentration C_n corresponding to maintenance dose D_n has been measured. Then substitution can be made into Eq. 5 to calculate another concentration C_{n+1} corresponding to a second maintenance dose D_{n+1}; and then by joining the points on semilogarithmic graph paper and extrapolating, the estimating line can be produced, which will have the appropriate S = ln b.

With respect to (c), predictions based on Eq. 6, when applied to the phenytoin data of Murphy et al. (21), had a mean absolute error of 5.1%; whereas when those predictions were applied to the propranolol data of Silber et al. (19), the mean absolute error was 12–13% of that based on use of all the data. Thus the use of a population value of the parameter b and one measured steady-state concentration allows the prediction of a dose needed to produce a desired steady-state concentration with satisfactory error for therapeutic drug monitoring.

There is another advantage of the semilogarithmic plots of data obeying simple Michaelis-Menten kinetics. The coefficients of variation of the parameters a and b in Tables 1, 3, and 5 indicate that intersubject variation of a is much greater than variation of b. The parameter a is analogous to the "initial capital" of the compound interest function, while the parameter b is analogous to the sum of unity and the "interest fraction." In pharmacokinetics, the value of a would be determined by the fraction of the dose reaching the circulation, the dose, the dosage interval, and the clearance. The parameter b would be expected to be related to the clearance, dose, and dosage interval, although future studies may modify these "guesses." Hence, this study suggests that the parameter a in relation to the initial dose contributes considerably more than the parameter b to the variability of C_{ss} in relation to the dose rate from subject to subject. Such concepts are not evident from the parameters V_m and K_m of the Michaelis-Menten equation. Hence, the semilogarithmic plots have revealed insights not apparent from simple Michaelis-Menten kinetics per se.

A word of caution is necessary. The linearity of such semilogarithmic plots holds only in the range of concentration 0.3–3 K_m. As can be seen from the examples, this is frequently the range of observations seen with therapeutic drug monitoring. The semilogarithmic plots exhibit marked curvature when the concentrations are $<0.3\ K_m$ or $>3\ K_m$. This range of concentrations correspond to a dose rate range 25–

TABLE 6. *Accumulation percentages[a] per milligram of maintenance dose per day*

Phenytoin[b]		Propranolol		Nicardipine[c]		Adinazolam[d]	
Subject	Accumulation %	Subject	Accumulation %	Subject	Accumulation %	Subject	Accumulation %
1	0.554	A	1.25	1	2.65	1	7.13
2	0.939	B	1.17	2	2.71	2	5.22
3	0.532	C	0.957	3	2.81	3	5.32
4	0.859	D	0.828	4	2.06		
7	0.558			5	3.36		
8	1.074			6	2.78		
9	0.657						
11	1.161						
12	0.717						
13	0.752						
Mean	0.780		1.05		2.73		5.89
CV (%)	28.5		18.4		15.2		18.3

[a] Accumulation percentage = 100 (b − 1).
[b] Based on data of Murphy et al. (21), where plasma concentrations were measured at variable times after dosing at steady-state.
[c] Based on $\bar{C}_{ss}$ with dosing every 8 h (unpublished data).
[d] Maintenance dose was that per 12 h rather than per day as for the other three drugs.

75% of V_m. Hence the situation is analogous to log dose–response plots in pharmacology.

REFERENCES

1. Koup JR, Sack CM, Smith AL, Gibaldi M. Hypothesis for the individualization of drug dosage. *Clin Pharmacokinet* 1979;4:460–9.
2. Slattery JT, Gibaldi M, Koup JR. Prediction of maintenance dose required to attain a desired drug concentration at steady-state from a single determination of concentration after an initial dose. *Clin Pharmacokinet* 1980;5:377–85.
3. Koup JR, Sack CM, Smith AL, Neely NN, Gibaldi M. Rapid estimation of chloramphenicol clearance in infants and children. *Clin Pharmacokinet* 1981;6:83–8.
4. Gerber N, Wagner JG. Explanation of dose-dependent decline of diphenylhydantoin plasma levels by fitting to the integrated form of the Michaelis-Menten equation. *Res Commun Chem Pathol Pharmacol* 1972;3:455–66.
5. Richens A, Dunlop A. Serum phenytoin levels in management of epilepsy. *Lancet* 1975;2:247–8.
6. Ludden TM, Allen JP, Valutsky WA, et al. Individualization of phenytoin dosage regimens. *Clin Pharmacol Ther* 1977;21:287–93.
7. Martin E, Tozer TN, Sheiner LB, Riegelman S. The clinical pharmacokinetics of phenytoin. *J Pharmacokinet Biopharm* 1977;5:579–95.
8. Mullen PW. Optimal phenytoin therapy: a new technique for individualizing dosage. *Clin Pharmacol Ther* 1978;23:228–32.
9. Chiba K, Ishizaki T, Miora H, Minagawa K. Michaelis-Menten pharmacokinetics and diphenylhydantoin and application in the pediatric age patient. *J Pediatr* 1980;96:479–84.
10. Rambeck B, Boenigk HE, Dunlop A, Mullen PW, Wadsworth J, Richens A. Predicting phenytoin dose—a revised nomogram. *Ther Drug Monit* 1979;1:325–33.
11. Grasela TH, Sheiner LB, Rambeck B, et al. Steady-state pharmacokinetics of phenytoin from routinely collected patient data. *Clin Pharmacokinet* 1983;8:355–64.
12. Vozeh S, Muir KT, Sheiner LB, Follath F. Predicting individual phenytoin dosage. *J Pharmacokinet Biopharm* 1981;9:131–47.
13. Sheiner LB, Rosenberg B, Marathe VV. Estimation of population characteristics of pharmacokinetic parameters from routine clinical data. *J Pharmacokinet Biopharm* 1977;5:445–79.
14. Sheiner LB, Beal SL. Evaluation of methods for estimating population pharmacokinetics parameters. I. Michaelis-Menten model: routine clinical pharmacokinetic data. *J Pharmacokinet Biopharm* 1980;8:553–71.
15. Wagner JG, Szpunar GJ, Ferry JJ. Commentary: exact mathematical equivalence of the venous equilibration ("well-stirred") model, the sinusoidal perfusion ("parallel-tube") model, and a specific two-compartment open model. *Drug Metab Dispos* 1984;12:385–8.
16. Wagner JG, Szpunar GJ, Ferry JJ. Michaelis-Menten elimination kinetics: areas under curves, steady-state concentrations and clearances for compartment models with different types of input. *Biopharm Drug Dispos* 1985;6:177–200.
17. Wagner JG, Sackellares JC, Donofrio PD, Berent S, Sakmar E. Nonlinear pharmacokinetics of CI-912 in adult epileptic patients. *Ther Drug Monit* 1984;6:277–83.
18. Wagner JG. Propranolol: pooled Michaelis-Menten parameters and the effect of input rate on bioavailability. *Clin Pharmacol Ther* 1985;37:481–7.
19. Silber BM, Holford NHG, Riegelman S. Dose-dependent elimination of propranolol and its major metabolites in humans. *J Pharm Sci* 1983;72:725–32.
20. Wilkinson GN. Statistical estimation in enzyme kinetics. *Biochem J* 1961;80:324–32.
21. Murphy JE, Bruni J, Stewart RB. Clinical utility of six methods of predicting phenytoin doses and plasma concentrations. *Am J Hosp Pharm* 1981;38:348–54.
22. Günsberg M, Bochner F, Graham G, Imhoff D, Passons G, Cham B. Disposition of and clinical response to salicylates in patients with rheumatoid disease. *Clin Pharmacol Ther* 1984;35:585–93.
23. Massey KL, Gotz VP, Russell WL. Dose-dependent kinetics of theophylline in adults with pulmonary disease. *Ther Drug Monit* 1984;6:284–9.
24. Wagner JG. *Fundamentals of clinical pharmacokinetics*. Hamilton, Illinois: Drug Intelligence Publications, Inc., 1975: 265–7.

Therapeutic Drug Monitoring
7:387–390 © 1985 Raven Press, New York

Serum Concentrations of Valproic Acid: Influence of Dose and Comedication

T. May and B. Rambeck

Department of Biochemistry, Gesellschaft für Epilepsieforschung, Bielefeld-Bethel, F.R.G.

Summary: The influence of valproate (VPA) dose, VPA preparation used, comedication (phenobarbital, phenytoin, carbamazepine) and factors such as age, weight, height, and sex on the concentration of VPA in serum was investigated. Nonlinear regression analysis showed that about 63% of the variance in the VPA morning concentrations of 259 inpatients could be explained by the following variables: dose, body weight, sex, and comedication. Age, height, and kind of preparation had no important influence on the VPA concentration. The relationship between dose and concentration of VPA is nonlinear, as the concentration does not increase proportionally with the dose but increases to a lesser extent. The serum concentration of VPA is clearly lower when the drug is given in combination with phenytoin (49.5%), carbamazepine (66.2%), or phenobarbital (76.3%) than when given alone (100%). **Key Words:** Valproic acid—Drug interactions.

Valproic acid (VPA) is an important anticonvulsant drug with a broad spectrum of activity against severe seizure disorders (1,2). Specification of a therapeutic range for VPA is more difficult than for other antiepileptic drugs, but some studies (3) suggest that the best therapeutic effect will be achieved within a concentration range of 40–100 μg/ml.

Several studies (4–7) have shown that other antiepileptic drugs may decrease VPA concentrations in serum. This effect is clinically relevant insofar as successful treatment with VPA may sometimes be achieved only after discontinuing comedication (5,8). The number of patients in most of these studies was small, however, and the relative effects of different, simultaneously given drugs could not be specified. Likewise, investigations of the relationship between dose and concentration of VPA have given contradictory results (9–12).

Address correspondence and reprint requests to Dr. B. Rambeck at Biochemisches Labor, der Gesellschaft für Epilepsieforschung, Maraweg 13, D-4800 Bielefeld 13, F.R.G.

We have studied the influence of the VPA dose and of phenytoin (PT), phenobarbital (PB), and carbamazepine (CZ), alone or in combination, on the VPA concentration in a large number of inpatients with supervised medication. Furthermore, the possible influence of certain physiological factors (age, weight, height, and sex) and the preparation used (Orfiril, Ergenyl) was taken into consideration.

PATIENTS AND METHODS

The patient group consisted of 259 inpatients (146 men, 113 women) in an epilepsy center (von Bodelschwinghsche Anstalten, Bielefeld-Bethel, F.R.G.). The intake of drugs was supervised. The mean VPA dose per body weight was 29.6 ± 15.1 mg/kg, the mean body weight was 59.5 ± 18.9 kg, and the mean age was 26.0 ± 13.6 years. 32 patients were on VPA monotherapy, 33 were also given PB, 17, CZ; 37, PT; 36, PB with PT; 40, PB with CZ; 18, PT with CZ; and 46, PB with PT and CZ. The patients were given VPA as enteric-coated tablets of the sodium salt. The preparations were Orfiril (Desitin, Hamburg, F.R.G.) or Ergenyl (Labaz, Munich, F.R.G.).

Only serum samples that were taken in the morning (between 7 a.m. and 8 a.m.) were examined. In order to keep random fluctuations of the VPA concentrations low, a mean VPA value obtained from at least two serum samples was used for each of the 259 patients.

The serum concentration of valproic acid was determined by gas chromatography according to the method of Dijkhuis and Vervloet (13).

A nonlinear regression model (Eq. 1) was used to examine the influence of the various factors on the VPA concentration. The model parameters b_1 to b_4 thereby determine if VPA dose (VPAD), weight (W), age (A), or height (H) have an increasing, decreasing, or no effect ($b = 0$). Using the model, it can in particular be determined whether the VPA concentration/dose relationship is linear ($b_1 = 1$) or whether it can be more suitably described by a curvilinear relationship ($0 < b_1 < 1$).

$$\text{VPA concentration} = b_0 \cdot \text{VPAD}^{b_1} \cdot W^{b_2} \cdot A^{b_3} \cdot H^{b_4} \cdot F_1 \cdot F_2 \cdot F_3 \quad (1)$$

Where VPAD is VPA dose (mg/d), W is body weight (kg), A is age (yr), H is height (cm), F_1 is sex, F_2 is preparation, and F_3 is type of comedication.

For F_1, F_2, and F_3, which have two or more distinct levels, dummy variables (14) were defined as follows:

$$F_1 = \begin{cases} 1 \text{ for men} \\ b_5 \text{ for women} \end{cases}$$

$$F_2 = \begin{cases} 1 \text{ for Orfiril} \\ b_6 \text{ for Ergenyl} \end{cases}$$

$$F_3 = \begin{cases} 1 \text{ for mono} \\ b_7 \text{ for PT} \\ b_8 \text{ for PB} \\ b_9 \text{ for CZ} \\ b_{10} \text{ for PT + PB} \\ b_{11} \text{ for PT + CZ} \\ b_{12} \text{ for PB + CZ} \\ b_{13} \text{ for PB + PT + CZ} \end{cases}$$

The model parameters b_5 to b_{13} show by which factor the VPA concentration is raised or lowered with respect to the corresponding reference groups. For example, $b_7 = 0.50$ means that patients receiving VPA with PT have, on the average, VPA concentrations 50% lower than patients on VPA monotherapy.

The model parameters were estimated according to the method of least squares (14) for different subsets of factors, using subprograms from the program library BMDP (15). Starting from a submodel with the factors VPA dose, body weight, and simultaneously given drugs, it was tested whether eliminating one of these factors, or including one of the other factors, significantly affected the VPA concentration. In case a factor did not show any significant effect on the VPA concentration at the 5% level (using the F test) it was not included in the regression equation or eliminated.

RESULTS AND DISCUSSION

Before examining the influence of comedication and physiological factors on the VPA level, the stability of the morning serum concentrations of 17 patients was studied over a period of five to 73 weeks. For each patient, seven to 13 morning concentrations of VPA were measured. The coefficients of variance were between 7.5 and 28.7%, with a mean value of 15.2 ± 5.2%. They correlated negatively ($r = -0.67$) with the serum concentration.

The VPA dose, comedication, body weight, and sex had a significant influence on the VPA concentration, whereas age, height, and the preparation used (Orfiril, Ergenyl) had not. The estimated parameters for the relevant factors and their interpretation are listed in Table 1. Inclusion of the relevant factors in the model equation gave a correlation between measured and estimated VPA concentrations of $r = 0.791$. These factors can thus explain 62.6% of the variance. The mean absolute deviation of the estimated VPA concentration from the measured concentration was 11.15 ± 9.04 μg/ml.

In many studies (3,6,10,16), only a weak correlation was found between VPA concentration and dose. Thus, it could not be decided whether there was a linear or a nonlinear dose/level relationship. Some of the studies, however, did not differentiate between patients on VPA monotherapy and those on polytherapy. Likewise, the serum samples were taken at different times of the day. Only a few authors found a high linear correlation between the VPA dose and concentration [e.g., Klotz (12), $r = 0.88$] or yet, a clearly nonlinear dose/level relationship [e.g., Vajda et al. (11)].

Our results demonstrate that the relationship between the VPA dose and VPA concentration is not linear. The VPA concentration does not increase proportionally with the VPA dose but increases to a lesser extent.

The cause of the nonlinearity of the dose/level relationship may be an increase in the free fraction of

TABLE 1. *Estimated parameters for the significant factors in Eq. 1*

Parameters	Estimates[a]	Remarks
b_0	2.561 ± 0.801	Constant factor
b_1 (VPA dose)	0.539 ± 0.041	Relation between the VPA dose and the serum concentration is not linear
b_2 (body weight)	−0.122 ± 0.049	Serum concentrations are lower when the body weights are high
b_5 (sex)	0.073 ± 0.039	Women have higher serum concentrations (+7.3%) than men
b_7 (PT)	49.5 ± 3.4	Estimated parameters are expressed as percentages: VPA serum concentrations of patients on comedication in comparison with patients on VPA monotherapy (100%).
b_8 (PB)	76.3 ± 4.1	
b_9 (CZ)	66.2 ± 4.9	
b_{10} (PT + PB)	51.1 ± 3.3	
b_{11} (PT + CZ)	49.8 ± 4.3	
b_{12} (PB + CZ)	60.8 ± 3.4	
b_{13} (PT + PB + CZ)	44.0 ± 2.9	

Inclusion of age (b_3), body height (b_4) or preparation (b_6) had no significant influence on the VPA concentration (using the *F* test). This means that b_3 and b_4 were not significantly different from 0, and b_6 was not significantly different from 1. VPA, valproic acid; PT, phenytoin; PB, phenobarbital; CZ, carbamazepine.

[a]Parameter estimates ± asymptotic standard deviations.

VPA with a rising VPA concentration (3,17). The clearance increases with the free plasma fraction. The convex relationship between the VPA dose and concentration could thus be explained. A decrease in bioavailability on increasing the VPA dose is unlikely because of the high water solubility of sodium valproate.

Our results show that the serum concentration of VPA is clearly lower when VPA is given in combination with PB, CZ, or PT than when VPA is given alone. This result is in agreement with other studies (4 to 7). Our results show, furthermore, that PT appears to reduce the VPA concentration most of all (by ~50%), whereas the additional influence of PB or CZ is only relatively slight. The VPA concentration seems to be lowered more by a combination of PB and CZ than by PB or CZ alone. The lowest VPA concentrations occur when PB, CZ, and PT are administered together. An examination of the residuals showed, furthermore, that the kind of comedication, but not the level of serum concentrations of the respective codrugs, appeared to influence the VPA concentration. The correlation of the residuals with the serum concentrations of PB, PT, or CZ was only very low (r = 0.015, 0.035, −0.069, respectively) and not significant in the respective groups.

The decrease of the VPA concentration by comedication is probably due to hepatic microsomal enzyme induction and a thereby increased clearance (7).

Our results thus show that the total VPA level can be considerably lowered by PB, CZ, and especially PT and combinations of these drugs. Furthermore, a nonlinear relationship of VPA concentration to dose has been demonstrated.

Acknowledgments: The authors are indebted to Mr. G. S. Macpherson, B.Sc., for translating the paper and to Mr. H. Jung for compiling the data.

REFERENCES

1. Simon D, Penry JK. Sodium di-n-propylacetate (DPA) in the treatment of epilepsy. A review. *Epilepsia* 1975;16:549–73.
2. Bruni J, Wilder J. Valproic acid. Review of a new antiepileptic drug. *Arch Neurol* 1979;36:393–8.
3. Wilder BJ, Karas BJ. Valproate—relation of plasma concentration to seizure control. In: Woodbury DM, Penry JK, Pippenger CE, eds. *Antiepileptic drugs*. New York: Raven Press, 1982:591–9.
4. Sackellares JC, Sato S, Dreifuss FE, Penry JK. Reduction of steady-state valproate levels by other antiepileptic drugs. *Epilepsia* 1981;22:437–41.
5. Henriksen O, Johannessen SI. Clinical and pharmacokinetic observations on sodium valproate—a 5-year follow-up study in 100 children with epilepsy. *Acta Neurol Scand* 1982;65:504–23.
6. Mesdjian E, Dravet C, Roger J. Sodium valproate plasma levels (total level and free fraction level) in epileptic patients: influence of dose, age, and associated therapy. In: Levy RH, Pitlick WH, Eichelbaum M, Meijer JWA, eds. *Metabolism of antiepileptic drugs*. New York: Raven Press, 1984:115–25.
7. Mattson RH. Valproate—interactions with other drugs. In: Woodbury DM, Penry JK, Pippenger CE, eds. *Antiepileptic drugs*. New York: Raven Press, 1982:579–89.
8. Covanis A, Gupta AK, Jeavons PM. Sodium valproate: monotherapy and polytherapy. *Epilepsia* 1982;23:693–720.
9. Gram L, Flachs H, Würtz-Jørgensen A, Parnas J, Andersen B. Sodium valproate, serum level and clinical effect in epilepsy: a controlled study. *Epilepsia* 1979;20:303–12.
10. Turnbull DM, Rawlins MD, Weightman D, Chadwick DW. Plasma concentrations of sodium valproate: their clinical value. *Ann Neurol* 1983;14:38–42.
11. Vajda FJE, Drummer OH, Morris PM, McNeil JJ, Bladin PF. Gas chromatographic measurement of plasma levels of sodium valproate: tentative therapeutic range of a new anticonvulsant in the treatment of refractory epileptics. *Clin Exp Pharmacol Physiol* 1978;5:67–73.
12. Klotz U. Pharmacokinetic studies with valproic acid in man. *Arzneimittelforsch/Drug Res* 1977;27:1085–8.
13. Dijkhuis I, Vervloet E: Rapid determination of the antiepileptic drug di-n-propylacetic acid in serum. *Pharmaceutisch Weekblad* 1974;109:42–5.

14. Draper NR, Smith H. *Applied regression analysis*. New York: Wiley and Sons, 1981.
15. Dixon WJ, Brown MB. BMDP-77 Biomedical computer programs, P-series. Berkeley: University of California Press, 1977:380–499.
16. Minns RA, Brown JK, Blackwood DHR, McQueen JK. Valproate levels in children with epilepsy. *Lancet* 1982;1:677–8.
17. Levy RH, Lai AA. Valproate—absorption, distribution, and excretion. In: Woodbury DM, Penry JK, Pippenger CE, eds. *Antiepileptic drugs*. New York: Raven Press, 1982:555–65.

Therapeutic Drug Monitoring
7:391–400 © 1985 Raven Press, New York

A New Approach to Establishing Individualized Maintenance Doses of Phenytoin

*K. Bachmann, *T. J. Sullivan, †J. Schwartz, and †L. Jauregui

**The University of Toledo College of Pharmacy and †St. Vincent Medical Center, Toledo, Ohio, U.S.A.*

Summary: A new method for arriving at individualized doses of phenytoin (PHT) is described. This method, designated the η method, operates on two measurements of unbound plasma PHT. One plasma sample is collected 48 h after a single, oral PHT dose (~4.5 mg/kg). From the single dose, single sample measurements of plasma unbound PHT individual estimates of intrinsic unbound PHT clearance (CL_{uint}) can be made. With the use of CL_{uint} and weight-adjusted mean population values of V_{max} predicted plasma concentrations of unbound PHT for 11 subjects exhibited a mean prediction error (mpe) of 0.07 mg/L with 95% confidence limits of −0.11 to 0.26 mg/L and an error coefficient of variation [root mean squared error (rmse)/mean unbound concentration at steady state (C_{uss})] of 0.4. The second plasma unbound PHT is collected at steady state. From CL_{uint} and one C_{uss} measurement, $\hat{V}_{max}$ and K_m can be directly calculated. Doses calculated by the η method to produce plasma unbound PHT concentrations of ~1.0 mg/L were identical to those calculated by the Bayesian method to yield plasma total PHT concentrations of ~10 mg/L. When those doses were administered to six subjects, the plasma unbound PHT concentrations predicted by the η method exhibited a mpe of −0.13 mg/L, with 95% confidence limits ranging from −0.33 to 0.06 mg/L and an error coefficient of variation of 0.2. The plasma PHT concentrations predicted by the Bayesian method exhibited an mpe of −1.30 mg/L, with 95% confidence limits of −4.02 to 1.42 mg/L and an error coefficient of variation of 0.3. Values of V_{max} and doses of PHT calculated to produce a C_{uss} of 1.0 mg/L calculated by the η method were nearly identical to V_{max} values and doses of PHT calculated by Bayesian double feedback (based on two different C_{ss} values) to produce a C_{ss} of 10.0 mg/L. **Key Words:** Phenytoin—Dosing adjustment—Unbound plasma concentrations—η Method—Single sample method.

Starting patients on maintenance doses of phenytoin (PHT) that will give rise to safe and effective plasma PHT concentrations is a difficult task owing to the nonlinear nature of PHT disposition kinetics. Fundamentally, doses can be optimized once individual estimates of the pharmacokinetic parameters, V_{max} and K_m, are known. Several methods for estimating these parameters are available, including nomograms (1,2), estimates from two or more different steady-state concentrations (3), and Bayesian feedback (4). All of these methods are based on measures of total (bound plus unbound) plasma concentrations of PHT at steady state. The measurement of plasma unbound PHT has been recently advocated for monitoring purposes (5–7).

We describe a new method for achieving desirable concentrations of plasma unbound PHT based on two measurements of unbound PHT: a pre–steady-state measurement of plasma unbound PHT following a test dose, and one steady-state measurement of plasma

Address correspondence and reprint requests to Dr. K. Bachmann at The University of Toledo College of Pharmacy, 2801 W. Bancroft, Toledo, OH 43606, U.S.A.

unbound PHT. This method derives from earlier observations that demonstrated the suitability of using a single salivary PHT measurement for assessing host factor influences on PHT clearance (8).

METHODS

Subjects

Eleven male Caucasian subjects participated after giving written informed consent. Each underwent a physical examination and the usual chemistry tests, and all were in good health. Their ages ranged from 20 to 27 years (mean 22.5 yr) and their weights ranged from 66.2 to 116.1 kg (mean 79.2 kg). All subjects were nonsmokers, and none took chronic medication. All abstained from ethanol consumption beginning at least 48 h prior to receiving PHT and throughout the sample collection periods.

Treatments

The experiments were conducted in three phases. In the first phase each subject was given a test dose of PHT of either 300 or 400 mg (~4.5 mg/kg). All doses of PHT were taken by mouth after an overnight fast and followed with 120 ml of tap water. Forty-eight hours after the test dose, a 5 ml blood sample was collected in a heparinized tube for the determination of total plasma PHT and plasma unbound PHT.

In the second phase each subject was dosed to steady state with low daily doses (225–425 mg) of PHT. The formulation (Infatabs; Parke Davis) was tableted and scored, which permitted the rounding of dosages to the nearest 25-mg increment. Doses were administered at 8-h intervals (7 a.m., 3 p.m., and 11 p.m.) with divided doses either identical to or within 25 mg of one another. Drug administration continued for 10 days. Eight hours after the last dose, another blood sample was collected for analysis of plasma total PHT and plasma unbound PHT concentrations.

Six of the 11 subjects participated in the third phase. This phase was otherwise identical to the preceding phase except that the PHT doses administered were individualized to produce plasma unbound PHT concentrations of ~1.0 mg/L in each subject and were calculated on the basis of individualized estimates of V_{max} and K_m derived from the data of the first two phases (vide infra).

Assay

Ultrafiltration of plasma was performed as previously described (9). The concentration of PHT in plasma (total PHT) and plasma ultrafiltrates (unbound PHT) was measured by a fluorescence polarization immunoassay using a TDx analyzer (Abbott) as previously described (8). Coefficients of variation (CVs) for the method were 1.7 and 3.1% for total and unbound PHT, respectively.

Steady-state unbound PHT concentrations were referenced to values for 37°C to account for the effect of temperature on PHT binding (10). This adjustment was made by dividing unbound PHT concentrations in samples ultrafiltered at room temperature by 0.65 (see also reference 7).

Pharmacokinetic Analysis

Intrinsic unbound PHT clearance (CL_{uint}) was estimated from measurements of unbound PHT in plasma ultrafiltrates collected 48 h after a single test dose of PHT (Phase 1).

Estimates of V_{max} and K_m (or K_{mapp} when referenced to total PHT measurements) were made in several different ways for comparison.

(a) V_{max} and K_{mapp} were estimated from total plasma PHT concentrations at steady state at the end of Phase 2 (C_{uss1}) using a Bayesian algorithm programmed for the T159 calculator (4).

(b) V_{max} and K_{mapp} were estimated from total plasma PHT concentrations at steady state following both Phase 2 (C_{ss1}) and Phase 3 (C_{ss2}; double feedback) using a Bayesian algorithm.

(c) $\hat{V}_{max}$ and K_m were estimated from CL_{uint} and plasma unbound PHT concentrations at steady state at the end of Phase 2 (C_{uss1}). (See Appendix for these calculations.)

(d) V_{max} was estimated from a mean weight-adjusted population value (11).

$$V_{max} = \left[415 \cdot \left(\frac{W}{70}\right)^{0.6}\right]/W \qquad (1)$$

where W represents an individual weight in kg, and 415 represents the population mean V_{max} of PHT expressed in units of mg/day.

(e) K_m was estimated from single sample data (Phase 1) using the following expression:

$$K_m = \frac{V_{max}}{CL_{uint}} \qquad (2)$$

where V_{max} was the a priori weight-adjusted population value.

(f) K_m was estimated from a mean population value referenced to plasma total PHT (K_{mapp}, see reference 11) as follows:

$$K_m = 0.1\ K_{mapp} \qquad (3)$$

where 0.1 is the nominal value for PHT free fraction.

Single dose PHT elimination was simulated using a Michaelis-Menten elimination model running on an Apple IIe computer. The purpose of those simulations was to determine the robustness of the method to widely varying pharmacokinetic parameters.

Simulations of single dose PHT elimination were modified from a previously published algorithm (12). For these simulations, the dose of PHT used was 300 mg. V_{max} values were 325, 415, and 500 mg/day. K_m values (referenced to unbound PHT) were set at 0.29, 0.57, or 0.86 mg/L. Extremes for both V_{max} and K_m values are ± 1 SD from the population means reported by Grasela et al. (11). Weight was held constant at 70 kg. Volume of distribution, V, referenced to unbound PHT, was set at 12, 15, and 18 L/kg. Apparent intrinsic unbound PHT clearance was calculated from the 48-h plasma unbound PHT concentrations ($\hat{CL}'_{int}$) just as it was for human subjects (see Appendix, eq. A1). A correction divisor, η, for calculating CL_{uint} from $\hat{CL}'_{int}$ was calculated for various combinations of dose, V_{max}, and K_m values by taking the ratio of ($\hat{CL}'_{int}$)/ (V_{max}/K_m), since:

$$CL_{uint} = \frac{V_{max}}{K_m} \qquad (4)$$

The influence of errant volume assumptions on simulated single sample estimates of CL_{uint} was assessed by comparing mean η values (see Appendix, Eq. A3) for each set of volume assumptions.

Data obtained from Phases 1 through 3 of studies involving healthy subjects were evaluated in several ways. (a) Estimates of V_{max} were obtained from measurements of unbound PHT 48 h following the test dose and from C_{uss1} (see Appendix, Eqs. A1 and A2; this two-step approach involving a pre–steady-state measurement and one steady-state measurement of unbound PHT is hereafter referred to as the η method). Such estimates were designated as $\hat{V}_{max}$ and were compared with Bayesian estimates of V_{max} derived from C_{ss1}. (b) Doses, R, designed to achieve a C_{uss2} of 1.0 mg/L were calculated for η method parameters. Doses designed to achieve a C_{ss2} of 10 mg/L were calculated for Bayesian parameters. Dose predictions by both methods were plotted against one another. (c) Doses were also predicted for achieving a steady-state concentration of 1.0 mg/L using weight-adjusted population V_{max} values (Eq. 1) and K_m values calculated as shown in Eq. 2. CL_{uint} was calculated from the single 48-h plasma unbound PHT concentration after the test dose (see Appendix, Eqs. A1 and A2). This method for calculating maintenance doses is hereafter referred to as the single sample method. Doses predicted by the single sample method were plotted against doses predicted by the Bayesian method.

The effectiveness with which predicted C_{uss1} levels were achieved in Phase 2, based on the actual doses used and the single sample estimates of V_{max} and K_m, was assessed as described by Sheiner and Beal (13). The effectiveness with which predicted η method doses and Bayesian doses actually elicited targeted plasma unbound PHT (C_{uss2}) and total PHT levels (C_{ss2}), respectively, was similarly analyzed. Finally, η method estimates of V_{max} ($\hat{V}_{max}$) were compared with Bayesian double feedback estimates of V_{max} (from C_{ss1} and C_{ss2}), and η method doses predicted to achieve 1.0 mg/L PHT plasma unbound concentrations were compared with doses derived from Bayesian double feedback predicted to achieve 10 mg/L PHT concentrations.

RESULTS

Predicted and actual plasma concentrations of unbound PHT based on estimates of CL_{uint} from the single sample procedure and from weight-adjusted mean population values for V_{max} are shown in Table 1. Low doses which engendered a mean (± SD) plasma unbound PHT concentration of 0.68 (± 0.22) mg/L were used. The mean prediction error (mpe) was 0.07 mg/L, with 95% confidence limits of − 0.11 to 0.24 mg/L and a root mean squared error (rmse) of 0.26 mg/L. Individual η method estimates of $\hat{V}_{max}$, K_m, and doses calculated to produce steady-state unbound PHT concentrations of 1.0 mg/L are shown in Table 2.

The mean (± SD) $\hat{V}_{max}$ estimated by the η method was 0.252 (±0.035) mg kg^{-1} hr^{-1}. Individual $\hat{V}_{max}$ estimates by the η method are plotted in Fig. 1a against individual V_{max} estimates from the Bayesian method operating on a single steady-state concentration of plasma total PHT (C_{ss1}). Doses calculated by the η method that are intended to achieve steady-state concentrations of unbound PHT of 1.0 mg/L are plotted against Bayesian doses intended to achieve steady-state concentrations of plasma total PHT of 10 mg/L. Exact doses by both methods are shown in Fig. 1b, and doses are rounded to the nearest 25-mg increment, i.e., doses that would actually be given, because of the constraints of the formulation, are shown in Fig. 1c. In Fig. 1d, doses predicted by the single sample method to achieve steady-state concentrations of 1.0 mg/L of unbound PHT are plotted against Bayesian doses predicted to produce a total plasma

TABLE 1. *Predicted concentrations of unbound phenytoin (PHT) based on single sample estimates of* CL_{uint}, *dose* (R), *and weight-adjusted population* V_{max}

Subject	CL_{uint}[a] (L h^{-1} kg^{-1})	V_{max}[b] (mg kg^{-1} h^{-1})	R (mg kg^{-1} h^{-1})	Predicted[c] C_{uss} (mg/L)	Actual C_{uss} (mg/L)
KF	0.899	0.258	0.166	0.52	0.40
DB	0.679	0.245	0.160	0.68	0.58
CN	0.615	0.230	0.149	0.68	0.65
EC	0.461	0.251	0.140	0.69	1.23
LB	0.549	0.252	0.142	0.60	0.49
EM	0.391	0.234	0.131	0.78	0.75
MD	0.566	0.245	0.146	0.64	0.57
TM	0.675	0.243	0.158	0.67	0.71
PN	0.404	0.246	0.132	0.70	0.82
KM	0.600	0.202	0.152	1.03	0.63
TB	0.700	0.207	0.163	1.10	0.63

[a] CL_{uint} was calculated by dividing $\hat{CL}'_{int}$ by 0.67.
[b] Weight-adjusted population V_{max} was calculated by Eq. 1.
[c] Predicted C_{uss} concentrations were calculated from Eq. A4.

PHT concentration of 10 mg/L. Doses in Fig. 1d are rounded to the nearest 25-mg increment. It is apparent that individual estimates of V_{max} by both methods (Bayesian and η) are quite similar, and predicted doses (rounded) by both methods are identical.

Predicted and actual plasma PHT concentrations are shown in Table 3 for the six subjects who completed Phase 3 of the investigation. These subjects were dosed to steady state using doses (rounded to the nearest 25-mg increment) that were calculated by the η method to produce plasma unbound PHT levels of approximately 1.0 mg/L and by the Bayesian method to produce PHT levels of 10 mg/L. Doses calculated by either method were identical (see Fig. 1C). That steady state had been reached in all subjects after 10 days was determined by calculating the time to reach 90% of steady-state values (14). For the η method, mpe referenced to unbound PHT was −0.13 mg/L with 95% confidence limits of −0.33 to 0.06 mg/L and an rmse of 0.22 mg/L. For the Bayesian method, which is referenced to total plasma PHT, the mpe was −1.30 mg/L with 95% confidence limits ranging from −4.02 to 1.42 mg/L, and rmse was 2.70 mg/L. These values are also shown in Fig. 2, along with analogous values for the single sample method. In Fig. 2 the mpe and 95% confidence limit is depicted for each method. Also shown are the error CVs (rmse/mean plasma concentration), which allow a more direct comparison of the precision of each method despite differing target concentrations for each of them.

It was possible to calculate a second set of V_{max}-K_m pairs for each of the six subjects who participated in Phase 3 from C_{ss1} and C_{ss2} using the Bayesian method (double feedback). As for the single feedback case, individual estimates of V_{max} (Bayesian) were compared with individual estimates of $\hat{V}_{max}$ calculated by the η

TABLE 2. *Individual estimates of* V_{max} *and* K_m *by the η method*

Subject	Weight (kg)	$\hat{V}_{max}$ (mg kg^{-1} h^{-1})	K_m (mg/L)	R (mg kg^{-1} h^{-1})	R (mg/day)
KF	62.6	0.309	0.34	0.231	346
DB	71.7	0.270	0.40	0.193	332
CN	83.9	0.237	0.39	0.171	344
EC	67.1	0.186	0.40	0.133	214
LB	66.2	0.301	0.55	0.194	309
EM	79.8	0.236	0.61	0.146	281
MD	71.2	0.267	0.47	0.182	310
TM	72.6	0.236	0.35	0.175	305
PN	70.8	0.220	0.54	0.143	243
KM	116.1	0.254	0.42	0.179	498
TB	108.9	0.259	0.37	0.189	494
Mean		0.252	0.44		
± SD		0.035	0.09		

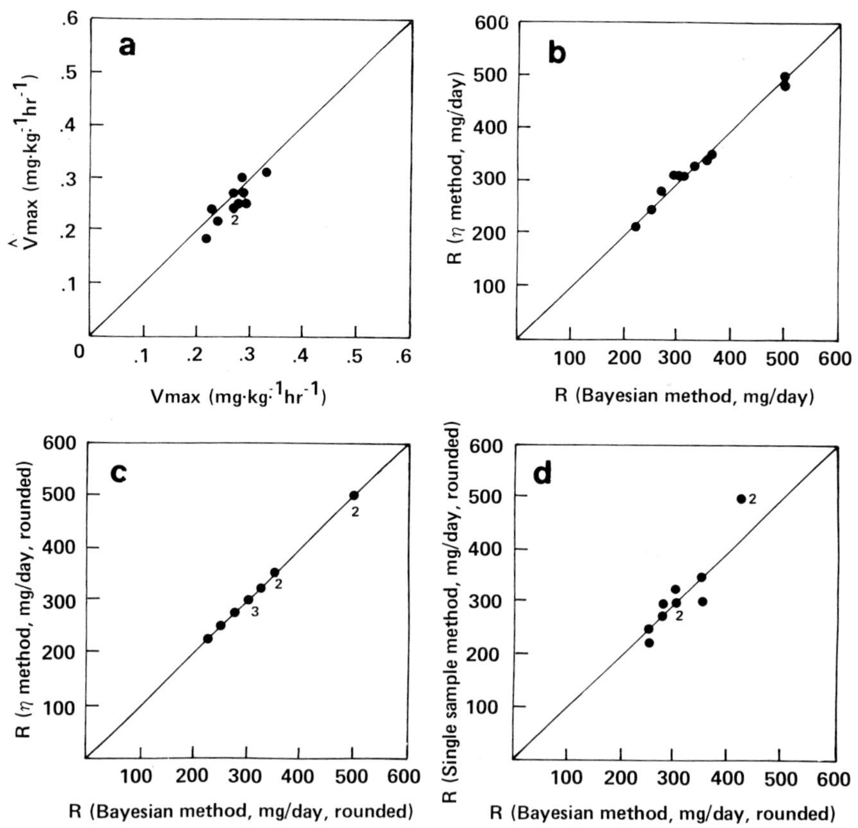

FIG. 1. a: η Method estimates of V_{max} vs. Bayesian estimates of V_{max}. **b:** Exact phenytoin (PHT) doses calculated from η method parameters to achieve plasma unbound PHT concentrations of 1.0 mg/L vs. exact PHT doses calculated from Bayesian parameters to achieve plasma total PHT concentrations of 10.0 mg/L. **c:** Doses from Fig. 1b rounded to the nearest 25-mg increment. **d:** PHT doses (rounded to the nearest 25-mg increment) calculated from single sample estimates of V_{max} and K_m to achieve plasma unbound PHT concentrations of ~1.0 mg/L vs. doses (rounded to the nearest 25-mg increment) calculated from Bayesian estimates of V_{max} and K_{mapp} to achieve plasma total PHT concentrations of ~10.0 mg/L. Numbers by plotting symbols depict the number of superimposed data points. Lines shown are identity lines.

method. These comparisons are shown in Fig. 3a. Also shown are the exact doses (Fig. 3b) and rounded doses (Fig. 3c, nearest 25-mg increment) of PHT

TABLE 3. *Predicted steady-state concentrations of phenytoin (PHT)[a] based on Bayesian and η method estimates of* V_{max} *and* K_m[b]

Subject	Predicted C_{ss} (mg/L) η	Predicted C_{ss} (mg/L) Bayesian	Actual C_{ss} (mg/L) η	Actual C_{ss} (mg/L) Bayesian
EC	1.22	10.60	1.26	12.25
LB	0.93	11.40	0.97	9.27
MD	0.91	10.17	1.40	15.32
PN	1.09	10.16	1.26	13.19
DB[c]	0.67	6.86	0.65	6.27
TM	0.94	9.10	1.02	9.80

[a]PHT concentrations are referenced to unbound PHT for the η method and to total PHT for the Bayesian method.
[b]K_m for η method; K_{mapp} for Bayesian method.
[c]DB had seven tablets of PHT remaining after Phase 3. His daily dose, therefore, was estimated as the difference between the total amount dispensed and total amount remaining, prorated over 10 days. By this method it was estimated that DB took the equivalent of 290 mg/day rather than the 325 mg/day that was calculated to produce a 1.0 mg/L concentration. Predicted concentrations for DB (both methods) assume a daily dose of 290 mg.

predicted to produce a steady-state plasma concentration of 10 mg/L (total PHT, Bayesian parameters) or 1.0 mg/L (unbound PHT, η parameters). There is good agreement between dosage predictions by the η method and by the Bayesian approach (double feedback).

In view of the concordance of $\hat{V}_{max}$ and V_{max} estimates and predicted dosages by both methods for the six subjects completing Phase 3, a prediction was made of the effect of using PHT doses derived from a population mean value for K_m (0.57 mg/L referenced to unbound PHT) and a weight-adjusted population value for V_{max} under the assumption that $\hat{V}_{max}$ and K_m estimates by the η method closely approximated true V_{max} and K_m values. That is, doses of PHT derived from population V_{max} and K_m values and designed to produce ~1.0 mg/L unbound PHT concentrations were calculated. Then the effect of those doses on PHT unbound concentrations was calculated assuming that individual K_m and $\hat{V}_{max}$ estimates according to the η method represented true V_{max} and K_m values. Predicted steady-state plasma concentrations of unbound PHT for both conditions are shown in Table 4. As expected, use of population mean values would yield a wide range of plasma concentrations (0.58–2.0 mg/L; CV 58%).

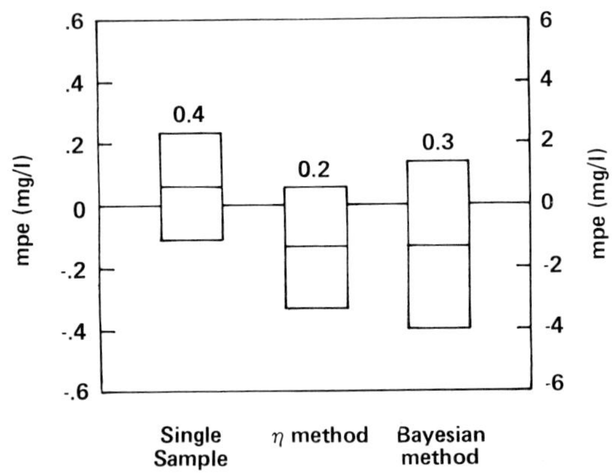

FIG. 2. Mean prediction errors for steady-state phenytoin (PHT) concentrations predicted from K_m and V_{max} values derived by three different methods. Horizontal lines denote mean prediction error (mpe). Extremes of each bar represent 95% confidence limits for mpe. Numbers atop each bar depict error coefficients of variation (root mean squared error/mean plasma PHT concentration).

Table 5 shows the impact of volume assumptions (referenced to unbound volume of distribution) on the ratio of $(\hat{CL}'_{int})/(V_{max}/K_m)$. All data in Table 5 are derived from simulations in which the "true" value for V is either 12, 15, or 18 L/kg but the assumed value is 12 L/kg. For the V_{max}-K_m-V combinations tested, the average ratio was practically independent of changes in "true" volume of distribution (0.722, 0.730, and 0.753 for 12, 15, and 18 L/kg, respectively). However, as the "true" volume deviates from the "assumed" volume of 12 L/kg, the variability in the ratio with changing V_{max}-K_m pairs increases. CVs of 7.6%, 13.7%, and 19.3% were observed for volumes of 12, 15, and 18 L/kg, respectively.

DISCUSSION

This investigation was directed toward determining the effectiveness with which either a single plasma concentration measurement of unbound PHT following a test dose by itself or in combination with one steady-state concentration measurement of unbound PHT could be used in establishing maintenance doses of PHT designed to elicit specified steady-state plasma unbound concentrations.

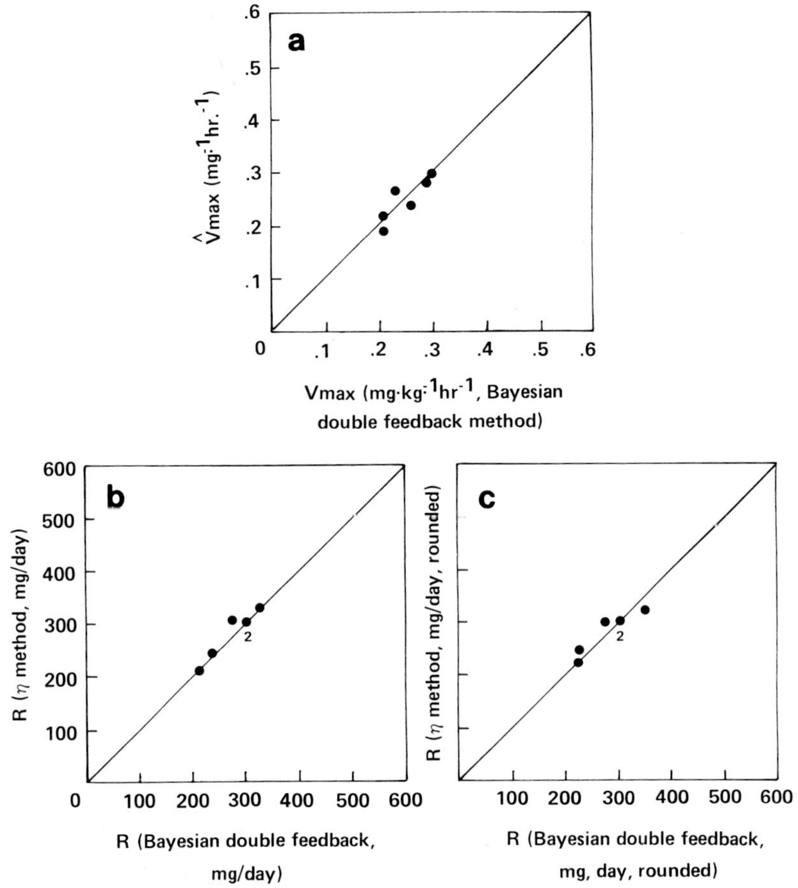

FIG. 3.a: η Method estimates of V_{max} vs. Bayesian double feedback estimates of V_{max}. **b:** Exact phenytoin (PHT) doses calculated from η method parameters to achieve plasma unbound PHT concentrations of 1.0 mg/L vs. exact PHT doses calculated from Bayesian double feedback parameters to achieve plasma total PHT concentrations of 10.0 mg/L. **c:** Doses from both methods rounded to the nearest 25 mg increment. Numbers by plotting symbols depict the number of superimposed data points. Lines shown are identity lines.

TABLE 4. *Effect of using phenytoin (PHT) doses derived strictly from population mean values of* V_{max} *and* K_m *when individualized* V_{max} *and* K_m *values deviate from population means*[a]

Subject	R^b (mg kg^{-1} h^{-1})	$V_{max}{}^c$ (mg kg^{-1} h^{-1})	$K_m{}^c$ (mg/L)	Population $C_{uss}{}^d$ (mg/L)	η^e C_{uss} (mg/L)
EC	0.155	0.186	0.40	2.00	1.22
LB	0.157	0.301	0.55	0.60	0.93
PN	0.162	0.220	0.54	1.50	1.09
TM	0.158	0.236	0.35	0.71	0.94
MD	0.161	0.267	0.47	0.72	0.91
DB	0.160	0.270	0.40	0.58	0.93

[a]Weight-adjusted V_{max} as calculated in footnote of Table 1. K_m set at 0.57 mg/L.
[b]Doses calculated to produce 1.0 mg/L unbound PHT based on population V_{max} and K_m values.
[c]η Method values assumed to represent true values on the basis of Phase 3 outcomes.
[d]Unbound PHT concentrations based on R, but assuming η method parameters represent true V_{max} and K_m values.
[e]Unbound PHT concentrations based on η method V_{max} and K_m derived doses (rounded) designed to achieve concentrations ~1.0 mg/L.

TABLE 5. *Effect of changes in* V_{max} *and* K_m *on estimates of η as determined by computer simulation*

V^a (L/kg)	V_{max} (mg kg^{-1} h^{-1})	K_m (mg/L)	$V_{max}/K_m{}^b$ (L h^{-1} kg^{-1})	$\hat{CL}'_{int}{}^c$ (L h^{-1} kg^{-1})	η^d
12	0.297	0.86	0.346	0.273	0.789
	0.297	0.57	0.522	0.392	0.751
	0.297	0.29	1.026	0.725	0.707
	0.247	0.86	0.287	0.222	0.774
	0.247	0.57	0.433	0.316	0.729
	0.247	0.29	0.852	0.567	0.666
	0.193	0.86	0.225	0.171	0.759
	0.193	0.57	0.339	0.239	0.704
	0.193	0.29	0.667	0.412	0.617
15	0.297	0.86	0.346	0.280	0.809
	0.297	0.57	0.522	0.378	0.723
	0.297	0.29	1.026	0.645	0.629
	0.247	0.86	0.287	0.239	0.833
	0.247	0.57	0.433	0.317	0.732
	0.247	0.29	0.852	0.522	0.613
	0.193	0.86	0.225	0.197	0.878
	0.193	0.57	0.339	0.255	0.752
	0.193	0.29	0.667	0.400	0.599
18	0.297	0.86	0.346	0.292	0.844
	0.297	0.57	0.522	0.376	0.719
	0.297	0.29	1.026	0.601	0.585
	0.247	0.86	0.287	0.258	0.896
	0.247	0.57	0.433	0.325	0.750
	0.247	0.29	0.852	0.499	0.586
	0.193	0.86	0.225	0.223	0.990
	0.193	0.57	0.339	0.273	0.804
	0.193	0.29	0.667	0.398	0.597

[a]Simulations were performed using a "true" V of 12 L/kg, 15 L/kg, or 18 L/kg, but for estimating $\hat{CL}'_{int}$ a constant value of 12 L/kg for V was assumed.
[b]V_{max}/K_m is the same as the actual CL_{uint}.
[c]Estimated from single 48-h plasma unbound PHT concentration.
[d]Calculated as the ratio of $(\hat{CL}'_{int})/(V_{max}/K_m)$.

The underpinning of these two approaches is the single dose, single sample procedure for estimating PHT $\hat{CL}'_{int}$ (8) from which accurate estimates of CL_{uint} can be made. Under the conditions specified by Bachmann et al. (8), estimates of $\hat{CL}_{int}/F$ (equivalent to $\hat{CL}'_{int}$ as reported herein) underestimated actual intrinsic unbound clearance. The reason cited was that F was ~0.7. However, as shown by Jusko et al. (15), the error in intrinsic clearance estimates actually derives from a misapplication of linear assumptions to a nonlinear process. Thus, the term in the denominator is more appropriately a model misspecification correction term, which we have chosen to call η. An important issue to resolve was whether or not the value for η would remain constant over a wide range of V_{max}-K_m combinations. Both the simulated data and the actual subject data suggest that for usual values of V, η is quite constant, exhibiting a CV of only 7.6%. Average values of η appear to remain constant over a wide range of changes in volume of distribution. Single sample estimates of antipyrine clearance appear to be quite robust to errors in assumptions about volume of distribution, V (16), and have been shown to deviate by no more than 1.5% from true clearance values even when the assumed value for V is 50% greater than the actual value (17). Unfortunately, the variability in CL_{uint} estimates for PHT is relatively sensitive to assumptions about V. This is not an unexpected finding, since CL_{uint} is equivalent to V_{max}/K_m, and the volume of distribution is concealed in V_{max}. For subjects belonging to subpopulations with abnormal V values (significantly >13 L/kg), as might be the case for individuals taking valproic acid (18) or uremic patients (19), care must be taken when applying this method. The suitability of this method in such patient groups must be demonstrated.

The use of a weight-adjusted population V_{max} value with a K_m derived from that V_{max} and from CL_{uint} to calculate initial maintenance doses should be adequate (see Fig. 2), providing that those weight-adjusted population V_{max} values are reasonable ones for the individuals to whom they are applied. We used a fairly homogeneous sample of subjects (young, healthy, Caucasian males of European descent) to optimize the probability that population V_{max} values from Grasela et al. (11) would be appropriate. It bears emphasis that the single sample method, itself, should be invoked only if the foregoing conditions are met.

No assumptions about V_{max} need to be made in order to apply the η method for establishing maintenance PHT doses. For the η method, $\hat{V}_{max}$ and K_m are calculated from a single 48-h measurement of unbound PHT after a test dose of ~4.5 mg/kg and one steady-state measurement of unbound PHT. The former measurement is used to calculate CL_{uint} (i.e., V_{max}/K_m); the latter measurement then permits calculation of both $\hat{V}_{max}$ and K_m. One might, however, employ the single sample approach in structuring the initial maintenance doses that will give rise to the steady-state unbound PHT measurement used in the η method. With the η method values for $\hat{V}_{max}$ and K_m, one can refine maintenance doses of PHT to achieve desirable steady-state concentrations of unbound drug. Providing that subjects exhibit relatively normal PHT plasma protein binding, our data suggest that doses derived from the η method will be at least as good as those derived from either Bayesian single or double feedback methods applied to one or two steady-state measurements, respectively, of plasma total PHT concentrations. Data from computer simulations suggest that the η method might also work for individuals exhibiting abnormal PHT protein binding once population values for V and η have been prospectively determined for various subpopulations, i.e., uremic and cirrhotic patients, and those taking valproic acid.

As with any procedure for establishing individualized doses, the assets and liabilities of the η method cannot be fully tallied until more subjects and epileptic patients have had their doses set by it. At this point, perceived advantages or disadvantages are only speculative. We are careful to note that the η method has been shown only to be comparable to the Bayesian method of establishing PHT maintenance doses in a small number of healthy male young adults. Whether, in fact, it will be widely applicable will depend upon the robustness of the use of specified values for η to actual extremes of V_{max} and K_m values. Both our computer-based and in vivo data suggest that setting η at ~0.7 for conditions in which PHT binding is relatively normal (i.e., V is ~13 L/kg) should suffice. This suggestion is also supported by the data of Gugler et al. (20) and Jusko et al. (15). Whether or not the η method can be applied to individuals exhibiting abnormal (i.e., decreased) PHT plasma protein binding will also depend upon the establishment of appropriate subpopulation values of V. It is apparent that the η method would be suitable only for those patients just being started on PHT and not in need of a loading dose, since a test dose must first be given and maintenance doses withheld for 48 h after the test dose.

However, the η method can potentially provide refined individualized PHT maintenance doses within a week or so, and a good approximation of an initial maintenance dose can be made within 48 h if the single sample method is first judiciously applied. Thus, for PHT-naive patients, the successive application of the single sample and η methods should allow a more rapid focusing of safe and effective PHT doses than other methods that operate on one or more steady-state levels of PHT. Finally, the η method invokes measures of plasma unbound PHT only, not unbound and total PHT. For the purpose of therapeutic drug monitoring, there is a growing recognition that monitoring unbound PHT concentrations may be preferable to monitoring total PHT concentrations (5–7).

APPENDIX

Intrinsic unbound PHT clearance estimated from a single plasma concentration of unbound PHT taken 48 h after a test dose is designated as $\hat{CL}'_{int}$ and is the same as $\hat{CL}_{int}/F$ of Bachmann et al. (8), where F is unity. $\hat{CL}'_{int}$ is calculated as follows:

$$\hat{CL}'_{int} = [\ln(D/V) - \ln C_{u48}] \cdot (V/t) \qquad (A1)$$

where V is a volume term (L/kg) which is set at 13 L/kg and is equivalent to V/F of Bachmann et al. (1985), D is the test dose of PHT (mg/kg), C_{u48} is the concentration of unbound PHT at 48 h after the test dose, and t is the sampling time (48 h).

CL_{uint} is the intrinsic unbound PHT clearance corrected for model misspecification by dividing $\hat{CL}'_{int}$ by η.

$$CL_{uint} = \hat{CL}'_{int}/\eta \qquad (A2)$$

This corrects for the underestimate of CL_{uint} following a low dose of PHT when CL'_{int} is calculated from a linear rather than a nonlinear model. The value for η used in this investigation was 0.67. This value represents the ratio of $\hat{CL}'_{int}/(V_{max}/K_m)$. That is

$$\eta = \hat{CL}'_{int}/(V_{max}/K_m) \qquad (A3)$$

where V_{max} and K_m are true values and CL'_{int} is derived from Eq. A1.

Average steady-state unbound PHT concentrations, C_{uss}, can be predicted from

$$C_{uss} = \frac{K_m \cdot R}{(V_{max} - R)} \qquad (A4)$$

where K_m and V_{max} are the Michaelis-Menten parameters for PHT and R is the dosing rate.
Since

$$CL_{uint} = V_{max}/K_m \qquad (A5)$$

where CL_{uint} is intrinsic unbound PHT clearance, then

$$K_m = V_{max}/CL_{uint} \qquad (A6)$$

Substituting into Eq. A4, C_{uss} can be defined as

$$C_{uss} = \frac{(V_{max}/CL_{uint}) \cdot R}{(V_{max} - R)} \qquad (A7)$$

Solving for V_{max}, one can write

$$V_{max} = \frac{R \cdot C_{uss}}{C_{uss} - (\frac{R}{CL_{uint}})} \qquad (A8)$$

Thus, if one has a single sample estimate of CL_{uint} (see Eqs. A1 and A2) and a steady-state measurement of C_{uss}, one can estimate V_{max} ($\hat{V}_{max}$) according to Eq. A8.

Application of Eqs. A1 and A2 to a 48-h measurement of unbound PHT after a test dose and Eq. A8 to a subsequent steady-state concentration of unbound PHT is designated as the η method for estimating $\hat{V}_{max}$.

K_m can then be estimated from Eq. A6.

Acknowledgment: The authors gratefully acknowledge the technical assistance of Mary Martin, B.S.N. This work was funded by a grant from the F.M. Douglass Foundation.

REFERENCES

1. Mullen PW. Optimal phenytoin therapy: a new technique for individualizing dosage. *Clin Pharmacol Ther* 1978; 23:228–32.
2. Richens A, Dunlop A. Phenytoin dosage nomogram. *Lancet* 1975;2:1305–6.
3. Ludden TM, Allen JP, Valutsky WA, et al. Individualization of phenytoin dosage regimens. *Clin Pharmacol Ther* 1977;21:287–93.
4. Vozeh S, Muir KT, Sheiner LB, Follath F. Predicting individual phenytoin dosage. *J Pharmacokinet Biopharm* 1981;9:131–46.
5. Rowland M. Plasma protein binding and therapeutic drug monitoring. *Ther Drug Monit* 1980;2:29–37.
6. Greenblatt DJ, Sellers EM, Koch-Weser J. Importance of protein binding for the interpretation of serum or plasma drug concentrations. *J Clin Pharmacol* 1982;22:259–63.
7. Kilpatrick CJ, Wanwimolruk S, Wing LMH. Plasma concentrations of unbound phenytoin in the management of epilepsy. *Br J Clin Pharmacol* 1984;17:539–46.
8. Bachmann K, Schwartz J, Forney R Jr., Jauregui L. Phenytoin as a probe of drug metabolism: predicting clearance with a salivary sample. *Pharmacology* 1985;30:145–52.
9. Bachmann K, Forney R Jr, Voeller K. Monitoring phenytoin in salivary and plasma ultrafiltrates of pediatric patients. *Ther Drug Monit* 1983;5:325–9.
10. Lunde PK, Rave A, Yaffe S, Lund L, and Sjoqvist F. Plasma protein binding of diphenylhydantoin in man: interaction with other drugs and the effect of temperature and plasma dilution. *Clin Pharmacol Ther* 1970;11:846–55.
11. Grasela TH, Sheiner LB, Rambeck B, et al. Steady-state pharmacokinetics of phenytoin from routinely collected patient data. *Clin Pharmacokinet* 1983;8:355–64.
12. Sullivan T, Wunderly D. A package of computer programs

designed to simulate pharmacokinetics monitoring of drug therapy. *Comput Programs Biomed* 1980;12:85–95.
13. Sheiner LB, Beal S. Some suggestions for measuring predictive performance. *J Pharmacokinet Biopharm* 1981;9:503–12.
14. Tozer T, Winter M. Phenytoin. In: Evans W, Schentag J, Jusko W, eds. *Applied pharmacokinetics*. Spokane, Washington. Applied Therapeutics, Inc. 1980:275–314.
15. Jusko W, Koup J, Alvan G. Nonlinear assessment of phenytoin bioavailability. *J Pharmacokinet Biopharm* 1976;4:327–36.
16. Dossing M, Poulsen H, Andreasen PB, Tygstrup N. A simple method for determination of antipyrine clearance. *Clin Pharmacol Ther* 1982;32:392–6.
17. Pilsgaard H, Poulsen H. A one-sample method for antipyrine clearance determination in rats. *Pharmacology* 1984;29:110–6.
18. Knott C, Hamshaw-Thomas A, Reynolds F. Phenytoin-valproate interaction: importance of saliva monitoring in epilepsy. *Br Med J* 1982;284:13–16.
19. Depner T, Stanfel L, Jarrad E, Gulyassy P. Impaired plasma phenytoin binding in uremia. Effect of in vitro acidification and anion-exchange resin. *Nephron* 1980;25:231–7.
20. Gugler R, Manion C, Azarnoff D. Phenytoin: pharmacokinetics and bioavailability. *Clin Pharmacol Ther* 1976;19:135–42.

Therapeutic Drug Monitoring
7:401–404 © 1985 Raven Press, New York

Effect of Phenothiazines on Serum Antiepileptic Drug Concentrations in Psychiatric Patients with Seizure Disorder

Dan Haidukewych and Ernst A. Rodin

Epilepsy Center of Michigan, Detroit, Michigan, U.S.A.

Summary: The intrapatient effect of starting (group A, n = 16), increasing (group B, n = 19), decreasing (group C, n = 23), and discontinuing (group D, n = 34) the phenothiazines (PHZs) thioridazine, chlorpromazine, or mesoridazine on serum phenytoin (PHT), phenobarbital (PB), and primidone (PRI) was studied at a constant antiepileptic drug regimen and between two consecutive steady-state concentration determinations in 92 institutionalized epileptic patients with psychiatric disorders. For PHZ initiation or dosage increase (groups A and B), serum PHT and PHT concentration-to-dose ratio (C/D) decreased by 44 ($p < 0.001$) and 41.6% ($p < 0.001$) in group A, and 32.9 ($p < 0.001$) and 35.3% ($p < 0.005$) in group B, respectively. For PHZ dosage decrease or discontinuation (groups C and D), serum PHT and C/D ratio increased by 54.8 ($p < 0.001$) and 51.3% ($p < 0.01$) in group C, and 71.2 ($p < 0.001$) and 69.2% ($p < 0.001$) in group D, respectively. The changes for PB were in the same direction, although to a lesser extent. No statistically significant differences were noted for PRI. For groups A and B, the clinical trend was for increase in number of seizures when PHZs were started or dosage increased. For groups C and D, a clear trend for PHT intoxication was evident when PHZ dosages were decreased or discontinued. **Key Words:** Antiepileptics—Phenothiazines—Interactions—Statistical correlations.

One of the difficult problems in the treatment of epilepsy is to achieve seizure control in epileptic patients institutionalized in psychiatric hospitals. These patients are usually suffering from epilepsy, either secondary to trauma or associated with psychoses. Combined use of antiepileptic drugs (AEDs) and phenothiazines (PHZs) is common, particularly in the mentally retarded where the incidence of both seizure disorders and behavior problems is high.

The literature reports on interactions of PHZs with AEDs are sparse and controversial. Several authors have reported that PHZs caused an increase in serum phenytoin (PHT) concentration (1,2). Others have found no significant changes (3), whereas still others found a decrease in serum PHT (4) and phenobarbital (PB) (5) concentration in association with PHZ comedication. The conclusion appears to be that in the majority of patients, PHZs do not cause significant changes in AED serum concentrations (6).

In the past decade our facility has been used in a consulting capacity for patients institutionalized at Caro Regional Mental Health Center, Caro, Michigan, U.S.A. Along with the mailed serum specimens, we received information regarding time of blood drawing, age, sex, weight, dosages of all prescribed medications, and data on the clinical status of the patients. After AED concentrations were determined, the consulting epileptologist (E.A.R.) advised the institutional staff

Address correspondence and reprint requests to Dr. D. Haidukewych at Epilepsy Center of Michigan, 3800 Woodward Avenue, Detroit, MI 48201, U.S.A.

TABLE 1. *Effect of added or increased phenothiazine (PHZ) medications on serum antiepileptic drug (AED) concentrations*[a]

Parameters	No. of patients	AED	AED + PHZ	AED + Increased PHZ	Percent difference	Significance
Group A: PHZ added to constant AED regimen (n = 16)						
PHZ (mg/day)	16	None	159.4 ± 76.9	—	100	p < 0.001 (T = 8.2951)
PHZ (mg/kg/day)	16	None	3.20 ± 1.69	—	100	p < 0.001 (T = 7.3362)
PHT (mg/day)	15	330.0 ± 79.2	330.0 ± 79.2	—	None	—
PHT (mg/kg/day)	15	6.56 ± 1.58	6.56 ± 1.64	—	None	—
PHT (μg/ml serum)	15	22.40 ± 4.87	12.55 ± 4.21	—	−44	p < 0.001 (T = 5.9406)
PHT (C/D ratio[b])	15	3.58 ± 1.06	2.09 ± 1.01	—	−41.6	p < 0.001 (T = 3.9551)
PB (mg/day)	5	106.0 ± 47.8	106.0 ± 47.8	—	None	—
PB (mg/kg/day)	5	2.14 ± 0.87	2.20 ± 1.00	—	2.8	NS
PB (μg/ml serum)	13[c]	34.29 ± 12.37	24.38 ± 6.15	—	−29.1	p < 0.02 (T = 2.6152)
PB (C/D ratio)	5	14.27 ± 3.75	10.81 ± 1.63	—	−24.2	NS
PRI (mg/day)	8	628.1 ± 116.1	628.1 ± 116.1	—	None	—
PRI (mg/kg/day)	8	12.54 ± 2.73	12.21 ± 2.31	—	−2.6	NS
PRI (μg/ml serum)	8	6.16 ± 1.86	5.34 ± 2.43	—	−13.3	NS
PRI (C/D ratio)	8	0.53 ± 0.22	0.46 ± 0.21	—	−13.2	NS
Time interval (mo) to AED reassay	16	—	6 ± 3	—	—	—
Group B: PHZ increased at constant AED regimen (n = 19)						
PHZ (mg/day)	19	—	186.4 ± 112.2	315.8 ± 167.3	69.4	p < 0.01 (T = 2.7896)
PHZ (mg/kg/day)	19	—	3.16 ± 2.13	5.04 ± 3.02	59.5	p < 0.025 (T = 2.4394)
PHT (mg/day)	18	—	344.7 ± 60.2	344.7 ± 60.2	None	—
PHT (mg/kg/day)	18	—	5.76 ± 1.23	5.73 ± 1.24	−0.5	NS
PHT (μg/ml serum)	18	—	18.92 ± 4.69	12.70 ± 4.63	−32.9	p < 0.001 (T = 4.5781)
PHT (C/D ratio)	18	—	3.65 ± 1.26	2.36 ± 1.19	−35.3	p < 0.005 (T = 3.5596)
PB (mg/day)	8	—	101.3 ± 20.3	101.3 ± 20.3	None	—
PB (mg/kg/day)	8	—	1.77 ± 0.59	1.79 ± 0.61	−1.1	NS
PB (μg/ml serum)	13[c]	—	22.81 ± 7.61	18.05 ± 5.35	−20.9	NS
PB (C/D ratio)	8	—	12.61 ± 3.06	10.56 ± 1.73	−16.3	NS
PRI (mg/day)	5	—	800.0 ± 189.6	800.0 ± 189.6	None	—
PRI (mg/kg/day)	5	—	11.36 ± 1.22	11.11 ± 1.65	−2.2	NS
PRI (μg/ml serum)	5	—	7.46 ± 2.58	5.76 ± 1.23	−22.8	NS
PRI (C/D ratio)	5	—	0.63 ± 0.23	0.55 ± 0.22	−12.7	NS
Time interval (mo) to AED reassay	19	—	—	4.8 ± 1.6	—	—

Group A = 10 women and 6 men; aged 30.9 ± 7.1 yr, thioridazine (n = 7), chlorpromazine (n = 6), and mesoridazine (n = 3). Group B = 10 women and 9 men; aged 34.5 ± 10.9 yr, thioridazine (n = 11), chlorpromazine (n = 1), and mesoridazine (n = 7). PHT, phenytoin; PB, phenobarbital; PRI, primidone.

[a]All characteristics are means ± SD.

[b]C/D ratio = μg/ml serum per mg/kg/day dose.

[c]Includes phenobarbital derived from primidone.

on the most appropriate pharmaceutical intervention. Retrospectively, manual search through our records identified those patients for whom PHZ comedication was started, dosages were increased or decreased, or PHZs were discontinued. Most importantly, these patients were selected because the changes in PHZs were made at constant AED dosages and between two consecutive steady-state AED concentration determinations.

Here we describe preliminary results on interactions of PHT, PB, and primidone (PRI) with PHZs: thioridazine (Mellaril), chlorpromazine (Thorazine), and mesoridazine (Serentil).

MATERIALS AND METHODS

Ninety-two epileptic patients (44 women, 48 men) with a mean age of 32 years (range 15–66 years) were involved in the study. The mean interval between the two consecutive AED concentration determinations at constant AED dosages was 6 months (range 1–9 months). Either PHZs were added (n = 16) to the antiepileptic drug regimen or dosages were increased (n = 19), decreased (n = 23), or discontinued (n = 34) at some unspecified time within the indicated limiting interval. Blood was drawn after an overnight food and drug fasting state.

Therapeutic Drug Monitoring
7:405–410 © 1985 Raven Press, New York

Michaelis-Menten Kinetics and the Steady-State Serum Phenytoin/Hydroxyphenytoin Ratio

Blaise F. D. Bourgeois and Nils Wad

Swiss Epilepsy Center, Zurich, Switzerland

Summary: The effect of nonlinear kinetics on the steady-state ratio of serum phenytoin (PHT) to total 5-(*p*-hydroxyphenyl)-5-phenylhydantoin (*p*-HPPH) was studied in epileptic patients. In each patient, the ratio increased in a nonlinear fashion in relation to both the PHT dose and the PHT serum level. Patients with longer apparent PHT half-lives ($t_{50\%}$) had a higher PHT/*p*-HPPH ratio. The $t_{50\%}$ was either measured directly and found to correlate well with the patient's calculated Michaelis-Menten parameters (V_{max} and K_m), or was calculated from V_{max} and K_m values. A close linear correlation was found between the steady-state PHT/*p*-HPPH ratio and $t_{50\%}$ values, interindividually and intraindividually, i.e., as the $t_{50\%}$ increased with increasing PHT concentration in a given patient, the PHT/*p*-HPPH ratio increased in the same proportion. This indicates a good correlation between the overall Michaelis-Menten kinetics of PHT elimination and the PHT/*p*-HPPH ratio. A close linear correlation between a wide range of PHT doses and steady-state serum total *p*-HPPH levels was found, suggesting that when the PHT dose is lower than V_{max}, the fraction of PHT undergoing parahydroxylation is constant. It is concluded that if, in a given patient, the *p*-HPPH level corresponds to the value expected from the PHT dose, it can be assumed that compliance and bioavailability are adequate and that the dose does not exceed V_{max}. In that case, the PHT/*p*-HPPH ratio will provide a good estimate of the $t_{50\%}$ of PHT at that particular PHT level. **Key Words:** Serum phenytoin—Serum 5-(*p*-hydroxyphenyl)-5-phenylhydantoin—Phenytoin half-life—Urinary excretion.

Hydroxylation to 5-(*p*-hydroxyphenyl)-5-phenylhydantoin (*p*-HPPH) is the major pathway in the enzymatic biotransformation of phenytoin (PHT), since urinary *p*-HPPH conjugated with glucuronic acid accounts for 60–80% of the PHT dose (1–6). Unchanged PHT is also excreted in the urine, but it represents in most cases <2% of the dose (5,6). The urinary *p*-HPPH/PHT ratio reflects the rate of metabolism and can be used to distinguish between fast and slow hydroxylators (7,8). In serum or plasma, *p*-HPPH is present mainly in its conjugated form as a glucuronide (5,9–11). Using total *p*-HPPH levels, Glazko et al. (6) demonstrated a relationship between PHT elimination half-life and plasma PHT/*p*-HPPH ratio after 15 days of PHT administration in volunteers. Because of nonlinear kinetics, PHT has only an apparent half-life ($t_{50\%}$), since the $t_{50\%}$ is dependent upon the initial concentration at which it is determined, and its value increases with increasing PHT concentrations in adults (12,13) as well as in children (14) and newborns (15). If the PHT/*p*-HPPH ratio is proportional to the apparent $t_{50\%}$ of PHT, this ratio must be concentration-dependent. We have investigated the effect of nonlinear PHT kinetics on the steady-state PHT/*p*-HPPH ratio in epileptic patients on chronic PHT therapy.

Address correspondence and reprint requests to Dr. B. F. D. Bourgeois at Swiss Epilepsy Center, Bleulerstrasse 60, CH-8008 Zurich, Switzerland.

METHODS

Subjects included in the study were epileptic inpatients of the Swiss Epilepsy Center. All were taking at least one antiepileptic drug in addition to PHT, with no change in drug regimen during the study period. The daily dose of PHT was divided in three doses, and all PHT doses were calculated in terms of PHT acid. Drug compliance was ascertained by the nursing staff. Patients were selected randomly or because of suspected slow or fast PHT metabolism. All patients had normal blood urea nitrogen values and no history of renal dysfunction. Blood samples for the determination of PHT and total *p*-HPPH were obtained in the morning prior to the first dose of the day in a total of 21 patients, whose ages ranged from 11.5 to 60 years (mean 26.6 years; SD, ± 13.4). In 10 patients, blood samples were obtained at two or three different doses. All patients were considered to be under steady-state conditions, either on the basis of repeated PHT levels or because a minimum of 2 weeks had elapsed after any change in PHT dosage (4 weeks in patients with relatively slow elimination). Collection of 24-h urine at steady state for the determination of PHT and *p*-HPPH was carried out in 11 patients (in one patient at two different PHT doses). In seven patients, the nonlinear kinetics of PHT were defined by determining the apparent V_{max} (maximum rate of elimination, mg/kg/day) and the apparent K_m (Michaelis constant or serum concentration at which $V_{max}/2$ is achieved). The determination of apparent V_{max} and K_m was based on the fact that at steady-state concentrations (C_{ss}, mg/L), the enzymatic reaction velocity v is equal to the rate of administration R (mg/kg/day) (16):

$$v = R = \frac{V_{max} \cdot C_{ss}}{K_m + C_{ss}} \tag{1}$$

V_{max} and K_m were calculated with two or three C_{ss}-dosage pairs, using the equation (16,17):

$$\frac{R}{C_{ss}} = \frac{V_{max}}{K_m} - \frac{1}{K_m} \cdot R \tag{2}$$

and least-squares regression analysis of R/C_{ss} versus R. In the same seven patients, the $t_{50\%}$ of PHT was measured under steady-state conditions (see Table 1). The $t_{50\%}$ value is defined as the time required for the concentration to decrease from an initial value (C_i) to $C_i/2$ during the elimination phase. In the case of Michaelis-Menten kinetics, $t_{50\%}$ is concentration-dependent, and the following equation for $t_{50\%}$ is rearranged from an equation derived by Gerber and Wagner (18; see also 19):

$$t_{50\%} = \frac{0.5\ C_i}{V_{max}} + \frac{K_m}{V_{max}} \cdot \ln 2 \tag{3}$$

TABLE 1. *Pharmacokinetic data of seven patients in whom the apparent half-life ($t_{50\%}$) of phenytoin was measured at steady state*

Subject no.	C_{ss} (=C_i)[a] (μM)	$t_{50\%}$ (h)	Serum PHT/ *p*-HPPH	K_m (mg/L)	V_{max} (mg/kg/day)
1	43	38.5	10.2	6.76	3.83
2	52	22.3	5.1	2.43	7.40
3	78	48.2	11.1	5.20	4.86
4	33	23.7	4.3	5.74	5.31
5	78	78.3	19.5	22.70	5.54
6	78	35.5	7.7	4.90	7.04
	26	17.0	3.2		
7	29	14.3	2.7	5.16	10.35

[a] C_{ss}, steady-state serum phenytoin level prior to the first dose of the day. C_i, initial concentration at which the apparent elimination $t_{50\%}$ of phenytoin was measured. C_i is equal to C_{ss} in all cases.

The initial serum level of PHT (C_i) used for the determination of $t_{50\%}$ was always the steady-state level prior to the first dose of the day (C_{ss}), and the lowest level used was the one closest to $C_{ss}/2$. The $t_{50\%}$ value was calculated by linear regression analysis of the logarithm of the concentrations versus time, using a minimum of four points. In one patient, $t_{50\%}$ was determined at a second C_{ss} while PHT was being discontinued. In the other patients, determining $t_{50\%}$ at a second C_{ss} was considered to be an excessive interference with therapy, and therefore, estimates of $t_{50\%}$ were calculated by using Eq. 3. For this purpose, V_{max} was converted from mg/kg/day to mg/L/h under the assumption of complete bioavailability and a volume of distribution of 0.65 L/kg (20).

Serum and urinary concentrations of PHT were determined by high performance liquid chromatography according to a method published previously (21). The same method was used for the determination of total (unbound + conjugated) *p*-HPPH. Urine samples (100 μl) and serum samples (500 μl) for the determination of total *p*-HPPH were incubated overnight at 37°C with 150 units of β-glucuronidase. The day-to-day coefficient of variation of *p*-HPPH was 5.1% in serum and 4.8% in urine. All results were expressed in μ*M* but converted to mg/L (conversion factor 3.97) when used in Eq. 1, 2, and 3. For statistical analysis, least-squares regression analysis was carried out with a programmable calculator (Texas Instruments 59), using the *t* statistic to test significance of the correlation.

RESULTS

The relationship between the PHT dose and the steady-state serum PHT/*p*-HPPH ratio is shown in

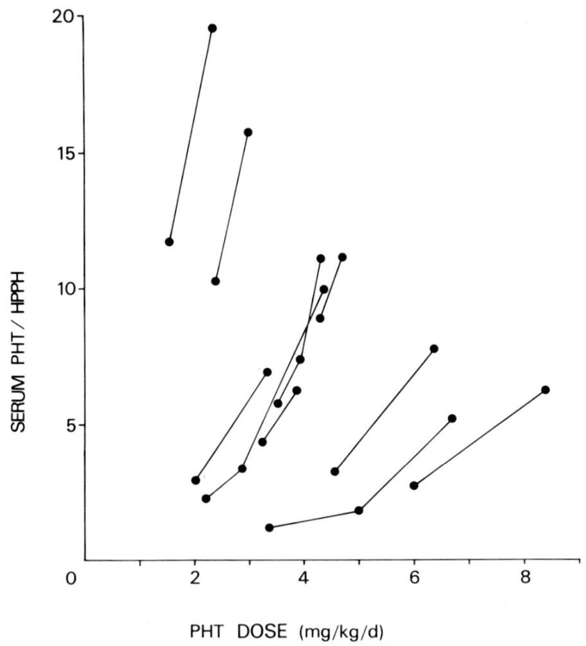

FIG. 1. Relationship between phenytoin (PHT) dose and serum PHT/5-(*p*-hydroxyphenyl)-5-phenylhydantoin (*p*-HPPH) ratio. Data pairs from the same patient are connected by a line.

Fig. 1. Although there is no apparent relationship for the entire group of patients, in each patient the ratio increases in a nonlinear manner. A similar nonlinear relationship between serum PHT level and PHT/*p*-HPPH ratio is shown in Fig. 2. The values for the $t_{50\%}$

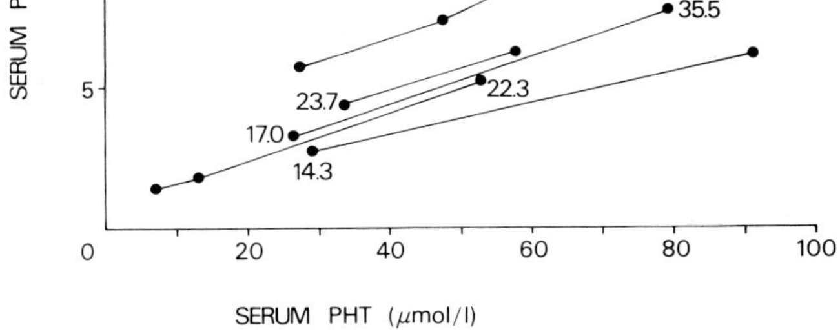

FIG. 2. Relationship between phenytoin (PHT) steady-state serum level and serum PHT/5-(*p*-hydroxyphenyl)-5-phenylhydantoin (*p*-HPPH) ratio. Numbers indicate apparent PHT half-life measured at the corresponding PHT level. Data pairs from the same patient are connected by a line.

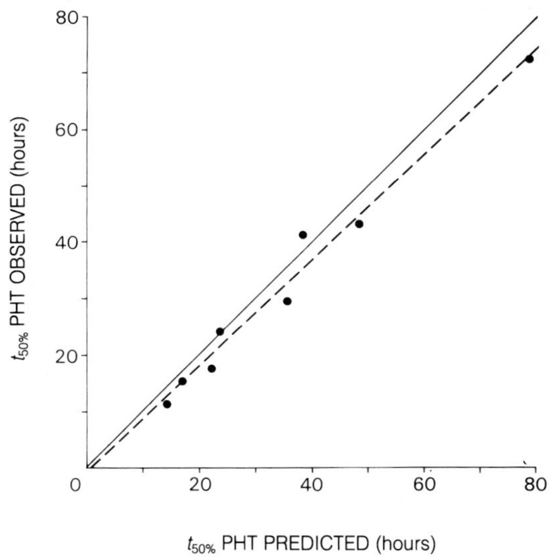

FIG. 3. Relationship between observed apparent phenytoin (PHT) half-life ($t_{50\%}$) and half-life predicted by using Eq. 3. The solid line is the line of identity, the dashed line is the regression line (n = 8; $r = 0.989$; $p < 0.001$; $y = 0.94x - 1.20$).

of PHT shown in this figure indicate that two factors are associated with a higher PHT/*p*-HPPH ratio: higher PHT levels and longer PHT $t_{50\%}$. The latter is particularly apparent in the three patients in whom the $t_{50\%}$ was determined at an initial concentration of 78 μM. In a group of seven patients, the relationship between the PHT/*p*-HPPH ratio and $t_{50\%}$ was therefore analyzed interindividually as well as intraindividually, i.e., in the same patient at different PHT levels. The pharmacokinetic data of the seven patients are indicated in Table 1. In six of the seven patients, a second $t_{50\%}$ value at a different C_i was predicted by using Eq. 3. Figure 3 illustrates the correlation between measured $t_{50\%}$ and $t_{50\%}$ predicted from Eq. 3 at the same C_i, using the patient's V_{max} and K_m values. Overall predicted $t_{50\%}$ were slightly lower than measured $t_{50\%}$, perhaps because V_{max} and K_m determinations were based on morning C_{ss} values and not on average C_{ss} values, which tends to give an overestimation of V_{max} and underestimation of K_m. As shown in Fig. 4, there is a close linear relationship between the serum PHT/*p*-HPPH ratio and the $t_{50\%}$ of PHT, not only among different patients, but also within a given patient at different PHT concentrations.

When the relationship between PHT dose and steady-state serum total *p*-HPPH levels was analyzed, a significant linear correlation was found for the entire group of data pairs, and individual patients showed a fairly constant ratio at different doses (Fig. 5). The corresponding relationship between dose and PHT level

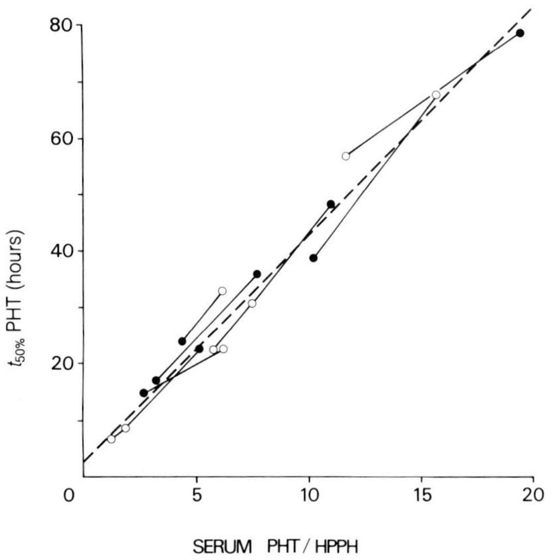

FIG. 4. Relationship between steady-state serum phenytoin (PHT))/5-(*p*-hydroxyphenyl)-5-phenylhydantoin (*p*-HPPH) ratio and apparent PHT half-life ($t_{50\%}$) at the same PHT level. Data pairs from the same patient are connected by a line. Measured $t_{50\%}$ values are represented by full circles, predicted values by open circles. The dashed line is the least-squares regression line (n = 16; $r = 0.986$; $p < 0.001$; $y = 4.0x + 2.8$).

for the same serum samples was not significant (n = 34; $r = 0.114$). Because of the heterogeneity of drug regimens, no difference between various drug combinations and the relationship between PHT dose and *p*-HPPH levels or PHT/*p*-HPPH ratios could be found.

Urinary PHT and *p*-HPPH values were obtained for comparison. There was a significant linear relation-

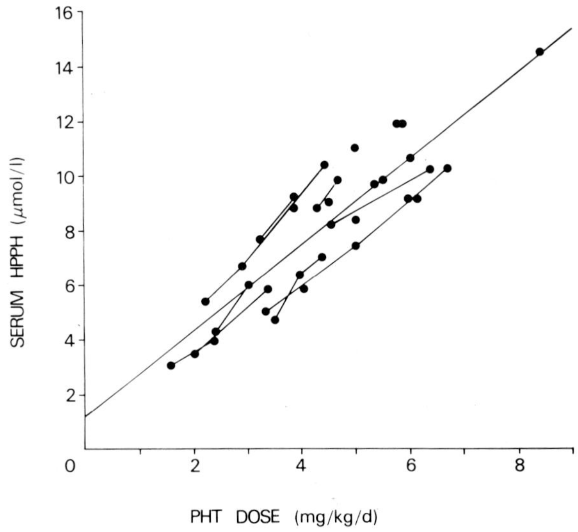

FIG. 5. Relationship between phenytoin (PHT) dose and steady-state serum 5-(*p*-hydroxyphenyl)-5-phenylhydantoin (*p*-HPPH) level. Data pairs from the same patient are connected by a line (n = 34; $r = 0.888$; $p < 0.001$; $y = 1.56x + 1.25$).

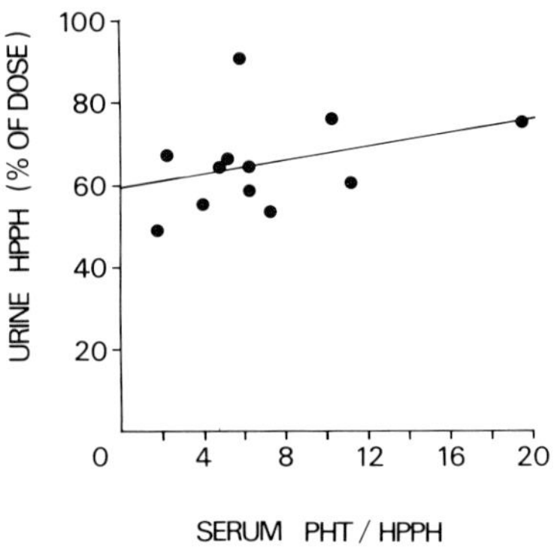

FIG. 6. Relationship between steady-state serum phenytoin (PHT)/5-(*p*-hydroxyphenyl)-5-phenylhydantoin (*p*-HPPH) ratio and corresponding 24-h urinary excretion of *p*-HPPH as percent of the dose. The relationship is not statistically significant (n = 12; $r = 0.345$).

ship between the serum and urine PHT/*p*-HPPH ratio (n = 12; $r = 0.970$; $y = 194.1x + 1.3$), as well as between $t_{50\%}$ and urinary PHT/*p*-HPPH (n = 6; $r = 0.983$; $y = 709.2x + 10.7$). The 24-h urinary excretion in percentage of the PHT dose was 1.7 ± 1.97 (mean ± SD) for PHT and 65.0 ± 12.3 for *p*-HPPH. There was no significant relationship between the 24-h urinary excretion of *p*-HPPH in the percentage of the PHT dose and either the PHT dose (n = 12; $r = 0.363$), the PHT $t_{50\%}$ (n = 6; $r = 0.524$) or the serum PHT/*p*-HPPH ratio (Fig. 6).

DISCUSSION

The purpose of the present study was to analyze the correlation between Michaelis-Menten kinetics and the steady-state serum ratio between PHT and total *p*-HPPH. Although there is no apparent relationship between the PHT dose and the serum PHT/*p*-HPPH ratio for the patient population as a whole, the finding of a nonlinear increase of the ratio with increasing PHT dose for each patient individually is consistent with nonlinear kinetics. Hoppel et al. (11) found no correlation between the PHT dose and the ratio of PHT to unconjugated or conjugated *p*-HPPH, and their suggestion that this may be due to interindividual differences is confirmed by the present results. The present study also shows an increase of the PHT/*p*-HPPH ratio at higher PHT steady-state levels in every patient. Comparison with $t_{50\%}$ values at different PHT steady-state levels indicates that two factors contribute to an increase of the PHT/*p*-HPPH ratio: longer $t_{50\%}$ values as shown by Glazko et al. (6) as well as higher PHT levels. Since, in any given patient, $t_{50\%}$ is itself concentration-dependent, these results suggest a direct relationship between $t_{50\%}$ and the PHT/*p*-HPPH ratio, not only in different patients, but also in a given patient at different concentrations. A direct linear correlation could be clearly demonstrated. This indicates that two patients showing the same $t_{50\%}$ will have a similar PHT/p-HPPH ratio, even if the $t_{50\%}$ was determined at different initial concentrations, and that in a given patient, the PHT/p-HPPH ratio will increase in the same proportion as $t_{50\%}$ with increasing PHT steady-state levels. This analysis was based not only on actually measured $t_{50\%}$ values, but also on values predicted according to Eq. 3, using the calculated Michaelis-Menten parameters V_{max} and K_m.

The fact that measured $t_{50\%}$ values correlate well with predicted values, and measured $t_{50\%}$ values as well as those predicted from Michaelis-Menten parameters correlate closely with the PHT/p-HPPH ratio, indicates that this ratio follows the overall Michaelis-Menten kinetics of PHT elimination in any given patient.

In the present study, a significant linear correlation between PHT dose and steady-state serum total p-HPPH level was found. At doses below V_{max}, such a relationship is in agreement with kinetic analysis. The serum steady-state level of unconjugated p-HPPH is determined by its rate of formation and its rate of elimination. The rate of formation is equal to the velocity v of PHT biotransformation (Eq. 1) multiplied by the fraction f of PHT undergoing parahydroxylation. At steady state, v is equal to the dose R, and the rate of formation of unconjugated p-HPPH is $R \cdot f$, i.e., proportional to the dose. The increased urinary losses of PHT at higher PHT levels are negligible, because only a small percentage of the PHT dose (average $<2\%$) is excreted unchanged by the kidneys. The elimination of unconjugated p-HPPH is determined by the rate of glucuronidation and by the renal clearance. A linear relationship between PHT dose and total p-HPPH levels can therefore be expected, but it implies, first, that the fraction f is not dose-dependent, and second, that all processes beyond the parahydroxylation of PHT (i.e., glucuroconjugation and renal excretion) are first-order processes without pronounced interindividual variability. The rate of glucuroconjugation can be expected to affect the total p-HPPH level, since the renal clearance has been shown to be higher for conjugated than for unconjugatd p-HPPH (5).

A linear relationship between p-HPPH concentration and its renal excretion has been demonstrated (9) and is suggested also by the good linear correlation found in the present study between serum and urine PHT/p-HPPH ratios. A lack of dose-dependency for f is suggested not only by the linear relationship between dose and p-HPPH level over a wide range of doses in several patients, but also by the fact that we found no correlation between the percentage of a PHT dose excreted in urine as p-HPPH and either the PHT dose, the PHT $t_{50\%}$, or the serum PHT/p-HPPH ratio. The relationship between PHT dose and serum p-HPPH seems to be particularly stable in a given patient (Fig. 5). Differences between patients could be due to interindividual variability with regard to the fraction of PHT undergoing parahydroxylation, the rate of glucuronidation, or the renal clearance. Impaired renal function is associated with a marked increase in serum p-HPPH levels (5,22). A relationship between the clearance of p-HPPH and the urine flow rate has been found in one study (23) but not in another (5). In conclusion to this analysis, since there is little renal elimination of unchanged PHT, there is no reason to expect nonlinearity between the p-HPPH level and the PHT dose at doses below V_{max}, despite Michaelis-Menten kinetics (Eq. 1), unless the fraction f decreases at higher PHT doses. Such a decrease of f would necessarily imply that the parahydroxylation of PHT is saturated at lower PHT levels than the other enzymatic pathways of PHT biotransformation. The results of the present study show no evidence of such selective saturation at therapeutic serum levels of PHT. In particular, in case of selective saturation, the relationship between $t_{50\%}$ and PHT/p-HPPH might not be linear, since $t_{50\%}$ reflects all processes involved in PHT elimination, and PHT/p-HPPH reflects parahydroxylation only.

All the correlations discussed in this article are valid only under strict steady-state conditions (i.e., when the PHT level as well as the p-HPPH level are at steady state) and when the dose is below V_{max}. When PHT reaches steady-state concentrations, p-HPPH has not yet reached its steady state, because only at this point does the rate of formation of p-HPPH reach a constant level. This is particularly important at high doses and in patients with slow PHT elimination. Prior to steady state, p-HPPH serum levels and urinary excretion will be lower in relation to the dose. When the PHT dose is above V_{max}, the rate of formation of p-HPPH has reached its maximum, and its level will no longer be proportional to the PHT dose. Also, the percentage of a PHT dose excreted as urinary p-HPPH will decrease. Doses near or above V_{max} might explain such reported decreases (24). We found no such trend in patients whose dose could be assumed to be below V_{max} (either because V_{max} was determined or because PHT reached a plateau level and did not accumulate).

On the basis of the present results, PHT and *p*-HPPH levels determined on a single blood sample obtained at steady-state in a patient with normal renal function can provide the following information: if the *p*-HPPH level corresponds to the value expected from the PHT dose, compliance and bioavailability are good, and the dose does not exceed V_{max}. In that case, the PHT/*p*-HPPH ratio will provide a good estimate of the $t_{50\%}$ of PHT at that particular PHT level. In case of impaired renal function, a urinary collection will be necessary in order to obtain the same information.

Acknowledgment: Dr. Bourgeois is the recipient of Research Grant No. 3.357-0.82 from the Swiss National Science Foundation. The authors wish to thank Mrs. H. Andai for secretarial help.

REFERENCES

1. Glazko AJ, Chang T, Baukema J, Dill WA, Goulet JR, Buchanan RA. Metabolic disposition of diphenylhydantoin in normal human subjects following intravenous administration. *Clin Pharmacol Ther* 1969;10:498–504.
2. Borofsky LG, Louis S, Kutt H. Diphenylhydantoin in children. Pharmacology and efficacy. *Neurology* 1973;23:967–72.
3. Maschner J, Bernhardt W. Ueberwachung der Langzeitmedikation mit Diphenylhydantoin. Gaschromatographische Bestimmung von Diphenylhydantoin und Hydroxy-Diphenylhydantoin. *Z Neurol* 1973;204:179–92.
4. Karlén B, Garle M, Rane A, Gutova M, Lindborg B. Assay of the major (4-hydroxylated) metabolites of diphenylhydantoin in human urine. *Eur J Clin Pharmacol* 1975;8:359–63.
5. Borga O, Hoppel C, Odar-Cederlöf I, Garle M. Plasma levels and renal excretion of phenytoin and its metabolites in patients with renal failure. *Clin Pharmacol Ther* 1979;26:306–14.
6. Glazko AJ, Peterson FE, Chang T, Dill WA, Smith TC, Buchanan RA. Phenytoin metabolism in subjects with long and short plasma half-lives. *Ther Drug Monit* 1982;4:281–92.
7. Albani M, Gabriel M, Toseland PA. The HPPH/phenytoin ratio in urine (phenytoinindex) as a parameter for phenytoin requirement prediction in childhood. In: Johannessen SI, Morselli PL, Pippenger CE, Richens A, Schmidt D, Meinardi H, eds. *Antiepileptic therapy: advances in drug monitoring*. New York: Raven Press, 1980:41–6.
8. de Wolff FA, Vermeij P, Ferrari MD, Buruma OJS, Breimer DD. Impairment of phenytoin parahydroxylation as a cause of severe intoxication. *Ther Drug Monit* 1983;5:213–5.
9. Dill WA, Baukema J, Chang T, Glazko AJ. Colorimetric assay of 5,5-diphenylhydantoin (Dilantin) and 5-(p-hydroxyphenyl)-5-phenylhydantoin. *Proc Soc Exp Biol Med* 1971;137:674–9.
10. Wilson JT, Höjer B, Rane A. Loading and conventional dose therapy with phenytoin in children: kinetic profile of parent drug and main metabolite in plasma. *Clin Pharmacol Ther* 1976;20:48–58.
11. Hoppel C, Garle M, Rane A, Sjöqvist F. Plasma concentrations of 5-(4-hydroxyphenyl)-5-phenylhydantoin in phenytoin-treated patients. *Clin Pharmacol Ther* 1977;21:294–300.
12. Arnold K, Gerber N. The rate of decline of diphenylhydantoin in human plasma. *Clin Pharmacol Ther* 1970;11:121–35.
13. Houghton GW, Richens A. Rate of elimination of tracer doses of phenytoin at different steady-state serum concentrations in epileptic patients. *Br J Clin Pharmacol* 1974;1:155–61.
14. Dodson WE. Phenytoin elimination in childhood: effect of concentration-dependent kinetics. *Neurology* 1980;30:196–9.
15. Bourgeois BFD, Dodson WE. Phenytoin elimination in newborns. *Neurology* 1983;33:173–8.
16. Ludden TM, Allen JP, Valutsky WA, et al. Individualization of phenytoin dosage regimens. *Clin Pharmacol Ther* 1977;21:287–93.
17. Martin E, Tozer TN, Sheiner LB, Riegelman S. The clinical pharmacokinetics of phenytoin. *J Pharmacokinet Biopharm* 1977;5:579–96.
18. Gerber N, Wagner JG. Explanation of dose-dependent decline of diphenylhydantoin plasma levels by fitting to the integrated form of the Michaelis-Menten equation. *Res Commun Chem Pathol Pharmacol* 1972;3:455–66.
19. Dodson WE. Pharmacology and therapeutics of epilepsy in childhood. In: Klawans HL, ed. *Clinical neuropharmacology*, vol. 4. New York: Raven Press, 1979:1–29.
20. Kostenbauder HB, Rapp RP, McGovern JP, et al. Bioavailability and single-dose pharmacokinetics of intramuscular phenytoin. *Clin Pharmacol Ther* 1975;18:449–56.
21. Wad N. Simultaneous determination of eleven antiepileptic compounds in serum by high-performance liquid chromatography. *J Chromatogr* 1984;305:127–33.
22. Letteri JM, Mellk H, Louis S, Kutt H, Durante P, Glazko AJ. Diphenylhydantoin metabolism in uremia. *N Engl J Med* 1971;285:648–52.
23. Bochner F, Hooper W, Tyrer J, Eadie M. Clinical implications of certain aspects of diphenylhydantoin metabolism. *Proc Aust Assoc Neurol* 1973;9:171–8.
24. Eadie MJ, Tyrer JH, Bochner F, Hooper WD. The elimination of phenytoin in man. *Clin Exp Pharmacol Physiol* 1976;3:217–24.

Therapeutic Drug Monitoring
7:411–414 © 1985 Raven Press, New York

Plasma Flupentixol Concentrations and Clinical Response in Acute Schizophrenia

A. E. Balant-Gorgia, R. Eisele, J. M. Aeschlimann, L. P. Balant, and G. Garrone

Unité de Monitoring Thérapeutique, Department of Psychiatry, University of Geneva, Geneva, Switzerland

Summary: Twenty-three acutely psychotic inpatients treated with flupentixol were included in the study. Steady-state plasma concentrations were compared with therapeutic outcome in a routine clinical setting. The threshold concentration for satisfactory antipsychotic effect appeared to be ~2 ng/ml. Controlled studies are needed to establish the existence and exact limits of a therapeutic window.
Key Words: Flupentixol—Plasma concentrations—Schizophrenia.

The active principle of Fluanxol, *cis*(Z)-flupentixol, a thioxanthene derivative, is a powerful neuroleptic with few sedative or cardiovascular side effects.

Unlike many other antipsychotics, flupentixol has no clinically active metabolites, and it is therefore a good probe drug for studying the relationship between plasma concentration and clinical response. We have performed such a study in 23 acutely psychotic inpatients undergoing routine clinical treatment. All subjects were hospitalized and treated independently by psychiatrists who were not part of the study.

METHODS

Patient Selection and Clinical Assessment

The 23 patients (Table 1) had a diagnosis of schizophrenia, paranoid type (n = 17), schizophrenia, undifferentiated type (n = 5), and schizophreniform disorder (n = 1) according to the *Diagnostic and Statistical Manual of Mental Disorders*, third edition (DSM-III) (1). The ages of the 16 male and seven female patients ranged from 18 to 54 years. The patients were hospitalized for acute psychotic relapse, and all were drug-free when they entered the study to be treated with flupentixol orally. Dosages were adjusted according to standard clinical criteria and ranged from 6 to 12 mg/day. The oral form of flupentixol, Fluanxol tablets or drops, is a 1:1 mixture of the active *cis*(Z)- and inactive *trans*(E)-isomer. Sedative medications were administered when necessary, and biperiden hydrochloride (Akineton) was used when needed to control extrapyramidal symptoms (Table 1).

Patients were evaluated by the Brief Psychiatric Rating Scale (BPRS) (2) on admission and subsequently at 10-day intervals.

Responders were defined, using the criteria of Magliozzi and co-workers (3), as those patients who experienced ≥50% improvement in ≥10 days.

Blood Sampling

Blood samples for assay of steady-state plasma levels of flupentixol were drawn by venipuncture into Venoject tubes containing EDTA as anticoagulant. Steady-state levels (4) were defined as those obtained at 8 a.m., 10 h after administration of the last dose of flupentixol, the identical dosage having been administered for at least 5 to 7 days.

Gas-Liquid Chromatographic Analysis

Plasma concentrations were analyzed by gas-liquid chromatography (5) on a Hewlett-Packard model 5880

Address correspondence and reprint requests to Dr. A. E. Balant-Gorgia at Unité de Monitoring Thérapeutique, Department of Psychiatry, University of Geneva, C. M. U.-CH-1211-Geneva 4, Switzerland.

TABLE 1. *Demographic data, percentage improvement, and flupentixol plasma concentrations*

DSM III diagnosis	Age	Sex	BPRS improvement (day 20) (%)	BPRS final improvement (days 30–60) (%)	Steady-state flupentixol plasma concentrations (ng/ml)	Antiparkinsonian drug	Sedative drug
Schizophrenia paranoid type							
1	52	M	18	47	3.6	—	Flurazepam[a] Levomepromazine[b]
2	54	M	64	64	2.9	Biperiden[c]	Flunitrazepam
3	25	M	53	53	2.2	—	—
4	23	M	46	46	1.7	Biperiden	—
5	19	M	18	44	1.5	Biperiden	Flurazepam
Schizophrenia undifferentiated type							
6	34	M	8	45	1.2	Biperiden	Levomepromazine
7	32	F	45	59	5.2	Biperiden	Flunitrazepam Oxazepam
Schizophrenia paranoid type							
8	37	F	43	43	1.8	Biperiden	Levomepromazine
9	24	M	53	53	1.8	—	Flurazepam Levomepromazine
Schizophrenia undifferentiated type							
10	22	F	3	61	2.9	Biperiden	—
Schizophrenia paranoid type							
11	28	M	—	49	1.8	Biperiden	—
12	45	M	45	55	4.2	—	Flunitrazepam Levomepromazine
13	28	M	—	28	2.1	—	—
14	40	F	—	66	1.9	—	—
15	28	F	18	65	1.5	—	Levomepromazine
16	26	F	50	50	2.3	—	—
Schizophrenia undifferentiated type							
17	30	M	19	32	1.7	Biperiden	—
Schizophreniform disorder							
18	27	M	—	49	1.5	—	—
Schizophrenia undifferentiated type							
19	23	M	52	52	1.9	Biperiden	Oxazepam
Schizophrenia paranoid type							
20	38	F	49	49	1.9	Biperiden	Bromazepam
21	30	M	30	48	1.8	—	Levomepromazine
22	24	M	42	52	2.8	—	Levomepromazine
23	18	M	27	27	3.5	Biperiden	Lormetazepam

BPRS, Brief Psychiatric Rating Scale, DSM III, Diagnostic and Statistical Manual of Mental Disorders (1).
[a]Benzodiazepines were administered at standard doses.
[b]Levomepromazine (Nozinan) was administered in small doses (between 25 and 100 mg/d) for its sedative effect.
[c]Doses of the antiparkinsonian drug biperiden hydrochloride (Akineton) varied from 2 to 4 mg/d.

or 5790 gas chromatograph equipped with a nitrogen-phosphorous detector. Separation was obtained with a 0.9 m column (2 mm internal diameter) packed with 2% OV-101 on Supelco port 80–100 mesh at a temperature of 260°C. A 2-ml sample of plasma was extracted with heptane-2-propanol. After centrifugation and evaporation to dryness at 40°C under a gentle stream of nitrogen, the samples were acetylated at 40°C during a 40-min period, and 5μl was then directly injected for the analysis.

A flupentixol analogue (Lu-9) or perphenazine was added as the internal standard. Calibration standards for flupentixol were prepared daily by adding 1, 2.5, 5, 7.5, and 10 ng of the active drug (*cis*(Z)-flupentixol) and 15 ng of Lu-9 or 25 ng of perphenazine to drug-free plasma. The lower limit of the method was 0.5 ng/ml (using a 2-ml extracted plasma sample). The within-day coefficients of variation (%) for identical samples were 9.30 at 1 ng/ml and 6.60 at 5 ng/ml. The measured values are divided by 2 to take into account the presence of inactive *trans*(E)-flupentixol (5).

Pilot Phase

In order to evaluate the relationship between the oral dose of Fluanxol and steady-state *cis*(Z)-flupentixol plasma concentrations, 40 plasma samples (including those obtained from our 23 patients) were selected from the routine monitoring data.

Statistical Methods

The total BPRS score, resulting from the summation of 18 items, was analyzed as a relative improvement of the score between the end of the treatment and the baseline value, as follows:

$$d(\text{BPRS}) = \frac{1 - \text{final (BPRS)}}{\text{Baseline BPRS}}$$

The stratification of the patient population was done according to the steady-state plasma concentrations. Two groups of equivalent size (i.e., 12 and 11 patients, respectively) were formed using a cutoff point of 2 ng/ml. The relationship between clinical response and plasma concentration range (i.e., below or above 2 ng/ml) was calculated using Fisher's exact test (6). Bilateral values under 0.05 were considered significant.

Pearson's correlation coefficient was used to assess the relationship between the orally administered dose and the measured steady-state plasma concentration.

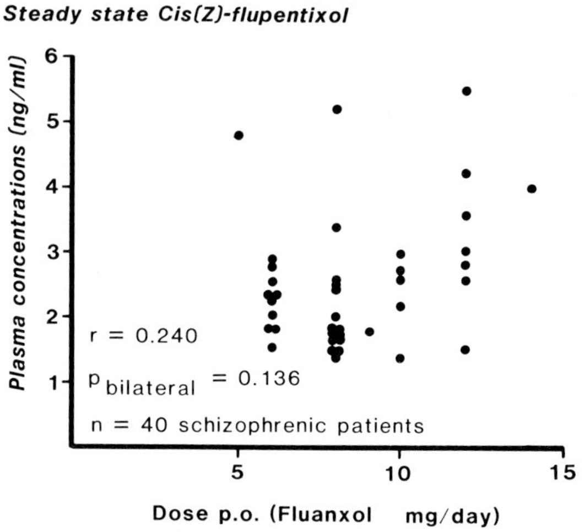

FIG. 1. Relationship between the prescribed oral dose of flupentixol in 40 schizophrenic patients and the measured steady-state plasma concentration.

RESULTS

There was a weak correlation ($r = 0.240$, $p_{\text{bilateral}} = 0.136$; 38*df*) between the oral dose of Fluanxol and the steady-state plasma concentrations of *cis*(Z)-flupentixol (Fig. 1), showing interindividual variability at all doses.

The distribution of the patients according to clinical response and steady-state plasma concentration is given in Tables 2 and 3 in Fig. 2. The value for Fisher's exact test in Table 3 (response vs. concentration) is $p = 0.026$, which is significant according to the chosen criteria.

DISCUSSION

Flupentixol undergoes extensive first-pass elimination (4), and its absolute bioavailability after oral administration is ~50%, with a range of ~20–70% (7).

Interindividual variability in the kinetics of the drug is pronounced, giving rise to fivefold differences in plasma concentrations at fixed dosages (8). The re-

TABLE 2. *Steady-state concentration and patient stratification*

Steady-state concentration (ng/ml)	n	Age (yr) Mean	Range	Sex M	F	End of treatment (days) 10	20	30	40	50	60
≤2	13	29.3	19–40	9	4	2	5	3	0	1	2
>2	10	35.7	22–54	7	3	0	4	4	1	0	1
Total (mean)	23	(32.8)		16	7	2	9	7	1	1	3

TABLE 3. *Steady-state concentration and clinical response*

Steady-state concentration (ng/ml)	No. of responders	No. of nonresponders (%)
1.2–1.9	4	9 (69)
2.1–5.2	8	2 (20)

p = 0.026, Fisher's exact test.

sults of our pilot study (Fig. 1) confirm these observations.

Flupentixol is a drug with a narrow therapeutic range, and extrapyramidal side effects are not uncommon, especially at higher doses (8).

The usefulness of the measurement of haloperidol plasma concentrations is now well documented (3,9–11) but data on flupentixol are relatively scarce. We intended to define the minimal steady-state plasma concentrations needed to optimize therapy, using an experimental protocol as close as possible to common clinical use of flupentixol.

Since intraindividual variations of flupentixol steady-state plasma concentrations (C_{ss}) were low, we used a "mean C_{ss}" for patients whose concentrations were measured at different occasions on the same oral dosage.

From our results (Table 3 and Fig. 2), it appears that the dose of Fluanxol should be individualized in order to reach a minimum C_{ss} of 2 ng/ml of the active

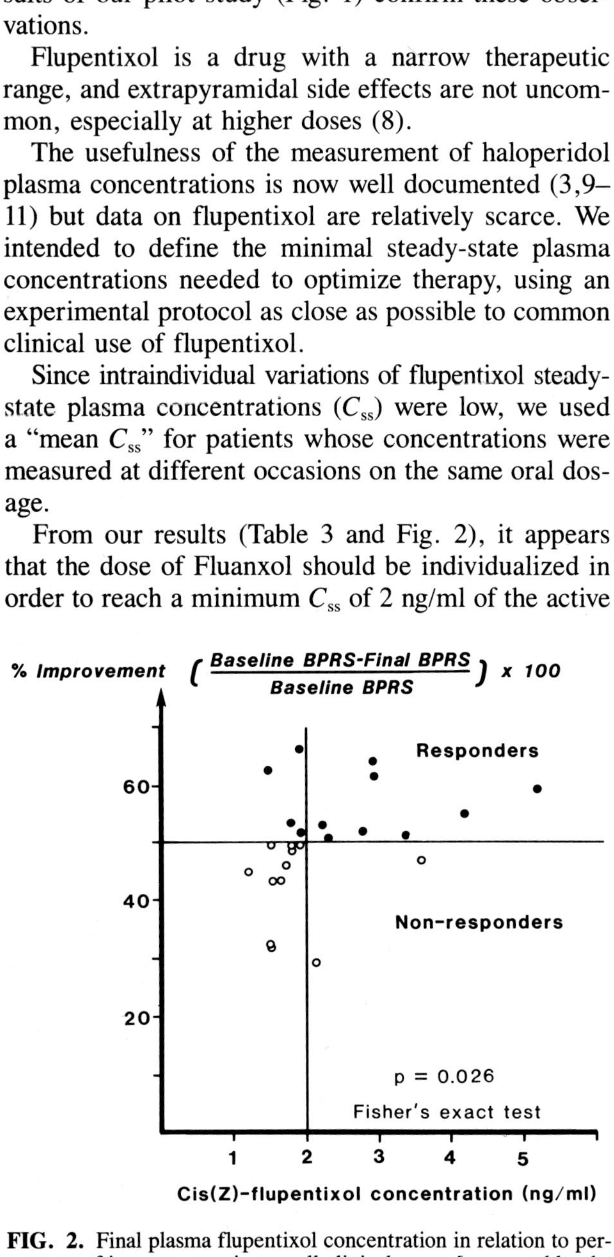

FIG. 2. Final plasma flupentixol concentration in relation to percentage of improvement in overall clinical status [measured by the Brief Psychiatric Rating Scale (BPRS)].

cis(Z)-flupentixol isomer. The fact that our patients were given an antiparkinsonian drug as soon as extrapyramidal side effects were observed does not allow us to define the maximally tolerated concentration of the drug to avoid these side effects.

Obviously, further data must be obtained in larger patient populations to define the therapeutic ranges of flupentixol plasma concentrations. The present study indicates, however, that plasma level monitoring of flupentixol might have a role in optimizing the clinical use of this potent antipsychotic drug. The cutoff point that best differentiated responders from nonresponders was 2 ng/ml, suggesting that this might be the minimum effective level of the drug. Controlled clinical studies are needed to verify this hypothesis.

Acknowledgment: The authors wish to thank Dr. A. Jørgensen and Dr. F. Schneller (Lundbeck) for the gift of the two isomers of flupentixol and the internal standard (Lu-9). They are also grateful for the skilled technical help of the technicians (I. Bandiera, Ch. Genet, and F. Piotton) of the Monitoring Laboratory.

REFERENCES

1. American Psychiatric Association. *Diagnostic and statistical manual of mental disorders*. 3rd ed. (French translation). Masson, Paris: 1983.
2. Overall JE, Gorhaus DR. The Brief Psychiatric Rating Scale. *Psychol Rep* 1962;10:799–812.
3. Magliozzi JR, Hollister LE, Arnold KV, Earle GM. Relationship of serum haloperidol levels to clinical response in schizophrenic patients. *Am J Psychiatry* 1981;138:365–7.
4. Jørgensen A. Pharmacokinetic studies in volunteers of intravenous and oral *cis*(Z)-flupentixol and intramuscular *cis*(Z)-flupentixol decanoate in Viscoleo. *Eur J Clin Pharmacol* 1980;18:355–60.
5. Balant-Gorgia AE, Balant LP, Genet Ch, Eisele R. Comparative determination of flupentixol in plasma by gas chromatograph and radioimmunoassay in schizophrenic patients. *Ther Drug Monit* 1985;7:229–35.
6. Fisher RA. The logic of inductive inference. *J Roy Stat Soc* (Series A) 1935;98:39–54.
7. Jørgensen A, Andersen J, Bjorndal N, Dencker SJ, Lundin L, Malm U. Serum concentrations of *cis*(Z)-flupentixol and prolactin in chronic schizophrenic patients treated with flupentixol and *cis*(Z)-flupentixol decanoate. *Psychopharmacology* 1982;77:58–65.
8. McCreadie RG, Flanagan WL, McKnight J, Jørgensen A. High dose flupentixol decanoate in chronic schizophrenia. *Br J Psychiatry* 1979;135:175–9.
9. Erickson SE, Hart SW, Chang S. Haloperidol dose plasma levels and clinical response: a double-blind study. *Psychopharmacol Bull* 1978;14:15–6.
10. Extein I, Augusthy KA, Gold MS, Pottash ALC, Martin D, Potter WZ. Plasma haloperidol levels and clinical response in acute schizophrenia. *Psychopharmacol Bull* 1982;18:156–8.
11. Miller DD, Hershey LA, Duffy JP, Abernethy DR, Greenblatt DJ. Serum haloperidol concentrations and clinical response in acute psychosis. *J Clin Psychopharmacol* 1984;4:305–10.

Therapeutic Drug Monitoring
7:415–420 © 1985 Raven Press, New York

Simultaneous Estimation of Serum Concentrations of Dapsone, Monoacetyldapsone, and Pyrimethamine in Chinese Men on Maloprim for Malaria Prophylaxis Using Reversed-Phase High Performance Liquid Chromatography

*H. S. Lee, *T. Y. Ti, †P. S. Lee, and †C. L. Yap

**Department of Pharmacology, Medical Faculty, National University of Singapore, and †Ministry of Defense, Singapore*

Summary: A reversed-phase high performance liquid chromatography method was developed to simultaneously estimate serum concentrations of dapsone (DDS), monoacetyldapsone (MADDS), and pyrimethamine (PYR) in 34 young adult Chinese men after they had taken the sixth weekly dose of Maloprim for malaria prophylaxis. Serum concentrations of DDS, MADDS, and PYR after 24 h were (mean ± SEM) 374 ± 31.3, 310 ± 30.4, and 121 ± 7.9 ng/ml, respectively. The 72-h serum concentrations of DDS, MADDS, and PYR were (mean ± SEM) 134 ± 21.6, 115 ± 17.9, and 80 ± 7.2 ng/ml, respectively. Serum concentrations of DDS and MADDS in many subjects after 120 h were <20 ng/ml, while mean ± SEM concentration of PYR was 53 ± 5.6 ng/ml. Acetylator phenotyping of the subjects showed that there were 31 (91%) fast acetylators, three (9%) intermediate acetylators, and no slow acetylators. **Key Words:** Reversed-phase high performance liquid chromatography—Dapsone—Monoacetyldapsone—Pyrimethamine—Malaria prophylaxis—Serum concentrations—Acetylator phenotype.

Dapsone (DDS) and pyrimethamine (PYR) is one of the drug combinations that may be used for chemoprophylaxis against chloroquine-resistant strains of *Plasmodium falciparum* (1). This combination is available as Maloprim (100 mg dapsone and 12.5 mg pyrimethamine per tablet).

Maloprim is used by the Singapore Armed Forces (SAF) for malaria chemoprophylaxis against chloroquine-resistant strains of *P. falciparum*. To study the serum concentrations of DDS and PYR, blood specimens were drawn from soldiers on chemoprophylaxis with Maloprim. We attempted to use the normal-phase high performance liquid chromatography (HPLC) analytical method reported by Jones and Ovenell (2) but found the method unsatisfactory for the following reasons: (a) Ammonium hydroxide and diisopropyl ether, present in the mobile phase, were volatile and hazardous; (b) Ammonium hydroxide did not mix well in the mobile phase, and it did not consistently maintain the pH of the mobile phase; and (c) A large serum peak, which could not be separated from PYR, was observed.

Therefore, a new reversed-phase HPLC method was developed to simultaneously estimate DDS and PYR in serum. A major metabolite, monoacetyldapsone (MADDS), was also estimated at the same time and from it the acetylator status of the individuals was determined. Philip et al. (3) had advocated the use of DDS as the drug of choice for acetylation phenotyping.

Address correspondence and reprint requests to Dr. H. S. Lee at Department of Pharmacology, Medical Faculty, National University of Singapore, Kent Ridge, Singapore 0511

MATERIALS

All reagents used were of chromatographic or analytical grade (E Merck, Darmstadt, or BDH Ltd). DDS [4,4′-diaminodiphenyl sulphone], MADDS [4-*N*-acetylamino-4′-aminodiphenyl sulphone], PYR [2,4-diamino-5-(4-chlorophenyl)-6-ethylpyrimidine], and metoprine [2,4-diamino-5-(3,4-dichlorophenyl)-6-methylpyrimidine] were supplied by the Wellcome Research Laboratory, Beckenham, Kent.

METHODS

Human Subjects

In the SAF, the routine schedule for taking Maloprim was as follows: one tablet before entering the malarious area, one tablet weekly during the stay in the malarious area, and one tablet weekly for 4 weeks after leaving the malarious area. To ensure compliance, a weekly parade for the administration of Maloprim was held. The regimental sergeant-major personally administered the Maloprim tablet to each soldier and inspected his oral cavity following the swallowing of the tablet. On the above schedule, blood samples were taken from 34 subjects at 24, 72, and 120 h following the sixth weekly dose of Maloprim. The blood samples were spun down immediately, and the separated serum samples were stored at −20°C until assayed.

The 34 Chinese male soldiers had a mean ± SEM age of 20.4 ± 0.2 years (range 20–26 years) and their mean ± SEM weight was 60 ± 0.75 kg (range 51–75 kg).

Extraction of Serum Samples

The extraction method used was a modification of that used by Jones and Ovenell (2); and Ahmad and Rogers (4). Metoprine 700 ng as the internal standard was routinely added to each 2 ml sample or calibrator, which was then alkalinized with 0.2 ml of 8 N NaOH. 12 ml of 1:2 dichloroethane was added, and the mixture was vortex-mixed for 1 min and centrifuged for 10 min at 900 *g*. The aqueous layer was aspirated off, and the organic layer was transferred to a conical tube. The organic extract was evaporated to dryness under a stream of nitrogen at 40°C. The residue was redissolved in 50 μl of mobile phase mixture just before injection into the HPLC. To prepare control calibrators, normal drug-free serum samples spiked with standard calibrators of DDS, MADDS, PYR, and the internal standard were subjected to the same extraction procedure. Results from these control calibrators were also compared with pure calibrators containing standards and the internal standard in water so as to determine the percentage recovery from the extraction procedure.

HPLC Assay Method

A Perkin Elmer Model Series 2 liquid chromatograph with a Perkin Elmer LC75 spectrophotometric detector was used. Concentration of the drugs and metabolite were determined by peak area (for DDS and MADDS) or peak height (for PYR) ratios of the drugs or metabolite with the internal standard. A Hewlett-Packard 3392A integrator was employed to obtain peak area ratios.

Samples were injected via a Rheodyn 7105 injector into the column (Hibar Lichrosorb RPC18, 10 μm, 250 × 4 mm). The mobile phase consisted of methanol (A) and 0.02 *M* phosphate buffer at pH 7.5 (B). Both solutions were filtered through 0.5- and 0.45-μm filters, respectively, and then degassed. The gradient elution program started at 32% methanol (A) in buffer (B) for 3 min, then increased at 2.5% per minute until the mixture contained 53% of (A) in (B) and was kept at this mixture until the end of the chromatogram. The flow rate of mobile phase was 1.5 ml/min. The UV detector wavelength used was 290 nm, which was optimum for all the components. Samples of chromatograms are shown in Fig. 1.

RESULTS

Using the internal standard method of calibration, it was found that the percentage recovery of the peak area or peak height ratios obtained for the whole range of control calibrators after extraction was about 94%. Specifically, they were 91 and 87% for DDS and MADDS, respectively, where the standards used ranged from 20 to 800 ng/ml. For PYR it was 103% where the range was from 20 to 375 ng/ml. The correlation coefficients between the peak area or peak height ratios and the serum concentrations were ≥0.9996 (Fig. 2). The calibration curves of DDS and MADDS were almost identical. The mean day-to-day coefficients of variation (CVs) of peak area or peak height ratios of calibrators from 8 calibration series were 13.8, 15.8, and 12.9% for DDS, MADDS, and PYR, respectively. The within-day CVs of four injections were 2.9 and 1.8% for 100 ng/ml DDS and MADDS, respectively, and 1.4% for 80 ng/ml PYR.

The chromatogram from the unspiked serum sample (Fig. 1a) showed a serum peak eluting at 5.94

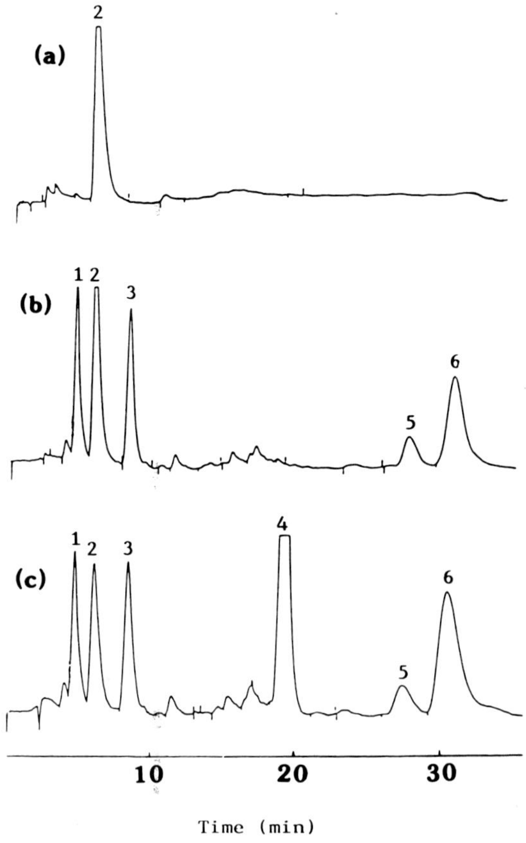

FIG. 1. Chromatograms of **(a)** extract of control human serum, **(b)** extract of control human serum spiked before extraction with calibration standards and internal standard, and **(c)** extract of subject serum spiked before extraction with internal standard. High performance liquid chromatography conditions as in text. Peaks: 1, dapsone; 2, serum peak; 3, monoacetyldapsone; 4, unknown metabolite; 5, pyrimethamine; 6, metoprine (internal standard).

min. This peak could be separated from DDS, eluting at 4.53 min, and MADDS, eluting at 8.41 min. PYR peaked at 28.32 min just before the internal standard, which eluted at 31.42 min (Fig. 1b). A very large peak, eluting at 19.7 min, was observed in every serum sample obtained from the subjects (Fig. 1c).

Table 1 shows the serum concentration of DDS, MADDS, and PYR in each individual 24, 72, and 120 h after the sixth weekly dose of Maloprim. Individual variations in serum concentrations of DDS, MADDS, and PYR were considerable. The mean ± SEM serum concentrations (ng/ml) of DDS, MADDS, and PYR after 24 h were 374 ± 31.3 (range 103–1,025), 310 ± 30.4 (range 90–840), and 121 ± 7.9 (range 37–228), respectively. After 72 h the serum concentrations of DDS, MADDS, and PYR were lower, and a number of the subjects had concentrations of <20 ng/ml. The mean ± SEM concentrations (ng/ml) of DDS, MADDS, and PYR were 134 ± 21.6 (range <20–532), 115 ± 17.9 (range <20–480) and 80 ± 7.2 (range <20–152), respectively. Serum concentrations fell with time, and by 120 h, i.e., the fifth day of the week, many subjects had DDS and MADDS concentrations <20 ng/ml, whereas concentrations of PYR in most subjects were still above the 20 ng/ml level with a mean ± SEM of 53 ± 5.6 ng/ml.

Using the 24- and 72-h serum concentrations, the calculated MADDS/DDS ratios resulted in values ranging from 0.29 to 1.45. The average ratios from these two different time samples were also obtained, and they ranged from 0.34 to 1.36 (Table 2). Based on other reports (5–7), MADDS/DDS ratios of <0.3 and >0.35 were used as criteria for slow and rapid acetylators, respectively. Our data showed that none of our subjects could be considered as a slow acetylator. Subject 8 had a ratio of 0.4 at the 24-h sample but 0.36 at the 72-h sample; subject 13 had a ratio of 0.34 at the 24-h sample, but the serum concentrations

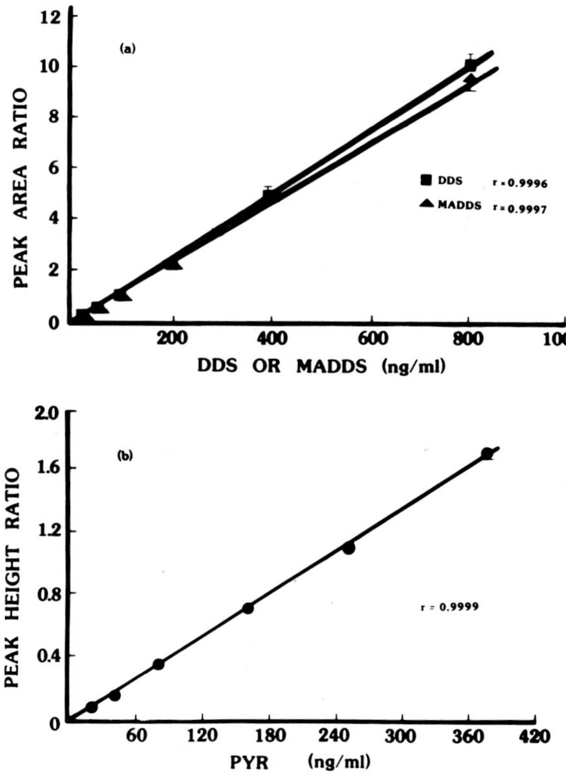

FIG. 2. Calibration curves of **(a)** dapsone (DDS) monoacetyldapsone (MADDS) (peak area ratios vs. concentrations) and **(b)** pyrimethamine (PYR) (peak height ratios vs. concentrations). Each point represents the mean ± SEM from eight sets of calibration curves.

TABLE 1. *Serum concentrations (ng/ml) of dapsone (DDS), monoacetyldapsone (MADDS), and pyrimethamine (PYR) in Chinese men 24, 72, and 120 h after the sixth weekly oral dose of Maloprim*

	24 h			72 h			120 h		
Subject	DDS	MADDS	PYR	DDS	MADDS	PYR	DDS	MADDS	PYR
1	405	400	150	105	113	90	72	72	65
2	375	300	177	150	140	110	63	38	70
3	305	305	NV	102	126	NV	<20	<20	NV
4	365	265	NV	87	110	NV	<20	20	NV
5	362	255	NV	55	80	<20	<20	<20	<20
6	237	180	73	50	36	<20	<20	<20	20
7	103	100	37	<20	<20	27	<20	<20	<20
8	650	262	82	360	129	76	142	57	29
9	291	194	113	178	100	42	38	<20	22
10	222	192	105	<20	20	43	<20	<20	29
11	170	198	40	<20	<20	19	<20	<20	<20
12	472	680	177	236	316	126	<20	<20	113
13	392	132	136	20	<20	<20	<20	<20	<20
14	472	502	228	64	75	130	<20	<20	90
15	444	512	164	65	68	100	<20	<20	86
16	186	110	137	<20	<20	112	<20	<20	97
17	186	224	182	20	50	152	<20	<20	61
18	210	90	141	34	<20	135	24	<20	115
19	228	200	185	26	34	127	<20	<20	82
20	530	590	118	380	300	108	<20	<20	102
21	593	840	156	377	480	137	97	160	62
22	1025	547	118	532	265	85	254	160	42
23	553	275	90	208	100	55	60	<20	33
24	435	330	138	162	130	96	<20	<20	71
25	435	525	112	160	192	85	92	122	47
26	557	335	100	240	175	96	95	90	70
27	258	235	120	105	100	96	<20	<20	52
28	408	417	130	197	242	113	50	80	61
29	360	105	129	132	55	72	<20	<20	72
30	188	228	90	35	33	58	<20	<20	33
31	263	250	76	68	87	44	<20	<20	24
32	568	288	101	200	106	85	50	28	63
33	298	332	73	118	128	45	58	63	<20
34	175	138	76	68	50	55	<20	<20	40
Range	103–1,025	90–840	37–228	<20–532	<20–480	<20–152	<20–254	<20–160	<20–115
Mean	374	310	121	134	115	80	38	33	53
SEM	31.3	30.4	7.9	21.6	17.9	7.2	8.7	7.4	5.6
n	34	34	31	34	34	32	34	34	32

Serum concentration <20 was taken to be 10 ng/ml for calculation of means ± SEM. NV, not valid.

at 72 h were too low to obtain the ratio; and subject 29 had a ratio of 0.29 at the 24-h sample but 0.42 at the 72-h sample. We considered these three subjects, of the total of 34 (3/34 = 9%), to be intermediate acetylators. The remaining 31 subjects (31/34 = 91%) were considered to be rapid acetylators. There were 14 subjects (41%) with ratios >1.00.

To investigate whether the rate of acetylation would affect the serum concentrations of DDS, we arbitrarily used the MADDS/DDS ratio of 0.7 to separate our subjects into two groups. We could not use the ratio 0.3 because all our subjects were either rapid or intermediate acetylators. Twenty-four subjects with MADDS/DDS ratios of >0.7 were considered to be in the faster (F) group, and the slower (S) group was made up of 10 subjects with MADDS/DDS ratios <0.7. It was found that the serum concentrations of DDS in the 24-h sample of the (F) group were statistically significantly lower ($p = 0.028$, analysis of variance using general linear model, statistical analysis system) when compared with the (S) group. The 72-h sample still showed a similar trend, but the difference was not statistically significant ($p = 0.095$). There was, however, no linear correlation between MADDS/DDS ratios and the serum DDS concentrations at the 24-h sample ($y = 0.00036x + 1.0222$, $r = -0.2177$, $p = 0.216$) or the 72-h sample ($y = 0.00033x + 0.9318$, $r = -0.1387$, $p = 0.434$). This finding is similar to that reported by Peters et al. (8).

TABLE 2. *Acetylator status determined from serum monoacetyldapsone/dapsone (MADDS/DDS) ratios at 24 and 72 h after the sixth weekly oral dose of Maloprim*

Subject	MADDS/DDS ratio		Average ratio	Acetylator status
	24 h	72 h		
1	0.99	1.27	1.13[a]	Rapid
2	0.80	0.93	0.87	Rapid
3	1.00	1.24	1.12[a]	Rapid
4	0.73	1.26	1.00	Rapid
5	0.70	1.45	1.08[a]	Rapid
6	0.76	0.72	0.74	Rapid
7	0.97	1.00	0.99	Rapid
8	0.40	0.36	0.38	Intermediate
9	0.67	0.56	0.62	Rapid
10	0.86	—	0.86	Rapid
11	1.16	—	1.16[a]	Rapid
12	1.44	1.34	1.39[a]	Rapid
13	0.34	—	0.34	Intermediate
14	1.06	1.17	1.12[a]	Rapid
15	1.15	—	1.15[a]	Rapid
16	0.59	—	0.59	Rapid
17	1.20	—	1.20[a]	Rapid
18	0.43	—	0.43	Rapid
19	0.88	—	0.88	Rapid
20	1.11	0.79	0.95	Rapid
21	1.42	1.30	1.36[a]	Rapid
22	0.53	0.50	0.52	Rapid
23	0.50	0.48	0.49	Rapid
24	0.76	0.80	0.78	Rapid
25	1.21	1.20	1.20[a]	Rapid
26	0.60	0.73	0.67	Rapid
27	0.91	0.95	0.93	Rapid
28	1.02	1.23	1.13[a]	Rapid
29	0.29	0.42	0.36	Intermediate
30	1.21	—	1.21[a]	Rapid
31	0.95	1.28	1.12[a]	Rapid
32	0.51	0.53	0.52	Rapid
33	1.11	1.08	1.10[a]	Rapid
34	0.79	0.74	0.77	Rapid

[a]Ratios >1.00, very rapid acetylators.

DISCUSSION

Our method, using the reversed-phase column and simple gradient mobile phase system, was less hazardous and more reproducible than the method of Jones and Ovenell (2), although each chromatogram took 35 min to complete. The serum peak that eluted at 5.94 min was well separated from DDS and MADDS. This serum peak was most probably caffeine, which was found to elute at exactly the same time. With this system, another major peak eluting at 19.70 min was observed. Since it was found in every serum sample of subjects who had taken Maloprim and not in the serum calibrators spiked with standards, it could be another major metabolite of either DDS or PYR. The nature of this metabolite is, however, not yet elucidated, but we are in the process of doing so. Recently, Edstein (9) published a method for the estimation of the components of Maloprim in plasma using reversed-phase ion-pair chromatography with pentane sulphonic acid as the counter ion. The method seemed simple and rapid, but the unknown major metabolite was not observed.

Although our group of subjects was quite uniform with regard to ethnic group, age, sex, and weight, we found tremendous variation in their serum concentrations of both DDS and PYR after the sixth weekly oral dose. The DDS concentrations were generally lower, especially the 24-h samples, when compared with those reported by Jones and Ovenell (2), whose subjects were three Caucasians from England and nine male Indians from Malaysia, all slow acetylators who had taken only one dose of Maloprim. Perhaps the very high percentage of rapid acetylators in our subjects could have contributed to the low serum concentrations of DDS. This possibility was further supported by our data that the serum DDS concentrations were significantly lower in our faster group (MADDS/DDS >0.7) of acetylators when compared with that in our slower group of acetylators. The rate of clearance, and the effect of multidosing on the rate of clearance of DDS and MADDS from the plasma in our subjects, were not known. If clearance was rapid, it could contribute to the low DDS levels as well. The difficulty with DDS is that its serum concentration could be further affected by the deacetylation of strongly protein bound MADDS back to DDS, even though this process was thought to be slower than the acetylation of DDS (10).

We have determined the acetylator phenotype of our subjects using the 24- and 72-h serum samples, but some of the concentrations of DDS at the 72-h samples were <20 ng/ml, and we could not use this sample for acetylator phenotyping for all the subjects. For those where the MADDS and DDS concentrations were >20 ng/ml at the 72-h sample, the MADDS/DDS ratios were similar to that of the 24-h sample for most subjects except for subjects 4 and 5. The differences in ratios obtained from different time samples of these two subjects did not, however, change their phenotype. In our group of Chinese males, 91% were rapid acetylators; this was indeed close to the 80–90% that was reported for the Oriental population by others (11,12). Nine percent of our subjects were intermediate acetylators, and there were no slow acetylators. It is not known whether the multidosing of Maloprim could have affected the serum concentrations of DDS and MADDS differently, thereby affecting the acetylator phenotyping.

The serum PYR concentrations in our subjects were considerably higher than those reported by Jones and Ovenell (2). This result was expected because the half-life of PYR is long and accumulation would have taken place in our multidosed subjects.

This reversed-phase HPLC method could be used to study the pharmacokinetics of Maloprim in different individuals, including the separation and isolation of the unknown major metabolite detected by this method. It can also be used to investigate whether there is any correlation between efficacy of chemoprophylaxis or manifestation of adverse drug reactions and serum drug concentration in the use of Maloprim and nonmalarial use of DDS.

Acknowledgment: We would like to thank Wellcome Research Laboratory for the supply of pure dapsone, monoacetyldapsone, pyrimethamine, and metoprine; Miss Y. M. Law, Miss G. H. Tan, and Mr. H. Lee for technical assistance; and Mrs. R. Lim for typing.

REFERENCES

1. Report of Meetings convened by The Ross Institute. Malaria prevention in travellers from the United Kingdom. *Br Med J* 1981;283:214–8.
2. Jones CR, Ovenell SM. Determination of plasma concentrations of dapsone, monoacetyldapsone and pyrimethamine in human subjects dosed with Maloprim. *J Chromatogr* 1979;163:179–85.
3. Philip PA, Roberts MS, Rogers HJ. A rapid method for determination of acetylation phenotype using dapsone. *Br J Clin Pharmacol* 1984;17:465–9.
4. Ahmad RA, Rogers HJ. Pharmacokinetics and protein binding interactions of dapsone and pyrimethamine. *Br J Clin Pharmacol* 1980;10:519–24.
5. Reidenberg MM, Drayer D, DeMarco AL, Bello CT. Hydralazine elimination in man. *Clin Pharmacol Ther* 1973;14:970–7.
6. Carr K, Oates JA, Nies AS, Woosley RL. Simultaneous analysis of dapsone and monoacetyldapsone employing high performance liquid chromatography: a rapid method for determination of acetylator phenotype. *Br J Clin Pharmacol* 1978;6:421–7.
7. Hanson A, Melander A, Wahlin-Boll E. Acetylator phenotyping: a comparison of the isoniazid and dapsone tests. *Eur J Clin Pharmacol* 1981;20:233–4.
8. Peters JH, Ross Gordon G, Ghoul DC, Tolentino JG, Walsh GP, Levy L. The disposition of the antileprotic drug dapsone (DDS) in Philippine subjects. *Am J Trop Med Hyg* 1972;21:450–7.
9. Edstein M. Quantification of antimalarial drugs. II. Simultaneous measurement of dapsone, monoacetyldapsone and pyrimethamine in human plasma. *J Chromatogr* 1984;307:426–31.
10. Gelber R, Peters JH, Ross Gordon G, Glazko AJ, Levy L. The polymorphic acetylation of dapsone in man. *Clin Pharmacol Ther* 1971;12:225–38.
11. Lunde PKM, Frislid K, Hansteen V. Disease and acetylation polymorphism. *Clin Pharmacokinet* 1977;2:182–97.
12. Ellard GA, Gammon PT. Acetylator phenotyping of tuberculosis patients using matrix isoniazid or sulphadimidine and its prognostic significance for treatment with several intermittent isoniazid-containing regimens. *Br J Clin Pharmacol* 1977;4:5–14.

Therapeutic Drug Monitoring
7:421–425 © 1985 Raven Press, New York

Computer Prediction of Serum Theophylline Concentrations in Ambulatory Patients

Paul A. Deci, *Larry M. Lopez, †J. Daniel Robinson, and †Ken Grauer

*Departments of Community Health, †Family Medicine, and *Pharmacy Practice, University of Florida Colleges of Medicine and Pharmacy, Gainesville, Florida, U.S.A.*

Summary: This study assessed the ability of a computer program Simulated Kinetics (SIMKIN) to predict serum theophylline concentrations in ambulatory patients receiving oral theophylline. Data were collected by retrospective review of prospectively obtained data. A total of only 20 measured serum theophylline concentrations could be included in the study, although records of 195 patients were reviewed. An estimated patient compliance of 90–110% was required and was computed using prescription refill information. Predicted serum theophylline concentrations were generated for each patient by entering into the SIMKIN program the characteristics pertinent to theophylline disposition and the patient's theophylline dosing regimen. Actual and SIMKIN-predicted theophylline concentrations were compared by using simple linear regression and by constructing a 95% confidence interval around the mean prediction error and root mean squared error. The ability of SIMKIN to predict therapeutic category, i.e., subtherapeutic, therapeutic, or toxic, was assessed using Fisher's exact test. SIMKIN predictions of individual theophylline concentration were insufficiently accurate to replace confirmatory followup monitoring of actual levels. However, SIMKIN was able to predict the therapeutic category with 70% accuracy. We conclude that SIMKIN may be useful for categorizing a dose regimen of theophylline as therapeutic, but that it is of little use in predicting individual concentrations in outpatients when literature-averaged pharmacokinetic parameters are the sole criteria for prediction, and compliance cannot be accurately assessed. **Key Words:** Asthma—Theophylline—Aminophylline—Pharmacokinetics.

Theophylline has a narrow range of therapeutic serum concentrations. Consequently, serum theophylline assays should be monitored periodically from patients receiving long-term theophylline treatment in order to maximize therapeutic benefits and minimize toxic effects (1). Serum theophylline assays are inconvenient, expensive, and uncomfortable for the patient. A more convenient and less costly way of evaluating a patient's serum theophylline concentration is needed. Computer programs that simulate drug serum concentrations as a function of time may partially fulfill this need.

SIMKIN (Simulated Kinetics) is an example of such a computer program, and it can be used in all ages of patients. It is an improved two-compartment (central-peripheral) computerized system with increased flexibility in modifying pharmacokinetic variables (2,3). Each of nine commonly monitored drugs has a preparatory program that allows the operator to enter age; sex; height; weight; pertinent laboratory parameters; and concomitant drugs, diseases, and social habits. Based upon these entries, pharmacokinetic parameters are set to the literature averages for each subgroup. This information, together with dose regi-

Address correspondence and reprint requests to Dr. L. M. Lopez at Box J-4; JHMHC, University of Florida, College of Pharmacy, Gainesville, FL 32610, U.S.A.

men of the drug in question, is subsequently passed to a simulation program, which graphically depicts change of serum drug concentration with time. Dose changes are recommended, which are designed to achieve the therapeutic range, but any dose may be entered for evaluation.

SIMKIN will also allow the operator to enter actual serum drug concentrations and fit data to further refine estimates of half-life and volume of distribution (4). Once these data are altered, SIMKIN recommends new dosage guidelines, which are also designed to attain the target concentration selected by the operator. The system operates on an IBM Personal Computer or an HP7470A Hewlett-Packard plotter.

Before such a system can be recommended for routine use in ambulatory practice, it is necessary to assess its ability to predict serum drug concentrations. Therefore, the goal of this study was to compare measured and SIMKIN-predicted serum theophylline concentrations (utilizing literature-averaged pharmacokinetic parameters only) from ambulatory patients receiving oral theophylline for chronic obstructive pulmonary disease.

METHODS

Subjects selected for the study were ambulatory patients treated by the Family Practice Medical Group, Inc. [(FPMG) Gainesville, FL, U.S.A.] All subjects were receiving oral theophylline for the treatment of chronic obstructive pulmonary disease, defined as asthma, chronic bronchitis, or emphysema. Each patient had at least one serum theophylline concentration measured by the FPMG Pharmacokinetic Service, using the enzyme multiplied immunoassay technique (EMIT). Each patient's compliance to prescribed theophylline was estimated as 90–110% for the month during which the serum theophylline concentration was obtained. Compliance was assessed by obtaining the following information from each patient's pharmacy: theophylline prescription refill dates, dosing regimen, and number of theophylline tablets dispensed for the stated time period. The number of theophylline doses purchased was divided by the number of theophylline doses prescribed, and the quotient was multiplied by 100%. Patients were excluded from the study if they had missed one or more theophylline doses during the 48 h before determination of the measured serum theophylline concentration.

Data were collected prospectively at the time of sample analysis. Retrospective review of all these medical records occurred after a sufficient sample size was obtained. Tabulated information from each patient included weight, sex, height, age(s), theophylline product (6,7), theophylline interactions, and measured serum theophylline concentrations. Dates, hours after previous dose, dosing regimen, and estimated patient compliance were also documented. Theophylline interactions adjusted for by SIMKIN are diet [high carbohydrate diet, high protein diet (8)], drugs [erythromycin (5,9), phenobarbital (10), propranolol (11), cimetidine (12), and phenytoin (13)], diseases [controlled or uncontrolled congestive heart failure (5), acute hepatitis (14), cholestasis (14), compensated or decompensated liver cirrhosis (14), and acute pulmonary edema (15)], and social habits [current smoker of marijuana or cigarettes, nonsmoker who stopped 6 to 12 months previously, nonsmoker who stopped less than 6 months previously (5,16,17)].

SIMKIN predicted serum theophylline concentrations were generated for each patient by entering required patient information into SIMKIN. SIMKIN, using mean pharmacokinetic parameters from medical literature, then generated a predicted serum theophylline concentration corresponding to the same time post-dose and dosing regimen of the measured concentration (4). Actual serum theophylline concentrations were measured using EMIT as described previously (18).

DATA ANALYSIS

Mean actual and predicted theophylline concentrations were compared using Student's t test for paired data. Individual values were compared using simple linear regression analysis. Multiplicative and additive biases were evaluated, respectively, by comparing observed slope with unity and observed y-intercept with zero using Student's t test. Bias and precision of SIMKIN-predicted values were further evaluated by constructing a 95% confidence interval around the mean prediction error (mpe) and root mean squared error (mse) for each group (19). The ability of SIMKIN to predict therapeutic or nontherapeutic concentrations was evaluated using Fisher's exact test. In all instances, observed differences in data were considered significant if the corresponding p value was <0.05.

RESULTS

One hundred ninety-five patients with a total of 337 serum theophylline concentrations were considered for the study. Twenty patients (10.2%) met selection criteria and were included in the study. One level was randomly selected from each of these patients and

TABLE 1. *Summary of patients*

Females	12
Males	8
Age (yr) (mean ± SD)	56 ± 15
Smokers	13
Heart failure	5
Hepatic cirrhosis	1
Total number	20

used for analysis. All but one patient were receiving an oral sustained-release theophylline product (Theo-Dur; Key Pharmaceuticals, Miami, FL, U.S.A.). One patient was taking another oral time-release theophylline product (Slo-Phyllin Gyrocaps; William H. Rorer, Inc., Fort Washington, PA, U.S.A.). Table 1 is a summary of patients entered in the study.

The ability of SIMKIN to predict actual serum theophylline concentrations based on literature-averaged pharmacokinetic parameters is summarized in Fig. 1 and Table 2. Data were analyzed for all patients and for previously identified subsets of the same patients. The observed differences between mean actual and predicted theophylline concentrations failed to achieve statistical significance for the entire group and for all subgroups analyzed.

Evaluation of predictive performance using linear regression revealed significant differences between *y*-intercept and zero for the entire group and for one subgroup, non-smokers. Significant differences between slope of regression lines and unity were noted for the entire group and four of the subgroups.

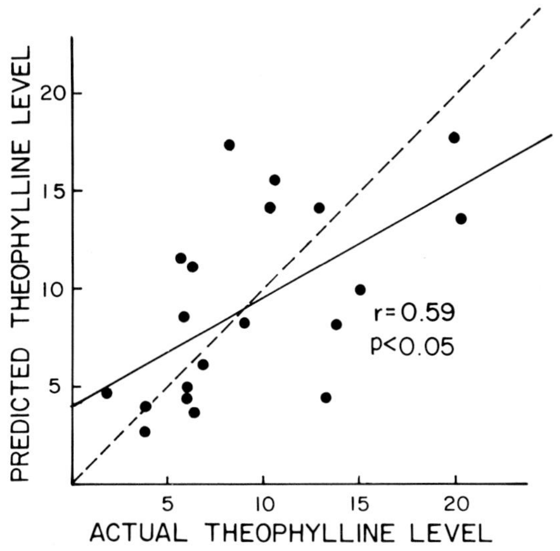

FIG. 1. Comparison of predicted and actual serum theophylline concentrations from 20 ambulatory patients. Solid line represents line of best fit. Dashed line represents line of perfect fit.

Correlation between actual and predicted theophylline concentrations for all patients was 0.59. Correlation coefficients for the various subgroups ranged from 0.39 for smokers to 0.91 for patients with congestive heart failure. Correlation coefficients for three subgroups were >0.71.

Further evaluation of bias and precision revealed subtle differences between actual and SIMKIN-predicted theophylline concentrations. Bias, i.e., mpe, of SIMKIN for all levels considered was in a positive direction. This direction, however, was variable when subgroups were analyzed, although all confidence intervals encompassed zero and overlapped with one another. Precision of SIMKIN, i.e., smallest rmse, was greatest in the subgroup of patients with controlled congestive heart failure. Confidence intervals for rmse encompassed zero in only three subgroups and not when all patients were considered. There was also considerable intergroup overlap in this parameter.

SIMKIN correctly predicted nine concentrations as subtherapeutic and five as therapeutic for a total of 14 correct predictions of 20 (70%). The program further predicted two concentrations of 20 (10%) as subtherapeutic when the concentrations were actually therapeutic, three concentrations of 20 (15%) as therapeutic when the concentrations were actually subtherapeutic, and one concentration of 20 (5%) as therapeutic when the concentration was toxic (20.2 μg/ml). The difference between this value and the upper end of the therapeutic range for theophylline is less than the sensitivity of the Syva EMIT theophylline assay (20). If this measured concentration is considered therapeutic instead of toxic, then SIMKIN correctly categorized 15 of 20 (75%) concentrations ($p < 0.05$).

DISCUSSION

SIMKIN accurately predicted group mean serum theophylline concentrations in adult patients. The program will accept patients of all ages, but no children were included in this study. All observed means of measured and predicted concentrations did not differ significantly. This finding may support use of mean pharmacokinetic values, which SIMKIN employs, but apparently is of little use in predicting individual theophylline levels in ambulatory patients using only literature-averaged pharmacokinetic parameters. This conclusion assumes that patient history and refill dates represent accurate determinants of compliance. Most studies indicate that, other than direct observation, there are no accurate methods of assessing compliance (21).

TABLE 2. *Comparison of actual and SIMKIN-predicted theophylline concentrations*

Groups analyzed (number of levels)	Theophylline levels (μg/ml) Actual	Theophylline levels (μg/ml) Predicted	Correlation coefficient	y-intercept (μg/ml)	Slope	mpe (μg/ml)	95% confidence interval for mpe (μg/ml)	rmse (μg/ml)	95% confidence interval—rmse (μg/ml)
One level/patient (20)	9.3	9.3	0.59	4.10[a]	0.56[a]	0.12	−2.01–2.25	4.44	2.12–6.76
Females (12)	10.7	10.9	0.60	3.90	0.65	−0.25	−3.29–2.79	4.57	1.47–7.67
Males (8)	8.3	8.0	0.64	3.30	0.56	0.38	−3.56–4.32	4.28	−0.47–9.03
Age 18–60 years (10)	9.1	8.8	0.44	3.60	0.58	0.23	−3.34–3.80	4.75	0.68–8.82
Age >60 years (10)	10.3	10.6	0.75	3.84	0.65	−0.23	−3.35–2.89	4.15	1.05–7.25
Smokers (13)	7.7	6.7	0.39	3.90	0.37[a]	1.37	−1.27–4.01	4.36	1.09–7.63
Nonsmokers (7)	13.7	15.4	0.50	12.6[b]	0.21[b]	−1.77	−6.17–2.63	4.75	0.42–9.08
Congestive heart failure, controlled (5)	12.0	12.8	0.91	0.18	1.05	−0.84	−4.53–2.85	2.80	−0.78–6.38
No congestive heart failure (15)	9.4	8.8	0.51	4.34	0.47[a]	1.61	−0.92–4.14	4.68	1.72–7.64
Level <3 hours after last dose (5)	10.4	13.9	0.82	1.20	1.20	−3.50	−8.27–1.27	4.91	−2.39–12.2
Level >3 hours after last dose (15)	9.7	8.9	0.62	3.70	0.53[a]	0.80	−1.40–3.00	4.22	1.89–6.55

[a] $p < 0.05$.
[b] $p < 0.01$.

SIMKIN did not accurately predict individual serum theophylline concentrations, as evidenced from linear regression analysis. Correlation coefficient for all levels evaluated was considerably <0.71, the minimal value necessary to account for 50% of observed variation in data. Also, multiplicative and additive biases were unacceptably high. Although these parameters improved significantly in some patient subgroups, firm conclusions from such subgroup analysis would be inappropriate because of the small sample size.

When bias and precision of SIMKIN are assessed by consideration of mpe and rmse, a similar conclusion can be reached. Observed mpe and corresponding confidence intervals suggest that SIMKIN prediction bias is minimal but variable. If, however, precision within ± 5.0 μg/ml for 95% of predictions is desired, then SIMKIN fails in this regard. Although the rmse is less than this value, its corresponding confidence interval exceeds it in all instances.

Although SIMKIN was unable to predict individual serum theophylline concentrations, it was better able to categorize dosing regimens as therapeutic or nontherapeutic. The ability of SIMKIN to predict toxic concentrations of theophylline could not be evaluated because of a lack of data. These results suggest that SIMKIN may be clinically useful in determining whether an ambulatory patient's theophylline dose regimen is likely to produce a therapeutic or nontherapeutic concentration, a feature of major interest to clinicians. These data do not, however, support the use of SIMKIN without appropriate followup determination of theophylline concentrations.

Of particular interest was the observation that SIMKIN over-predicted serum theophylline concentrations drawn <3 h after dose, as shown by comparison of means of the measured and predicted concentrations. This observation supports findings of other investigators that patients who are taking a sustained-release theophylline product may have a lag time after taking a dose before serum theophylline concentrations begin to rise (2). Consideration is now being given to include a programmed lag time for these products in the SIMKIN program.

SIMKIN has the ability to adjust clearance value of theophylline in a patient if at least one serum theophylline concentration is known. Volume of distribution and elimination half-life in a patient can be estimated if at least one serum theophylline concentration is known. Theoretically, this feature should enable SIMKIN to more accurately predict subsequent serum theophylline concentrations. This study did not evaluate this feature because of an insufficient number of compliant patients with multiple serum theophylline concentrations. This SIMKIN feature needs to be evaluated in ambulatory patients.

Previous investigators (19) have criticized evaluation of predictive performance using linear regression. Regression analysis was labeled as misleading, since it assesses degree of association and overestimates precision of a predictor. Instead, bias and precision should be evaluated by analysis of mpe and rmse. These points, which are critical of regression analysis, are appropriate if predictive performance is evaluated only by consideration of a correlation coefficient. When multiplicative and additive biases are quantitatively evaluated, as was done for this investigation, the results and conclusions should be equivalent for the two methods of data analysis. These data suggest, however, that consideration of mpe and rmse may not be sensitive enough to evaluate predictive performance. It appears that confirmation with regression analysis is necessary when these latter analyses suggest acceptance of a predictor.

An important limitation of this investigation was the limited number of patients who met established compliance criteria. This suggests that physicians and pharmacists should more vigorously encourage and monitor ambulatory patient compliance to theophylline by such means as checking prescription refill information. Since absolute compliance could not be determined in our patient population, noncompliance may also explain some of the variability between actual and predicted serum theophylline concentrations (21). The fact that only 10.2% of patients were found to be compliant may actually be the most important finding of this study. Such a finding suggests that predicting theophylline concentrations in patients is less important than developing ways to persuade patients to take their medication.

In summary, we evaluated the ability of a simulated pharmacokinetic computer program to predict serum theophylline concentrations in ambulatory patients. The computer program did not accurately predict individual patient concentrations, although it was able to correctly categorize a dose regimen as therapeutic or nontherapeutic. The predictive ability of the program after either a known theophylline concentration or in the presence of multiple diseases was not evaluated because of a small sample size. We conclude that computerized use of literature-averaged pharmacokinetic parameters may be useful for categorizing a dose regimen of theophylline as therapeutic, but that it is of little use in predicting individual concentrations if no prior concentrations are known. Further work is necessary to determine the usefulness of SIMKIN in predicting subsequent theophylline concentrations after an initial concentration has been obtained.

Acknowledgment: This investigation was supported by Grant 5T35 HL07489 from the National Institute of Health.

REFERENCES

1. Hendeles L, Weinberger M. Theophylline: a "state of the art" review. *Pharmacotherapy* 1983;3:2–44.
2. Hatton RC, Gotz VP, Robinson JD, et al. Conversion from intravenous aminophylline to sustained-release theophylline: computer simulation versus in vivo results. *Clin Pharm* 1983;2:347–52.
3. Iafrate RP, Gotz VP, Robinson JD, et al. Computer-simulated conversion from intravenous to sustained-release oral theophylline. *Drug Intell Clin Pharm* 1982;16:19–25.
4. Robinson JD, Hatton RC, Russell WL, Klapp D, Lopez LM. Accuracy of serum gentamicin concentration predictions generated by a personal-computer software system. *Clin Pharm* 1984;3:509–16.
5. Hendeles L, Weinberger M, Johnson G. Theophylline. In: Evans WE, Schentag JJ, Jusko WJ, eds. *Applied pharmacokinetics.* San Francisco: Applied Therapeutics, 1980:95–138.
6. Weinberger M, Hendeles L, Wong L, et al. Relationship of formulation and dosing interval to fluctuation of serum theophylline concentration in children with chronic asthma. *J Pediatr* 1981;99:145–52.
7. Upton RA, Thiercelin JF, Guentert TW, et al. Evaluation of the absorption of some commercial sustained-release theophylline products. *J Pharmacokinet Biopharm* 1980;8:131–49.
8. Weinberger M, Smith G, Milavetz G. Diet and theophylline. *Pediatrics* 1981;68:600–1.
9. Renton KW, Gray JD, Hung DR. Depression of theophylline elimination by erythromycin. *Clin Pharmacol Ther* 1981;30:422–6.
10. Landay RA, Gonzalez MA, Taylor JC. Effect of phenobarbital on theophylline disposition. *J Allergy Clin Immunol* 1978;62:27–9.
11. Conrad KA, Nyman DW. Effects of metoprolol and propranolol on theophylline elimination. *Clin Pharmacol Ther* 1980;28:463–7.
12. Roberts RK, Grice J, Wood L, et al. Cimetidine impairs the elimination of theophylline and antipyrine. *Gastroenterology* 1981;81:19–21.
13. Marquis JF, Caruthers SG, Spence JD, et al. Phenytoin-theophylline interaction. *N Engl J Med* 1982;307:1,189–90.
14. Staib AJ, Schuppan D, Lissner R, et al. Pharmacokinetics and metabolism of theophylline in patients with liver disease. *Int J Clin Pharmacol Ther Toxicol* 1980;18:500–2.
15. Piafksy KM, Sitar DS, Rangno RE, et al. Theophylline kinetics in acute pulmonary edema. *Clin Pharmacol Ther* 1977;21:310–6.
16. Powell JR, Thiercelin J, Vozeh S, et al. The influence of cigarette smoking and sex on theophylline disposition. *Am Rev Resp Dis* 1977;116:17–23.
17. Jusko WJ, Schentag JJ, Clark JH, et al. Enhanced biotransformation of theophylline in marijuana and tobacco smokers. *Clin Pharmacol Ther* 1978;24:406–10.
18. Robinson JD, Steeves RA. EMIT theophylline assay at reduced cost. *Ther Drug Monit* 1982;4:427–31.
19. Beal SI, Sheiner LB. Scientific commentary. Some suggestions for measuring predictive performance. *J Pharmacokinet Biopharm* 1981;9:503–12.
20. Fisher Diagnostics. TheraChem anticonvulsants/theophylline controls package insert. Orangeburg, New York: 1981.
21. Haynes RB, Taylor DW, Sackett DL, eds. *Compliance in health care.* Baltimore: Johns Hopkins University Press, 1979.

Therapeutic Drug Monitoring
7:426–434 © 1985 Raven Press, New York

Cimetidine-Theophylline Interaction: Effects of Age and Cimetidine Dose

Ira A. Cohen, Cary E. Johnson, Rosemary R. Berardi, Martha L. Hyneck, and *Sami R. Achem

*College of Pharmacy, The University of Michigan, Ann Arbor, Michigan and *The University Hospital, Jacksonville, Florida, U.S.A.*

Summary: Influences of cimetidine dose and age on the cimetidine-theophylline interaction were evaluated. Group Y consisted of nine young adults, aged 22–35 years, and Group O of nine elderly adults, aged 60–74 years. Each subject completed three study phases in this randomized crossover study. During Phase A, oral dosing of 5 mg/kg theophylline was followed by 14 serial blood samples drawn over 36 h. Phases B and C involved the same procedures, but with oral cimetidine treatment of either 200 or 300 mg every 6 h, respectively. Theophylline pharmacokinetic parameters for Group Y, Group O, and Groups Y + O were calculated. Analyses of variance (ANOVA) for crossover design were performed for each variable. Intragroup interphase ANOVA results were interpreted using multiple range tests (Tukey's Q). Comparisons between groups were performed using two-sided Student's *t* tests ($\alpha = 0.05$). Within each phase, the area under the concentration–time curve (AUC), elimination half-life ($t_{1/2\ el}$), clearance (Cl_p), and volume of distribution (V_d) of theophylline for the elderly subjects were not significantly different from those of the younger adults. Mean changes in AUC, $t_{1/2\ el}$, and Cl_p between Phases A and B for both Groups Y and O were highly significant (29.2 vs. 40.4, 36.7 vs. 44.8, and 25.9 vs. 29.8%, respectively). Further significant changes in those parameters were associated with 1.2 g/day of cimetidine (Phase C). Alterations of theophylline pharmacokinetics by cimetidine appear to be dose-related and are of similar magnitude in elderly and young healthy adults. **Key Words:** Cimetidine—Theophylline—Interaction—Dosage—Age—Pharmacokinetics.

The H_2-antagonist cimetidine has been found to interact with a variety of drugs and other chemicals through several mechanisms (1–5). Since 1980, a number of studies and reports have addressed the ability of cimetidine to inhibit the metabolism of theophylline (6–27). The inhibitory effect, which has been demonstrated in both animal and human livers, appears to be secondary to a direct competitive and reversible binding of cimetidine to hepatic microsomal mixed-function oxidases (28–31).

Antipyrine, like theophylline, has a low hepatic extraction and is metabolized by microsomal mixed-function oxidases (32). When used as a marker for factors altering the intrinsic hepatic clearance of drugs, antipyrine is affected by cimetidine similarly to theophylline (6,17,21,33,34).

The influence of cimetidine on hepatic clearance is probably related to the imidazole ring structure of cimetidine rather than to its interference with H_2-receptors (6,15–17,26,28–31,35). Metabolic pathways for theophylline predominantly inhibited by cimeti-

Address correspondence and reprint requests to Dr. I. A. Cohen at St. Joseph Mercy Hospital, Department of Pharmacy, P.O. Box 995, Ann Arbor, MI 48106, U.S.A.

Presented in part at the American Gastroenterological Association meeting, New Orleans, Louisiana, May 20, 1984.

dine are those responsible for *N*-demethylation, while the 8-oxidation metabolism is not significantly affected (23).

Since the binding of cimetidine to hepatic microsomal enzymes seems to be competitive and reversible, it would be expected that the magnitude of the drug interaction between cimetidine and theophylline would be related to the concentration of cimetidine present and, hence, to cimetidine dose. In vitro and animal data support this hypothesis (36), as do the results of a study examining the influence of cimetidine dose on the clearance of antipyrine (33). However, the only study that prospectively examined the influence of cimetidine dose on the interaction found that the clearance of theophylline in 12 healthy subjects was comparably diminished by daily doses of 1.2 and 2.4 g of cimetidine (26). Although the authors concluded that the interaction is dose-independent, it is highly possible that they masked a dose-response relationship by choosing too high a starting dose of cimetidine. If microsomal enzyme binding sites were nearly saturated when cimetidine was dosed at 1.2 g/day, the administration of 2.4 g/day (a dose rarely used in clinical practice) would not be expected to cause significant additional changes in theophylline metabolism. Yet, a dose-dependent relationship might be found if relatively lower doses commonly utilized in clinical practice (e.g., 800 and 1,200 mg/day) were studied.

The influence of age on the existence and magnitude of the cimetidine-theophylline interaction is also poorly defined. Studies in humans and animal models have suggested aging-related alterations in the intrinsic metabolizing capacity of the liver, resulting in decreased liver microsomal enzyme concentrations and subsequent impaired metabolism of some drugs (37–39). The exact mechanism by which the elderly may lose their capacity to metabolize those agents remains unclear. The influence of aging on enzyme inhibition is even less well studied. One investigation found that the influence of cimetidine on the clearance of antipyrine was similar in both young and elderly humans (33). To our knowledge, there have been no previous controlled trials prospectively examining the influence of aging on the magnitude of cimetidine-theophylline drug interaction. Cimetidine is primarily eliminated as unchanged drug in the urine (40). Therefore, it is not unexpected that populations of healthy elderly subjects have been shown to have diminished clearance of cimetidine, resulting in higher concentrations of the drug, compared with a population of young adults receiving the same daily dose (40). Current cimetidine dosing guidelines do not recommend dosage adjustment until the creatinine clearance falls below 40 ml/min (40). The elderly, who have relatively diminished creatinine clearance as a function of aging, are likely to receive full doses of cimetidine. Therefore, it seems likely that the higher serum concentrations of cimetidine achieved in the general population of elderly subjects would lead to alterations in theophylline clearance of a comparable and probably higher magnitude than that achieved by a matched population of younger adults. To our knowledge, however, a prospective controlled study evaluating the influence of age on the cimetidine-theophylline drug interaction has not previously been reported.

Therefore, the objective of this study was to evaluate the influences of both cimetidine dose and age on the magnitude of the cimetidine-theophylline drug interaction.

METHODS

Subjects

A total of 18 volunteers completed the study. All subjects gave their informed consent, and the study was approved by the Human Studies Committee of the University of Michigan and by the Operating Subcommittee of the University's Clinical Research Center (CRC). Subjects were divided into two groups on the basis of age (Table 1). Group Y consisted of nine volunteers between the ages of 22 and 35 years (mean 28.0 ± 4.5 years), weighing between 56.8 and 84.1 kg (mean 71.1 ± 9.2 kg). Group O consisted of nine volunteers between the ages of 60 and 74 years (mean 67.2 ± 4.4 years), weighing between 59.1 and 92.7 kg (mean 74.4 ± 10.4 kg). All volunteers were healthy as determined by a complete medical history, screening physical examination and a battery of laboratory tests, including an electrocardiogram and determinations of serum creatinine, total bilirubin, albumin, electrolytes, blood urea nitrogen, and liver enzymes. A minimal baseline creatinine clearance of 40 ml/min as estimated by the method of Cockcroft and Gault (41) was required for inclusion into the study population. Cigarette smokers and users of other tobacco products, as well as persons exposed to known inhibitors or inducers of hepatic microsomal enzyme activity within 6 months of the study, were excluded. The ingestion of alcoholic beverages, medications, charcoal-broiled foods, and xanthine-containing foods and beverages was prohibited for 1 week prior to the study and throughout the study period (a total of ≈6 weeks).

TABLE 1. *Subject age, weight, and treatment schedule*

Group	Subject	Age (yr)	Weight (kg)	Treatment subgroup	Phase sequence		
					1st phase	2nd phase	3rd phase
Y	1	29	61.4	I	A[a]	B[b]	C[c]
	2	31	62.3	I	A	B	C
	3	35	84.1	III	C	A	B
	4	24	77.3	III	C	A	B
	5	25	80.0	II	B	C	A
	6	34	71.4	III	C	A	B
	7	26	56.8	I	A	B	C
	8	26	75.0	II	B	C	A
	9	32	71.8	II	B	C	A
O	10	65	64.1	I	A	B	C
	11	74	59.1	I	A	B	C
	12	67	85.9	II	B	C	A
	13	68	72.3	III	C	A	B
	14	60	92.7	I	A	B	C
	15	73	70.5	II	B	C	A
	16	63	80.0	III	C	A	B
	17	68	72.7	II	B	C	A
	18	67	72.7	III	C	A	B

[a]Phase A, theophylline control phase without cimetidine treatment.
[b]Phase B, theophylline with cimetidine 200 mg orally every 6 h.
[c]Phase C, theophylline with cimetidine 300 mg orally every 6 h.

Treatments, Schedules, and Sampling

Subjects within each age group were randomly assigned to one of three study sequence subgroups (I, II, and III) in this three-way crossover study (Table 1). During Phase A (control phase) subjects fasted overnight (from 12 midnight) until 4 h after receiving a single 5 mg/kg oral dose of theophylline elixir (Elixophyllin, 80 mg anhydrous theophylline per 15 ml, lot W10659, exp. 8/86; Berlex Laboratories, Inc., Wayne, NJ, U.S.A.) at 8 a.m. The dose was administered with 120 ml of water. Fourteen blood samples were taken from a forearm vein through an indwelling heparin lock or (for later drawings) by separate venipunctures immediately before dosing with theophylline and at 0.25, 0.5, 0.75, 1, 1.5, 2, 3, 4, 6, 8, 12, 24, and 36 h after dosing with theophylline. Blood samples were transferred to silicone-coated, rubber-stoppered, 10-ml glass tubes (Venoject, lot 13294; Terumo Medical, Elkton, MD, U.S.A.) and upon clotting were centrifuged. The separated serum fractions were transferred to coded polypropylene plastic tubes (Falcon, 12 × 75 mm with caps, lot 20834935; Becton Dickinson Co., Oxnard, CA, U.S.A.) and frozen at −20°C (42) until just prior to assay. Lunch and dinner conforming to the protocol guidelines were provided to subjects by the CRC at 4 and 10 h, respectively, after dosing with theophylline.

Phase B entailed repeating the same procedures described for Phase A but included "lower dose" cimetidine, 200 mg (Tagamet, lot 49 1T12, exp. 11/30/84; Smith Kline & French Laboratory Co., Carolina PR) administered orally every 6 h (6 a.m., 12 p.m., 6 p.m., 12 a.m.) starting 3 days prior to the dosing of theophylline and continuing throughout the 36-h post-theophylline period of blood sampling.

Phase C was identical to Phase B except that the "higher dose" cimetidine, 300 mg (Tagamet, lot 1110 1T13, exp. 11/30/84) every 6 h, was utilized.

A 10-day drug-free period separated each study phase from the next. The treatment schedules for each of the 18 subjects are shown in Table 1.

Assay for Theophylline and Cimetidine

Samples were analyzed for theophylline concentration by a fluorescence polarization immunoassay system (TDx: Theophylline Reagent Pack, lot 50-785-HQ, exp. 4/84; Theophylline Controls, lot 49-585-HQ, exp. 5/84; Theophylline Calibrators, lot 46-139-HQ, exp 1/84; Abbott Laboratories Diagnostics Division, North Chicago, IL, U.S.A.) according to the guidelines of the manufacturer (43). Frozen serum was allowed to equilibrate to room temperature and was vortex-mixed prior to assay. Two internal controls with known theophylline concentrations of 14.6 and 24.2 μg/ml (Level I, lot 4N416, exp. 5/84; Level II, lot 4N415, exp. 5/84; General Diagnostics, Morris Plains, NJ, U.S.A.) were assayed with each run of samples.

Aliquots of frozen serum from Phases B and C corresponding to 1 and 2 h after the administration of the 6 a.m. dose of cimetidine were also allowed to equilibrate to room temperature, vortex-mixed, and assayed for cimetidine utilizing a modification (44) of a high pressure liquid chromatography procedure originally described by Mihaly et al. (45). The resultant cimetidine concentration data were indicative of approximate post-dosing peak cimetidine concentrations and were utilized as indirect indicators of compliance with the cimetidine dosing regimen and to allow for the correlation of cimetidine concentration with pharmacokinetic parameters to be assessed.

Statistical Analysis

Theophylline serum concentration–time data were utilized to calculate the area under the serum concentration–time curve (AUC, μg/ml/h) from 0 through 36 h and from 0 to infinity, the elimination half-life (h), the apparent volume of distribution for fraction of dose absorbed (V_d/F, where F for theophylline elixir is 1), the absorbed dose (100%) divided by the volume of distribution for the one-compartment open model (FD/V_d, μg/ml), and the clearance of theophylline from serum. For Groups O, Y, and Y + O, analysis of variance (ANOVA) for crossover design was performed for the aforementioned variables as well as for plasma concentrations at each sampling time (μg/ml), peak plasma concentration (μg/ml), and time of peak plasma concentration (h). Intragroup interphase results from the ANOVA were interpreted using multiple range tests (Tukey's Q). Comparisons of parameters between Groups Y and O were performed using two-sided Student's *t* tests between two means. The confidence level for significance was $\alpha = 0.05$.

RESULTS

Subjects

The body weight of Groups Y and O were not significantly different as determined by Student's *t* tests between the two means. The mean body surface areas (1.89 ± 0.17 and 1.92 ± 0.14 m^2) and mean theophylline dosage administered during each of the three study phases (355.4 ± 46.0 and 372.4 ± 52.3 mg) were not significantly different between Groups Y and O, respectively. As expected on the basis of age-related changes in renal function for the healthy elderly subjects, both the weight-adjusted and non–weight-adjusted mean creatinine clearances for Group O subjects were significantly lower than those of the younger adults (52.9 ± 7.9 vs. 100.8 ± 17.7 and 55.8 ± 9.9 vs. 100.7 ± 11.1 ml/min, respectively; $p < 0.001$).

Assay

The between-run coefficient of variation for the TDx assay of theophylline was 3.1% at 14.6 μg/ml and 2.4% at 24.2 μg/ml. These results reflect the repeated assay of the controls with each of the 54 assay runs performed over an 18-h period. The between-run coefficient of variation for the cimetidine assay was 4.6% at 1 μg/ml as determined by the analysis of eight replicate samples.

Theophylline Pharmacokinetic Parameters

Mean concentration–time data for the three phases of each study group (Groups Y, O, and Y + O) and ANOVA for between-phase differences within each group were determined (Table 2), and log concentration versus time were plotted for Groups Y and O (Fig. 1). For each data set, the correlation coefficients for the least-squares linear regression of the terminal elimination points approached unity ($r^2 > 0.999$).

Mean theophylline pharmacokinetic parameters for each phase of each group and results of between-group statistical comparisons within each study phase were calculated (Table 3). The only comparison of pharmacokinetic parameters between Groups Y and O that indicated a statistically significant difference was for the peak concentrations of theophylline during Phase C where the mean concentration was greater for the elderly subjects ($p = 0.045$). Within each of the three phases, the mean for time to reach the peak theophylline concentration, AUC, elimination half-life of theophylline, theophylline serum clearance, and apparent volume of distribution for the healthy elderly subjects were not found to differ significantly from those of the younger adults.

Between-phase differences for mean pharmacokinetic parameters expressed as percentage change for each group were estimated, and statistical comparisons for between-group data were statistically analyzed (Table 4). Although the mean peak theophylline concentrations attained during the cimetidine treatment phases were significantly higher than those noted in the control phase (Phase A) in both the elderly subjects and for the overall population, the increase in mean theophylline peak between the lower cime-

TABLE 2. *Summary of mean theophylline concentration–time data*

		Serum concentrations for phase and time indicated						Significance of difference by analysis of variance		
		Phase A		Phase B		Phase C				
Group	Serum sampling time (h)	Mean	CV[a] (%)	Mean	CV (%)	Mean	CV (%)	Phase A vs. Phase B	Phase B vs. Phase C	Phase A vs. Phase C
Y (n = 9)	0.25	6.76	79.7	5.44	86.5	2.76	64.1	NS[b]	NS	$p < 0.05$
	0.50	8.87	45.7	8.41	45.8	8.87	47.8	NS	NS	NS
	0.75	10.12	30.1	9.70	26.7	9.49	41.1	NS	NS	NS
	1.0	9.62	25.2	9.43	27.5	9.30	36.2	NS	NS	NS
	1.5	9.17	17.4	9.07	16.1	9.21	22.5	NS	NS	NS
	2.0	9.15	9.5	9.03	12.7	9.25	11.9	NS	NS	NS
	3.0	8.58[c]	9.3	9.01	10.1	9.05	10.3	NS	NS	NS
	4.0	7.88[c]	9.0	8.68[c]	11.4	8.62[c]	9.7	$p < 0.05$	NS	$p < 0.05$
	6.0	6.53[c]	15.9	7.32[c]	11.0	7.60[c]	14.3	$p < 0.05$	NS	$p < 0.05$
	8.0	5.45[c]	19.3	6.60[c]	11.1	6.86[c]	16.2	$p < 0.05$	NS	$p < 0.05$
	12.0	3.99[c]	31.7	4.88[c]	11.2	5.20[c]	18.6	$p < 0.05$	NS	$p < 0.05$
	24.0	1.47[c]	54.3	2.42[c]	25.5	2.76[c]	32.5	$p < 0.05$	NS	$p < 0.05$
	36.0	0.50[c]	104.1	1.09[c]	35.3	1.49[c]	46.8	$p < 0.05$	$p < 0.05$	$p < 0.05$
O (n = 9)	0.25	5.76	68.7	7.71	97.4	5.91	95.9	NS	NS	NS
	0.50	8.61	46.1	9.81	53.3	9.05	52.0	NS	NS	NS
	0.75	10.32	30.3	9.98	28.1	10.30	31.8	NS	NS	NS
	1.0	9.76	24.2	10.80	11.5	11.21	19.5	NS	NS	NS
	1.5	9.13	23.2	10.95	10.8	10.79	10.6	NS	NS	NS
	2.0	9.28	17.4	10.05	7.5	9.90	9.6	NS	NS	NS
	3.0	8.73[c]	12.4	9.22[c]	7.7	9.28	9.9	NS	NS	NS
	4.0	7.87[c]	14.6	8.68[c]	7.4	8.83[c]	8.5	$p < 0.05$	NS	$p < 0.05$
	6.0	6.54[c]	19.9	7.61[c]	11.0	7.63[c]	11.0	$p < 0.05$	NS	$p < 0.05$
	8.0	5.29[c]	22.9	6.57[c]	13.9	6.70[c]	13.2	$p < 0.05$	NS	$p < 0.05$
	12.0	3.45[c]	33.5	4.81[c]	19.0	5.17[c]	17.8	$p < 0.05$	NS	$p < 0.05$
	24.0	1.16[c]	70.8	2.13[c]	48.4	2.63[c]	39.0	$p < 0.05$	$p < 0.05$	$p < 0.05$
	36.0	0.35[c]	135.8	0.90[c]	87.1	1.32[c]	64.4	$p < 0.05$	$p < 0.05$	$p < 0.05$
Y + O (n = 18)	0.25	6.26	73.7	6.58	94.2	4.33	101.1	NS	NS	NS
	0.50	8.74	44.6	9.11	49.5	8.96	48.5	NS	NS	NS
	0.75	10.22	29.3	9.84	26.6	9.89	35.6	NS	NS	NS
	1.0	9.69	24.0	10.12	20.7	10.25	28.5	NS	NS	NS
	1.5	9.15	19.9	10.01	16.1	10.00	18.1	NS	NS	NS
	2.0	9.21	13.7	9.54	11.3	9.57	11.0	NS	NS	NS
	3.0	8.65[c]	10.7	9.11[b]	8.7	9.16[c]	9.9	$p < 0.05$	NS	$p < 0.05$
	4.0	7.88[c]	11.8	8.68[c]	9.3	8.73[c]	8.9	$p < 0.05$	NS	$p < 0.05$
	6.0	6.54[c]	17.5	7.46[c]	10.9	7.62[c]	12.4	$p < 0.05$	NS	$p < 0.05$
	8.0	5.37[c]	20.6	6.59[c]	12.2	6.78[c]	14.4	$p < 0.05$	NS	$p < 0.05$
	12.0	3.72[c]	32.5	4.85[c]	15.1	5.19[c]	17.6	$p < 0.05$	NS	$p < 0.05$
	24.0	1.31[c]	60.9	2.27[c]	36.8	2.70[c]	34.8	$p < 0.05$	$p < 0.05$	$p < 0.05$
	36.0	0.42[c]	115.2	0.99[c]	61.0	1.40[c]	54.0	$p < 0.05$	$p < 0.05$	$p < 0.05$

[a] CV (%), coefficient of variation for each mean as percentage.
[b] NS, not significant as determined by three-way crossover ANOVA using Tukey's allowable difference for comparison of treatment averages.
[c] Considered within terminal elimination phase for calculation of elimination rate constant (K_{el}) and elimination half-life ($t_{1/2\,el}$).

tidine dosing phase (Phase B) and the higher cimetidine dosing phase (Phase C) was negligible. Highly significant increases in AUC over those in the control phase were found for all subject groups during Phase B, and a further significant increase in AUC was found between B and C when the cimetidine dose was increased. Similarly, significant increases in theophylline elimination half-life between Phases A and B occurred in both the young and the elderly; further (although less dramatic) increases in theophylline half-life were associated with higher doses of cimetidine when Phases B and C were compared. Significant decreases in clearance of theophylline during the cimetidine treatment phases paralleled the increases in AUC and elimination half-life. Changes in theophylline clearance between Phases B and C were significant for both the overall population and the subpopulation of elderly subjects. Small but consistent

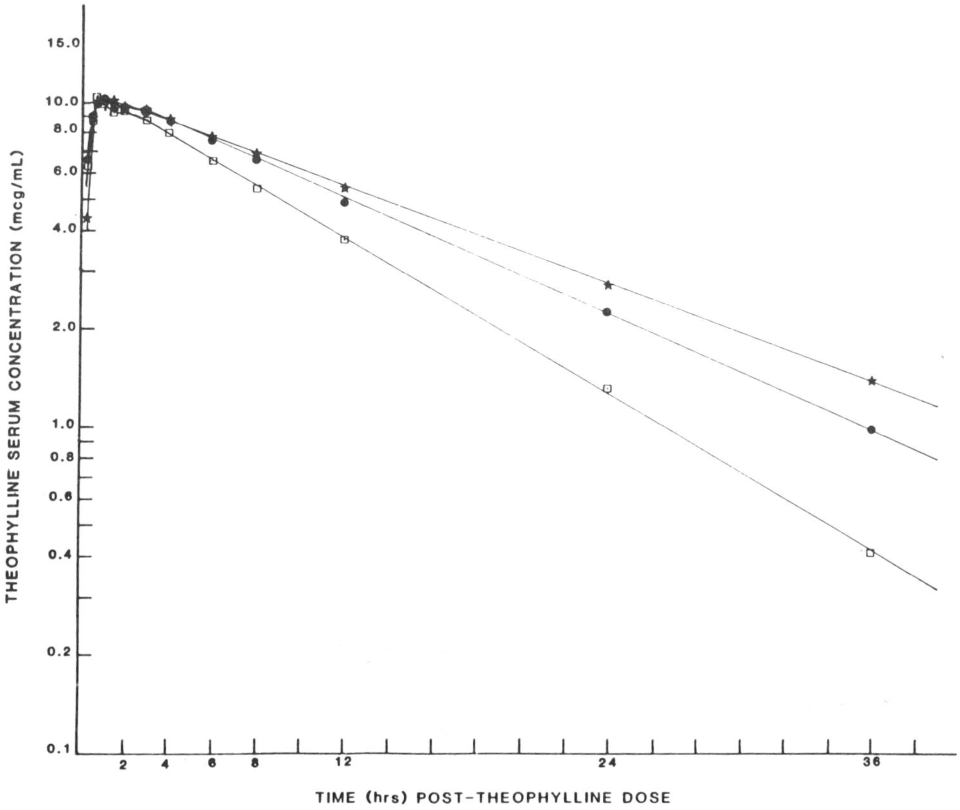

FIG. 1. Theophylline serum concentration versus time for Groups Y + O. Phase A (squares), theophylline without cimetidine; Phase B (circles), theophylline with cimetidine 200 mg every 6 h; Phase C (stars), theophylline with cimetidine 300 mg every 6 h.

TABLE 3. *Comparison of group means of theophylline (TH) pharmacokinetic parameters for each treatment phase*

Parameter	Group	Phase A	Phase B	Phase C
Peak TH concentration	Y	11.63 ± 2.89	11.41 ± 2.41	11.48 ± 2.31
(μg/ml)	O	11.13 ± 2.07[a]	13.50 ± 3.24[a]	13.58 ± 2.62[b]
	Y + O	11.38 ± 2.45	12.46 ± 2.97	12.53 ± 2.63
Time to peak TH	Y	1.22 ± 0.90	1.53 ± 1.40	1.39 ± 1.26
concentration (h)	O	1.42 ± 0.99[a]	0.83 ± 0.54[a]	0.89 ± 0.44[a]
	Y + O	1.32 ± 0.93	1.18 ± 1.09	1.14 ± 0.95
Area under conc–time	Y	131.54 ± 37.44	169.91 ± 27.78	191.08 ± 47.66
curve (AUC^{∞})	O	119.93 ± 40.31[a]	168.44 ± 50.48[a]	189.43 ± 57.11[a]
	Y + O	125.74 ± 38.21	169.17 ± 39.54	190.25 ± 51.04
TH elimination half-	Y	7.93 ± 2.25	10.84 ± 1.85	12.62 ± 2.80
life ($t_{1/2\ el}$) (h)	O	6.97 ± 2.54[a]	10.09 ± 3.60[a]	11.96 ± 4.05[a]
	Y + O	7.45 ± 2.38	10.46 ± 2.80	12.29 ± 3.39
TH plasma clearance	Y	2.86 ± 0.75	2.12 ± 0.28	1.96 ± 0.51
(Cl_p) (L/h)	O	3.36 ± 1.00[a]	2.36 ± 0.65[a]	2.11 ± 0.60[a]
	Y + O	3.11 ± 0.90	2.24 ± 0.50	2.03 ± 0.55
TH volume of	Y	0.44 ± 0.03	0.46 ± 0.05	0.48 ± 0.06
distribution (V_d)	O	0.42 ± 0.03[a]	0.43 ± 0.05[a]	0.45 ± 0.03[a]
(L/kg)	Y + O	0.43 ± 0.03	0.45 ± 0.05	0.47 ± 0.05

See Table 1 for definition of Phases A, B, and C.

[a]NS ($p > 0.05$) when differences between means for Groups Y and O for this parameter and treatment phase are compared by two-tailed Student's *t* test.

[b]$p = 0.045$ for two-tailed Student's *t* test between means of Groups Y and O.

TABLE 4. *Analyses of between-phase differences of group means for theophylline pharmacokinetic parameters*

Parameter	Group	Phase A → Phase B		Phase A → Phase C		Phase B → Phase C	
		% Δ	Significance	% Δ	Significance	% Δ	Significance
Peak concentration	Y	−1.9	NS[a]	−1.3	NS	+0.6	NS
	O	+21.3	$p < 0.05$[b]	+22.0	$p < 0.05$	+0.6	NS
	Y + O	+9.5	$p < 0.05$	+10.1	$p < 0.05$	+0.6	NS
Time to peak	Y	+25.4	NS	+13.9	NS	−9.2	NS
	O	−41.5	$p < 0.05$	−37.3	$p < 0.05$[b]	+7.2	NS
	Y + O	−10.6	NS	−13.9	NS	−3.4	NS
Area under curve (AUC^{∞})	Y	+29.2	$p \ll 0.05$	+45.3	$p \ll 0.05$	+12.5	$p \ll 0.05$
	O	+40.4	$p \ll 0.05$	+58.0	$p \ll 0.05$	+12.5	$p \ll 0.05$
	Y + O	+34.5	$p \ll 0.05$	+51.3	$p \ll 0.05$	+12.5	$p \ll 0.05$
Elimination half-life ($t_{1/2\ el}$)	Y	+36.7	$p \ll 0.05$	+59.1	$p \ll 0.05$	+16.4	$p < 0.05$
	O	+44.8	$p \ll 0.05$	+71.6	$p \ll 0.05$	+18.5	$p \ll 0.05$
	Y + O	+40.4[c]	$p \ll 0.05$	+65.0[d]	$p \ll 0.05$	+17.5	$p \ll 0.005$
Clearance (Cl_p)	Y	−25.9	$p \ll 0.05$	−31.5	$p \ll 0.05$	−7.5	NS
	O	−29.8	$p \ll 0.05$	−37.2	$p \ll 0.05$	−10.6	$p < 0.05$
	Y + O	−28.0[e]	$p \ll 0.05$	−34.7[f]	$p \ll 0.05$	−9.4	$p < 0.05$
Volume of distribution (V_d)	Y	+4.5	$p < 0.05$	+9.1	$p \ll 0.05$	+4.3	NS
	O	+2.4	NS	+7.1	$p < 0.05$	+4.7	$p < 0.05$
	Y + O	+4.7	$p < 0.05$	+9.3	$p \ll 0.05$	+4.4	$p < 0.05$

[a] Between-phase means not significantly different when analyzed by three-way crossover analysis of variance (ANOVA) using Tukey's Q test and/or paired Student's *t* test.
[b] Between-phase means significantly different ($p < 0.05$ or $p \ll 0.05$) when compared by three-way crossover ANOVA using Tukey's Q test or by paired Student's *t* test.
[c] Range for individual subjects, 12.3–101.2%.
[d] Range for individual subjects, 26.6–124.6%.
[e] Range for individual subjects, 4.98–48.2%.
[f] Range for individual subjects, 16.0–50.2%.

and statistically significant increases in the apparent volume of distribution for theophylline between Phases A and B and between Phases B and C were found for the overall population of elderly and younger adults.

Concentrations of cimetidine from serum obtained from each subject at ~2 h following the patients' scheduled 6 a.m. dose of cimetidine during both Phases B and C were in excess of 0.5 μg/ml for all subjects, indicating relative compliance with cimetidine administration. Comparisons of mean serum cimetidine concentrations between the elderly and the young adults revealed no significant differences for either Phase B or Phase C.

DISCUSSION

Both the healthy elderly subjects in Group O and the younger healthy adults in Group Y manifested significant alterations in theophylline clearance, elimination half-life, and area under the plasma concentration–time curve. These changes in theophylline pharmacokinetic parameters were enhanced significantly when the daily dose of cimetidine was increased from 800 mg to 1.2 g. The magnitude of the drug interaction between cimetidine and theophylline, therefore, appears to be dose-related and, in healthy human subjects, is not significantly influenced as a function of age.

The mean changes in theophylline clearance and half-life over the control phase when this population (Groups Y and O) received 1.2 g/day of cimetidine are comparable to those reported by Powell et al. (26) when the same daily cimetidine dose was administered to 12 healthy men (34.7 vs. 36%, and 65.0 vs. 61.4%, respectively). However, Powell et al. utilized 1.2 g cimetidine as the starting daily dose and did not find further significant alterations in theophylline pharmacokinetic parameters when that dose was doubled. It is evident from our results that the magnitude of the cimetidine-theophylline interaction is not linear and is probably saturable, since increases in dose from 800 to 1,200 mg/day yielded alterations in AUC, elimination half-life, and clearance of 12.5, 17.5, and 9.4%, respectively. It is, therefore, probable that the starting dose of cimetidine used by Powell et al. was too high to allow detection of an interaction that is possibly dose-related up to the point of saturating microsomal binding sites with cimetidine.

Results confirming comparable influences of cimetidine on theophylline pharmacokinetics in both the young and the elderly, and the dose-magnitude correlation for the drug interaction, are comparable to those reported by Feely et al. (33) for the interaction of cimetidine with antipyrine. On the basis of our results and those of Feely et al., it seems apparent that healthy elderly subjects are affected comparably to younger healthy adults by the interactions of cimetidine with both theophylline and antipyrine. It is also of interest to note that the baseline theophylline pharmacokinetic parameters, including half-life and clearance, for the healthy elderly subjects in our study are comparable to those of the younger subjects.

It was expected that the magnitude of the interaction was dose-dependent and, therefore, might correlate with cimetidine concentrations achieved. In spite of possessing significantly lower creatinine clearances, the serum concentrations of cimetidine achieved by Group O subjects were comparable to those for Group Y. The serum assayed for cimetidine was drawn 2 h after the previous scheduled dose of the drug. It is likely that concentrations achieved at that time may not reflect the true peak concentrations and that this factor may account for the failure to confirm the expected correlations of serum cimetidine concentration and creatinine clearance with the magnitude of the drug interaction. It is also possible that concentrations of cimetidine within hepatocytes is a better correlate of the dose-dependent nature of the drug interaction than is serum concentration. Further research is required to resolve this issue.

The small but statistically significant increases in the volume of distribution for theophylline are notable. Previous investigations have found no alteration in that parameter. Since the volume of distribution is inversely related to clearance, it is possible that increases in theophylline volume of distribution may slightly blunt changes in clearance. However, should this finding be confirmed by subsequent clinical studies, it is still unlikely that such minor alterations in theophylline volume of distribution are of clinical importance.

CONCLUSIONS

This study confirms the dose-dependent relationship of cimetidine on pharmacokinetic alterations associated with the cimetidine-theophylline drug interaction. In addition, the study results show that the magnitude of the interaction in healthy elderly subjects is comparable to that manifested in healthy younger adults.

Acknowledgment: This study was funded by the Clinical Research Center, The University of Michigan Hospitals, under grant no. 5M01-RR00042 and by grant no. 2S07-RR05571-18 of the Biomedical Research Support Grant Program, Division of Research Resources, National Institutes of Health.

REFERENCES

1. Somogyi A, Gugler R. Drug interactions with cimetidine. *Clin Pharmacokinet* 1982;7:23–41.
2. Bauman JH, Kimelblatt BJ. Cimetidine as an inhibitor of drug metabolism: therapeutic implications and review of the literature. *Drug Intell Clin Pharm* 1982;16:380–6.
3. Mangini RJ. Clinically important cimetidine drug interactions. *Clin Pharm* 1982;1:433–40.
4. Sorkin EM, Darvey DL. Review of cimetidine drug interactions. *Drug Intell Clin Pharm* 1983;17:110–20.
5. Freston JW. Cimetidine. II. Adverse reactions and patterns of use. *Ann Intern Med* 1982;97:728–34.
6. Henry DA, MacDonald IA, Kitchingman G, Bell GD, Langman MJS. Cimetidine and ranitidine: comparison of effects on hepatic drug metabolism. *Br Med J* 1980;281:775–7.
7. Jackson JE, Plachetka JR. More on cimetidine-theophylline interaction. *Drug Intell Clin Pharm* 1981;15:809–10.
8. Jackson JE, Powell JR, Wandell M, Bentley J, Dorr R. Cimetidine decreases theophylline clearance. *Am Rev Respir Dis* 1981;113:615–7.
9. Reitberg DP, Bernhard H, Schentag JJ. Alteration of theophylline clearance and half-life by cimetidine in normal volunteers. *Ann Intern Med* 1981;95:582–5.
10. Ambrose PJ, Harralson AF. Lack of effect of cimetidine on theophylline clearance. *Drug Intell Clin Pharm* 1981;15:389–90.
11. Bauman JH, Kimelblatt BJ. Comment on effect of cimetidine on theophylline clearance. *Drug Intell Clin Pharm* 1981;15:808.
12. Campbell MA, Plachetka JR, Jackson JE, Moon JF, Finley PR. Cimetidine decreases theophylline clearance. *Ann Intern Med* 1981;95:68–9.
13. Hendeles L, Weinberger M, Smith G, Milavetz G. The interaction of cimetidine and theophylline. *Drug Intell Clin Pharm* 1981;15:808–9.
14. Bauman JH, Kimmelblatt BJ, Caraccio TR, Silverman HM, Simon AT, Beck GJ. Cimetidine-theophylline interaction: report of four patients. *Ann Allerg* 1982;48:100–2.
15. Dal Negro R, Pomari C, Zoccatelli O, Trevisan F, Carloni C, Turco P. Pharmacokinetics of theophylline and the H_2-antagonist drugs cimetidine and ranitidine. *Int J Clin Pharmacol Ther Toxicol* 1984;22:221–6.
16. Schwartz JI, Bachmann KA, Bond LW, Mahajan VK. Impact of cimetidine on the pharmacokinetics of theophylline. *Clin Pharm* 1982;1:534–8.
17. Breen KJ, Bury R, Desmond PV, et al. Effects of cimetidine and ranitidine on hepatic drug metabolism. *Clin Pharmacol Ther* 1982;31:297–300.
18. Lalonde RL, Koob RA, McLean WM, Balsys AJ. The effects of cimetidine on theophylline pharmacokinetics at steady state. *Chest* 1983;83:221–4.
19. DeAngelis C, Walker SE, Bartle WR. Effect of low-dose

cimetidine on theophylline metabolism. *Clin Pharm* 1983;2:563–7.
20. Mulkey PM, Murphy JE, Shleifer NH. Steady-state theophylline pharmacokinetics during and after short-term cimetidine administration. *Clin Pharm* 1983;2:439–41.
21. Roberts RK, Grice J, Wood L, Petroff V, McGuffie C. Cimetidine impairs the elimination of theophylline and antipyrine. *Gastroenterology* 1981;81:19–21.
22. Vestal RE, Thummel KE, Musser B. Cimetidine inhibits theophylline clearance in patients with chronic obstructive pulmonary disease: a study using stable isotope methodology during multiple oral dose administration. *Br J Clin Pharmacol* 1983;15:411–8.
23. Grygiel JJ, Miers JO, Drew R, Birkett DJ. Differential effects of cimetidine on theophylline metabolic pathways. *Eur J Clin Pharmacol* 1984;26:335–40.
24. Gugler R, Wolf M, Hansen HH, Jansen JC. The inhibition of drug metabolism by cimetidine in patients with liver cirrhosis. *Klin Wochenschr* 1984;62:1126–31.
25. Hsu K, Garton A, Sproule BJ, Tam YK, Legatt D, Herbert FA. The influence of orally administered cimetidine and theophylline on the elimination of each drug in patients with chronic airway obstruction. *Am Rev Resp Dis* 1984;130:740–3.
26. Powell JR, Rogers JF, Wargin WA, Cross RE, Eshelman FN. Inhibition of theophylline clearance by cimetidine but not ranitidine. *Arch Intern Med* 1984;144:484–6.
27. Roberts RK, Grice J, McGuffie C. Cimetidine-theophylline interaction in patients with chronic obstructive pulmonary disease. *Med J Aust* 1984;140:279–80.
28. Puuruncn J, Pelkonen O. Cimetidine inhibits microsomal metabolism in the rat. *Eur J Pharmacol* 1979;55:335–6.
29. Rendic S, Sunjic V, Toso R, Kajfez F, Ruf H. Interaction of cimetidine with liver microsomes. *Xenobiotica* 1979;9:555–64.
30. Puurunen J, Sotaniemi E, Pelkonen O. Effect of cimetidine on microsomal drug metabolism in man. *Eur J Clin Pharmacol* 1980;18:185–7.
31. Knodell RG, Holtzman JL, Crankshaw DL, Steele NM, Stanley LN. Drug metabolism by rat and human hepatic microsomes in response to interaction with H_2-receptor antagonists. *Gastroenterology* 1982;82:84–8.
32. Breckenridge A. Antipyrine half-life and drug elimination. *Clin Pharmacokinet* 1980;5:301–3.
33. Feely J, Pereira L, Guy E, Hockings N. Factors affecting the response to inhibition of drug metabolism by cimetidine-dose response and sensitivity of elderly and induced subjects. *Br J Clin Pharmacol* 1984;17:77–81.
34. Rollinghoff W, Paumgartner G. Inhibition of drug metabolism of cimetidine in man: dependence on pretreatment microsomal liver function. *Eur J Clin Invest* 1982;12:429–32.
35. Wilkinson CF, Hetnarski K, Hicks IJ. Substituted imidazoles as inhibitors of microsomal oxidation and insecticide synergists. *Pesticide Biochem Physiol* 1973;4:299–312.
36. Speeg KV, Patwardhan RV, Avant GR. Inhibition of microsomal drug metabolism by histamine H_2-receptor antagonists studied in vivo and in vitro in rodents. *Gastroenterology* 1982;82:89–96.
37. Birnbaum LS, Baud MB. Induction of hepatic mixed function oxidases in senescent rodents. *Exp Gerontol* 1978;13:299–303.
38. Crooks J, O'Malley K, Stevenson IH. Pharmacokinetics in the elderly. *Clin Pharmacokinet* 1976;1:280–96.
39. Richey DP, Bender D. Pharmacokinetic consequences of aging. *Annu Rev Pharmacol Toxicol* 1977;17:49–65.
40. Abate MA, Hyneck ML, Cohen IA, Berardi RR. Cimetidine pharmacokinetics. *Clin Pharm* 1982;1:225–33.
41. Cockcroft DW, Gault MH. Prediction of creatinine clearance from serum creatinine. *Nephron* 1976;16:31–41.
42. Johnson CE, Cohen IA, Bickley SK, Hyder DM. Stability of theophylline in human serum and whole blood. *Am J Hosp Pharm* 1984;41:2065–8.
43. Abbott Laboratories, Diagnostics Division. TDX therapeutic drug monitoring system. Sections: theory of measurement, principles of operation, antiasthmatic drug assays. North Chicago, Illinois, August 1982.
44. Berardi RR, Cohen IA, Hyneck ML, et al. Comparative bioavailability of two tablet formulations of cimetidine. *Biopharm Drug Dispos* 1984;5:169–76.
45. Mihaly GW, Cockbain S, Jones DB, Hansen RG, Smallwood RA. High pressure liquid chromatographic determination of cimetidine in plasma and urine. *J Pharm Sci* 1982;71:590–2.

Therapeutic Drug Monitoring
7:435–438 © 1985 Raven Press, New York

Effects of Salsalate (Nonacetylated Salicylate) and Aspirin on Serum Prostaglandins in Humans

H. G. Morris, N. A. Sherman, C. McQuain, *M. B. Goldlust, *S. F. Chang, and *L. I. Harrison

*National Jewish Hospital and Research Center, Denver, Colorado; and *Riker Laboratories, 3M Center, St. Paul, Minnesota, U.S.A.*

Summary: Prostaglandin E_2 (PGE_2), thromboxane B_2 (TXB_2), and salicylic acid were measured in blood samples from 10 healthy men after administration of antiinflammatory doses of aspirin (3.9 g/day) or salsalate (3.0 g/day). Each medication was given for 3 days, followed by an observation period of 13 days. Plasma salicylate concentrations were slightly, but generally insignificantly, higher during aspirin dosing, although both drugs produced salicylic acid levels in the antiinflammatory range. Serum levels of PGE_2 and TXB_2, which reflected synthesis of cyclo-oxygenase products by platelets, were minimally affected by salsalate but profoundly suppressed by aspirin. When medication was discontinued, the effects of salsalate on serum PGE_2 and TXB_2 were readily reversible within 36 h, whereas the recovery from aspirin was still incomplete after 13 days of observation. These results indicate that the two orally administered salicylates have differential effects on prostaglandin synthesis in platelets and may also differ in their therapeutic and adverse effects. **Key Words:** Prostaglandins—Thromboxane—Salsalate—Aspirin.

Salsalate, an important member of the salicylate group of nonsteroidal antiinflammatory agents, provides the physician with a safer alternative to aspirin. Salsalate is similar to aspirin in therapeutic effectiveness against arthritic conditions (1–2) but causes no platelet dysfunction (3) and produces less gastrointestinal bleeding and gastric erosion than aspirin (4–5).

Numerous reports have been published on the in vitro and in vivo effects of aspirin on prostaglandin synthesis and metabolism (6–8); to our knowledge, this is the first report on the clinical effects of salsalate on indices of prostaglandin metabolism. In this study, antiinflammatory doses of salsalate and aspirin were administered orally to healthy subjects for 3 days, and the effects on two indices of prostaglandin metabolism were monitored serially in blood specimens before, during, and after therapy. The results demonstrated that aspirin had a profound effect on prostaglandin synthesis in platelets, while salsalate caused minimal suppression. These results suggest that these salicylate derivatives may have differential effects, which may influence the beneficial and adverse effects of therapy.

Address correspondence and reprint requests to Dr. L. I. Harrison at Riker Laboratories, Inc., 3M Center 270-3S-05, St. Paul, MN 55144, U.S.A.

Presented in part at the American Society for Clinical Pharmacology and Therapeutics 84th Annual Meeting, San Diego, California, U.S.A., March 9–11, 1983.

METHODS

Ten healthy male volunteers (aged 24–34 years) entered and completed the study. Subjects were required to abstain from all medications for 2 weeks prior to the study and to have high (≥90 ng/ml) serum thromboxane B_2 (TXB_2) levels at the time of study initiation. The mean serum TXB_2 concentration (mean ± SE) for the group was 257 ± 28 ng/ml.

The study protocol was reviewed and approved by the Human Experimentation Committee of the National Jewish Hospital and Research Center.

Subjects were assigned to two treatment groups according to a randomized schedule. Medications were given for periods of 3 days, with 13 days of observation following treatment. Aspirin tablets were given in doses of 1,300 mg orally every 8 h (3.9 g/day). Salsalate (500 mg tablets Disalcid; Riker Laboratories, Inc, St. Paul, MN, U.S.A.) was administered in doses of 1,500 mg orally every 12 h (3.0 g/day). Because of greater gastrointestinal tolerance, salsalate was administered in two divided doses each day, whereas aspirin was given in three divided doses. Subjects were seen daily during the period of dosing and for the 2 days following. Thereafter, they were seen at intervals of 2–3 days.

Venous blood samples were used to monitor drug concentrations and cyclo-oxygenase metabolites during the course of the study. Heparinized blood samples were collected for drug measurements before and 3 h after medication on days 1 and 3, and 36–40 h after the last dose of medication on the morning of day 5. Plasma was separated by centrifugation at 4°C, and the plasma samples were frozen at − 20°C until assayed. Plasma concentrations of salicylic acid and salsalate were determined by a high pressure liquid chromatographic method (9). The assays of salsalate and salicylic acid were linear over the concentration range of 1–150 μg/ml. The relative standard deviations for replicate analyses of the 5.0-, 20.0-, and 50.0-μg/ml concentration standards for both salsalate and salicylic acid were ≤4% (9).

For serum TXB_2 and PGE_2 determinations, duplicate venous blood samples were obtained at the times noted above, and also periodically during the treatment and observation periods. These samples were incubated at 37°C for 30 min. The serum was separated by centrifugation at 4°C and frozen at − 20°C until assay. Assays were performed in duplicate with 0.2 ml serum. A double-antibody radioimmunoassay procedure was used for both analyses (10). The assay sensitivities for TXB_2 and PGE_2 were 5–10 pg/tube, with coefficients of variation for repetitive assays of 10% (10). The antisera have minimal cross-reactivity with other cyclo-oxygenase metabolites in plasma or serum.

For each subject, the percentage of suppression of serum TXB_2 and PGE_2 was calculated by comparing the control value obtained just prior to the first dose of drug with the value obtained 3 h after the morning dose on day 3. An unpaired *t* test was used to determine whether there were significant differences between drugs. Salicylic acid levels were similarly compared by a *t* test. For all statistical evaluations, $p \leq 0.05$ was considered significant.

RESULTS

Plasma Drug Concentrations

Plasma concentrations of salicylic acid were within the therapeutic range for antiinflammatory therapy by the third day of dosing with either 3.0 g/day salsalate or 3.9 g/day aspirin. Plasma salicylic acid concentrations, on the average, tended to be higher following aspirin than following salsalate (Table 1). However, the plasma level differences were statistically significant for the predose level on day 3 only.

Three hours after administration of salsalate, plasma also contained small amounts of unchanged salsalate; levels were similar on days 1 and 3 (Table 1). No unchanged drug was detectable 12 h after dosing, as shown by the predose level on day 3.

Serum Prostaglandins

Figures 1 and 2 show the serial changes in serum TXB_2 and PGE_2. Administration of aspirin caused a precipitous drop in both cyclo-oxygenase metabolites to almost undetectable levels. Complete suppression of these metabolites was evident within 3 h after the first dose of aspirin, persisted throughout the period

TABLE 1. *Mean plasma concentrations (±SD) of salicylic acid and salsalate*

	Aspirin treatment		Disalcid treatment			
	Salicylic acid (μg/ml)		Salicylic acid (μg/ml)		Salsalate (μg/ml)	
	Predose	3 h	Predose	3 h	Predose	3 h
Day 1	0	82 ± 11	0	84 ± 11	0	18 ± 5
Day 3	148 ± 25[a]	186 ± 32	117 ± 11[a]	164 ± 14	0	16 ± 7
Day 5	35 ± 40	—	7 ± 9	—	0	—

[a]Significantly different ($p < 0.05$); other differences between salicylic acid levels not significant.

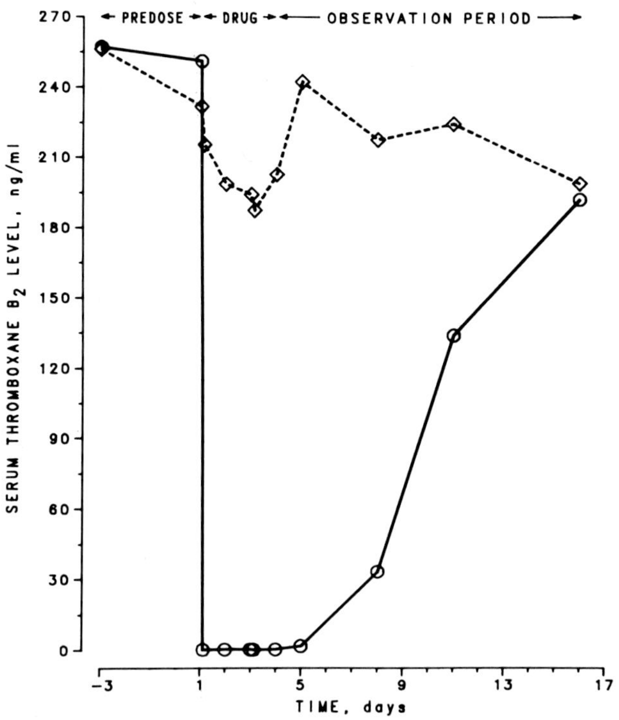

FIG. 1. Mean serum thromboxane B_2 levels in five subjects who received aspirin (circles) or salsalate (diamonds). Standard deviations were ~50% or less of the mean values in all but one case.

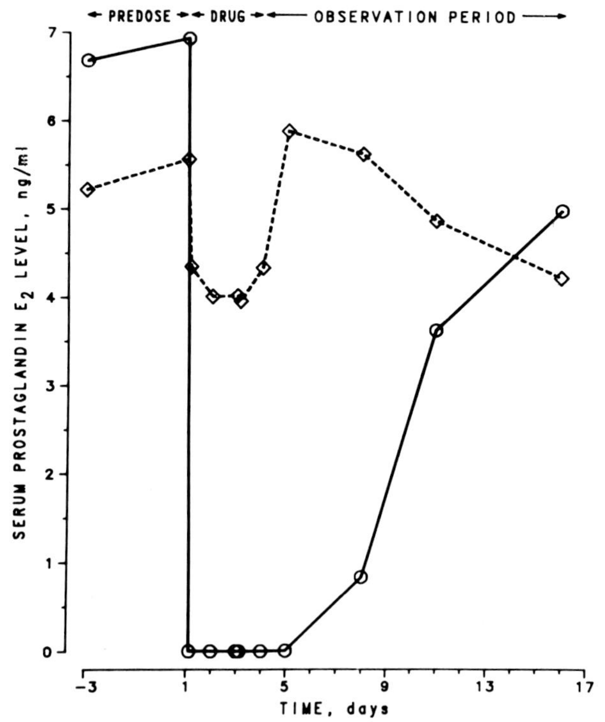

FIG. 2. Mean serum prostaglandin E_2 levels in five subjects who received aspirin (circles) or salsalate (diamonds). Standard deviations were ~50% or less of the mean values in all cases.

of treatment, and was followed by a very slow return to control levels. Thirteen days after discontinuation of aspirin, serum TXB_2 and PGE_2 were still significantly lower than control levels ($p < 0.05$).

Conversely, the response to salsalate treatment was variable, with some subjects showing only small decreases in serum concentrations of TXB_2 and PGE_2, whereas other subjects showed no suppression. Thus, although the mean values of TXB_2 and PGE_2 after the third day of treatment were 7.9 and 20.6% lower than the control values, the differences were not significant (Table 2). The subsequent slight decline in values during the 13-day observation period appeared to be due to random variation (not significantly different than the control values) and did not represent drug effect.

Salsalate caused significantly less suppression of serum TXB_2 and PGE_2 than did aspirin ($p < 0.01$). Calculations based on the maximum suppression during treatment suggested that the suppressive activity of aspirin was 3–5 times greater than that of salsalate. However, the difference in potency was even greater when considered in relation to the marked differences in duration of suppression induced by the two medications.

DISCUSSION

The measurements of TXB_2 and PGE_2 in serum largely reflect prostaglandin synthesis by platelets during blood clotting. The marked differences observed in the effects of aspirin and salsalate on serum prostaglandins indicate that salicylate, per se, has relatively little influence on platelet cyclo-oxygenase. Rather, the profound suppression of serum prostaglandins induced by aspirin stems from the acetylation of platelet cyclo-oxygenase during the brief period before orally administered aspirin is completely hydrolyzed (11). We have previously observed that small doses of aspirin, considerably lower than those needed for antiinflammatory effect, also cause significant suppression of serum prostaglandins (12).

The differences in magnitude of suppression induced by the two medications reflects the relative potencies of salicylic acid versus acetylsalicylic acid on these parameters. Furthermore, whereas the suppression with aspirin approached 100% (11), suppression with salsalate was low and not statistically significant. The modest effects of salsalate are readily reversible, as is shown by the marked differences in rates of recovery of serum TXB_2 and PGE_2 to control levels after discontinuation of medication.

TABLE 2. *Comparative effects of aspirin and salsalate on serum thromboxane B_2 (TXB_2) and prostaglandin E_2 (PGE_2)*

Parameter	Drug-to-baseline comparison Mean percentage suppression (range): Aspirin	Salsalate	Drug-to-drug comparison: Aspirin to salsalate
Serum TXB_2	100.0[a] (99.9–100.0)	7.9 (−22.1–37.2)	$p \leq 0.01$
Serum PGE_2	100.0[a] (100.0–100.0)	20.6[b] (−5.3–49.8)	$p \leq 0.01$

[a] $p \leq 0.01$ compared with baseline.
[b] Not significant compared with baseline.

Salsalate doses of 3.0 g/day and aspirin doses of 3.9 g/day theoretically yield the same amounts of salicylic acid. However, in the body, about 13% of a salsalate dose is not converted to salicylic acid (13). The slight differences in plasma salicylic acid levels cannot account for the large differences in the effects of the two drugs on magnitude and duration of suppression of platelet synthesis of cyclo-oxygenase products. Both drugs maintained salicylic acid levels >100 μg/ml after 2 days of dosing.

This study provides additional in vivo evidence that salicylate derivatives differ in their effects on certain tissues. Similar conclusions based on studies of platelet function have been reported previously for salsalate, aspirin, salicylic acid, sodium salicylate, and diflunisal (3,14). Our data suggest that the differences in function stem from the differential effects of salicylate derivatives on platelet synthesis of cyclo-oxygenase products. These differences may influence the benefits and risks of therapy.

Acknowledgment: This study was supported by a grant from Riker Laboratories, Inc. The authors wish to thank the following staff members of Riker Laboratories for their contributions to this study: T. M. Welscher, B. P. Ekholm, C. R. Kehe, and D. C. Kvam.

REFERENCES

1. Singleton PT. Salsalate: its role in the management of rheumatic disease. *Clin Ther* 1980;3:80–102.
2. McPherson TC. Salsalate for arthritis: a clinical evaluation. *Clin Ther* 1984;6:388–403.
3. Estes D, Kaplan K. Lack of platelet effect with the aspirin analog, salsalate. *Arthritis Rheum* 1980;23:1303–7.
4. Edmar D. Effects of salicylates on the gastric mucosa as revealed by roentgen examination and the gastrocamera. *Acta Radiol* 1971;11:57–66.
5. Mielants H, Veys EM, Verbruggen G, Schelstraete K. Comparison of serum salicylate levels and gastro-intestinal blood loss between salsalate (Disalcid) and other forms of salicylates. *Scand J Rheumatol* 1981;10:169–73.
6. Shen TY. Prostaglandin synthetase inhibitors I. In: Vane JR, Ferreira SH, eds. *Handbook of experimental pharmacology.* New York: Springer-Verlag, 1979:316–7. (Antiinflammatory Drugs; vol. 51/II).
7. Patrignani P, Filabozzi P, Patrono C. Selective cumulative inhibition of platelet thromboxane production by low-dose aspirin in healthy subjects. *J Clin Invest* 1982;69:1366–72.
8. Lorenz R, Siess W, Weber PC. Effects of very low versus standard dose acetylsalicylic acid, dipyridamole and sulfinpyrazone on platelet function and thromboxane formation in man. *Eur J Pharmacol* 1981;70:511–8.
9. Harrison LI, Funk ML, Ober RE. High-pressure liquid chromatographic determination of salicylsalicylic acid, aspirin, and salicylic acid in human plasma and urine. *J Pharm Sci* 1980;69:1268–71.
10. Morris HG, Sherman NA, Shepperdson FT. Variables associated with radioimmunoassay of prostaglandins in plasma. *Prostaglandins* 1981;21:771–88.
11. Granstrom E. On the metabolism of prostaglandin E_1 in man. Prostaglandins and related factors. *Prog Biochem Pharmacol* 1967;3:89–93.
12. Spector SL, Morris HG, Selner JC. Clinical responses and serum prostaglandin levels in aspirin idiosyncrasy: effect of aspirin and a new non-steroidal anti-inflammatory agent. *Chest* 1981;80:676–81.
13. Dromgoole SH, Cassell S, Furst DE, Paulus HE. Availability of salicylate from salsalate and aspirin. *Clin Pharmacol Ther* 1983;34:539–45.
14. Nitelius E, Brantmark B, Fredholm B, et al. Actions and interactions of acetylsalicylic acid, salicylic acid and diflunisal on platelet aggregation. *Eur J Clin Pharmacol* 1984;27:165–8.

Therapeutic Drug Monitoring
7:439–441 © 1985 Raven Press, New York

Sensitive High Performance Liquid Chromatographic Analysis of Ethmozin in Plasma

J. M. Poirier

Department of Pharmacology, Saint-Antoine Hospital, Paris, France

Summary: A sensitive high performance liquid chromatographic procedure for the quantitative determination of ethmozin is described. Following a one-step extraction of the drug and the internal standard, protriptyline, by diethylether at pH 9.0, the organic solvent is evaporated and the residue is reconstituted in the mobile phase and injected into the chromatograph. The separation is obtained using a CN-bonded column with a methanol-propanol-2-perchloric acid 1.16 *M* mobile phase. Ethmozin is detected at 268 nm. Under these conditions, the lower limit of detection is 11 n*M*, and the lower limit of quantification is 22 n*M* (10 ng/ml) for ethmozin. The procedure is linear between 0 and 8,620 n*M*. **Key Words:** High performance liquid chromatographic assay—Ethmozin.

Ethmozin, the ethyl ester hydrochloride of 10-(3-morpholinopropionyl)phenothiazine-2-carbamic acid, is a new antiarrhythmic drug, which is potentially effective for the control of atrial and ventricular arrhythmias (1–3). Two methods have been previously reported for the high performance liquid chromatography (HPLC) determination of ethmozin in plasma. The first, with a silica column (4), has the chromatographic stability problems of unbounded column materials, and the other, using a cation-exchange column (5), provides better results compared with the reversed-phase column. The disposition kinetics of ethmozin are not well known, and prior to investigating the pharmacokinetics and pharmacodynamics in humans, we have developed a simple HPLC assay for ethmozin in plasma, using a CN-bounded phase column.

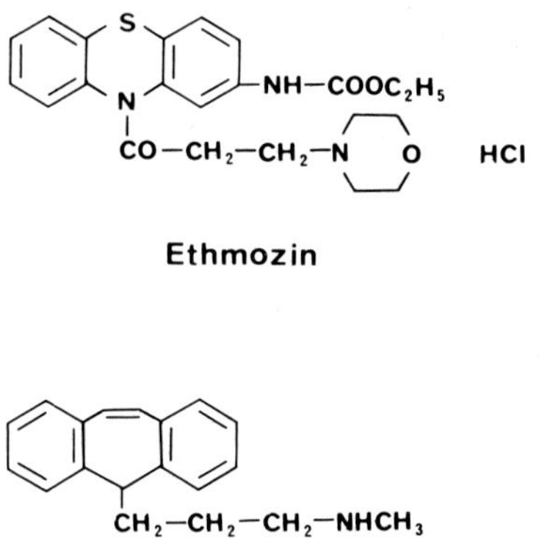

FIG. 1. Molecular structure of ethmozin and protriptyline (internal standard).

MATERIALS AND METHODS

Chemicals and Reagents

Stock solutions of ethmozin hydrochloride (216 μ*M*) and the internal standard protriptyline (380 μ*M*) (Fig. 1) were prepared in methanol. These stock solutions, stored at 4°C, were stable for at least 1 month without observable degradation. Diethylether, methanol, perchloric acid (70%), and sodium hydroxide were obtained from Prolabo (RP Normapur). The 2 *M* *N*-*N*-bis(2-hydroxyethyl)glycine buffer (Sigma) was prepared by adjusting the pH of the corresponding weighed amount to 9.0 with 10 *M* sodium hydroxide.

HPLC

The solvent delivery system was a constant-flow pump (M 45; Waters Associates), and sample injection was performed using an automatic injector (WISP 710

Address correspondence and reprint requests to Dr. Poirier at Saint-Antoine Hospital, 184 Rue du Faubourg Saint-Antoine, 75012 Paris, France.

B, Waters Associates). The chromatograms were obtained from an integrator (SP 4270; Spectra Physics). The analytical column was a Lichrosorb CN 10 μm (Hibar RT; E. Merck), which was used at ambient temperature. The column effluent was monitored with a variable wavelength absorbance detector at 268 nm (M 480; Waters Associates). The mobile phase was methanol-propanol-2-perchloric acid 1.16 *M* (70:30:0.25) vol/vol, and the flow rate was 2.0 ml/min for a back pressure of 90 bars.

Sample Preparation

One milliliter of plasma was pipetted into a 10-ml capped glass tube, and 10 μl of stock solution of internal standard, 500 μl of buffer solution pH 9.0, and 6 ml of diethylether were added. The tube was capped and shaken vigorously for 10 min, after which it was centrifuged for 5 min at 3,500 rpm. The organic phase was removed, transferred to a conic tube, and evaporated under a stream of nitrogen at 40°C. All of the residue was dissolved in 200 μl of mobile phase, and an aliquot was injected (≤150 μl).

Instrument Calibration

Standard solutions containing ethmozin at 216, 431, 1,078, 2,155, and 4,311 n*M* (100–2,000 ng/ml) were prepared using a 1:5 dilution in methanol of the stock solution of ethmozin. Then, 5–100 μl was placed in 10-ml glass tubes, evaporated to dryness under a stream of nitrogen, and redissolved in 1 ml of blank plasma.

These standards were extracted and analyzed by this procedure, and a standard curve was prepared by plotting the ethmozin/protriptyline peak area ratio from the extracted plasma samples versus the plasma ethmozin concentrations. A curve calculated by the least-squares method was used to calculate unknown plasma levels.

RESULTS AND DISCUSSION

In the present method, pretreatment of the sample is very simple, involving a one-step solvent extraction at pH 9.0 by diethylether. Therefore the time required is shorter than in the other methods described (4–5).

It was found that 83% of ethmozin was extracted from plasma (mean ± SD: 83.5 ± 3.0%, n = 5), and the recovery was not affected if a 2-ml plasma sample was employed (mean ± SD: 84.0 ± 2.2%, n = 5).

Using a CN-bounded phase column, the endogenous components from plasma are eluted in the solvent front, and the chromatographic analysis of one sample is achieved in <15 min. Under the chromatographic conditions described, protriptyline and ethmozin were eluted from the column in 9.2 and 11.2 min, respectively. Representative chromatograms from blank plasma and spiked human plasma extracted are shown in Fig. 2.

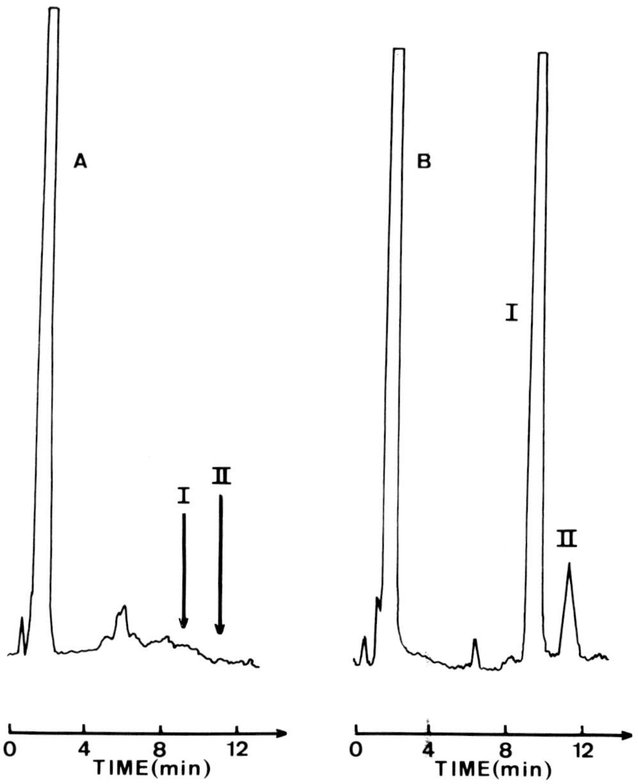

FIG. 2. Chromatograms of extracted human plasma. **A:** 2 ml of blank plasma extracted, residue redissolved in 200 μl of mobile phase, 150 μl injected. **B:** 1 ml of blank plasma spiked with 108 n*M* of ethmozin and 3.80 μ*M* of protriptyline (internal standard), after extraction. Peak I: protriptyline 9.2 min. Peak II: ethmozin 11.2 min.

Linear Range

Standards consisting of 12 samples ranging from 0 to 8,621 n*M* (0–4,000 ng/ml) were prepared using human plasma, extracted, and analyzed by HPLC. A least-squares linear regression was used to calculate a linear equation relating peak area ratio and ethmozin concentration. The method of analysis is linear up to the highest concentration tested, 8,621 n*M*. The correlation coefficient obtained was good (r^2 = 1,000), and no significant difference from the origin was observed.

TABLE 1. *Reproducibility*

Added concentration of ethmozin[a] (n*M*)	Measured concentration (n*M*)	± SD (n*M*)	CV (%)
22	22	3.93	18.2
108	105	12.61	12.0
216	217	8.04	3.7
431	433	10.60	2.5
2,155	2,156	29.12	1.4

[a]As the hydrochloride salt.

Reproducibility

The reproducibility of this procedure was evaluated by analyzing several samples at known plasma concentrations the same day along a series of standards. Drug concentrations were calculated from the obtained linear regression and used to determinate the mean, standard deviation, and CV (%) for each concentration. The results are presented in Table 1.

The intra-assay precision of this method, as evaluated by the CV (%), ranged from 18.2 at 22 n*M* (10 ng/ml) to 1.4 at 2,155 n*M* (1,000 ng/ml) for the ethmozin.

In order to determine low concentrations of ethmozin, we have tested the linearity of the method between 0 and 431 n*M* (200 ng/ml) of plasma on 3 different days in calculating and comparing the least-squares linear regression obtained. Each point of concentration was the mean of five determinations. The interassay precision of standard curves was <3%.

Specificity

The chromatographic system used in this assay can separate and quantify ethmozin with no interference from the extractable components of plasma (see Fig. 2). The retention times of extracts from patient samples taking ethmozin are not different from standard samples, and no metabolite was found.

Limits of Detection and Quantification

The Waters M 480 detector and Spectra Physics SP 4270 integrator are capable of detecting slight deviations from the baseline, and the limit of detection for ethmozin is 11 n*M* (5 ng/ml) of plasma when the residue is redissolved in 200 μl of mobile phase and 150 μl is injected. The limit of quantification is established as 22 n*M* (10 ng/ml) for ethmozin (150 μl of the extract injected).

Acknowledgment: Ethmozin and protriptyline were generously supplied by Du Pont de Nemours and Merck Sharp & Dohme-Chibret, respectively.

REFERENCES

1. Votchal BE, Lozinskii LG. Effectiveness of the new antiarrhythmic compound ethmozin. *Klin Med* 1971;10:16–21.
2. Kaverina NV, Senova ZR, Mitrofavov VS, Runova MF. Pharmacology of ethmozin: a new antiarrhythmic drug. *Farmakol Toksikol* 1972;2:182–5.
3. Morganroth J, Pearlman AS, Dunkman WB, Horowitz LN, Josephson ME, Michelson EL. Ethmozin: a new antiarrhythmic agent developed in the USSR: efficacy and tolerance. *Am Heart J* 1979;98:621–8.
4. Whitney CC, Weinstein SH, Gaylord JC. High-performance liquid chromatographic determination of ethmozin in plasma. *J Pharm Sci* 1981;70:462–3.
5. Piotrovski VK, Metelitsa VI. Ion-exchange high-performance liquid chromatography in drug assay in biological fluids. I. Ethmozin. *J Chromatogr* 1982;231:205–9.

Therapeutic Drug Monitoring
7:442–446 © 1985 Raven Press, New York

Comparison of High Pressure Liquid Chromatography and Fluorescence Polarization Immunoassay Methods in a Theophylline Pharmacokinetic Study

*Richard L. Lalonde, *Michael B. Bottorff, and †Arthur B. Straughn

**Departments of Clinical Pharmacy and †Pharmaceutics, College of Pharmacy, University of Tennessee Center for the Health Sciences, Memphis, Tennessee, U.S.A.*

Summary: High pressure liquid chromatography (HPLC) and fluorescence polarization immunoassay (FPIA) were compared in a theophylline pharmacokinetic study. Eight healthy subjects received single 600-mg oral doses of two different sustained-release theophylline formulations. Fourteen blood samples were collected over 57 h after each dose, and the serum was analyzed for theophylline using both HPLC and FPIA methods. In comparing the two formulations using HPLC, there was no statistical difference in the area under the curve (AUC), terminal rate constant (k), or time of peak. However, there was a 13% difference in peak theophylline concentration ($p < 0.05$). The same statistical conclusions were made for all parameters when using FPIA. When comparing the kinetic parameters determined with each assay, the AUC was 12% greater and the k was 17% smaller with FPIA ($p < 0.05$). Orthogonal regression of all serum theophylline concentrations showed that FPIA = 1.04 HPLC + 0.20; $r = 0.987$, $p < 0.001$. Stratification of serum theophylline concentrations into different ranges showed that FPIA overestimated the HPLC results in each range, but the percentage of overestimation was greater at lower concentrations ($p < 0.05$). The use of FPIA seems appropriate in comparative studies of theophylline pharmacokinetics; however, the calculated kinetic parameters may differ slightly from those obtained with HPLC. **Key Words:** Theophylline—Assays—Pharmacokinetics.

After many years of clinical use, theophylline is still considered an effective bronchodilator and is commonly prescribed for patients with acute and chronic obstructive pulmonary disease. In view of the numerous factors known to alter the pharmacokinetics of theophylline and its narrow therapeutic index, the monitoring of serum theophylline concentrations has become common practice (1).

Several different assay methods are now available for theophylline. Among these, high pressure liquid chromatography (HPLC) has gained broad acceptance in research laboratories because of its sensitivity, accuracy, and ability to measure theophylline and its metabolites separately. Conversely, fluorescence polarization immunoassay (FPIA) and other immunoassay methods are now widely used in clinical and hospital laboratories because they can be automated to deal with a large number of samples rapidly. Since immunoassays are very versatile, some investigators are now using them for theophylline pharmacokinetic studies when information on theophylline metabolites is not deemed necessary.

The FPIA method for theophylline has been shown to be comparable in precision and accuracy to HPLC

Address correspondence and reprint requests to Dr. R. L. Lalonde at Department of Clinical Pharmacy, University of Tennessee Center for the Health Sciences, 26 South Dunlap Street, Suite 202, Memphis, TN 38163, U.S.A.

and other methods (2–4). However, to our knowledge, no systematic evaluation of FPIA as a research tool in pharmacokinetics has been reported. The purpose of this study was to compare the results obtained by FPIA with those of an accepted standard (HPLC) in a theophylline pharmacokinetic study.

METHODS

Eight healthy male subjects ranging in age from 22 to 31 years and in weight from 73 to 89 kg participated. All subjects were nonsmokers and had no evidence of significant past or current illnesses, based on a medical history, electrocardiogram, and clinical chemistry tests. The subjects were not receiving any other medications and were instructed to abstain from alcohol and xanthine-containing foods for 48 h prior to and during the study. Written informed consent was obtained from each volunteer, and the protocol was approved by the university's Institutional Review Board.

On two occasions 1 week apart, each subject received in randomized order a single 600-mg oral dose of one of the two sustained-release theophylline formulations. The doses were administered with 240 ml water after a 9-h overnight fast. The subjects fasted for another 5 h and then received a standard lunch followed 5 h later by a standard dinner.

Ten-milliliter blood samples were collected via an indwelling catheter or by direct venipuncture just prior to and at 2, 4, 6, 8, 10, 12, 14, 16, 25, 30, 35, 49, and 57 h after the dose. Blood samples were allowed to clot at ambient temperature and were then centrifuged, and the serum was frozen at −20°C until the time of analysis.

Each serum sample was analyzed for theophylline using FPIA (TDx; Abbott Laboratories, Irving, TX, U.S.A.) and HPLC methods. The latter consisted of a reversed-phase liquid chromatography system with a μBondapack C18 column (30 cm × 4 mm), a WISP model 710 B autoinjector, a model 6000 A pump, and a model 440 detector (254 nm), all from Waters Associates, Inc., (Milford, MA, U.S.A.). Detector response from the 1-V output was integrated using a Hewlett-Packard 3350 series laboratory automation system. The mobile phase [0.05 *M* tetrabutylammonium chloride in acetate buffer: acetonitrile (96:4) adjusted to a pH of 4.3 with glacial acetic acid] was passed through the column at a rate of 2.0 ml/min. Serum samples (0.5 ml) were prepared for chromatography by addition of internal standard (β-hydroxypropyltheophylline), followed by extraction with 5 ml of 3% isopropranol/chloroform. The organic phase was evaporated to dryness under a stream of nitrogen, reconstituted with mobile phase, and transferred to WISP vials for injection. For each set of subject samples assayed, a standard curve was prepared using serum fortified to contain 0.25, 1.0, 5.0, and 10.0 μg/ml of theophylline. This method is specific for theophylline in the presence of 3-methylxanthine, paraxanthine, xanthine, 1–2 dimethyluric acid, 1-methyluric acid, uric acid, theobromine, and caffeine. The coefficients of variation (%) for this assay were 10.9 at 0.25, 5.8 at 1.0, 3.1 at 5.0, and 1.5 at 10.0 μg/ml. All standard curves were linear with correlation coefficients >0.998.

The FPIA procedure utilized the Theophylline-II reagents (monoclonal antibodies), calibrators, controls, and autoanalyzer according to the manufacturer's protocol, without any modification. The standard curve was prepared using calibrators with 0.0, 2.5, 5.0, 10.0, 20.0, and 40.0 μg/ml of theophylline. The coefficients of variation (%) were 13 at 1.2, 3.2 at 5.0, and 2.4 at 10.0 μg/ml. Two controls were included with each carousel of serum samples. All serum samples were assayed in duplicate, with the mean of the two concentrations used in calculations.

Data Analysis

The terminal first-order rate constant *(k)* was determined by linear least-squares regression of the terminal log-linear portion of the theophylline concentration–time curve. The area under the curve (AUC) was calculated by the linear trapezoidal rule up to the last concentration used in the linear regression (C_{last}), then extrapolated to infinity with the ratio C_{last}/k. The peak theophylline concentration (C_p) and the time of that peak (T_p) were determined directly from the serum concentration–time curves. The pharmacokinetic parameters were compared using an analysis of variance (ANOVA), which was designed to study the effects of subjects, order of treatments, theophylline formulations, and assay methods.

The serum theophylline concentrations were stratified for descriptive analytical purposes into four groups: <3, 3 to <6, 6 to <9, and 9 to <12 μg/ml. Grouping of the serum theophylline concentration pairs was accomplished using the HPLC values. A total of 199 concentration pairs had measurable theophylline concentrations with each assay. Within each group, the numerical difference in theophylline concentrations (FPIA-HPLC) and the percentage difference (FPIA-HPLC)·100/HPLC were determined for each serum theophylline concentration pair. Since normal distri-

TABLE 1. *Pharmacokinetic parameters [$\bar{x}$(SD)] for two theophylline formulations as determined by HPLC*

	AUC (μg · h/ml)	k (h^{-1})	C_p (μg/ml)	T_p (h)
Product 1	208 (71)	0.080 (0.022)	8.9 (1.4)[a]	9.3 (1.8)
Product 2	231 (67)	0.075 (0.015)	10.1 (1.6)[a]	8.8 (2.4)

HPLC, high pressure liquid chromatography; AUC, area under the curve; k, terminal rate constant; C_p, peak concentration; T_p, time of peak concentration.
[a]$p < 0.05$.

bution was not observed, the numerical differences within each group were compared with a zero difference using the nonparametric Wilcoxon one-sample test. The percentage differences were compared between the four groups using the Kruskal-Wallis and the conservative multiple comparison tests (5). The above statistical analyses were performed with the use of the Statistical Analysis System (SAS Institute, Inc., Cary, NC, U.S.A.). Correlation between the serum theophylline concentrations as obtained by the two assay methods was determined by Pearson's product moment correlation coefficient. In addition, weighted perpendicular (orthogonal) least-squares regression was used to describe the relationship between the HPLC and FPIA concentration pairs (6,7). In all statistical analyses, the 5% level of confidence was used to reject the null hypothesis.

RESULTS

The results of the bioavailability comparison using HPLC are presented in Table 1. Although there was an 11% difference in the AUC, it did not achieve statistical significance. Only with C_p was there a statistical difference between the two theophylline products ($p < 0.05$). The bioavailability comparison using FPIA (Table 2) led to the same statistical conclusions for each parameter as when the data were analyzed using HPLC. A similar trend was observed with both

TABLE 2. *Pharmacokinetic parameters [$\bar{x}$(SD)] for two theophylline formulations as determined by FPIA*

	AUC (μg · h/ml)	k (h^{-1})	C_p (μg/ml)	T_p (h)
Product 1	238 (91)	0.068 (0.028)	9.2 (1.4)[a]	9.8 (2.3)
Product 2	253 (49)	0.063 (0.013)	10.6 (1.3)[a]	8.8 (2.1)

FPIA, fluorescence polarization immunoassay; AUC, area under the curve; k, terminal rate constant; C_p, peak concentration; T_p, time of peak concentration.
[a]$p < 0.05$.

TABLE 3. *Comparison of pharmacokinetic parameters [$\bar{x}$(SD)] as determined by HPLC and FPIA*

	AUC (μg · h/ml)	k (h^{-1})	C_p (μg/ml)	T_p (h)
HPLC	220 (68)[a]	0.078 (0.018)[a]	9.5 (1.6)	9.0 (2.1)
FPIA	246 (71)[a]	0.065 (0.022)[a]	9.9 (1.5)	9.3 (2.2)

HPLC, high pressure liquid chromatography; FPIA, fluorescence polarization immunoassay; AUC, area under the curve; k, terminal rate constant; C_p, peak concentration; T_p, time of peak concentration.
[a]$p < 0.05$.

assay methods for product differences in AUC, k, and T_p. The power of the ANOVA for AUC was similar for both assay methods (0.44 and 0.49 for HPLC and FPIA, respectively). When the results for each product were pooled and compared between HPLC and FPIA (Table 3), differences were observed for AUC and k ($p < 0.05$). Therefore, even if similar differences between formulations were observed with the two assay methods, the absolute values of the kinetic parameters were different.

A comparison of the theophylline concentration pairs as determined by HPLC and FPIA is illustrated in Fig. 1. The correlation coefficient was 0.987 ($p < 0.001$), while the results of the orthogonal regression analysis show a slope of 1.04 and intercept of 0.20, indicating that FPIA overestimated the HPLC results in the range of concentrations studied. Figures 2 and 3 illustrate the distribution of numerical differences observed between the two assay methods in different concentration ranges. Again, the trend is for

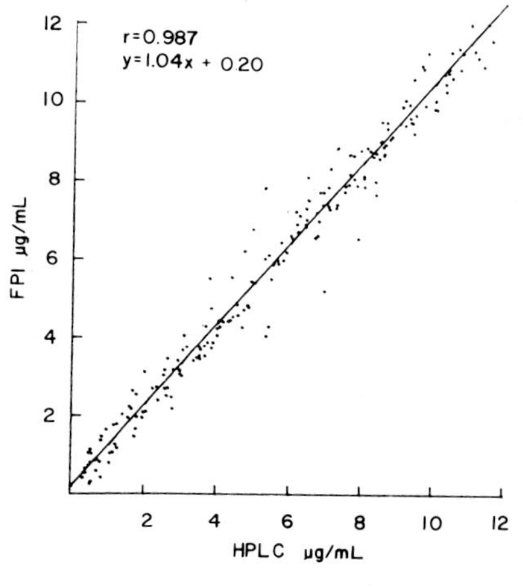

FIG. 1. Comparison of the serum theophylline concentration pairs as determined by high pressure liquid chromatography (HPLC) and fluorescence polarization immunoassay (FPI).

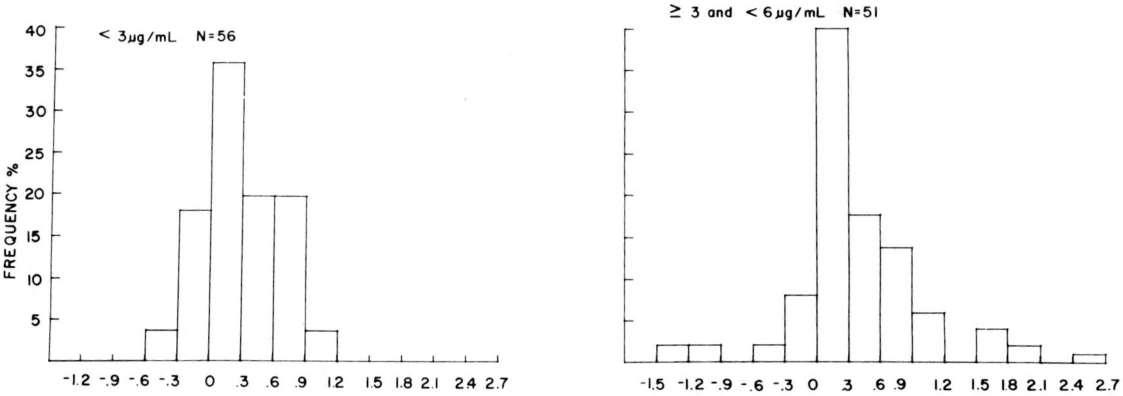

FIG. 2. Observed differences in serum theophylline concentrations between fluorescence polarization immunoassay and high pressure liquid chromatography (FPIA-HPLC) at concentrations <3 (left) and ⩾3 through <6 (right) µg/ml.

the FPIA results to be higher. This trend is confirmed with the data from Table 4, showing numerical differences greater than zero in all four concentration ranges ($p < 0.05$). Furthermore, the percentage of overestimation by FPIA was greater at the lowest concentrations than at the highest one ($p < 0.05$).

DISCUSSION

In this comparative bioavailability study, the same statistical conclusions were reached regardless of the assay method used. The differences in AUC, k, and T_p between formulations were not statistically significant; however, similar trends were observed with each assay method.

Overall, the mean AUC was 12% greater and the mean k 17% smaller with FPIA in comparison with HPLC. These parameters are not independent of each other since the same theophylline concentrations are used to estimate them and k is used to extrapolate the AUC to infinity. The observed differences are explained by the higher serum theophylline concentrations measured by FPIA in each concentration range (leading to a higher AUC) and the larger percentage of overestimation by FPIA at the lowest concentration range (leading to a smaller k and a larger extrapolated portion of AUC).

The percentage of overestimation by FPIA was smaller at serum theophylline concentrations >3 µg/ml; however, it increased to a median of 18.4% at concentrations <3 µg/ml. The source of this relative bias is unclear, but it could be related to theophylline metabolites. However, the available data suggest little or no interference from metabolites with FPIA (8–10). Another source of error comes from the larger coefficients of variation at the lower concentration with both assays. Recently, some investigators have reported falsely elevated theophylline concentrations measured with FPIA in patients with renal impairment (9,10). This apparent interference can be ruled out in this study, since our subjects were young, healthy volunteers with normal renal function. It should also

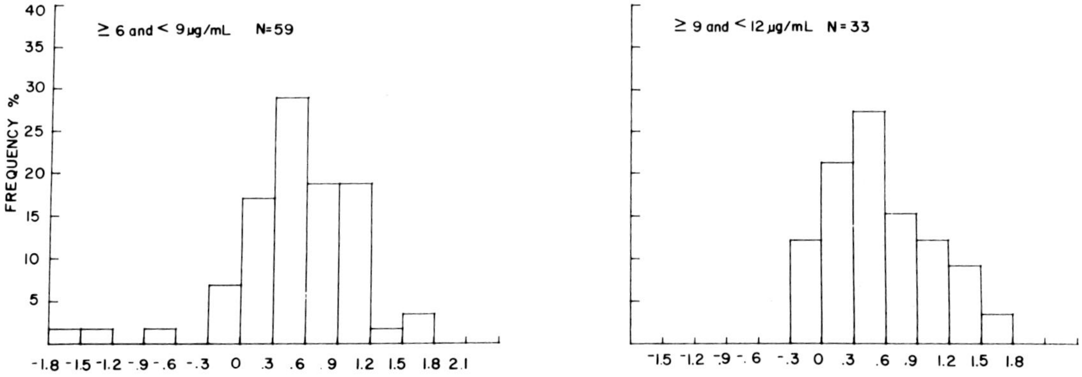

FIG. 3. Observed differences in serum theophylline concentrations between fluorescence polarization immunoassay and high pressure liquid chromatography (FPIA-HPLC) at concentrations of ⩾6 through <9 (left) and ⩾9 through <12 (right) µg/ml.

TABLE 4. *Theophylline concentrations as obtained by HPLC and FPIA in four concentration ranges*

	0–3 μg/ml (n = 56)	3–6 μg/ml (n = 51)	6–9 μg/ml (n = 59)	9–12 μg/ml (n = 33)
HPLC[a]	1.5 (0.9)[b]	4.4 (0.9)[b]	7.5 (0.8)[b]	10.1 (0.7)[b]
FPIA[a]	1.8 (1.0)[b]	4.8 (1.1)[b]	8.0 (0.9)[b]	10.6 (0.7)[b]
Percent difference[c]	+ 18.4[d]	+ 5.0	+ 7.5	+ 4.3[d]

HPLC, high pressure liquid chromatography; FPIA, fluorescence polarization immunoassay.

[a] $\bar{x}$ (SD).

[b] $p < 0.05$ (differences between FPIA and HPLC values are >0).

[c] Median values.

[d] $p < 0.05$ between lowest and highest concentration ranges.

be emphasized that the assay bias observed in this study is a relative one and could be due to an error in the HPLC and/or FPIA methods.

Usually, new assay methods are evaluated and compared with an established method using correlation and linear least-squares regression analysis. Ordinary least-squares regression of y on x, however, assumes that there is no error in the x (abscissa) values. This is clearly not the case when comparing two assay methods. Riggs et al. (6) showed that use of ordinary least-squares regression when both variables are subject to error will lead to erroneous estimates of the true slope and intercept. Although several other techniques have been evaluated, the weighted perpendicular (orthogonal) least-squares regression method has been recommended and found to give better estimates of regression parameters when both variables are subject to experimental error (6,7).

Inherent differences between assay methods may explain some of the observed discrepancies. One method is based on liquid chromatography and the other on an antigen-antibody reaction. Furthermore, different concentrations of theophylline were used to prepare the standard curves for each method.

In the present study, the assay methods were compared over a serum theophylline concentration range of 0–12 μg/ml. Therefore, the results should not be extrapolated to the higher concentrations that are often measured in patients receiving theophylline therapy. The lower concentrations evaluated in this study are those usually obtained in single-dose pharmacokinetic studies with theophylline.

In this relative bioavailability study, identical statistical conclusions were drawn from the results from HPLC and FPIA methods. The use of the FPIA method, therefore, seems appropriate in comparative studies of theophylline pharmacokinetics. Since differences were observed in the pharmacokinetic parameters calculated with each assay method, these differences may also be apparent when comparing studies that used HPLC and FPIA. However, such study comparisons are often limited by significant differences in study populations and methodologies.

REFERENCES

1. Hendeles L, Weinberger M. Theophylline: a state of the art review. *Pharmacotherapy* 1983;3:2–44.
2. Hill HD, Jolley ME, Wang CHJ, et al. Fluorescence polarization immunoassay (FPIA) for theophylline: clinical correlation and reagent stability [Abstract]. *Clin Chem* 1981;27:1086.
3. Landesman PW, Walters MI, Even L. A comparison of six methods for theophylline [Abstract]. *Clin Chem* 1983;29:1238.
4. Wong SHY, DellaFera SS, Fernandes RM. Antiepileptics and theophylline monitoring by fluorescence polarization immunoassay (FPIA) [Abstract]. *Clin Chem* 1983;29:1157.
5. Hollander M, Wolfe DA, eds. *Nonparametric statistical methods.* New York: John Wiley and Sons, 1973.
6. Riggs DS, Guarnieri JA, Addelman S. Fitting straight lines when both variables are subject to error. *Life Sci* 1978;22:1305–60.
7. Jusko WJ. Guidelines for collection and pharmacokinetic analysis of drug disposition data. In: Evans WE, Schentag JJ, Jusko WJ, eds. *Applied pharmacokinetics.* San Francisco: Applied Therapeutics Inc., 1980:639–80.
8. Theophylline II Monograph. Diagnostics Division, Abbott Laboratories: North Chicago, Illinois. 1984.
9. Patel JA, Clayton LT, LeBel CP, McClatchey KD. Abnormal theophylline levels in plasma by fluorescence polarization immunoassay in patients with renal disease. *Ther Drug Monit* 1984;6:458–60.
10. Nelson KM, Mathews SE, Bowers LD. Theophylline concentrations may be falsely high in serum of uremic patients. *Clin Chem* 1983;29:2125–6.

Therapeutic Drug Monitoring
7:447–450 © 1985 Raven Press, New York

Stability of Bupropion and its Major Metabolites in Human Plasma

S. Casey Laizure and C. Lindsay DeVane

Departments of Pharmacy Practice and Psychiatry, Colleges of Pharmacy and Medicine, University of Florida Gainesville, Florida, U.S.A.

Summary: Bupropion (BUP) is a new, monocyclic, second-generation antidepressant with efficacy comparable with that of the tricyclics but possessing a more favorable side-effect profile. Therapeutic drug monitoring services are expected to be widely available following the marketing of BUP, yet relatively little has been published on its clinical pharmacokinetics. The purpose of this study was to assess the drug's plasma stability and to determine the best storage conditions for conducting pharmacokinetic studies of BUP and its major metabolites. Human plasma was spiked with known concentrations of BUP and its major basic metabolites, threo-amino alcohol (TB), erythro-amino alcohol (EB), and hydroxy metabolite (HB), and incubated under varying conditions of temperature and pH. BUP showed a log linear degradation that was both temperature and pH dependent. BUP half-life in pH 7.4 plasma stored at 22 and 37°C was 54.2 and 11.4 h, respectively. Incubation at 37°C, pH 2.5 to 10, for 48 h had minimal effect on metabolite concentrations. These results indicate that drug degradation must be considered in studies involving the incubation of plasma for protein binding determinations and the collection and storage of plasma samples for drug concentration analysis during therapeutic drug monitoring. **Key Words:** Bupropion—Pharmacokinetics—Metabolites.

Measurement of plasma or serum concentrations of psychoactive drugs has become a valuable research tool and clinical aid in psychiatry (1,2). With the advent of modern technologies such as high performance liquid chromatography (HPLC) to quantitate the relatively low plasma concentrations of antidepressants and antipsychotics, commercial laboratories have extended analytical services beyond the research institution to the office practitioner. Precisely quantitating the concentration of these drugs in plasma samples has presented no difficulty because of drug instability.

Though the tricyclic antidepressants and their metabolites may be stable in human plasma (3), this stability does not assure that the second-generation antidepressants have the same characteristics. Unlike the tricyclics, that constitute a class of drugs with a similar three-ring structure, the second-generation antidepressants are a diverse group of compounds, that include monocyclic, bicyclic, tetracyclic, and heterocyclic ring systems. With the introduction of newer antidepressants and other psychoactive drugs, there is increasing interest in determining their plasma concentrations for research and clinical applications. Already, some laboratories are offering plasma concentration measurements of second-generation antidepressants before some of these compounds have been marketed.

Bupropion (BUP) is a structurally novel, nontricyclic antidepressant whose efficacy has been established in open and double-blind, placebo-controlled studies (4,5). Its low side-effect profile suggests that this agent will have important clinical advantages over

Address correspondence and reprint requests to Dr. C. L. DeVane at Box J-4, College of Pharmacy, University of Florida, Gainesville, FL 32610, U.S.A.

the widely used tricyclic antidepressants (6,7). BUP is a highly metabolized compound in humans (Fig. 1). The major metabolites are threo-amino alcohol (TB), erythro-amino alcohol (EB), and hydroxy metabolite (HB). After single oral doses and at steady state, these metabolites achieve plasma concentrations much higher than those of BUP (8 and S. C. Laizure et al., unpublished observations). Future pharmacokinetic studies should account for the presence of these metabolites. Therefore, it is important to document the plasma stability of these compounds in order to generate valid pharmacokinetic data. The purpose of this study was to determine the stability of BUP and its major metabolites in plasma under varying storage conditions.

MATERIALS AND METHODS

Blood was collected from drug-free healthy volunteers by venipuncture of antecubital veins. The blood samples were centrifuged and the plasma transferred to volumetric flasks containing known amounts of BUP and its three major metabolites. The final concentrations were chosen to approximate drug and metabolite concentrations observed during chronic dosing (8). Two to three 1-ml aliquots were separated and stored under varying conditions of pH and temperature to serve as treatment groups. Plasma pH was adjusted using either sodium hydroxide, 1 *M*, or concentrated phosphoric acid. Control samples were kept frozen at − 17°C. All samples were shielded from light during storage.

The first experiment included samples of pH 2.5, 5, 7.4, 8.5, and 10 stored at 37°C. For each pH group, the drug concentration in two samples was compared with results from two control samples following a 48-h storage. In additional experiments performed at pH 7.4, sample groups were stored at room temperature (22°C) and at 37°C for various time intervals as long as 96 h. To assess long-term stability (>6 months), reassay was performed on frozen samples (− 17°C, pH 7.4) that had been taken from subjects who had participated in a previous pharmacokinetic study of the oral disposition of bupropion (S. C. Laizure et al., unpublished observations). All samples had been stored following initial assay for 6 months to a year.

All BUP and metabolite concentrations were determined with the HPLC method developed by Cooper et al. (8). The samples for each experiment were extracted and analyzed during the same chromatographic procedure.

In the first experiment, which assessed the effect of pH, Student's *t* test was used for comparison of control and treatment groups. The level of significance was set at $p < 0.01$ according to Bonferroni's adjustment to compensate for the use of multiple *t* tests for comparison of means (9). In the experiments of drug decay over time, linear regression using standard techniques was performed on the log of drug concentration versus time values to determine a drug disappearance half-life ($t_{1/2}$). The reassay of stored subject samples was evaluated using the *t* statistic for paired comparisons (10).

RESULTS

BUP was the only compound of the four tested that degraded extensively in human plasma under the treat-

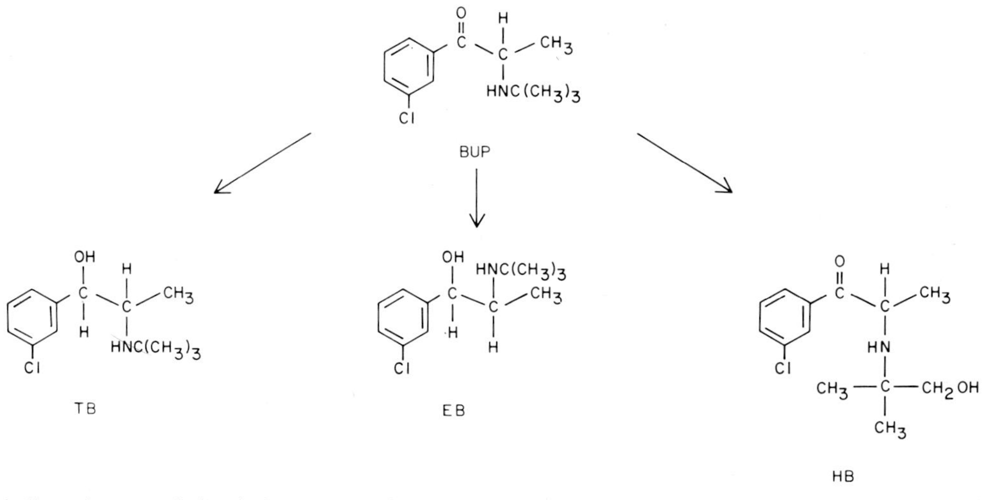

FIG. 1. Metabolic pathways and chemical structures of bupropion (BUP) and its major basic metabolites, erythro-amino alcohol (EB), threo-amino alcohol (TB), and hydroxy metabolite (HB).

TABLE 1. *Change in mean concentration of bupropion and its major metabolites when stored at 37°C, pH 2.5–10, over 48 h*

pH	BUP 0 h	BUP 48 h	HB 0 h	HB 48 h	EB 0 h	EB 48 h	TB 0 h	TB 48 h
2.5	180.3	181.6	741.9	751.0	183.8	188.9	728.5	752.2
5	188.7	30.3[a]	740.4	804.5	202.5	191.1	726.4	786.0
7.4	200.1	53.6[a]	845.1	790.3	205.9	194.2	827.2	800.0
8.5	197.8	49.7[a]	850.8	819.5	201.9	189.6	795.8	784.4
10	192.4	21.5[a]	791.0	785.3	197.7	172.5[a]	783.0	730.8

Each value is the mean from assay of two 1-ml plasma aliquots. BUP, bupropion; HB, hydroxy metabolite; EB, erythro-amino metabolite; TB, threo-amino metabolite.
[a]Significantly different compared with 0-h sample; $p < 0.01$.

ment conditions. Table 1 summarizes the results of test sample incubation at 37°C at pH values from 2.5 to 10. BUP concentrations decreased from 73 to 89% at pH values from 5 to 10. At pH 2.5, BUP degradation was inhibited and no significant change in plasma concentration resulted after 48 h of incubation at 37°C. The mean EB concentration at 0 and 48 h for pH 10 showed a significant decline (Table 1), but represented only a 13% reduction compared with the zero-time concentration. Further study of BUP alone was conducted, as it represented the most labile compound in the handling of analytical plasma samples (Table 1).

In order to characterize the rate of BUP decay, test samples were incubated over various time intervals as long as 96 h, and decay curves were constructed from the data. The results of incubating plasma from one volunteer are shown in Fig. 2. BUP degradation appeared to occur in a log linear fashion at 22 and 37°C with a $t_{1/2}$ of 54.2 ($r^2 = 0.9546$) and 11.4 h ($r^2 = 0.9895$), respectively, (Fig. 2). In plasma taken from a second volunteer, BUP disappeared with a $t_{1/2}$ of 41.9 h at 22°C and pH 7.4.

The long-term stability of BUP plasma samples stored at − 17°C was evaluated by the reassay of old subject samples from another study. Plasma samples from four subjects, two samples from each subject, were reassayed and the results were compared with those from the initial plasma concentration determinations. The samples had been stored at − 17°C for 131–326 days (mean 233 days). The means of the BUP plasma concentrations from the original analyses and from subsequent reanalyses were 103.2 and 97.9 ng/ml, respectively. A paired comparison (10) did not show a statistical difference between BUP concentrations ($p > 0.1840$) or any of the three metabolites, HB ($p > 0.1311$), EB ($p > 0.2810$), and TB ($p > 0.3562$).

DISCUSSION

The implications of this study are relevant to both the clinical practitioner and the researcher. Blood samples obtained for therapeutic plasma concentration monitoring should be collected and centrifuged, and the plasma frozen just after collection. If plasma samples must be mailed to a distant laboratory for anal-

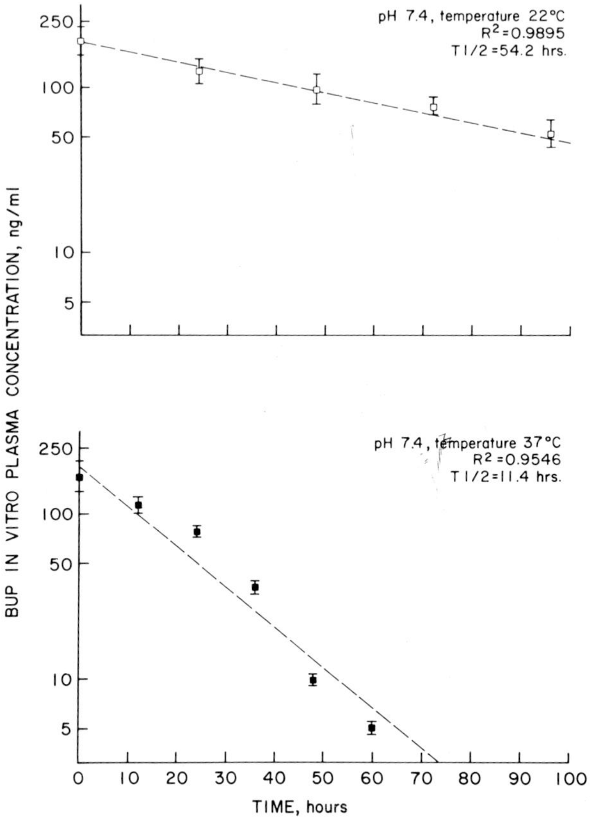

FIG. 2. In vitro degradation of bupropion in human plasma at pH 7.4. Each point represents the mean (SD) of three plasma aliquots. R^2, correlation coefficient; $T_{1/2}$, half-life.

TABLE 2. *Theoretical loss of bupropion in plasma at room temperature (22°C) and at 37°C based on degradation curves from Fig. 2*

Time (h)	Amount remaining (%)	
	22°C	37°C
0	100	100
2	97	88
4	95	78
8	90	61
16	81	38
24	74	23
48	54	5

ysis, then preferably they should be shipped in a frozen state.

While the freezing of samples is not immediately crucial, allowing exposure at room temperature (22°C) for 4 h or longer could result in significant degradation. This can be appreciated by observing the percentage of BUP remaining after various time intervals of room temperature exposure in Table 2. These data were calculated using the $t_{1/2}$ obtained from linear regression of the data shown in Fig. 2.

The researcher's knowledge of the stability of BUP is essential for the planning of valid kinetic studies. If large volumes of plasma samples are rethawed several times to obtain small aliquots, then lowered concentrations of BUP can be expected if this procedure is repeated several times. The study of plasma protein binding by equilibrium dialysis presents special problems because it usually requires incubation of plasma samples containing drug for several hours at 37°C. As can be appreciated from Table 2, the degradation of BUP would be considerable in this situation. In the only published protein binding study of BUP of which we are aware (11), dialysis was performed at 37°C for 5 h. The extent of the plasma protein binding of BUP needs reevaluation in light of the present findings.

Determination of the mechanism of BUP degradation in human plasma was beyond the scope of this study, but some speculation is possible from the available data. BUP did not degrade into any of the three major basic metabolites. The degradation of BUP at pH 7.4, 22, and 37°C was performed with only BUP present in plasma samples. No quantifiable metabolites appeared in the plasma at any time points despite almost complete BUP disappearance at the later time points. Also, the degradation of BUP was a spontaneous process. A similar degradation occurred when BUP was incubated in isotonic normal saline buffered to pH 7.4 with phosphate buffer. This observation, coupled with the fact that an extremely low pH (2.5) inhibited degradation (protonation at the amine group), indicates a spontaneous hydrolysis reaction involving the carbon-nitrogen bond of the amine group (Fig. 1). The resulting products are most likely acidic and would require a different extraction method to isolate and chromatograph. Acidic degradation products of BUP would most likely not retain antidepressant activity; however, these breakdown products may have other unforeseen pharmacologic activities.

In summary, BUP is an unstable compound in plasma. Biological samples for drug concentration analysis should be frozen soon after collection to maintain drug stability. This instability is not a major concern with the three major basic metabolites of BUP. BUP plasma samples may be stored frozen for 6 months or longer without appreciable degradation.

REFERENCES

1. Anonymous. Monitoring drug concentrations in neuropsychiatry. *Br J Clin Pharmacol* 1979;8:291–2.
2. Task force on the use of laboratory tests in psychiatry; tricyclic antidepressants—blood level measurements and clinical outcome: an APA task force report. *Am J Psychiatry* 1985;142:155–61.
3. Zetin M, Rubin R, Rydzewski R. Tricyclic antidepressant sample stability and the vacutainer effect. *Am J Psychiatry* 1981;138:1247–8.
4. Fabre LF, McLendon D. Double-blind placebo-controlled study of bupropion hydrochloride (Wellbutrin) in the treatment of depressed in-patients. *Curr Ther Res* 1978;23:393–402.
5. Fann WE, Schroeder DH, Mehta NP, Soroko FE, Maxwell RA. Clinical trial of bupropion HCl in treatment of depression. *Curr Ther Res* 1978;23:222–9.
6. Farid FF, Wenger TL, Tsai SY, Singh BN, Stern WC. Use of bupropion in patients who exhibit orthostatic hypotension on tricyclic antidepressants. *J Clin Psychiatry* 1983;44:5(sec 2):170–3.
7. Halaris AE, Stern WC, van Wyck Fleet J, Rochelle MR. Evaluation of the safety and efficacy of bupropion in depression. *J Clin Psychiatry* 1983;44:5(sec 2):101–3.
8. Cooper TB, Suckow RF, Glassman A. Determination of bupropion and its major basic metabolites in plasma by liquid chromatography with dual-wavelength ultraviolet detection. *J Pharm Sci* 1984;73:1,104–7.
9. Miller RG. *Simultaneous statistical inference.* New York: McGraw Hill Book Company, 1966:66–70.
10. SAS Institute. *Statistical analysis system (SAS) user's guide.* Cary, North Carolina: SAS Institute, 1982:220–1.
11. Findlay JWA, Rogers JZ, Smith PG, et al. Pharmacokinetics of bupropion, a novel antidepressant agent, following oral administration to healthy subjects. *Eur J Clin Pharmacol* 1981;21:127–35.

Therapeutic Drug Monitoring
7:451–454 © 1985 Raven Press, New York

Determination of Serum Theophylline by Apoenzyme Reactivation Immunoassay System

Mario Plebani and Angelo Burlina

Department of Clinical Chemistry and Clinical Microscopy, Ospedale Civile, Padova, Italy

Summary: A reagent strip for the quantitative analysis of theophylline in serum or plasma was evaluated. The strip is based on the apoenzyme reactivation immunoassay system (ARIS) technique and is intended for use with the Ames Seralyzer reflectance photometer. The method gave CVs at three theophylline levels ranging from 3.8 to 6.3% (within run) and from 2.8 to 6.9% (day to day). The regression lines obtained from the correlation studies were $y = 0.959x + 0.51$ ($n = 105$, $r = 0.9906$, $S_{y/x} = 0.56$) for the comparison ARIS *(y)* versus Syva enzyme multiplied immunoassay *(x)* methods, and $y = 0.986x + 0.32$ ($n = 105$, $r = 0.9832$, $S_{y/x} = 0.62$) for the comparison ARIS *(y)* versus Abbott TDx fluorescence polarization immunoassay *(x)* methods. The interference from triglycerides, hemoglobin, bilirubin, and ascorbic acid, and the cross-reactivity of 8-chlorotheophylline, caffeine, 1,3-dimethyluric acid, theobromine, and 1,7-dimethylxanthine, were also investigated and discussed. The method was found to be reliable, simple, and rapid. It provides a practicable solution for immediate determinations of theophylline. **Key Words:** Theophylline—Apoenzyme reactivation immunoassay system—Enzyme multiplied immunoassay system—Fluorescence polarization immunoassay.

Theophylline has been used in both emergency and chronic treatment of asthma for more than 50 years. However, the narrow therapeutic index of the drug requires monitoring of serum levels (1,2). Accurate methods for measuring theophylline have been available for many years, but they do not always provide a convenient solution for assaying urgent specimens and small batches of samples. Recently a quantitative reagent strip assay for serum or plasma theophylline, based on the principle of the apoenzyme reactivation immunoassay system (ARIS), was described (3–7).

It is a colorimetric, homogeneous, competitive binding assay, and employs the prosthetic group flavin adenine dinucleotide (FAD) as label. Theophylline in the sample competes with the FAD-theophylline conjugate for a limited number of antibody binding sites. Unbound conjugate combines with glucose oxidase apoenzyme to regenerate the holoenzyme, whose activity is measured by means of a color reaction. All components necessary for the assay are incorporated into the reagent area of the strip. For quantitation, changes in reflectance during the reaction are monitored by means of a reflectance photometer, whose use in the assay of blood constituents has already been reported (8–10). We have evaluated the analytical performance of this method in relation to other comparative methods.

MATERIALS AND METHODS

Samples

Blood samples were collected from inpatients and outpatients receiving oral or intravenous theophylline. The sera were separated without delay, divided into

Address correspondence and reprint requests to Prof. A. Burlina at Laboratorio Centrale di Chimica e Microscopia Clinica, Ospedale Civile, 35128 Padova, Italy.

three portions for determination by each method, and stored at −20°C until assayed.

For the precision study, three serum pools at different theophylline levels were prepared, subdivided in aliquots, and frozen.

Seralyzer ARIS Reagent Strip Method

The materials used were from Ames Division, Miles Laboratories, Inc., Elkhart, IN, U.S.A., and were supplied by Miles Italiana S.p.A., Cavenago Brianza, Italy.

The reagent strips contain the following active ingredients in dry form: FAD-theophylline conjugate, monoclonal antibody to theophylline, apoglucose oxidase, glucose, peroxidase, and 3,3′,5,5′-tetramethylbenzidine.

Low and high calibrators (5 and 25 mg/L theophylline, respectively) and control (15 mg/L theophylline) are solutions of the drug in normal human serum.

Instructions for the test are contained in a preprogrammed test module, which also includes the optical filter (740 nm). This module is for use with the Ames Seralyzer, a reflectance photometer designed for the quantitative analysis of blood analytes by reagent strips.

In the theophylline assay, 30 μl of a diluted sample (30 μl serum plus 800 μl distilled water) is pipetted onto the reagent pad of the strip, which is then pushed into the reflectance photometer. The rate of development of the blue color generated is measured between 60 and 80 sec. A two-point calibration line, which is stored in the photometer's memory, allows the instrument to display the theophylline concentration directly.

This sample dilution allows measurement of theophylline concentrations in the range of 3.0–30.0 mg/L; higher values require a further sample dilution.

Comparative Methods

Theophylline assays were performed according to the manufacturer's directions by the following two methods: (a) homogeneous enzyme immunoassay (EMIT) kits operated on the Emit Autolab 5000 System (reagents and apparatus from Syva Co., Palo Alto, CA, U.S.A., supplied by Bracco S.p.A., Milano, Italy) and (b) fluorescence polarization immunoassay (FPIA) carried out with TDx reagents and analyzer (Abbott Laboratories, Diagnostic Division, North Chicago, IL, U.S.A., supplied by Abbott S.p.A., Roma, Italy).

TABLE 1. *Precision of the Seralyzer apoenzyme reactivation immunoassay system (ARIS) strip test for serum theophylline*

	Human serum pools		
	1	2	3
Within run (n = 16)			
Mean (mg/L)	4.7	14.8	23.0
SD (mg/L)	0.29	0.56	1.30
CV (%)	6.3	3.8	5.6
Between run (n = 11)[a]			
Mean (mg/L)	4.8	15.1	21.3
SD (mg/L)	0.33	0.45	0.60
CV (%)	6.9	3.0	2.8

[a]Eleven days.

Chemicals

Theophylline used for the recovery study was from Sigma Chemical Company, St. Louis, MO, U.S.A. The influence of ascorbic acid on the test was evaluated using ascorbic acid from Farmitalia-Carlo Erba, Milano, Italy. The substances used in the cross-reactivity studies were: 8-chlorotheophylline (Janssen Chimica, Beerse, Belgium), caffeine (Merck, Darmstadt, West Germany), 1,3-dimethyluric acid (Fluka AG, Buchs, Switzerland), theobromine, and 1,7-dimethylxanthine (Sigma).

RESULTS

The precision of the Seralyzer ARIS reagent strip test for theophylline was assessed by replicate measurements of three human serum pools at subtherapeutic, therapeutic, and toxic theophylline levels. The within-run precision (16 replicates) and the between-run precision (single assays in 11 days with daily calibration) are shown in Table 1.

For the recovery study, a clinical serum pool at therapeutic theophylline level was diluted with equal volumes of seven serum-based theophylline solutions prepared by the addition of theophylline to drug-free serum. The data obtained are reported in Table 2. The mean percentage recovery was 101.4% (range, 100.0–103.8%).

The linearity was evaluated in the range of 4.5–22.3 mg/L by diluting human serum at a high theophylline level with drug-free serum. Each of the five dilutions was tested in duplicate; the regression line parameters were $y_{(found)} = 0.994x_{(expected)} - 0.13$, $S_{y/x} = 0.12$, $r = 0.9996$ ($p < 0.001$).

For the correlation study, 105 clinical serum specimens were assayed with the Seralyzer ARIS reagent strip method *(y)* and with the EMIT and FPIA TDx

TABLE 2. *Analytical recovery for Seralyzer ARIS strip test*

Theophylline (mg/L)		
Added[a]	Expected	Found[b]
1.25	7.15	7.30
2.5	8.40	8.40
5.0	10.90	11.15
7.5	13.40	13.40
10.0	15.90	16.50
12.5	18.40	18.40
20.0	25.90	26.40

[a]Serum-based solutions mixed 1:1 with a clinical serum pool at 11.8 mg/L theophylline.
[b]Mean of duplicates.

methods *(x)*. Plots of the data are shown in Figs. 1 and 2, respectively.

The interference study was performed by mixing two serum-based theophylline solutions with equal volumes of drug-free clinical sera containing ascorbic acid, bilirubin, triglycerides, or hemoglobin. While ascorbic acid was added to the clinical serum, the other substances tested for interference were present in the native sera. Theophylline concentration was determined in each sample in duplicate by the Seralyzer ARIS reagent strip method.

The cross-reactivity of 8-chlorotheophylline, caffeine, 1,3-dimethyluric acid, theobromine, and 1,7-dimethylxanthine in the theophylline assay by the Seralyzer ARIS method was evaluated by mixing a serum-based theophylline solution with equal volumes of drug-free clinical sera supplemented with increasing quantities of each cross-reacting substance, so as to obtain final concentrations of 7.5 mg/L theophylline, 0.37–6 mg/L 8-chlorotheophylline, 3.8–62 mg/L caffeine, 1.5–12 mg/L 1,3-dimethyluric acid, 5.0–50 mg/L theobromine, and 4.5–70 mg/L 1,7-dimethylxanthine. The concentrations of compound that caused the measured theophylline value to increase by 20% (9 instead of 7.5 mg/L) are reported in Table 3.

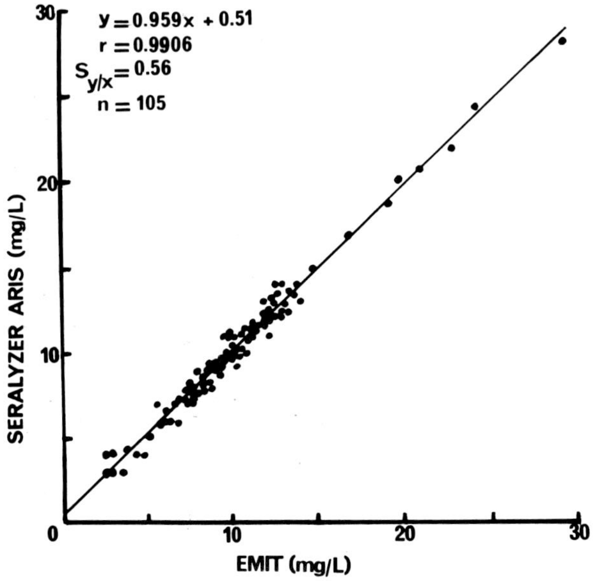

FIG. 1. Correlation between Seralyzer apoenzyme reactivation immunoassay system (ARIS) reagent strip and enzyme multiplied immunoassay technique (EMIT) methods for the determination of serum theophylline.

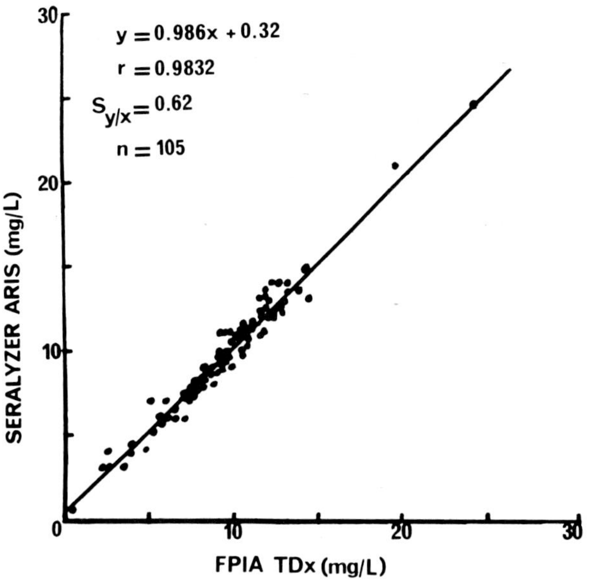

FIG. 2. Correlation between Seralyzer apoenzyme reactivation immunoassay system (ARIS) reagent strip and fluorescence polarization immunoassay (FPIA) TDx methods for the determination of serum theophylline.

Bilirubin (35.5 and 96.5 m*M*), triglycerides (1.67 and 2.65 m*M*), and hemoglobin (1.5 and 3.0 g/L) did not interfere with the assay. Ascorbic acid at 0.57 m*M* did not interfere but at 1.14 m*M* reduced the apparent theophylline concentration by 11%.

TABLE 3. *Cross-reactivity*

	Concentration[a]
8-Chlorotheophylline	1.2
Caffeine	16.3
1,7-Dimethylxanthine	13.1
Theobromine (3,7-dimethylxanthine)	13.5
1,3-Dimethyluric acid	4.8

[a]Concentration (mg/L) required to produce a 20% increase in the measured theophylline value in a sample containing 7.5 mg/L theophylline.

DISCUSSION

The Seralyzer ARIS reagent strip method showed a satisfactory precision and a good recovery and linearity. We found a good correspondence between this method and the EMIT and FPIA TDx methods. Recently, other authors have reported a satisfactory correlation between the results obtained by the present method and by liquid chromatography (11,12). Triglycerides, hemoglobin, and bilirubin at the tested concentrations did not interfere in the theophylline assay. No interference was obtained with ascorbic acid at a concentration of 0.57 m*M* which is seldom found in serum, even following ingestion of high doses of the vitamin (13).

The use of a monoclonal antibody has allowed a reduction of the influence of potential cross-reactants within acceptable limits, also in a particular situation such as the dry phase immunochemistry.

Caffeine, theobromine, and 1,7-dimethylxanthine significantly interfered only at concentrations higher than those expected following ingestion of caffeine-containing beverages and methylxanthine drugs (14–16).

1,3-Dimethyluric acid is not present in the serum of patients during theophylline therapy (15); however, this theophylline metabolite has been recently found at concentrations higher than that indicated in Table 3, in the serum of uremic patients receiving theophylline (17).

8-Chlorotheophylline, which is present in the drug dimenhydrinate, interfered with the assay.

The ready-to-use reagent strips and liquid calibrators, along with the storage of the calibration line in the instrument memory, are features that make the Seralyzer ARIS method easy and rapid to perform, besides reducing the cost of the analysis when the assay of a single sample is required. Therefore, this method provides a practical solution for determining theophylline concentration in emergency situations and also in the clinical laboratory when small batches of samples are to be routinely processed.

Acknowledgment: We are grateful to Miles Italiana, S.p.A., for the provision of the ARIS theophylline reagents. Thanks are also due to Dr. A. Imbasciati and Dr. G. Tarenghi for technical assistance.

REFERENCES

1. Jacobs MH, Senior RM, Kessler G. Clinical experience with theophylline: relationships between dosage, serum concentration and toxicity. *JAMA* 1976;235:1983–6.
2. Woodcock AA, Johnson MA, Geddes DM. Theophylline prescribing, serum concentrations and toxicity. *Lancet* 1983;2:610–3.
3. Morris DL, Ellis PB, Carrico RJ, et al. Flavin adenine dinucleotide as a label in homogeneous colorimetric immunoassays. *Anal Chem* 1981;53:658–65.
4. Tyhach RJ, Rupchock PA, Pendergrass JH, et al. Adaptation of prosthetic-group-label homogenous immunoassay to reagent-strip format. *Clin Chem* 1981;27:1499–504.
5. Burd JF, Ellis PB, Greenquist AC, et al. Measurement of theophylline with the substrate-labeled fluorescent immunoassay and apoenzyme reactivation immunoassay system in solution and in solid phase reagent strips. In: Avrameas S, Druet P, Masseyeff R, Feldmann G, eds. *Immunoenzymatic techniques*. Amsterdam: Elsevier Science, 1983:239–46.
6. Pippenger CE, Terrentine SJ. Quantitative strip test analysis of theophylline in plasma or serum by dry phase immunochemistry. *Clin Chem* 1984;30:1016.
7. Rupchock PA, Sommer RG, Greenquist AC. A dry reagent ARIS immunoassay for the determination of theophylline with the Ames Seralyzer reflectance photometer. *Clin Chem* 1984;30:1014.
8. Greyson J. Problems and possibilities of chemistry on dry reagent carriers. *J Automatic Chem* 1981;3:66–71.
9. Zipp A. Development of dry reagent chemistry for the clinical laboratory. *J Automatic Chem* 1981;3:71–5.
10. Karmen A, Lent R. Clinical chemistry testing with the Ames Seralyzer dry reagent system. *J Clin Lab Autom* 1982;2:284–96.
11. Lindberg R, Ivaska K, Irjala K, Vanto T. Demonstration of theophylline in serum with the Seralyzer Aris reagent strip test evaluated. *Clin Chem* 1985;31:613–4.
12. Rupchock P, Sommer R, Greenquist A, Tyhach R, Walter B, Zipp A. Dry reagent strips used for determination of theophylline in serum. *Clin Chem* 1985;31:737–40.
13. Levin S, ed. *Vitamin C: its molecular biology and medical potential*. New York: Academic Press, 1976:150–1.
14. Rall TW. Central nervous system stimulants. The xanthines. In: Gilman AG, Goodman LS, Gilman A, eds. *The pharmacological basis of therapeutics*. 6th ed. New York: MacMillan, 1980:594–5, 603.
15. Li TM, Benovic JL, Buckler RT, Burd JF. Homogeneous substratelabeled fluorescent immunoassay for theophylline in serum. *Clin Chem* 1981;27:22–6.
16. Wilson JF, Marshall RW, Williams J, Richens A. Accuracy and precision of gas-liquid chromatographic, high-pressure liquid chromatographic, and enzyme immunoassay techniques for the measurement of theophylline concentrations in serum: a comparison based on external quality assurance measurements. *Ther Drug Monit* 1984;6:243–50.
17. Opheim KE, Ainardi V, Raisys VA. Increase in apparent theophylline concentration in the serum of two uremic patients as measured by some immunoassay methods (caused by 1,3-dimethyluric acid?). *Clin Chem* 1983;29:1968–9.

Therapeutic Drug Monitoring
7:455–460 © 1985 Raven Press, New York

Loop-Column Extraction and Liquid Chromatographic Analysis of Doxorubicin and Three Metabolites in Plasma

Cynthia A. Riley, William R. Crom, and William E. Evans

Clinical Pharmacokinetics Laboratory, Pharmaceutical Division, St. Jude Children's Research Hospital, Memphis, Tennessee, U.S.A.

Summary: A sensitive and specific high performance liquid chromatographic method for the separation and quantitation of doxorubicin and three metabolites is described. The new method involves isocratic reversed-phase separation of these compounds, with quantitation by either electrochemical or fluorescence methods. A novel loop-column method was used to extract the compounds of interest from plasma, eliminating the need for organic extraction of biological samples before injection into the chromatographic system. The limit of sensitivity with the fluorescence method was about 2.3 ng on column. Sensitivity with electrochemical detection was better, although there was more interference by early eluting plasma components. The between-run CV (%) for replicate analysis of doxorubicin in identical plasma samples was 2.0 at 112.5 ng/ml, 5.4 at 40.0 ng/ml, and 9.9 at 14.0 ng/ml. Precision for each of the three metabolites was comparable. Accuracy for doxorubicin and each metabolite ranged from 93 to 107% at concentrations of 14.0, 40.0, 65.0, 112.5, and 140.0 ng/ml. The new loop-column extraction method, with injection of plasma samples directly onto the chromatograph, is simpler and more efficient than previous methods requiring organic extraction, making it more feasible for routine processing of clinical samples. **Key Words:** Doxorubicin—High performance liquid chromatography—Loop column—Extraction—Adriamycin.

Doxorubicin (Adriamycin; Adria Laboratories Inc., Columbus, OH, U.S.A.) is an anthracycline antibiotic that is an effective antitumor agent for numerous solid tumors and leukemia (1,2). It is generally accepted that doxorubicin exerts its effects by intercalation between base pairs in the DNA helix in the cell nucleus, thereby preventing replication (3), although there is still uncertainty concerning the precise mode of action of the drug (4); its distribution and metabolism in plasma, tissue, and leukemia cells; and the possible cytotoxic role of intermediate metabolites (5,6). Thus, additional clinical pharmacokinetic and pharmacodynamic studies of doxorubicin are needed.

Previous pharmacokinetic studies have used high performance liquid chromatographic (HPLC) methods that require organic extraction of the drugs and metabolites from biological fluids prior to injection onto the chromatographic system (7–10). However, all of the previously reported extraction procedures suffer from one or more major shortcomings, as previously outlined by Robert (11). For example, extraction by organic methods is labor-intensive and time-consuming, requiring partition between the organic and aqueous phases, with careful removal, drying, and reconstitution of the organic layers. The recovery is frequently inefficient, ranging from 50 to 70%, and is not comparable for all anthracyclines and metabolites, since

Address correspondence and reprint requests to Dr. W. E. Evans at Clinical Pharmacokinetics Laboratory, Pharmaceutical Division, St. Jude Children's Research Hospital, 332 North Lauderdale, P.O. Box 318, Memphis, TN 38105, U.S.A.

the extent of recovery depends upon the partition coefficients of the compounds and the pH of the extraction medium. Other limitations include handling the large volume of organic solvent required to extract plasma efficiently, and the concentration-dependent effects on extraction efficiency. Because of these limitations, Robert (11) developed a technique involving C-18 Sep-Pak cartridges (Waters Associates Inc., Milford, MA, U.S.A.) to extract anthracyclines from serum or plasma. Although that method overcomes some of the limitations of previous extraction methods, it still requires collection, evaporation, and reconstitution of an organic eluate from the disposable cartridges, is expensive unless the disposable cartridges are regenerated, and is not amenable to automation. In an effort to overcome these limitations, we have developed a selective and sensitive isocratic HPLC-fluorescence method for separating and quantitating doxorubicin and three potential metabolites; it is simple and rapid, requires no organic pre-extraction of plasma, and meets accepted standards for precision and accuracy. We also describe the electrochemical quantitation of doxorubicin and its metabolites, offering an alternative to measuring the fluorescence of the parent drug and metabolites.

METHODS

Doxorubicin hydrochloride was obtained from Aldrich Chemical Co. (Milwaukee, WI, U.S.A.). Doxorubicin metabolites (doxorubicinol, 7-deoxydoxorubicinol aglycone, 7-deoxydoxorubicin aglycone, and doxorubicin aglycone) were kindly provided by Dr. Mervyn Israel (University of Tennessee Center for the Health Sciences, Memphis, TN, U.S.A.). Pharmaceutical grade daunorubicin hydrochloride was obtained from the National Cancer Institute, National Institutes of Health, (Bethesda, MD, U.S.A.) and was used as an internal standard. Distilled water was purified by a Milli-Q water purification system (Millipore Corporation, Bedford, MA, U.S.A.). HPLC-grade acetonitrile was used as purchased from Burdick and Jackson Laboratories (Muskegon, MI, U.S.A.). Reagent-grade glacial acetic acid and certified sodium acetate (Fisher Scientific Co., Pittsburgh, PA, U.S.A.) were used as received.

The chromatographic system consisted of a Constametric III HPLC pump (Laboratory Data Control, Riviera Beach, FL, U.S.A.) with a Rheodyne model 7125 injector valve. The loop column was a 3.9-mm internal diameter × 2.3-cm column (Waters Associates), dry packed with μBondapak phenyl 37–50 μm

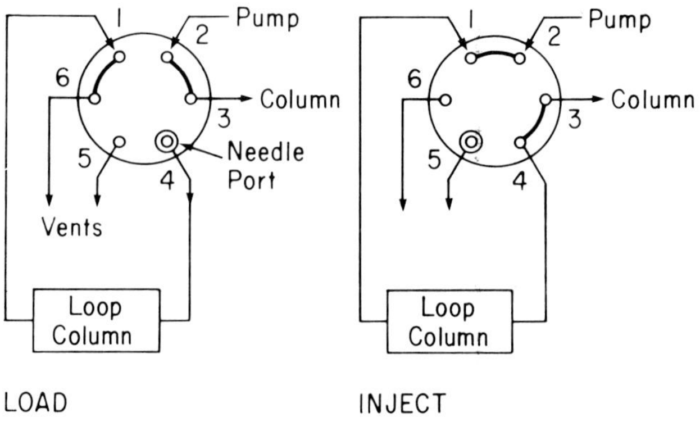

FIG. 1. Rheodyne Model 7125 flow diagram of the injector configuration, fitted with a loop column.

packing (Waters Associates), attached where the standard volumetric sample loop is normally connected (Fig. 1). A 3.9-mm internal diameter × 2.3-cm guard column, packed with μBondapak phenyl packing, was attached proximal to the analytical column and changed periodically to protect the analytical column, since plasma was injected directly into the system. Column effluent was monitored with a Gilson Spectra/Glo Filter Fluorometer (model FL-1A) equipped with a 45-μl flow cell, a 480-nm excitation filter, and a 560-nm emission filter (Doxorubicin filters; Gilson Medical Electronics, Inc., Middleton, WI, U.S.A.). Integration of peak heights, calculation of multilevel calibration curves, and computations for quantitation of unknowns were carried out with an S/P 4100 computing integrator (Spectra-Physics Inc., Mountain View, CA, U.S.A.).

To achieve adequate isocratic separation of components of interest, the mobile phase consisted of a solution of distilled water, acetonitrile, and glacial acetic acid (volumes of 69:30:1). The distilled water and acetic acid mixture was first adjusted to pH 4 with a 20% solution of sodium acetate (≃40 ml/L), then filtered (Millipore vacuum filtration system), and degassed by sparging with helium followed by about 2 min of vacuum degassing. The mobile phase flow rate was 2 ml/min. Operating pressure with this system was ~1,000 psi with a new analytical column and daily changes of filter inserts of the loop column. The initial equilibration of column with mobile phase was ~30 min. The maximum sensitivity settings of the fluorescence detector were used.

Removal of gross particulate matter from plasma samples prior to injection was necessary to prevent clogging of the loop column. This was accomplished by high-speed centrifugation (Microfuge; Beckman Instruments Inc., Fullerton, CA, U.S.A.). Daunorub-

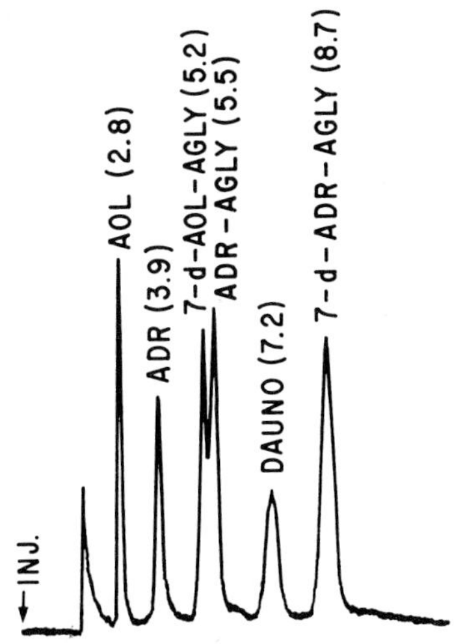

FIG. 2. High performance liquid chromatographic-fluorescence chromatogram of spiked plasma showing resolution of doxorubicinol (AOL), doxorubicin (ADR), 7-deoxydoxorubicinol aglycone (7-d-AOL-AGLY), doxorubicin aglycone (ADR-AGLY), daunorubicin (DAUNO), and 7-deoxydoxorubicin aglycone (7-d-ADR-AGLY). Retention times (min) are shown in parentheses.

icin, 20.00 μl (25 ng), as internal standard, was added after centrifugation to each volumetrically measured sample to be injected. The sample (50–500 μl) was vortex-mixed well and introduced directly with a gas-tight glass syringe into the chromatographic system through port 4 with the injector in the load position (Fig. 1). The sample volume in excess of the loop column capacity left the system through the appropriate injector vent while the compounds of interest remained adsorbed on the loop column because of their affinities for the column packing. With the injector still in the load position, the loop column was washed with 0.5 ml of filtered deionized water to remove potentially interfering substances such as proteins or other polar compounds. The components of interest were then eluted from the loop column, and subsequently the analytical column, by the mobile phase after the injector was switched to the inject position. After the last compound had eluted from the column, as evidenced by the chromatogram, the injector was returned to the load position and the loop column was prepared to receive another sample by washing with ~0.5 ml of filtered deionized water.

RESULTS

The new HPLC system resolved doxorubicin and three human metabolites (Fig. 2). The potential to resolve doxorubicin aglycone is evident, but since it probably is not a doxorubicin metabolite detectable in human plasma (6), it was not routinely included in the multilevel calibration standards. Daunorubicin was also resolved from doxorubicin and metabolites, permitting its use as an internal standard. The retention times and capacity factors of all six components of the chromatogram are summarized in Table 1.

TABLE 1. *Separation of doxorubicin and potential metabolites by reversed-phase HPLC*

Compound	Retention time (min)	Capacity factor (K′)
Doxorubicinol	2.82	0.75
Doxorubicin	3.93	1.5
7-Deoxydoxorubicinol aglycone	5.21	2.25
Doxorubicin aglycone	5.53	2.5
Daunorubicin (internal standard)	7.17	3.5
7-Deoxydoxorubicin aglycone	8.71	4.5

HPLC, high performance liquid chromatography.

The calibration curves for doxorubicin and metabolites, using fluorescence detection, were linear from at least 9.4 to 150 ng/ml (Fig. 3). The smallest detectable quantity of doxorubicin, defined as at least three times the baseline fluorescence noise signal was ≈2.3 ng on column. This amount corresponds, for 250 μl of plasma injected onto the loop column, to a concentration of ≈9.4 ng/ml of plasma. Lower concentrations could be quantitated by injecting larger sample volumes (i.e., up to 500 μl). Responses with electrochemical detection were more than 10 times higher than those obtained by fluorescence for some of the compounds (Fig. 4). However, plasma components produced electrochemical peaks early in the chromatogram, and were not completely resolved from the compounds of interest with the separation conditions described. Since there were no interfering fluorescent peaks, and adequate sensitivity was achieved with fluorescence detection using the described HPLC conditions, further modifications to allow routine use of electrochemical detection were not necessary. However, we have previously reported that this method of detection has proved useful for daunorubicin and its metabolites (12) and offers an alternative method for quantitation of potentially nonfluorescent anthracycline metabolites.

As summarized in Tables 2 and 3, the new method of loop-column extraction, isocratic reversed-phase separation, and fluorescence detection is precise and accurate over the concentration range evaluated. To determine between-run precision and accuracy of the assay (defined as a percentage of the spiked value), five samples of known concentrations of each compound were assayed in triplicate on 4 different days. Five determinations at three concentrations for each

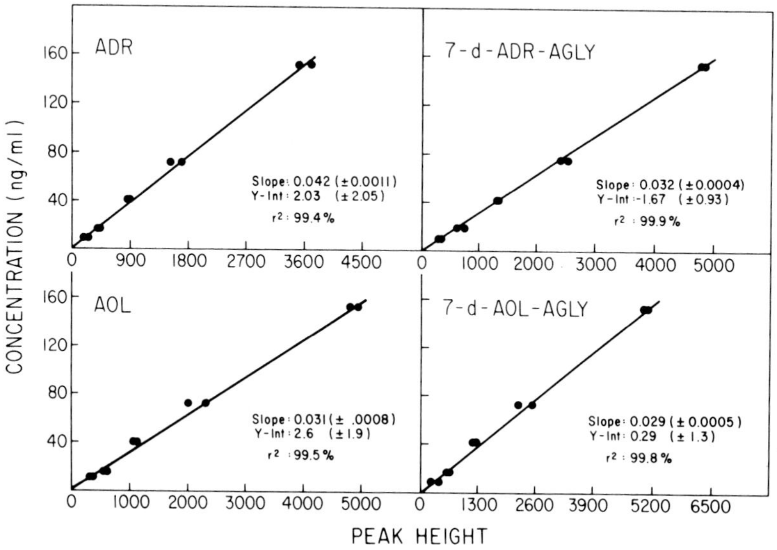

FIG. 3. Linear calibration curves for doxorubicin (ADR), 7-deoxydoxorubicin aglycone (7-d-ADR-AGLY), doxorubicinol (AOL), and 7-deoxydoxorubicinol aglycone (7-d-AOL-AGLY). Slopes and y-intercepts ($\pm$ SD) were generated from linear regression of serum concentrations vs. peak heights.

compound were performed within a day to assess within-run precision and accuracy. These data are summarized in Table 3.

Using the loop-column extraction method, the mean (CV%) extraction efficiencies for doxorubicin, doxorubicinol, 7-deoxydoxorubicin aglycone and 7-deox-

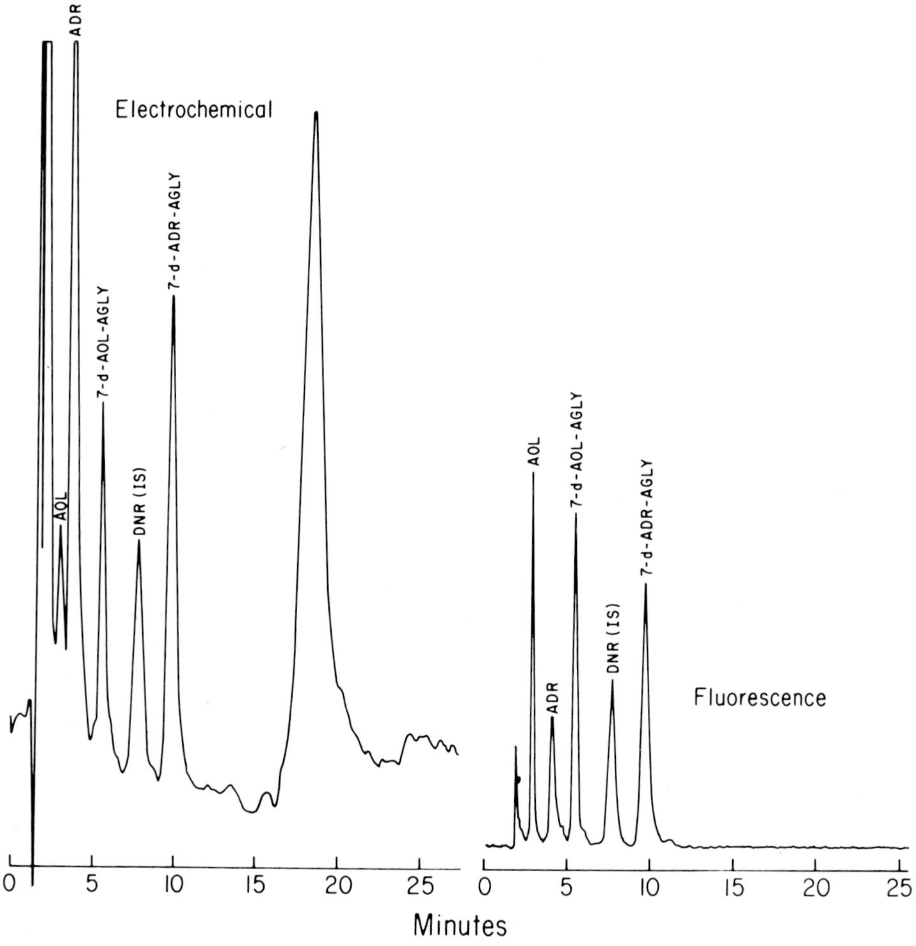

FIG. 4. High performance liquid chromatography chromatograms generated from a single spiked plasma sample injection with serial fluorescence and electrochemical detection. AOL, doxorubicinol; ADR, doxorubicin; 7-d-AOL-AGLY, 7-deoxydoxorubicinol aglycone; DNR(IS), daunorubicin; 7-d-ADR-AGLY, 7-deoxydoxorubicin aglycone.

TABLE 2. *Within-run precision and accuracy of doxorubicin and metabolites*

Compound	n	Actual concentration (ng/ml)	Measured mean (SD) (ng/ml)	Accuracy (%)	CV (%)
Doxorubicin	5	14.0	14.8 (1.3)	105.6	8.9
	5	40.0	37.9 (1.7)	94.8	4.5
	5	112.5	107.1 (5.7)	95.2	5.3
Doxorubicinol	5	14.0	15.3 (1.7)	109.1	11.2
	5	40.0	39.4 (1.4)	98.4	3.5
	5	112.5	110.2 (5.3)	97.9	4.8
7-Deoxydoxorubicinol aglycone	5	14.0	13.2 (0.5)	94.3	4.0
	5	40.0	37.3 (1.0)	93.3	2.7
	5	112.5	101.9 (3.4)	90.6	3.4
7-Deoxydoxorubicin aglycone	5	14.0	14.8 (0.4)	105.7	2.7
	5	40.0	38.4 (2.4)	96.0	6.2
	5	112.5	106.3 (5.3)	94.5	5.0

ydoxorubicinol aglycone were 76 (6), 78 (7), 73 (8), and 74 (17), respectively, over a concentration range of 15–200 ng/ml.

Figure 5 shows the plasma concentration–time profile of doxorubicin and metabolites measured by the new method in a patient with osteosarcoma, who was treated with 75 mg/m² of doxorubicin. Figure 6 is a typical patient chromatogram.

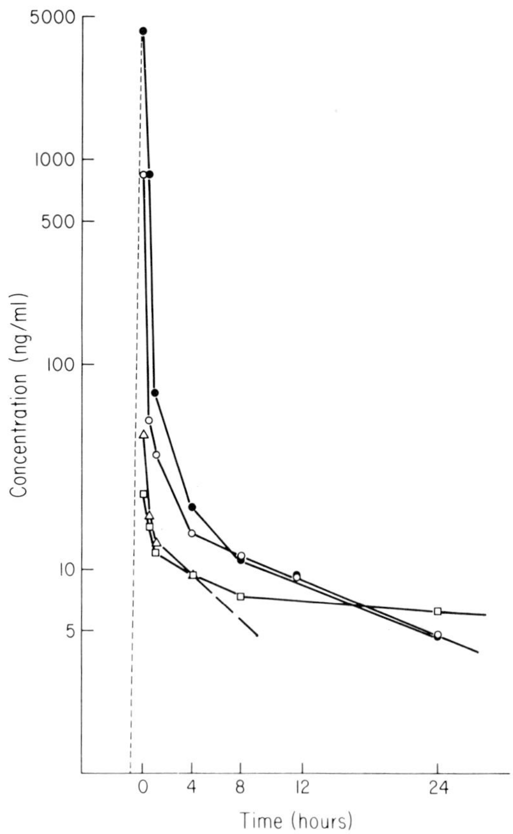

FIG. 5. Semilogarithmic plot of doxorubicin (filled circles), doxorubicinol (opened circles), 7-deoxydoxorubicinol aglycone (squares), and 7-deoxydoxorubicin aglycone (triangles) plasma concentrations versus time following a 30-min i.v. infusion of 75 mg/m² doxorubicin, administered to a patient with osteosarcoma (broken line represents theoretical concentration of doxorubicin during infusion).

DISCUSSION

The current study demonstrates that doxorubicin and three of its metabolites can be simultaneously separated and quantitated by a new chromatographic technique that requires no organic pre-extraction of plasma. The loop-column extraction method is simple and easy to perform, and overcomes most of the variability and inefficiencies of previously described organic extraction procedures (7–11). Moreover, the simplicity of the loop-column extraction method makes it easier to adapt to routine clinical laboratory procedures. The loop column requires a minimal amount of trouble-shooting. To avoid clogging of the loop column, which was manifested by increased pressure, the frits were changed daily and samples were closely monitored for particulate matter. The loop column packing lasted through ~100 injections of plasma, at which time it was repacked.

Although fluorescence detection proved to be an acceptable method for quantitation, the electrochem-

TABLE 3. *Between-run precision and accuracy of doxorubicin and metabolites*

Compound	n	Actual concentration (ng/ml)	Measured mean (SD) (ng/ml)	Accuracy (%)	CV (%)
Doxorubicin	12	14.0	13.5 (1.4)	96.7	9.9
	12	40.0	40.5 (2.2)	101.1	5.4
	12	65.0	65.6 (4.2)	100.9	6.4
	12	112.5	112.7 (2.2)	100.2	2.0
	12	140.0	134.2 (5.5)	95.9	4.1
Doxorubicinol	12	14.0	14.0 (1.0)	99.8	7.2
	12	40.0	42.2 (1.8)	105.0	4.1
	12	65.0	69.4 (3.6)	106.7	5.2
	12	112.5	115.4 (3.5)	102.5	3.0
	12	140.0	147.0 (4.0)	105.0	2.7
7-Deoxydoxorubicinol aglycone	12	14.0	13.2 (1.1)	94.4	8.6
	12	40.0	39.0 (1.7)	97.5	4.3
	12	65.0	65.1 (4.5)	100.1	6.9
	12	112.5	110.0 (3.2)	97.8	2.9
	12	140.0	132.3 (5.6)	94.5	4.3
7-Deoxydoxorubicin aglycone	12	14.0	13.1 (1.9)	97.5	14.6
	12	40.0	37.4 (2.2)	93.4	6.0
	12	65.0	66.0 (6.0)	101.5	9.1
	12	112.5	109.2 (6.1)	97.1	5.6
	12	140.0	131.8 (7.0)	94.2	5.3

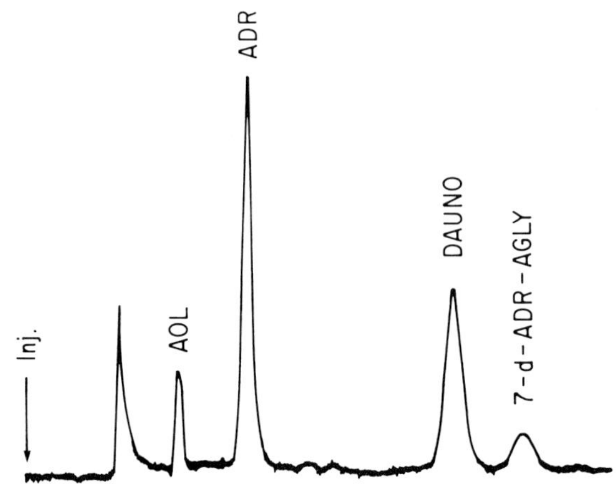

FIG. 6. Typical patient chromatogram 15 min after the end of a 30-min i.v. infusion of 35 mg/m² doxorubicin. Inj, injection; AOL, doxorubicinol; ADR, doxorubicin; DAUNO, daunorubicin; 7-d-ADR-AGLY, 7-deoxydoxorubicin aglycone.

ical detector displayed high sensitivity for some of the compounds of interest. The change in relative size of the peak heights for doxorubicin and doxorubicinol (Fig. 4) demonstrates a difference in fluorescence and electrochemical detector responses for these two compounds, but the feasibility of determining concentrations of doxorubicin and metabolites by nonfluorescent HPLC methods is demonstrated. Alternatively, these two detection methods may be combined, and peak height ratios may be used to confirm the identity of peaks.

The chromatographic data from patient plasma samples, following a 75 mg/m² i.v. infusion, indicate extensive metabolism of doxorubicin, which could result in significant differences in plasma and leukemia cell exposure to the parent drug and its principal cytotoxic metabolite (doxorubicinol). More extensive studies to establish the pattern of accumulation of doxorubicin and metabolites in plasma and leukemia cells are needed, since previous work with daunorubicin suggests that intracellular metabolism may relate to clinical efficacy (13), and studies with doxorubicin suggest that the risk of cardiotoxicity may be influenced by peak concentrations of the drug (14). The method described herein should prove useful for such studies.

Acknowledgments: Supported in part by NIH Grant CA24176, NIH Cancer Center Support Grant CA21765, and the American Lebanese Syrian Associated Charities. The authors wish to gratefully acknowledge the assistance of Drs. Joseph A. Sinkule and Mervyn Israel and the development of this method, and Fabrienne Holloway, Marlene Jacks, Linda Rawlinson, and Betsy Williford for assistance with preparation of the manuscript.

REFERENCES

1. Blum RH, Carter SK. A new anticancer drug with significant clinical activity. *Ann Intern Med* 1974;80:259–68.
2. Carter SK. Adriamycin—a review. *J Natl Cancer Inst* 1975;55:1265–70.
3. DiMarco A. Adriamycin: the therapeutic activity of experimental tumors. In: Carter SK, ed. *International symposium on adriamycin*. New York: Springer-Verlag, 1972:53–6.
4. Tritton TR, Yee G. The anticancer agent adriamycin can be actively cytotoxic without entering cells. *Science* 1982;217:248–50.
5. Goodman J, Hochstein P. Generation of free radicals and lipid peroxidation by redox cycling of adriamycin and daunomycin. *Biochem Biophys Res Commun* 1977;77:797–801.
6. Bachur NR. Anthracycline antibiotic pharmacology and metabolism. *Cancer Treat Rep* 1979;63:817–21.
7. Israel M, Pegg WJ, Wilkinson PM, Garnick MB. Liquid chromatographic analysis of adriamycin and metabolites in biological fluids. *J Liquid Chromatogr* 1978;1:795–800.
8. Hulhovan R, Desager JD. Quantitative determinations of low levels of daunomycin and daunomycinol in plasma by high-pressure liquid chromatography. *J Chromatogr* 1976;125:369–77.
9. Shimozawa S, Mimaki Y, Arcki Y, Oda T. Determination of the concentration of adriamycin and its metabolites in the serum and tissues of Ehrlich carcinoma-bearing mice by high performance liquid chromatography. *J Chromatogr* 1980;196:463–71.
10. Peters JH, Murray JF. Determination of adriamycin and aclacinomycin-A in plasma by high-pressure liquid chromatography and spectrophotofluorography. *J Liquid Chromatogr* 1974;2:15–20.
11. Robert J. Extraction of anthracyclines from biological fluids for HPLC evaluation. *J Liquid Chromatogr* 1980;3:1561–72.
12. Akpofure C, Riley CA, Sinkule JA, Evans WE. Quantitation of daunorubicin and metabolites by high-performance liquid chromatography with electrochemical detection. *J Chromatogr (Biomed Appl)* 1982;232:377–83.
13. Green W, Huffman D, Wiernik PH, Schimpff S, Benjamin R, Bachur NR. High-dose daunorubicin therapy for acute nonlymphocytic leukemia. Correlation of response and toxicity with pharmacokinetics and intracellular daunorubicin reductase activity. *Cancer* 1972;30:1419–27.
14. Legha SS, Benjamin RS, Mackay B, et al. Reduction of doxorubicin cardiotoxicity by prolonged continuous intravenous infusion. *Ann Intern Med* 1982;96:133–40.

Therapeutic Drug Monitoring
7:461–465 © 1985 Raven Press, New York

Ultrafiltration Compared with Equilibrium Dialysis in the Determination of Unbound Phenytoin in Plasma

Yuichi Koike, Anita Magnusson, Eugen Steiner, Anders Rane, and Folke Sjöqvist

Department of Clinical Pharmacology at Karolinska Institute, Huddinge University Hospital, Huddinge, Sweden

Summary: Protein binding of phenytoin (PHT) was studied in 36 patients with normal kidney function and six uremic patients. We compared a newly introduced ultrafiltration (UF) technique (EMIT Free Level System I) for measuring unbound PHT in plasma with an equilibrium dialysis (ED) method. The precision of the UF method was satisfactory (the CV within samples was 4.2%, and between days, 3.4%). PHT concentrations were measured with both homogeneous enzyme immunoassay and high performance liquid chromatography using plasma samples from epileptic patients. The values obtained agreed well. Unbound concentrations of PHT determined by the UF technique and ED were identical in both normal and uremic plasma obtained from patients under treatment. Unbound concentrations of PHT correlated significantly to total concentrations in both groups of patients. The investigated UF technique thus appears to be accurate for measuring unbound concentrations of PHT in plasma. Controlled clinical studies are required to show that this is a cost-effective clinical service. **Key Words:** Phenytoin—Unbound level—Enzyme multiplied immunoassay technique—Ultrafiltration—Equilibrium dialysis.

Monitoring of phenytoin (PHT) in plasma is a well-documented laboratory service for patients with grand mal seizures. A therapeutic plasma concentration range has been established (1,2) referring to total concentrations of PHT in plasma. It is generally considered that only the unbound fraction of a drug will exert the pharmacological effects (3).

The binding of PHT to albumin is markedly decreased in uremia (4) but is also affected by factors such as hyperbilirubinemia (5,6), levels of free fatty acids (7), hepatic diseases (6,8,9), and displacing drugs such as acetylsalicylic acid (10) and valproic acid (11). In these cases, measurement of the unbound PHT concentration in plasma might be more valuable than assay of the total concentrations, but this postulate has not yet been proved by controlled clinical studies.

Address correspondence and reprint requests to Dr. Y. Koike at Department of Clinical Pharmacology, Karolinska Institute, Huddinge University Hospital, S-141 86 Huddinge, Sweden.

There are several techniques to measure protein binding of drugs, such as equilibrium dialysis (ED) and ultrafiltration (UF). The latter method has been simplified by a recently developed separating device (EMIT Free Level System I). We have compared this new UF method with ED, which has been used so far in our laboratory for measuring unbound PHT in plasma. PHT was analyzed by enzyme immunoassay technique (EMIT) and more specifically by high performance liquid chromatography (HPLC), since it has been reported that the major metabolite 5-(4-hydroxyphenyl)-5-phenylhydantoin (HPPH) might interfere with the immunoassay (12–16).

MATERIALS AND METHODS

Plasma Samples

For the comparison of UF and ED, we obtained single plasma samples from 36 nonuremic epileptic patients and 14 samples from six uremic epileptic patients who were treated with PHT.

Twelve plasma samples from uremic patients and seven samples from nonuremic epileptic patients were analyzed with HPLC and EMIT. Spiked plasma was used in order to evaluate factors affecting the UF method.

Methods

Plasma samples were divided into two parts, one being prepared for UF and the other for ED. Each experiment was performed in duplicate. Some factors that might affect the UF method (sample volume, centrifugation time, *g* force, temperature, and total concentration of PHT) were tested.

UF was performed with the EMIT Free Level System I filled with 1 ml of plasma. The filter was centrifuged at 1,000 *g* for 15 min at room temperature (25 ± 3°C). About 200 μl of ultrafiltrate was collected into the cup and used for assay. Total and unbound PHT concentrations were determined by EMIT. All values are expressed as μ*M*.

In the ED method we used Teflon chambers with two compartments separated by a dialysis membrane (Technicon, Solna, Sweden). Before use, the membranes were soaked for 1 h in distilled water. The chambers were provided with 0.5 ml of patient plasma containing ^{14}C-labeled PHT in one compartment and 0.5 ml of isotonic phosphate buffer (pH 7.35, ion strength 0.168) in the other (17). The Teflon chambers were rotated, and equilibrium was reached after 5 h.

HPLC analysis was performed according to the method of Dolan et al. (18). Two hundred microliters of plasma was applied on a Clin-Elute column (Analytichem International, Inc., Harbour City, CA, U.S.A.). Enphenemal (methylphenobarbitone), 50 μl of 100 μ*M*, was used as an internal standard, and 150 μl of 0.02 *M* phosphate buffer (pH 7.4) was added. Then, the sample was eluted with 3 ml of a mixture of 95 ml of dichloromethane and 5 ml of isopropanol, and the organic phase was evaporated. The residue was dissolved in 100 μl of the mobile phase (39% methanol/61% 0.02 *M* phosphate buffer) and 25 μl was injected on the HPLC. The chromatographic system consisted of a ConstaMetric III pump, SpectroMonitor III detector, and Supelcosil LC-18 reversed-phase column.

Calculation of the Percentage of Unbound Phenytoin

With UF the percentage of unbound PHT was calculated as the ratio between the PHT concentration in the ultrafiltrate and that in plasma. In ED, the percentage of unbound PHT was calculated by dividing the radioactivity in buffer by that in plasma after dialysis.

Factors Affecting PHT Binding

The effect of the following factors on PHT binding was studied experimentally: sample volume (0.5–1.2 ml), centrifugation time (5–30 min), *g* force (1,000–2,500), temperature (10–37°C), and PHT concentration (30–90 μ*M*).

Statistical Analysis

One-way analysis of variance (ANOVA) was used in order to assess factors affecting unbound levels of PHT as determined with the EMIT Free Level System I. Student's two-tailed *t* test was used to compare the UF and ED methods. The relationship between variables was tested by using linear least-squares regression analysis. The predetermined level of significance was $p < 0.05$.

RESULTS

Within the experimental conditions chosen, centrifugation time, *g* force, and sample volume had no significant effect on the estimated unbound fraction of PHT. As expected, the percentage of unbound PHT increased significantly as the temperature or total PHT concentration was raised.

In order to determine the precision of the UF and ED methods, the binding in plasma spiked with PHT, 60 μ*M*, was assayed repeatedly. With both methods, the CVs between samples and between days were satisfactory (Table 1).

TABLE 1. *Precision of ultrafiltration and equilibrium dialysis methods for phenytoin binding in spiked plasma*

	Within samples		Between days
	UF	ED	UF
Mean (μ*M*)	4.3	4.3	4.4
SD	0.18	0.16	0.15
CV (%)	4.2	3.7	3.4
No. of samples	10	12	7

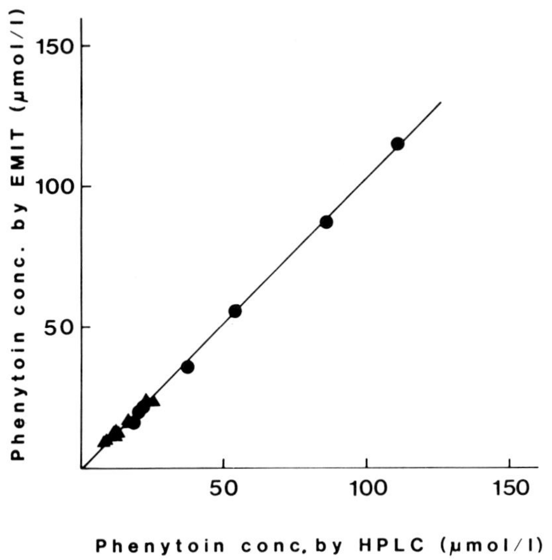

FIG. 1. Comparison of plasma concentrations of phenytoin determined by high performance liquid chromatography (HPLC) and enzyme multiplied immunoassay technique (EMIT) from seven normal epileptic patients (circles) and 12 uremic patients (triangles) treated with PHT. Slope of the regression line was 1.03, intercept 0.42, and $r = 0.99$.

The values obtained with HPLC and EMIT based on analysis of plasma from normal epileptic patients and from uremic patients agreed well (Fig. 1).

Student's two-tailed t test revealed no significant difference between the UF and ED methods (Table 2).

In patients with normal kidney function, total concentrations ranged from 14 to 118 μ*M*. The unbound concentration (fraction) measured by UF varied between 1.1 and 10.4 μ*M* (7.5–13.8%). In the uremic patient group, total PHT concentrations ranged from 9 to 24 μ*M*, and unbound concentrations (UF) from 1.6 to 5.9 μ*M*. The mean unbound concentrations were similar in the two groups, confirming the original observations (19).

Figure 2 shows the relationship between unbound PHT concentration and the corresponding total PHT concentrations in plasma from normal and uremic patients. In both groups, unbound PHT concentrations significantly correlated to total PHT concentrations, but the slopes of the two regression lines differed.

Figure 3 compares the unbound PHT concentrations determined with UF and ED methods in 50 samples, including uremic patient samples. There was little difference between the values obtained with the two methods. Similarly, there was a strong correlation between the percentage of unbound PHT determined with the two methods.

DISCUSSION

Although the unbound drug concentration is theoretically more closely related to the pharmacological effects than total drug in body fluids (3), unbound drug levels are seldom measured routinely, for two reasons. First, such measurements are technically more demanding; and second, there is poor evidence that they are cost-effective in terms of improving the quality of drug therapy. The first problem has been partly resolved by the development of simplified UF methods such as the EMIT Free Level System I.

We have compared this method with ED in measurements of free PHT concentrations in plasma. Several factors that might affect the performance of the ultrafiltration method were evaluated. Among these factors, sample volume, centrifugation time, and g force had no effect on the measurement of PHT unbound fraction. On the other hand, the unbound fraction was significantly increased from 6.7 to 8.7% when the temperature was increased from 10 to 37°C.

TABLE 2. *Phenytoin concentrations in plasma samples from patients with normal kidney function and uremic patients*

	Total concentration EMIT (μ*M*)	Unbound concentration UF (μ*M*)	Percentage unbound fraction UF	Unbound concentration ED (μ*M*)	Percentage unbound fraction ED
Patients with normal kidney function (n = 36)					
Mean	49.5	4.6	9.7	4.8	9.8
SD	25.6	2.5	1.4	2.5	1.3
Range	14–118	1.1–10.4	7.5–13.8	1.3–10.3	7.3–12.8
Uremic patients (n = 14)					
Mean	15.4	3.2	20.0	3.0	18.8
SD	5.5	1.5	3.6	1.4	3.2
Range	9.0–24.0	1.6–5.9	14.2–28.8	1.6–5.8	14.3–28.4

EMIT, enzyme multiplied immunoassay technique; UF, ultrafiltration; ED, equilibrium dialysis.

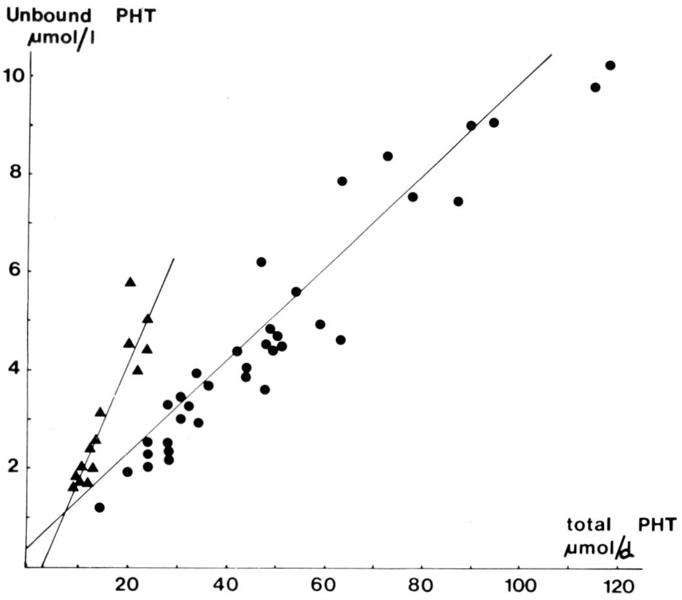

FIG. 2. Relationship between unbound concentrations of phenytoin (PHT) in ultrafiltrate and total concentrations in normal (circles) and uremic (triangles) plasmas. $r = 0.94$ ($p < 0.001$) and 0.93 ($p < 0.001$), respectively.

All of the following UF and ED measurements were carried out at room temperature.

There was a small but significant increase in the unbound fraction of PHT with increasing total concentrations. These results are in accordance with previous reports (20). Lunde et al. (10) also found that the unbound fraction increased with increasing total PHT concentrations within the clinical concentration range (20–200 µ*M*). Our results confirm these observations, but their clinical importance is probably small in most patients.

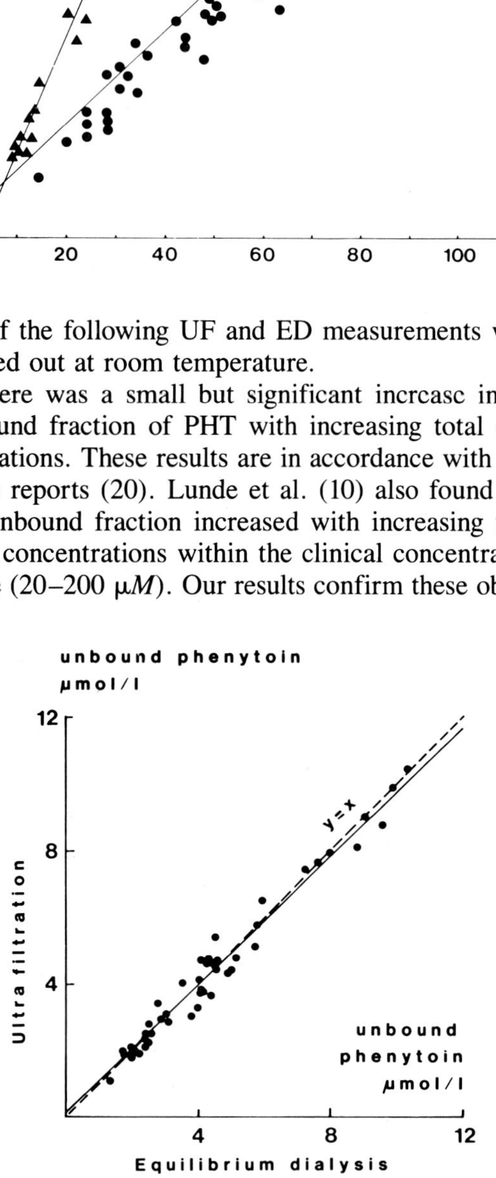

FIG. 3. Relationship between the unbound phenytoin concentrations determined by ultrafiltration and equilibrium dialysis in 50 samples, including uremic patient samples. Slope was 0.97, intercept 0.06, and $r = 0.99$ ($p < 0.001$).

With respect to quality control, the CV in each intra- and inter-assay change was <5% for the UF method. The precision of the ED method was similar to that of the UF method.

It has been reported that total PHT concentrations measured with EMIT might be higher than those obtained with chromatographic methods (12–16). Interference by PHT metabolites (14), such as HPPH in conjugated and unconjugated forms (12,16) has been proposed to account for these differences (21). Therefore, uremic patient samples were also assayed with HPLC. Using EMIT reagent kits with lot numbers of recent date, we found no discrepancy between measurements of PHT with EMIT and HPLC. The high correlation between the HPLC and EMIT methods indicates that no metabolites were comeasured in the latter method. However, the number of uremic patients was small, and we did not actually measure PHT metabolites in the samples.

In our study of 36 epileptic patients with normal kidney function, interpatient variability of the percentage of free fraction was about twofold. This result is in accordance with previous reports concerning interindividual variation in plasma protein binding in nonuremic patients (22–25). As expected (19), the average free fraction of uremic patient samples was higher than in the normal patient group, whereas the mean unbound concentrations were similar in the two groups.

From a pharmacokinetic point of view, measurement of unbound concentration is preferable in therapeutic drug monitoring (26–28). There was a significant correlation between UF and ED measurements in both unbound concentration and unbound fraction. The ultrafiltration method with the new separation device has a great potential for measurements of unbound concentrations of PHT because of its rapidity and reliability. Continued investigations are necessary to evaluate whether such measurements will improve the quality of treatment of patients with epilepsy. Such studies must adhere to the principles of controlled clinical trials.

Acknowledgment: This study was supported by grants from the Swedish Medical Research Council 04X-03902. Filters and DPH EMIT assay reagent kits were kindly provided by Syva, Sweden (Dr. J. Öhman).

REFERENCES

1. Lund L. Anticonvulsant effect of diphenylhydantoin relative to plasma level. A prospective three year study in ambulant patients with generalized epileptic seizures. *Arch Neurol* 1974;31:289–94.
2. Reynolds EH, Chadwick D, Galbraith A. One drug (phenytoin) in the treatment of epilepsy. *Lancet* 1976;1:923–6.
3. Koch-Weser J, Sellers EM. Binding of drugs to serum albumin. *N Engl J Med* 1976;294:311–6; 526–31.
4. Reidenberg MM, Odar-Cederlöf I, von Bahr C, Borgå O, Sjöqvist F. Protein binding of diphenylhydantoin and desmethylimipramine in plasma from patients with poor renal function. *N Engl J Med* 1971;285:264–7.
5. Rane A, Lunde PKM, Jalling B, Yaffe SJ, Sjöqvist F. Plasma protein binding of diphenylhydantoin in normal and hyperbilirubinaemic infants. *J Pediatr* 1971;78:877–82.
6. Hooper WD, Bochner F, Eadie MJ, Tyrer JH. Plasma protein binding of diphenylhydantoin. Effects of sex hormones, renal and hepatic disease. *Clin Pharmacol Ther* 1974;15:276–82.
7. Fredholm BB, Rane A, Persson B. Diphenylhydantoin binding to proteins in plasma and its dependence on free fatty acid and bilirubin concentration in dogs and newborn infants. *Pediatr Res* 1975;9:26–30.
8. Blaschke TF, Meffin PJ, Melmon KL, Rowland M. Influence of acute viral hepatitis on phenytoin kinetics and protein binding. *Clin Pharmacol Ther* 1975;17:685–91.
9. Kurata D, Wilkinson GR. Erythrocyte uptake and plasma binding of diphenylhydantoin. *Clin Pharmacol Ther* 1974;16:355–62.
10. Lunde PKM, Rane A, Yaffe SJ, Lund L, Sjöqvist F. Plasma protein binding of diphenylhydantoin in man. *Clin Pharmacol Ther* 1970;11:846–55.
11. Mattson RH, Cramer JA, Williamson PD, Novelly RA. Valproic acid in epilepsy: clinical and pharmacological effects. *Ann Neurol* 1978;3:20–5.
12. Nandedkar AKN, Williamson R, Kutt H, Fairclough GFF Jr. A comparison of plasma phenytoin level determinations by EMIT and gas-liquid chromatography in patients with renal insufficiency. *Ther Drug Monit* 1980;2:427–30.
13. Burgess ED, Friel PN, Blair AD, Raisy VA. Serum phenytoin concentrations in uremia. *Ann Intern Med* 1981;94:59–60.
14. Matzke GR, Sawchuk RJ. Elevated serum phenytoin concentrations in a uremic patient when measured by enzyme-multiplied immunoassay. *Drug Intell Clin Pharm* 1981;15:386–8.
15. Aldwin L, Kabakoff DS. Metabolite interference in homogenous enzyme immunoassay of phenytoin [Letter]. *Clin Chem* 1981;27:770–1.
16. Sawchuk RJ, Matzke GR. Contribution of 5-(4-hydroxyphenyl)5-phenylhydantoin to the discrepancy between phenytoin analysis by EMIT and high-pressure liquid chromatography. *Ther Drug Monit* 1984;6:97–103.
17. Ehrnebo M, Agurell S, Boréus L-O, Gordon E, Lönroth U. Pentazocine binding to blood cells and plasma proteins. *Clin Pharmacol Ther* 1974;16:424–9.
18. Dolan JW, van der Wal SJ, Bannister SJ, Snyder LR. On-line liquid chromatographic analysis for drugs with the technicon "FAST-LC" system: performance data for theophylline and for four commonly used anticonvulsants and their metabolites. *Clin Chem* 1980;26:871–80.
19. Odar-Cederlöf I, Borgå O. Kinetics of diphenylhydantoin in uremic patients: consequences of decreased plasma protein binding. *Eur J Clin Pharmacol* 1974;7:31–7.
20. Friel P. Methods for free drug level analysis. *Am Assoc Clin Chem* 1983;1–6.
21. McClellan AC, Chan K-M, Lichti DA, Meltzer VN, Ladenson JH. Comparison of the EMIT phenytoin procedure with old and new antibodies. *Clin Chem* 1984;30:808–9.
22. Barth N, Alvan G, Borgå O, Sjöqvist F. Two-fold interindividual variation in plasma protein binding of phenytoin in patients with epilepsy. *Clin Pharmacokinet* 1976;1:444–52.
23. Yacobi A, Lampmann T, Levy G. Frequency distribution of free warfarin and free phenytoin fraction values in serum of healthy human adults. *Clin Pharmacol Ther* 1977;21:283–6.
24. Rimmer EM, Buss DC, Routledge PA, Richens A. Should we routinely measure free plasma phenytoin concentration? *Br J Clin Pharmacol* 1984;17:99–102.
25. Petersen GM, McLean S, Aldous S, von Witt RJ, Millingen K. Plasma protein binding of phenytoin in 100 epileptic patients. *Br J Clin Pharmacol* 1982;14:298–300.
26. Rowland M. Plasma protein binding and therapeutic drug monitoring. *Ther Drug Monit* 1980;2:29–37.
27. Greenblatt DJ, Sellers EM, Koch-Weser J. Importance of protein binding for the interpretation of serum or plasma drug concentrations. *J Clin Pharmacol* 1982;22:259–63.
28. Sjöqvist F. Therapeutic drug monitoring—twenty years experience. In: Lemberger L, Reidenberg MM, eds. *Proceedings of the Second World Conference on Clinical Pharmacology and Therapeutics*. Washington, 1983: Am Soc Pharmacol Exp Ther, Bethesda, Maryland, 1984:38–63.

Therapeutic Drug Monitoring
7:466–471

Determination of Free Disopyramide Plasma Concentrations Using Ultrafiltration and Enzyme Multiplied Immunoassay

Gursharan Raghow, Marvin C. Meyer, and Arthur B. Straughn

Department of Pharmaceutics, College of Pharmacy, University of Tennessee Center for the Health Sciences, Memphis, Tennessee, U.S.A.

Summary: Disopyramide is an antiarrhythmic drug that exhibits nonlinear binding to plasma proteins. As a result, the total body clearance increases with increasing total drug plasma concentration. A rapid and sensitive method for the determination of free (unbound) disopyramide plasma concentrations is described. The procedure employs an ultrafiltration system (Centrifree), which can be used for basic drugs, along with an enzyme multiplied immunoassay system (EMIT) for the measurement of free disopyramide concentrations in plasma water filtrate. The EMIT method was adapted to permit measurement of disopyramide in plasma over a concentration range of 0.02–1.2 μg/ml. Plasma storage at − 20°C, filtration volume, or the presence of buffer and mono-*N*-dealkylated metabolite in plasma did not affect the binding determinations. There was no loss of drug during the filtration process. A good correspondence was found between the EMIT assay and a high performance liquid chromatography method, when applied to plasma samples obtained from a human subject who had ingested disopyramide. Furthermore, the extent of protein binding determined by the ultrafiltration system and by equilibrium dialysis were in good agreement. The binding of disopyramide in fortified human plasma decreased from 64 to 52% over a total drug concentration range of 1–5 μg/ml. **Key Words:** Disopyramide—Binding—Ultrafiltration—Enzyme multiplied immunoassay technique—Dialysis.

Recent studies have demonstrated that the pharmacokinetics of disopyramide, an antiarrhythmic drug, are nonlinear (1–7). The result is that plasma concentrations of the drug do not increase in proportion to the administered dose. It has also been found that the binding of disopyramide to plasma proteins is nonlinear, and the fraction of drug bound decreases with increasing drug concentration. Since the apparent clearance of disopyramide is dependent on free rather than total drug concentration, clearance will increase as a function of increasing free drug concentration. In addition, cardiac activity is better correlated to free disopyramide plasma concentrations (3). The implications of these findings are that monitoring of disopyramide plasma concentrations during therapy should include a determination of free drug concentrations. Furthermore, pharmacokinetic studies, as well as bioavailability studies comparing different dosage forms, should also measure free disopyramide.

Protein binding determinations are frequently done by equilibrium dialysis, although this method may require 5–24 h for equilibration. In addition, the procedure may require corrections for volume shifts between the compartments of the dialysis cell for accurate measurements (8–10). The use of ultrafiltration is a

Address correspondence and reprint requests to Dr. M. C. Meyer at Department of Pharmaceutics, College of Pharmacy, University of Tennessee Center for the Health Sciences, Memphis, TN 38163, U.S.A.

more rapid method, although loss of drug during the filtration process can result in significant errors (11,12).

Several high performance liquid chromatography (HPLC) methods have been reported for the determination of disopyramide in plasma (13–16). In addition, assays involving the enzyme multiplied immunoassay (EMIT) system (17) and fluorescence immunoassay (18) (Ames TDA) are also available. However, the HPLC and EMIT assays are not sufficiently sensitive to measure the low free plasma disopyramide concentrations. Thus, the present work evaluated an ultrafiltration system designed for basic drugs. In addition, the EMIT assay was modified to gain the sensitivity required for free disopyramide in plasma filtrates.

METHODS

EMIT Assay of Free and Total Plasma Disopyramide

The assay of total disopyramide plasma concentration employed the EMIT assay kit (Syva Co.), which consisted of calibrators containing 0, 0.5, 1, 2, 4, and 8 μg/ml of disopyramide; a pH 8, Tris HCl buffer solution; and reagents A and B. A 50-μl aliquot of each calibrator or unknown plasma sample was aspirated and delivered, along with a 250-μl aliquot of buffer, into a 2-ml beaker. A 50-μl aliquot of this dilution was further combined with 250 μl of buffer, along with 50-μl aliquots of reagent A and B. A portion of the mixture was then aspirated into a Gilford Stasar III spectrophotometer set at 340 nm and equipped with a Syva CP-5000 EMIT Clinical Processor and printer. The sample dilutions were prepared with a model 1500 pipettor-dilutor (Syva Co.).

The assay of free disopyramide plasma concentrations, as determined after ultrafiltration or equilibrium dialysis, employed calibrators over a concentration range of 0.02–1.2 μg/ml. These calibrators were prepared from a 10 μg/ml solution of disopyramide (Searle Pharmaceuticals, Inc.) in 0.01 *M* phosphoric acid, diluted with pH 7.4, 0.055 *M* Tris-HCl-buffer. The final concentrations were 0, 0.02, 0.05, 0.08, 0.2, 0.4, 0.8, and 1.2 μg/ml of disopyramide. The assay of the calibrators and unknown plasma samples for free disopyramide concentration, after filtration or dialysis, followed the procedure outlined above for total disopyramide concentration, except that the samples were only diluted once with 250 μl of buffer.

A comparison was made between the EMIT assay for total disopyramide and the HPLC method described later, using plasma samples obtained from a subject 0, 0.5, 1, 2, 3, 4, 6, 8, and 12 h after he had received a single 100-mg dose of disopyramide in solution. The precision and accuracy of the EMIT assay for free disopyramide plasma concentrations was assessed by separately prepared fortified control plasma samples containing 0.1 and 0.6 μg/ml of disopyramide, along with calibration standards on several different days.

HPLC Assay of Disopyramide and Metabolite in Plasma

The HPLC assay, based on the work of Meffin et al. (15), was employed to assess the performance of the EMIT assay described above. The disopyramide, mono-*N*-dealkylated metabolite and internal standard (*p*-chlorodisopyramide) were provided by G. D. Searle, Inc. Standard solutions were prepared in 0.01 *M* phosphoric acid, containing 0.2, 0.5, 1, 2, 3, or 5 μg/ml of disopyramide and 0.1, 0.25, 0.5, 1, 1.5, or 2.5 μg/ml of metabolite. The internal standard was also prepared in 0.01 *M* phosphoric acid, at a concentration of 4 μg/ml. Mixtures of 1 ml of plasma, 0.5 ml of disopyramide/metabolite solution, 0.5 ml of internal standard, 0.5 ml of 1 N sodium hydroxide, and 5 ml of ether were placed in 20-ml centrifuge tubes with poly-tef-lined screw caps, and gently shaken on a platform shaker for 15 min. After centrifugation, the ether layer was transferred to a 15-ml silanized conical tube, and 50 μl of 0.1 N sulfuric acid was added. The contents of the tube were vortex-mixed for 30 s and centrifuged at 3,000 rpm for 15 min at − 10°C. The ether layer was aspirated, and the aqueous layer was transferred to autosampler vials for injection. The assay used a Waters Associates C-18 μBondapak column, a 6000A pump, a WISP 710B autosampler, and a 440 UV detector. A 10–30 μl sample was loaded onto the column and eluted with the mobile phase consisting of 32% acetonitrile/68% [0.11% sodium 1-heptanesulfonic acid (Eastman) and 1% glacial acetic acid in water], with a flow rate of 1.8 ml/min. The eluent was monitored at 254 nm, attenuated at 0.01 absorbance units full scale, and recorded at a chart speed of 0.1 inches per minute with a 10 mV Fisher recorder.

Protein Binding Studies

Ultrafiltration

Amicon micropartitioning system filters (Centrifree) were used for separation of free and protein-bound disopyramide. The plasma samples were placed on the filters and centrifuged at 3,000 rpm (DAMON IEC-CRU-5000) using a fixed angle rotor (model 831-A). Preliminary studies indicated more rapid and uniform filtration with a fixed angle rotor, compared with a swinging-bucket rotor.

Initial studies were conducted to determine any loss of disopyramide, e.g., by binding to the filtration device, during the filtration process. One-milliliter solutions containing 0.5 μg/ml of disopyramide in deionized water or in plasma water were placed onto the filters and centrifuged. The filtrate was assayed using the previously described HPLC assay.

Plasma samples are often stored frozen before analysis. Thus, it was important to determine the effect of storage on the stability of disopyramide and on the binding of disopyramide to plasma proteins. Furthermore, the binding of disopyramide has been reported to increase slightly with a decrease in plasma pH (M. Brinkley, unpublished observations). Preliminary studies demonstrated that 50 μl of pH 7.6 1 *M* phosphate buffer per milliliter of plasma resulted in a stable final pH of 7.6. This pH was selected to permit a comparison with earlier work (M. Brinkley, unpublished observations). A 75-ml portion of human pooled plasma was combined with 3.75 ml of the phosphate buffer, and 25-ml aliquots were fortified with disopyramide, resulting in final concentrations of 0, 0.5, and 2.5 μg/ml. These mixtures were further divided into four 6-ml portions to be assayed for total and free disopyramide by the EMIT assay, immediately, and after storage at −20°C for 1 and 3 weeks.

It was also necessary to establish that the addition of the small quantity of phosphate buffer did not affect the binding of the disopyramide to plasma proteins. To evaluate this potential, two 12-ml portions of pooled human plasma were fortified to contain 2.5 μg/ml of disopyramide. A 600-μl aliquot of 1 *M* phosphate buffer (pH 7.6) was added to one sample, and the pH of the other sample was adjusted to pH 7.6 by bubbling in a 5:95 mixture of CO_2/O_2 gas. Nine 1-ml aliquots of each of the two plasma samples were then added to the Centrifree filters and centrifuged for 15 min at 3,000 rpm to obtain ~0.15 ml of filtrate. The filtrate was assayed for free disopyramide concentration using the EMIT assay. The effects of buffer and metabolite were also evaluated by determining the percentage of free disopyramide in plasma samples containing no buffer, buffer, and buffer with 1 μg/ml of metabolite. A 4.75-ml portion of pH 7.6 plasma was combined with (a) 250 μl of deionized water containing 50 μg/ml of disopyramide, (b) 250 μl of pH 7.6 buffer containing 50 μg/ml of disopyramide, or (c) 250 μl of pH 7.6 buffer containing 50 μg/ml of disopyramide and 20 μg/ml of metabolite. The final concentrations of disopyramide and metabolite in these solutions were 2.5 and 1.0 μg/ml, respectively. Three 1-ml aliquots of each of these three solutions were then filtered through the Centrifree filters, and a portion of the filtrate and initial solution was assayed for free and total disopyramide, respectively, using the EMIT assay.

A study was also conducted to determine if the volume of plasma water filtered could affect the disopyramide binding. Duplicate 1-ml portions of plasma, fortified with 2 μg/ml of disopyramide, were placed on separate Centrifree filters and were centrifuged for 5, 10, 15, and 20 min at 3,000 rpm at room temperature. The filtrates were assayed for free disopyramide using the EMIT assay.

Equilibrium Dialysis

In order to validate the protein binding results obtained with the ultrafiltration system, equilibrium dialysis was employed as a reference method. Dialysis cells (Technilab Instruments) were used with a cellulose membrane (Bel-art Products, No. 40299) having a molecular weight cut-off of 6,000. The membranes were prepared by boiling in deionized water for three 1-h periods, with an exchange of water after each hour. The membranes were stored for a least 24 h at 4°C in pH 7.4 phosphate buffer containing 4.1 g/L sodium chloride, with an ionic strength of 0.26 (10). A 3.6 cm^2 membrane was inserted between the halves of the dialysis cell after the surface moisture had been removed from the membrane. Human plasma samples were fortified to contain ~1–5 μg/ml of disopyramide, and 1.5-ml aliquots were placed on one side of the membrane. A 1.5-ml aliquot of pH 7.4 phosphate buffer was placed on the other side of the membrane, and the dialysis cells were shaken in a 37°C water bath for 24 h. A 1-ml portion of the protein solution side of the dialysis cell was then placed on Centrifree filter and centrifuged for 15 min at 3,000 rpm, and the filtrate was assayed for free disopyramide. In addition, portions of both protein solution and buffer solution removed from the dialysis cell were assayed for total and free disopyramide, respectively, using the EMIT assay.

TABLE 1. *Accuracy and precision of the enzyme multiplied immunoassay technique for disopyramide as determined from control samples run along with seven different standard curves*

	Measured disopyramide in controls (μg/ml)	
Standard curve no.	0.1 μg/ml	0.6 μg/ml
1	0.10	0.58
	0.09	0.58
2	0.10	0.57
3	0.09	0.56
	0.10	0.59
4	0.10	0.59
5	0.09	0.58
	0.10	0.58
6	0.09	0.58
7	0.10	0.62
Mean	0.10	0.58
CV (%)	5.4	2.7

RESULTS AND DISCUSSION

EMIT and HPLC Assay Methods

The HPLC method demonstrated good standard curve linearity over a plasma concentration range of 0.1–2.5 μg/ml for disopyramide (r = 0.999) and 0.05–1.25 μg/ml for metabolite (r = 0.998), for plots of peak height ratio (drug or metabolite/internal standard) versus drug or metabolite concentration. The assay exhibited a precision ranging from a CV (%) of 2.3–6.8 for the highest and lowest concentration of disopyramide, and a CV (%) of 3.9–10.8 for the highest and lowest metabolite concentration, respectively. The recovery of drug and metabolite from extracted plasma samples was in excess of 90%. The metabolite, drug, and internal standard were well separated chromatographically, with elution times of 3.8, 5.0, and 7.5 min, respectively. No interfering peaks were observed when drug-free plasma samples were carried through the assay procedure.

The good precision of the EMIT assay, using pooled human plasma fortified to contain 0.1 and 0.6 μg/ml of disopyramide, is shown in Table 1. Table 2 summarizes the results obtained using the HPLC and the EMIT assay for plasma samples from a human subject who had ingested a 100-mg solution dose of disopyramide. The results with the two methods are in excellent agreement, and both are satisfactory for the determination of total plasma disopyramide concentrations over the concentration range found in these samples. However, the EMIT assay is much more rapid. Furthermore, the lower limit of sensitivity of the HPLC assay (0.05 μg/ml) would not be adequate to characterize the total disopyramide concentrations much longer than 16–20 h after dosing, nor would it be capable of determining free plasma disopyramide concentrations at the lower total drug concentrations.

Ultrafiltration

The preliminary studies demonstrated no loss of disopyramide during the filtration process when aqueous or plasma-water solution containing 0.5 μg/ml of disopyramide were passed through the filter. These findings are in contrast to the significant filter binding of disopyramide noted by others (11,12), who employed a filtration system developed for acidic anticonvulsant drugs. These authors note that interactions between the filtration system and the filtered drug could result in an overestimation of the extent of binding.

The effect of plasma sample storage at −20°C on the stability of the disopyramide and the extent of protein binding was also evaluated using the Centrifree filters. No significant change in plasma pH was found during storage for a 3-week period, using pooled human plasma initially treated with 50 μl of pH 7.6 buffer per milliliter of plasma. In addition, the percentage of disopyramide bound for samples containing a total disopyramide plasma concentration of 0.5 μg/ml was 81.2 and 77.4% after 1 and 3 weeks of storage, respectively, compared with an initial determination of 80.2%. Similarly, 63.6 and 60.5% binding was observed in samples containing 2.5 μg/ml disopyramide after 1 and 3 weeks, respectively, compared with an initial binding of 64.3%. Thus, it appeared that free disopyramide concentrations could be deter-

TABLE 2. *Concentrations of total disopyramide in duplicate plasma samples of a human subject obtained after a 100-mg dose, by enzyme multiplied immunoassay technique (EMIT) and high performance liquid chromatography (HPLC)*

	Concentration of disopyramide (μg/ml)	
Sample (h)	EMIT (mean)	HPLC (mean)
0.5	1.50, 1.54 (1.52)	1.60, 1.21 (1.41)
1.0	1.65, 1.66 (1.65)	1.67, 1.65 (1.66)
2.0	1.48, 1.51 (1.50)	1.55, 1.55 (1.55)
3.0	1.27, 1.30 (1.28)	1.32, 1.32 (1.32)
4.0	1.21, 1.24 (1.22)	1.16, 1.21 (1.19)
6.0	0.98, 0.96 (0.97)	0.94, 0.95 (0.95)
8.0	0.71, 0.73 (0.72)	0.68, 0.72 (0.70)
12.0	0.35, 0.36 (0.36)	— — —[a]

[a]Not available for analysis.

TABLE 3. *Comparison of disopyramide binding using equilibrium dialysis and filtration*

Initial total disopyramide (μg/ml)[a]	Equilibrium total disopyramide (μg/ml)[b] (Mean)	Equilibrium free disopyramide (μg/ml)[c] (Mean)	Dialysis percentage bound disopyramide[d] (Mean)	Filtration free disopyramide (μg/ml)[e] (Mean)	Filtration percentage bound disopyramide[d] (Mean)
0.92	0.68	0.25	63.2	0.25	63.2
	0.74 (0.69)	0.25 (0.25)	66.2 (63.5)	0.26 (0.26)	64.9 (61.4)
	0.64	0.25	61.0	0.28	56.0
1.94	1.42	0.48	66.2	0.50	64.8
	1.49 (1.46)	0.52 (0.51)	65.0 (65.1)	0.56 (0.54)	62.0 (62.6)
	1.47	0.53	64.0	0.57	61.0
2.99	2.13	0.85	60.1	0.80	62.4
	2.15 (2.14)	0.80 (0.80)	62.8 (62.3)	0.81 (0.81)	62.3 (62.2)
	2.14	0.76	64.0	0.81	62.0
4.74	3.32	1.47	55.7	1.46	56.0
	2.98 (3.10)	1.49 (1.45)	50.0 (53.2)	1.54 (1.48)	48.0 (52.0)
	3.00	1.38	54.0	1.44	52.0

[a]Sample placed on protein side of dialysis cell.
[b]Assay of protein side of dialysis cell, after equilibration.
[c]Assay of buffer side of dialysis cell, after equilibration.
[d](Total concentration-free concentration)/total concentration.
[e]Assay after filtration of protein side of dialysis cell.

mined in samples that had been initially frozen prior to the time the protein binding determinations were conducted.

Studies to evaluate the effect of the pH 7.6 buffer and metabolite in the plasma indicated no significant influence of these variables on the protein binding measurements. The mean (n = 9) percentage of disopyramide bound in plasma adjusted to pH 7.6 with 50 μl of pH 7.6 buffer per milliliter of plasma was 79.5% (CV 10.6%) compared with a mean of 82% binding (CV 7.0%) for the plasma adjusted to pH 7.6 with CO_2/O_2 gas. In addition, the mean percentage of disopyramide bound in plasma, at a total concentration of 2.5 μg/ml, was 82.7, 82.5, and 82.8% when the drug was added in water, in pH 7.6 buffer, or in pH 7.6 buffer containing 1 μg/ml of metabolite, respectively.

Finally, no differences were found in the fraction of drug recovered in filtrates obtained with the Centrifree filters, when the centrifugation was stopped after 5, 10, 15, or 20 min. These results are consistent with those of other workers (11,19), who found that the use of ultrafiltration to determine protein binding was not sensitive to the volume of the filtrate.

Comparison of Ultrafiltration and Equilibrium Dialysis

Table 3 provides a direct comparison between the percentage of disopyramide binding using ultrafiltration and equilibrium dialysis. As noted by others (1–7), the percentage binding decreased with increasing disopyramide concentration, using both methods. In addition, the percentage binding found using equilibrium dialysis was essentially the same as that determined when the solution on the protein side of the dialysis cell was subsequently filtered.

In conclusion, the use of the Centrifree filters, which can be employed for acidic or basic drugs, along with the EMIT assay modified to permit quantitation of low concentrations of disopyramide in plasma filtrate, provides a rapid and accurate means to assess free disopyramide plasma concentrations.

REFERENCES

1. Hinderling PH, Garrett ER. Pharmacokinetics of the antiarrhythmic disopyramide in healthy humans. *J Pharmacokinet Biopharm* 1981;4:199.
2. Karim A, Nissen C, Azarnoff DL. Clinical pharmacokinetics of disopyramide. *J Pharmacokinet Biopharm* 1982;10:465.
3. Lima JJ, Boudoulas H, Blanford M. Concentration-dependence of disopyramide binding to plasma protein and its influence on kinetics and dynamics. *J Pharmacol Exp Ther* 1981;219:741.
4. Meffin PJ, Robert EW, Winkle RA, Harapat S, Peters FA, Harrison DC. Role of concentration-dependent plasma protein binding in disopyramide disposition. *J Pharmacokinet Biopharm* 1979;7:29.
5. Giacomini KM, Swezey SE, Turner-Tamiyasu K, Blaschke TF. The effect of saturable binding to plasma proteins on the pharmacokinetic properties of disopyramide *J Pharmacokinet Biopharm* 1982;10:1.
6. Haughey DB, Lima JJ. Influence of concentration-dependent protein-binding on serum concentrations and urinary excre-

tion of disopyramide and its metabolite following oral administration. *Biopharm Drug Dispos* 1983;4:103.
7. Lima JJ, Haughey DB, Leier CV. Disopyramide pharmacokinetics and bioavailability following the simultaneous administration of disopyramide and ^{14}C-disopyramide. *J Pharmacokinet Biopharm* 1984;12:289.
8. Tozer TN, Gambertoglio JG, Furst DF, Avery DS, Holford, NHG. Volume shifts and protein binding estimates using equilibrium dialysis-application to prednisolone binding in man. *J Pharm Sci* 1983;72:1,442–6.
9. Giacomini KM, Abany A, Blaschke TF. Calculation of drug concentration in plasma after equilibrium dialysis. *Br J Clin Pharmacol* 1982;14:752–3.
10. Lima JJ, MacKichan JJ, Libertin N, Sabino J. Influence of volume shifts on drug binding during equilibrium dialysis: correction and attenuation. *J Pharmacokinet Biopharm* 1983;11:5.
11. David BM, Tjokrosetio R, Ilett KF. Plasma protein binding of disopyramide by equilibrium dialysis and ultrafiltration. *Ther Drug Monit* 1983;5:81–6.
12. Norris RLG, Ahokes JT, Rovenscroft PJ. Determination of unbound fraction of disopyramide in plasma: a comparison of equilibrium dialysis, ultrafiltration through dialysis membrane and ultrafree anticonvulsant drug filters. *J Pharmacol Methods* 1982;7:7–14.
13. Ilett KF, Hackett LP, Tjokrosetio R. Disopyramide determination by gas chromatography, liquid chromatography and mass spectrometry. *Clin Chem* 1979;25:1900–4.
14. Lima JJ. Liquid chromatographic analysis of disopyramide and its mono-N-dealkylated metabolite. *Clin Chem* 1979;25:405–8.
15. Meffin PJ, Harapat SR, Harrison DC. High-pressure liquid chromatographic analysis of drugs in biological fluids: III. Analysis of disopyramide and its mono-N-dealkylated metabolite in plasma and urine. *J Chromatogr* 1977;132:503–10.
16. Swezey CB, Ponzo JL. Determination of disopyramide phosphate in serum by high-performance liquid chromatography. *Ther Drug Monit* 1984;6:211–4.
17. Pape BE. Enzyme immunoassay of disopyramide in serum. *Clin Chem* 1981;27:2038–40.
18. Lima JJ, Shields BJ, Howell LH, MacKikhan JJ. Evaluation of fluorescence immunoassay for total and unbound serum concentrations of disopyramide. *Ther Drug Monit* 1984;6:203–10.
19. Whitlam JB, Brown KF. Ultrafiltration in serum protein binding determinations. *J Pharm Sci* 1981;70:146–50.

Therapeutic Drug Monitoring
7:472–477 © 1985 Raven Press, New York

Therapeutic Monitoring of Chlorpromazine II: Pitfalls in Whole Blood Analysis

G. McKay, J. K. Cooper, E. M. Hawes, J. W. Hubbard, M. Martin, and K. K. Midha

College of Pharmacy, University of Saskatchewan, Saskatoon, Saskatchewan, Canada

Summary: Pooled whole blood from healthy volunteers was spiked with pure, synthetic chlorpromazine, chlorpromazine sulfoxide, or chlorpromazine *N*-oxide and then made alkaline with either sodium hydroxide or sodium carbonate. The addition of alkali causes lysis of red cells, the contents of which spill into the plasma. The lysed samples were allowed to stand at room temperature for various timed intervals before extraction with organic solvents and analysis by high performance liquid chromatography. It was found that a portion (10–14%) of the chlorpromazine spike was oxidised to chlorpromazine sulfoxide, whether the blood was made alkaline with sodium hydroxide or sodium carbonate. Chlorpromazine *N*-oxide added to whole blood was entirely destroyed in the presence of alkali. The chlorpromazine *N*-oxide was rapidly reduced to chlorpromazine, a portion of which subsequently underwent oxidation to chlorpromazine sulfoxide. We have found that chlorpromazine *N*-oxide resides almost entirely in the plasma with only a small portion (<4%) distributed into the red cells. Hence, it is essential that red cells and plasma be separated before analysis. Chlorpromazine and chlorpromazine *N*-oxide can then be extracted from plasma by a method that does not lead to reduction of chlorpromazine *N*-oxide. Alkaline extraction methods must be avoided in the analysis of chlorpromazine in the red cell fraction.
Key Words: Chlorpromazine—Chlorpromazine sulfoxide—Chlorpromazine *N*-oxide.

In recent years, there has been an increasing emphasis on the measurement of neuroleptic drugs in red blood cells or whole blood (1–5). It has been suggested that neuroleptic concentrations in red blood cells may be a better reflection of drugs in the central nervous system than are plasma levels (6,7). Drug analysis in whole blood or red blood cells requires more careful consideration than in plasma or serum, because red blood cells contain reactive molecules such as glutathione, cysteine residues of hemoglobin, and other reductive systems that can cause artifacts in analysis (8–10). For example, Bickel et al. (11) have reported interconversions between imipramine and its *N*-oxide in whole blood. On the other hand, Powis and De Graw (12) suspected that indicine *N*-oxide was reduced by hemoglobin that had been denatured by contact with chloroform during the extraction process. Hemoglobin was also implicated in the oxidation of chlorpromazine (CPZ) to chlorpromazine sulfoxide (CPZSO) in one study (13); however, other researchers (14) were unable to detect any CPZSO when CPZ was incubated with hemoglobin under the same conditions that gave CPZSO in red blood cells or red blood cell lysate.

Recently, we have found that chlorpromazine *N*-oxide (CPZNO) can undergo reduction to CPZ in clinical plasma samples made alkaline with sodium hydroxide (15). This leads to the measurement of spuriously high plasma concentrations of CPZ and correspondingly low levels of CPZNO. By contrast,

Address correspondence and reprint requests to K. K. Midha at College of Pharmacy, University of Saskatchewan, Saskatoon, Saskatchewan, S7N 0W0, Canada.

we found no reduction of CPZNO in plasma samples alkalinized with sodium carbonate. Consequently, we carried out the present study to investigate the stability of CPZ, CPZSO, and CPZNO during alkaline extraction procedures from whole blood.

METHODS

Materials

CPZ and CPZSO were kindly supplied by Poulenc Limited, Montreal, Quebec, Canada. CPZNO was synthesized in our laboratories by oxidation of CPZ with peroxybenzoic acid (details to be reported elsewhere). The synthetic sample was identical by thin-layer chromatography, chemical ionization mass spectrometry (TLC, CI-MS) with a reference sample kindly supplied by Dr. A. A. Manian (Department of Health and Human Services, Alcohol, Drug Abuse, and Mental Health Administration, National Institute of Mental Health, Rockville, MD, U.S.A.). The purity and structural integrity of all three compounds were confirmed by TLC, CI-MS, nuclear magnetic resonance (NMR), infrared (IR), and elemental analysis. All other chemicals were commercial analytical grade.

High Performance Liquid Chromatography (HPLC)

High performance liquid chromatographic equipment, mobile phase, and operating conditions were as reported previously (16) except that the column was packed with 5 μm Spherisorb CN, not 10 μm Spherisorb CN. HPLC and all other operations were carried out in subdued light and at ambient temperature.

Collection of Whole Blood

Samples from three healthy volunteers were collected by venipuncture into evacuated heparinized tubes (Vacutainers; Becton-Dickinson, Mississauga, Ontario, Canada), care being taken not to allow the blood to contact the rubber stopper. Blood from the three volunteers was decanted into a beaker and mixed (mean packed cell volume 0.41). Freshly drawn blood was used in all experiments and was collected as required from the same three volunteers.

Preparation of Samples

One milliliter of double-distilled water was added to 2.0 ml whole blood, followed by 40 μl acetonitrile containing 200 ng CPZ, CPZSO, or CPZNO. The sample was mixed and the pH adjusted either by the addition of 0.5 ml saturated sodium carbonate (condition 1) or by the addition of 0.5 ml 10 *M* sodium hydroxide (condition 2). The alkalinized samples were then allowed to stand at ambient temperature for the appropriate time before extraction (0, 15, 30, 45, 60, 90, and 120 min). Three samples were prepared for each time point.

Extraction of Samples

The lysed whole blood samples were extracted with 5.0 ml *n*-pentane containing 3% isopropanol (PIP), by shaking (IKA Vibrax Shaker; Terochem Laboratories Limited, Edmonton, Alberta, Canada) for 15 min. The mixture was then centrifuged (1,500 *g*). The aqueous layer was separated and subjected to a second extraction with PIP as described above. The aqueous layer was then set aside for subsequent extraction with methylenedichloride (MDC).

To the combined PIP extracts were added an anti-bumping granule and 50 ng prochlorperazine in 1.0 ml PIP as external standard. The mixture was then evaporated at 65°C (Thermolyne Dri-Bath; Fisher Scientific Company, Edmonton, Alberta, Canada). The tube containing the residue was sealed and stored at − 20°C until analyzed, at which time the residue was mixed with 200 μl acetonitrile (Vortex-Genie; Fisher Scientific Company). The acetonitrile solution (100 μl) was injected into the HPLC.

The aqueous layer from the second extraction with PIP was transferred to a clean tube to which 5.0 ml MDC was added. The aqueous and MDC layers were mixed on a Multipurpose Rotator (Canlab, Edmonton, Alberta, Canada) for 30 min and then centrifuged (1,500 *g*). The MDC layer was separated and mixed with 1.0 ml PIP containing 50 ng prochlorperazine as external standard. The solution was then evaporated (Thermolyne Dri-Bath) at 40°C in a stream of dry nitrogen, care being taken not to allow the residue to dry out completely. The tube containing the moist residue was sealed and stored at − 20°C until analysis, at which time the residue was dissolved by mixing (Vortex-Genie) with 200 μl acetonitrile. Aliquots (100 μl) of acetonitrile solution were injected into the HPLC.

CALCULATIONS

All calculations for these absolute recovery-type experiments were based on the absolute injection technique. The peak height of CPZ (or metabolite) was compared with the peak height of the corresponding standard in acetonitrile (100 μl). The external standard (prochlorperazine) was used to assure consistency in the relative retention times of CPZ and metabolites. The absolute recoveries of CPZ and CPZSO are expressed as totals recovered in the PIP and MDC extracts. CPZNO was not extracted by PIP and its recoveries are, therefore, from MDC only.

RESULTS

In these experiments, CPZ, CPZSO, or CPZNO were each added separately to samples of pooled human whole blood, which were subsequently made alkaline by the addition of sodium carbonate (condition 1) or sodium hydroxide (condition 2). The samples were allowed to stand at room temperature for various timed intervals. The blood was then extracted with PIP and subsequently with MDC. The PIP and MDC extracts were analyzed separately for CPZ, CPZSO, and CPZNO by HPLC. Table 1 shows absolute percentage recoveries of CPZ and CPZSO in the two solvents. For convenience, however, data for CPZ and CPZSO will be presented as total absolute percentage recovery values in PIP plus MDC. CPZNO was not extracted significantly by PIP, but previous studies (15) have shown it to be extracted from aqueous media by MDC.

In experiments in which CPZ was added to whole blood that was subsequently made alkaline by either condition 1 or condition 2, a peak was observed in the HPLC traces that corresponded in retention time to CPZSO (8.6 min), in addition to the expected peak for CPZ (2.7 min). HPLC eluates for the peak at 8.6 min were collected from several runs, bulked, and evaporated, and the residue was subjected to direct probe chemical ionization mass spectrometry using ammonia as reagent gas. The mass spectrum, which contained quasi-molecular ions at m/z 335/337 and other diagnostic ions, was very similar to that of an authentic reference sample of CPZSO. It was concluded that a portion of the CPZ spike had undergone oxidation to CPZSO in the alkaline whole blood.

TABLE 1. *Composite mean (n = 21) percentage absolute recovery values for CPZ and CPZSO (±SD) after successive extractions of blood with PIP and then MDC*

Spike	Alkali condition	First solvent PIP	Second solvent MDC	Total PIP + MDC
CPZ	1	62.0 ± 2.4	3.3 ± 0.5	65.3 ± 2.0
CPZ	2	62.7 ± 2.4	9.6 ± 1.6	72.3 ± 1.7
CPZSO	1	26.1 ± 1.7	25.2 ± 1.2	51.3 ± 2.4
CPZSO	2	20.9 ± 1.1	45.9 ± 1.6	66.8 ± 1.9

CPZ, chlorpromazine; CPZSO, chlorpromazine sulfoxide; PIP, *n*-pentane with 3% ispropanol; MDC, methylenedichloride.

Figure 1 shows CPZ and CPZSO recovered from whole blood spiked with CPZ and alkalinized under condition 1. Note that the recoveries were not affected by the time interval during which the alkalinized samples were allowed to stand before extraction (incubation time). Therefore, results can be reported as composite mean percentage recoveries (Table 2). This shows that similar results were obtained whether the samples were alkalinized under condition 1 or condition 2. In both cases, a portion of the CPZ spike was recovered as CPZSO (PIP plus MDC).

When CPZSO was added to whole blood, however, only unchanged CPZSO was recovered from whole blood alkalinized under condition 1 or condition 2. No other chlorpromazine-related peaks were detected in the HPLC chromatograms. Again, the recoveries of CPZSO were unaffected by the incubation time and are reported as composite mean percentage absolute recoveries (Table 2).

Pure, synthetic CPZNO was added to whole blood that was subsequently alkalinized by condition 1 or condition 2 and extracted as described in Methods. According to previous experience (15), CPZNO can be extracted from aqueous media into MDC. There was no peak for CPZNO, however, at the appropriate retention time (6.5 min) in HPLC traces of the MDC extracts. Instead, the HPLC traces of both PIP and MDC extracts contained two peaks, which corre-

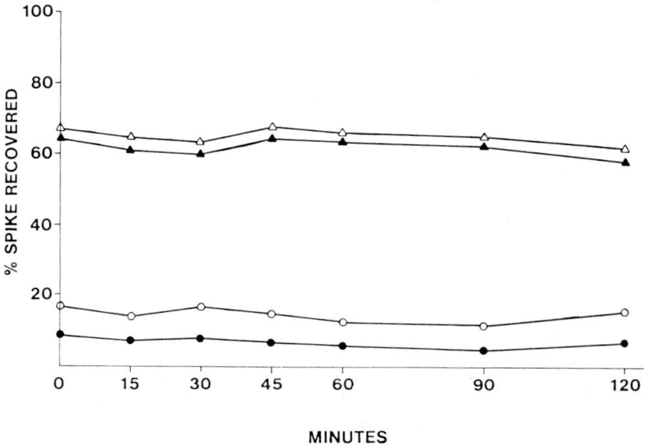

FIG. 1. Recovery of chlorpromazine (CPZ) (triangles) and chlorpromazine sulfoxide (circles) from whole blood spiked with CPZ, alkalinized (condition 1), and allowed to stand at room temperature for various time intervals before extraction. Closed symbols represent mean (n = 3) recoveries in *n*-pentane with 3% isopropanol (PIP). Open symbols represent mean (n = 3) recoveries in PIP plus methylenedichloride.

TABLE 2. *Composite mean (n = 21) percentage absolute recoveries in PIP plus MDC (± SD)*

Spike	Alkali condition	CPZ ± SD (%)	CPZSO ± SD (%)	CPZNO ± SD (%)[a]	Total ± SD (%)
CPZ	1	65.3 ± 2.0	13.9 ± 1.9	0	79.2 ± 2.3
CPZ	2	72.3 ± 1.7	9.7 ± 1.5	0	82.0 ± 2.4
CPZSO	1	0	51.3 ± 2.4	0	51.3 ± 2.4
CPZSO	2	0	66.8 ± 1.9	0	66.8 ± 1.9
CPZNO	1	58.7 ± 2.7[b]	11.4 ± 1.3	0	70.1 ± 3.7
CPZNO	2	59.7 ± 4.1[c]	17.5 ± 3.3	0	77.2 ± 6.1

CPZ, chlorpromazine; CPZSO, chlorpromazine sulfoxide; CPZNO, chlorpromazine *N*-oxide; PIP, *n*-pentane with 3% isopropanol; MDC, methylenedichloride.
[a]Recovery of 0% indicates less than the detection limit.
[b]49.1 ± 1.8% recovered in PIP; the remainder in MDC.
[c]48.1 ± 3.1% recovered in PIP; the remainder in MDC.

sponded in retention times to CPZ (2.7 min) and CPZSO (8.7 min). The HPLC eluates corresponding to these peaks were collected from several runs. The appropriate fractions were bulked and evaporated, and the respective residues were subjected to ammonia gas chemical ionization mass spectrometry by direct insertion probe. The mass spectra obtained were identical to those of authentic reference samples of CPZ and CPZSO. It was concluded that CPZNO spike had been converted into a mixture of CPZ and CPZSO in the alkaline whole blood.

Figure 2 shows that the length of the incubation period had no effect on the amounts of CPZ and CPZSO produced from CPZNO in whole blood alkalinized under condition 1. Similar results were obtained from blood alkalinized under condition 2. Note

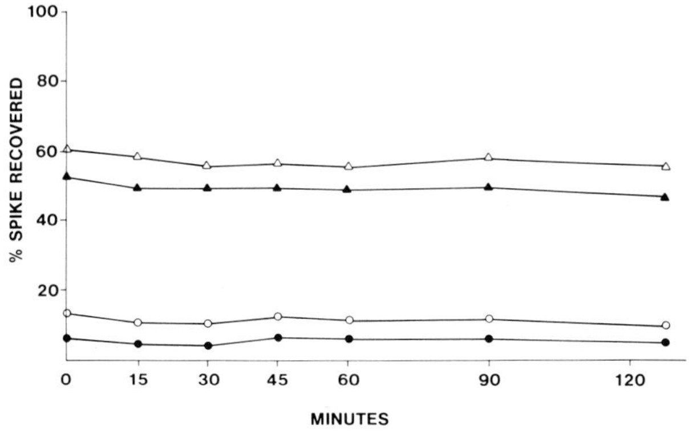

FIG. 2. Recovery of chlorpromazine (triangles) and chlorpromazine sulfoxide (circles) from whole blood spiked with chlorpromazine *N*-oxide, alkalinized (condition 1), and allowed to stand at room temperature for various timed intervals before extraction. Closed symbols represent mean (n = 3) recoveries in *n*-pentane with 3% isopropanol (PIP). Open symbols represent mean (n = 3) recoveries in PIP plus methylenedichloride.

that in each case, 70% or more of the spike was accounted for in terms of CPZ and CPZSO (Table 2), even though no unchanged CPZNO was detected.

DISCUSSION

The present experiments were designed to investigate potential interconversions between CPZ, CPZSO, and CPZNO during extraction from alkalinized whole blood. In a previous study, we found that CPZNO was reduced to CPZ during extraction from plasma made alkaline with sodium hydroxide, although alkalinization with sodium carbonate did not induce the interconversion. Consequently, for the sake of consistency in the present study, we chose to use the exact same alkalinization conditions and the same terminology (conditions 1 and 2) as used in our earlier work (15).

Data are reported here as absolute recoveries because we wished to avoid any correction for losses during extraction and concentration of solvents. The use of recoveries relative to a true internal standard would incorporate some correction for such factors. Furthermore, there was also the possibility that an internal standard might itself undergo chemical changes in alkalinized whole blood, making results very difficult to interpret. The absolute recovery method, on the other hand, enabled us to sum the amounts of CPZ, CPZSO, and CPZNO actually recovered and to indicate the total percentage of spike accounted for in each experiment (Table 2). Note that the total absolute recoveries were 70% or higher in all experiments except those involving a CPZSO spike.

The use of two solvents was appropriate for two reasons. First, whereas CPZ was very efficiently extracted by shaking with two successive aliquots of PIP, this solvent system did not extract significant amounts of CPZNO. The latter can be extracted into MDC, provided conditions that reduce the *N*-oxide function are avoided (15). CPZSO was extracted from whole blood by both solvents, although MDC was the more efficient solvent under condition 2 (Table 1). Second, we wished to investigate the suggestion that reduction of *N*-oxide might occur as a result of changes to hemoglobin brought about by the use of chlorinated hydrocarbon solvents (12). In fact, we found that 83% of the CPZ formed from CPZNO in alkaline whole blood (in either condition) was recovered in PIP, and only about 17% in MDC (Fig. 2). Note that the samples were extracted with PIP before MDC, which indicates that factors other than the use of chlorinated hydrocarbon solvents must also be involved in the reduction of *N*-oxide in alkalinized whole blood.

The technique of extraction with two successive aliquots of PIP is extremely efficient for the extraction of CPZ, but it is a very lengthy procedure because of the number of transfer and centrifugation steps involved (15). During this time, drug and metabolites remain exposed to oxidation/reduction systems present in the alkaline whole blood. This is undoubtedly why the time interval between alkalinization and extraction had no apparent effect on recovery in the present experiments. Note that Figs. 1 and 2 include percentage recoveries in PIP alone. This shows that the oxidation of CPZ to CPZSO, and the reduction of CPZNO to CPZ, can occur during an extraction procedure of a type commonly used in the analysis of CPZ in clinical samples. Furthermore, similar results were obtained whether the blood was made alkaline with sodium hydroxide or with sodium carbonate. This is in contrast to earlier studies with plasma, in which reduction of CPZNO occurred only in the presence of sodium hydroxide (15). Thus, it appears that conventional methods of analysis of CPZ in whole blood samples from patients mediated with CPZ are particularly prone to yield spurious results.

Another key point is that the addition of alkali causes lysis of red blood cells. Consequently, the contents of the red blood cells pour into the plasma when whole blood is made alkaline. This is of vital importance because, in subsequent studies, we have found that CPZNO resides almost entirely in the plasma, and only a small portion (<4%) is distributed into the red blood cells (unpublished data). This means that the problem of the facile reduction of CPZNO can largely be avoided by separating the red blood cells from plasma before analysis. CPZNO can then be measured in the plasma fraction, where it occurs in considerable quantities in clinical samples (15,17).

In contrast to the *N*-oxide metabolite, CPZ is distributed into the red blood cells to a considerable extent (18). Hence, spurious oxidation of CPZ to CPZSO is likely to occur in separated red blood cells, especially when alkaline extraction methods are used in the analysis. Our data suggest that other researchers (13,14) who reported conversion of CPZ into CPZSO in red blood cells observed, in fact, an artifact brought about by their use of alkali in contact with red blood cell material. In subsequent work (unpublished), we found that very little CPZ was oxidized to CPZSO (1%) after incubation in whole blood under physiological conditions and subsequent analysis by a method that did not promote the oxidation of CPZ.

CONCLUSIONS

CPZNO is readily reduced to CPZ, and CPZ is oxidized to CPZSO in whole blood made alkaline before extraction. It is essential that red blood cells and plasma be separated before analysis. Alkaline extraction methods should be avoided in the analysis of CPZ and CPZSO in red blood cells.

Acknowledgment: The authors gratefully acknowledge the Medical Research Council of Canada for Grant No. DG 248 to J. W. H. and Grant No. MT 7838 to K. K. M. Messrs. T. J. Jaworski and P. K. F. Yeung are thanked for their technical assistance.

REFERENCES

1. Schvarksburd A, Nwokeafor V, Smith RC. Red blood cell and plasma levels of thioridazine and mesoridazine in schizophrenic patients. *Psychopharmacology* 1984;82:55–61.
2. Smith RC, Vroulis G, Shvarksburd A, et al. RBC and plasma levels of haloperidol and clinical response in schizophrenia. *Am J Psychiatry* 1982;139:1054–6.
3. Casper R, Garver DL, Dekirmenjian H, Chang S, Davis JM. Phenothiazine levels in plasma and red blood cells. *Arch Gen Psychiatry* 1980;37:301–5.
4. Smith RC, Tamminga CA, Crayton JW, Dekirmenjian H, Davis JM. Relationship of butaperazine blood levels to plasma prolactin in chronic schizophrenic patients. *Psychopharmacology* 1979;66:29–33.
5. Smith RC, Crayton JW, Dekirmenjian H, Klass D, Davis JM. Blood levels of neuroleptic drugs in non-responding chronic schizophrenic patients. *Arch Gen Psychiatry* 1979;36:579–84.
6. Garver DL, Dekirmenjian H, Davis JM, Casper R, Ericksen S. Neuroleptic drug levels and therapeutic response: preliminary observations with red blood cell bound butaperazine. *Am J Psychiatry* 1977;134:304–7.
7. Garver DL, Davis JM, Dekirmenjian H, Jones FD, Casper R, Haraszti J. Pharmacokinetics of red blood cell butaperazine and clinical effects. *Arch Gen Psychiatry* 1976;33:862–6.
8. Eyer P, Lierheimer E. Biotransformation of nitrosobenzene in the red cell and the role of glutathione. *Xenobiotica* 1980;10:517–26.
9. Diepold C, Eyer P, Kampffmeyer H, Reinhardt K. Reactions

of aromatic nitroso compounds with thiols. *Adv Exp Med Biol* 1982;136B:1173–81.
10. Dolle B, Topner W, Neumann HG. Reactions of arylnitroso compounds with mercaptans. *Xenobiotica* 1980;10:527–36.
11. Bickel MH, Weder HJ, Aebi H. Metabolite interconversions between imipramine, its *N*-oxide and its desmethyl derivative in rat tissues in vivo. *Biochem Biophys Res Commun* 1968;33:1012–8.
12. Powis G, De Graw CL. N-oxide reduction by hemoglobin, cytochrome C and ferrous ions. *Res Commun Chem Pathol Pharmacol* 1980;30:143–50.
13. Traficante LJ, Sakalis G, Siekierski J, Rotrosen J, Gershon S. Rapid in vitro sulfoxidation of chlorpromazine by human blood: inhibition by an endogeneous plasma protein factor. *Life Sci* 1979;24:337–46.
14. Kaul PN, Chopde C, Clark ML. Complications in chlorpromazine level determination contributed by blood components. In: Usdin E, Eckert H, Forrest S, eds. *Phenothiazines and structurally related drugs.* New York: Raven Press, 1980:159–62.
15. Hubbard JW, Cooper JK, Hawes EM, et al. Therapeutic monitoring of chlorpromazine I: pitfalls in plasma analysis. *Ther Drug Monit* 1985;7:222–8.
16. Cooper JK, McKay G, Midha KK. Subnanogram quantitation of chlorpromazine in plasma by high performance liquid chromatography with electrochemical detection. *J Pharm Sci* 1983;72:1259–62.
17. Craig JC, Gruenke LD, Hitzeman BA, Holaday J, Loh HH. Simultaneous determination of chlorpromazine and its major metabolites in plasma and red blood cells by a GLC/MS method: clinical implications. In: Usdin E, Eckert H, Forrest IS, eds. *Phenothiazines and structurally related drugs.* New York: Raven Press, 1980:129–32.
18. Lund A. The distribution of chlorpromazine between plasma and erythrocytes. *Acta Pharmacol Toxicol* 1983;47:300–4.

Therapeutic Drug Monitoring
7:478–480 © 1985 Raven Press, New York

Short Communication

Extremely Rapid Hydroxylation of Debrisoquine: A Case Report with Implication for Treatment with Nortriptyline and Other Tricyclic Antidepressants

*Leif Bertilsson, ‡Anna Åberg-Wistedt, *Lars L. Gustafsson, and †Conny Nordin

*Departments of *Clinical Pharmacology and †Psychiatry, Karolinska Institute, Huddinge Hospital, Huddinge; and ‡Department of Psychiatry, Danderyds Hospital, Danderyd, Sweden*

The benzylic E-10-hydroxylation of the tricyclic antidepressant nortriptyline (NT) is genetically regulated (1,2) and is closely related to the polymorphic hydroxylation of debrisoquine (3) in healthy subjects (4) and depressed patients (5). Poor hydroxylators develop high plasma levels of NT (5,6) and such patients may experience adverse reactions even on low doses of NT (6). We have previously described a poor hydroxylator with a debrisoquine metabolic ratio of 43 (6). This patient was successfully treated with 20 mg NT daily, which is much lower than the usually recommended daily dose (150 mg) for treatment of depression.

Several recent debates (7–9) have concerned strategies involved in treating poor hydroxylators of debrisoquine with various drugs. However, as shown in the present report, there are also problems in treating patients at the other extreme of the distribution, i.e., the extremely rapid hydroxylators.

CASE REPORT

A 41-year-old woman, a nonsmoker, had been treated since 1972 for long periods with high doses of NT (300–500 mg/day, Sensaval; Pharmacia) to achieve therapeutic plasma levels (200–600 nM = 50–150 μg/L (10). During the years 1982–1983 she was treated with NT 300 mg/day (100 + 200 mg) in addition to lithium sulfate (18 + 18 mmol/day Lithionit; Astra) and promethazine hydrochloride (50 mg at bedtime Lergigan; Recip). During these 2 years the concentration of NT was analyzed in seven plasma samples using high performance liquid chromatography (HPLC) (11). The levels ranged between 210 and 350 nM (mean ± SD 291 ± 56). In one sample drawn in August, 1983, the plasma level of unconjugated 10-hydroxy-NT determined by mass fragmentography (12) was 2,730 nM, while that of NT was 350 nM. During NT and lithium treatment the patient remained depressed for long periods of time. Anticholinergic side effects were only slight, if present at all.

During April–June, 1984, the patient was given amitriptyline (AT) hydrochloride (50 mg × 3 Tryptizol; Merck Sharp and Dohme) instead of NT. In two samples taken 3 and 5 weeks after starting AT treatment, plasma levels of AT were 130 and 110 nM and 50 and <75 nM of NT, respectively, as determined by HPLC (11). After an initial short improvement of the depression during AT treatment, the patient became depressed again.

After nine sessions of electroconvulsive treatment during June–July, 1984, with a slight effect only, the patient has been treated since September, 1984, with zimelidine hydrochloride (Zelmid; Astra) with relatively good results.

A debrisoquine hydroxylation phenotyping test (3) was performed as previously described (4) in both January, 1983, during NT treatment and August, 1984, when the patient was drug-free. The urinary ratios of debrisoquine/4-hydroxydebrisoquine on these two occasions were 0.10 and 0.07, respectively (Fig. 1).

DISCUSSION

This patient is clearly an extremely rapid hydroxylator of both nortriptyline and debrisoquine. She had

Address correspondence and reprint requests to Dr. L. Bertilsson at Department of Clinical Pharmacology, Huddinge Hospital, S-141 86 Huddinge, Sweden.

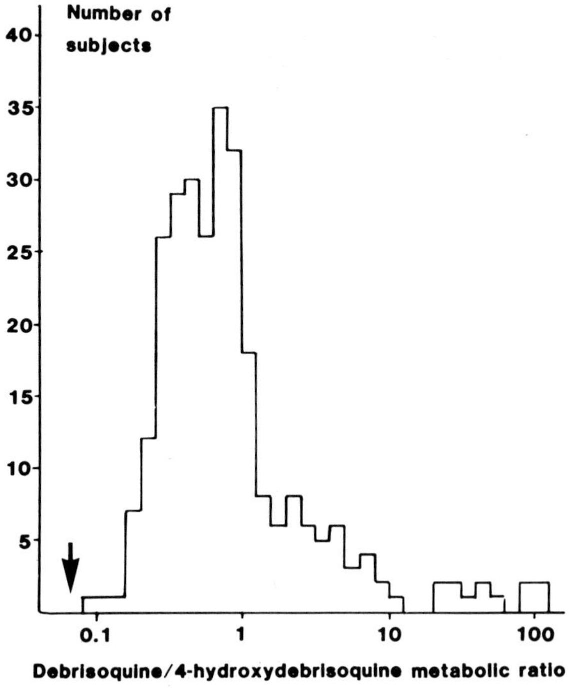

FIG. 1. Distribution of the debrisoquine metabolic ratio (debrisoquine/4-hydroxydebrisoquine in urine) (log scale) in 327 healthy Swedish subjects (shown by the courtesy of Drs. J. Säwe and E. Steiner). The debrisoquine metabolic ratio in the patient reported here was 0.07 (arrow), when the patient was not treated with any other drugs.

a debrisoquine metabolic ratio of 0.07, which was lower than those in all of 327 healthy Swedish subjects phenotyped in our department (Fig. 1). To compensate for the fast metabolism of NT the patient was treated with high doses of the drug, and therapeutic plasma levels of NT (200–600 nM) could then be attained. However, 10-hydroxy-NT accumulated in plasma to very high levels (2,730 nM; 692 nM per dose unit of mg/kg body weight). As a comparison, the mean level of unconjugated 10-hydroxy-NT in 33 depressed patients treated with NT was 265 ± 81 nM per mg/kg body weight (range 137–472). The level of this unconjugated metabolite is not determined by renal function (13), and, in addition, the patient had a normal renal function as shown by a Cr-EDTA test. Thus, the high levels of 10-hydroxy-NT were determined by the very rapid and extensive hydroxylation of NT.

10-Hydroxy-NT is about 50% as potent as NT in the contribution of neuronal uptake inhibition of noradrenaline (14). But why then did the patient not have a better response to the NT treatment? High levels of NT have less antidepressant effect than intermediate levels (10). One mechanism might be that high NT levels block a postsynaptic receptor; this possibility is supported experimentally (15). Whether extremely high levels of 10-hydroxy-NT also have this effect is unknown, but it may be possible. There is, at present, too little information about the properties of 10-hydroxy-NT to answer this question.

Our patient had very high levels of unconjugated 10-OH-NT with only slight or no anticholinergic side effects. This result confirms in vitro studies (16) indicating that 10-hydroxy-NT has much less anticholinergic side effect than the parent drug.

This case report suggests that there may be greater problems in the treatment of depression with NT for extremely rapid hydroxylators than for poor hydroxylators. The latter group could simply be treated with reduced doses (6). The metabolism of several tricyclic antidepressants, e.g., NT (4,5), AT (17,18), chlorimipramine (19), and desipramine (20,21), is interrelated and regulated in a manner similar to the hydroxylation of debrisoquine. In line with this process is that our patient developed low plasma levels of both AT and NT when she was treated with AT. There seem to be difficulties in optimizing the treatment of extremely rapid hydroxylators with all tricyclic antidepressants. In such cases it may be warranted to try a nontricyclic antidepressant, which is not metabolized by the debrisoquine hydroxylase. The serotonin uptake blocker zimeldine was successfully used to treat our patient. This drug might be used in certain patients in spite of its side effects (22).

Acknowledgment: This study was supported by grants from the Swedish Medical Research Council (3902) and from the Karolinska Institute.

REFERENCES

1. Alexanderson B, Evans DAP, Sjöqvist F. Steady-state plasma levels of nortriptyline in twins: influence of genetic factors and drug therapy. *Br Med J* 1969;2:764–8.
2. Åsberg M, Evans DAP, Sjöqvist F. Genetic control of nortriptyline kinetics in man—a study of relatives of propositi with high plasma concentrations. *J Med Genet* 1971;8:129–35.
3. Mahgoub A, Idle JR, Dring LG, Lancaster R, Smith RL. Polymorphic hydroxylation of debrisoquine in man. *Lancet* 1977;2:584–6.
4. Mellström B, Bertilsson L, Säwe J, Schulz H-U, Sjöqvist F. E- and Z-10-hydroxylation of nortriptyline—relationship to polymorphic debrisoquine hydroxylation. *Clin Pharmacol Ther* 1981;30:189–93.
5. Nordin C, Siwers B, Benitez J, Bertilsson L. Plasma concentrations of nortriptyline and its 10-hydroxy metabolite in depressed patients—Relationship to the debrisoquine hydroxylation metabolic ratio. *Br J Clin Pharmacol* 1985;19:832–5.
6. Bertilsson L, Mellström B, Sjöqvist F, Mårtenson B, Åsberg M. Slow hydroxylation of nortriptyline and concomitant poor

debrisoquine hydroxylation: clinical implications. *Lancet* 1981;1:560–1.
7. Idle JR, Oates NS, Shah RR, Smith RL. Protecting poor metabolisers, a group at high risk of adverse drug reactions. *Lancet* 1983;1:1388.
8. Lennard MS, Ramsay LE, Tucker GT, Woods HF. Protecting the poor metabolisers: clinical consequences of genetic polymorphism of drug oxidation. *Pharm Int* 1983;4:53–7.
9. Jack DB, Wilkins MR. Protecting the poor metaboliser—from what? *Br J Clin Pharmacol* 1984;17:488–9.
10. Åsberg M. On the relationship between plasma concentrations of tricyclic antidepressant drugs and therapeutic response. In: Clayton PJ, Barrett JE, eds. *Treatment of depression: old controversies and new approaches.* New York: Raven Press, 1983:85–104.
11. Mellström B, Braithwaite R. Ion-pair liquid chromatography of amitriptyline and metabolites in plasma. *J Chromatogr* 1978;157:379–85.
12. Borgå O, Palmér L, Sjöqvist F, Holmstedt B. Mass fragmentography used in quantitative analysis of drugs and endogenous compounds in biological fluids. *Proceedings of the 5th International Congress on Pharmacology.* Basel, Switzerland: S. Karger, 1972 (vol III):56–68.
13. Dawling S, Lynn K, Rosser R, Braithwaite R. Nortriptyline metabolism in chronic renal failure: metabolite elimination. *Clin Pharmacol Ther* 1982;32:322–9.
14. Bertilsson L, Mellström B, Sjöqvist F. Pronounced inhibition of noradrenaline uptake by 10-hydroxy-metabolites of nortriptyline. *Life Sci* 1979;25:1285–92.
15. Haefely W, Hürlimann A, Thoesen H. Scheinbar paradoxe Beeinflussung von peripheren Noradrenalinwirkungen durch einige Thymoleptika. *Helv Physol Acta* 1964;22:15–33.
16. Wägner A, Ekqvist B, Bertilsson L, Sjöqvist F. Weak binding of 10-hydroxymetabolites of nortriptyline to rat brain muscarinic acetylcholine receptors. *Life Sci* 1984;35:1379–83.
17. Mellström B, Bertilsson L, Lou Y-C, Säwe J, Sjöqvist F. Metabolism of amitriptyline—relationship to polymorphic debrisoquine hydroxylation. *Clin Pharmacol Ther* 1983;24:516–20.
18. Balant-Gorgia AE, Schulz P, Dayer P, et al. Role of oxidation polymorphism on blood and urine concentrations of amitriptyline and its metabolites in man. *Arch Psychiatr Nervenkr* 1982;232:215–22.
19. Mellström B, Bertilsson L, Träskman L, Rollins D, Åsberg M, Sjöqvist F. Intraindividual similarity in the metabolism of amitriptyline and chlorimipramine in depressed patients. *Pharmacology* 1979;19:282–7.
20. Bertilsson L, Åberg-Wistedt A. Debrisoquine hydroxylation test predicts steady-state plasma levels of desipramine. *Br J Clin Pharmacol* 1983;15:388–90.
21. Spina E, Birgersson C, von Bahr C, et al. Phenotypic consistency in the hydroxylation of demethylimipramine and debrisoquine in healthy volunteers and human liver microsomes. *Clin Pharmacol Ther* 1984;36:677–82.
22. Nilsson BS. Adverse reactions in connection with zimelidine treatment—a review. *Acta Psychiatr Scand* 1983;68(suppl 308):115–9.

Therapeutic Drug Monitoring
7:481–484 © 1985 Raven Press, New York

Case Report

Phenytoin/Clonazepam Interaction

Ivan N. Saavedra, *Ledda I. Aguilera, *Evelyng Faure, and *Daniel G. Galdames

*Departments of Biochemistry and Chemistry, Medicine Faculty, University of Chile, and *Departments of Neurology and Neurosurgery, Jose Joaquin Aguirre Hospital, Santiago, Chile*

Summary: An interaction between phenytoin (PHT) and clonazepam (CZP) occurred in an epileptic patient, who had been treated with PHT with partial seizure control. The addition of CZP brought about a significant decrease of PHT plasma levels (from 24.8 to 16 μg/ml) in spite of increases in the PHT dose. Gradual reduction of CZP, without modifying the PHT dosage, caused significant increases in PHT plasma levels to 42.4 μg/ml with signs of intoxication. A review of the literature shows contradictions: some authors state that there is no interaction between the drugs; other authors state either an increase or decrease in PHT plasma levels. These paradoxical results could be explained by the bidirectional effect of these drugs in hepatic enzyme metabolism. The importance of monitoring plasma levels of antiepileptic drugs is emphasized when several medications are required in the treatment of epilepsy. **Key Words:** Drug interactions—Antiepileptic drugs—Phenytoin plasma levels—Phenytoin intoxication—Clonazepam.

Contradictory evidences have been shown by Shader et al. (1) with regard to the effect of clonazepam (CZP) on phenytoin (PHT) metabolism. In recent literature, the clinical significance of interaction between the two drugs has tended to be denied. Perucca (2) concludes that there is no convincing evidence to show that benzodiazepines can significantly stimulate the hepatic enzyme metabolism of the drug in human beings. Dreifuss et al. (3) state that there is not enough evidence to show a clinically significant interaction between CZP and PHT.

We present a clinical case in which a CZP/PHT interaction was clearly demonstrated, with a marked clinical repercussion.

CLINICAL CASE

The patient was a 20-year-old man weighing 63 kg. He was single, right-handed, and a third-grade student in a boarding school for mentally ill individuals. According to his medical history, at the age of 4 months he had had epileptic seizures, that were considered to be infantile spasms of undetermined cause and were treated with adrenocorticotropic hormone, PHT, and phenobarbital. He was mentally retarded, with an I.Q. of 50–65, and experienced generalized tonic-clonic epileptic seizures from the age of 4 months.

When the patient was 19 years old, he went to another hospital where he was treated by one of the authors (L. I. Aguilera). PHT, 300 mg/day, was prescribed, resulting in a plasma level of 24.80 μg/ml. Partial remission of seizures was obtained, and CZP, 1.5 mg/day, was included in the treatment. The addition of CZP coincided with an increase in seizures and a decrease in PHT plasma levels from 22 to 16 μg/ml.

At that time, the patient was sent to our Pharmacokinetic unit, where neurological examination showed mental retardation, the results of the general exami-

Address correspondence and reprint requests to Dr. I. Saavedra at P.O. Box 70086, Santiago-7, Chile.

nation being within normal limits. The results of an electroencephalogram were compatible with subcortical epilepsy in an intercritical period. A cerebral computerized tomographic scan was normal. Psychometric evaluation showed mental retardation (I.Q. 50–65). The results of hematologic, hepatic, renal, and osseous humoral examinations were normal.

RESULTS

The gradual decrease in PHT plasma levels from 24.8 to 16 μg/ml in the absence of any other drug except CZP and in spite of the increasing PHT dose, together with the rigorous medical follow-up and absence of other concurrent pathologies, led us to postulate a CZP/PHT pharmacokinetic interaction. At that time, the patient was hospitalized in our service without modification of the antiepileptic drug treatment. At the time of his admission, and in the first and second week after hospitalization, PHT plasma levels were monitored. They fluctuated from 16 to 18 μg/ml. CZP was gradually decreased by 0.5 mg/week and finally discontinued, while a 375 mg/day PHT dose was maintained. Then, signs of intoxication, a permanent vertiginous sensation, diplopia, lateral nystagmus, Romberg's sign, and dissymmetry were found. Those signs disappeared when the PHT dose was decreased to 325 mg/day, with corresponding decreases in the plasma level to 24 μg/ml (Fig. 1).

DISCUSSION

Plasma levels inconsistent with those expected in an epileptic patient usually lead to suspicion of prescription noncompliance, in this case, the very fact of hospitalization and monitoring of drug administration can result in dramatic, frequent increase in plasma levels and symptoms of intoxication (6,7).

This explanation did not apply to our patient, since he daily attended a special school where rigorous rules for proper drug ingestion were prescribed to the students, and where plasma levels were appraised during the first stage of hospitalization.

The patient had always received the same pharmaceutical formulation of PHT (F. N. Laboratorio, Chile), which has a bioavailability analogous to that of dilantin (Parke Davis, Detroit, MI, U.S.A.), according to Cid et al. (8). The work of Pippenger et al., (9), concerning the variability of various analytical techniques for determining the plasma levels of antiepileptic drugs, is already classic. All of the patient's PHT plasma levels were determined in our unit, which is a National Reference Center.

The determination of PHT plasma levels was carried out through gas liquid chromatography using the Saavedra et al. (4) on column methylation technique applied to PHT by Galdames et al. (5). It had recently tested against an enzyme multiplied immunoassay system (10), and the result led us to conclude that the former is reliable and reproducible, as has also been demonstrated by the empirical evidence of 8 years of use.

Samples of plasma were always taken before the first daily dose of PHT and once steady state was achieved when there was dose change, so that obtained values were comparable ones.

Systemic diseases, which can alter PHT kinetics, have not been found during patient follow-up. The periodic humoral evaluation we usually perform to search for precocious adverse reactions has remained within standard limits, clearly excluding hepatic and renal pathology, malnutrition, and gastrointestinal disturbances.

Other than the antiepileptic drugs, the patient did not receive any drug that could have interacted with PHT, so that the only reasonable explanation is the CZP/PHT pharmacokinetic interaction.

Little information is found in the scientific literature about CZP/PHT interaction, and the existing information leads to contradictory conclusions. Johannessen et al. (11) and Nanda et al. (12) did not find any CZP influence on PHT metabolism. Huang et al. (13) and Windorfer et al. (14) described a significant increase in PHT plasma levels; whereas Edwards and Eadie (15) found a meaningful decrease, in full agreement with the clinical case described here.

Although Browne (16), in his study of CZP, concludes that there is no evidence that benzodiazepine derivates cause a relevant clinical enzymatic microsomal induction in human beings, a bidirectional interaction, as suggested by Eadie et al. (17), may occur, in which CZP may stimulate the enzymatic system to metabolize PHT in some patients and may inhibit it in others, producing either a decrease or an increase, respectively, in drug plasma levels.

We have not undertaken technological research of the above-mentioned hypothesis, but we can suggest that even though this interaction is not frequent, it must be taken into account in patients who receive PHT and CZP simultaneously when both drugs are essential, and PHT plasma levels should be determined regularly.

Recently, Lambie and Johnson (18) have stated that CZP plasma levels tend to decrease under the influence of antiepileptic drugs, and have emphasized the

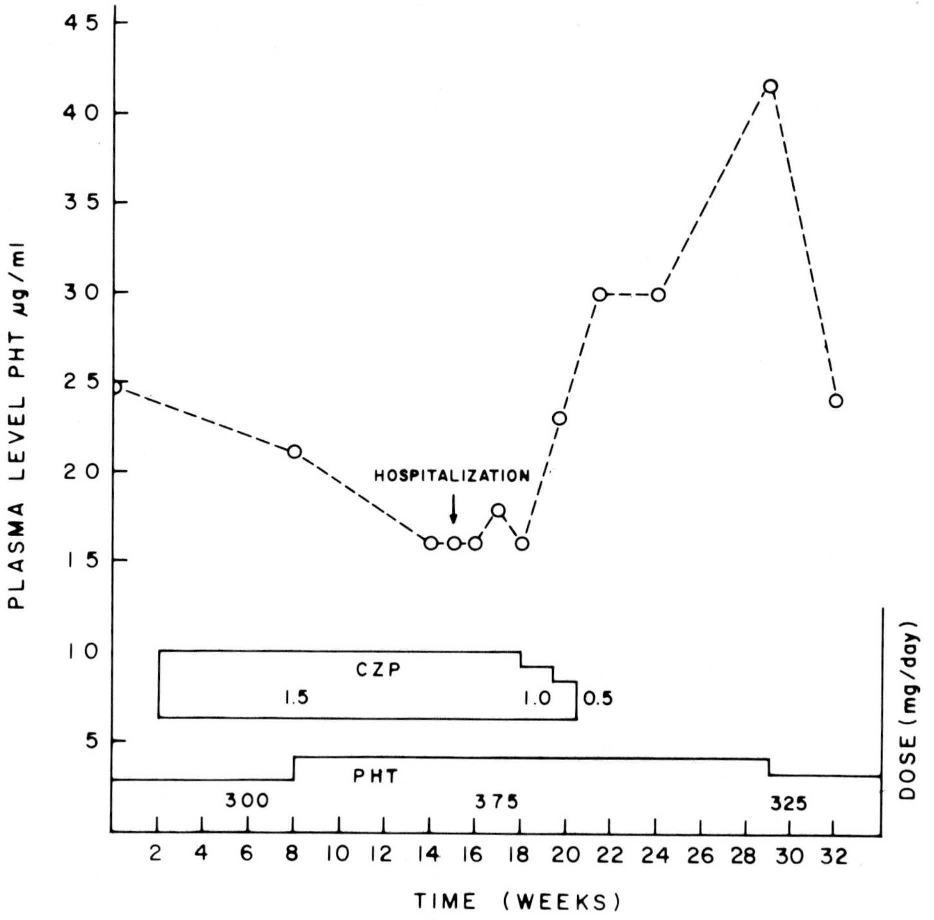

FIG. 1. Antiepileptic treatment with phenytoin (PHT) and clonazepam (CZP) showing plasma levels of PHT.

importance of monitoring drug levels in the blood when several drugs are used simultaneously.

Acknowledgment: This work was supported by grant B-1445-835-5 project of the Development and Bibliotecs Department of the University of Chile. The authors are grateful to Mr. Santiago Leyton for his technical assistance.

REFERENCES

1. Shader RJ, Wemberger DR, Greenblatt DJ. Problems with drug interactions in treating brain disorders. In: Hendrie HG, ed. Symposium on brain disorders: clinical diagnosis and management. *Psychiatr Clin North Am* 1978;1:51–69.
2. Perucca E. Drug interaction. 2nd ed. In: Laidlaw J, Richens A, eds. New York: Churchill Livingstone, 1982:358–71.
3. Dreifuss FE, Susumu S. Clonazepam. In: Woodbury DM, Penry JK, Pippenger CE, eds. *Antiepileptic drugs.* 2nd ed. New York: Raven Press, 1982:737–52.
4. Saavedra I, Concha G, Valenzuela A, Galdames D, et al. Determinación de 5,5 difenilhidantoina y fenobarbital en plasma, por cromatografía en fase líquido-gaseosa. Rev. Méd. Chile 106:217–220, 1978.
5. Galdames D, Saavedra I, Ortiz M, Aguilera L, et al. Plasma levels of Diphenylhydantoin and the control of adult epileptic seizures: Chilean experience. Epilepsia 21:467–74, 1980.
6. Blackwell B. Patient compliance. *N Engl J Med* 1973;289:249–52.
7. Lund M, Jorgensen RS, Kuhl V. Serum diphenylhydantoin in ambulant patients with epilepsy. *Epilepsia* 1964;5:51–8.
8. Cid E, Moran I, Monaris M, Lasserre CH, Vidal V. Bioavailability of four brands of phenytoin. *Biopharm Drug Dispos* 1981;2:391–4.
9. Pippenger CE, Penry JK, White BG, Daly DD, Buddington R. Interlaboratory variability in determination of plasma antiepileptic drug concentration. *Arch Neurol* 1976;33:351–5.
10. Galdames D, Saavedra I. Estudio de correlacion entre la determinación de drogas antiepilépticas por inmunoensayo enzimático homogeneo (EMIT) y cromatografía líquido gaseosa. X Congreso Neurológico de Argentina, Mar Del Plata, Argentina, Marzo de 1985.
11. Johannessen SI, Strandjord RE, Munthe-Kaas AW. Lack of effect of clonazepam on serum levels of diphenylhydantoin, phenobarbital and carbamazepine. *Acta Neurol Scand* 1977;55:506–12.
12. Nanda RN, Johnson RH, Keogh HJ, et al. Treatment of epilepsy with clonazepam and its effect on other anticonvulsants. *J Neurol Neurosurg Psychiatry* 1977;40:538–43.
13. Huang CY, McLeod JG, Sampson D, et al. Clonazepam in the treatment of epilepsy. *Proc Aust Assoc Neurol* 1973;10:67–74.
14. Windorfer A Jr, Saner W. Drug interaction during anticonvulsant therapy in childhood: diphenylhydantoin, primidone, phenobarbital, clonazepam, nitrazepam, carbamazepine and dipropylacetate. *Neuropediatrics* 1977;8:29–41.
15. Edwards VE, Eadie MJ. Clonazepam: a clinical study of its

effectiveness as an anticonvulsant. *Proc Aust Assoc Neurol* 1973;10:61–6.
16. Browne TR. Clonazepam. A review of a new anticonvulsant drug. *Arch Neurol* 1976;33:326–32.
17. Eadie MJ, Tyrer JH. *Hydantoin anticonvulsant therapy. Pharmacological basis and practice.* 2nd ed. New York: Churchill Livingstone, 1980:45–131.
18. Lambie DG, Johnson RH. Serum concentration of clonazepam and the therapeutic effect of the drug. *Acta Neurol Scand* 1983;67:97–102.

Therapeutic Drug Monitoring
7:485–487 © 1985 Raven Press, New York

Case Report

Hemodialysis Clearance of Pentobarbital During Continuous Infusion

*Daniel Wermeling, *Kenneth Record, †Richard Bell, ‡William Porter, and *Robert Blouin

**College of Pharmacy, and †Department of Surgery, and ‡Division of Clinical Chemistry, Department of Pathology, College of Medicine, University of Kentucky, Lexington, Kentucky, U.S.A.*

Summary: The hemodialysis clearance of pentobarbital during continuous infusion was determined in a 34-year-old man in acute renal failure. Pentobarbital specimens were obtained simultaneously from arterial blood entering and leaving the dialysis machine at five 1-h intervals. The mean hemodialysis clearance of pentobarbital was 22.3 ml/min. Pentobarbital concentration was relatively unaffected throughout the dialysis period, because of the high dose and continuous infusion of a drug with low hepatic intrinsic clearance and a short dialysis period. A large contribution to total body clearance was not evident, and dosage adjustment would have been unwarranted. **Key Words:** Pentobarbital—Hemodialysis—Continuous infusion.

Pentobarbital, an ethyl-1-methylbutyl derivative of barbituric acid, has been used extensively as a central nervous system (CNS) depressant. Various levels of CNS depressant activity are seen, from sedation to general anesthesia, depending upon the dose (1). High concentrations of pentobarbital are known to depress other physiologic functions such as respiration, hemodynamics, and gastrointestinal tone (1–4). The therapeutic uses of pentobarbital include induction of coma for treatment of elevated intracranial pressure, induction of anesthesia, and use as an anticonvulsant. Pentobarbital, as many other barbiturates, is not used as extensively as in the past. Safer and less toxic agents, namely, the benzodiazepines, have taken their place in some medical practices.

The purpose of this study was to reexamine the hemodialysis clearance rate of pentobarbital as a therapeutic modality in a patient with renal failure.

Address correspondence and reprint requests to Dr. K. Record at Albert Chandler Medical Center, 800 Rose Street, Room C-117, Lexington, KY 40536-0084, U.S.A.

CASE REPORT

A 34-year-old black man sustained a fractured liver, right perinephric and retroperitoneal hematoma, right and left multiple rib fractures with right hemopneumothorax, mediastinal widening, and other multiple injuries following a motor vehicle accident. Initial treatment at a community hospital had included placement of a right thoracostomy tube, exploratory celiotomy with control of the hepatic hemorrhage by suture, and closure of the superficial lacerations. Decreasing urinary output, a rising serum urea nitrogen (BUN 84 mg/dl), a rising serum creatinine (5.4 mg/dl), and progressive adult respiratory distress syndrome 6 days following injury prompted transfer of the patient to the regional trauma center. The progressive renal failure (BUN 107 mg/dl, serum creatinine 7.3 mg/dl) prompted placement of a double lumen Uldall catheter and institution of hemodialysis. Five 1-h hemodialysis periods were assessed during hemodialysis using a single needle method, a Gambro type DEM 10-D1 parallel flow machine equipped with a Gambro flat plate, and cuprophan membrane. A standard dialysate fluid was utilized, with a flow rate of 500 ml/min.

Eleven days following his injury, the patient sustained a brief cardiac arrest, presumably the result of an arrythmia induced by hyperkalemia (serum potassium 6.9 mEq/L). He was promptly resuscitated but remained neurologically unresponsive. In an effort to manage the development of post-arrest seizures and reduce the metabolic demands on the central nervous system, the patient was placed in a pentobarbital coma. A pentobarbital infusion of 100 mg/h was maintained for 4 days, after which he was gradually weaned. His neurologic status had improved to the point where he would obey commands and move all four extremities.

There was little improvement in the patient's adult respiratory distress syndrome, and he manifested ongoing signs of clinical sepsis. Reexploration of his abdomen failed to control the septic process. The patient died 47 days following his original injuries.

METHODS

Pentobarbital specimens were obtained simultaneously from arterial blood entering and leaving the hemodialysis machine at five 1-h intervals. The patient's hematocrit, blood flow, and dialysate flow were recorded for each hour. Serum samples were frozen at − 5°C until the time of analysis.

Pentobarbital determinations were performed on a Hewlett-Packard 5790A gas chromatograph equipped with a 12.5 m cross-linked dimethyl silicone capillary column and a nitrogen selective thermionic detector. The column was operated isothermally at 185°C for 4.5 min and then temperature programmed at 15°C/min to a final temperature of 245°C. Nitrogen was used as the carrier gas.

Serum samples were buffered with ½ vol of 0.225 *M* phosphate buffer, pH 7.5, and then double extracted with 5-ml portions of anhydrous diethyl ether. The combined ether extracts were evaporated to dryness at 50°C. The residue was reconstituted in 50 μl of anhydrous ether, and 1 μl was introduced into the chromatograph using the split injection mode (split ratio 40:1).

For quantitation, 5-ethyl-5-*p*-tolybarbituric acid was used as the internal standard, and peak heights were automatically computed with a Hewlett-Packard 3390A reporting integrator.

Pentobarbital dialysis clearance was calculated using the following formula:

$$CL_d = Qb \times (1\text{-Hct}) \times (C_a - C_v)/C_a$$

TABLE 1. *Pentobarbital hemodialysis clearance data*

Sampling time (h)	Extraction ratio[a]	Hct (%)	Qb (ml/min)	CL_d (ml/min)
1	0.274	30	150	28.77
2	0.238	30	150	24.99
3	0.110	33	150	11.05
4	0.230	32	150	23.56
5	0.227	32	150	23.15
Mean	0.216	31.4	150	22.30
SD	0.062	1.3	0	5.96

[a]Extraction ratio $C_a - C_v/C_a$.

where CL_d is the hemodialysis plasma clearance of pentobarbital, Qb is bloodflow through the dialysis machine, C_a is the pentobarbital concentration entering the dialysis machine, C_v is the pentobarbital concentration leaving the dialysis machine, and Hct is the patient's hematocrit.

RESULTS

The hemodialysis clearance values of pentobarbital are found in Table 1. The mean hemodialysis clearance was 22.3 ml/min for the five 1-h periods.

DISCUSSION

The effect of hemodialysis on the pharmacokinetics of pentobarbital has not been well described. In the early 1960s, hemodialysis was utilized to remove barbiturates from the bloodstream of severely overdosed patients (5–8). Setter et al. found that the serum half-life of short-acting barbiturates was reduced from 30 h to 14 h during dialysis (6). Hudson et al. found the hemodialysis clearance of pentobarbital to be 27 ml/min in a single patient (5). Data presented in this case study demonstrated a mean dialysis clearance of 22.3 ml/min. Although sampling time No. 3 has a lower extraction ratio and clearance, the mean pentobarbital clearance corroborates the Hudson data.

The primary route of pentobarbital elimination from the body is via hepatic oxidation and glucuronidation. The drug has a low hepatic intrinsic clearance of 20–50 ml/min (9). Several investigators have found that hepatic metabolism of certain drugs can be accelerated by uremia, which was a condition our patient suffered (10,11). Reidenberg et al. found no difference in the total body clearance of pentobarbital in uremic patients (33 ml/min) versus a control group (27 ml/min) (9). Thus, changes in pentobarbital clearance would not be expected in this renal failure patient.

Previous studies of patients with pentobarbital overdose show that hemodialysis can effectively increase total body clearance of pentobarbital by 50–75%. However, in this case, there was little difference in the pentobarbital concentration entering the dialysis machine at each sampling hour because of the high dose and continuous infusion of pentobarbital, a drug with low hepatic intrinsic clearance. Also, the dialysis period in this case is much shorter than the usual dialysis treatment of an overdose. Although a hemodialysis clearance of 22.3 ml/min was demonstrated, a large contribution by hemodialysis to total body clearance was not evident, and dosage adjustment would have been unwarranted.

REFERENCES

1. Harvey SC. Hypnotics and sedatives. In: Goodman LS, Gilman A. *The pharmacological basis of therapeutics.* 6th ed. New York: Macmillan, 1980:349–61.
2. Traeger SM, Henning RJ, Dobbin W, Giannotta S, Weil MH, Weiss M. Hemodynamic effects of pentobarbital therapy for intracranial hypertension. *Crit Care Med* 1983;11:697–700.
3. Marshall LF, Smith RW, Shapiro HM. The outcome with aggressive treatment in severe head injuries. Part II: Acute and chronic barbiturates administration in the management of head injury. *J Neurosurg* 1979;50:26–30.
4. Lafferty JJ, Keykhah MM, Shapiro HM, Van Horn K, Behar MG. Cerebral hypometabolism obtained with deep pentobarbital anesthesia and hypothermia. *Anesthesiology* 1978;49:159–64.
5. Hudson JB, Dennis AJ, Hobbs DR, Sussman HC. Extended hemodialysis in short acting barbiturates poisoning: case report. *South Med J* 1969;62:457–60.
6. Setter JG, Maker JF, Schreiner GE. Barbiturate intoxication. *Arch Intern Med* 1966;117:224–35.
7. Iversen BM, Willassen Y, Bakke OM, Wallem G. Assessment of barbiturate removal by charcoal hemoperfusion in overdose cases. *Clin Toxicol* 1979;15:139–47.
8. Pond S, Rosenberg J, Benowitz NL, Takki S. Pharmacokinetics of hemoperfusion for drug overdose. *Clin Pharmacokinet* 1979;4:329–54.
9. Reidenberg MM, Lowenthal DT, Buggs W, Gasporo M. Pentobarbital elimination in patients with poor renal function. *Clin Pharmacol Ther* 1976;20:67–70.
10. Letteri JM, Mellk H, Louis S, et al. Diphenylhydantoin metabolism in uremia. *N Engl J Med* 1971;285:648–52.
11. Oder-Cederlof L, Borgia O. Kinetics of diphenylhydantoin in uremic patients: consequences of decreased plasma protein binding. *Eur J Clin Pharmacol* 1974;7:31–7.

Therapeutic Drug Monitoring
7:488–490 © 1985 Raven Press, New York

Letters to the Editor

An Interactive Opinion on the Rationalization of Therapeutic Cyclosporine Monitoring

To the Editor: When your editorial on cyclosporine (1) was published, we were just completing our review article on the clinical pharmacokinetics of cyclosporine (CSA) (R. Camsonne and M. A. Monline, unpublished observations). We appreciate fully your call, and the efforts of Moyer (2), to promote a rational approach to standardize and thus improve the precision of CSA therapeutic monitoring.

According to our understanding, the following points must be considered with respect to the monitoring of CSA: (a) The concentration of CSA at receptor sites, necessary not only for initiating a therapeutic response (at the level of T-lymphocyte subpopulation) but also for inducing side effects (at the level of other immunosystem components or at specific sites within strategic target organs such as the kidney (3), determines the therapeutic effectiveness or toxicity of the drug in individual patients. (b) The peculiar stereoregulation induced-temperature–dependent partition of CSA between red blood cells and plasma (4) make it worthwhile to use only plasma separated at 37°C for therapeutic monitoring of CSA in controlling clinical outcomes. (c) When plasma or serum is separated from blood cells at 37°C, CSA concentration most accurately reflects the in vivo CSA concentration in serum with respect to the following equilibration: stored or sequestered CSA $\rightleftarrows$ plasma protein binding CSA (90%) $\rightleftarrows$ freely diffusible CSA $\rightleftarrows$ receptor sites for both therapeutic effects and side effects. (d) The equivalent in vivo equilibrium state oversimplifies numerous simple or complex transport mechanisms that regulate CSA distribution between all tissues (skin, fat, brain; and with high concentrations, liver, pancreas, lymphoid organs, and kidney (3,5)). Red blood cell CSA concentrations are just a single facet of CSA storage mechanisms in the body. The measurement of CSA in blood with or without hematocrit corrections (6), or in plasma at temperature conditions other than 37°C (6), seems simply to add extra variables, which are difficult to control except for academic purposes.

The proper choice of analytical methods is also a difficult decision. It has been suggested that one or more of the metabolites present in blood at high concentrations (7) may be active immunosuppressants or may play an active role in producing toxicity. Therefore, in our opinion, a radioimmunoassay that quantitates both CSA and some of its 17 metabolites might be advantageous in comparison to the first generation of high performance liquid chromatography (HPLC) assays, which quantitate only the parent drug. HPLC assays able to separately quantitate CSA and each of its metabolites (8) in plasma would be welcome and would enhance our understanding of which metabolites are pharmacologically active.

Since CSA is currently administered once or twice a day, the pertinent steady-state trough blood or plasma CSA concentration might vary twofold, as do the troughs of digoxin administered to either adults or newborns (9). For these reasons, there has been increased confusion and misunderstanding among practitioners with respect to the interpretation of CSA concentrations in the clinical environment. Therefore, the therapeutic range of CSA in our laboratory is precisely defined, at the present time, as follows: 200–750 ng/ml trough steady-state level after twice-daily dose, determined by the Sandoz radioimmunoassay (the specificity of antibody may vary from one antiserum to another) on the whole blood. The corresponding figure for plasma separatd at 37°C is ~100–375 ng/ml. However that may be, this last therapeutic range is still too wide and should be reevaluated with specific methods that quantitate CSA and metabolites of interest. There is still one point worth remembering: the very high concentration of CSA in kidneys, the main target organ for development of side effects and T subsets, the main pharmacological target site of white blood cells where the CSA concentration is 1,000 times greater than that of red blood cells (4), requires that we establish a clear understanding of tissue pharmacokinetics in relation to the plasma (separated at 37°C) drug concentrations.

R. Camsonne
X.Troussard
Laboratoire de Pharmacologie et Exploration Fonctionnelle B
Caen, France

REFERENCES

1. Pippenger CE. Cyclosporine: right or wrong? [Editorial]. *Ther Drug Monit* 1985;7:1.
2. Moyer TP. Measurement of cyclosporine: a challenge to the professional laboratory organizations. *Ther Drug Monit* 1985;7:123–4.
3. Atkinson K, Biggs JC, Britton K. Distribution and persistence of cyclosporin in human blood. *Lancet* 1982;X:1165–9.
4. Atkinson K. Britton K, Biggs JC. Distribution and concentration of cyclosporin in human blood. *J Clin Pathol* 1984;37:1167–71.
5. Von Willevrand E, Hayry P. Cyclosporin A deposition in renal allografts. *Lancet* 1983;X:1983–92.
6. Yatscoff RW, Rush DN, Jeffrey JR. Effects of sample preparation of cyclosporin A measured in plasma. *Clin Chem* 1984;30:1,812–4.
7. Robson S, Neuberger J, Keller HP, et al. Pharmacokinetic study of cyclosporin A in patients with primary cirrhosis. *Br J Clin Pharmacol* 1984;18:627–31.
8. Lensymer G, Field BL. Improved liquid chromatographic determination of cyclosporine with concomitant detection of a cell-bound metabolites. *Clin Chem* 1985;31:196–201.
9. Moulin MA, Muller G, Letellier PH, et al. Traitement d'une tachyarythmie foetale et posologie de la digoxine. *Therapie* 1983;38:67–9.

Caffeine Interference with the CANAM-Theophylline Reagent Kit

To the Editor: The CANAM-Theophylline reagent (CANAM Diagnostic Company, Garland, TX, U.S.A.) is a fluorescence polarization reagent, marketed as an economical alternative for use on the Abbott Laboratories TDx analyzer (Abbott Diagnostics, Inc., North Chicago, IL, U.S.A.). A comparison of samples from 70 patients, submitted to our laboratory for theophylline determinations, resulted in a correlation coefficient of 0.983, a slope of 0.835, and a *y*-intercept of +0.29. The mean theophylline value of the 70 patients was 12.6 μg/ml with the CANAM reagent and 11.1 μg/ml with the Abbott reagent. The bias was 1.5 μg/ml, which is statistically significant. The between-run precision of the trilevel Abbott controls ranged from 1.06 to 2.17% and was judged acceptable.

Retention samples from the AACC-TDM Quality Control Program, sent to our laboratory monthly as part of our ongoing quality control program, were also assayed with the CANAM reagent. The results obtained are shown in Table 1.

The CANAM-Theophylline reagent package insert indicates that the reagent has a cross-reactivity of <7% with caffeine. However, the above data suggest that the cross-reactivity is >7%. We performed a cross-reactivity study by adding different concentra-

TABLE 2. *Theophylline concentrations after the addition of various concentrations of caffeine to theophylline-free serum*

Amount of caffeine added (μg/ml)	Values obtained (μg/ml)		Percentage of cross-reactivity with CANAM reagent
	Abbott reagents	CANAM reagents	
22.5	None detected	1.5	6.67
45.0	None detected	3.1	6.89
97.0	0.07	6.7	6.91
196.0	0.4	12.8	6.53

TABLE 1. *Serum theophylline concentrations and target values of theophylline and caffeine of the monthly AACC-TDM samples*

Month/Year	Mean value reported by all laboratories (μg/ml)	Values obtained with CANAM reagents (μg/ml)	Target values (μg/ml)	
			Theophylline	Caffeine
January 1984	25.4	23.7	25.0	0.0
February 1984	15.3	16.4	14.5	6.0
March 1984	12.2	14.0	11.0	15.0
April 1984	15.2	17.9	12.5	30.0
May 1984	39.9	43.3	37.0	20.0
June 1984	5.8	6.2	5.0	5.0
July 1984	7.9	8.4	7.0	10.0
August 1984	11.2	12.0	11.6	10.0
October 1984	13.2	16.4	11.8	30.0
December 1984	7.5	8.5	8.0	3.0
January 1985	43.6	48.5	50.0	5.0
February 1985	16.3	19.2	17.0	6.0
March 1985	10.5	11.0	10.0	0.0
April 1985	4.7	7.5	5.0	15.0
May 1985	13.1	14.0	14.0	4.0

TABLE 3. *Theophylline concentrations after the addition of various concentrations of caffeine to a pooled serum containing 9.5 μg/ml theophylline*

Amount of caffeine added (μg/ml)	Values obtained (μg/ml) Abbott reagent	CANAM reagent	Percentage of cross-reactivity with CANAM reagents
22.5	9.4	15.5	26.67
45.0	9.5	17.8	18.44
97.0	9.6	23.9	14.85
196.0	9.8	37.4	14.23

tions of caffeine (1,3,7-trimethylxanthine) to theophylline-free serum and to a pooled sample containing 9.5 μg/ml of theophylline. The caffeine was obtained from the Sigma Chemical Company, St. Louis, MO, U.S.A. The results of this study are presented in Tables 2 and 3.

The data in Tables 1 and 3 suggest that the cross-reactivity with caffeine is greatly enhanced when theophylline is present in the sample. It should also be noted that a significant elevation in the theophylline value can be expected with therapeutic caffeine concentrations (4–15 μg/ml). Laboratories should also be aware that unacceptable results are likely to be obtained when the CANAM-Theophylline reagent is used to assay survey samples such as those supplied by the AACC-TDM Quality Control Program, since caffeine is frequently added to these samples. Therefore, it is prudent to investigate this observed enhanced interference from caffeine whenever an alternative reagent for fluorescence polarization is used for theophylline determinations. It should also be noted that the CANAM reagent is marketed under different label(s).

Ingo S. Kampa
Jean I. Jarzabek
Department of Pathology
The Valley Hospital
Ridgewood, New Jersey, U.S.A.

Therapeutic Drug Monitoring
7:491 © 1985 Raven Press, New York

Announcement

Quality Assessment in Therapeutic Drug Monitoring

April 3–4, 1986

A two-day conference, "Quality Assessment in Therapeutic Drug Monitoring," will be held on April 3–4, 1986, at the University of Surrey, Guildford, United Kingdom. The conference is designed to provide a forum where problems involved with quality assessment in therapeutic drug monitoring are discussed. The aim of the conference is to examine methods of assessment of the quality of drug analysis not only during therapeutic drug monitoring but also during research and development. Discussion will also be held on ways in which both the analyzing laboratory and the persons interpreting the results can best benefit from these schemes. The meeting hopes to attract clinical biochemists, pharmacists, and clinical pharmacologists. The conference is organized by Dr. G. Mould, Clinical Pharmacokinetic Unit, St. Luke's Hospital, Guildford, Surrey, GU2 5XH, U.K. Address all enquires to Dr. Mould at the preceding address.

Therapeutic Drug Monitoring
7:492–497 © 1985 Raven Press, New York

Therapeutic Drug Monitoring
Volume 7, 1985

Subject Index

Acetaminophen
  and oral contraceptive interaction (review), 26
  pediatric overdose (review), 148
  pediatric pharmacology, 2
Age effects
  cimetidine and theophylline interaction, 426
Alcohol
  pediatric overdose (review), 148
Allopurinol
  HPLC, plasma and urine, 324
Amikacin
  automated substrate-labeled fluorescent immunoassay, 108
  overview (review), 12
Aminoglycoside
  computer estimation of pharmacokinetics, 258
  TDM, peak concentrations, 303
Amitriptyline
  pharmacokinetics during peritoneal dialysis, 255
Ammonia. *See* Hyperammonemia.
Antibiotics
  and oral contraceptive interactions (review), 26
Antibodies
  monoclonal, fluorescence polarization immunoassay of theophylline, 355
Anticonvulsant drugs
  CI-912 blood–brain barrier transport, 247
  and oral contraceptive interactions (review), 26
  steady-state serum levels, Chinese epileptic patients, 83
Antidepressant drugs
  bupropion stability in plasma, 447
  debrisoquine rapid hydroxylation (case report), 478
  desmethylimipramine overdose, nonlinear kinetics in slow hydroxylator (case report), 239
  specific request form for TDM, 299
  tricyclic
    pediatric overdose (review), 148
    in serum and plasma, 242
Antiepileptic drugs
  phenothiazine effect, psychiatric patients with seizure disorder, 401
  and valproate-induced hyperammonemia, 185
Antipyretic drugs
  pediatric, clinical pharmacology (review), 2
Aspirin
  liquid chromatography, 216
  pediatric pharmacology, 2
  and serum prostaglandins, 435
Atrial fibrillation
  digoxin interaction with nifedipine, 372

Bayesian forecasting
  lidocaine pharmacokinetics, 66
  prothrombin response to warfarin therapy, 174
Benzodiazepines
  and oral contraceptive interactions (review), 26
Bioavailability
  carbamazepine and carbamazepine-epoxide, 36
  clonidine radioimmunoassay, 344
  phenytoin, urinary excretion of *p*-hydroxyphenytoin, 283
Blood
  collection systems, propranolol HPLC, 358
Blood levels
  chloroquine and desethyl metabolite, HPLC microassay, 207, 211
  chlorpromazine TDM, 472
  cyclosporin A distribution, 61
  phenytoin, in paroxysmal choreoathetosis, 81
Blood–brain barrier
  CI-912 transport, 247
Body fat
  and theophylline distribution, 197
Book Reviews
  Applications of Optimal Control Therapy in Biomedicine, 128
  Benzodiazepine Recognition Site Ligands: Biochemistry and Pharmacology, 244
  Compendium of Pharmaceuticals and Specialities, 19th Ed., 245
  Free Radicals in Molecular Biology, Aging, and Disease, 244
  Guide to Clinical Studies and Developing Protocols, 246
  Marihuana in Science and Medicine, 128
  Neurotransmitters, Seizures and Epilepsy II, 246
  Practical Immunoassay, The State of the Art, 127
Brain
  erythrocyte transport of CI-912, 247
Bretylium
  dose nomogram, in renal impairment, 265
Bupropion
  and metabolites, stability in plasma, 447

Carbamazepine
  automated substrate-labeled fluorescent immunoassay, 108
  and epoxide metabolite
    lateral gaze nystagmus in epileptics, 277
    pharmacokinetic and bioavailability studies, 36
    serum protein binding in newborn infants, 274
  and phenytoin interaction, 51
  protein binding and disposition, in pregnancy, 269
  saliva concentrations, 41
  total and free, EMIT and HPLC, 46
Case reports
  Desmethylimipramine Overdose: Nonlinear Kinetics in Slow Hydroxylator, 239
  Evidence Supporting 3(S)-3-Hydroxyquinidine-Associated Cardiotoxicity, 308
  Extremely Rapid Hydroxylation of Debrisoquine: Case Report with Implication for Treatment with Nortriptyline and Other Tricyclic Antidepressants, 478
  Hemodialysis Clearance of Pentobarbital During Continuous Infusion, 485
  Influence of High-Dose Pentobarbital on Theophylline Pharmacokinetics, 181
  Phenytoin/Clonazepam Interaction, 481
Children and infants
  chloramphenicol, clinical pharmacology (review), 159
  clinical pharmacology of antipyretic drugs (review), 2
  newborn, carbamazepine and carbamazepine-epoxide protein binding, 274
  sulfonamide pharmacokinetics, and maturing kidney function (review), 130
  TDM in acute drug intoxication (review), 148

TDM consultation service in pediatric hospital, 295
Chloramphenicol
clinical pharmacology in pediatrics (review), 159
HPLC, interference by dobutamine, 121
Chloroquine
and desethyl metabolite, HPLC microassay, 207, 211
Chlorpromazine
plasma analysis, 222
whole blood, 472
Choline salicylate
pediatric pharmacology, 2
Chronic obstructive pulmonary disease
theophylline serum levels, 168
CI-912
blood–brain barrier transport, 247
Cimetidine
and theophylline interaction, age effects, 426
Clinical studies
anticonvulsant drugs in Chinese epileptic patients, 83
antiepileptic drugs, and valproate-induced hyperammonemia, 185
aspirin and nonacetylated salicylate effects on serum prostaglandins, 435
blood collection systems, propranolol HPLC, 358
carbamazepine protein binding and disposition in pregnancy, 269
cimetidine and theophylline interaction, age effects, 426
cyclosporin A in whole blood and plasma, 61
digoxin interaction with nifedipine, atrial fibrillation, 372
flupentixol in acute schizophrenia, 411
liver disease, false-positive digoxin, 202
phenothiazine effect on antiepileptic drugs, in psychiatric patients with seizure disorders, 401
phenytoin blood levels in paroxysmal choreoathetosis, 81
phenytoin dosing methods, 74
phenytoin metabolism, 283
phenytoin-hydroxyphenytoin steady-state ratio in epileptics, 405
red blood cell electrolytes, digoxin TDM, 191
theophylline, in chronic obstructive pulmonary disease, 168
theophylline distribution, role of body fat, 197
Clonazepam
and phenytoin interaction (case report), 481
Compliance
in epileptic patients, phenobarbital TDM, 87
Computer
drug assay, Bayesian forecasting, lidocaine pharmacokinetics, 66
pharmacokinetic estimation, 258
theophylline serum level prediction, 421
Contraceptives, oral
drug interactions (review), 26
Cyclosporin A
in whole blood and plasma, 61

Dapsone
reverse phase HPLC, and malaria prophylaxis, 415
Debrisoquine
rapid hydroxylation (case report), 478
Dentistry
local anesthesia, plasma lidocaine, 369
Desmethylimipramine
overdose, nonlinear kinetics in slow hydroxylator (case report), 239
Diclofenac
pediatric pharmacology, 2
Digoxin
false-positive results, in liver disease, 202
and nifedipine interaction, atrial fibrillation, 372
TDM, red blood cell electrolytes, 191
Disopyramide
ultrafiltration and EMIT, 466
Dobutamine
interference in HPLC of chloramphenicol, 121
Dosage
amikacin (review), 12
anticonvulsant drugs, Chinese epileptic patients, 83
bretylium, nomogram for renal impairment, 265
pediatric antipyretic drugs (review), 2
phenytoin comparison, 74
phenytoin, individual maintenance, 391
prediction, drugs with simple Michaelis-Menton elimination kinetics, 377
valproic acid, 387
Doxorubicin
and metabolites, loop-column extraction and HPLC, 455
Doxycycline
and theophylline pharmacokinetics, 92
Drug interactions
amikacin activity (review), 12
antiepileptic drugs, and valproate-induced hyperammonemia, 185
carbamazepine
and phenobarbital, in epilepsy, lateral gaze nystagmus, 277
and phenytoin, 51
doxycycline and theophylline, 92
nifedipine and digoxin, atrial fibrillation, 372
oral contraceptives, 26
pentobarbital and theophylline (case report), 181
phenothiazines and antiepileptic drugs, psychiatric patients with seizure disorder, 401
phenytoin and clonazepam (case report), 481
theophylline and cimetidine, age effects, 426
valproic acid, 387
Drug overdose
TDM in children, 148

Editorials
Cyclosporine Quality Control Program, 371
Cyclosporine Quality Control Program is a Reality, 129
Cyclosporine: Right or Wrong?, 1
Electrolytes
red blood cell, digoxin monitoring, 191
Electromyography
perhexiline maleate, long-term treatment, 54
EMIT (enzyme multiplied immunoassay technique)
and automated substrate-labeled fluorescent immunoassay comparison, 108
carbamazepine, total and free, plasma levels, 46
disopyramide in plasma, 466
theophylline
in chronic obstructive pulmonary disease, 168
comparison with apoenzyme reactivation immunoassay, 451
comparison with PETINIA, 95
Epilepsy
Chinese, steady-state serum levels of anticonvulsant drugs, 83
lateral gaze nystagmus, with carbamazepine treatment, 277
noncompliance, phenobarbital TDM, 87
and psychiatric disorders, phenothiazine effect on antiepileptic drugs, 401
valproic acid therapy, and hyperammonemia, 290
Equilibrium dialysis
and ultrafiltration, free phenytoin in plasma, 461
Erythrocytes
blood–brain barrier transport of CI-912, 247
electrolytes, digoxin monitoring, 191
Ethmozin
HPLC of plasma, 439

Fluoroimmunoassay
primidone and phenobarbital dual assay, 101
valproic acid, comparison with gas liquid chromatography, 236
Flupentixol
in acute schizophrenia, 411
plasma levels, gas chromatography and radioimmunoassay, in schizophrenia, 229

Gas chromatography
flupentixol, plasma levels, in schizophrenia, 229

Gas liquid chromatography
valproic acid
comparison with fluoroimmunoassay, 236
in plasma or serum, 336
Gentamicin
automated substrate-labeled fluorescent immunoassay, 108
Glucocorticoids
and oral contraceptive interactions (review), 26

Hemodialysis
pentobarbital clearance (case report), 485
High pressure liquid chromatography (HPLC)
allopurinol and oxypurinol, plasma and urine, 324
carbamazepine
and carbamazepine-epoxide, 36
total and free, plasma levels, 46
chloramphenicol, interference by dobutamine, 121
chloroquine and desethyl metabolite in whole blood, microassay, 207, 211
chlorpromazine, plasma analysis, 222
with electrochemical detection, vitamin E in plasma and serum, 364
ethmozin in plasma, 439
and fluorescence polarization immunoassay comparison, theophylline pharmacokinetics, 442
and loop-column extraction, doxorubicin and metabolites, 455
6-mercaptopurine in serum or plasma, 315
propranolol, blood collection systems, 358
reverse phase
nifedipine in plasma, 321
simultaneous estimation of dapsone, monoacetyldapsone, and pyrimethamine in malaria prophylaxis, 415
theophylline
comparison with PETINIA, 95
doxycycline effect, 92
warfarin in plasma, 329
p-Hydroxyphenytoin
urinary excretion, phenytoin bioavailability, 283
3(S)-3-Hydroxyquinidine
cardiotoxicity (case report), 308
Hyperammonemia
valproate-induced, effect of antiepileptic treatment, 185
valproic acid therapy, 290

Ibuprofen
pediatric pharmacology, 2
Immunoassay
apoenzyme reactivation, serum theophylline, 451
automated substrate-labeled fluorescent, comparison with EMIT, 108
fluorescence polarization
and HPLC comparison, theophylline pharmacokinetics, 442
serum salicylates, 351
theophylline monoclonal antibodies, 355
fluoro-
primidone and phenobarbital, 101
valproic acid, comparison with gas liquid chromatography, 236
particle-enhanced turbidimetric inhibition (PETINIA), for theophylline, 95
valproic acid in serum or plasma, 336
See also EMIT (enzyme multiplied immunoassay technique); Radioimmunoassay.
Iron
pediatric overdose (review), 148

Kidney
acute failure, hemodialysis clearance of pentobarbital (case report), 485
bretylium nomogram for dosing, in renal impairment, 265
end-stage failure, theophylline monoclonal antibodies, fluorescence polarization immunoassay, 355
maturing function in children, and sulfonamide pharmacokinetics, 130

Letters to the Editor
Caffeine Interference with CANAM-Theophylline Reagent Kit, 489
Extraction of Interfering Substance from Sera of Uremic Subjects Prior to Homogeneous Enzyme Immunoassay, 124
On the Interaction Between Phenytoin and Antineoplastic Agents, 123
Interactive Opinion on the Rationalization of Therapeutic Cyclosporine Monitoring, 488
Measurement of Cyclosporine: A Challenge to the Professional Laboratory Organizations, 123
Leukemia
acute lymphoblastic, HPLC of 6-mercaptopurine, 315
Lidocaine
pharmacokinetics, Bayesian forecasting, 66
plasma levels, during local anesthesia in dentistry, 369
Liquid chromatography
plasma aspirin and salicylate, 216
Liver disease
digoxin, false elevations, 202
Liver function tests
perhexiline maleate, long-term treatment, 54

Malaria prophylaxis
reverse phase HPLC of dapsone, monoacetyldapsone, and pyrimethamine, 415
6-Mercaptopurine
HPLC of serum or plasma, 315
Monoacetyldapsone
reverse phase HPLC, and malaria prophylaxis, 415

Naproxen
pediatric pharmacology, 2
Nifedipine
and digoxin interaction, atrial fibrillation, 372
plasma, reverse phase HPLC, 321
Nomogram
bretylium dosing in renal impairment, 265
Nystagmus
lateral gaze, in carbamazepine-treated epileptics, 277

Oxypurinol
HPLC, plasma and urine, 324

Paroxysmal choreoathetosis
phenytoin blood levels, 81
Penicillin
amikacin inactivation (review), 12
Pentobarbital
hemodialysis clearance (case report), 485
high dose, and theophylline pharmacokinetics (case report), 181
Perhexiline maleate
long-term treatment, TDM and electromyography, 54
Peritoneal dialysis
amitriptyline pharmacokinetics, 255
PETINIA. *See* Immunoassay, particle-enhanced turbidimetric inhibition.
Pharmacokinetics
aminoglycoside TDM, peak levels, 303
amitriptyline, during peritoneal dialysis, 255
aspirin and salicylate, 216
bupropion in plasma, 447
carbamazepine
and carbamazepine-epoxide, 36
in saliva, 41
chloramphenicol, in pediatrics (review), 159
computer estimation, 258
desmethylimipramine overdose (case report), 239
lidocaine, Bayesian forecasting, 66
Michaelis-Menton, phenytoin-hydroxyphenytoin steady-state serum ratio, 405
in pediatric drug overdose (review), 148
prothrombin response to warfarin therapy, 174

simple Michaelis-Menton elimination kinetics, prediction of drug dosage, 377
sulfonamides, in children, and maturing kidney function (review), 130
theophylline
computer prediction, 421
doxycycline effect, 92
and high-dose pentobarbital (case report), 181
HPLC comparison with fluorescence polarization immunoassay, 442
Pharmacology
amikacin (review), 12
chloramphenicol, in pediatrics (review), 159
pediatric antipyretic drugs (review), 2
Phenobarbital
automated substrate-labeled fluorescent immunoassay, 108
noncompliance in epileptic patients, 87
pediatric overdose (review), 148
and primidone, dual-label fluoroimmunoassay, 101
steady-state serum levels, Chinese epileptics, 83
Phenothiazines
and serum antiepileptic drugs, psychiatric patients with seizure disorder, 401
Phenytoin
automated substrate-labeled fluorescent immunoassay, 108
blood levels, in paroxysmal choreoathetosis, 81
and carbamazepine interactions, 51
and clonazepam interaction (case report), 481
dosage methods, 74
free plasma levels
ultrafiltration comparison with equilibrium dialysis, 461
ultrafiltrate protein, 313
and hydroxyphenytoin steady-state ratio, Michaelis-Menton kinetics, 405
individual maintenance doses, 391
pediatric overdose (review), 148
steady-state serum levels, Chinese epileptics, 83
urinary excretion of *p*-hydroxyphenytoin, 283
Photodiode array detector
warfarin in plasma, 329
Plasma levels
allopurinol and oxypurinol HPLC, 324
aspirin and salicylate, liquid chromatography, 216
carbamazepine, total and free, 46
chlorpromazine TDM, 222
clonidine radioimmunoassay, 344
cyclosporin A, 61
disopyramide, ultrafiltration and EMIT, 466
doxorubicin and metabolites, loop-column extraction and HPLC, 455
ethmozin HPLC, 439
flupentixol
in acute schizophrenia, 411
in schizophrenia, gas chromatography and radioimmunoassay, 229
lidocaine, during local anesthesia in dentistry, 369
6-mercaptopurine HPLC, 315
nifedipine, reverse phase HPLC, 321
phenobarbital, noncompliance in epileptic patients, 87
phenytoin
with carbamazepine comedication, 51
ultrafiltration comparison with equilibrium dialysis, 461
tricyclic antidepressants, 242
valproic acid, solid-phase column extraction and gas liquid chromatography, 336
vitamin E HPLC, 364
warfarin, HPLC and photodiode array detector, 329
Pregnancy
carbamazepine protein binding and disposition, 269
Primidone
automated substrate-labeled fluorescent immunoassay, 108
and phenobarbital, dual-label fluoroimmunoassay, 101
Propranolol
HPLC, blood collection systems, 358
Prostaglandins
serum, effects of nonacetylated salicylate and aspirin, 435
Protein binding
carbamazepine
and carbamazepine-epoxide, in newborn infants, 274
in pregnancy, 269
Prothrombin
warfarin effects, Bayesian forecasting, 174
Pyrimethamine
reverse phase HPLC, and malaria prophylaxis, 415

Quinidine
automated substrate-labeled fluorescent immunoassay, 108

Radioimmunoassay
clonidine, solid phase second antibody separation, 344
digoxin, false elevations in liver disease, 202
flupentixol, in schizophrenia, 229
Reviews
Chloramphenicol: Clinical Pharmacology in Pediatrics, 159
Clinical Pharmacokinetics of Sulfonamides in Children: Relationship Between Maturing Kidney Function and Renal Clearance of Sulfonamides, 130
Clinical Pharmacology of Pediatric Antipyretic Drugs, 2
Oral Contraceptive Drug Interactions, 26
Overview of Amikacin, 12
Therapeutic Drug Monitoring in Pediatric Acute Drug Intoxications, 148
Rifampin
and oral contraceptive interactions, 26

Salicylate
nonacetylated, and serum prostaglandins, 435
pediatric overdose (review), 148
plasma levels, liquid chromatography, 216
serum, fluorescence polarization immunoassay, 351
Saliva
carbamazepine concentrations, 41
Schizophrenia
acute, plasma flupentixol, 411
flupentixol, plasma levels, 229
Serum levels
anticonvulsant drugs, Chinese epileptic patients, 83
6-mercaptopurine HPLC, 315
salicylates, fluorescence polarization immunoassay, 351
theophylline
apoenzyme reactivation immunoassay, 451
in chronic obstructive pulmonary disease, 168
computer prediction, 421
tricyclic antidepressants, 242
valproic acid
dose and comedication, 387
solid-phase column extraction and gas liquid chromatography, 336
vitamin E HPLC, 364
Side effects
amikacin (review), 12
antiepileptic treatment and valproate-induced hyperammonemia, 185
cardiotoxicity with 3(S)-3-hydroxyquinidine (case report), 308
chloramphenicol, in pediatrics (review), 159
lateral gaze nystagmus in carbamazepine-treated epileptics, 277
perhexiline maleate, long-term treatment, 54
Solid-phase column extraction
valproic acid in plasma or serum, 336
Spectrophotofluorometry
chloroquine and desethylchloroquine, 211
Statistics
Bayesian forecasting, lidocaine pharmacokinetics, 66
Sulfonamides
pharmacokinetics, in children, and maturing kidney function (review), 130

Theophylline
apoenzyme reactivation immunoassay, 451
automated substrate-labeled fluorescent immunoassay, 108
in chronic obstructive pulmonary disease, 168
and cimetidine interaction, age effects, 426
distribution, role of body fat, 197
Du Pont immunoassay adapted to centrifugal analyzer, 95
and oral contraceptive interactions (review), 26
pediatric overdose (review), 148
pharmacokinetics
doxycycline effect, 92
high-dose pentobarbital effects (case report), 181
HPLC comparison with fluorescence polarization immunoassay, 442
serum, computer prediction, 421
Therapeutic drug monitoring (TDM)
aminoglycosides, peak concentrations, 303
antidepressant drugs, specific request form, 299
bretylium nomogram, renal impairment, 265
carbamazepine
and carbamazepine epoxide, lateral gaze nystagmus in epileptics, 277
saliva concentrations, 41
chloramphenicol HPLC, interference by dobutamine, 121
chlorpromazine
plasma analysis, 222
whole blood analysis, 472
clonidine radioimmunoassay, 344
consultation service in pediatric hospital, 295
digoxin, and red blood cell electrolytes, 191
dosage prediction, drugs with simple Michaelis-Menton elimination kinetics, 377
noncompliance in epileptic patients, 87
pediatric acute drug intoxications (review), 148
perhexiline maleate long-term treatment, 54
phenytoin
individual maintenance doses, 391
ultrafiltrate protein, 313
primidone and phenobarbital, dual-label fluoroimmunoassay, 101
Tobramycin
automated substrate-labeled fluorescent immunoassay, 108

Ultrafiltration
Amicon micropartition MPS-1 system, free valproic acid concentration, 115
disopyramide in plasma, 466
and equilibrium dialysis, unbound phenytoin in plasma, 461
protein-bound and free phenytoin, 313
Urine
allopurinol and oxypurinol HPLC, 324
clonidine radioimmunoassay, 344
p-hydroxyphenytoin, 283

Valproic acid
chronic therapy, and hyperammonemia, 290
fluoroimmunoassay, comparison with gas liquid chromatography, 236
free concentration, Amicon micropartition MPS-1 ultrafiltration system, 115
hyperammonemia, and antiepileptic treatment, 185
plasma and serum, solid-phase column extraction and gas liquid chromatography, 336
serum levels, dose and comedication, 387
Vitamin E
HPLC with electrochemical detection, 364

Warfarin
HPLC and photodiode array detector, 329
prothrombin response, Bayesian forecasting, 174

Author Index

Aberg-Wistedt A, 478
Achem SR, 426
Adir J, 265
Aeschlimann JM, 411
Agarwal RP, 61
Aguilera LI, 481
Albani F, 46, 123, 277
Albertini A, 236
Alván G, 207, 211
Ambrosetto G, 277
Aoyama T, 87
Arnetoli G, 185

Bachmann K, 258, 391
Baciewicz AM, 26
Bakst AW, 245
Balant LP, 229, 411
Balant-Gorgia AE, 229, 411
Bartelli M, 185
Baruzzi A, 46, 123, 277
Bauer LA, 181
Beightol LA, 351
Bell R, 485
Berardi RR, 426
Bertilsson L, 478
Blanke RV, 115
Blaser J, 303
Blouin RA, 181, 485
Boeckx RL, 95
Bootman JL, 168
Bottorff MB, 442
Bourgeois BFD, 405
Bowers LD, 308
Brandon RA, 216
Bredon JW, 168
Breimer DD, 372
Bruguerolle B, 369
Buice RG, 321
Burlina A, 451

Campbell SC, 168
Campostrini R, 185
Camsonne R, 488
Caron G, 108
Castle MC, 364
Casto DT, 274
Chang SF, 435
Chang Y-C, 81
Chou D, 128
Chow CT, 344
Cohen IA, 426
Coleman RW, 174
Connor R, 308
Contin M, 46, 277
Cooke WJ, 364
Cooper JDH, 54
Cooper JK, 222, 472
Cornford EM, 247
Crom WR, 455
Cunha BA, 12

Dauphin A, 324
Deci PA, 421
DeVane CL, 447
Dickinson RG, 36, 41, 283

Eadie MJ, 36, 41, 216, 283
Eisele R, 229, 411
Ekman L, 207
Eleborg L, 239
Ensom RJ, 197
Ericsson O, 242, 207, 211
Esber HJ, 344
Evans WE, 455

Failler JM, 324
Farina PR, 344
Farinotti R, 324
Faure E, 481
Fernandes R, 358
Flint N, 74
Forney R, Jr., 258
Fraser AD, 299
Friedman D, 246
Friel PN, 269
Frölich JC, 202
Furner RL, 121

Gal P, 274
Galdames DG, 481
Garrons G, 411
Genet C, 229
Gibson GA, 181
Goldlust MB, 435
Gonzenbach HR, 303
Grauer K, 421
Greenberg M, 315
Greenblatt DJ, 244
Groce JB, III., 274
Gronau G, 258
Gupta MK, 127
Gurley BJ, 321
Gustafsson LL, 211, 478

Haidukewych D, 51, 290, 401
Harrison LI, 435
Haughey DB, 355
Hawes EM, 222, 472
Hekster YA, 130
Hempenius J, 92
Henthorn TK, 239
Hillers J, 372
Hillman R, 66
Hoek FJ, 191
Holden R, 358
Holtkamp A, 92
Homon CA, 344
Hooper WD, 36, 41, 283
Hubbard JW, 222, 472
Hyneck ML, 426

Isnardon R, 369

Jarzabek JI, 489
Jauregui L, 391
Jenden DJ, 222
Jewesson PJ, 197
John G, 290
Johnson CE, 426
Jones WN, 168
Jonkman JHG, 92
Josselson J, 265

Kampa IS, 489
Karnes HT, 351
Keirns JJ, 344
Kelly AR, 336
King AR, 36, 41
Kleinbloesem CH, 372
Koike Y, 461
Koopmans R, 191
Koren G, 295
Kraft CJ, 355
Krauss E, 308
Kurokawa T, 87
Kvalheim G, 329
Kvinnsland S, 329

Lai M-L, 83
Lais CJ, 308
Laizure SC, 447
Lalonde RL, 442
Landon J, 101
Landon KP, 247
Lee HS, 415
Lee MH, 355
Lee PS, 415
Leheta BJ, 51
Lesser RP, 246
Lin FC, 358
Lin W-N, 336
Lindström B, 207, 211
Lippens RJJ, 130
Lockhart JDF, 54
Lønning PE, 329
Lopez LM, 74, 421
Ludden TM 66, 174
Lüthy R, 303

MacLeod SM, 295
Magnusson A, 461
Maguire B, 283
March C, 115
Martin M, 222, 472
Matenga J, 54
May PRA, 222
May T, 389
McGhan WF, 168
McKay G, 222, 472
McPherson RA, 61
McQuain C, 435
Messori A, 185
Meyer MC, 466
Midha KK, 222, 472
Miller DQ, 269
Milligan T, 313
Moolenaar AJ, 372
Moroni F, 185
Morris HG, 435
Moyer TP, 123
Mungall DR, 174
Munson ST, 95

Narang PK, 265
Narayanan S, 358
Nelson KM, 308
Nordin C, 239, 242, 478

Oosterhuis B, 191
Opheim KE, 148

Paganini M, 185
Patterson M, 36, 283
Paul R, 54
Perrier DG, 168
Perucca E, 46, 277
Pesce AJ, 255
Pilcher J, 54
Pippenger CE, 1, 129, 371
Plebani M, 451
Poirier JM, 439
Pongsin V, 258
Porter W, 485
Powel MB, 121
Procaccianti G, 277

Raghow G, 466
Rais M, 207
Raisys VA, 148
Rambeck B, 389
Rane A, 461
Rapp RP, 181
Record K, 485
Riley CA, 455
Ristuccia AM, 12, 159
Riva R, 46, 123, 277
Robinson CA, 121
Robinson JD, 74, 421
Rodin EA, 290, 401
Rombo L, 207, 211
Rosenkranz B, 202
Ross CA, 355
Rundell CA, 124

Saavedra IN, 481
Salem RB, 74
Santucci M, 277
Säwe J, 239
Schoenmaker R, 92
Schwartz J, 391
Shamberger RJ, 244
Sheehan M, 108
Sheiner L, 66
Sherman NA, 435
Sidhu P, 321
Sidki AM, 101
Signorini C, 236
Simmen HP, 303
Singh S, 255
Sjöqvist F, 207, 211, 461
Smith DS, 101
Smith MT, 216
Soldin SJ, 295, 315
Sonnabend W, 303
Spina E, 239, 242
Steiner E, 461
Straughn AB, 442, 466
Sullivan TJ, 391
Sunshine I, 128
Svec JM, 174

Takaki S, 87
Tamary H, 315
Tasset JJ, 255
Threatte GA, 61
Ti TY, 415
Tibbs PA, 181
Tosoni S, 236
Troussard X, 488
Tupper SE, 124
Turley CP, 313
Turnell DC, 54

Ueland PM, 329

Valenza T, 185
van Boxtel CJ, 191
van Brummelen P, 372
van der Boon WJV, 92
Van Putten T, 222
Vozeh S, 66
Vree TB, 130

Wad N, 405
Wagner JG, 377
Wandell M, 66
Wang B-J, 81
Wermeling D, 485
Whalen CE, 315
White WB, 358
Williams C, 74
Wilson JT, 2
Wong SHY, 358

Yap CL, 415
Yerby MS, 269

Zaccara G, 185
Zappoli R, 185
Zavorskas PA, 344
Zielinski JJ, 51, 290
Zipursky A, 315

Subscription Problems?

Most subscription problems are actually a need for information. It is hoped that the following will answer any questions you may have.

1 Please attach a current mailing label when sending an inquiry about your journal subscription (or at least the exact name and address to which the journal is sent).

2 All subscriptions are available on a calendar year basis only. If you send in a subscription in the middle of the year, issues already published in that year's volume will be mailed to you as a separate package.

3 Please allow us 6 to 8 weeks for correct processing of your change of address. It is important that you send a copy of your most recent mailing label AND your new address. Changes cannot be made without both addresses. Please send this information to:

RAVEN PRESS, Subscription Dept.
P.O. Box 2046
Mahopac, NY 10541 USA

4 All other correspondence should be sent to:

RAVEN PRESS
Journal Customer Service
P.O. Box 2046
Mahopac, NY 10541 USA

5 Claims for non-receipt of issues will be honored if we are notified within two months (four months for foreign) of publication. We cannot honor requests made after these time limits.

6 Please remember that in order to qualify for the individual subscription rate, your order must be paid with a personal or P.C. (professional corporation) check.

Our objective is to provide the best possible service to you. Following the above procedures will enable us to do this. Your assistance and understanding will be appreciated.

U.S. Postal Service

STATEMENT OF OWNERSHIP, MANAGEMENT AND CIRCULATION
Required by 39 U.S.C. 3685.

1A. TITLE OF PUBLICATION: Therapeutic Drug Monitoring

1B. PUBLICATION NO.: 6 5 7 7 7 0

2. DATE OF FILING: Sept. 30, 1985

3. FREQUENCY OF ISSUE: Quarterly

3A. NO. OF ISSUES PUBLISHED ANNUALLY: 4

3B. ANNUAL SUBSCRIPTION PRICE: $75.00

4. COMPLETE MAILING ADDRESS OF KNOWN OFFICE OF PUBLICATION *(Street, City, County, State and ZIP+4 Code) (Not printers)*
Raven Press Books Ltd., Inc. 1140 Ave. of the Americas, New York, NY 10036

5. COMPLETE MAILING ADDRESS OF THE HEADQUARTERS OF GENERAL BUSINESS OFFICES OF THE PUBLISHER *(Not printer)*
Raven Press Books Ltd., Inc. 1140 Ave. of the Americas, New York, NY 10036

6. FULL NAMES AND COMPLETE MAILING ADDRESS OF PUBLISHER, EDITOR, AND MANAGING EDITOR *(This item MUST NOT be blank)*

PUBLISHER *(Name and Complete Mailing Address)*
Dr. Alan E. Edelson, Raven Press, 1140 Ave. of the Americas, New York, NY 10036

EDITOR *(Name and Complete Mailing Address)* C.E. Pippenger, Ph.D., Dept. Biochemistry, The Cleveland Clinic Foundation, 9500 Euclid Ave., Cleveland, OH 44106 and Folke Sjoqvist, M.D., Karolinska Institute, Huddinge University Hospital, S-141 86 Huddinge, Sweden.

MANAGING EDITOR *(Name and Complete Mailing Address)*
Ed Barnas, Raven Press, 1140 Ave. of the Americas, New York, NY 10036

7. OWNER *(If owned by a corporation, its name and address must be stated and also immediately thereunder the names and addresses of stockholders owning or holding 1 percent or more of total amount of stock. If not owned by a corporation, the names and addresses of the individual owners must be given. If owned by a partnership or other unincorporated firm, its name and address, as well as that of each individual must be given. If the publication is published by a nonprofit organization, its name and address must be stated.) (Item must be completed.)*

FULL NAME	COMPLETE MAILING ADDRESS
Raven Press Books Ltd., Inc. (Corp.)	1140 Ave. of the Americas, NY, NY 10036
Dr. Alan E. Edelson (stockholder)	16 Washington Ave., Irvington, NY 10533
Carol Edelson (stockholder)	16 Washington Ave., Irvington, NY 10533
New Yorker Magazine (stockholder)	25 West 43rd St., New York, NY 10036

8. KNOWN BONDHOLDERS, MORTGAGEES, AND OTHER SECURITY HOLDERS OWNING OR HOLDING 1 PERCENT OR MORE OF TOTAL AMOUNT OF BONDS, MORTGAGES OR OTHER SECURITIES *(If there are none, so state)*

FULL NAME	COMPLETE MAILING ADDRESS
NONE	

9. FOR COMPLETION BY NONPROFIT ORGANIZATIONS AUTHORIZED TO MAIL AT SPECIAL RATES *(Section 423.12 DMM only)*
The purpose, function, and nonprofit status of this organization and the exempt status for Federal income tax purposes *(Check one)*

☐ (1) HAS NOT CHANGED DURING PRECEDING 12 MONTHS
☐ (2) HAS CHANGED DURING PRECEDING 12 MONTHS
(If changed, publisher must submit explanation of change with this statement.)

10. EXTENT AND NATURE OF CIRCULATION *(See instructions on reverse side)*	AVERAGE NO. COPIES EACH ISSUE DURING PRECEDING 12 MONTHS	ACTUAL NO. COPIES OF SINGLE ISSUE PUBLISHED NEAREST TO FILING DATE
A. TOTAL NO. COPIES *(Net Press Run)*	1,739	1,645
B. PAID AND/OR REQUESTED CIRCULATION 1. Sales through dealers and carriers, street vendors and counter sales	--	--
2. Mail Subscription *(Paid and/or requested)*	1,257	1,192
C. TOTAL PAID AND/OR REQUESTED CIRCULATION *(Sum of 10B1 and 10B2)*	1,257	1,192
D. FREE DISTRIBUTION BY MAIL, CARRIER OR OTHER MEANS SAMPLES, COMPLIMENTARY, AND OTHER FREE COPIES	108	108
E. TOTAL DISTRIBUTION *(Sum of C and D)*	1,365	1,300
F. COPIES NOT DISTRIBUTED 1. Office use, left over, unaccounted, spoiled after printing	374	345
2. Return from News Agents	--	--
G. TOTAL *(Sum of E, F1 and 2—should equal net press run shown in A)*	1,739	1,645

11. I certify that the statements made by me above are correct and complete

SIGNATURE AND TITLE OF EDITOR, PUBLISHER, BUSINESS MANAGER, OR OWNER: Circulation Dir.

PS Form 3526, July 1984

(See instruction on reverse)